Robotics in Genitourinary Surgery

Ashok K. Hemal · Mani Menon

Editors

Robotics in Genitourinary Surgery

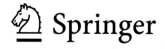

Springer

Editors
Prof. Dr. Ashok K. Hemal
Department of Urology, Comprehensive
    Cancer Center
Institute for Regenerative Medicine
Robotics and Minimally Invasive Surgery
Baptist Medical Center
Wake Forest University School
    of Medicine
Wake Forest University Health Sciences
Winston-Salem, NC, USA

Dr. Mani Menon
Professor of Urology
Columbia University
New York Director
Menon-Vattikuti Center
New York Presbyterian Hospital
USA

ISBN 978-1-84882-113-2   e-ISBN 978-1-84882-114-9
DOI 10.1007/978-1-84882-114-9
Springer London Dordrecht Heidelberg New York

British Library Cataloguing in Publication Data
A catalogue record for this book is available from the British Library

Library of Congress Control Number: 2011920995

Printed on acid-free paper

Springer is part of Springer Science+Business Media (www.springer.com)

Preface

It has been a privilege for us to write the preface for this book, *Robotics in Genitourinary Surgery*. The da Vinci robot is a staggeringly sophisticated tool, although it has been around for only a decade and has witnessed a logarithmic increase in numbers of robot-assisted surgeries since its inception. This is particularly true in the USA, with other parts of the world closely following.

Patients have accepted the technology at breathless pace. Urological surgeons have been slower to do so. This is human nature, and it is always difficult to learn and apply new technologies. Already the field of urological oncology has been turned on its head, and the signature oncological procedure, the radical prostatectomy is overwhelmingly performed with robotic assistance. Several years ago, *The New York Times* published an article looking at how new technology has disseminated across the USA within the years after its introduction. At an acceptance rate of over 60% at 5 years, robotic radical prostatectomy exceeded the penetration of electricity, cell telephones, or the personal computer!

Yet there are controversies about the robot-assisted technique. Nay sayers, who share the common quality of never having seriously tried doing robotic surgery, complain that there is no real benefit from robotic surgery and that it is slick marketing that has resulted in the acceptance of the robot. They say that the learning curve is steep, that surgeons are attempting robotics without proper training, and that the robotic manufacturer is responsible for most of this. There is some truth to all of this. As among the pioneers of these procedures, we have heard it all, at symposia, in the hallways, in editorials, and in rejections of early (and some not-so-early) manuscripts. These are the slings and arrows of outrageous fortune. As newer generations of surgeons have embraced robotics, these protestations are becoming less vociferous, and robotic surgery will find its appropriate place. The technology is wonderful, in the proper hands the da Vinci robot is an incredibly sophisticated tool, and the learning issues will be resolved as robotic surgery becomes mainstream training in residencies.

This textbook aims to provide comprehensive, state-of-art information about the various topics dedicated to robotic urologic procedures. Our intention on the one hand has been to make our urologic colleagues at large aware of the eclectic varieties of urologic surgeries that are being done with robotic assistance and at the same time provide details of robotic setup, instrumentation, and surgical nuances of different procedures. The contributors to the book are truly pioneers and experts in the field of robotic surgery across the world. They could have written just about any topic in robotics, but they helped us in writing this book. This book contains nine sections (History; Basics and Development of Program; Training and Research; the

Prostate; Adrenal, Kidney and Ureter; Bladder; Pediatric Urology; Female Urology and Infertility; Patient's Perspective and Future) with 60 chapters tailored to address the history, technique, research, and experience in the field of robotic urologic surgery. We thank the pioneers and innovative urological surgeons who have developed and nurtured robotic urologic surgery from its infancy to maturity to serve our patients and community.

When the history of robotics is written, the authors of the chapters will stand out among the great surgeons in urology.

The editors are eternally grateful to all the individual contributors of this book in helping to lay the foundations of robotic surgery. Every one is a hero in their own right. We hope that Intuitive Surgical, the manufacturer of the robot, recognizes this and, more importantly, makes the technology more affordable and the training more structured.

NC, USA   Ashok K. Hemal
MI, USA   Mani Menon

Contents

Contributors

Claude Abbou Department of Urology, Henri Mondor Hospital, Creteil, France

Piyush K. Agarwal Vattikuti Urology Institute, Henry Ford Hospital, Detroit, MI, USA

Thomas E. Ahlering Department of Urology, University of California Irvine, Irvine, CA, USA

David M. Albala Division of Urologic Surgery, Duke Prostate Center, Duke University Medical Center, Durham, NC, USA

Paul E. Andrews Mayo Clinic, Urology, Phoenix, AZ, USA

Shadie R. Badaan Urology Robotics Laboratory, James Buchannan Brady Urological Institute, Johns Hopkins Medicine, Baltimore, MD, USA

Ketan K. Badani Columbia University Medical Center/NY Presbyterian Hospital, New York, NY, USA

John M. Barry Division of Urology, Oregon Health and Science University, Portland, OR, USA

Brian M. Benway Division of Urologic Surgery, Washington University School of Medicine, St. Louis, MO, USA

Akshay Bhandari Vattikuti Urology Institute, Henry Ford Health System, Detroit, MI, USA

Sam B. Bhayani Division of Urologic Surgery, Department of Surgery, Washington University School of Medicine, St. Louis, MO, USA

Georges A. de Boccard Robot-Assisted Laparoscopic Surgery Center, Clinic Generale Beaulieu, Geneva, Switzerland

Ralph W. deVere White UC Davis Cancer Center, Sacramento, CA, USA

Ronald S. Boris Urologic Oncology Branch, National Cancer Institute, National Institutes of Health, Bethesda, MD, USA

Ugur Boylu Department of Urology, Center for Minimally Invasive and Robotic Surgery, Tulane University School of Medicine, New Orleans, LA, USA

Alberto Briganti Department of Urology, Vita-Salute University, San Raffaele Hospital, Milano, Italy

Arthur Caire Division of Urologic Surgery, Department of Surgery, Duke Prostate Center, Duke University Medical Center, Durham, NC, USA

Umberto Capitanio Urology Department, Vita-Salute San Raffaele, Milano, Italy

Paul Carpentier Department of Urology, Onze-Lieve-Vrouw (OLV) Clinic, Aalst, Belgium

Peter R. Carroll Department of Urology, UCSF - Helen Diller Family Comprehensive Cancer Center, University of California, San Francisco, CA, USA

Pasquale Casale Children's Hospital of Philadelphia, University of Pennsylvania School of Medicine, Philadelphia, PA, USA

Erik P. Castle Mayo Clinic, Department of Urology, Phoenix, AZ, USA

Ben Challacombe The Urology Centre, Guy's Hospital, London, UK

Karim Chamie David Geffen School of Medicine, University of California, Los Angeles, CA, USA

Sanket Chauhan Global Robotics Institute, Celebration Health/Florida Hospital, Celebration, FL, USA

Jed-Sian Cheng Department of Urology, SUNY Upstate Medical University, Syracuse, NY, USA

Rafael E. Coelho Global Robotics Institute, Celebration Health/Florida Hospital, Celebration, FL, USA

Matthew R. Cooperberg Department of Urology, UCSF - Helen Diller Family Comprehensive Cancer Center, University of California, San Francisco, CA, USA

Anthony J. Costello Division of Surgery, Department of Urology, The Royal Melbourne Hospital, University of Melbourne, Melbourne, Australia

Prokar Dasgupta The Urology Centre, Guy's Hospital, London, UK

Cole Davis Department of Urology, UCSF - Helen Diller Family Comprehensive Cancer Center, University of California, San Francisco, CA, USA

Geert de Naeyer Department of Urology, Onze-Lieve-Vrouw (OLV) Clinic, Aalst, Belgium

Harveer S. Dev Cambridge University Clinical School, St John's College, Cambridge, UK

Pierre Dubernard Centre Urologie Bellecour, Lyon, France

Stacey Dusik-Fenton Vattikuti Urology Institute, Henry Ford Health System, Detroit, MI, USA

Jack S. Elder Vattikuti Urology Institute, Henry Ford Hospital, Children's Hospital of Michigan, Detroit, MI, USA

Daniel S. Elliott Department of Urology, Mayo Clinic, Rochester, MN, USA

Daniel D. Eun Division of Urology, Penn Urology at Pennsylvania Hospital, University of Pennsylvania, Philadelphia, PA, USA

Michael D. Fabrizio Endourology/Laparoscopy Program, Eastern Virginia Medical School, Norfolk, VA, USA

Randy Fagin The Prostate Center of Austin, Austin, TX, USA

Michael N. Ferrandino Division of Urologic Surgery, Department of Surgery, Duke Prostate Center, Duke University Medical Center, Durham, NC, USA

Robert S. Figenshau Surgery, Washington University School of Medicine, St. Louis, MO, USA

David S. Finley UCLA Department of Urology, Clark Urology Center, Los Angeles, CA, USA

John M. Fitzpatrick Department of Surgery, Mater Misericordiae University Hospital, Dublin, Ireland

Thomas Frede Department of Urology, Helios-Kliniken, Müllheim, Germany

Andrea Gallina Department of Urology, Vita-Salute San Raffaele University, Milano, Italy

Prasanna Sooriakumaran ACMI Corp. Endourological Society Fellow, James Buchanan Brady Foundation Department of Urology, Weill Cornell Medical College, Institute for Prostate Cancer, Lefrak Center of Robotic Surgery, New York Presbyterian Hospital, New York, NY, USA

Gagan Gautam Section of Urology, Department of Surgery, University of Chicago Medical Center, Chicago, IL, USA

Matthew T. Gettman Department of Urology, Mayo Clinic, Rochester, MN, USA

Ahmed Ghazi Division of Laparoscopy and Robotic Surgery, University of Rochester Medical Center, Rochester, NY, USA

David A. Gilley Department of Urology, Indiana University School of Medicine, Indianapolis, IN, USA

Rita Gobet Leitende Aerztin für Kinderurologie, Universitäts-Kinderspital, Zurich, Switzerland

Ali Serdar Gözen Department of Urology, SLK-Kliniken Heilbronn, University of Heidelberg, Heidelberg, Germany

Sonal Grover Lefrak Center of Robotic Surgery and Prostate Cancer Institute, Brady Foundation Department of Urology, Weill Medical College of Cornell University, New York, NY, USA

Khurshid A. Guru Urologic Oncology Roswell Park Cancer Institute, Buffalo, NY, USA

Gabriel P. Haas Astellas Global Development, Inc., Deerfield, IL, USA

Matthew H. Hayn Urologic Oncology, Roswell Park Cancer Institute, Buffalo, NY, USA

Ashok K. Hemal Department of Urology, Comprehensive Cancer Center, Institute for Regenerative Medicine, Robotics and Minimally Invasive Surgery, Baptist

Medical Center, Wake Forest University School of Medicine, Wake Forest University Health Sciences, Winston-Salem, NC, USA

Elias Hyams Department of Urology, Langone Medical Center, New York University, New York, NY, USA

A. Karim Kader Department of Urology, Comprehensive Cancer Center, Center for Cancer Genomics, Winston-Salem, NC, USA

Ty T. Higuchi Department of Urology, Mayo Clinic, Rochester, MN, USA

Santiago Horgan Minimally Invasive Surgery, University of California San Diego, San Diego, CA, USA

Abolfazl Hosseini Section of Urology, Department of Molecular Medicine and Surgery, Karolinska Institutet, Stockholm, Sweden

J. Hubert Department of Urology, University Hospital of Nancy, CHU Nancy – Brabois Vandoeuvre les Nancy, France

Martin N. Jonsson Section of Urology, Department of Molecular Medicine and Surgery, Karolinska Institutet, Stockholm, Sweden

Jean Joseph Section of Laparoscopic and Robotic Surgery, University of Rochester Medical Center, Rochester, NY, USA

Mark H. Katz Urology, Boston School of Medicine, Boston, MA, USA

Sanjeev A. Kaul Vattikuti Urology Institute, Henry Ford Hospital, Children's Hospital of Michigan, Detroit, MI, USA

Kirk A. Keegan Urology, Vanderbilt University, Nashville, TN, USA

Yoshiyuki Kojima Department of Nephro-urology, Nagoya City University Graduate School of Medical Sciences, Children's Hospital of Philadelphia, University of Pennsylvania, Philadelphia, PA, USA

Rajeev Kumar Department of Urology, All India Institute of Medical Sciences, New Delhi, India

M. Ladrière Department of Nephrology, University Hospital of Nancy, CHU Nancy – Brabois Vandoeuvre les Nancy, France

David I. Lee Presbyterian Medical Center, University of Pennsylvania, Philadelphia, PA, USA

John B. Malcolm Eastern Virginia Medical School/Urology of Virginia, Norfolk, VA, USA

Barry B. McGuire Department of Urology, Mater Misericordiae University Hospital, Dublin, Ireland

Ben R. McHone Urologic Oncology Branch, National Cancer Institute, National Institutes of Health, Bethesda, MD, USA

Pierre Mendoza Department of Urology, Penn Presbyterian Medical Center, University of Pennsylvania, Philadelphia, PA, USA

Mani Menon Professor of Urology, Columbia University, New York Director, Menon-Vattikuti Center, New York Presbyterian Hospital, USA

Francesco Montorsi Department of Urology, Vita-Salute San Raffaele, Milano, Italy

Michael E. Moran Southwestern Urology, Tucson, AZ, USA; Department of Urology, University of Florida, Gainesville, FL, USA; American Urological Association's William P. Didusch Center for Urologic History, Linthicum, MD, USA

Alexander Mottrie Urology Department, Onze Lieve Vrouw Hospital, Aalst, Belgium

Phillip Mucksavage University of Pennsylvania Medical Center, Philadelphia, PA, USA

Patrick Mufarrij Department of Urology, Langone Medical Center, New York University, New York, NY, USA

Vinod Narra Department of Surgery, Henry Ford Hospital, Detroit, MI, USA

David E. Neal Department of Oncology, University of Cambridge, Addenbrookes Hospital, Cambridge, UK

Rafael Nuñez-Nateras Mayo Clinic, Department of Urology, Phoenix, AZ, USA

Michael A. Olympio Departments of Anesthesiology and Urology, Baptist Medical Center, Wake Forest University Health Sciences, Winston-Salem, NC, USA

Kenneth J. Palmer Department of Urology, College of Medicine, University of Central Florida, Florida, USA

Manish N. Patel Department of Robotic Urologic Surgery, Vattikuti Urology Institute, Detroit, MI, USA

Vipul R. Patel Global Robotics Institute, Celebration Health/Florida Hospital, Celebration, FL, USA

James O. Peabody Department of Urology, Vattikuti Urology Institute, Henry Ford Health System, Detroit, MI, USA

Craig A. Peters Division of Surgical Innovation, Technology and Translation, Sheikh Zayed Institute for Pediatric Surgical Innovation, Children's National Medical Center, Washington, DC, USA

Peter A. Pinto Urologic Oncology Branch, National Cancer Institute, National Institutes of Health, Bethesda, MD, USA

Raj S. Pruthi Division of Urologic Surgery, The University of North Carolina at Chapel Hill, Chapel Hill, NC, USA

Jens Rassweiler Urologische Klinik, SLK Klinikens, Heilbronn, Germany

Jamil Rehman Urology, SUNY-Stony Brook University/Brandon Regional Hospital, Centereach, New York, USA

Chad R. Ritch Department of Urology, Columbia University Medical Center – New York Presbyterian, New York, NY, USA

Charles-Henry Rochat Robot-Assisted Laparoscopic Surgery Center, Clinic Generale Beaulieu, Geneva, Switzerland

Craig G. Rogers Vattikuti Urology Institute, Henry Ford Hospital, Detroit, MI, USA

Leticia Ruiz Department of Urology, Social Security Metropolitan Hospital, Panama, Republic of Panama

Andrea Salonia Urology Department, Vita-Salute San Raffaele, Milano, Italy

Mattia N. Sangalli Department of Urology, Onze-Lieve-Vrouw (OLV) Clinic, Aalst, Belgium

Peter Schatteman Department of Urology, Onze-Lieve-Vrouw (OLV) Clinic, Aalst, Belgium

Paul F. Schellhammer Sentara Medical Group, Eastern Virginia Medical School, Urology of Virginia, Norfolk, VA, USA

Martin C. Schumacher Section of Urology, Department of Molecular Medicine and Surgery, Karolinska Institutet, Stockholm, Sweden

Usha Seshadri-Kreaden Department of Clinical Affairs, Intuitive Surgical, Sunnyvale, CA, USA

Nimish C. Shah Department of Urology, Cambridge Urology, Cambridge, UK

Arieh L. Shalhav University of Chicago Medical Center, Chicago, IL, USA

Saurabh Sharma Department of Urology, Penn Presbyterian Medical Center, University of Pennsylvania, Philadelphia, PA, USA

Mark S. Shimko Department of Urology, Mayo Clinic, Rochester, MN, USA

Sameer Siddiqui Vattikuti Urology Institute, Henry Ford Health System, Detroit, MI, USA

Iqbal Singh Department of Urology, Clinical Instructor, Urology, Wake Forest Baptist Medical Centre, Wake Forest University Medical School, Winston-Salem, NC, USA

Michael Stifelman Langone Medical Center, New York University, New York, NY, USA

Dan Stoianovici Urology Robotics Laboratory, James Buchannan Brady Urological Institute, Johns Hopkins Medicine, Baltimore, MD, USA

Nazareno Suardi Urology Department, Vita-Salute San Raffaele, Milano, Italy

Yinghao Sun Department of Urology, Changhai Hospital, Second Military Medical University, Shanghai, China

Chandru P. Sundaram Department of Urology, Indiana University School of Medicine, Indianapolis, IN, USA

Gyung Tak Sung Department of Urology, Dong-A University Hospital, Busan, South Korea

Atsushi Takenaka Division of Urology, Kobe University Graduate School of Medicine, Kobe, Japan

Gerald Y. Tan Lefrak Center of Robotic Surgery and Prostate Cancer Institute, Brady Foundation Department of Urology, Weill Medical College of Cornell University, New York, NY, USA; Department of Urology, Tan Tock Seng Hospital, Singapore, Singapore

Dogu Teber Department of Urology, University of Heidelberg, Heidelberg, Germany

Ashutosh K. Tewari Lefrak Center of Robotic Surgery and Prostate Cancer Institute, Brady Foundation Department of Urology, Weill Medical College of Cornell University, New York, NY, USA

Raju Thomas Department of Urology, Center for Minimally Invasive and Robotic Surgery, Tulane University School of Medicine, New Orleans, LA, USA

Kari J. Thompson Division of Minimally Invasive Surgery, University of California San Diego, San Diego, CA, USA

Matthew E. Nielsen Department of Urologic Surgery, University of North Carolina at Chapel Hill, Chapel Hill, NC, USA

Pankaj Wadhwa Department of Urology, RG Stone Urology and Laparoscopy Hospital, B-1, Vishal Enclave, Rajouri Garden, New Delhi, India

Eric M. Wallen Division of Urologic Surgery, The University of North Carolina at Chapel Hill, Chapel Hill, NC, USA

David S. Wang Boston University Medical Center, Boston, MA, USA

N. Peter Wiklund Department of Urologic Surgery, Karolinska University Hospital, Stokholm, Sweden

Howard N. Winfield Division of Robotic and Minimally Invasive Surgery, Department of Urology, DCH Regional Medical Center, Tuscaloosa, AL, USA

Michael E. Woods Urology, Loyola University Medical Center, Maywood, IL, USA

Kevin C. Zorn Department of Urology, Division of Robotic Surgery, University of Montreal Medical Center, Montreal, QC, Canada

Part I
History, Basics, and Development of Program

Chapter 1

The History of Robotic Surgery

Michael E. Moran

1.1 Introduction

> If you will have the precision out of them, and make their
> fingers measure degrees like cog-wheels, and their arms
> strike curves like compasses, you must inhumanize them.
> (J. Ruskin, The Stones of Venice[1])

We stand at the threshold of the *information age*
rapidly integrating the next technologic wonders into
our everyday lives.[2] For instance, who would have
thought that with little difficulty, we can go *online*,
purchase an airline ticket halfway around the world,
and return before the weekend is over. Certainly no
one would have considered this even a remote possibility at the turn of the twentieth century or even by
the end of World War II. Think about this for 1 min, *to
go online* implies that we can immediately communicate to a travel agent or directly with the airline carrier,
reserve and pay for our ticket, select our seat and any
dietary preferences without leaving the office or home.
Coupled to this is the fact that the aviation has come
a long way from Orville and Wilbur's sensational but
expected powered flight at Kitty-Hawk, SC, just over
100 years ago!

For millennia, one of humanity's fondest dreams
was to fly like birds. Aeronautics engineering has not
only allowed this to happen but also exceeded anything possible from nature in a span of less than a
century. Certainly, the primitive notions by such brilliant men as Leonardo da Vinci thought that powered
flight might be possible by flapping wings; however,
wind tunnel experimentation and wing designs coupled
to innovations in jet propulsion have made supersonic
flight a reality. The technology of flight is now an
everyday expectation and no one could foresee going
backward. We have landed a man on the moon with
computer technology that is equivalent to an Intel®
286 processor which many younger urologists cannot
now remember; we have an autonomous, robotic rover
on Mars, and our expectations of continued advances
in aeronautics remains undaunted. Robots are another
one of humanity's dreams.

The definition of the word "robot" can be debated,
but according to The Robot Institute of America
(1979), it is defined as follows: "a reprogrammable,
multifunctional manipulator designed to move materials, parts, tools, or specialized devices through various programmed motions for the performance of a
variety of tasks." Webster's dictionary states: "an automatic device that performs functions normally ascribed
to humans or a machine in the form of a human."
Mankind has been enthralled by the possibility of
mechanizing human actions from the earliest recorded
times; in fact some evidence for this is seen in Homer's
Iliad. A historical perspective on the coming of age of
robotics is appropriate for any knowledgeable discussion and forms a basis for understanding the intense
perceptions our patients have about this form of therapy. Consider this is an intellectual introduction to a
rapidly expanding research effort that is applying the
power of computer technology to the engineering of
mechanical actuators with a significant past. In fact, the
history of robotic technology is almost as compelling
as the technology itself.

M.E. Moran (✉)
Southwestern Urology, Tucson, AZ, USA; Department
of Urology, University of Florida, Gainesville, FL, USA;
American Urological Association's William P. Didusch
Center for Urologic History, Linthicum, MD, USA
e-mail: memoran2@juno.com

A.K. Hemal, M. Menon (eds.), *Robotics in Genitourinary Surgery*,
DOI 10.1007/978-1-84882-114-9_1, © Springer-Verlag London Limited 2011

1.2 History of Robotics

> Any sufficiently advanced technology is indistinguishable from magic. (Arthur C. Clarke[122])

The word *robot* was introduced from a play written by the Czech author Karel Capek in the work *Rossum's Universal Robots* (RUR) in 1920. In this satire, all unpleasant manual labor is performed by manufactured biologic beings.[3] Robots have gradually morphed into our machines and have assumed a more human mantra, even undergoing anthropomorphitization, such as the computer HAL in Stanley Kubrick's interpretation of Arthur C. Clarke's tale *2001: A Space Odyssey*.[4] Isaac Asimov in fact goes much further in his classic work *Runaround*. Here he generates three basic laws of robots: first law—a robot must not harm a human being or, through interaction, allow one to come to harm; second law—a robot must always obey human beings unless it is in conflict with the first law; third law—a robot must protect itself from harm unless it is in conflict with the first or the second law. Asimov first explored the notion of robotic potential in the short story *Runaround* in 1942 but later added his zeroth law—a robot may not injure humanity or, through inaction, allow humanity to come to harm.[5] The recent motion picture adaptation of the science fiction potential for robotics was seen in *Bicentennial Man*, where Robin Williams plays the robot seeking to become human, or in *The Terminator*, where Arnold Schwarzenegger (governor of the State of California!) is a robot out to change the future.[6,7] These highly publicized but currently erroneous expectations of robots have an intriguing history and several recent books have discussed early prototypic robots, or automatons. These will be presented in detail because it allows the user of current systems to better understand their implications and to better understand human robotic interactions and mankind's desire or attraction/repulsion toward robotic technologies. Uniquely, there are two quite distinct histories that lead to different cultural perceptions of robots, the Western and the Eastern historic legacies. They will be presented separately.

1.3 Western Robotics

About 3.4 billion years ago, an anaerobic organism developed the capacity to reproduce and life arrived on this Earth, the third planet from the sun. The earliest solution to storing data, replicating information, and developing along a pathway of growth potential to self-awareness commenced. Deoxyribonucleic acid (DNA) became a biomolecular method of storing vast amounts of genomic data that allowed for adaptive proliferation of life forms.[8] The Cambrian explosion possibly represents the most unprecedented time where the potential of this biomolecular database was allowed full expression. At the inception of the Paleozoic era, an intense period of biologic diversification occurred producing a massive outpouring of multicellular animals about 530 million years ago.[9] Our subspecies *Homo sapiens* probably arrived geologic moments ago, perhaps 40,000 years or so, and tool making was one of our distinguishing features. Our earliest accounts of technology are based upon our mythologies and religious beliefs. According to Hebrew Scripture, the first human being, Adam, was created by God on the sixth day of creation. In rabbinic lore, Adam begins his existence as a golem. On the third hour of the sixth day, God assembles virgin dirt from all corners of the Earth, thus linking the first human to all of the planets. In the fourth hour, God kneads the dirt and in the 5th hour shapes the form of man. In the sixth hour, God makes this lump of clay into a golem. By the seventh hour, God breathes a soul into the creature and the golem becomes a self-aware human being.[10] This in ancient Judeic context suggests that the act of creation itself is infused into humanity. "If the righteous desired it, they could create worlds, for it is written, 'your iniquities have distinguished between you and your God' " [Isaiah 59:2].

Greek mythology tells us that Prometheus stole fire from Zeus to give to mankind and was punished for this. Icarus flew with wings made of lightweight wax that melted as he arose closer to the sun. Dedalus is also known to have animated statues so that they could move about and appeared lifelike. These mythical illustrations reinforce the contention that mankind has always been interested in technology and augmented function with inventions. In 250 BC, Ctesibius of Alexandria, a Greek physician and inventor, developed a mechanical water clock, or clepsydra.[11] In the thirteenth century, Albertus Magnus, a Dominican monk who is most well known as Thomas Aquinas's mentor, probably built an artificial man that apparently could move.[12]

It was not until 1495 that one of the least known inventions of Leonardo da Vinci was drawn and the first real automaton can be verified. Leonardo was in his late 20s about this time and was experimenting with his painting technique on wet plaster. In the 1950s a researcher interested in the rare drawings and writings of this Renaissance master noted what appeared to be mechanical notations on one of Leonardo's works. At the Florence Museum of the History of Science, they have now shown that this drawing is a scale version of a mechanized, armored knight. It should be noted that at this time, there was no method of rendering mechanical drawings for craftsmen to work from, there were no motors, no electricity, no steam engines, and springs were only in their infancy. In fact, rubber had not yet been found by the French explorers in Honduras. From da Vinci's writings it appears he was aware of the writings of Homer and a "mechanized cart" enthralled him. He had developed a mobile automaton that could be programmed to turn and had rack-and-pinion front wheel drive. This foundation became the basis for another of his famous automatons, a mobile, movable lion that was used to welcome King Francis I from France.[13] Though da Vinci's discoveries would not come to light for centuries, there is strong evidence that his drawings were widely distributed. Another tinkerer and inventor from Spain Gianello Torriano mechanized an automaton referred to as the Japanese tea server.

In the early eighteenth century, Jacques de Vaucanson (1709–1782) would follow in the path of the ancients but improved the mechanisms of animation and would become world renowned. He was thought of as the master "toy maker" of Europe and attracted the royal attention of Louis XV. His finest creation was a mechanical duck with hundreds of moving parts. This duck could eat, drink and apparently "digest," and excrete although this is known to have been a preformed paste. He went on to construct musical automatons, the most famous being the "drummer and fife" player and a "flutist." What is remarkable about these automatons was the anatomical similarity they had to the real things (humans). In fact, the flutist could be seen to breathe, with a bellows-like device inserted into the chest cavity that would draw in air and express it toward the devices' mouth so that it could play the flute. Vaucanson had studied the anatomy of animals and humans extensively and created in his "flutist's" mouth all representations of a normal human. His machines were unparalleled in their complexity and decades would

pass before anyone could duplicate his efforts.[14] René Descartes, the father of the Enlightenment, believed that animals, man included, were nothing more than biologic machines. His disquisitions on consciousness is related in his "*cogito ergo sum.*" There now is no sure proof, but it has been recounted that during his last trip to the Norway, he took with him a mechanical doll, thought to look like his dead daughter Francine.[15]

Largely due to the success of Vaucanson, other machinists and watchmakers became interested in making mechanical automatons. In fact, it had become quite fashionable for the aristocracy to collect sophisticated mechanical devices for entertainment. Particularly to our discussion, two more European individuals deserve mention. Jaquet-Droz, a Swiss inventor, in the 1770s made moving and musical androids. In fact, some of these machines still enchant audiences in Neuchâtel, Switzerland. Mary Shelly, the author of *Frankenstein: The Modern Prometheus*, was delighted by these automatons.[16,17] These devices appeared like children and were mechanized only to draw (usually king's portraits) or write (commonly would quote Descartes). But Jaquet-Droz was most interested in musical automatons. He had one automaton that could play the harpsichord and appeared to consider the audience and breathe. The other Frenchman was Roulet-Descamps, who became famous for his intricate, smaller mechanical pieces. Collectors vied with each other to obtain his most sophisticated automata. By the 1800s there were whole shows of such "mechanical wonders."[18]

In what was then thought as the ultimate attempt at automata, von Kempelen developed a sophisticated machine that could play chess against a human opponent. It widely toured all of Europe and eventually made its way to the New World. The *Turk*, as it was referred to, was an immediate sensation. His touring would make von Kempelen famous and wealthy, for crowds of people would pay just to observe this mechanical device usually beat the most gifted chess players of the time. In fact, it is known that Benjamin Franklin played against the *Turk* and lost.[19] Scholars were attracted to these shows in an attempt to understand the inner workings of this automaton but were never able to figure how it was done. A book published in 1773 about this mechanical device was titled *Inanimate Reason*. Recall that this device appeared just as the "Industrial Revolution" was beginning. The average person of that period had almost unlimited expectations of mechanical wonders. The steam engine was on the horizon and mechanized factories were being discussed. The mechanical workings of this machines' left arm were extraordinary, but in reality, it was indeed a magic trick with von Kempelen's accomplices coming from the best chess players of the age. Maelzel, another tinkerer, eventually bought this machine and brought it to America. Here, as was true in Europe, it attracted large crowds and prompted Edgar Allen Poe to write a famous essay on the impossibility of a mechanical device to reason or think.[20] It would be another 200 years before Poe's essay would be proven false when IBM's computer, Deep Blue, beat Garry Kasparov, the world's Master chess player, in 1997.[21]

Between 1805 and 1871, Jean Robert-Houdin, the father of modern magic, became well known. One of his passionate interests was automata. He became famous for his ingenious gadgets and machines, many of which would be used in his magic shows. He eventually developed a whole "menagerie" of these devices including a moving pasty cook, "Fantastic Orange Tree," "Diavaolo Antonio," and "the Writer."[22] People would come to his shows and would remain spellbound when these mechanical devices would perform in ways that even trained animals could not. Many of his creations were later used by Georges Méliès, the father of modern cinematography and master of special effects, and are now in museums in Paris.[23]

At the onset of the twentieth century, the famous inventor Nikola Tesla, who developed alternating current, generators, the radio, and many other devices, also turned his attention to automata.[24] He proposed that autonomous mechanical devices could be used to eliminate the need for soldiers in war. He designed, built, patented, and demonstrated the first autonomous, programmable, remote-controlled submarine. Tesla's device was mobile, autonomous, interactive with its human controllers via radio and so advanced that it did not even attract the interest of the armed services or any other scientists of the time.[25] Tesla's main contemporary Thomas Edison was likewise at work upon an early mechanized device, the Edison talking doll. Unlike Tesla's huge expectations, Edison thought only to sell the product to the huge doll market at the turn of the century. The idea was to incorporate his new phonograph into a realistic appearing doll that could talk. His prototype device appeared on the cover of

Scientific America in April 1890. Edison created a whole division near his research facility in New Jersey, but like Tesla, this product was not ready for the time and the Edison doll was quickly withdrawn from the market.[15]

Approximately 20 years and one World War later, Karel Capek, the Czech playwright, wrote *Rossum's Universal Robots* which became a success playing throughout Europe, England, and the United States in 1921.[3] Capek probably took a suggestion from his brother to use the Czech word "robot" meaning peasant or worker as a title for his automata. In *RUR*, the brilliant scientist Rossum manufactures a line of biologic humanoids designed to save mankind from work. The plot becomes sinister when the robots are used in a war to kill humans. The robots are given emotions and become no longer tolerant of humans and wipe mankind from the face of the earth, except one. Capek's word "robot" has stuck and has replaced all others in discussing such machines.[3]

In May of 1950, W. Grey Walter and his wife built a mobile robot to investigate the way it learns. *An Imitation of Life* appeared in *Scientific America* in May 1950 (pp. 42–45) describing his first two efforts to build robots.[26] He stated that the human brain has 10,000 million cells, but his robotic "tortoises" had only two miniature radio tubes. In addition, these little machines that he gave mock biologic names *Machina speculatrix* were mobile and sought light. These robots had two sense organs, two motors, and an onboard 6-V hearing aid battery. Later, Walter built more advanced circuits for his robots because he wanted them to learn.[27] He called the advanced machines *Machina docilis* that demonstrated conditioned reflex learning and he published his second paper "A Machine that Learns" (Sci. Am. Aug 1951, 60–63). During the 1940s, electronic data processors were just beginning to be investigated. Vannevar Bush published his classic work "As We May Think" in July's *Atlantic Monthly*. Bush was a well-known scientist who essentially spells out the coming of the *Informational Age*. In this article, he predicts the rise of computers, digital photography, the FAX machines, the Internet, digital word processors, voice recognition, automatic language translation, scanners, advanced mathematics programs, cellular phones, and much more.[28] Ted Nelson in 1965, the father of "hypertext," credits most of his ideas to Bush from having read "As We May Think."

1.4 Eastern Robotics

There is little doubt that the ancient Chinese were culturally adept and developed many technologic advances. Mechanical engineering was quite advanced as early as the empire of King Wu (976–922 BC) of the Western Zhou Dynasty. It is written that one such skilled artisan named Yan Shi made a humanoid robot that could sing and dance like a real human being.[29] This device is said to have possessed lifelike organs such as bones, muscles, joints, skin, and hair. At the beginning of Emperor Tang Xuan Zhong's rule and the Tang Dynasty, there were numerous accounts of such fetes of automation. One other gifted designer was Daifeng Ma, who built and repaired lead carriages, drums that recorded the mileage of the carriage on journeys, and birds that measured the wind's direction. His most famous automated device was a dresser for the queen. Through ingenious levers and switches, when the queen opened the mirror, the doors beneath automatically opened as well. He devised a robotic woman servant for the queen that would bring washing paraphernalia and towels. When the towel was removed from the servant's arm, it automatically triggered the machine to back away back into the closet.

One later Chinese book, *Stories of Government and the People* or *Chao Ye Qian Zai*, contains several accounts of other robotic technologies during the Tang Dynasty.[30] King Lan Ling (550–577 AD) is said to have possessed a humanoid robot that looked like a non-Chinese ethnicity that could both dance and serve drinks. Ling Zhao was a monk from the northern regions of China who is reported to have built a pool for the Emperor Wu Cheng. Ling in addition built a miniature boat that self-propelled itself to the Emperor and automatically served wine. Detailed accounts of the boat include a little wooden man that could clap its hands and the boat would start to play music. Another skilled mechanical engineer was Yin Wenliang from Luozhou. He created an automated man that could propose a toast to his guests at banquets. He also animated a wooden woman that could play the sheng (a Chinese pipe with 13 reeds) and sing. The final artisan of note was Yang Wulian, who created a wooden monk in Qinzhou City. The monk held a wooden bowl to collect alms. Amazingly, when the bowel had been filled, it triggered the monk to proclaim "alms solicited!"[30]

The most well documented of all of the automata comes from Han Zhile, who was actually a Japanese craftsman who moved to China between 806 and 820 AD.[31] He is known to have created mechanical birds, phoenixes, cranes, crows, and magpies. Though made of wood, some of the ornithologic prototypes could be made to pretend to eat, drink, chirp, and warble like real birds. He is reported to have installed mechanical devices inside some of the birds to drive their wings to make them fly. He is reported to have also created a mechanical cat. One of the most marvelous creatures was an automated bed for the Emperor Xianzong named "a dragon on demand." It was activated by someone applying their weight to the bed, thus triggering the release of an intricately carved dragon.

Arising much later than the ancient Chinese automata were the Japanese Karakuri. The word Karakuri means a mechanical device to tease, trick, or take a person by surprise.[32] There are three main categories of Karakuri. Butai Karakuri are puppets used to entertain people in theaters. Zashiki Karakuri are small and used to entertain people in rooms and small groups. Dashi Karakuri are automatons that performed on wooden floats and could be much larger. The Japanese typically used these automata for religious festivals for performing re-enactments of Japanese myths and legends as a form of entertainment. There are several museums in Japan with collections of these intricate mechanical devices such as the Arashiyama Orgel Museum outside of Kyoto. In addition, many of these truly beautiful devices can be viewed "online" with brief descriptions of the device, how they worked, who built them, and what they represent to the Japanese people. Most were built in the seventeenth century.[33]

By the twelfth century, tales of Konjaku Monogatari Shu had developed crude robotic devices for irrigating rice paddies. The most famous nearly modern robotic device from Japan is the 1927 Gakutensoku.[34] It was presented from the people of Japan for the International Exposition that was supposed to have a diplomatic role. Therefore, it was designed to exhibit features from all races. It was actuated by compressed air and could write fluidly and raise its eyelids. Gakutensoku means "learning from divine reason" and was not designed as a laborer but to think, write, and entertain.

By the 1950s, Japanese cultural infatuation with robots underwent an epiphany from the unlikely source of a comic book character.[35] This character would become a cultural icon and eventually spawn enough resolve by these people to spur the Japanese government into funding future robotic research on a scale only comparable to the effort the US government used in the Apollo program. The cartoon character is the Mighty Atom, or better known to the West as Astro Boy. His first black and white appearance occurred on Japanese television in 1963. Many of Japan's top roboticists grew up immersed in the Astro Boy era and can relate their interests in this career from early exposure to this cartoon character.

Osamu Tezuka, the creator of Astro Boy, could not have predicted the outcome of his little cartoon boy would have on the ideals and future of the Japanese people. First conceived and printed in 1951, the series begins with the death of roboticist Dr. Boynton's son Aster in a car accident set in the year 2000. The distraught Boynton sets out to make the robot boy in his son's image, but disappointed with his creation, he soon disowns him. The robot boy is passed off but is found by Dr. Elefun, who schools him in humanity and trains him to battle against anything that might threaten mankind.[34]

Most importantly, Dr. Elefun teaches Astro Boy human feelings such as love, courage, compassion, friendship, and self-doubt. But Astro Boy is not human and struggles with finding the bridges between being a robot and trying to be human. Tezuka's portrayal of this robot boy who struggles with being a partner with his human colleagues continues throughout the series. The robot is never a drone or pure worker for the whim of humanity but assists with his own abilities. This more closely parallels the Japanese vision of the future of intelligent technologies in general. Corporate Japan echoes these themes to this day; robots are an immensely worthwhile endeavor to companies and they expect their robotic products to be helpmates to their human counterparts, not slaves or potential threats as we saw from Western versions. This modern example can best be seen in Sony's newest entertainment robot QRIO (pronounced CURIO).[35]

The first industrial robot was introduced into Japan in 1967. It was a Versatran robot from American Machine and Foundry (AMF). The following year, Kawasaki licensed the hydraulic robot designs from Unimation and started production in Japan. From that time onward, Japan has rapidly become the global leader in the design, development, and distribution of robots of all types (particularly industrial). The whole of the now European Union did bypass Japan in the number of industrial robotic installations in 2001. But, no single country even comes close to Japan in the number of robotic applications. The International Federation of Robotics estimates that Japan (approximately the size of California) installed three times the number of industrial robots than did the US in 2001 (28,369 vs. 10,824). Germany which is also a very industrialized country installed 12,524 robots in the same year. According to the World Fact Book 2002, Japan possesses 410,000 of the world's 720,000 "working robots." These trends highlight a fundamental difference that technology is perceived from East to West.

But don't stop there, Sony Corp. unleashed a robotic dog in 1999 named Aibo. They have since sold approximately 100,000 of these robotic companions. Humanoid robots are the next major desire of the Japanese corporate giants. The Japanese government recently planned to spend ¥30 billion (about $258 million) annually on a 30-year program to develop a humanoid robot with the same mental, physical, and emotional capacities of a 5-year-old human; it is called the Atom Project.[36]

This commitment to this technology is already bearing fruit. Every year, Japan hosts ROBODEX, an exposition that exposes corporate prototypes to the people and the media. The third event, ROBODEX 2003, was held on April 3–6. In 4 days, 66,264 people attended; there were 393 press, 29 speakers, 24 vendors, and 13 universities at the event. There were 90 types of robots exhibited at ROBODEX 2003, most of which were personal assist-type machines. Most of these robots were humanoid in appearance, were small, unimposing, with large heads and eyes. If speech was added, it was usually high-pitched and childlike. The goal according to some technologic enthusiasts is that Japan expects to have a robot in every household in the twenty-first century. If robots can be made to be intelligent, feeling and mobile, they can be more interactive and become personal partners. Some feel that Japan's market for human-friendly robots will soon outstrip the domestic PC market, which generated ¥1.67 trillion ($14.3 billion) in shipments in 2002. Japan's current robot market, ¥400 billion, could grow to ¥3 trillion by 2010 and 8 trillion by 2025 according to some projections.[37]

1.5 Engineering Modern Robots

When a scientist states that something is possible, he is most certainly right. When he states that something is impossible, he is very probably wrong. (Arthur C. Clarke's three laws of technology[122])

1.5.1 From Greek Myths to Reality

Our modern Western thought is inexplicably linked to ancient Greek civilization and thought. Greek mythology represents some of the earliest writings that have been preserved as were the folk tales written by Homer. One needs to look no further to the implications of technology and society than the myths recounted by him and the events surrounding the Greek gods. Hephaestus was the Greek god of fire, particularly the blacksmith's fire, as he would become the patron of craftsmen, artisans, and manufacturers. He was depicted in ancient works of sculpture and paintings as the lame god, born from Hera, who despised him because of his weak and crippled form. As the story goes, he is cast out of Mount Olympus by the repulsed Hera and falls for an entire day before landing in the sea. He is rescued by nymphs, who carry him to the island of Lemnos where he builds a palace and his forges under a volcano. Hephaestus creates a golden thrown as a present to Hera, but his intentions are sinister and she becomes entrapped. Dionysus is sent by Zeus to intoxicate and bring Hephaestus back to Mount Olympus in order to entreat him to release his mother. This is of course attended to with a bribe and Aphrodite is promised to Hephaestus as his wife.[38]

Hephaestus was the great craftsman for the gods and supposedly created many wonderful devices out of metal. His primary helpers were the Cyclopes, who assisted him as workmen. He made weapons and armor for the gods and their heroes. He made Athena's shield and Aros' arrows. He manufactured the chariot for the sun god Helios and the invincible armor for Achilles. In the Greek creation myth, it is Hephaestus who is given the ingenuity of creating the female gender by shaping Pandora (meaning, "all gifts") out of clay. It is also Hephaestus who is ordered by Zeus to chain Prometheus to the rock in Mount Caucasus. "Against my will, no less than yours, I must rivet you with brazen bonds... Such is the prize you have gained for your championship of man."[39] In addition, some of Hephaestus other creations include an animated bull given to King Aeetes that could breathe fire from its mouth. He wrought the famed necklace of Harmonia and Oengrioun's fabulous underground house. But for the sake of our discussion here, his most poignant creation was Talos.[38] Zeus asks Hephaestus to create a bronze humanoid creature for Europa (Zeus' lover), the queen of Crete. Talos is a gigantic automaton whose task is the warder of Crete. He guards this island country by running around it three times daily to drive pirates or invaders off with volleys of stones. But Talos is no ordinary automaton. His secret for life is apparently an infusion of god's blood, or ichor by Hephaestus. Talos, the man of bronze, had beneath the metallic sinew of his ankle "a red vein with its issues of life and death" covered by his skin. It is this part of his invulnerable body where a nail was used to fashion the cover and protect its secret vitality. The Argonauts from Homer's Odyssey were to be the downfall of the mythical creation. Medea, who was with Jason on his return trip from Troy, enchants Talos promising to make him immortal. While enchanted by her, the nail is removed allowing the ichor to gush out toppling the mechanical man.[39]

The first encounter with technology is as a robot, or an automaton infused with some god-like fluid for animation. This first robot is meant to be a guardian or a protector to the people of Crete. But there is another ancient Greek myth, just as powerful technologically speaking, that continues to have influence on our modern era, the story of Pygmalion. These myths, as we shall see, can have a profound effect on human psyche, society's expectations, and the creative spirit, at least by Western standards.

Pygmalion is either a gifted Cyprian sculpture or a king, or both. As the myth is told, Pygmalion finds the women of Cyprus so impossibly flawed that he resolves to create a statue of his ideal woman.[40] He embodies this statue with every feminine grace and virtue he can devise and sculptures his masterpiece from the finest virgin ivory (or perhaps marble). After months of labor, he completes the most exquisite art ever created and, of course, he falls in love with it. He is depicted standing in his studio kissing its ivory lips, holding the stone hands, dressing, and grooming the figure like a large doll.[41] But Pygmalion becomes despondent as the lifeless statue could not return his affections and the cold stone could not fathom his love.

It is lost in the mists of time, but Pygmalion's statue eventually assumes a name, Galatea (sleeping love). Pygmalion presents gifts and prayers to Aphrodite, who hears and animates his statue. He goes on to marry his statue and is blessed by Aphrodite with a long life and a son, Paphros.[42]

Both of these ancient Greek myths have founded their modern technologic legacies, respectively. Talos has created the image of an automaton being constructed for the benefit of humanity. This myth will be recreated and changed throughout the history of the Western world. When Sir Artegall fell under the power of Radigund, the queen of the Amazons, it is Talus that brings Britomart to the rescue.[43] This word also finds itself evolved to the word talismans. The four talismans from the *Oriental Tales* (1743) were a little golden fish, which could get from the sea anything that it was bidden; a poniard, which made the person wearing it invisible; a ring of steel, which allowed the wearer to read the secret desire of men's hearts; and the fourth a bracelet, which protected the wearer from poisons.[44] The current iteration of the Greek myth of Talos, the protector, is utilized in the US Department of Defenses modern missile defense system.[45]

The Pygmalion myth is much more ingrained into our modern psyches. William Schwenk Gilbert, better known as the first half of the great operatic comedy duo, Gilbert and Sullivan, wrote a three-act comedy called Pygmalion and Galatea. In addition, a great deal of modern Hollywood stereotypic activity has gone into a Pygmalion-like movie theme. Pygmalion fantasies abound in Hollywood images and in literature. Whenever man seeks to make the woman of their lives into the likeness thought to be archetypical, the myth of Pygmalion is perpetuated.

The roots of artificial intelligence, however, can be found linked to the myth of Pygmalion. The first programming by demonstration research was David Smith's Pygmalion, which was inspired by the question: "Can a programming environment be constructed to stimulate creative thought?" He identified various aspects of creative thought and concluded that programming systems should support visual and analogical aspects of creative thought and that programming should be less tedious. The design of Pygmalion was inspired by the ease of use of text editors, especially in comparison with programming languages. Pygmalion became that system. Unlike later systems which tried to add programming to otherwise typical user interfaces, Smith constructed a special user interface which contained the typical operations of a programming language. This user interface was the first to make use of *icons*, which he used to subsume the notions of variable, reference, data structure, function, and picture. Icons have since become Smith's most well-known contribution to computer science and represent his attempt to bring computer programming to life. This represents modern computing's symbol of its Pygmalion legacy.[46]

This urge to create something living is common among artists. Artists have consistently reported an exhilaration during the act of *creation*, followed by depression when the work is completed. "For it is then that the painter realizes that it is only a picture he is painting. Until then he had almost dared to hope that the picture might spring to life." This is also the lure of programming, except that unlike other forms of art, computer programs do "come to life" in a sense.[47]

By the fourth century, Aristotle postulated that mechanical contrivances could reduce the amount of human labor. "If every instrument could accomplish its own work, obeying or anticipating the will of others...if the shuttle could weave, and the pick touch the lyre, without a hand to guide them, chief workmen would not need servants, nor masters slaves." This classic thinker of ancient Greece would have known of the story of Daedalus, the master craftsman of classic lore, who is said to have animated dolls and statues. Daedalus was also the designer and builder of the fantastic mazes on Crete. In order to escape, he built wings for his son Icarus and himself to fly away from the land where they were held hostage. Of course, Icarus would fly close to the sun and fall to his death, as would most "would-be" inventors of mechanized flight until the Montgolfier brothers flew aloft in a hot air balloon in 1783.[48] And even they were predicted to do so by Professor Black at the University of Edinburgh in 1767, who announced to his class that a vessel, filled with hydrogen, would rise naturally into the air.[49] Aeschylus wrote about such "living statues" and no less of an authority than Socrates is quoted "that if they were left untethered they might take off, giving you the slip like a runaway slave." A remarkably creative individual who lived during Plato's lifetime was Archytas of Tarentum. He designed great cranes that could help in building magnificent structures with less human effort. He is thought to have constructed wooden pigeons that could fly using power from steam. The most amazing reference to the ancient world might be applied to Hero of Alexandria around 150 BC. Hero is credited with the invention of the syringe in medicine. He is also thought to have created a humanoid automaton that had a head that could not be severed from its neck. It achieved motion by utilizing an ingenious system of cogs and wheels. The most widespread technical wonders of that long-ago era were the complex water clocks or clepsydra that could be found in many of the city centers.[50]

But the Greek's greatest contribution to the advancement of technology was recorded in the works of Ctesibius, Philon, and Heron regarding hydraulic machines. Ctesibius is given the credit for inventing the hydraulic organ. This is an ingenious method for using water power through pipes to create music. Fabulous fountains with enchanting statuaries could also produce music and provide power to animate moving sculptures.[51] Heron would eclipse even these with his works on hydraulics and pneumatics. These masters of engineering would vanish for about 1500 years but their work was transcribed and propagated by Arabs and the Byzantines.[52] In fact, one Arab engineer is credited with several hydraulic mechanized devices, but also the modern flush toilet, Al-Jazari. By 1501, Heron's works on hydraulics and pneumatics were translated into Latin by Giorgio Valla. Future mechanical enthusiasts would find numerous wonders from these ancient Greek thinkers, and the rise of complex mechanical automata would follow directly.[53,54]

Lastly, one cannot finish a tale about Greek lore without ending with the great, blind poet–laureate Homer. In his *Iliad*, Homer recounts the use of automated carts that could be used by the gods:

> …since he was working on 20 tripods which were to stand against the wall of his strong-founded dwelling. And he had set golden wheels underneath the base of each one so that of their own motion they could wheel into the immortal gathering, and return to his house: a wonder to look at. (Homer the *Iliad*, book 18[123])

1.5.2 *World's Fair Robots*

It is possible that in the recent history of the world, only wars have had a more dramatic impact upon our society than expositions. The first industrial exposition occurred in Paris in 1798 and allowed the public to witness progress and technologies that could change the lives of everyone.[55] Steam-powered machines became all of the rage during the Industrial Revolution.[56] In short order, fictional writers began to concoct stories with steam-powered men, *The Steam Man of the Prairies*.[57] The Columbian Exposition presented the first steam engine-powered version of this type of robot built by Professor George Moore from Canada.[58] Within 5 years, Zadock Deddrick, a machinist from Newark, developed a working "Steam Man" that pulled a carriage.[59] This process continued into the nineteenth century when the extraordinary potential of remote-controlled robotic devices was clearly demonstrated to an unsuspecting public at the 1898 Electrical Exhibition in Madison Square Garden, New York City.[24] Nicola Tesla was at the height of his inventive prowess when he brought upon the unprepared world a fully automated, remote-controlled robotic submersible boat. "Teleautomata will ultimately be produced, capable of acting as if possessed of their own intelligence, and their advent will create a revolution."[25]

It would be 37 years and one World War later at the San Diego Exposition that the next robotic device would greet the public. A little known and not widely regarded demonstration of a 2,000-lb mechanical man was demonstrated by its inventor Professor Harry May. Alpha, the robot's name, was 6′2″ tall and could roll its eyes, open and close its mouth, sit and stand, move its arms, and fire a revolver.[60] By 1939, the super secret and far more popular mechanical man was introduced at the New York World's Fair by the electronics giant Westinghouse. Elektro was a spectacular hit at the Westinghouse Pavilion. Elektro would stand high above the audience on a platform and supposedly respond to English-spoken commands. Elektro was able to perform far more complex tasks than Alpha; he was able to move about on the stage with a strange sliding gate. Elektro was about 7 feet in height and costs several hundred thousand dollars for the Westinghouse Corporation to make in Mansfield, Ohio. Records of the company show that they in fact manufactured eight robots from 1931 to 1940. These robots could all move actuated arms and walk. Elektro used a 78-rpm record player to simulate conversation and had a vocabulary of more than 700 words.[61] Elektro was captivating; he enthralled millions of visitors and went on tour following the World's Fair and even appeared in a bad "B" movie, "Sex Kittens Go to College," subtitled Beauty and the Robot.[62] Most curious of all, these mechanical men were not called robots yet, because Karel Capek's play *Rossum's Universal Robots* had not achieved the notoriety and cultural conversion of this word at this time.[3]

The electronics in these early metal men were primitive with loud electrical motor drivers and vacuum tube relays. They would be replaced with microcircuits and far more rapid, efficient, and quiet mechanics in the not too distant future. The World's Fair phenomenon and robots continue to this day. The last Worlds Expo 2005 was held in Aichi, Japan, and closed in September with over 22,000,000 in attendance.[63] The theme was "Nature's Wisdom," but the technology was definitely center stage. The robot assumed a key role with "We Live in a Robot Age." Working robots roved around the grounds and performed routine chores about the grounds including the following: sanitation, garbage collection, security, guide robots, child care duties, and handicapped aid robots. Multiple prototype robots were demonstrated for 11 days in June. In addition, the exhibition had a "Robot Station" where visitors were able to interact with a whole host of robotic-based venues. As is the core of most such industrial expositions, manufacturers were present to show off their future technologies, including Toyota, Honda, SONY, Mitsubishi, and Brother Industries.[63]

1.5.3 The Legacy of Raymond C. Goertz

At this midpoint in discussing engineered robots, it is appropriate to give credit to the engineer who perhaps has done more for modern robotic development than any other, but who is seldom, if ever mentioned, Raymond C. Goertz.[64] Almost every graduate textbook on robotics mentions Goertz, yet surgical papers fail to recognize this man's truly monumental influence on this field.[65]

Ray Goertz was part of the World War II effort euphemized as the Manhattan Project. As a young engineer, he worked at Enrico Fermi's experimental site outside of Chicago called Argonne National Laboratories (ANL). Part of Goertz's obscurity relates to the politically volatile issues surrounding nuclear materials. In September 1944, Manhattan Project's 100-B plutonium reactor began outputting enough of this substance to achieve criticality at Hanford and Ray Goertz developed the first unilateral manipulator to handle this hazardous material for the Atomic Energy Commission. By 05:29:45 AM, Mountain War Time on July 16, 1945, the successful results of "handling" this material culminated in the explosive crescendo called the Trinity test. Goertz and co-workers at ANL demonstrated the first mechanical, bilateral master–slave manipulator device (MSM) in 1949.[66] Goertz had become acutely aware that the haptic senses were necessary to manipulate delicate objects and had incorporated force-feedback systems that greatly improved deftness of the human–machine combination.[67] By the height of the Cold War years, 1954, Goertz had improved the teleoperations by applying principles of cybernetics and constructing the first electronic master–slave manipulator systems.[68]

Goertz applied modern engineering skills with an ancient mechanical device, the pantograph, to create the first MSM. He also codified the terms that university and industrial developers could follow. Not only did Goertz improve his master–slave manipulators, he also performed the primordial research regarding degrees of freedom necessary for smooth motion by remote manipulation. He developed teleoperated systems that are the direct forerunner of modern robotic surgical systems. He even developed one of the first head-mounted displays as a prototype for virtual reality. Goertz incorporated nautical terms such as pitch, yaw, and roll into the lexicon of robotics. Finally, the efforts of this incredibly prolific individual led to the creation of a spin-off company, Central Research Labs (CRL) in Red Wing, Minnesota. By 1953, Ray Goertz was ultimately replaced by Demetrius Jelatis at CRL which has made over 8000 MSMs for over 26 different countries.[69] Goertz's legacy lives on and his first principles of an MSM are as applicable to our own robotic surgical systems.[64] They are as follows:

– The motion of the slave arm must possess six independent degrees of freedom, three of translation and three of rotation to position gripping devices, and a tong squeeze motion to grip items.
– The motion of the slave arm must be coupled to the master arm so that the position and the direction of the two arms correspond.

– The coupling of the two arms must be bilateral. This important concept means that forces at the slave end must be reflected to the master end and displacements produced at the slave end must be able to produce a displacement at the master end. Another way to state this important concept is to say the manipulator must be back-drivable or compliant. This means that the slave arm must be able to align itself in response to the constraints imposed by the task being done. A classic example of this concept is the ability of an MSM to rotate a crank which follows a constrained path.

1.5.4 The University of Robotics

Concurrent with the revolution in computer technology, the robotics effort gained momentum especially in our centers of higher learning. Early robotic prototypes arose in research laboratories at some US universities, particularly Stanford (SRI), Carnegie Mellon, and MIT. Others were industrial, such as General Electric's prototype "walking vehicle" or colloquially referred to as the "elephant" by Ralph Mosher.[70] Others were developed for the dangerous environments of US nuclear-powered facilities. But serious federal funding for Stanford's mobile robot "Shakey" evolved from an Advanced Research Projects Agency (ARPA) grant for artificial intelligence and from these humble beginnings a whole network of robotic centers would evolve. Shakey was a mobile, intelligent robot that could search for objects within its environment.[71] It had an "off-board" PDP-10 computer linked to the robot by radio. It certainly had difficulty working independently and was incredibly slow. One of the early investigators from this SRI team was a young Australian, Rodney Brooks. He would move on to MIT's Artificial Intelligence Laboratories to continue building and investigating robotics. Brook's labs now have many prototypes utilizing computer strategies that were significantly different to any type of previously available programming. Based upon an investigational autonomous robot called "Genghis," Brook's new computerized algorithms were termed subsumption programs. The idea was to build robots with programs that were intelligent, situated, embodied agents that could interact with their environment. The computation is organized asynchronously with network active elements in a layered architecture. Sensors and actuators are connected to this control program so as to modify the robot's "behavior." Genghis thus became a hunter-seeker. Some of the first sensors given to these robots were sonar and light sensors. Genghis demonstrated surprising adaptability to his environment and a life-like quality not previously accorded to advanced robots (except the Turk). Genghis weighed just about 1 kg., had six legs for mobility, walked, and sought all under its subsumption programming. It could negotiate even rough terrain using 12 motors, 12 force sensors, 6 pyroelectric sensors, 1 inclinometer, and 2 whiskers.[72]

The MIT program sought to investigate the known robotic dogma. Do complex robotic behaviors need to be a product of complex control systems? They believed that things should be simple, interface systems and subsystems. Do robots need to be expensive? They sought to build cheap robots that worked in human environments. The world is 3D and the robot must function in 3D. Do coordinate systems have to be very sophisticated? They noted that coordinate systems for robots are the source of a large number of errors. The real world is not constructed of simple polyhedra. They noted that visual data are necessary for high-level tasks, but sonar might be good for low-level tasks such as object avoidance. Their robots must perform even if one or more of its sensors fail or give erroneous information. To quote Brooks, "we are interested in building 'artificial beings'—robots that survive for days, weeks and months without human assistance, in a dynamic and complex environment. Such robots must be self-sustaining."[72] The MIT robotics labs came up with a method to solve this complex control problem that had faced roboticists since the beginning. Their method is nothing like human neurologic control systems; it is organized asynchronously with network-active elements. They called their robotic control systems subsumption programs. The computations are fixed topology of unidirectional connections. Messages are sent over connections with semantics of small numbers (typically 8–16 bits) with dynamics designed into both the sender and the receiver. Sensors and actuators are connected to this via asynchronous two-sided buffers. "Allen" was their first subsumptive robot and it was almost entirely reactive—using sonar readings to keep away from people and other objects. Allen also had a non-reactive higher level which attempted to head toward a goal. Next came Genghis, whose primary program is to search for a moving object and track and chase it. It is amazingly insect-like and really interacts with the environment to complete its programmed task. The laboratory has pursued more sophisticated behaviors and have begun to downsize the robots (recall their goal of reducing cost). "Herbert" uses a laser scanner to find soda cans, infrared proximity sensors to navigate, and a magnetic compass to maintain its global sense of orientation. Its task is to wander around the laboratory looking for things to clean up and bring them back to where Herbert started. "Squirt" followed with a diminutive weight of 50 g and measured only 5/4 cubic inches. Squirt incorporates an 8-bit onboard computer, battery, three sensors, and a propulsion system. Its normal activity is bug-like hiding in dark corners and venturing out to investigate noises. Squirt's control system fits 1,300 bytes of code into its computer.[72]

There are many problems with subsumption systems, especially when adaptive learning is necessary for the robot. More research into sensors, computational algorithms, and actuators are all necessary, but as with computing costs are dropping. There are now sophisticated robotic kits that your children can purchase from LEGO[TM]. Multiple parallel fields of research are beginning to merge with robotics technologies. More degrees of freedom are possible from robotic systems.[73] More computer horsepower is available, to make even the most sophisticated interactive systems work smoothly. The roles of robotic systems are beginning to be systematically evaluated. Robots are proving vital in the hazardous industry sector. Robots are used routinely in nuclear reactor facilities. Robots are expected to play a significant role in precursor missions to Mars. Robotic morphology is being evaluated. Vehicular-mobile-payload-carrying devices are just beginning to be utilized. Humanoid devices are planned for future space shuttle missions. Robotic control systems are tackling such problems as balance of control issues. Can a single human control many robots at once? Robots can be used to augment human functions. Funding and vigorous research is ongoing to alleviate the handicaps of deafness, blindness, and motor dysfunction from limb loss or nerve damage. Robotic exoskeleton devices are being investigated, robotic "prosthetic" wheelchairs that interact with the environment are being tested, and cochlear implant

technology is advancing.[74] Robotic systems are gradually creeping into our daily lives with toys such as the "My Real Doll," AIBO, and smart appliances (vacuum cleaner and lawnmowers). Human–robot relationships are being investigated. AIBO, Sony's first robotic pet, has already generated many interesting observations by observing responses from its owners. Robotic appearance will establish the social expectations of these systems in our society. Honda, the auto company, is investing millions of dollars into its automated, walking robotic system, named Asimo walked to the grave of Karel Capek. Robotics programs at universities are increasing at a rapid rate. Born of Stanford's Shakey work, Brooks went to MIT, Moravec joined the team at Carnegie Mellon, and the modern run to advanced machines ensued. Some researchers are working on matching robotic morphology with task and environment. The most significant work is being done at MIT and in Japan using humanoid facial expressions to study robotic–human interactions.[75]

1.5.5 Out of the Laboratory

George Devol and Joe Engelberger in the early 1950s thought that machines could be manufactured that could take the place of skilled workers in factories.[76] They developed the first modern industrial robots, called "unimates." Engelberger went on to develop the first robotics company, called "Unimation." Robots in the workplace are thought to have many potential advantages. The robot can work in a potentially dangerous place without risk of injury. Thus, the mechanical worker is safer. In addition, the robot's program makes each movement always with the same specifications and it can perform very fast depending upon the servo-motors. The machines are reliable and can perform for prolonged periods of time before requiring service. When parts wear out, they are simply replaced. Some types of industrial robots can be reconfigured and redeployed to perform several tasks.[77]

In 1961, the UNIMATE was introduced to the automotive industry as the first industrial robot. In 1971, the first microprocessor was introduced, allowing computer mass to be reduced to postage stamp-sized circuits that cost about as much as dinner. By 1996, 6 million components were placed upon a single silicon chip adding to the speed and power of the integrated circuit. In 1997, Sojourner, the first automated, autonomous robotic space rover, explored the surface of Mars.[2]

Finally, surgical applications of robotics are just beginning to be realized. Our expectations for robots is somewhat jaded by our Hollywood stereotypes.[78] This burgeoning technology is in its infancy and the future will probably not be quite as we have thought to be.

1.6 Surgical Robotics

His latest achievements in the substitution of machinery, not merely for the skill of the human hand, but for the relief of the human intellect, are founded on the use of tools of a still higher order. (Charles Babbage[79])

Technology and microelectronics are revolutionizing every aspect of our society. Polymer science, microcomputerization, optical engineering, bio-engineering, and many other technologic arenas are being focused upon advanced health-care delivery.[2] Surgery has not been immune to such technologic advancement. But as we have already seen, there exists a great deal of historical precedent. At the dawn of the Enlightenment, technology began to focus upon healthcare, and surgeons in particular attempted to simulate surgery using machines. Jacques de Vaucanson, Francois Quesnay, and Claude-Nicolas LeCat represent seventeenth century proponents of simulators in medical education; but there is no evidence that any of these three luminaries had any substantive success. De Vaucanson whom we have already mentioned actually presented some type of mechanical device to the Royal Academie.[80] LeCat, a noted lithotomists, also devised a crude surgical simulator. But a little known midwife outdid all of these great inventors. Le Boursier du Coudray epitomized the enlightenment attitudes toward broadening knowledge to the common man. She ceaselessly sought to bring education to the woman in villages and towns throughout France in response to the population crisis and the very high birth morbidity and mortality (approx. 200,000 infant mortalities in France in 1729, some areas reached 25%).[81] Her original textbook *Abrégé* utilized some of the first color anatomical illustrations, her method of teaching complex birthing techniques to peasant woman throughout France, and her birthing simulator was a complex machine, complete

with fluids [*wet ware*] to aid learning. Her techniques and methods are surprisingly modern in context and her plan to use every method available to improve the performance of her pupils is poignant. The color illustrations in *Abrégé* remain profoundly effective but the only existent models of her simulator are even more remarkable.[82] She developed influential support from the likes of lithotomist Frére Côme. Her teaching methods affected untold thousands of medical practitioners, from midwives to surgeons, and she received royal support from Louis XV. Voltaire wrote about her and she became an icon of progressive France, but remained ostracized by much of the conventional medical practitioners. She continued to educate midwives and physicians for 23 years before retiring at the age of nearly 70 after training an estimated 10,000 pupils.[83]

Automation represents the most advanced capacity for minimal access intra-abdominal surgery. In 1985, a robotic engineer began to develop feasibility studies into the possibility of a neurologic robot in the Department of Mechanical Engineering of Imperial College in London.[84] Brian Davies joined the urologic team headed by J.E.A. Wickham and turned his attention to the prostate. By 1987, this team collaborated with Roger Hibberd and guided by Anthony Timoney proceeded from the laboratory to clinical trials with a six-axis Unimate PUMA robot. They called their device the PROBOT.[85] Pneumatic robotic arms were already available for holding the laparoscope better than can the trusted medical student by the mid-1980s.[86] Precision, computerized response devices that interact with the human hand–eye coordination capacity are utilized by the military for weaponry. Children's games are already utilizing this same technology for amazing games of video skill. It is foreseeable that this same capacity will evolve into microrobotic intra-abdominal devices that will work on remote radio-signal commands. Such systems for surgical intervention are already being developed. Complete, remote surgical interaction with the endoscopic camera and robotic instruments coupled with computer-mediated feedback (auditory, visual, and tactile) provides a near "virtual reality" for the surgeon. Robodoc[TM] is one such computer-controlled, robotic, interactive orthopedic device. It can rapidly and reproducibly make total joint replacement a precision-tooled, automated procedure.[87] But this represents just the initial surgical application of a whole host of robotic technology. The Massachusetts Institute of

Technology is proposing new computerized intelligence chips that allow small, mobile robotic devices to learn and interact. Such GNAT robots combine distributed real-time control with sensor-triggered behavior. Currently, insect-like mobile robots have been constructed but are limited in their capacity to perform dexterous surgical maneuvers by inadequacies of the microengines. The University of California, Berkeley, and AT&T Bell laboratories are independently investigating microengines that could power small robotic devices. Nippondenso, one of the world's largest automanufacturers, has devised an electromagnetic wave engine, utilizing microwave energy "beamed" into it from a distance. Where this technology shall lead no one can quite predict. These microrobotic, computer-controlled, intra-abdominal surgical devices are sure to become more advanced.[88] This leads us to our current state of robotic surgery.

1.6.1 Complete Robotic Surgery

The United States Department of Defense has long been interested in the development of frontline methods of improving care to injured soldiers. Life-threatening injuries occurring immediately during battle might be salvageable if surgical care could be instantly instituted. In addition, after George Bush's announcement of the United States' intention of getting a man on Mars, the National Aeronautics and Space Administration (NASA) Ames Research Center began to fund proposals for the eventual need for possible surgical intervention on astronauts remote from a hospital.[2] A team of investigators led by Michael McGreevey and Stephen Ellis began to investigate computer-generated scenarios that could be perceived on head-mounted displays (HMDs).[89] To this team eventually came Scott Fisher, who added 3D audio and came up with the concept of "telepresence." This was the notion that one person could be projected with the immersive experience of another (real or imaginary). Joseph Rosen, a plastic surgeon at Stanford University, began to experiment with Philip Green from Stanford Research Institute (SRI) to develop dexterity-enhancing robots for telemanipulation.[90] These two teams would eventually collaborate, and together Joe Rosen and Scott Fisher produced the fundamentals of telepresence surgery. This combined the dexterity-enhancing robotics of Green and the "virtual reality" systems of NASA for an immersive surgical experience. The initial systems conceived that the surgeon would be in a helmeted immersive sight/sound environment wired electronically to "data gloves" that would digitally track the surgeon's motions and reproduce them at remote robotic instruments. The notion of the data glove came from Jaron Lanier, a computer scientist interested in virtual reality. The initial targeted surgery was on the hand.

Many of the initially designed features of Green's Telepresence System were at the time unworkable from an engineering standpoint. The HMD was subsequently replaced with monitors, and the data gloves were replaced with handles for controllers at the surgeon's console. Since the imperative at this time was for space and/or military application for acute surgical care, the end effectors were substantially similar to open surgical instruments. This was all occurring in the late 1980s. By 1989, then Colonel Richard Satava stationed at Silas B. Hayes Army Hospital in Monterey became involved in this project and more Federal aid became available.[91] Serendipitously, that same year found Jacques Perissat of Bordeaux presenting on the technique of laparoscopic cholecystectomy at the Society of American Gastrointestinal Endoscopic Surgeons (SAGES) in Atlanta. Upon returning from this meeting, the team of investigators began to consider developing a system that could be applied to minimally invasive laparoscopic surgery. Satava presented a videotape of a bowel anastomosis using the telepresence surgery system to the Association of Military Surgeons of the United States. The results of this single demonstration of this technology resulted in a July 1992 Defense Advanced Research Projects Agency (DARPA) grant for further investigation and development. In addition, Satava became the program manager for Advance Biomedical Technologies to aid funding of technologically advanced projects. With the funding now possible, by 1995, the robotic system was in prototype mounted into an armored vehicle (the Bradley 557A) that could "virtually" take the surgeon to the front lines and immediately render surgical care to the wounded, called MEDFAST (Medical Forward Area Surgical Team).[91] The technology caught the attention of Alan Alda (aka Hawkey Pierce from the TV drama M.A.S.H.), now the voice of *Discovery Channel*, who filmed a piece on this technology.

The primordial "team" began to split apart; however, Satava was transferred to DARPA, Joe Rosen left Stanford for a position in plastic surgery at Dartmouth-Hitchcock Hospital and an engineering affiliation with the department of engineering. Jon Bowersox was recruited to join the team as replacement for Rosen and furthered the research by performing the first remote telesurgical procedure, another intestinal anastomosis, in an ex vivo porcine model in 1994. He later turned his attention to vascular surgical research interests.[91] Also in 1993, Yulyn Wang, Ph.D., from the University of California, Santa Barbara, developed software for control motion of robotic systems and founded a company called Computer Motion. Wang succeeded in developing a robotic camera holder called automated endoscopic system for optimal positioning (AESOP). He became interested in complete robotic surgery and obtained DARPA funding and money from the entrepreneurs to develop ZEUS, a modular robotic system to be integrated with AESOP. HERMES was the integrated operating room control system that allowed the complete integration of Computer Motion's robotic system.[92] It was the ZEUS robotic system that made history during the performance of the first remote surgery across the Atlantic Ocean (surgeon in New York City, patient in Brussels).[93]

In 1995, surgical entrepreneur Frederic H. Moll, MD (formerly started three other successful surgical enterprises, but then medical director of Guident), Rob Younge (an engineer who had co-founded Acuson), and John Freund (an MBA from Harvard) became interested in the potential of the "telepresence" work from SRI. Fred saw that this technology could be applied specifically to the area of burgeoning laparoscopic surgeries with some modifications. They arranged a group of scientists from the SRI group, from International Business Machines (IBM), and the Massachusetts Institute of Technology (MIT) in a fledgling company. Two people particularly would influence the design and development of the robotic surgical instrument, J. Ken Salisbury, who was working in Rodney Brooks' Artificial Intelligence Laboratory, and graduate student Akhil J. Madhani both left to join the start-up company of Moll's called *Intuitive Surgical*.[94] From the outset, they formed the belief that the focus of robotic-assisted surgery should be compatible with minimally invasive surgery and they licensed the rights to patents to build a system with three basic components:

1. A master–slave software-driven system that would provide intuitive control of a suite of seven-degree-of-freedom robotic instruments.
2. A computerized vision system that would be three dimensional and immersive (Green's legacy).
3. A redundant method for insuring safety consisting of sensors to allow maximum safety during the robotic procedure.

The team now at Intuitive Surgical experimentally chose to locate the surgeon's hands below the console as the optimum position. Next, the tip-to-tip control idea was evolved to get maximum dexterity from the surgeon's fingers at the master console to the virtual jaws of the instruments themselves. It was felt that the tip-to-tip method allowed the surgeon to always remain oriented to the jaws of the robotic via a software interface allowed true surgical intention.[95]

Intuitive tested the first prototype in March of 1997 using their robotic system with a then available stereo endoscope. By 15 April 1997 the first robotic surgery was performed by Jacques Himpens and Guy Cardiere of Brussels, Belgium, a robotic cholecystectomy.[96]

For the bulk of 1998, Intuitive focused intensely upon the development of a better binocular, computer-enhanced imaging system so as to achieve superior resolution and three-dimensional perception for the advanced robotic surgical procedures intended. In 1999, the company developed the system architecture for the da Vinci Surgical System[TM]. da Vinci was equipped with an elaborate safety system that checks its position every 750 μs, using at least one motherboard for each active arm and another for the imaging systems.[94] The first 200-patient trial was completed on cholecystectomy and Nissen fundoplications leading to Food and Drug Administration (FDA) approval of this robotic system in July 2000. In December 2002, the FDA also approved the use of the next generation da Vinci System with the addition of a fourth robotic arm to the tower. This fourth arm is identical to the other two and the surgeon can toggle with a foot pedal between control of any two of the three surgical instrument robotic arms. Late in 2003, Intuitive also introduced a new highly magnifying panoramic computer-enhanced digital video system that toggles with a foot switch from close-up, 3D view and wide-angle 2D views to aid in the surgery of complex sutured repairs. In addition, the company is actively investigating "downsizing" of their current 8-mm robotic actuators to 5 mm and smaller.[94] The FDA currently requires that the American surgeon performs the telerobotic operation within the same operating room as the patient, but this is not necessary with this technology as we have already seen.

1.6.2 Microrobotic Surgery

Scale down the size of the robots, add more intelligent software, and the microrobotic systems become possible. The technology for creating working clinical devices is in its infancy but such devices are already available in children's toys. Clinical interest for such systems already exists for stereotactic brain surgery. In one futuristic system, Wieneke and Lutze utilize a microendoscopic trocar system with miniaturized electronically orienting instruments with outer diameters of 0.63 mm.[97] New steering mechanisms such as microfluidics (no cables or mechanical structures) allow the device to be electronically steered toward the site of the pathology. The optics were produced micro-technically by the LIGA process for fabrication of freely movable microstructures. A host of electronically controllable microinstruments from graspers to scissors have been made from super-elastic behavior of materials such as nickel–titanium alloys or plastics.[98]

One can envision the basic robotic surgical instrument of the future that will be introduced through very tiny portals or via an endoluminal route. The head of the device will be similar to an insect with small, paired optical sensors for guiding the robotic intervention. The end effectors will be mounted upon the "head" with other sensors much like feelers that will monitor the local–regional environment.[99] The mouthparts will be dexterous darning apparatus to reapproximate any structure that needs to be repaired. There will be retractable-powered devices such as laser fibers for hemostasis or soldering.

1.6.3 Autonomous Microrobotic Surgery

One step further removed from the microrobots just mentioned are the autonomous microrobots that interest basic scientists around the world. These will have the capacity to learn from mistakes and might be capable of self-replication and recruitment. If more than one device is needed, it will attract another. They will be capable of orienting themselves for purposeful cooperative behavior and controlling the environment to accomplish whatever task is given to them.[100] Sound too far-fetched, think again. The ability to micromanufacture component parts and integrate intelligent technologies is in its infancy. Autonomous robotic technologies are rapidly advancing and medical/surgical applications will be sought.[101,102]

1.6.4 Nano-robotic Surgery

Go one final step and you come to the realm of nanotechnology. This shall be discussed in the final section of this chapter.

1.7 Human–Robot Interface (Cyborgs)

> My robots were machines designed by engineers, not pseudo-men created by blasphemers. (Asimov, 1994[124])

The exact beginning of cybernetics is perhaps difficult to ascertain, but the article *An Essay on the Origins of Cybernetics* from a 1959 article by D.L. Stewart is the best place to start.[103] He notes that the word *cybernetics* was derived from the Greek *kubernetes* or "steersman" and was coined by Norbert Wiener, a professor of mathematics at MIT. In 1948, Wiener started meeting with other young scientists monthly at Vanderbilt Hall in the early 1940s. One of the first investigators he met was a Harvard Medical School professor of physiology Arturo Rosenblueth. This pair would later team up during the war years to investigate a machine's ability to predict voluntary control (desperately needed for wartime anti-aircraft design systems). By 1943 these investigations were published in the *Philosophy of Science* called *Behavior, Purpose and Teleology*.[125] They specifically defined behavior as any change of an entity with respect to its surroundings. This began the scientific understanding of mechanized actions or the understanding of human behavior with mechanized processes. Their first classification separated *active behavior*, in which the object is itself the source of energy in the output, and *non-active behavior* or *passive behavior*, in which all the energy in the output come from the immediate output. The essence of their theories was based upon feedback loops for control; the mathematics was just beginning at this time. They stated, "the broad classes of behavior are the same in machines and in living organisms...while the behaviouristic analysis of machines and living organisms is largely uniform, their functional study reveals deep differences." Wiener and Rosenblueth's ideas would begin to stimulate formal scientific investigation when the Josiah Macy, Jr. Foundation organized a series of scientific meetings to fertilize new methods of investigation throughout the 1940s. By the 1950s, the term *cybernetics* was increasingly utilized to describe much of the scientific investigation of control mechanisms, digital processing, and of course computer technologies and intelligent systems.[103]

Artificial intelligence (AI) uses computer technology to strive toward the goal of machine intelligence and considers implementation as the most important result; cybernetics uses epistemology (the limits to how we know what we know) to understand the constraints of any medium (technological, biological, or social) and considers powerful descriptions as the most important result.[104] The computer chip comes from germanium or silicon solid-state transistors that were the first of two Nobel Prizes for John Bardeen.[105] In 1950, ENIAC at the Moore School of Electrical Engineering at the University of Pennsylvania was the first modern electronic computer with the essential features found on current computers. By the early 1950s, microprocessors began to be conceptualized and computers began to make their way into scientific and business accounting. In the summer of 1956, John McCarthy, who founded the Stanford Artificial Intelligence Laboratory (SAIL) along with Marvin Minsky, started a 6-week workshop at Dartmouth College on "Artificial Intelligence." There were 12 original participants in this prophetic group. The field of AI came into being when the concept of universal computation,[126] the cultural view of the brain as a computer, and the availability of digital computing machines were combined. The field of cybernetics came into being when concepts of information, feedback, and control [Wiener 1948] were generalized from specific applications (e.g., in engineering) to systems in general, including systems of living organisms, abstract intelligent processes, and language. We have already talked about Vannevar Bush's vital

contributions with his view of the information revolution (1945 article *As We May Think*). In the early 1960s, Ted Nelson conceived and designed hypertext and the systems for storing and transferring information. Tim Berner-Lee followed by delivering the World Wide Web to his employers, built it, and placed it upon the nascent Internet of the early 1990s.[2]

It has been said that computers will be 1,000 times more powerful than they are currently within 20 years.[106] At that point, it is expected that our electronic machines will be more intelligent than us. What will we be able to do with so much computing power? Let us explore just some of the intriguing possibilities in light of some of today's cutting edge, fusion work on man and machines.[107] Cochlear implants were some the first fusions of electronics engineering and human neurophysiologic function. The pioneering work of Georg von Bekesy in 1950 demonstrated that the basilar membrane in the inner ear was responsible for analyzing signal input into different frequencies. William House working closely with 3 M company had developed a working unit consisting of three mechanisms: signal processor, signal transmitter/receiver, and implanted electrodes. By the 1980s, the Technical University of Vienna, also working with 3 M, improved this design and added automatic gain controls. Multichannel implants became available in the mid-1980s.[108]

The next obvious digital–neurobiologic interface would help correct blindness. Such advanced technologies are rapidly progressing in such labs at Johns Hopkins University and the University of Tübingen. There are currently two types of retinal implants, subretinal and epiretinal. These electronic microchip processors such as the *Optobionics* 2-mm device are composed of tiny electrodes, powered by 3,500 microscopic solar cells. Thus the light coming into the eye both powers the chip and transfers the signal for processing to the brain.[109]

Now go one step further into amputees and spinal cord-injured patients and the next possible cybernetic applications can be appreciated.[110] Miguel Nicolelis at Duke University published a classic article in *Nature Neuroscience* in 1998. He implanted multi-site neural ensemble electrophysiology monitors into the cerebral cortex of three adult owl monkeys (*Aotus trivirgatus*).[111] He studied and sought specific cortical areas that had neuronal responses to tactile stimulation, particularly on the animals' hands and arms. He developed a computerized artificial neural network to train and derive the responses. Once the computer's neural network was trained (after 360 stimulus runs with derived values from linear discriminant analysis), they were able to replicate the same responses as predicted from the monkey's cortex. For 2 years, they monitored the signals and modeled them using the computer's neural network. Taking this a step further, they were next able to attach the computer's neural network to a robotic arm. Whenever the monkey would reach for food, the robotic arm would now reach for food in a similar fashion. Wired via the Internet to a similar arm at Boston's MIT, the monkey could also perform the same task in both places at once.[112]

Using the human nervous system and fusing information transfer with digital technologies is in its infancy. There is ongoing work with robotic artificial legs and arms that can connect or communicate with nerve endings from the stump of a lost limb.[113] In addition, computer–brain interface technologies that can directly interpret EEG brain waves are already functionally being tried at advanced research centers. At MIT, a select group of handicapped individuals are being trained to directly interface with a computer's mouse-like device to aid these individuals with connecting to the Internet, writing, controlling other mechanical devices within their environments, and generally trying to improve their existence.[114] Many of these advanced technologies can be expected to have "spin-off" devices that could become widely available in the next 10 years. Man–machine interface issues will become an increasingly sophisticated issue in the very near future.

1.8 Future Considerations (Nanotechnology)

In 1997, one of the seminal battles between the human brain and artificial intelligence was fought and lost...the world shivered. (TIME[21])

The Nobel physicist Richard Feynman predicted in a 1959 talk entitled "There's plenty of room at the bottom" that the theoretical possibility of manipulating things on a molecular scale.[115] Prior to this prophetic lecture, Albert Einstein as part of his doctoral dissertation calculated that the size of a single

sugar molecule was about 1 nm in diameter (for scale imagine that 10 hydrogen atoms side by side, it is one thousandth the length of a typical bacterium, one millionth the size of a pinhead).[116] The first living cells housing nanoscale biomachines evolved 3.5 billion years ago. In 400 BC, Democritus coined the word "atom," which was thought to be the basis of all matter. In 1905 Albert Einstein calculated the diameter of the sugar molecule described previously. In 1931 Max Knoll and Ernst Ruska developed the electron microscope for sub-nanometer imaging. In 1959 Richard Feynman gave the prophetic lecture predicting the rise of nanotechnologies. In 1968 Alfred Y. Cho and John Arthur of Bell Labs invented molecular-beam epitaxy, to deposit single atomic layers on a surface. In 1974 Norio Taniguchi conceived the word "nanotechnology." In 1981 Gerd Binnig and Heinrich Rohrer created a scanning tunneling microscope, which can image individual atoms. By 1985 Robert F. Curl Jr., Harold W. Kroto, and Richard E. Smalley discovered buckminsterfullerenes, also known as buckyballs, which measure about 1 nm in diameter. D. Eric Drexler published his futuristic book *Engines of Creation* in 1986 that popularizes nanotechnology. In 1989, Donald M. Eigler of IBM wrote the company's name using individual xenon atoms. In 1991, Sumio Iijima of NEC in Tsukuba, Japan, discovered nanotubes. In 1993, Warren Robinett of the University of North Carolina and R. Stanley Williams of the University of Southern California at Los Angeles devised a virtual-reality system connected to a scanning tunneling microscope that lets the user see and touch atoms. In 1998 Cees Dekker's group at the Delft University of Technology created a transistor from a carbon nanotube. In 1999, James M. Tour at Rice University and Mark A. Reed of Yale University demonstrated that single molecules can act as molecular switches. In 2000 the Clinton administration announced the National Nanotechnology Initiative, which provided a big boost in funding to nanoresearch. Later in that same year, Eigler and others devised a quantum mirage with a magnetic atom, proving a possible means of transmitting information without wires at a molecular level.[2]

Currently there are several proposals to the National Nanotechnology Initiative for medical applications. Some are for diagnostic possibilities including the use of artificial magnetic crystals that detect particular biologic entities such as pathogens. Other applications include the use of semiconductor nanocrystals, a quantum "dot." These dots owe their special properties to quantum mechanics and emit photons of light in only one specific wavelength. These quantum "dots" can be attached to DNA sequences which when scanned can act like a genetic bar code, looking for flaws. A dendrimer is a branching molecule roughly the size of a protein that has a large internal surface area. They can be created in a variety of sizes and might be able to transmit DNA sequences into cell's nuclei much safer than virus particles. Other dendrimers might be able to act as microdrug delivery vectors. Nanoshells are small beads of glass coated with gold that can absorb light, particularly near-infrared which can be beamed into the body. These nanoshells could then be induced from an extracorporeal strong infrared source to be heated. Buckyballs can be made from just a few dozen carbon atoms. The potential for the future of nanotechnology like many other futuristic applications to medicine is unknown. But it is intriguing to speculate about the possibilities. Using artificial scaffolds that nanotechnology might conceive cancerous tumors at the cellular range might be identifiable and destroyed. Using synthetic scaffolds, we might be able to regenerate bones, cartilage, skin, or more complex organs.[117]

1.9 Conclusions

At the dawn of the next millennium and the rise of the information age, intelligent technologies (ITs) are beginning to effect every aspect of surgical practice. It will be expected that products of this age will be essential in areas of diagnosis, therapy, and education. The same three aspects of medical science that have been thought to be essential for the advancement of medicine will be strongly influenced by intelligent technologies: computers, telecommunications, robotics, microrobotics, and virtual reality simulation. Diagnosis is already beginning to show signs of the intelligent technology invasion with virtual colonoscopy, 3D imaging systems, microendoluminal probes, real-time teleconferencing and consultation, and telementoring and teleproctoring. Therapy cannot be far behind these initial diagnostic endeavors. The tools to perform surgery remotely already exist and are being refined, miniaturized, and increasingly more autonomous. The trend in the surgical realm includes

a paradigm shift from minimally to noninvasive procedures (i.e., percutaneous lithotripsy to shock wave lithotripsy); from direct hands-on to direct hands-off (i.e., laparoscopic, catheter stenting, robotic assisted to robotic performed) procedures; and from single modal therapy to multimodal therapies (i.e., resection and reconstruction to biologically tagged, image guided, dexterity enhanced). Education will be substantially aided by the infusion of ITs by the creation of computer-aided skill development. One would hope that an acceptable degree of surgical error could rival or improve upon the current standards accepted by the aviation industry (FAA) for pilots trained continuously on flight simulators (<0.0001%).[118]

Some other trends might be expected from this technologic influx. There will be more procedures performed with endoscopic guidance. There probably will be a trend toward interdisciplinary cooperation. Much of the ability to minimize the trauma of surgery further will require fusion image processing. The pathology identified with advanced magnetic image devices and computerized tomography will be targeted similarly to stereotactic brain surgery currently. The endoscopic view will provide a stable position to monitor the robotic ablation or reconstruction necessary to obviate the patient's pathologic process. Newer imaging modalities will likely exist such as MR/PET hybrid devices. MRI already possesses the ability to observe thermal gradients within tissues. Image-guided thermal ablation or cryoablation might not even require endoscopic control. Most likely, patients will be diagnosed at even earlier stages of disease processes, thanks to advances in proteomics.[119] Therefore, the extent of disease to be treated will likely be less, and the interventions might not need to be as drastic but the precision robotic controls will be mandatory and such robots are in pipeline research stages.[120]

The explosive and sometimes experimental development of laparoscopic surgery has certainly not been all straightforward. In urology, the early 1990s were all enthusiasm over laparoscopic pelvic lymphadenectomy and varicocelectomy. Interest waned by 1993–1994. Only those urologic laparoscopists comfortable with the more complex types of laparoscopic surgeries pursued the technology and general surgery rapidly became the leader of technologically advanced surgery where it currently remains. But as technologies come, so might they go as predicted by F. Mosteller in 1980. New technology has an apparent life cycle with five stages: (1) feasibility (technical performance, applicability, safety complications, morbidity, mortality); (2) efficacy (benefit for the patient demonstrated in centers of excellence); (3) effectiveness (benefit for the patient under normal conditions, reproducible with widespread application); (4) costs (benefit in terms of cost effectiveness); and (5) gold standard.[121]

To understand how humanity will deal with the coming maelstrom of technologic wonders that our science is about to spew forth into our lives, we must as Winston Churchill once advised, "the further backwards you look, the further forward you see." The relevance of looking to the myths and lore that are the foundations of modern thoughts and perceptions is where to begin to understand technology and the changes that will affect *all* aspects of our civilization and not just the way we practice urology. The history of robotics is almost as intriguing as the robots themselves, almost!

References

1. Ruskin J. *Selected Writings*. London: JM Dent-Everyman; 1995.
2. Moran ME. Law of accelerating returns. *J Endourol*. 2006;20(6):1–8.
3. Moran ME. Rossum's universal robots: not the machines. *J Endourol*. 2007;21(12):1399–1402.
4. 2001: A Space Odyssey. 1968. Stanley Kubrick and Arthur C. Clarke, MGM.
5. Moran ME. Three laws of robotics and surgery. *J Endourol*. 2008;22(8):1–4.
6. Bicentennial Man. Isaac Asimov and Chris Columbus. 1492 Pictures; 1999.
7. The Terminator. James Cameron and Gale Anne Hurd. Hemdale Film; 1984.
8. Watson JD. *The double helix: a personal account of the discovery of the structure of DNA*. New York: Touchstone; 1986.
9. Gould SJ. Wonderful life. *The burgess shale and the nature of history*. New York: W.W. Norton & Co; 1989.
10. Sherwin BL. *Golems among us. How a Jewish legend can help us navigate the biotech century*. Chicago, IL: Ivan R. Dee Publ.
11. Firoozi F, Moran ME, Capello S, Belarmino J, Kolios E, Perrotti M. Robotics in urology – the inevitable heritage of Hellenism. *J Endourol*. 2005;19(7):A118, 906.
12. Moran ME. Out of the darkness – two monks, two mythical humanoid machines. *J Endourol*. 2006;20(1):A228.
13. Moran ME. The da Vinci robot. *J Endourol*. 2006;20(12):986–990.
14. Moran ME. Jacques de Vaucanson: the father of surgical simulation. *J Endourol*. 2007;21(7):679–683.
15. Wood G. *Edison's Eve. A Magical History of the Quest for Mechanical Life*. New York: Anchor Books; 2002.
16. Shelley M. *Frankenstein*. New York: Dell Publ; 1975.
17. The National Library of Medicine. Frankenstein: Penetrating the Secrets of Nature. http://www.nlm.nih.gov/hmd/frankenstein/franktable.html. Accessed June 14, 2009.
18. Bedini SA. The Role of Automata in the History of Technology. http://xroads.virginia.edu/~DRBR/b_edini.html. Accessed June 14, 2009.
19. Standage T. *The turk. The life and Times of the Famous Eighteenth-Century Chess-Playing Machine*. New York: Berkley Books; 2002.
20. Poe EA. Von Kempelen and His Discovery; 1850.
21. Christopher J. Game over: Kasparov and the machine. *TIME*. 2004;Jan 22.
22. Edmonds IG. *The Magic Man; The Life of Robert-Houdin*. Nashville: T. Nelson Pub; 1972.
23. http://www.geocities.com/Hollywood/Academy/9657/GMelies.html. Accessed June 14, 2009.
24. Cheney M. *Tesla. A Man Out of Time*. New York: Simon & Schuster; 2001.
25. Belarmino J, Moran ME, Firoozi F, Capello S, Kolios E, Perrotti M. Tesla's robot and the dawn of the current era. *J Endourol*. 2005;19(7):A214, 915.
26. Walter WG. *An imitation of life*. Scientific American, 42–50. May 1950.
27. Walter WG. *A machine that learns*. Scientific American, 60–63. August 1951.
28. Bush V. 1945. As We May Think. The Atlantic Monthly. www.press.umich.edu/jep/works/vbush/vbush0.shtml. Accessed June 14, 2009.
29. Xin M. Ancient Science and Technology: Tang Dynasty. http://www.pureinsight.org/pi/articles. Accessed June 14, 2009.
30. Xin M. Ancient Chinese Technology: Robots. http://www.pureinsight.org/pi/articles. Accessed June 14, 2009.
31. Ran S. Ancient Chinese Technology: Han Zhihe, Ingenious Craftsman Who Created Flying Mechanical Birds. http://www.pureinsight.org/pi/articles. Accessed June 14, 2009.
32. www.csvohio.edu/history/japan/karakuri.html. Accessed June 14, 2009.
33. http://en.wikipedia.org/wiki/karakuri. Accessed June 14, 2009.
34. www://cjn.or.jp/karakuri. Accessed June 14, 2009.
35. Kara D. A Culture of Robots. http://www.roboticstrends.com. Accessed June 14, 2009.
36. Matthews J. Sony Spring Festival 2004 at Dediage. www.generation5.org/content/2004/mediage.asp. Accessed June 14, 2009.
37. Matus D. A Robot in Every Home. http://www.hawaiibusiness.cc/hb72003/default.cfm. Accessed June 14, 2009.
38. http://homepage.mac.com/cparada/GML/Hephaestus.html. Accessed June 14, 2009.
39. http://www.theoi.com/Tartaros/Talos.html. Accessed June 14, 2009.
40. http://www.pygmalion.ws/stories/greek1.htm. Accessed June 14, 2009.

41. http://www.Keirsey.com/pygmalion/mirroroffiction.html. Accessed June 14, 2009.
42. http://www.dl.ket.org/latin1/mythology/3fables/love/pygmalion.htm. Accessed June 14, 2009.
43. Spenser H. Faerie queene.v.1: 1596.
44. http://www.bibliomania.com. Accessed June 14, 2009.
45. Adams BD. Ballistic missile defense. New York: Elsevier; 1971.
46. http://www.cs.umd.edu/hcil/pda/thesis/pda/node22.html. Accessed June 14, 2009.
47. http://www.pygmalion.ws/stories/blackboard.htm. Accessed June 14, 2009.
48. Hart C. A. Directory of Heavier-than-Air Flying Machines in Western Europe, 850 BC–1783 AD from The Prehistory of Flight. http://www.cabinetmagazine.org/issues/11/assets/flight_chart.html. Accessed June 14, 2009.
49. Marion F. Attempts in Ancient Times to Fly in the Air. http://www.worldwideschool.org/library/books/tech/engineering/WonderfulBalloonAscnent. Accessed June 14, 2009.
50. Firoozi F, Moran ME, Capello S, Belarmino J, Kolios E, Perrotti M. Robotics in urology – the inevitable heritage of Hellenism. *J Endourol*. 2005;197:A118, 906.
51. http://www.fusionanomaly.net/ctesibius.html. Accessed June 14, 2009.
52. http://www.history.rochester.edu/steam/hero/translators.html. Accessed June 14, 2009.
53. http://www.ubr.com/clocks/pub/clep/clep.html. Accessed June 14, 2009.
54. Curtis JR. 2000. The Water Organ and Other Related Sound-Producing Automata. http://cfaonline.asu.edu/haefer/classes/564/464.papers/curtisjwaterorgan.html. Accessed June 14, 2009.
55. Chappell U. History of World's Fairs. http://www.expomuseum.com. Accessed June 14, 2009.
56. Belarmino J, Moran ME, Faroozi F, Capella S, Kolios E, Perrotti M. Technology of robotics: rapidly changing methods. *J Endourol*. 2005;19(1):A69.
57. Ellis ES. The Steam Man of the Prairies. *Beadle's American Novel*. 1868:No. 45.
58. A mechanical man. 1893. *New York Times*, 15 April.
59. Buckley D. 1868. Dederick's Steam Man. http://www.davidbuckley.net/DB/HistoryMakers/1868DederickSteamMan.htm. Accessed June 14, 2009.
60. http://www.davidbuckley.net/DB/HistoryMakers/Alpha1932.htm. Accessed June 14, 2009.
61. Szondy D. http://davidszondy.com/future/robot/elektro1.htm. Accessed June 14, 2009.
62. Sex Kittens Go to College. 1960. Albert Zugsmith Productions.
63. http://www.expo2005.com. Accessed June 14, 2009.
64. Moran ME. Raymond Goertz – legacy to robotics. *J Endourol*. 2007;21(1):A141–A142.
65. Angelo JA Jr. *Robotics: A Reference Guide to New Technology*. New York: Greenwood Press; 2006.
66. Goertz RC. Fundamentals of general purpose remote manipulators. *Nucleonics*. 1952;1011:36–42.
67. Goertz R, Thompson R. Electronically controlled manipulator. *Nucleonics*. 1954;12(11):46–47.
68. Goertz R. Some work on manipulators systems at ANL: Past, present, and a look at the future. *ROSE Seminar*. 1964;May 26–27.
69. Central Research Laboratories. History of Telemanipulator Development. http://www.centres.com/nuclear/manip/maniphis.htm. Accessed June 14, 2009.
70. Debut of a metal giant. 1969. *TIME* April 11.
71. Aylett R. *Robots bringing intelligent machines to life?* New York: Quarto Publishing; 2002.
72. Brooks RA. Flesh and machines: how robots will change us. Boston, MA: Vintage Books; 2003.
73. Menzel P, D'Aluisio F. *Robo Sapiens Evolution of a New Species*. Cambridge: MIT Press; 2000.
74. Perkowitz S. *Digital People from Bionic Humans to Androids*. Washington, DC: Joseph Henry Press; 2004.
75. Moran ME, Belarmino J, Firoozi F, Capello S, Kolios E, Perrotti M. Humanoid robotic surgery. *J Endourol*. 2005;191:A69.
76. Devol G. U.S. Patent 2,988,237. Programmed Article Transfer. Filed December 10, 1954 and issued June 13, 1961.
77. Engelberger J. *Robots in Service*. Cambridge: MIT Press; 1989.
78. Capella S, Moran ME, Belarmino J, Faroozi F, Kolios E, Perrotti M. Hollywood stereotypes and robotic surgery. *J Endourol*. 2005;197:A120, 907.
79. Morrison P, Morrison E. *Charles Babbage and His Calculating Engines: Selected Writings by Charles Babbage and Others*. New York: Dover Publications; 1961.
80. Moran ME, Marsh C, Perrotti M. Jacques de Vaucanson: father of surgical simulation. *J Endourol*. 2006;201:A1.
81. Moran ME. Enlightenment via simulation – "croneology's" first woman. *J Endourol*. 2010;24(1):5–8.
82. Le Boursier du Coudray AM. 1759. Abrégé de l'art des accouchements. Paris.
83. Rattner GN. The king's midwife. *A history and mystery of madame du coudray*. Berkeley, CA: Univ Calif Press; 1998.
84. Robot surgery pioneer receives professorship at Imperial College. http://www.imperial.ac.uk/P3176.htm. Accessed June 14, 2009.
85. Dasgupta P, Challacombe B, Murphy D, Khan MS. Coming full circle in robotic urology. *BJU Int*. 2006;97: 4–5.
86. Moran ME. Robotic surgery: urologic implications. *J Endourol*. 2003;17:695–708.
87. Paul HA, Bargar WL, Mittlestadt B, et al. Development of a surgical robot for cementless total hip arthroplasty. *Clin Orthop*. 1992;354:8–16.
88. Moran ME. Evolution of robotic arms. *J Robotic Surg*. 2007;1:103–111.
89. Fisher SS, McGreevy MM, Humphries J, Robinett W. Virtual environmental display system. In: Crow, F and Pizer, S (Eds) Proceedings of the Workshop on Interactive 3-D Graphics. 1986;1:1–12.
90. Green PS, Hill JH, Satava RM. Telepresence: dexterous procedures in a virtual operating field. *Surg Endosc*. 1991;57:192A.
91. Satava RM. History of Robotic Surgery. The Early Chronicles: A Personal Historical Perspective.

http://www.websurg.com/robotics/history.php. Accessed June 14, 2009.

92. Wang Y, Sackier J. Robotically enhanced surgery: from concept to development. *Surg Endosc*. 1996;8:63–66.

93. Marescaux J, Leroy J, Gagner M, Rubino F, Mutter D, Vix M, et al. Transatlantic robot-assisted telesurgery. *Nature*. 2001;413:379–380.

94. Moran ME, Marsh C, Perrotti M Under the hood: the da Vinci® surgical system™. *J Endourol*. 2006;201:A223.

95. Ballantyne GH, Moll F. The da Vinci telerobotic surgical system: the virtual operating field and telepresence surgery. *Surg Clin N Am*. 2005;83:1293–1304.

96. Himpens J, Leman G, Cardiere GB. Telesurgical laparoscopic cholecystectomy. *Surg Endosc*. 1998;12:1091.

97. Schurr MO, Heyn SP, Menz W, Buess G. Endosystems – future perspectives for endoluminal surgery. *Minimal Invas Ther Allied Technol*. 1998;7:37–42.

98. Buess G, Kipfmuller K, Hack D, Grussner R, Heintz A, Junginger A. Technique of transanal endoscopic microsurgery. *Surg Endosc*. 1988;2:71–75.

99. Schurr MO, Kunert W, Neck J, Voges U, Buess GF. Telematics and telemanipulation in surgery. *Minimal Invas Ther Allied Technol*. 1998;7:97–103.

100. Guber AE. Potential for microsystems in medicine. *Minimal Invas Ther*. 1995;4:267–275.

101. Goh PMY, Kok K. Microrobotics in surgical practice. *Br J Surg*. 1997;84:2–4.

102. Flynn AM, Udayakumar KR, Barrett DS, McLurkin JD, Frank DL, Shectman AN. Tomorrow's surgery: micromotors and microrobots for minimally invasive procedures. *Minimal Invas Ther Allied Technol*. 1998;7: 343–352.

103. Stewert DJ. An essay on the origins of cybernetics. http://www.hfr.org.uk/cybernetics-pages/origins.htm. Accessed June 14, 2009.

104. Fritz S and Editors of Scientific American. Understanding artificial intelligence. New York: Warner Books; 2002.

105. Hoddeson L, Daitch V True genius. The life and science of John Bardeen. The only winner of two Nobel Prizes in physics. New York: Joseph Henry Press; 2002.

106. Kurzweil R The age of spiritual machines. New York: Penguin Books; 1999.

107. Kheng NC. HIFU Robot. http://mrcas.mpe.ntu.edu.sg/ research/urobot/hifu.htm. Accessed June 14, 2009.

108. Wilson BS, Dorman MF Cochlear implants: a remarkable past and a brilliant future. *Hear Res*. 2008;242(1–2): 3–21.

109. Chow AY, Chow VY, Packo CH, Pollack JS, Peyman GA, Schuchard R. The artificial silicone retina microchip for the treatment of vision loss from retinitis pigmentosa. *Arch Opthalmol*. 2004;122:460–469.

110. Clarke A Natural born cyborg. Oxford: Oxford University Press; 2003.

111. Nicolelis MAL, Ghazanfar AA, Stambaugh CR, et al. Simultaneous encoding of tactile information by three primate cortical areas. *Nature Neurosci*. 1998;1:621–630.

112. Wessberg J, Stambaugh CR, Kralic JD, et al. Real-time prediction of hand trajectory by ensembles of cortical neurons in primates. *Nature*. 2000;408:361–365.

113. Mazlish B. The man–machine and artificial intelligence. http://www.stanford.edu/group/SHR/4-2/text/ mazlish.html. Accessed June 14, 2009.

114. Millan JR, Renkens F, Mourino J, Gerstner W. Noninvasive brain-actuated control of a mobile robot by human EEG. *IEEE Trans Biomed Eng*. 2004;516:1026–1033.

115. Feynman RP. *"Surely you're joking, Mr. Feynman!" Adventures of a curious character*. New York: W.W. Norton & Co; 1985.

116. Gribbin J, Gribbin M. *Annus mirabilis. 1905, Albert Einstein, and the theory of relativity*. New York: Chamberlin Bros; 2005.

117. Moran ME. From the bottom up – nanourology. *J Endourol*. 2007;211:A91.

118. Moran ME. Virtual reality – history and development. *J Endourol*. 2007;211:A150.

119. Check E. Proteomics and cancer. Running before we can walk. *Nature*. 2004;429:496–497.

120. Kheng NC. HIFU URObot. http://mrcas.mpe.ntu.edu. sg/research/urobot/hifu.htm

121. Mostellar F. *Assessing Medical Technologies*. Washington, DC: National Academy Press; 1985.

122. Clarke AC. *Hazards of prophecy: the failure of imagination. From collection "profiles of the future: an inquiry into the limits of the possible"*. New York: Harper & Row; 1962.

123. Homer. The Iliad. Fagles R, Tran. New York: Penguin Classics Edition; 1990.

124. Asimov I. I, Asimov: a Memoir. New York: Bantam Books; 1994.

125. Bosenblueth A. *Mind and Brain: Philosophy of Science*. Cambridge, MA: The MIT Press; 1967.

126. Minsky M. *The Society of the Mind*. New York: Simon & Schuster; 1985.

Chapter 2

Robotic Instrumentation and Operating Room Setup

Ty T. Higuchi and Matthew T. Gettman

Abbreviations

da Vinci© S	da Vinci© streamlined
da Vinci© Si	da Vinci© streamline integrated
HD	high definition
3D	three dimensional
LED	light-emitting diode
CCU	camera control units

2.1 Robotic Instrumentation

2.1.1 da Vinci® Surgical System

To date, four different da Vinci® Surgical Systems have been released – standard, streamlined (S), S-high definition (HD), and S integrated (Si) – HD. Each system is composed of a surgeon console, a patient cart, and a vision cart.[6,7] In addition, each system requires several sterile accessories and EndoWrist® instruments (Table 2.1). The standard system was released in 1999 and was available with one camera arm and two to three instrument arms. In 2006 the S system was introduced. This system has a similar platform to the standard system but added a motorized patient cart, color-coded fiber-optic connections, easier instrument exchanges, quick click trocar attachments, increased range of motion and reach of instrument arms, and an interactive video touch screen display. In 2007 the

M.T. Gettman (✉)
Department of Urology, Mayo Clinic, Rochester, MN 55905, USA
e-mail: gettman.matthew@mayo.edu

S system became available with an HD camera and video system. Recently, the Si-HD system was released with an upgraded surgeon console and dual console capability. The dual console feature connects two surgeon consoles to the same patient cart. This allows two surgeons to coordinate a surgical procedure by exchanging control over the endoscope and instrument arms throughout the procedure.

2.1.1.1 Surgeon Console

The surgeon console (Figs. 2.1 and 2.2) is the driver's seat for the da Vinci® Surgical System. From here the surgeon adjusts the system using the pod controls, views a three-dimensional (3D) image of the surgical field through the stereoviewer, and manipulates the instrument arms using the master controllers and foot pedals.[6,7] The standard and S systems have similar surgeon consoles, while the Si system was remodeled to increase ergonomics, working space, and integrate several controls into a central location (Fig. 2.2).

For the standard and S systems (Fig. 2.1), the pod controls are located adjacent to the arm rests. The right-side pod controls turn the system on and off and communicate any major system errors, while the left-side pod controls set the system configuration and troubleshoot system faults. On the outside of the left-side pod are adjustment buttons for raising and lowering the height of the surgeon console. The Si system integrates the right and left pod controls into a central touch pad located on the armrest and adds the ability to adjust the surgeon console in four different directions for increased ergonomics.

The stereoviewer projects a real-time magnified image of the surgical field. The 3D image is created

A.K. Hemal, M. Menon (eds.), *Robotics in Genitourinary Surgery*,
DOI 10.1007/978-1-84882-114-9_2, © Springer-Verlag London Limited 2011

Table 2.1 Instruments for robotic-assisted surgery

Laparoscopic instruments	Robotic instruments
• Veress needle	• da Vinci® Surgical System
• Visiport™ (Ethicon Endo-surgery, Cincinnati, OH)	• 8-mm robotic trocars (2–3 depending on the number of instrument arms)
• 12-mm Optiview™ and 12-mm Xcel™ (Ethicon Endo-surgery, Cincinnati, OH)	• EndoWrist® instruments
• 6-mm Ternamian EndoTIP trocars™ (Storz, Culver City, CA)	• Sterile drapes for camera and instrument arms, camera, and telemonitor
• Fascial closure device	• Sterile camera mount and camera trocar mount (depending on the system)
• 10-mm ENDOCATCH® entrapment sac (Covidien, Norwalk, CT)	• Sterile trocar mount (depending on the system)
• Curved Endo Metzenbaum scissors	• Sterile instrument adapter (comes attached to the drape for the S)
• Maryland dissector	• Sterile camera adapter
• Hook cautery	
• Needle driver	
• Endoscopic clip applier	
• Suction irrigator	
• 0 and 30° laparoscope lens	
• Camera and fiber-optic cords	
• 5- and 10-mm Hem-o-lock® clips (Teleflex Medical, Research Triangle Park, NC)	
• Hot water bath for endoscopes	

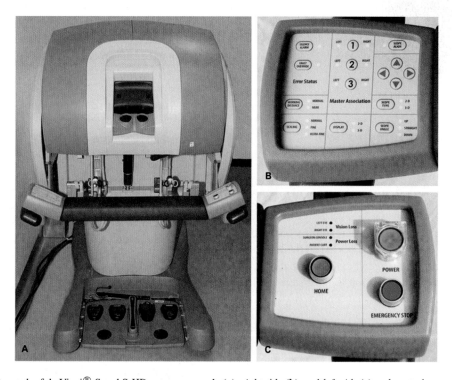

Fig. 2.1 Photograph of da Vinci® S and S-HD surgeon console (**a**), *right*-side (**b**), and *left-side* (**c**) pod controls

by capturing two independent views from two 5-mm endoscopes fitted into the stereo endoscope (Fig. 2.3). The images are then displayed into right and left optical channels in the stereoviewer to give the 3D image.[7] In addition, system status icons and messages are displayed in specific locations within the stereoviewer to alert the surgeon to any changes with the system or instruct them on how to correct system faults. The system also communicates to the surgical team any system errors (faults) through a series of beeps. Directly adjacent to the stereoviewer are infrared sensors that activate/deactivate the surgeon console and instruments

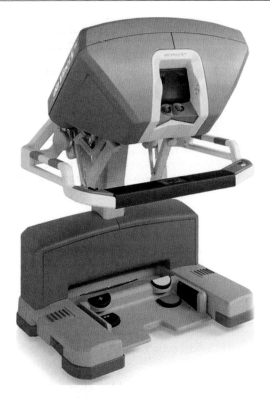

Fig. 2.2 Photograph of da Vinci Si-HD system with surgeon console. Courtesy of Intuitive Surgical, Inc., copyright 2009

when the surgeon's head is placed/removed between them. Below the stereoviewer are knobs to adjust the intraocular distance, intercom volume, brightness, and contrast. Some of these controls are not equipped on every model.

For all of the da Vinci® Surgical Systems the master controllers (Fig. 2.4) are the manual controls the surgeon uses to manipulate the robotic instruments and endoscope. The controllers are grasped with the index finger and thumb and movements are scaled, filtered, and relayed to the EndoWrist® instruments. There is no measurable delay between surgeon and robotic instrument movement.[6] This eliminates physiologic tremor and the system allows the surgeon to adjust a scale factor (2:1, 3:1, and 5:1) so that 2, 3, or 5 cm of movement in the masters translates into 1 cm of movement in the instrument arm.[3] The total working area for the master controllers in the standard and S systems is 1 ft^3, while the Si system is approximately 1.5 times larger. Surgeons adjust their working space using the master clutch (see below) to avoid collision with the walls of the working space or the other master, and to prevent stretching and fatigue. The Si-HD has a finger clutch on each of the master controllers that can also be used to adjust the working space. To activate the instrument arms during surgery, the surgeon

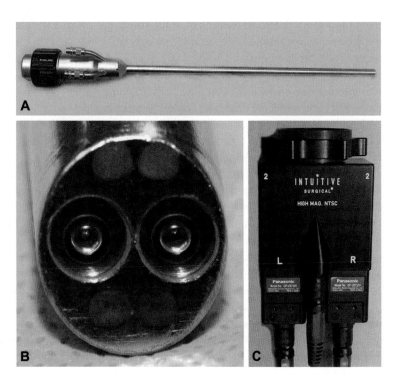

Fig. 2.3 Photograph of the da Vinci® stereo endoscope (**a**) showing the two individual 5-mm endoscopes (**b**) and camera (**c**) with *right* and *left* optical channels

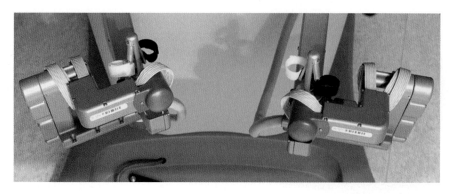

Fig. 2.4 Photograph of master controllers from the da Vinci® S system

must "match grips" by grasping the masters to match the position and grip of the instrument tip. This feature prevents accidental activation of the instrument arms and inadvertent tissue damage.

The foot switch panel has five pedals – clutch, camera, focus, bipolar/auxiliary, and cautery – used in conjunction with the master controllers to drive the surgery. The clutch pedal is used to adjust the working distance of the master controllers or shift to the third instrument arm. Completely depressing the clutch pedal disengages the master controllers from the instrument arms and the surgeon can readjust the controllers to a more comfortable working position. Adjusting the working distance of the masters is similar to moving a computer mouse when the limits of the mouse pad are reached. We generally recommend adjusting the working distance when your elbows start to lift off of the armrest or if the master controllers are colliding with each other or the side walls. Tapping the clutch pedal shifts the designated master controller to the third robotic arm. Tapping the clutch again will toggle back to the default settings. The camera pedal allows the surgeon to make adjustments to the camera and activate auxiliary visual channels. Completely depressing the camera pedal disengages the master controllers from the instrument arms and engages the endoscope. The endoscope may then be moved or rotated to the appropriate area of interest. Moving the master controllers together or apart on the S-HD systems with camera pedal depressed performs digital zoom (see below). Tapping the camera pedal on the S systems activates the auxiliary visual channels in the lower third of the stereoviewer. This channel can be connected to ultrasound or intraoperative monitors. In the center of the footswitch panel is a focus control pedal for the endoscope labeled +/–. The standard

system has an auxiliary pedal, while the S system has a bipolar pedal that can be connected to bipolar energy. The coagulation pedal is connected to a compatible electrosurgical unit. The Si-HD system has a completely remodeled foot panel with two tiers of pedals and pedals on the side of the panel. There are still clutch and camera pedals on the left side of the panel, while there is a cut and coagulation pedal on the right side. The pedals on the side of the panel are used to switch control between the two surgeons in dual console mode. In addition the side footswitch panel on the right can be used to change between the coagulation pedal and the bipolar mode. This feature prevents inadvertent electrosurgical activation of the wrong instrument arm. The back of the surgeon console houses the AC power connection, color-coded cable connections, bipolar and monopolar cautery inputs, and additional audio and visual connections.

2.1.1.2 Patient Cart

The patient cart for the standard and S systems (Fig. 2.5) houses the camera and instrument arms.[6,7] Each arm has several robotic arm clutch buttons that assist with the gross movements of the arm (Fig. 2.6). The clutch button must be depressed to move the arm, otherwise there will be resistance encountered and the arm will return to the original position. In addition, each arm also has a specific camera/instrument clutch button near the camera/instrument-mounting brackets that is used to adjust the trajectory of the arm during docking and to insert or withdraw instruments. Each camera/instrument arm requires several sterile accessories that are placed during the draping procedure (Fig. 2.7).

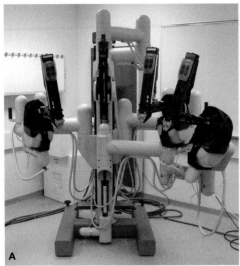
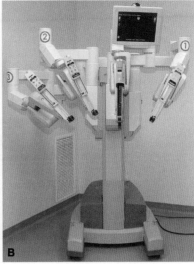

Fig. 2.5 Photograph of the da Vinci® standard patient cart with optional third instrument arm (**a**) and da Vinci® S patient cart (**b**)

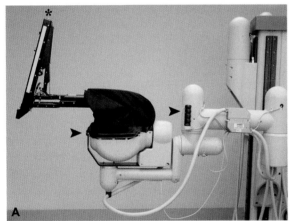

The standard system was originally offered with a camera arm and two instrument arms. Later an optional third instrument arm became available for new standard systems or could be added as an upgrade to existing systems. Each arm on the standard system is color coded with the camera arm (blue) and the instrument arms (yellow, green, and red). Similar to the standard system, the S systems have a camera arm and two instrument arms and are available with an optional third instrument arm. These models also added an LED light near the camera/instrument clutch. The LED light communicates the status of the arm to the surgical team using a preset color scheme. The S systems also have a touch screen monitor that can be mounted to the patient or the vision cart. It is synchronized with the stereoviewer and displays all of the system status icons and messages. The monitor can be used for endoscope alignment, to toggle between video inputs, or for telestration. Telestration allows the surgeon or the team member to draw real-time images on the screen that can be relayed to the stereoviewer. This feature is especially useful for training residents or fellows. The back of the patient cart houses cable connections and the S systems have a motor drive to assist docking the patient cart.

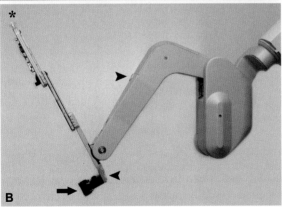

Fig. 2.6 Photograph of the da Vinci® standard instrument arm (**a**) showing the set-up clutch buttons (*arrowhead*) and instrument clutch button (*asterisks*). **b** Photograph of the da Vinci® S and HD instrument arm showing the set-up clutch buttons (*arrowheads*) and instrument clutch button with LED indicator (*asterisks*). Also seen is the trocar mount (*arrow*)

2.1.1.3 Vision Cart

The vision cart contains the light source, the video processing equipment, the camera focus control, and the

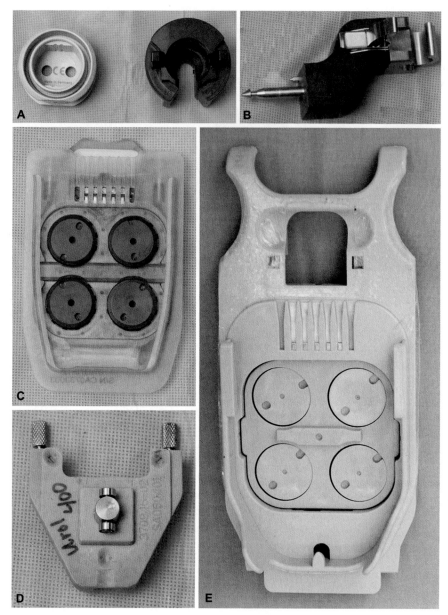

Fig. 2.7 Photographs of sterile accessories placed during the draping procedure. **a** Camera sterile adapter (*left*) and camera arm sterile adapter (*right*) and camera trocar mount (**d**). da Vinci® standard instrument arm sterile adapter (**c**) and trocar mount (**d**). The standard instrument arm adapter can be used 50 times before being discarded compared to the S models (**e**), which can be used only one time before being discarded

camera storage bin.[6,7] There are also several empty storage areas that can be used for insufflators, electrosurgical units, or a DVD recording device. A telemonitor may be placed on top of the tower. The light source is a xenon fiber-optic system with a lamp life of approximately 500 h. Typically this is connected to the endoscope by a sterile bifurcated cable to illuminate the right and left channels. On some of the standard systems, two light sources and two cables were required. The lamp on the S systems can be changed by a member from the surgical team, while the standard system requires a service visit.

The endoscope (Fig. 2.3) is available as a 0° and 30° lens. We typically use the 30° downward lens for most robotic procedures in the pelvis, while a variety of endoscopes are used for interventions of the upper urinary tract. The endoscope is connected to either a high-magnification ($15\times$ magnification with $45°$ view) or a wide-angle ($10\times$ magnification with $60°$ view) camera head with right and left optical channels. The right and left optical channels are connected to two three-chip camera control units (CCUs). The input from these CCUs is integrated in the surgeon console to produce the 3D image. The camera head is also connected to an automatic focus control that is linked to the focus control pedal on the surgeon console.

The S-HD system adds a high-definition camera and CCUs to increase resolution and aspect ratio. The first generation HD system has a resolution of 720p ($1,280\times720$) which is significantly increased from standard NTSC (720×480). The aspect ratio also increases to 16:9, which improves the viewing area by 20%. The system also has a digital zoom that allows the surgeon to magnify the tissue without moving the endoscope. This is done by pressing the left and right arrow keys on the left-side pod controls or depressing the camera pedal and moving the masters together or apart. With the Si-HD, the system increased resolution to 1080i ($1,920\times1,080$). The patient cart for the Si-HD was remodeled to integrate several of the cable connections into single connections: light source and camera control unit connections. In addition the camera adjustments and white balance are performed using the central touch pad or telemonitor.

2.1.1.4 EndoWrist® Instruments

The EndoWrist® instruments (Fig. 2.8) carry out the surgeon's motions that are relayed from the master controllers. These instruments restore the degrees of freedom (DOF) lost by conventional laparoscopy by adding three DOF at the end of the instrument, giving a total of seven DOF with $180°$ of articulation and $540°$ of rotation simulating a surgeon's hand.[3] Each instrument has a fixed number of uses before being discarded. The system automatically tracks the number of uses remaining on each instrument and communicates this in the stereoviewer. The instrument arm will not function if an outdated instrument is loaded.[6]

EndoWrist® instruments are composed of instrument housing with release levers, instrument shaft, wrist, and tip. The da Vinci® standard instruments are 52 cm with grey housing compared to the S systems being 57 cm with blue housing. The instruments are not interchangeable between the standard and S systems. Currently, there are more than 40 EndoWrist® instruments available in 8 or 5 mm shaft diameters and several have been designed specifically for urologic surgery. The 8-mm instruments operate on an "angled joint" compared to the 5 mm on a "snake joint." The angled joint allows the tip to rotate using a shorter radius compared to the snake joint (Fig. 2.9). We have consistently used the 8-mm prograsp forceps, hot shears, large needle driver, and Maryland bipolar forceps for our robotics practice.

2.2 Surgical Team

The surgical team consists of the surgeon, circulating nurse, surgical technician, and surgical assistant(s). Each member must be knowledgeable in robotic-assisted surgery and communication between each of these individuals is vital for successful outcomes.[8,9] Intuitive Surgical offers a training course for the surgical team and each member should complete the course

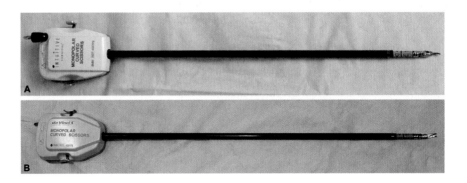

Fig. 2.8 Photograph of an EndoWrist® instrument for the standard (**a**) and S (**b**) systems

Fig. 2.9 Photograph of EndoWrist® needle drivers. On the *left* is a 5-mm needle driver with the "snake joint" compared to the 8-mm needle driver with an "angled joint"

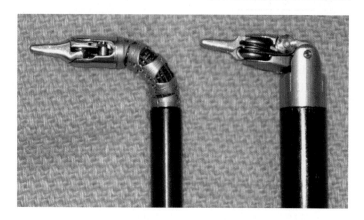

prior to starting on the surgical team. It is also important for the surgical team to remain consistent and it is generally recommended to have a dedicated team to work through the learning curve and if possible, all robotic cases.[8]

The surgeon will lead the team and should not only master driving the robot but also become familiar with the setup, basic operation, and troubleshooting the system. The circulating nurse and the surgical technician are critical for operating the robot and should become experts on system startup, draping, docking, instruments, troubleshooting, exchanging instruments, and turnover. The surgical assistant should have a similar knowledge but will also need to understand the basics of laparoscopic surgery and be comfortable assisting with trocar placement, clipping, suction, irrigation, retraction, and cutting.[8,10]

2.3 Operating Room Setup

The operating room should be able to accommodate all of the robotic components so that there is a clear view of the patient from the surgeon console, tension-free cable connections between the equipment, and clear pathways for operating room personnel to move freely around the room (Fig. 2.10). In addition the room should be able to facilitate docking of the robot from several different angles depending on the type of surgery being performed.

If the operating room is a standard operating room (Fig. 2.11a) that is converted to a robotics room on operative days, there may need to be additional laparoscopic towers to hold the insufflator, insufflation tank, electrosurgical units, video system, and extra monitors. In this situation, some of the equipment may also be placed on the vision cart. Ideally the operating room will be in a dedicated room designed for laparoscopic surgery with an integration system to allow DVD recording and telemedicine (Fig. 2.11b). In addition, flat panel monitors are mounted from the ceiling, CO_2 is piped directly into the room for insufflation, and ceiling-mounted equipment booms house insufflators, electrosurgical units, laparoscopic camera equipment, and lights sources.

2.4 Robotic-Assisted Surgery

Before the patient enters the room, the surgical team must prepare the da Vinci® Surgical System using the sterile accessories (Fig. 2.7), which is described in detail during the training sessions offered by Intuitive Surgical and by Bhandari et al.[6] Once the patient has been anesthetized and positioned properly, we secure a face shield plate (Fig. 2.12) to protect the patient's face and endotracheal tube from inadvertent damage or dislodgement from the endoscope. Robotic-assisted surgery can then begin with abdominal or retroperitoneal access. Pneumoperitoneum may be established using a Veress needle or with open trocar placement by the Hassan technique.[9,11,12] We typically gain transabdominal access by making a small incision and carrying it to the level of the fascia. The fascia is then elevated with tracheal hooks and the Veress needle is inserted.[13] Placement is verified with

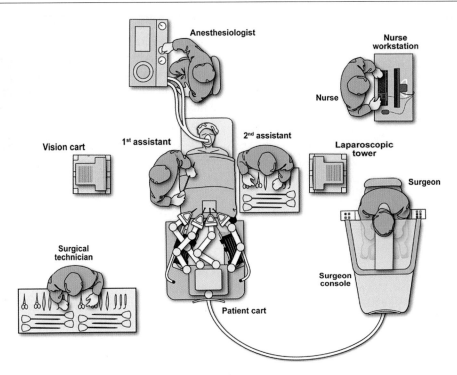

Fig. 2.10 Schematic of the operating room setup and surgical team for performing robotic-assisted surgery using the da Vinci® Surgical System

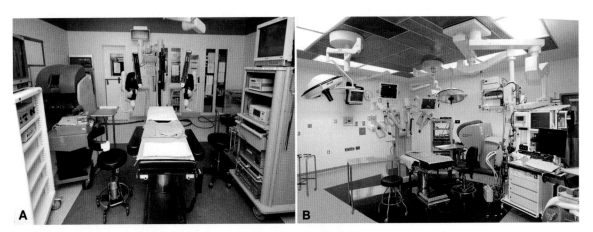

Fig. 2.11 Photograph of operating room for the da Vinci® standard (**a**) and S (**b**) systems. da Vinci® standard operating room (**a**) with an additional laparoscopic tower and seating for a second surgical assistant. da Vinci® S system operating room (**b**) where several telemonitors are mounted from the ceiling and a laparoscopic tower is mounted on a ceiling boom with the electrosurgical unit, insufflator, and light source. The room is also equipped with an integration system for DVD recording and telemedicine

the hanging drop test and the abdomen is insufflated to 15 mmHg. A 12-mm trocar is then placed with a Visiport™ (Ethicon Endo-surgery, Cincinnati, OH). This will serve as the trocar for the da Vinci® endoscope, and the robotic camera arm is compatible with most 12-mm laparoscopic trocars. The camera trocar should be placed 15–18 cm from the target anatomy to allow optimal visualization of the surgical field. For obese patients, the camera trocar may need to be placed closer to target anatomy to adjust for abdominal girth.

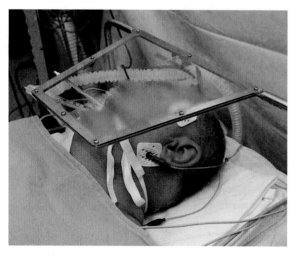

Fig. 2.12 Photograph of patient with face shield plate secured to the operating room table. This protects the patient's face and endotracheal tube from inadvertent damage or dislodgement by the endoscope

This is especially important when using the da Vinci® standard system.[12] After visual access is obtained, secondary trocars can be placed under laparoscopic vision.

The robotic instrument arms are compatible only with specific da Vinci® 8- or 5-mm metal trocars that can be placed using blunt or sharp obturators (Fig. 2.13). The robotic trocars need to be inserted with the thick black band at the level of the abdominal fascia. This acts as the pivot point for the trocar and the robotic instrument arm. It is recommended that

the robotic trocars be placed at least 8–10 cm away from the camera to avoid instrument arm collision and facilitate intracorporeal suturing. In addition, the angle created by the robotic and camera trocars should be greater than 90° to increase instrument arm maneuverability.[8,10] Other laparoscopic instruments may need to be available for lysis of adhesions prior to robot docking and for the first assistant to use during the procedure (Table 2.1).

2.4.1 Patient Cart Docking

After abdominal access is obtained, the surgical table is placed in the desired position (Trendelenburg, etc.), and the patient cart is maneuvered into position to align the patient cart tower, camera arm, and target anatomy. One member of the surgical team maneuvers the patient cart while another one guides the driver. To avoid any confusion during docking, it is recommended that the navigator uses anatomic or room references versus directional cues.

The standard system is pushed into position and the brakes at the base of the cart are hand tightened. The S systems have a motor drive to assist with docking; however, the use of the motor drive is not mandatory for the docking process. To operate the motor drive, the shift switches on the base of the cart are turned to the drive position. The motor drive is engaged by holding the throttle-enable switch on the left and turning the throttle forward or backward with the right

Fig. 2.13 Photograph of 8-mm trocar for the da Vinci® standard (**a**) and S systems (**b**). The trocars for the S systems also have a trocar that can be connected to the insufflator. Also shown are the sharp and blunt obturators used for trocar placement

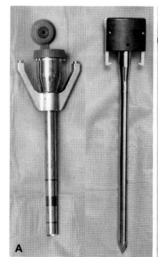

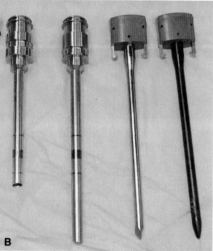

hand. To move the cart without the motor drive assist, the shift switches are placed into neutral. There is no mechanical brake like the standard system and once an instrument arm is connected to a trocar, the motor drive brakes lock automatically to keep the cart from moving.

The camera arm is the first one connected to the patient by locking the camera trocar mount to the camera trocar. It is important to use the robotic arm clutch buttons for gross movements of the camera arm and the camera clutch to adjust the final trajectory of the arm. Exclusively using the camera clutch may limit the range of motion of the camera during surgery. The instrument arms are then attached to the robotic trocars and screwed into place using a twist-lock device when using a standard system. If using the S systems, snap-mounted devices are used to engage the robotic trocars. The robotic arm clutch is used for gross movements and the instrument clutch is used for the final trajectory. Once all of the robotic arms are connected, the surgical team should check each of the arms for proper working distance and make sure the arms are not compressing the patient.

The endoscope is inserted by placing the lens into the trocar and locking it into the camera trocar mount. The endoscope can then be advanced into the surgical field using the camera clutch button. EndoWrist® instruments are inserted by straightening the instrument wrist and placing the tip into the trocar and sliding the instrument housing into the adapter. The instrument is then advanced into the surgical field using the instrument clutch button. Each instrument should be placed into the patient under direct vision. To remove an instrument, the surgeon should straighten the instrument wrist and the assistant squeezes the release levers and pulls the instrument out. The S systems feature a guided tool change where instruments can be placed to a depth of 1 mm short of the previous instrument position.

Once the robot is docked, the surgical team can take their positions for the procedure. The surgeon sits at the console, circulating nurse at their workstation, surgical technician on the patient's left, and the surgical assistant in the appropriate position. When using a robotics system with two instrument arms, a second surgical assistant or the surgical technician can assist with the procedure from the patient's other side. Using a third instrument arm eliminates the need for a second surgical assistant during the procedure. The cost and benefits of the third instrument arm must be weighed against the cost of a second assistant.

2.4.2 System Shutdown

Once robotic-assisted surgery is complete, the instruments and endoscope are removed. The arms are disconnected from the trocars and the patient cart is undocked from the patient. For the S systems the motor drive system cannot be activated until all the instruments are removed and the instrument and camera arms are disconnected. The specimen is delivered within a specimen retrieval bag by extending one of the incisions. This incision and any 12-mm trocars made with a cutting trocar require fascial closure to prevent incisional hernias. The 8- and 5-mm trocars generally do not require fascial closure.[8,9] Once the surgery is completed, the sterile accessories and drapes are removed and the system is cleaned. It is not necessary to power the system off between surgical procedures.

2.5 Conclusions

Numerous advances in technology have ultimately led to the development of robotic-assisted surgery using the da Vinci© Surgical System. To date robotic-assisted surgeries have been described for almost every genitourinary organ and the use of robotics continues to increase. Successful implementation of a robotics program hinges on a complete understanding of the robotics system, instrumentation, and operating room setup and a complete understanding of instrumentation required. In addition a knowledgeable and collegial surgical team is crucial for operating room dynamics and likely facilitates patient outcomes.

References

1. Davies BL, et al. A surgeon robot prostatectomy – a laboratory evaluation. *J Med Eng Technol*. 1989;13(6):273–277.
2. Davies BL, et al. The development of a surgeon robot for prostatectomies. *Proc Inst Mech Eng H*. 1991;205(1): 35–38.

3. Dasgupta P, Rose K, Challacombe B. Equipment and technology in robotics. In: Smith JA, Tewari A, eds. *Robotics in Urologic Surgery*. Philadelphia, PA: Saunders Elsevier; 2008:3–9.

4. Rovetta A, Sala R. Execution of robot-assisted biopsies within the clinical context. *J Image Guid Surg*. 1995;1(5):280–287.

5. Challacombe BJ, et al. The history of robotics in urology. *World J Urol*. 2006;24(2):120–127.

6. Bhandari A, Hemal A, Menon M. Instrumentation, sterilization, and preparation of robot. *Indian J Urol*. 2005;21(2):83–85.

7. Narula VK, Melvin SM. Robotic surgical systems. In: Patel VR, ed. *Robotic Urologic Surgery*. London: Springer; 2007:5–14.

8. Gettman MT, et al. Current status of robotics in urologic laparoscopy. *Eur Urol*. 2003;43(2):106–112.

9. Su LM, Smith JA Jr. Laparoscopic and robotic-assisted laparoscopic radical prostatectomy and pelvic lymphadenectomy. In: Wein AJ, Kavoussi LR, Novick AC, Partin AW, Peters CA, eds. *Campbell-Walsh Urology*. Philadelphia, PA: Saunders Elsevier; 2007:2985–3005.

10. Gettman MT, Cadeddu JA. Robotics in urologic surgery. In: Graham SD, Gleen JF, Keane TE, eds. *Glenn's Urologic Surgery*. Philadelphia, PA: Lippincott Williams & Wilkins; 2004:1027–1033.

11. Gettman MT, et al. Robotic-assisted laparoscopic partial nephrectomy: technique and initial clinical experience with da Vinci robotic system. *Urology*. 2004;64(5):914–918.

12. Gettman MT, et al. Laparoscopic radical prostatectomy: description of the extraperitoneal approach using the da Vinci robotic system. *J Urol*. 2003;170(2 Pt 1):416–419.

13. Joyce AD, Beerlage H, Janetscheck G. Urological laparoscopy for beginners. *Eur Urol*. 2000;38(3):365–373.

Chapter 3

Port Placement in Robotic Urologic Surgery

Chad R. Ritch and Ketan K. Badani

3.1 Introduction

In 2001, the da Vinci Surgical System (Intuitive Surgical, Inc., Sunnyvale, CA) was approved for use in urology (www.fda.gov) and the technological improvements have translated to a paradigm shift, especially in the field of urologic oncology. Robotic-assisted laparoscopic prostatectomy (RALP) has quickly become the minimally invasive surgical procedure of choice at most centers of excellence and robotic-assisted laparoscopic radical and partial nephrectomy (RALPN/RALN) and cystectomy (RALC) are also increasing in numbers. The impetus for the robotic approach to surgical management is based on a combined need for minimally invasive treatment with optimal surgical outcomes. Historically, conventional laparoscopy has been at the forefront of minimally invasive surgical technique and the fundamental principles of robotic surgery are founded upon those used in laparoscopic surgery. However, the advanced technology utilized in robotics has required modifications of these techniques to capitalize on the enhanced capabilities of robotic surgery. Whereas laparoscopic surgery is limited by counterintuitive movement, 2D visualization, and a decreased range of motion, robotic surgery offers 3D visualization, seven degrees of freedom, and is a natural reflection of the surgeon's movement. Robotic surgery therefore offers enhanced capabilities for visualization, surgical dexterity, and exposure to the surgical field but these

are ultimately dependent on the proper placement of the ports used for access. This chapter will provide a comprehensive overview of the standard techniques for access and port placement in a number of major robotic urologic procedures focusing on the nuances of prostate, renal, bladder, and female robotic urologic surgery.

3.2 General Principles of Port Placement

Pre-operative assessment and planning is critical and mastery of surgical anatomy is imperative to success as the exposure and access to the surgical field will dictate the progress and outcome of any operation. The majority of robotic urologic procedures are performed transperitoneally and are therefore based on the creation of pneumoperitoneum as done in laparoscopic surgery. A significant difference between laparoscopy and robotic port placement is the remote presence of the surgeon with only a single bedside assistant, whereas laparoscopy requires both surgeon and assistant at the bedside. In addition, the da Vinci Surgical System requires three (standard) or four (S model) ports for the robotic arms and, depending on the procedure, one or two assistant ports. Therefore, for a given procedure, one must consider a total number of ports ranging from 4 to 6 for placement. As with conventional laparoscopy, angulation toward the surgical site while preventing the crossing of instruments or "rolling" is essential. Special consideration is given to abdominal wall anatomical landmarks, particularly the rectus muscles and epigastric vessels. These landmarks can change with body habitus and prior abdominal surgery, therefore patient selection for

K.K. Badani (✉)
Columbia University Medical Center/NY Presbyterian
Hospital, New York, NY 10032, USA
e-mail: kb2388@columbia.edu

A.K. Hemal, M. Menon (eds.), *Robotics in Genitourinary Surgery*,
DOI 10.1007/978-1-84882-114-9_3, © Springer-Verlag London Limited 2011

robotic procedures should consider these pre-operative factors as well. In general, contraindications to laparoscopic procedures are the same as those for robotic procedures which include inability to tolerate pneumoperitoneum, extreme obesity, intestinal obstruction or distention, massive hemoperitoneum, generalized peritonitis, extensive prior abdominal surgery, abdominal wall hernias, and advanced intra-abdominal malignancy.[1] Location of the robotic system is another added variable to port placement when compared to that of conventional laparoscopy. The field must be accessible to the robotic system which, for a transperitoneal urologic procedure, typically requires the robot positioned at the foot of the operating table and the patient in dorsal lithotomy position with steep Trendelenburg. Other variations of robotic positioning will be discussed in detail with each procedure later in the chapter.

3.2.1 Establishing Pneumoperitoneum and Primary Access

The site of primary access for establishing pneumoperitoneum is periumbilical, approximately 1 cm away, though variations will exist for different procedures. The Veress technique utilizes a needle with a spring-loaded inner sheath that retracts as the needle advances through the tissue then springs forward once tension is released upon entering the peritoneal cavity. Once intra-peritoneal, the sheath covers the needle, thereby preventing injury to intra-abdominal organs. After identification of the site for primary access, an incision is made through the skin followed by cautery using the cutting current through the dermis. The abdominal wall is then raised away from the intra-abdominal organs by firmly grasping the skin and fat on either side of the incision and lifting upwards perpendicularly to the body with one hand (surgeon and assistant) (Fig. 3.1). With the other hand, the surgeon then places the Veress needle again ensuring a plane of entry that is perpendicular to the patient's body (Fig. 3.1). For patients in steep Trendelenburg, a common mistake is to enter perpendicular to the floor as opposed to the patient's body, thereby "skiving" the needle entry. During advancement of the Veress needle, one should hear three "clicks" which correspond to the sheath's spring slightly releasing with passage through the following abdominal wall layers: Scarpa's fascia, anterior rectus sheath, and posterior rectus sheath (Fig. 3.2). Occasionally there may be only two clicks, particularly below the arcuate line where the anterior and posterior rectus sheaths are fused. A recent Cochrane database review of the literature looking at 17 randomized controlled trials of laparoscopic access demonstrated no significant disadvantage of Veress needle access over other techniques except for an increase in extraperitoneal insufflation and increased rate of failed entry when compared to direct trocar access.[2] Following needle placement, there is a sequence of steps that must be performed

Fig. 3.1 Correct angle of entry for Veress needle insertion. The plane of entry for the Veress needle and an imaginary horizontal line corresponding to the patient's abdominal wall should be perpendicular. The surgeon and the assistant should simultaneously lift the abdominal wall up and away from the abdominal contents to prevent intra-abdominal injury from the Veress needle

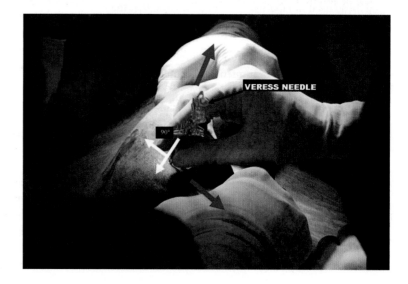

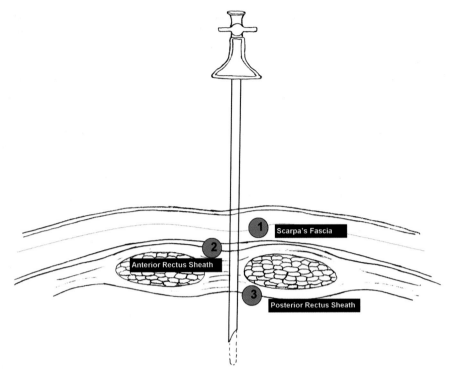

Fig. 3.2 Passage of the Veress needle through the abdominal wall. Three distinct clicks of the retractable spring-loaded needle can be heard as the Veress needle traverses: (*1*) Scarpa's fascia, (*2*) the anterior rectus sheath, and (*3*) the posterior rectus sheath then finally entering into the peritoneal cavity

ritually to confirm correct passage of the Veress needle and to prevent injury[3]:

(1) Aspiration of the needle – air should be easily aspirated. If blood or succus is aspirated, there may be vascular or bowel injury and the needle should *not* be removed so as to identify the site of injury. Bowel contents typically appear as small particles in the syringe. An alternative access site should then be attempted and location of the injury site sought out.

(2) Drop test – apply a drop of 1–2 mL of saline into the needle. If the saline drop falls easily and rapidly, then it is highly likely that the needle is correctly positioned in a low-pressure space. In performing the drop test, we prefer not to screw the needle onto the syringe as this may cause the needle to retract back into the tissue when the syringe is screwed off or disconnected.

(3) CO_2 insufflation and opening pressure – the insufflation cord is connected to the needle and the opening pressure is read aloud. Opening pressure should typically range from 2 to 7 mmHg and is

always <10 mmHg. If the pressure is >10 mmHg, then the needle should be withdrawn slightly as it may be up against intra-abdominal contents. If the pressure remains high, then the needle may be in the abdominal wall or an intestinal cavity. In the former case, remove the needle and restart the Veress algorithm. In the latter case, stop insufflation and aspirate to inspect for bowel contents. If the opening pressure remains low, then continue insufflation at 1–2 L/min for a total of 3–5 L and relax the grasp on the abdominal wall allowing intra-peritoneal pressure to reach 15 mmHg. The abdomen should appear uniformly distended and the patient's ability to tolerate pneumoperitoneum should be confirmed with the anesthesiologist. The Veress needle may then be withdrawn.

Primary access is then performed after pneumoperitoneum has been established and the patient stable. A trocar is the instrument used to establish primary access. Trocars vary in size and style and will be discussed in detail later in this chapter. The skin incision used for the Veress needle should be made sufficiently large enough for passage of the primary trocar. The trocar is held with two hands: the dominant hand is used for the driving force behind the trocar and the non-dominant hand is used to serve as a guard for smooth advancement through the tissue with the thumb and forefinger placed around its distal portion to gently guide and stabilize trocar insertion. The incision is engaged, as always, with the trocar tip at an angle perpendicular to the patient's body and a gentle twisting motion with steady pressure is applied until a slight release of tissue is felt. The stopcock is then opened and the "whoosh" of gas is used to confirm intraperitoneal placement. The insufflation cord is then connected to the trocar stopcock and pressure and flow are again noted. The camera is then inserted through the trocar and the abdominal viscera in the trajectory of the Veress insertion site is inspected for signs of injury followed by the surrounding organs and lastly the intra-abdominal cavity is inspected for adhesions.

Direct open access via the Hasson technique is another operative approach for primary access. A small infraumbilical incision is made and two stay sutures (typically 0 Prolene) are placed on opposite sides of the fascia. With the fascia tented, an incision is made through this layer exposing the peritoneum which is then grasped with a forceps and opened using a Metzenbaum scissors. A blunt-tipped trocar is then passed directly into the peritoneum and the stay sutures are secured to the arms of the trocar to hold it in place. A balloon trocar may also be used which has a small balloon around the trocar to secure it within the fascia once filled with air. The Hassan technique is typically used in patients with multiple prior abdominal surgeries or extremely obese patients.

3.2.2 Types of Trocars Used for Robotic Surgery Port Placement

There are two main classes of trocars: cutting trocars and dilating (axial or radial) trocars. Cutting trocars utilize a blade to simultaneously cut fascia while advancing through the tissue. Dilating trocars penetrate tissue without the use of a blade but have a sharp tip which helps with advancement through the tissue. The diameter of the defect created by a dilating trocar is one half the size of the trocar whereas the cutting

trocar creates a defect that is equal to the size of the defect and requires closure when trocars larger than 5 mm are used.[3] The coaxially dilating trocars employ a Veress needle passed through an expandable mesh. After Veress access into the intra-abdominal cavity, the needle is then removed and a blunt-tipped coaxially dilating trocar is passed through the mesh sheath. The advantage of this trocar is that after removal, the fascia contracts, thereby avoiding the need for closure.[2] The da Vinci robot has 5- and 8-mm dilating bladeless trocars available for the robotic arm ports.

3.2.3 Port Placement Troubleshooting

Port placement during robotic surgery is critical to the success of the procedure. If the ports are incorrectly placed, the robotic arms will collide externally making the operation extremely challenging. The goal of port placement is also to provide sufficient distance between the camera and working ports to prevent rolling and crossing of instruments internally. One particular challenge to robotic port placement is the obese patient as the anatomical landmarks are difficult to identify and the distance from the surgical site is challenging to estimate.[4] Typically, during RALP, the larger abdomen requires ports to be placed more cephalad from the pubic symphysis and deeper into the body with lateral deflection of the robot arms.[4]

During port placement, the correct angle for entry into the peritoneum is important as an incorrectly positioned port can impede movement of the robotic arm. The correct angle of entry is always perpendicular to the plane of the patient and, after entry is confirmed on camera, the angle is directed toward the surgical site away from bowel and adjacent organs. When using STEP trocars, a common mistake is to angle incorrectly on entry and puncture the mesh of the sheath with the trocar. If this occurs, remove the trocar and re-attempt placement at the correct angle. The port should always be inspected to ensure that it is freely mobile and not "skived" (inappropriately positioned at a fixed angle upward or downward away from the surgical site). If the port is "skived," then it should be removed and again repositioned with the help of the sharp-tipped trocar as previously described.

Adhesions and prior abdominal surgery pose another significant challenge to robotic port placement.

If the patient has visible external scars, care is taken to avoid placing the ports directly through the scar or in a trajectory that involves the scar when feasible. We recommend the use of the Hasson technique for placement of the camera port in patients with extensive prior abdominal surgery. After placement of the camera port, the abdominal cavity is inspected for adhesions. If adhesions are present, the first ports to be placed for any procedure would be those that are outside of the field of the adhesion but in a position that would permit manual laparoscopic adhesiolysis. After adhesiolysis, the remainder of the ports can then be safely placed. Occasionally, an alternative access port site may be necessary solely for adhesiolysis when there are extensive adhesions that block the position of all conventional port sites.

3.3 Robotic-Assisted Laparoscopic Radical Prostatectomy (RALP)

After the patient is prepped and draped and positioned in dorsal lithotomy with steep Trendelenburg, the bladder is drained with a 20-Fr Foley catheter to ensure that it is completely decompressed and outside of the field of port placement. For the four-arm da Vinci models, we typically place six ports: two assistant ports (12 and 5 mm) for suctioning, passing sutures, and retraction, three robotic ports (8 mm including the fourth arm for retraction), and the 12-mm camera port. For the three-arm standard da Vinci system, we omit the fourth arm robotic port for a total of five ports (Fig. 3.3). The 12-mm camera port is placed slightly left of the umbilicus using the Veress technique, as previously described. After pneumoperitoneum is established, primary inspection of the intraperitoneal cavity is performed to ensure that no injuries to the bowel or adjacent organs have occurred and attention is then turned to the lateral (assistant) port. The right anterior superior iliac spine (ASIS) is identified and a point which is approximately 2–3 finger breadths superior and 1–2 finger breadths medial to this landmark is marked out. The camera is then used to confirm, from an intra-peritoneal standpoint that there are no adhesions or bowel in the trajectory of the incision and port site. If there are any adhesions noted, contralateral port placement is then undertaken and laparoscopic adhesiolysis is performed as previously described.

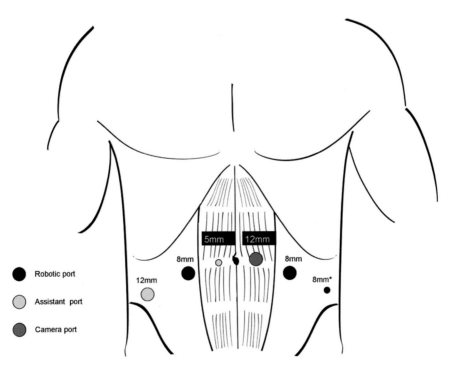

Fig. 3.3 Port placement for robotic-assisted laparoscopic prostatectomy. *The three-arm model uses a 5-mm assistant port as opposed to the 8-mm robot arm port used for the four-arm model

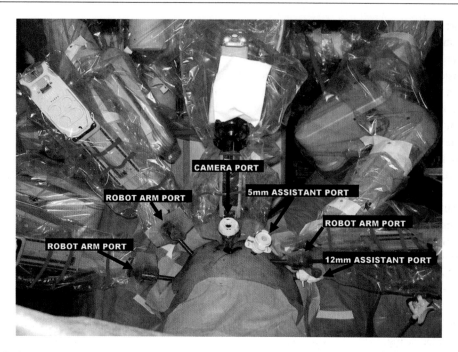

Camera port labels: CAMERA PORT, ROBOT ARM PORT, 5mm ASSISTANT PORT, ROBOT ARM PORT, ROBOT ARM PORT, 12mm ASSISTANT PORT

Fig. 3.4 The final appearance of ports after docking the robot for robotic-assisted radical prostatectomy

A skin incision is made parallel to Langer's lines to expose the dermis and the cutting current from the Bovie is then used to incise this layer. For assistant ports, we prefer to use the radially dilating STEP trocars. The STEP trocar is inserted via the Veress technique under direct visualization. A 12-mm blunt-tipped trocar is then inserted through the mesh sheath with special attention at aiming the trajectory toward the pelvis. After placement of the 12-mm port, the insufflation tube is then moved from the camera port to this port. Attention is then turned to the right-sided 8-mm robotic arm port, which is placed approximately 10 cm away from the midline camera port slightly below the level of the umbilicus and just lateral to the edge of the rectus muscle. The robotic arm port has a sharp plastic trocar which can directly pierce the fascia. After confirmation of the appropriate port site, the trocar is inserted, perpendicular to the plane of the patient and with gentle rotation and pressure, under the aid of direct visualization from the camera. After the sharp tip is visually identified on camera coming through the peritoneum, the port is angled toward the pelvis and the sharp trocar is removed and the robotic port is advanced to the level of the thick 1-cm black mark. For the second assistant suction port (5 mm), an imaginary line is drawn connecting the right-sided 8-mm robotic

port and the midline camera port and, at the midpoint of this line, the port is then inserted under visualization using a STEP trocar and Veress needle as described for the 12-mm assistant port. On the left side of the patient, for the fourth-arm model, an 8-mm fourth robotic arm port is placed using the same landmarks as the 12-mm right-sided lateral assistant port (2–3 fingerbreadths superior and 1–2 fingerbreadths medial to the ASIS). For the three-arm da Vinci model, a 5-mm assistant port may also be placed at this location for a second bedside assistant for retraction.[4] Finally, another 8-mm left-sided robotic working port is then placed in a position which is an exact mirror image to the 8-mm right-sided robotic port (lateral to the edge of the rectus muscle, approximately 10 cm and slightly inferior to the camera port). The final RALP port configuration has fan-like appearance with all ports aiming toward the pelvis and with sufficient distance between the robotic arms (Fig. 3.4).

3.3.1 Port Site Closure

After de-docking the robot, the robotic camera is manually placed through the lateral right-sided 12-mm assistant port and a laparoscopic grasper is then used to deliver the string of the endocatch bag containing the specimen through the midline camera port. It is then secured outside of the body with a Kelly clamp later for specimen extraction.

Removal of all ports is always performed in a sequential manner under direct visualization. We prefer to use the robotic fourth-arm port for placement of the Jackson–Pratt (JP) drain and this port is typically removed first. Care is taken to remove this port with a "one-to-one" motion so as not to disrupt the position of the JP drain. Each port site is directly visualized on removal to ensure that there is no bleeding internally so as to prevent port site hematomas which can be severe enough to warrant re-exploration. The camera port is the last to be removed as this is our extraction site for the surgical specimen. Using cautery we cut down on the skin and fascia over the port enough to insert an index finger into the defect. The external portion of the string on the endocatch bag is held in the non-dominant hand after the port is removed and using the dominant hand a gentle sweep with the index finger is performed to ensure that there is no bowel or omentum directly under the fascia. The fascia and skin are then incised down onto the index finger with cautery to a minimum estimated length necessary for specimen removal. After the specimen has been extracted and the all port sites inspected externally for hemostasis, we close the extraction site with a single fascial layer using the necessary number of figure of eight 0-Vicryl suture to ensure complete closure of the defect. The skin layer of the extraction and all other port sites are then closed with subcutaneous 4-0 Biosyn suture and dressed with Steri-Strips, gauze, and an occlusive biomembrane dressing (Tegaderm; 3 M Corporation).

3.4 Robotic-Assisted Radical Cystectomy (RARC) and Urinary Diversion

The patient is positioned and padded in the identical manner as that described for RALP (lithotomy position with steep Trendelenburg). Port placement for RALP is very similar to that of RARC, with some modification, and the reader should therefore refer to that section for details on how to properly place these ports. Particularly important during RARC is the ability to perform extended pelvic lymphadenectomy and mobilization of the ureters along with transferring the left ureter to the right under the sigmoid mesentery.[5]

The first port to be placed is that of the robotic camera. Pneumoperitoneum is established using the Veress technique and the 12-mm camera port is placed slightly to the left of the umbilicus. Under direct visualization, the robotic and assistant ports are then placed as outlined in Fig. 3.5. The assistant is positioned to the right of the patient and the first assistant port (12 mm) is placed approximately 2–3 fingerbreadths above the ASIS and 1–2 cm medial to the mid-axillary line using the Veress technique with a radially dilating STEP trocar. The next port to be placed is the 8-mm right-sided robotic camera port which is positioned approximately 2–3 cm below the level of the umbilicus and slightly lateral to the right rectus muscle. Attention is then turned to the 10-mm assistant port for suctioning, which is placed slightly cephalad and halfway between the camera and the right-sided robotic port. We prefer to use a 10-mm versus a 5-mm assistant port as the larger size permits easier passage of clips and energy devices for control of the vascular pedicles when needed. For the da Vinci fourth arm, an 8-mm robotic port is placed at a position 2–3 fingerbreadths above the left ASIS and 1–2 cm medial to the mid-axillary line. The final 8-mm robotic port is placed on the left side, in a mirror image to the right-sided 8-mm robotic port (2–3 cm below the umbilicus, lateral to the edge of the left rectus muscle). The robot is then docked as previously described.

At our institution, we prefer to perform extracorporeal urinary diversion. After completion of the dissection and complete mobilization of the ureters, the left ureter is tunneled underneath the sigmoid colon and the robot is dedocked and a 4- to 6-cm periumbilical midline incision is then made toward the pubic symphysis through which the specimen can be removed and a segment of ileum can be retrieved for extracorporeal urinary diversion. Through this extraction site, both ureters should have sufficient length to reach the abdominal wall after release of pneumoperitoneum. The ileal–cecal junction is identified and the ileum brought out through the incision. For ileal conduit diversions, our stoma site is typically the RLQ through the rectus muscle or, in select cases, we may

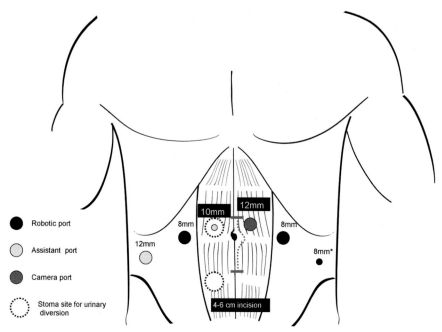

Fig. 3.5 Port placement for robotic-assisted radical cystectomy and urinary diversion. A 4–6-cm periumbilical incision is made going toward the symphysis pubis for the extracorporeal creation of the conduit or the neobladder. We routinely place the stoma in the right lower quadrant through the rectus muscle but, in select cases, we may utilize the 10-mm assistant port site for the stoma to improve cosmesis. *A 5-mm port may be placed for a second assistant in the three-arm model versus an 8-mm robot arm port for the fourth-arm

expand the 10-mm assistant port site for location of the stoma. In the case of orthotopic neobladder diversion, the ports remain in place and the segment of intestine is delivered via midline incision for creation of the reservoir extracorporeally. The neobladder is then placed back into the pelvis and the midline incision is closed and the robotic system is redocked in order to perform the urethroneovesicostomy.[6] It is sometimes beneficial to pre-place anastomotic sutures robotically in the urethra prior to creation of the neobladder. Intra-abdominal robotic urinary diversion has been described using a slightly different template for port placement.[7] Beecken et al.[7] utilize an initial three-port placement, using the standard da Vinci system, with the 12-mm paraumbilical camera port (via Hasson technique) and two 8-mm robotic arms placed lateral to the right and left rectus and slightly inferior to the umbilicus. Additionally, 10-mm assistant trocars are placed lateral to the robotic ports and above the ASIS.[7] These are used for passage of graspers, suctioning, clip appliers, and bowel stapler.

3.5 Robotic-Assisted Renal Procedures

3.5.1 Robotic-Assisted Radical Nephrectomy (RARN) and Partial Nephrectomy

The port placement for a robotic-assisted renal procedure is challenging due to the laterality of the surgery and the positioning of the patient. Enough space must be given between each port to permit freedom of movement for all arms while creating a working space for the bedside assistant. The operating room table orientation will need to be re-configured to accommodate the robot which is docked facing the dorsal aspect of the patient (in lateral decubitus position) and at an angle to the location of the renal hilum, particularly for partial nephrectomy.[8] The monitors, insufflation tower, and electrocautery stand are set up on the same side of the room as the robot and directly facing the bedside assistant (Fig. 3.6).

Fig. 3.6 Operating room setup and orientation for robotic renal procedures. The OR table is typically placed at an angle which allows the robot to approach the dorsal aspect of the patient (in lateral decubitus position) when being docked. The first assistant is then facing directly opposite to the robot and vision cart/monitors

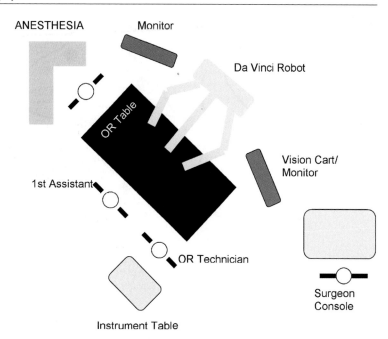

The patient is placed in the modified lateral decubitus position and the bed is flexed slightly to expose the space between the costal margin and the anterior superior iliac spine (ASIS). After the patient is prepped and draped, pneumoperitoneum is established by placing the Veress needle in a region slightly inferior to the ipsilateral subcostal margin and superior to the umbilicus. The following anatomical landmarks are then identified: ASIS, subcostal margin, anterior axillary line, mid-clavicular line, and posterior axillary line (Figs. 3.7 and 3.8). The 12-mm camera port is placed 2–3 finger breadths below the subcostal margin roughly in between the mid-clavicular line and the anterior axillary line. We typically use the 12-mm STEP trocar with Veress technique for our camera port. The 30° lens looking up is used for the placement of

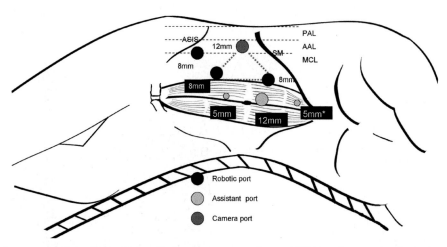

Fig. 3.7 Port placement for right-sided robotic radical nephrectomy. The 12-mm camera port and the 8-mm robot arm ports are triangulated toward the renal hilum. *A subxiphoid 5-mm port may be added for liver retraction during *right-sided* renal procedures. ASIS, anterior superior iliac spine; SM, subcostal margin; AAL, anterior axillary line; MCL, mid-clavicular line; PAL, posterior axillary line

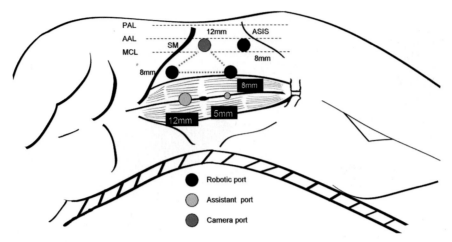

Fig. 3.8 Port placement for left-sided robotic radical nephrectomy. The 12-mm camera port and the 8-mm robot arm ports are triangulated toward the renal hilum. ASIS, anterior superior iliac

spine; SM, subcostal margin; AAL, anterior axillary line; MCL, mid-clavicular line; PAL, posterior axillary line

the remaining ports under direct visualization as previously described. For the robotic arms, two 8-mm ports are placed approximately 8–10 cm medially away from the camera port such that the three ports (camera and two robot ports) form a triangle (Fig. 3.9). With respect to robotic partial nephrectomy, the positioning of the robotic ports can be adjusted depending on the location of the tumor. For upper pole tumors (and patients with

a large body habitus), the ports may be shifted laterally and superiorly.[9] Use of the fourth arm is optional and may be used for retraction. This port is placed slightly below the ASIS, lateral and superior to the 8-mm robot assistant port.

The role of the bedside assistant is crucial to the success of robotic partial nephrectomy. The assistant is responsible for clamping and unclamping the artery

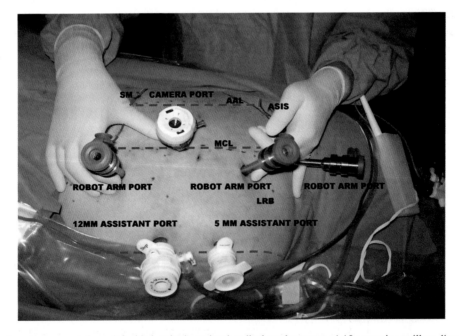

Fig. 3.9 Final port placement for a left-sided, robotic-assisted radical nephrectomy. AAL, anterior axillary line; MCL, mid-clavicular line; ASIS, anterior superior iliac spine; LRB, lateral rectus border; SM, subcostal margin

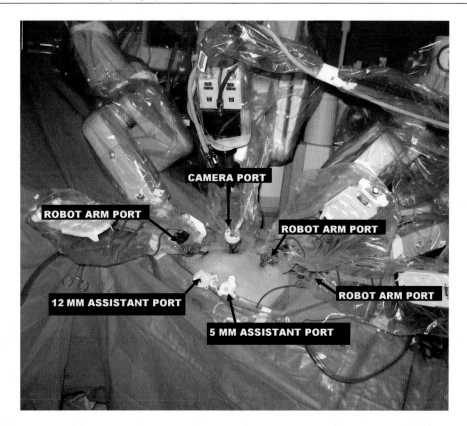

Fig. 3.10 Docking of the robot for *left-sided*, robotic-assisted radical nephrectomy. The patient is positioned in the right lateral decubitus position and the robot is docked facing the dorsal aspect of the patient

and vein to during warm ischemia as well as for passing the sutures needed for obtaining hemostasis in the surgical site. In addition, they may be required to retract the colon during dissection and for right-sided position, liver retraction is important as well.[10] One or two assistant ports may be used. These are typically placed in periumbilical midline, adjusting laterally if patient is obese. The 12-mm port is placed approximately 2 cm cephalad to the umbilicus and the optional 5-mm port is placed 2 cm caudal to the umbilicus and the robot is then docked facing the dorsal aspect of the patient (Figs. 3.9 and 3.10).

3.5.2 Robotic-Assisted Pyeloplasty and Pyelolithotomy

For most robotic-assisted renal procedures the positioning of the patient is fairly similar. As previously described for robotic-assisted radical and partial nephrectomy, the operating room table orientation will need to be re-configured to accommodate the robot which is docked facing the dorsal aspect of the patient. The patient is positioned in a modified 45–60° lateral decubitus position without raising the kidney rest. The robot, tower with monitors, insufflation, and electrocautery are all positioned on the same side of the room so that they are directly facing the bedside assistant (Fig. 3.6).

Our landmarks for port placement in the lateral decubitus position are the anterior superior iliac spine, (ASIS), subcostal margin, anterior axillary line, and mid-clavicular line (Figs. 3.7 and 3.8). Pneumoperitoneum is established with the Veress needle in a region slightly inferior to the ipsilateral subcostal margin and lateral to the umbilicus. The 12-mm camera port is placed laterally, three finger breadths below the subcostal margin between the mid-clavicular and anterior axillary line. Two 8-mm robotic arm ports are then placed under direct visualization. These ports are placed such that the robotic camera port and two robotic arms are triangulated toward the renal pelvis with approximately 8 cm between each robot port and the camera port (Fig. 3.9). Two assistant ports, 5 and 12 mm, are then placed in the midline, periumbilically for passing sutures and for suctioning. For liver retraction, an additional 5-mm port can be placed in the midline, subxiphoid area for a self-retaining retractor.[11,12]

3.6 Robotic-Assisted Laparoscopic Sacrocolpopexy (RALSC)

The open transabdominal approach for sacrocolpopexy has achieved high success rates for most patients; however, the morbidity of the operation and the length of post-operative stay are limiting factors.[13] The transvaginal approach is another option that is less invasive but has not demonstrated as uniformly successful outcomes as the transabdominal approach.[14]

Surgeons therefore developed laparoscopic sacrocolpopexy in an effort to strike a balance between providing good outcomes with a minimally invasive approach. Unfortunately, the laparoscopic technique is challenging and operative times are significantly longer than the transvaginal approach and its widespread use has been limited.[15] Recently, surgeons have turned to the da Vinci robot to perform robotic-assisted laparoscopic sacrocolpopexy (RALSC) so as to maximize the benefits of laparoscopy while decreasing the technical challenges of a straight laparoscopic approach using the improved visualization and increased range of motion of the robotic system.[16,17]

For this procedure, the patient is placed in Trendelenburg and dorsal lithotomy positions with the arms tucked on both sides. After she is prepped and draped, a Foley catheter is inserted to decompress the bladder. A standard periumbilical incision can be made for placement of the 12-mm camera port but occasionally we may place the camera port supraumbilically as an alternate site. We use a Veress technique

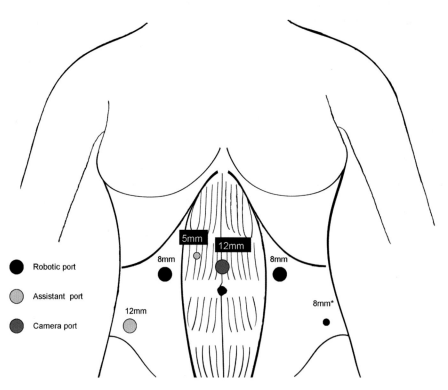

Fig. 3.11 Port placement for robotic-assisted laparoscopic sacrocolpopexy. The camera port may be placed supraumbilically as shown. In addition, the 8-mm robot arm ports are placed slightly more cephalad compared to those in a prostatectomy to allow better access to the sacral promontory. *The three-arm model utilizes a 5-mm assistant port versus 8-mm robot arm port used for the four-arm model

for insufflation followed by a 12-mm cutting trocar for insertion of the camera port once pneumoperitoneum has been established. The robotic camera is then used to inspect the abdominal viscera to ensure no injuries have been made and the intra-abdominal site for the first assistant port, on the patient's right side, is identified. This site is approximately 2–3 fingerbreadths above the ASIS and slightly lateral to the mid-clavicular line. Using the Veress technique and a radially dilating STEP trocar, a 12-mm port is then placed under direct visualization. This port is used for passage of sutures and synthetic mesh material. Attention is then turned to the first 8-mm robotic port which is placed lateral to the right rectus muscle and in line with the umbilicus. It should be noted that our positioning of the robotic ports for RALSC is similar to that for a RALP; however, they must be placed slightly more cephalad to allow for maximal access to the sacral promontory while still being able to reach the pelvis during sacrocolpopexy. Another 5-mm assistant port is placed midway between the right-sided robotic assistant port and the camera port and is used for suctioning and retraction. The second 8-mm robotic port is then placed on the left side, lateral to the rectus muscle and again in line with the umbilicus. The final configuration is shown in Fig. 3.11. We routinely employ the fourth arm, placed approximately three fingerbreadths cephalad to the iliac crest on the left lateral sidewall.

References

1. Gomella L, Pietrow P, Albala D. Basic laparoscopy. In: Graham S, Glenn J, Keane T, eds. *Glenn's Urological Surgery*. 6th ed. Philadelphia, PA: Lippincott, Williams and Wilkins; 2004:113.
2. Ahmad G, Duffy J, Phillips K, et al. Laparoscopic entry techniques. *Cochrane Database Syst Rev*. 2008;16(2): CD006583.
3. Collins S, Lehman D, McDougall E, et al. *AUA Handbook of Laparoscopic and Robotic Fundamentals*. 1st ed. Linthicum, MD: American Urological Association; 2007.
4. Mikhail A, Stockton B, Orvieto M, et al. Robotic assisted laparoscopic prostatectomy in overweight and obese patients. *Urology*. 2006;67:774–779.
5. Hemal A. Robotic and laparoscopic radical cystectomy in the management of bladder cancer. *Curr Urol Rep*. 2009;10:45–54.
6. Menon M, Hemal A, Tewari A. Robotic assisted radical cystectomy and urinary diversion in female patients: technique with preservation of the uterus and vagina. *J Am Coll Surg*. 2004;198:386–393.
7. Beecken W, Wolfram M, Engl T, et al. Robotic assisted laparoscopic radical cystectomy and intra-abdominal formation of an orthotopic ileal neobladder. *Eur Urol*. 2003;44:337–339.
8. Benway B, Wang A, Cabello J, et al. Robotic partial nephrectomy with sliding-clip renorrhaphy: technique and outcomes. *Eur Urol*. 2009;55:592–599.
9. Rogers C, Singh A, Blatt A, et al. Robotic partial nephrectomy for complex renal tumors: surgical technique. *Eur Urol*. 2008;53:514–523.
10. Kaul S, Laungani R, Sarle R, et al. da Vinci-assisted robotic partial nephrectomy: technique and results at a mean of 15 months of follow-up. *Eur Urol*. 2007;51: 186–192.
11. Badani K, Hemal A, Fumo M, et al. Robotic extended pyelolithotomy for treatment of renal calculi: a feasibility study. *World J Urol*. 2006;24:198–201.
12. Mufarrij P, Woods M, Shah O, et al. Robotic dismembered pyeloplasty: a 6-year, multi-institutional experience. *J Urol*. 2008;180:1391–1396.
13. Reddy K, Malik TG. Short-term and long-term follow-up of abdominal sacrocolpopexy for vaginal vault prolapse: initial experience in a district general hospital. *J Obstet Gynaecol*. 2002;22:532–536.
14. Benson J, Lucente V, McClellan E. Vaginal versus abdominal reconstructive surgery for the treatment of pelvic support defects: a prospective randomized study with long-term outcome evaluation. *Am J Obstet Gynecol*. 1996;176:1418–1421.
15. Ostrzenski A. Laparoscopic colposuspension for total vaginal prolapse. *Int J Gynaecol Obstet*. 1996;55:147–152.
16. Akl M, Long J, Giles D, et al. Robotic-assisted sacrocolpopexy: technique and learning curve. *Surg Endosc*. 2009;21:2390–2394.
17. Elliott D, Krambeck A, Chow G. Long-term results of robotic assisted laparoscopic sacrocolpopexy for the treatment of high grade vaginal vault prolapse. *J Urol*. 2006;176:655–659.

Chapter 4

Achieving Efficiency in the Operating Room: Step by Step

Randy Fagin

4.1 Introduction

Efficiency is essential to success in any activity. Whether at the robotic console, in the boardroom, or playing professional sports, efficiency is a key element that separates the highly successful from the average. The amazing thing is that becoming efficient is not all that hard once you have the tools. This chapter will focus on giving you the tools you need to become more efficient in the operating room than you ever thought possible. The model I created, and will share with you, has been implemented in hospitals across the United States. The results that have been achieved have been dramatic and sustainable across a wide diversity of hospital settings including small community hospitals, university centers, large private hospitals, union-based hospitals, and just about every hospital size and setting from coast to coast. By following the key principles in this model, operating rooms of all shapes and sizes have successfully improved their efficiency and in doing so have reduced the potential for errors, as well as improved the quality of the operation, increased the revenue generated, and created both success and growth of their centers and the surgeons that work there.

4.1.1 Efficiency Improves Quality, Revenue, and Success

When people think of efficiency, they often mistake efficiency for speed. They are *not* the same. Increasing efficiency is not about doing things faster. Although efficiency will improve the speed with which you perform tasks, speed is only the by-product and not the goal. Efficiency is about eliminating wasteful activities and focusing one's attention on patterns and beneficial tasks. Increasing efficiency in the operating room allows you to achieve improvements in three critical areas: quality, revenue, and success.

4.1.1.1 Quality

When you focus on the elimination of wasteful actions and activities and focus on patterns and beneficial tasks, the result is a reduction in the variability of your task execution. As surgeons, we are acutely aware that reducing variability reduces the potential for errors. This is why we perform procedures step by step, the same way every time. In the operating room, as is true in surgery, reducing variability increases attention to relevant details and creates a systematic approach to mistake proofing. Thus, efficiency in the operating room will improve the quality of care that is delivered by reducing the potential for errors.

4.1.1.2 Revenue

When we eliminate wasteful activities through improved efficiency, one of the by-products is

R. Fagin (✉)
The Prostate Center of Austin, Austin, TX 78746, USA
e-mail: rfagin@austin.rr.com

A.K. Hemal, M. Menon (eds.), *Robotics in Genitourinary Surgery*,
DOI 10.1007/978-1-84882-114-9_4, © Springer-Verlag London Limited 2011

increased speed of execution. By eliminating wasteful actions and activities, there is simply less to do, so the speed with which you can complete a task improves. For the surgeon and the hospital reimbursement is fixed, if you can complete an operation in less time with fewer complications, your revenue per unit time will increase. Therefore, efficiency in the operating room increases revenue generated per unit time.

4.1.1.3 Success

An interesting thing also happens when you improve efficiency, you actually improve your procedure credibility and branding. One example is that surgeons who consistently perform an equally successful procedure in less time with less variability are thought of as better surgeons than those who take longer and have more variability in their procedure. Although both surgeons may be equally talented and produce equivalent outcomes, the more efficient surgeon is thought of as better. The result of this is an increase in credibility and branding for the more efficient surgeon which increases their competitive advantage setting up long-term security and success. In this way, efficiency in the operating room significantly influences success.

4.2 Operating Room Efficiency Defined

When most surgeons think of operating room efficiency, they think of the time it takes to perform a procedure. Operating room efficiency, however, should really be defined as the time the operating room is in use and not available to perform other surgical procedures. When defined in this way, operating room efficiency includes the time it takes to

– set up the room
– get the patient into the room
– intubate and position the patient
– dock the robot
– perform the operation
– undock the robot
– close the patient
– get the patient to recovery

When defined in this way, the procedure time is only one element in improving efficiency and it is all the other activities that we will focus on as they are constant regardless of the procedure being performed.

4.3 Myths and Realities of Operating Room Efficiency

There are many myths and realities of operating room efficiency, so let's dispel the myths and focus on the realities that will allow you to apply this model and achieve success.

4.3.1 Myth #1: You Need More Manpower to Increase Efficiency

To turn the room over more efficiently, you believe that you need residents, fellows, more scrub techs, more circulators, more people. Because you are lacking the manpower many other efficient centers have, you cannot improve your efficiency.

4.3.1.1 Reality #1

You need five people to efficiently turn your room. You need

• two scrub techs
• one circulator
• one first assist
• one operating room attendant

With this core team of only five people, teams across the country are able to achieve turnover of less than 15 min from when one patient exits the room to when the next patient enters. If you have these five people, which I know you do, you have the manpower to improve your operating room efficiency.

4.3.2 Myth #2: You Need More Instrument Sets to Improve Your Efficiency

You believe that you are constantly delayed by central sterilization. Your hospital will not buy you more instrument sets, so you are at the mercy of sterilization and since you cannot speed up the sterilization process, you cannot improve your efficiency.

4.3.2.1 Reality #2

The reality is all you need are two instrument sets. No matter what procedure you are doing, your console time is longer than the reprocessing/sterilization time of the instruments. Since it takes you longer to perform an operation than it takes to sterilize your instruments, you have all the time you need while doing one case to have the next set of instruments sterilized in time to start the second case.

4.3.3 Myth #3: Our Room Turnover Times Are as Good as It Gets

In your hospital your turnover times are not your unique problem, they occur in every room with all different types of cases. Because it is a system problem that is not specific to robotics, this is completely out of your control and limits your ability to improve your efficiency.

4.3.3.1 Reality #3

The reality is that turnover times at your hospital are based on the case and the surgeon operating. There are surgeons in your hospital who perform identical procedures to other surgeons at your hospital but have much faster turnover times. The reality is that you can become one of those surgeons who consistently has the faster turnover times by applying this model.

4.4 Efficiency Theory and Implementation

Before we look at the specifics of a model for efficiency, let's first examine the big picture for improving efficiency, then we will move on to the practical tool you can use for implementation.

4.4.1 The Big Picture

The big picture is that there are two types of activities that occur in the operating room: external activities and internal activities:

4.4.1.1 External Activities

External activities are those elements that can be done while the operating room is actively engaged in a surgical procedure. They are external to the procedure being performed. An example would be the circulator's paperwork. This paperwork can be filled out while the patient is in the room and you are operating.

4.4.1.2 Internal Activities

Internal activities are those elements that must be done while the operating room is "down" and not engaged in a surgical procedure. An example would be mopping the floor. This must be done only after the procedure is over and the patient leaves the room.

To improve efficiency you must do two things: convert internal activities into external activities and create task overlap.

4.4.1.3 Convert Internal to External Tasks

First, you must convert internal activities to external activities. You must take tasks that are traditionally done while the patient is out of the room and convert them to tasks that are performed while the patient is in the room. An example would be draping the robot. This is traditionally done before the patient enters the room but can be performed while the patient is in the room.

4.4.1.4 Create Task Overlap

Second, you want to have tasks performed in parallel rather than in series. Traditionally, in the operating room, tasks are performed in series (Fig. 4.1). First the team works together to set up the back table, then they work together to drape the robot, then the patient is brought back. The reality is that tasks like these can and should be performed by one person. With one person performing these tasks, they can then be done simultaneously (Fig. 4.2). For example, one person can set up the back table at the same time that another person drapes the robot. By executing tasks in parallel, you will reduce the time it takes to get all these tasks finished. In addition, if you also take elements that are

Old Approach

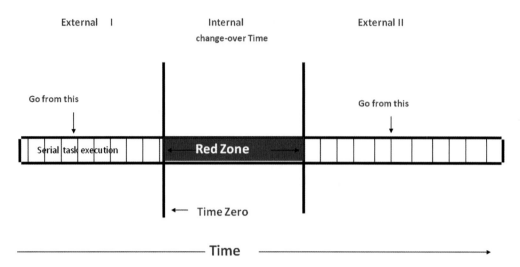

Fig. 4.1 Old approach to activities in the OR using serial task execution

New Approach

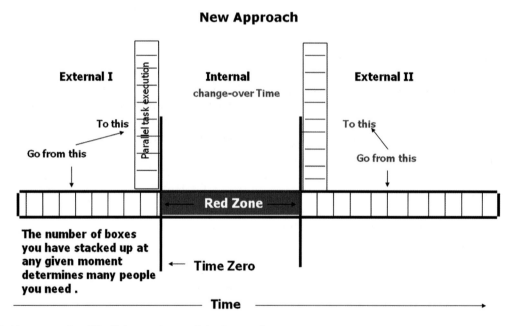

Fig. 4.2 New approach to OR efficiency using parallel task execution

traditionally done while the operating room is "down" (the "red zone" on Figs. 4.1, 4.2, and 4.3) and convert them to tasks done while the patient is still in the room, you will reduce the number of tasks that need to be done in the "red zone" and will reduce your room turnover time (Fig. 4.3).

4.5 The Operating Room Efficiency Model

Now that you know the basics, let's apply these key concepts in a model that you can implement in the operating room. We are going to go step by step with

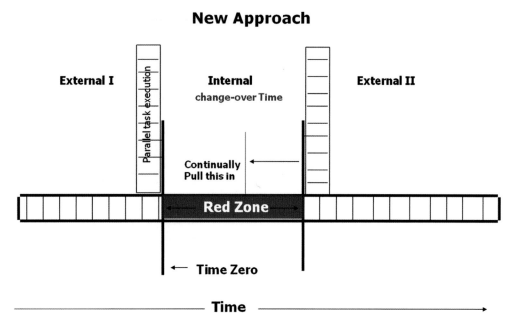

Fig. 4.3 New approach to OR efficiency using parallel task execution

each figure depicting the roles and parallel tasks for the five critical people in the room: surgeon, nurse circulator, scrub tech, surgical assistant, and anesthesia. Under each heading I will list the specific task overlap that is critical for that step in the robotic procedure.

Step 1: Setting up the back table (Fig. 4.4)

Task overlap: Go get the patient before the back table is set up

The key for efficiency at this stage of the procedure is that once the back table is opened, the circulator and anesthesia representative go to get the patient. The back table may look like a giant pile at this point but it takes 5–10 min to go to pre-op holding and return with a patient and that is more than enough time for the scrub (and in some places first assistant) to completely set up the back table. There is no need to wait for the back table to be set up to go get the patient. In addition, to make back table setup more efficient, minimize the instruments you open. You do not need a full open set opened and counted. If you choose, an open set can be in the room left unopened next to the back table and opened only in the case of the rare emergency.

Step 2: Patient enters the OR (Fig. 4.5)

Task overlap: Drape the robot while the patient is being intubated

When the patient enters the room, the surgeon and the circulator should be focused on positioning and prepping the patient, while the scrub tech is focused on draping the robot. Remember, anesthesia still needs to intubate the patient, then the patient will need to be positioned, prepped, and draped. These activities will take 5–15 min which gives the scrub more than enough time to drape the robot while the patient is in the room and these other activities are being performed.

Step 3: Patent draped (Fig. 4.6)

Task overlap: Team members need to anticipate the surgeon's needs, not react to them

Once the patient is draped, the surgeon will make his initial incision, insufflate the abdomen with CO_2, and place the ports. While the surgeon is doing this, the team should be anticipating his/her needs. The circulator should connect the bovie, then the gas in that order since this is the order in which the surgeon will need it (first incision, then insufflation). The assist's role at this time is to clean and prepare the scope since this is the next item needed. These steps are the same every case, so anticipating the needs of the surgeon should be easy and routine. By anticipating surgeon's needs instead of reacting to requests, efficiency is further improved.

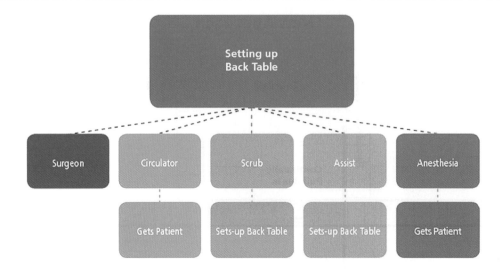

The Key: Create Task Overlap

• Circulator - Gets patient from pre-op while back table is set up.

• Anesthesia - Gets patient from pre-op while back table is set up.

TASK OVERLAP: NO NEED TO WAIT TO GET PATIENT UNTIL AFTER BACK TABLE SET UP.
Scrub and Assist - Set up back table:
   • Minimize the amount of instruments on the back table. Limit it to *da Vinci* instruments only.
   • Open surgical tray can remain unopened and placed to the side of back table.

PRE-SURGERY INSPECTION SHOULD BE CONDUCTED PRIOR TO THE ANESTHETIZATION OF PATIENT

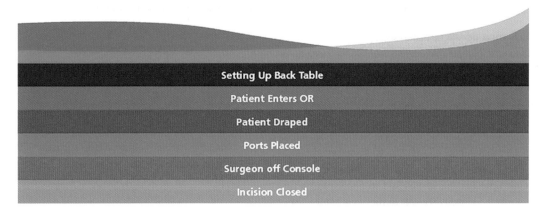

Fig. 4.4 Trigger point "opening back table" and associated parallel tasks

Step 4: Ports placed (Fig. 4.7)
Task overlap: Docking should be a team effort that includes the surgeon

Docking should be a team event that includes the surgeon. The surgeon is the only consistent person in the operating room, so he/she needs to be as facile with the docking procedure as the team. Because team members can change from day to day, the ability of the surgeon to complete simple tasks

like this will reduce variability and improve efficiency and consistency. Once the robot is docked, the surgeon will move to the console and it is at this point that the circulator should begin his/her paperwork. In many operating rooms the circulator will disrupt the workflow up to this point by trying to complete paperwork or make computer entries. The console time will be more than long enough for any circulator to complete all the necessary

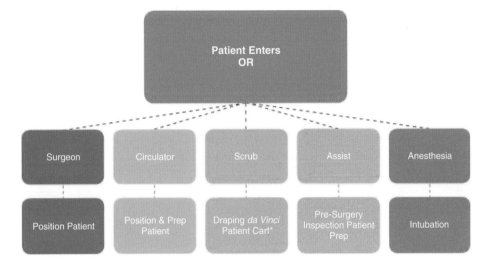

The Key: Create Task Overlap

- Surgeon - Positions patient and performs surgical site assessment

- Circulator - Positions patient, preps patient

- Scrub - Continues to drape *da Vinci* patient cart while patient is positioned and prepped

NO NEED TO WAIT FOR PATIENT CART TO BE DRAPED BEFORE PATIENT ENTERS ROOM

- Assist - Conducts pre-surgery inspection and assists in patient preparation

PRE-SURGERY INSPECTION SHOULD BE CONDUCTED PRIOR TO THE ANESTHETIZATION OF PATIENT.

* Drape kits designed to reduce OR turnover time are now available for the *da Vinci*. S** model. Ask your representative for more information.

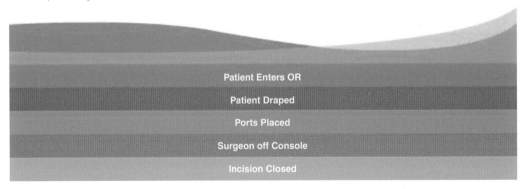

Fig. 4.5 Trigger point "Patient Enters OR" and associated parallel tasks

paperwork and make all the required computer entries and doing so while the surgeon is at the console does not disturb the workflow in the operating room and leads to improved efficiency.

Step 5: Surgeon off the console (Fig. 4.8)

Task overlap: While the surgeon closes the patient, the robot should be undraped and the back table cleared

When the surgeon stands up from the console, he/she is telling the room that they are done using the robot and all of the equipment associated with it. This means the robot should not just be rolled back but it should also be undraped and the robotic equipment (reposables, ports, etc.) should be cleaned up and removed from the room. By removing the drapes, cleaning up the robotic equipment, and sending it to central sterilization, you are performing part of the turnover while the patient is still in the room. The surgeon will take 10–20 min to

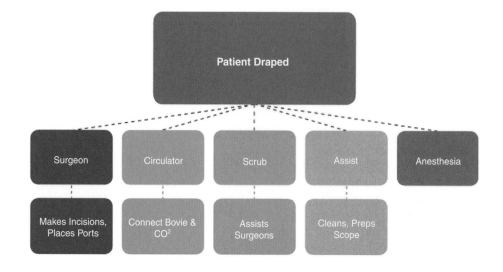

The Key: Create Task Overlap

- Surgeon - Insufflates, makes incisions, places camera and instrument ports

- Scrub - Assists surgeon with incision, port placement, instrumentation

- Circulator - Prepares auxiliary equipment (ESU, gas, etc.)

- Assist - Cleans and prepares scope for port placement visualization

TEAM MEMBERS SHOULD ANTICIPATE THE SURGEON'S NEED FOR INSTRUMENTS AND EQUIPMENT.

- Connect Bovie
- Gas tubing connected

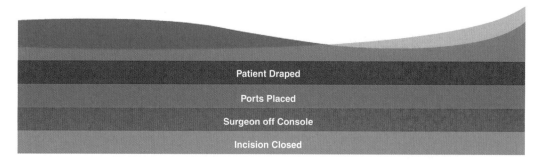

Fig. 4.6 Trigger point "Patient Draped" and associated parallel tasks

remove the specimen and close the abdomen which gives plenty of time for the team to begin stripping the room of unnecessary items.

Step 6: Patient exits the OR (Fig. 4.9)

Task overlap: While the patient heads to recovery, the scrub and the assist complete the room cleanup and begin to open for the next case

With the operation complete, the surgeon heads out to talk to the family of the patient he just operated on and the patient who he/she will be operating on next. The circulator and the anesthesia are bringing the patient to recovery and the scrub and the assist should be completing what little is left of room cleanup and then should immediately open for

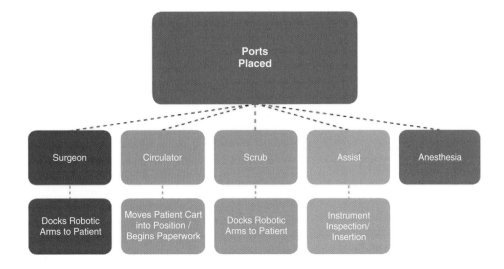

The Key: Create Task Overlap

- Circulator - Moves *da Vinci* patient cart into position. Once locked in place and surgery begins, paperwork can be started.

- Surgeon - Docks robotic arms to ports

- Scrub - Assists surgeon in docking of robotic arms to ports

- Assist - Gathers and inspects robotic instrumentation and auxiliary instrumentation and prepares for insertion

DOCKING AND DRIVING THE *DA VINCI* SYSTEM IS A TEAM EVENT THAT SHOULD BE PRACTICED CONTINUALLY. HAVING CONSISTENT TEAM MEMBERS FOR ALL CASES WILL ALSO INCREASE EFFICIENCY.

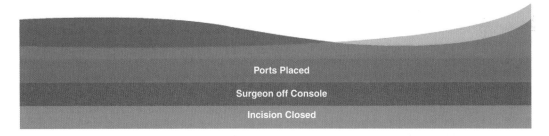

Fig. 4.7 Trigger point "Ports Placed" and associated parallel tasks

the next case. With the back table already cleared and the robot already undraped, all that is left to do is take out the garbage, mop, and open for the next case. These few remaining tasks take less than 15 min and should be the only "red zone" items to complete, minimizing the time turnover should take.

4.5.1 Implementing This Operating Room Efficiency Model

Implementing this model is a team effort that requires two things to be successful: everyone must play an active role and you need a coach.

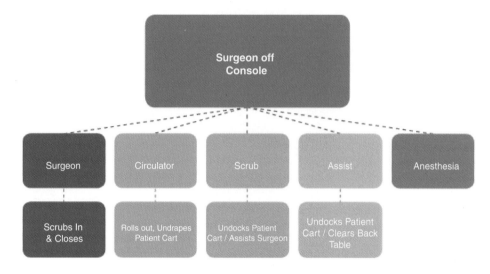

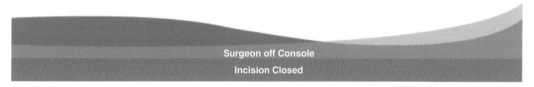

Fig. 4.8 Trigger point "Surgeon Off Console" and associated parallel tasks

4.5.2 Everyone Must Play an Active Role

When I say that everyone must play an active role, I truly mean everyone. All five team members including the surgeon must be actively involved. This model will not work if you hand your team their instructions and sit in the lounge waiting for it to happen. Regardless of your level of involvement, you may encounter team members who lack the ability or desire to be efficient. When this occurs, you need to get some new team members. This honestly can be as easy as asking your OR director for new team members. It never ceases to amaze me what you will get if you simply ask. Remember, everyone benefits from this efficiency model, so you and the OR director are on the same side here. An efficient team benefits both of you.

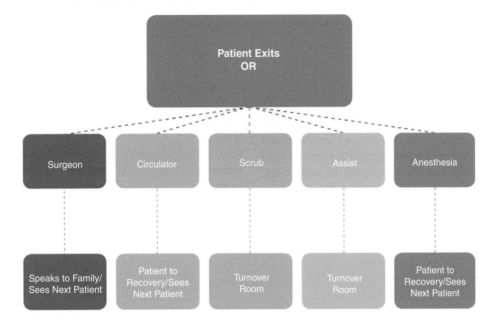

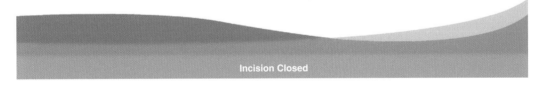

Fig. 4.9 Trigger point "Patient Exits OR" and associated parallel tasks

4.5.3 You Need a Coach

Every successful team needs a coach to motivate and guide the team. The coach needs to be someone with the following three qualities:

(1) Must be in a position of authority with respect to the team
(2) Must be respected by the team
(3) Must lead by example (needs to work with the team, not just direct them)

This means your coach can be the surgeon, the circulator, the robotic co-ordinator, or the OR director. You can be equally effective in implementing this model by choosing as your coach whichever individual in your institution best fits. The coach must set goals using this model, be actively involved in helping the team to achieve these goals, and reward the team for their achievements.

4.6 Conclusion

This operating room efficiency model has been used to successfully improve the efficiency of diverse operating rooms across the United States. The results are universally dramatic and sustainable and the performance improvements are significant and reproducible. I know what some of you are thinking "My situation is unique. I cannot implement this entire model because of (insert your reason here)". Let me tell you, I've heard it all and I guarantee you that you can create performance improvements using this model regardless of your situation. One of the unique aspects of this model is the ability to implement various fragments of it in part or in total. Regardless of the limitations and challenges your operating room faces, you can implement those part(s) of this model that you choose, eliminate those part(s) you simply cannot implement due to your unique situation, and still achieve significant benefits in performance improvement. So use this model and begin enjoying the improvements in quality, revenue, and success it can bring.

Chapter 5

Laparoscopy vs. Robotics: Ergonomics – Does It Matter?

Jens Rassweiler, Ali Serdar Gözen, Thomas Frede, and Dogu Teber

5.1 Introduction

Laparoscopy has brought many benefits to patients mainly by reducing the peri-operative morbidity. On the other hand, the distribution of the technique is handicapped by the difficulty of the procedure due to some significant limitations concerning the ergonomics of this surgical technique. Even more, it had been recognized, that laparoscopic surgery can also harm laparoscopic surgeons and this phenomenon is now under worldwide investigation.[1,2]

The disadvantages of laparoscopic procedures are mainly due to the nonergonomic design of surgical instruments and the outdated environment of the operating theatre. As laparoscopic surgery became more advanced and complex, the duration of the procedures expanded and, in proportion, so did the levels of mental and physical stress imposed to the surgical team.[3] Yet so far, only minor changes have been made to the operating room, which was originally designed for conventional operations, and also recently proposed designs by the manufacturers (i.e., OREST – Dornier; OR-1 – Karl Storz) are not based on ergonomic studies.[4,5]

Ergonomics, a relatively new science, gained wide popularity in the field of industrial engineering. Experts began to notice that when workers do their jobs under nonergonomic circumstances, they become stressed and fatigued, resulting in a drop of quality and quantity of production. As the advertising industry began to tout the "ergonomic design" of various cars and household utensils, ergonomics was respected as a serious factor influencing the sales of such products. Today, enormous sums are earmarked for ergonomic research into industrial design. In turn, new software tools have been developed to assess the ergonomic feature of new products. These tools are designed to measure the posture and movement of the human body very accurately, without using any markers.

Unfortunately, medicine did not get in on the ground floor of these ergonomic developments, because in this area, productivity and quality cannot be connected as directly to ergonomics as in industry, and the profit gained from ergonomic reorganization is difficult to quantify in financial terms.[6] Thus, the main reason for choosing a particular instrument represents its cost–quality ratio and not its ergonomic design.

However, based on recent efforts from general surgeons and urologists, the assessment of laparoscopic surgery is now under way (Table 5.1). We already have many objective data on the problems that arise in the course of everyday practice, and some attempts have been made to alter the operating environment accordingly.[7–9] On the other hand, the recently introduced da Vinci robot offers significantly improved ergonomics providing a console for the surgeon with 3D vision and instruments with seven degrees of freedom. But the device still also has some limitations compared to open surgery and even laparoscopy such as the complete loss of the tactile sense.[10–16]

In this chapter, we want to focus on the ergonomic problems of laparoscopy in comparison to the da Vinci system based on the current literature and personal long-term experience with both techniques.

J. Rassweiler (✉)
Urologische Klinik, SLK Klinikens, Heilbronn, Germany
e-mail: jens.rassweiler@slk-kliniken.de

A.K. Hemal, M. Menon (eds.), *Robotics in Genitourinary Surgery*,
DOI 10.1007/978-1-84882-114-9_5, © Springer-Verlag London Limited 2011

Table 5.1 Components of ergonomics (modified from Stone and McCloy)

To optimize system performance while maximizing human wellbeing and operational effectiveness, ergonomics embraces a range of human centered issues:
– Body size (anthropometry), motion, and strength capabilities (biomechanics)
– Sensory-motor capabilities – vision, hearing, haptics (force and touch), dexterity
– Cognitive processes and memory (including situational awareness)
– Training and current knowledge relating to equipment, systems, practices, and medical conditions (including emergencies)
– Expectations and cultural stereotypes related to operations and equipment
– General health, age, motivation, stress levels, and mental fatigue

Table 5.2 The ergonomic problems of laparoscopic surgery

Problem	Description
Reduction of range of motion	Only four degrees of freedom (instead of six)
Increase of tremor due to fulcrum effect	Inversion of instrument's motion with a varying scaling effect
Two-dimensional vision	No stereovision (3D camera and display)
Misalignment in eye–hand target	Misorientation between real and visible movements on the screen
Reduced haptic sense	Only minimal tactile feedback
Increased static stress	Musculo-skeletal problems (shoulder pain, gonarthrosis) due to rotated and bent position
Frequent physical discomfort	Musculo-skeletal problems (shoulder pain, gonarthrosis) due to rotated and bent position
Discomfort due to instruments	Surgeon's thumb

5.1.1 Limitations of Laparoscopy

Laparoscopic surgery in general is handicapped by the *reduction of the range of motion* because of the fixed trocar position determining the angle of the respective instrument to the working field[17,18](Table 5.2). The incision point acts like a spherical joint that *limits the degrees of freedom (DOF)* of the instrument from six to only four (Fig. 5.1): jaw, pitch, rotation, insertion plus the actuation of instrument. This also applies to the endoscope making it impossible to observe anatomic structures from different sides while keeping the viewpoint in focus.

Another problem is the *two-dimensional view of the telescope*. The absence of shadows, stereovision, and movement parallax in particular make it difficult for a surgeon to accurately determine spatial distance and movements and impair his eye–hand coordination (Fig. 5.2). The latter may be compensated by the experience of the surgeon, particularly if the working field is small and the camera can be put close to the object; however, particularly in the case of reconstructive surgery (pyeloplasty, urethro-vesical anastomosis), it may become a crucial handicap.[19]

5.1.2 Mental Stress

During laparoscopic operations, surgeons suffer from high levels of mental and physical stress. After a certain time (i.e., 4–5 h), the so-called *fatigue*

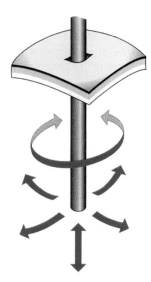

Fig. 5.1 Limited degrees of freedom (DOF) of laparoscopy

syndrome sets in characterized by mental exhaustion, reduced dexterity, and a reduced capacity for good judgment.[20]

Mental stress is caused by numerous factors.[21,22] The view of the operative situation is displayed on a monitor widely separated from the field of action, so the surgeon has to overcome the natural instinct to direct the eyes to the activity of the hands. Moreover,

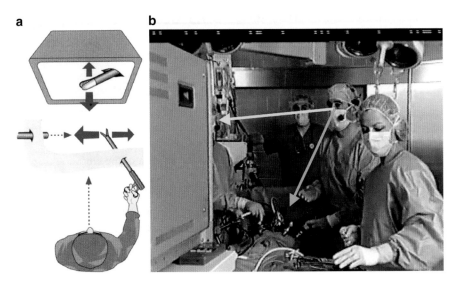

Fig. 5.2 The problem of impaired eye–hand coordination. **a** Movement on screen may differ from the axis of the instruments. **b** Dissociation of eye–target axis

he cannot reach the operative field directly with his hands. The two-dimensional viewing of a three-dimensional field has to be interpreted and synchronized to instrument movement by use of only .four4 degrees of freedom. In addition to performing the operation, the surgeon has to monitor constantly the different devices used during the procedure (i.e., insufflator, gas connection, suction device). In case of an inexperienced anesthetist, further factors may aggravate the situation (i.e., degree of relaxation, excessive fluid administration).

Although it is not easy to measure mental stress, there are early reports using physiologic measurement, such as skin conductance level or electro-oculography. Van der Schatte Olivier et al.[23] introduced the following three cardiologic stress parameters:

– The mean square of successive differences (MS-SDs) between consecutive heart beats
– The pre-injection period (PEP) corresponding to the time of isovolumetric contraction
– The average heart rate (HRA) recorded by an ambulatory monitoring system

The MSSD reflects the beat-to-beat variability of the heart rate and is highly linked to respiratory sinus arrhythmia (RSA). Changes in RSA can display changes in vagal activity. If vagal activity decreases RSA, MSSD will also be reduced because fewer oscillatory changes in heart rate occur. An increased stress level will therefore lead to a decrease in MSSD. In conclusion, high MSSD values reflect low stress level.

The PEP is the interval between the onset of ventricular depolarization and the opening of the semilunar valves. Changes in PEP correspond to changes in β-adrenergic inotropic drive to the left ventricle. The β-adrenergic tone can be manipulated by epinephrine infusion, adrenoreceptor blockade, exercise, and emotional stress.

It has been shown that mental stress can be compensated for with mental effort, but such efforts surely lead to earlier fatigue.

5.1.3 Physical Stress

Standing in a fixed position determined by the placement of trocars and the site of the screen causes static strain to eyes, head, neck, spine, and the joints of the knee and foot, which translates into eye strain, neck and shoulder pain, or stiffness. This type of stress can be measured by duration of the stressful postures and the degree of rotation of the joints respectively declination of the spine as compared to a comfortable position.[17,18,24–26] Further measurements include force plate measurements of the feet and motion analysis. Lee et al.[27] could demonstrate that the assistant also has to face a high-risk ergonomic situation being created by the assistant's left or caudal leg bearing 70–80% of body weight over time.

In order to pivot the instruments around the trocars, which are fixed to the abdominal wall, increased muscle activity and awkward movements of the upper limb are necessary. The force to control laparoscopic instruments can be six times greater than that needed for open surgery, and the problem is magnified further by the nonergonomic design of the handle. Badly designed hand instruments can even lead to damage of the nerves of the thumb and thenar, causing the so-called laparoscopist's thumb.[28]

To measure physical strain precisely, a wide array of sophisticated devices have to be used. The investigative tools for such cinematic studies are based on cinematography, video recording, optoelectronic systems, goniometers, and systems combining photocells, light beams, and timers. The movements (i.e., the posture) of the surgeon are recorded on standard or special (infrared) video cameras for evaluation.[29] In most cases, the individual being measured has to wear a special outfit with reflective markers, motion sensors, electrodes, etc., which is not easily accomplished during clinical cases. Markers attached to the surgeon may drift, and the view of the marker is often obscured during manipulation. It is also uncertain to what degree the wires and attached sensors may influence the surgeon's movement. For this reason, ergonomic studies are mainly done during laboratory experiments.

5.1.4 The Role of Questionnaires

Besides the objective evaluation of mental and physical stress during laparoscopic or robotic surgery, the analysis of the subjective assessment of ergonomic problems is important.[30,31] This is mainly based on questionnaires. Such studies have been able to provide information on prevalence, significance, and awareness associated with the different techniques. Hemal et al.[2] found that surgeons performing laparoscopy have indeed significant ergonomic problems resulting in frequent neck pain, shoulder stiffness, finger numbness, and eye strain in 13–22.4%. This was significantly more frequent compared to a control group of open surgeons who complained such problems only in 6–10.2%.

5.1.5 Geometrical Compensation

Basic studies on the principles of ergonomic handles defined the ergonomic ideal position for the laparoscopic surgeon as follows[28,32]:

20° abduction of the forearms with 40° internal rotation and 10° retroversion
90–120° flexion of the elbow
No rotation of the surgeon

The arm is slightly abducted, retroverted, and rotated inward at the shoulder level. The elbow is bent at about 90–120°, and the hand grasps the instrument in the basic position, with the wrist slightly extended; the metacarpophalangeal and the proximal interphalangeal joints are flexed at 30–50°; and the distal interphalangeal joints are almost extended. Fingers 2–5 are abducted by about 5–10°, and the thumb is opposed to the index finger.

An ideal grip for manipulating the functional elements and holding the laparoscopic instrument is a mixture of three different grips:

the contact grip characterized by touching an object with parts of the hand;
the seizing grip carried out by the thumb and one or all fingers;
the encircling grip employing two or more fingers mainly to perform strenuous work.

The *contact grip* is used for activating HF current, suction/irrigation buttons, or cogwheels for rotation of the instrument; *seizing grip* for opening/closing the effector; and *encircling grip* for holding the instrument. To support this, the instrument's handle must contact the hand at its most sensitive zones: the fingertips and the area between the thenar of the thumb and the inner surface of the hand. The instrument's shaft must represent an extension of the lower arm so as to transfer the turning movement directly to the effector.

With increasing training and analysis of the important geometrical factors, laparoscopic surgeons were able to deal with some of these problems, even in case of endoscopic suturing.[33–35] In principle, this means that the angle between the instruments should not be less than 25° and not more than 45°, and the angle between the operating field and the horizontal line should not exceed 55° (Fig. 5.3). Moreover, the

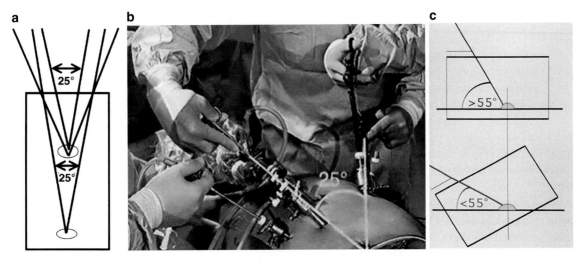

Fig. 5.3 Geometry of laparoscopic suturing. **a** Angle between the instruments (scheme). **b** Use of port beyond midline for suturing. **c** Angle between working field and instruments (scheme)

choreography of endoscopic suturing tries to overcome the limitations: by use of the almost perpendicular angle between the needle holders to adjust the position of the needle and by use of the non-dominant hand for passing the needle.

However, there is no doubt that even the experienced laparoscopic surgeon is still limited in his movements if compared to open surgeon. This becomes most evident when performing a complex procedure such as laparoscopic radical prostatectomy. There are several important steps during this operation which are significantly more difficult to carry out in comparison to open surgery, i.e., the control of the dorsal vein complex, the dissection of the lateral pedicles, the preservation of the neurovascular bundles, and most importantly the urethro-vesical anastomosis.

The correct adjustment of the table height and the use of stands to avoid the raising of shoulder during laparoscopic surgery are very important. In the survey of Wauben et al.[31] the chosen table height varied between 45 and 55 cm, with 60% of the surgeons preferring the table at pubic height. The lowering of the patient toward the surgeon may also compensate for insufficient lowering of the table and provide a better angle to the working field (Fig. 5.3b).

Eighty-seven percentage of the laparoscopic surgeons use a foot pedal to control diathermic or ultrasonic equipment.[31] Only a few (17%) use a hand-controlled device. The use of the foot pedals was found to be uncomfortable by more than a half of the respondents (53%). This concerned the lack of visual control, unbalanced position of the surgeon, and the use of too many pedals during laparoscopic surgery. On the other side, only 5% fully agreed that pedals cause discomfort in the legs and the foot. However, there is no doubt that the surgeon has to flex the foot to control a foot pedal, which requires to balance the body weight on the contralateral leg (Fig. 5.4).

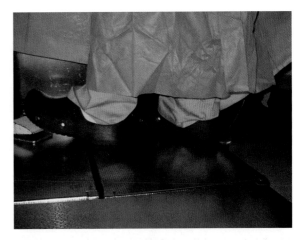

Fig. 5.4 Control of foot pedal during laparoscopic surgery with the right leg bearing 70–80% of body weight and 20° anteflexion of left foot

5.1.6 Technological Compensation

In the laparoscopic literature, a number of aids have been described to improve the surgeon's depth perception.[36] Shadows can be introduced by using illumination cannulae. Stereovision can be introduced by using a stereo-endoscopic system.[25] Comparisons between mono- and stereo-endoscopes, however, have demonstrated that with current technology, three-dimensional systems show no advantages for the experienced surgeon.[37,38] Another possibility would be the use of rotatable endoscopes and instruments.[36] However, the recent introduction of *HDTV technology* has significantly improved the depth perception, mainly due to the better resolution of the image (Fig. 5.5).

In the review of Wauben et al.[31] carried out in the year 2004, only 19% used a flat screen. Eighty-seven percentages of the monitors were placed on a tower without height adjustment and 10% on a movable arm without height adjustment. Even if the placement of the monitor below the eye level has been recommended in the ergonomic guidelines based on several randomized studies,[9,30,39] 77% of the respondents were not hindered by the actual monitor position and 64% even satisfied. This correlates with the personal experience of the authors.

Matern and Waller[28] focused on the requirements of an *ideal handle for laparoscopy*. Mostly in use are two types of handles: ring handle (like scissors) and shank handle, both with an in-line and angled version. Some needle holders have palm handles (i.e., in-line

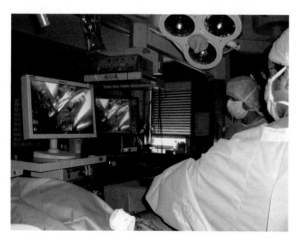

Fig. 5.5 The use of an HDTV monitor for laparoscopic surgery with excellent resolution and increased field of view

shank handles), and recently pistol handles have been introduced. Because of the symmetrical form, ring and shank handles can be used equally well by both right and left hands. They can be produced economically and are easy to clean. Ring and shank handles are suitable for one-handed manipulation of two instrument functions (i.e., opening/closing of the effector and rotation; dissector, scissors). Elements for further functions such as suctioning and cutting with coagulation have no place on these two-dimensional flat handles. For this reason, foot pedals have to be used.

Multifunctional instruments may reduce time-consuming instrument changes. Applying such functions (i.e., coagulation, irrigation/suction) requires special handles. Three-dimensional pistol handles allow the integration of several different elements because of the handle volume. Also motorized six-DOF instruments use such handles. However, there have been further modifications of ergonomic multifunctional handles, which can be found in the literature.[28,40,41] Unfortunately, most of them are still experimental.

Already in 1999, Schurr et al.[42] proposed a special chair (i.e., cockpit design) with pedal switches to improve the ergonomy of laparoscopic procedure. Since 4 years, we use a surgical support during laparoscopic radical prostatectomy (Fig. 5.6) mainly to reduce the stress on the knee joints suffering from arthroscopically proven gonarthrosis. This chair can be used only when the surgeon works with the ipsilateral trocars. For suturing we use the right medial port over the midline, which can be accomplished only in a standing position (Fig. 5.3b). Recently, Albayrak et al.[43] presented a specially designed ergonomic body support consisting of a platform with foot pedal, a semistanding support, a remote control, and a chest support. EMG results showed an average reduction of 44% for the erector spinae muscle, 20% for the semitendinosus muscle, and 74% for the gastrocnemius muscle when using the chest support. The average muscle reduction using the semistanding support was 5, 12, and 50%, respectively.

5.1.7 Telemanipulators

A more conceptional approach to these problems represents the development of computer-enhanced

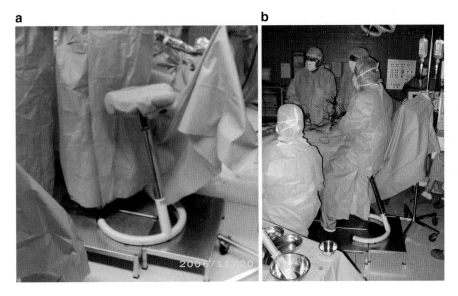

Fig. 5.6 The use of a chair/support **a** during laparoscopic radical prostatectomy **b**

telemanipulators. The concept of intelligent steerable surgical instrument system has been described by various authors. A first functional master–slave manipulator for surgery was introduced by Green et al.[44] in 1991. This manipulator was not designed for endoscopic use and had only four DOF in its first release. But it formed the basis for the industry to develop a marketable product providing six (seven) DOF: the da Vinci system.[10–15]

5.1.8 Telepresence Surgery

The da Vinci system is the first surgical system that addresses most of these problems sufficiently (Table 5.3):

- the problem of depth perception
- the problem of eye–hand coordination
- the problem of limited range of motion (i.e., DOF)

For this purpose, a computerized robotic system has been designed with stereo-endoscopic system, a computer-controlled mechanical wrist providing six DOF (plus actuation of the instrument), used from a console with handles that can be utilized at the console always in an ergonomic working position (Figs. 5.7 and 5.8).

Table 5.3 The ergonomic problems of robotic surgery

Problem	Description
No tactile feedback	Haptic sense has to be compensated by vision
Minimal control of grasping force	Force has to be adapted by experience (i.e., risk of suture rupture)
No direct access to assistant port	The surgeon is completely dependent on assistant (i.e., suction, clipping, suture insertion)
No direct communication with assistant	Only from console to OR table
Assistant limited by arms	Disturbed access, same problems of laparoscopy
Only 2D vision for assistant	View of surgeon may differ from the view of screen of assistant
Some physical discomfort	Musculo-skeletal problems at the neck and shoulder due to the anteflexed position and mental stress

5.1.9 The Surgeon's Console

The surgeon performs the procedure seated at the console holding specially designed instruments (Fig. 5.7). Highly specialized computer software and mechanics transfer the surgeon's hand movements exactly to the microsurgical movements of the manipulators at the operative site. The video image gathered from inside the abdomen provided by two parallely arranged three-chip cameras is projected so that it coincides with

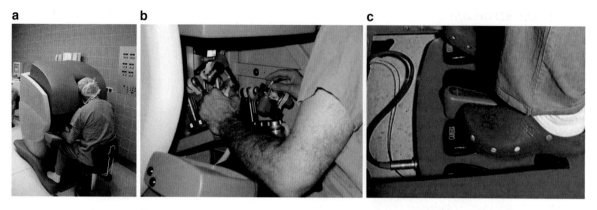

Fig. 5.7 Sitting at the da Vinci console **a** with hands in the loops, arms supported by armrest **b** and foot control of five pedals **c** with anteflexion of <20°

the workspace of the master manipulators. This overlap creates the visual illusion for the surgeon that his hands are holding onto tool tips inside the body (Surgical Immersion[R] Technology). As a result, the surgeon manipulates the tools as though he was holding onto the instruments directly.

5.1.10 The Surgical Arm Unit

Every motion of the handles is sensed by high-resolution motion sensors, processed, and transferred to the two surgical manipulators (Fig. 5.8). These slave manipulators (surgical arms) provide three degrees of freedom (pitch, jaw, insertion). The last element are the surgical instruments (i.e., end effector): At the tip of the instruments, a cable-driven mechanical wrist (Endo-Wrist[R] technology) adds three more DOF

(including rotation) and one motion for tool actuation (i.e., grip). The grip torque of the end effector (i.e., needle holder, forceps) was programmed to 1.0 N. Monopolar and bipolar electrocautery can be applied to one of the end effectors by using one of the 5-ft switches at the console if the respective instrument has been introduced. In order to enhance precision, the system allows for scaling of the master–slave motion relation. Accordingly, a motion scale of 3:1 will move the tool 1 mm inside the abdomen for every 3 mm of motion at the master console. Usually, a motion scaling of 2:1 is used. In addition the system filters unintended movements (i.e., by tremor) by applying a 6-Hz motion filter. Finally, it is possible to temporarily disconnect the end effectors from the master handles within its working space, while the position of the instruments remains unchanged (clutch function controlled by foot pedal).

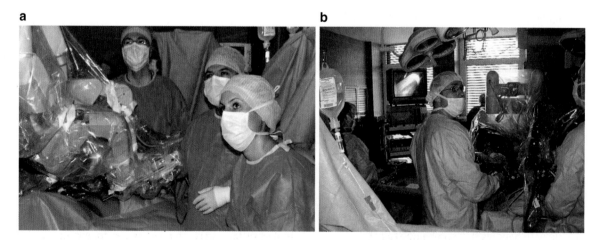

Fig. 5.8 Working at the OR table **a** surrounded by the robot arms interfering with the actions of the assistant **b**

5.1.11 The 3D Imaging System

The high-resolution 3D endoscope consists of two- to three-chip charge-coupled device cameras (InSite^R) with two high-intensity illuminators to ensure a bright image of the operative field. 0° as well as 30° lenses can be used; the 30° lenses can be additionally mounted either down or upside looking. The video image enables an up to 10-fold magnification according to the distance of the endoscope to the operative field. The endoscope – once inserted – is moved by the surgeon. Camera control is by pressing the footswitch that locks the slave-tool manipulators in place and gives the operator control of the camera through the master manipulators. The endoscope is then manipulated according to simultaneous movement of the two handles at the console. Another foot pedal can be also used for re-focusing the image.

5.1.12 Ergonomic Advantages of the da Vinci System

The main ergonomic advantage represents the introduction of a console (Table 5.4):

– The surgeon works in a seated position with a virtual 3D in-line view to the operating field.
– The elbows are supported by an arm rest.
– The surgeon has five different foot pedals to activate.
– The clutch function allows the surgeon always to work with his arms/hands in an ergonomic position.
– The surgeon moves the camera together with automatic correction of the adequate position of the instruments.

Table 5.4 Comparison of ergonomic advantages of laparoscopic vs. robotic surgery

Laparoscopy	Robotic Surgery
Use of all trocars	Excellent working ergonomy at console
Use of all instruments	Tremor filter, working scaling
HDTV technology for all	3D vision for surgeon
Six- to eightfold magnification	In-line view to (virtual) operative field six-degrees-of-freedom instruments 10-fold magnification

– The surgeon has two ergonomic handles (i.e., two loops) that transfer the activation of the seven-DOF instruments independent of the type of the instrument (i.e., forceps, needle holder).

The *seated position of the surgeon* with a virtual in-line view to the working field represents an innovation for surgical procedures, which has been realized only during microsurgery using an operative microscope. However, there is no need for the surgeon to exchange the instruments under the view of the operating field. He is able to activate different exchangeable instruments. As we know from penile surgery (i.e., hypospadia repair), the sitting position minimizes the physical stress of the surgeon and allows easy use of the foot pedals in contrast to the standing position of the surgeon during laparoscopy.

The *camera control by the surgeon* requires a certain learning curve, but after this it offers a stable and adequate view of the working field with automatic adaptation of the instruments. Moreover, the clutch function enables to work always in a centralized – per se most ergonomic – position at the console independent of the situation at the operating field. This represents a significant advantage of laparoscopy, where some steps of the operation may require an awkward position of the surgeon due to the fixed trocar arrangement.

The fact that the surgeon does not need to adapt to the handle (i.e., scissor-like, palm type) of the respective instrument (i.e., forceps, needle holder) represents another advantage over laparoscopy (and open surgery).

5.1.13 Ergonomic Disadvantages

The main disadvantage for the surgeon at the console represents the complete lack of haptic sense (i.e., tactile feedback). This has to be compensated by visual senses. Moreover, the surgeon depends completely on adequate assistance (i.e., suction, clipping) of the surgeon at the OR table. He can only demonstrate and communicate where a clip should be placed.

The ergonomics of the assisting surgeon are limited even more compared to standard laparoscopy.[14] This is due to the interference of the robotic arms, which may significantly reduce the dexterity of the assistant

(Fig. 5.8). Moreover, the surgeon cannot use the trocars of his assistant (i.e., to demonstrate correct use of the suction device; correction of a retracting instrument). With the use of a four-arm system the surgeon can control most of the functions attributed to the assistant (i.e., use of the telescope, retraction). Moreover, the surgeon has no easy access to parameters of auxiliary devices for laparoscopy (i.e., insufflator flow, pressure of pneumoperitoneum, setting of the HF generator) and the communication to the staff at the OR table might be disabled (i.e., noise of insufflator, respiratory device, patient warmer) causing significant mental stress.

Finally, disadvantages of the motion scaling (2:1) represent the fact that the surgeon may need moving long distances with his arms at the console for certain maneuvers (i.e., pulling on a suture/thread during continuous suturing), which is easily performed with the laparoscopic techniques.

5.1.14 Comparative Studies on Ergonomics of Laparoscopy and Robotics

There are only a few studies comparing the ergonomics of both techniques. Berguer and Smith[45] were the first to compare the ergonomics of both techniques in a sophisticated experimental study with novices and experienced laparoscopic surgeons. Overall, there was a lower stress level with the robot; however it did not reach statistical significance. However, they in their study used the ZEUS robot, which provides only four DOF. Interestingly, the seated position alone did represent an advantage. Due to the inferior ergonomy of the device, the authors measured a significantly higher arm abduction angle with the ZEUS system compared to laparoscopic technique despite the seated position. Since this finding was not accompanied by a higher Deltoid muscle activation, the authors concluded that it resulted from the placement of surgeon's arms on the padded armrest of the ZEUS system.

Similarly, Lee et al.[46] did not find any advantage of the ZEUS system over manual laparoscopy in their simulation study. In contrast, the time to completion was longer for the telerobotic technique with the ZEUS device. However, based on the rapid upper limb assessment (RULA) score and the job strain index (JSI),

they found that telerobotic surgery provides a more comfortable environment for the surgeon without any additional mental stress.

Van der Schatte Olivier et al.[23] presented a very interesting experimental trial with a surgically inexperienced population. They had to perform three different tasks (rope passing, needle copping, and bend dropping) using either laparoscopy or the three-armed da Vinci robot. Based on the introduction of objective parameters to measure mental discomfort (MSSD, PEP), they could clearly demonstrate the superiority of the robot-assisted group in terms of lower stress load and an increased work efficiency. However, these data may not reflect the clinical reality, where surgeons have adapted their performance to the well-known limitations of laparoscopy. Moreover, in actual surgical situations, with team work also playing a substantial role, the working environment can be more complex and demanding. Nevertheless, the authors could demonstrate the implementation of a robotic system for execution of laparoscopic tasks enhances performance and reduces cognitive stress levels as well as physical discomfort.

Bagrodia and Raman[47] presented a survey based on a questionnaire sent out via the Endourology Society and Society of Urologic Oncology to surgeons performing open, pure laparoscopic, or robot-assisted prostatectomy. Neck and/or back pain was experienced in 50, 56, and 23% of surgeons after open, laparoscopic, and robot-assisted prostatectomy. In the robotic group, neck pain was overwhelmingly more common than back pain (21 vs. 1%). This is due to the sitting position at the console. However, certain tasks are associated with more arm abduction bit but not concomitant increases in deltoid muscle activity, because the operators' arms are supported by padded arm rests. The high frequency of neck pain during robot-assisted surgery likely comes from straining to optimally visualize the high-resolution display, similar to what is experienced when reading a book on a table or working on a computer for long times.

5.1.15 The Impact of the Type of Procedure

The advantage of robotic-assisted surgery significantly depends on the type of the procedure. Back pain

Table 5.5 Steps to compensate for ergonomic limitations of laparoscopy and robotic surgery

Laparoscopy

Adjustment of table height to guarantee relaxed working (i.e., right angle of elbow)

Support for the surgeon enabling to operate temporarily in a seated position

Design of special chairs that incorporate pedal switches and body support (i.e., cockpit type) to reduce fatigue

Adjustment of the height of the monitor to avoid "chin-up" position

Placement of trocars (i.e., semilunar arrangement) to provide an adequate angle of the instruments (i.e., by changing their use)

Use of a motorized camera holder (i.e., AESOP) to improve the stability of the image

Insertion of instruments by the OR nurse enabling the surgeon to keep his eye on the monitor

Follow a trunk endurance training program

Robotics

Intensive training and standardization of the camera position, use of clutch function, position of fourth arm to reduce the mental stress (i.e., minimize the use of the foot pedals)

Use of the flexed position of the instrument (i.e., forceps) to apply it similar to a right-angle dissector

Standardization of the trocar position to minimize collision of the arms and disturbance of the assistant

represents the most common pain location after laparoscopic radical prostatectomy (i.e., 28%); however, in studies following laparoscopic cholecystectomy or splenectomy, back pain was not one of the most cited problems.[31] With appropriate patient positioning, most of these procedures can be performed with all trocar sites placed to one side of the midline similar to transperitoneal or retroperitoneal laparoscopic renal surgery. Such a configuration permits the surgeon to stand orthogonally to the patient, thus minimizing torque on the back (Fig. 5.3d). Consequently, the majority of surgeon strain is transmitted to the neck, which is hyperextended to look at the video display while working at a lower-than optimal height on tables that were initially designed for open procedures.[9]

Laparoscopic radical prostatectomy, however, is quite different, because it requires the surgeon to operate in a craniocaudal (or parallel) axis to the patient. Thus, ports are placed on both sides of the midline and operative work may necessitate reaching over the patient and across the midline (i.e., during urethrovesical anastomosis). Furthermore, the monitor is not located across the patient but positioned toward the

lower extremities, requiring secondary neck strain, while the back and the torso are already torqued toward the pelvis (i.e., torero position). Collectively, such positioning variable may be reflected in a higher rate of back discomfort in the reviewed literature.[2,25,48]

Indeed, the relevance of the ergonomic advantages of robot has to be balanced against the ease of performing the respective procedure by pure laparoscopy (Tables 5.4 and 5.5).

5.2 Discussion

Most of the laparoscopic procedures in urology are technically challenging. The experience in the United States has clearly demonstrated that the da Vinci system may significantly shorten the learning curve of these operations.[13] In Germany, however, based on a different reimbursement system, the device has not yet reached the same successful user rates (i.e., <10% vs. 80%). As a consequence, the rate of laparoscopic procedures (i.e., radical prostatectomy) is about 30%. It has to be emphasized that until now, there is no prospective randomized study comparing both techniques either clinically or technically.[16,49] Therefore, a more practice-oriented approach is used to evaluate the impact of the robot on the ergonomics.

At the beginning, some specific difficulties of the da Vinci system have been encountered[11]:

– interpretation of magnified anatomy
– lack of tactile feedback
– coordinated interaction between surgeon and assistants
– need of specific instruments for urological procedures

5.2.1 Interpretation of Magnified Anatomy

The first problem for a laparoscopic surgeon represents the interpretation of the respective anatomical structures (i.e., the dorsal vein complex, bladder neck, vas deferens) seen under stereoscopic vision with a 10-fold magnification. It proved to be difficult to adjust the new image to the known two-dimensional picture one has been using over the last decade. The same applies to identify small vessels.

5.2.2 Lack of Tactile Feedback

The lack of haptic sense aggravates the dissection technique in this novel situation. Even if "standard" laparoscopy does only provide a minimal amount of tactile sensation, the effect of training and experience finally enabled the surgeon to have a certain haptic sensation, i.e., to assess the shape of the prostate, the severity of adhesions, the strength of a suture or knot. The da Vinci system, actually, does not provide any tactile feedback. To avoid the injury to instruments, needles, and tissue, the device has a programmable grip torque that differs for the various end effectors (grasper, fine needle holder, etc.). Usually, a grip torque of 1 N is recommended for all instruments. Moreover, some force feedback is provided so that tissue contact (i.e., bony resistance), as well as external forces (collision of slaves), is reflected at the master.

Nevertheless, the surgeon has to compensate the missing tactile feedback by the improved stereoscopic vision (i.e., observing the deformation of tissue and the increasing tension on the suture). Indeed, with increasing experience, one is able to estimate the applied strength on the suture when performing a knot. It proved to be difficult only if some tension has to be applied to the suture (i.e., to control the DVC). Nevertheless, working remotely without tactile feedback requires new surgical skills, solely based on visual inputs. This of course increases the mental stress during surgery.

5.2.3 Coordinated Interaction Between Surgeon and Assistants

The complexity of the operation itself requires proper assistance and instrumentation. In contrast to a laparoscopic nephrectomy or adrenalectomy, a laparoscopic radical prostatectomy cannot be performed as solo-surgery. There is a need for retraction of the gland or adjacent structures. For vascular control, clips have to be placed, and sometimes suction is required to clear the operating field. All these have to be carried out by the assistant working under a deteriorated ergonomic situation (Fig. 5.8).

5.2.4 Prerequisites for a Successful Operation

Based on a correct indication, the success of any operation is based on the following factors:

the expertise of the surgeon
the expertise of the assistant
the interaction between surgeon and assistant
the working ergonomy
a proper instrumentarium

There is a general consensus that the *expertise of the surgeon* represents the key factor of the success of the operation, independent of the technique (i.e., open vs. laparoscopic vs. robotic[50]). However, besides the expertise of the assistant respectively the interaction between both an ideal working ergonomy may play an important role.

In *laparoscopy,* an experienced surgeon has accomplished facilities to overcome the drawbacks of the technique. Even more, he is able to compensate for some deficiencies of his assistant by taking over his part/port and adjusting the camera. This is based on the direct and uncomplicated interaction between surgeon and assistant. A significant advantage of laparoscopy represents the fact that the surgeon is able to apply every instrument (i.e., clips, staplers) and is not reduced to monopolar scissors, bipolar forceps, and needle drivers. However, even based on a large experience, there are steps during the operation, which still induce significant physical stress (i.e., suturing of the urethro-vesical anastomosis in a deep pelvis with a prominent pubic bone). Moreover, in the standing position, there is usually a slight rotation of the torso together with significant force on the standing leg (i.e., during bipolar coagulation using the foot pedal; Fig. 5.4).

In *robotic surgery,* the working ergonomy for the surgeon is optimized due to the seated position, the clutch function, the tremor filter, and the in-line 3D vision. It is important to note that the sitting position alone does not improve the performance as shown by Berguer and Smith with the ZEUS device lacking the seven DOF.[45] Moreover, in the da Vinci robot, the surgeon himself controls the camera. On the other hand, there is no tactile feedback, and the surgeon is very much dependent on optimal assistance (i.e., placement of clips). The working ergonomy for certain steps of the procedure can be even worse than during standard laparoscopy because of the robotic arms interfering with the manipulations of the assistant. The introduction of the fourth arm has improved this with respect to proper tissue retraction and exposure of the working field, but the situation for the assistant remains unchanged. Moreover, the mental stress on the surgeon at the console controlling five foot pedals and two arm handles (plus the fourth arm) should not be underestimated.

In conclusion, based on similar levels of expertise, laparoscopy has the advantage that the surgeon is able to use all instruments via all trocars. He can even use different instruments, which are not available for the surgeon at the console, such as peanuts, right-angle dissector, Ligasure. On the other hand, robotic surgery offers the optimal seated working position and ergonomy, but the lack of tactile feedback and a handicapped access for the assistant.

5.2.5 Perspectives

Evidently, manufacturers yet have insufficiently taken into consideration most of the aspects of ergonomics with respect to laparoscopy. In contrast to the enormous improvement of the video and camera systems (i.e., from one-chip, three-chip to HDTV technology), we are still using the same scissors, dissectors, and needle holders. Patents of ergonomic instrument design have been bought by the companies but not yet brought to clinical use.[32] Automated camera holders like the AESOP have been withdrawn from the market. The only significant improvement of the instruments is their ability to be cleaned for easy sterilization. Some ideas were realized to improve the control of the auxiliary devices (i.e., insufflator, HF generator) directly by the surgeon with OREST system (Dornier) or even the OR-1 (Karl Storz). However, all these improvements have no impact on the ergonomics of the procedure.

What is important for laparoscopy? Does the robot represent the final solution? Even if the da Vinci device has optimized the ergonomics of laparoscopic surgery, it also has some limitations and is not cost effective. Therefore, we still believe that a significant effort should be invested to improve the ergonomics of the pure laparoscopy. The geometry for a successful performance of the procedure has been analyzed sufficiently.[32–35] This concerns the angle between both instruments (i.e., 25–45°), the angle between the instruments and the working field (i.e., <55°), and the angle of the elbows (90–120°). The position of the table, the patient, and the surgeon (i.e., using a stand) has to accomplish this; however, the placement of the trocars may not be always adequate (i.e., due to the anatomy of the patient, intra-abdominal adhesions). Intraoperative navigation using the preoperative data of a CT scan may be helpful to determine the optimal position of the trocars[51](Fig. 5.9).

Some authors have focused on the adequate placement of the video monitor to avoid the "chin-up" position, e.g., below the eye level of the surgeon.[21,24] Even guidelines for ergonomics of laparoscopy have been formulated, but most of the laparoscopic surgeons are not aware of them.[9,31] Another alternative would be the use of helmets with integrated 3D vision (Viking System). However, according to our personal experience with device, the quality of the video display is still not reaching the standard of an HDTV monitor (Fig. 5.10). Moreover, the helmet induces additional physical and mental stress for the surgeon. Based on our large experience, the dissociation between the view on the screen and the working field can be very well compensated. The assisting nurse has to stabilize the position of the trocar during exchange of the instruments to allow the surgeon to keep his eyes on the monitor (Fig. 5.2).

On the other hand, particularly in the case of long-lasting procedure, a sitting position may be very helpful (Fig. 5.6). During laparoscopic radical prostatectomy, this is feasible only during some steps of the procedure, when only the ipsilateral ports are used (i.e., apical dissection, dissection at bladder neck). For suturing, the surgeon still has to stand up. Some authors have proposed to place the surgeon or the camera assistant in the midline close to the head. This might be inconvenient for the anesthetist and difficult in case of large or obese patients.[17,52,53] Some authors have proposed a specific OR chair with armrests and a foot bank for the pedals.[42,43] This seems to be a very interesting idea; however, such a chair would also require a change of the configuration of the OR table.

There is consensus that future operating theatres should be equipped with OR tables specifically designed for laparoscopic surgery. Such an ergonomic operating platform should not only be accompanied by a seated position of the surgeon but also minimize

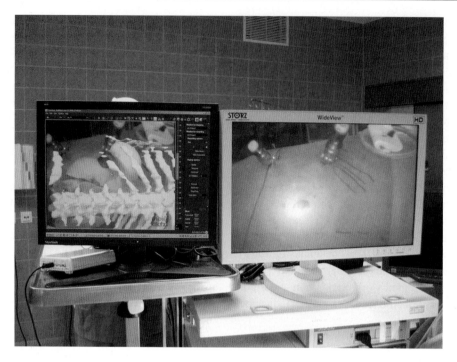

Fig. 5.9 Preoperative determination of optimal trocar placement based on segmented CT-scan images

any friction between the surgeon's leg and the table when using trocars beyond the midline and minimize the need of rotation (i.e., torque).

Finally, the ergonomy of the handles minimizing the applied force and maximizing the tactile ability has to be improved.[28] Needle holders with an integrated spring-loaded mechanism to open the branches, which require significant force to stabilize the instrument,

should be withdrawn from the market. The software to test newly designed instruments is available.

Recently, Tse et al.[48] could show that trunk muscle training significantly improved the discomfort and failure rate of laparoscopic surgery when randomizing medical students. Indeed, daily laparoscopic surgery may represent such a continuous training and contribute to the learning curve of the experts.

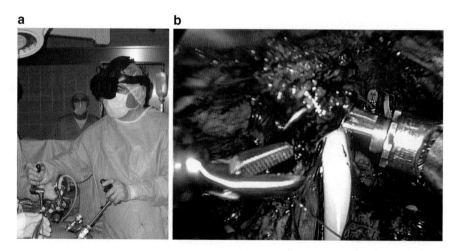

Fig. 5.10 Combined use of seven-DOF laparoscopic instruments (Radius System) with 3D video helmet. **a** External view. **b** Endoscopic view. Use of Radius device together with 3D helmet

In case of robotic surgery, further improvement should mainly aim at the development of devices offering haptic sense for the surgeon.[54]

5.3 Conclusions

There is a need to improve the ergonomics of laparoscopic surgery. The design of the da Vinci robot offers a variety of ergonomic advantages compared to pure laparoscopy. However, there are also some disadvantages, such as the lack of tactile feedback and restricted ergonomics for the assistant. The impact of these advantages also depends on the type of the procedure. On the other hand, efforts should be undertaken by all manufacturers being involved in the design of the operating theatre should focus on the improvement of ergonomics according to the existing guidelines. This concerns the design of not only armamentarium and instruments but also the OR table, platforms, OR chairs, arrangement of lines, and cables.

References

1. Vereczkei A, Bupp H, Feussner H. Laparoscopic surgery and ergonomics – it's time to think of ourselves as well. *Surg Endosc*. 2003;17:1680–1682.
2. Hemal AK, Srinivas M, Charles AR. Ergonomic problems associated with laparoscopy. *J Endourol*. 2001;15:499–503.
3. Berguer R, Forkey DL, Smith WD. Ergonomic problems associated with laparoscopic surgery. *Surg Endosc*. 1999;13:466–468.
4. Janetschek G, Rassweiler J. Future outlook. In: Janetschek G, Rassweiler J, Griffith D, eds. *Laparoscopic Surgery in Urology*. New York, NY: Thieme Stuttgart; 1996: 276–280.
5. Deinhardt M. Manipulators and integrated OR systems – requirements and solution. *Min Inv Ther Allied Technol*. 2003;12:284–292.
6. Stone R, McCloy R. Ergonomics in medicine and surgery. *BMJ*. 2004;328:1115–1118.
7. Seitz T, Balzuhat J, Bupp H. Anthropometry and measurement of posture and motion. *Int J Indus Ergonom*. 2000;25:447–453.
8. Koneczny S, Matern U. Instruments for the evaluation of ergonomics in surgery. *Min Inv Ther Allied Technol*. 2004;13:167–177.
9. Van Veelen MA, Jakimowicz JJ, Kazemir G. Improved physical ergonomics of laparoscopic surgery. *Min Inv Ther Allied Technol*. 2004;13:161–166.
10. Binder J, Kramer W. Robotically assisted laparoscopic radical prostatectomy. *BJU Int*. 2001;87:408–410.
11. Rassweiler J, Frede T, Seemann O, Stock C, Sentker L. Telesurgical laparoscopic radical prostatectomy – initial experience. *Eur Urol*. 2001;40:75–83.
12. Rassweiler J, Binder J, Frede T. Robotic and telesurgery: will they change our future? *Curr Opinion Urol*. 2001;11:309–320.
13. Hemal AK, Menon M. Robotics in urology. *Curr Opin Urol*. 2004;14:89–93.
14. Binder J, Bräutigam R, Jonas D, Bentas W. Robotic surgery in urology: fact or fantasy. *BJU Int*. 2004;94:1183–1187.
15. Dasgupta P, Jones A, Gill IS. Robotic urological surgery: a perspective. *BU Int*. 2005;95:20–23.
16. Rassweiler J, Hruza M, Teber D. Li-ming su: laparoscopic and robotic assisted radical prostatectomy – critical analysis of the results. *Eur Urol*. 2006;49:612–624.
17. Mitre AI, Duarte RJ, Arap MA, et al. Ergonomic aspects related to surgeon position in laparoscopic radical prostatectomy. *J Endourol*. 2009;23:259–262.
18. Gofrit ON, Mikahalil AA, Zorn KC, Zagaja GP, Steinberg GD, Shalhav AL. Surgeons' perceptions and injuries during and after urologic laparoscopic surgery. *Urology*. 2008;71:404–407.
19. Breedveld P, Stassen HG, Meijer DW, Stassen LPS. Theoretical background and conceptual solution for depth perception and eye–hand coordination problems in laparoscopic surgery. *Min Invas Ther Allied Technol*. 1999;8:227–234.
20. Matern U, Koneczny S. Safety, hazards and ergonomics in the operating room. *Surg Endosc*. 2007;21:1965-1969.
21. Berguer R. Ergonomics and laparoscopic surgery. *Laparosc Today*. 2005;4:8–11.
22. Reyes DAG, Tang B, Cushieri A. Minimal access surgery (MAS)-related surgeon morbidity syndromes. *Surg Endosc*. 2006;20:1–13.
23. Van der Schatte Olivier RH, van't Hullenaar CDP, Ruurda JP, Broeders IAMJ. Ergonomics, user comfort, and performance in standard and robot-assisted laparoscopic surgery. *Surg Endosc*. 2009;23:1365–1371.
24. Van Det MJ, Meijerink WJHJ, Hoff G, van Veelen MA, Pierie JPEN. Ergonomic assessment of neck posture in the minimally invasive surgery suite during laparoscopic cholecystectomy. *Surg Endosc*. 2008;22: 2421–2427.
25. Johnston WK III, Hollenbeck K, Wolf JS Jr. Comparison of neuromuscular injuries to the surgeon during hand-assisted and standard laparoscopic urologic surgery. *J Endourol*. 2005;19:377–381.
26. Wolf JS Jr, Marcovich R, Gill IS. Survey of neuromuscular injuries to the patient and surgeon during urologic laparoscopic surgery. *Urology*. 2000;55: 831–836.
27. Lee G, Lee T, Dexter D, et al. Ergonomic risk associated with assisting in minimally invasive surgery. *Surg Endosc Surg*. 2009;23:182–188.
28. Matern U, Waller P. Instruments for minimally invasive surgery. Principles of ergonomic handles. *Surg Endosc*. 1999;13:174–182.
29. Vereczkei A, Feussner H, Negele T, et al. Ergonomic assessment of the static stress confronted by surgeons

during laparoscopic cholecystectomy. *Surg Endosc*. 2004;18:1118–1122.

30. Van Det MJ, Meijerink WJHJ, Hoff C, Totté ER, Pierie JPEN. Optimal ergonomics for laparoscopic surgery in minimally invasive surgery suites: a review and guidelines. *Surg Endosc*. 2009;23:1279–1285.

31. Wauben ÖSGL, van Veelen MA, Gossor D, Goossens RHM. Application of ergonomic guidelines during minimally invasive surgery: a questionnaire survey of 284 surgeons. *Surg Endosc*. 2006;20:1268–1274.

32. Matern U. Ergonomic deficiencies in the operating room: examples from minimally invasive surgery. *Work*. 2009;32:1–4.

33. Frede T, Stock C, Renner C, Budair Z, Abdel-Salam Y, Rassweiler J. Geometry of laparoscopic suturing and knotting techniques. *J Endourol*. 1999;13:191–198.

34. Frede T, Stock C, Rassweiler JJ, Alken P. Retroperitoneoscopic and laparoscopic suturing: tips and strategies for improving efficiency. *J Endourol*. 2000;14:905–913.

35. Rassweiler J, Klein J, Teber D, Schulze M, Frede T. Mechanical simulators for training for laparoscopic surgery in urology. *J Endourol*. 2007;21:252–262.

36. Schurr MO, Kunert W, Arezzo A, Buess G. The role and future of endoscopic imaging systems. *Endoscopy*. 1999;71:557–562.

37. Pietrabissa A, Scarcello E, Carobbi A, Mosca F. Three dimensional versus two-dimensional video system for the trained endoscopic surgeon and the beginner. *Endosc Surg*. 1994;2:315–317.

38. McDougall EM, Soble JJ, Wolf JS, Nakada SY, Elashry OM, Clayman RV. Comparison of three-dimensional and three dimensional laparoscopic video systems. *J Endourol*. 1996;10:371–374.

39. Van Veelen MA, Jakimowicz JJ, Kazemir G. Improved physical ergonomics of laparoscopic surgery. *Min Invas Ther Allied Technol*. 2004;13:161–166.

40. Frede T, Hammady A, Klein J, et al. The radius surgical system – a new device for complex minimally invasive procedures in urology? *Eur Urol*. 2007;51:1015–1022.

41. Koneczny S, Mattern U. Instruments for the evaluation of ergonomics in surgery. *Min Invas Ther Allied Technol*. 2004;13:167–177.

42. Schurr MO, Buess GF, Wieth F, Saile H-J, Botsch M. Ergonomic surgeon's chair for use during minimally invasive surgery. *Surg Laparosc Endosc Percutan Tech*. 1999;4:244–247.

43. Albayrak A, van Veelen MA, Prins JF, Snijders CJ, de Ridder H, Kazemir G. A newly designed ergonomic body support for surgeons. *Surg Endosc*. 2007;21:1835–1840.

44. Green PE, Piantanida TA, Hill JW, Simon IB, Satava RM. Telepresence: dexterous procedures in a virtual operating field. *Am Surg*. 1991;57:192(abstract).

45. Berguer R, Smith W. An ergonomic comparison of robotic and laparoscopic technique: the influence of surgeon experience and task complexity. *J Surg Res*. 2006;134:87–92.

46. Lee EC, Rafiq A, Merrell R, Ackerman R, Dennerlein JT. Ergonomics and human factors in endoscopic surgery: a comparison of manual vs telerobotic simulations systems. *Surg Endosc*. 2005;15:1064–1070.

47. Bagrodia A, Raman JD. Ergonomics considerations of radical prostatectomy: physician perspective of open, laparoscopic, and robot-assisted techniques. *J Endourol*. 2009;23:627–633.

48. Tse MA, Masters S, Lo CY, Patil NG. Trunk muscle training, posture fatigue, and performance in laparoscopic surgery. *J Endourol*. 2008;22:1053–1058.

49. Kenngott HG, Müller-Stich BP, Reiter MA, Rassweiler J, Gutt CN. Robotic suturing: technique and benefit of advanced laparoscopic surgery. *Minim Invasive Ther Allied Technol*. 2008;17:160–167.

50. Ficarra V, Novara G, Artibani W, et al. Retropubic, laparoscopic, and robot-assisted radical prostatectomy: a systematic review and cumulative analysis of comparative studies. *Eur Urol*. 2009;55:1037–1063.

51. Baumhauer M, Feuerstein M, Meinzer H-P, Rassweiler J. Navigation in endoscopic soft tissue surgery: perspectives and limitations. *J Endourol*. 2008;22:751–766.

52. Stolzenburg JU, Truss MC, Do M, et al. Evolution of endoscopic extraperitoneal radical prostatectomy (EERPE)—technical improvements and development of a nerve-sparing, potency-preserving approach. *World J Urol*. 2003;22:147–152.

53. Guillonneau B, Vallancien G. *Laparoscopic radical prostatectomy: the Montsouris technique. J Urol*. 2000;163:1643–1949.

54. Lee DH, Choi J, Park JW, et al. An implementation of sensor-based force feedback in a compact laparoscopic surgery robot. *ASAIO J*. 2009;55:83–85.

Chapter 6

Anesthetic Considerations for Robotic Urologic Surgery

Michael A. Olympio

6.1 Introduction

This chapter will focus upon the complex physiology and implications of pneumoperitoneum (PPT) and the Trendelenburg position (TP) which challenges the anesthetic management through the neurologic, pulmonary, cardiovascular, hepatic, and renal systems. Robotic-assisted laparoscopic urologic surgery (RALUS) limits access to the limbs and hinders routine monitoring and its interpretation, primarily from hydrostatic gradients. Although the effects of capnoperitoneum (CPT) for laparoscopic cholecystectomy (Lap-C) have been well described, the added effects of TP have not. The predominant types of RALUS (prostatectomy, cystectomy, and nephrectomy) differ in anesthetic management secondary to position, complexity, organ function, duration, access, morbidity, length of stay, and postoperative recovery. The anesthesia team should know their surgeon's outcomes regarding these factors in order to best manage the anesthetic.

6.2 The Anesthetic Implications of Pneumoperitoneum and Positioning

6.2.1 Inflation Gas

Knowledge and consideration of alternatives to carbon dioxide (CO_2) are important because compromised

M.A. Olympio (✉)
Departments of Anesthesiology and Urology, Baptist Medical Center, Wake Forest University Health Sciences, Winston-Salem, NC 27157–1009, USA
e-mail: molympio@wfubmc.edu

patients may not tolerate hypercarbia, as it might lead to severe combined metabolic and respiratory academia.[1] Other types of inflation gas have been used for laparoscopy including nitrous oxide (N_2O), helium, argon, oxygen, air, and nitrogen[2] but the properties most desirable for laparoscopic surgery are (1) high solubility in the blood stream, (2) inability to support combustion, (3) lack of effect upon blood–gas equilibrium, (4) minimal hepatic, renal, hemodynamic, and respiratory effects, (5) capability to manage embolism of the gas into the bloodstream, and (6) minimal cost and ready accessibility.

CO_2 remains the most favorable in this regard, but its major disadvantage is the need to increase ventilation in compliance-reduced lungs. Hypercarbia is generally well tolerated or easily reduced,[2] but extreme hypercarbia may occur in patients with poor cardiac output, lung disease, obesity or impaired ventilation, necessitating post-op ventilation, or it might worsen a metabolic acidemia leading to myocardial depression and systemic vasodilation, or cause direct sympathetic stimulation.[3] End-tidal CO_2 ($EtCO_2$) increases over 8–10 min from onset and reaches a plateau over the next 15–20 min, whereas retroperitoneal insufflation will further increase CO_2 absorption from higher vascularity and spread to other spaces.[4,5] CPT lowers intraperitoneal pH causing abdominal or shoulder tip pain[6] and increases cerebral blood flow (CBF) and intracranial pressure (ICP) through impedance of lumbar venous drainage; TP worsens these effects.[7] Isothermic (37° vs. 21°) CO_2 will improve pulmonary function and perhaps UOP in the postoperative period.[8]

Helium is a clinical alternative,[9] with little effect on the respiratory and cardiovascular systems. It has a favorable diffusion capability like CO_2, was favorably

A.K. Hemal, M. Menon (eds.), *Robotics in Genitourinary Surgery*,
DOI 10.1007/978-1-84882-114-9_6, © Springer-Verlag London Limited 2011

tested in patients with COPD, and is associated with lower catecholamines, mean arterial pressure (MAP), and ICP.[10] and acidosis. Embolization of any alternative gas may be more dangerous, since it is not as soluble as CO_2 or not readily exhaled.[11] Air, oxygen, and N_2O support combustion and are not very soluble, but some authors advocate N_2O without a clear risk of combustion in vivo.[2]

6.2.2 Intra-abdominal Pressure

Higher degrees of IAP may cause adverse effects[12] (Table 6.1), and these may be eliminated by the abdominal wall lift procedure (AWL).[13,14] The European Association for Endoscopic Surgery (EAES)[14] recommends, "...to use the lowest IAP allowing adequate exposure... to avoid an IAP of more than 12 mmHg combined with TP because it reduces pulmonary compliance ... and there is ventilation-perfusion impairment." EAES defines low-pressure PPT as 5–7 mmHg and normal as 12–15 mmHg with a transient 15 mmHg considered high. They conclude that the hemodynamic effects of PPT are without consequences and are mostly overcome by volume loading, particularly in reverse TP (r-TP). Regardless, the anesthesiologist may struggle to achieve stability and to prevent complications.

Table 6.1 Adverse effects of higher intra-abdominal pressure (12–15 mmHg vs. 5–7 mmHg)

Increased	Decreased
Shoulder-tip pain	Venous return
Heart rate	Preload
Mean arterial pressure	Cardiac output
Pulmonary vascular resistance	Pulmonary compliance
Systemic vascular resistance	Renal blood flow
Renin–aldosterone	Urine production
Angiotensin	Hepatoportal circulation
Vasopressin	Splanchnic microcirculation
Airway resistance	Gastric mucosal pH
pCO$_2$	
Liver enzymes	
Central venous pressure	
Shunt	
Intraocular pressure	
Intracranial pressure	
Catheline[12]	

6.2.3 Cerebral, Ocular, Facial, and Laryngeal Effects

PPT and TP will increase hydrostatic pressure in the face and sclera, leading to edema or plethora, and may cause edema of the glottis and vocal cords affecting the course of extubation. Both hypercarbia and IAP will increase ICP, which may occur early and also with helium gas.[10] These effects are mediated through compression of the inferior vena cava (IVC), increased CVP, impaired venous drainage of the lumbar venous plexus, and subsequently impaired CSF resorption.[7,15,16] Pre-emptive hyperventilation does not significantly decrease ICP. Postoperative headache, nausea, and vomiting are attributed to this ICP, and not to hypercarbia.[17] Concomitant MAP elevations may be caused primarily by the release of vasopressin which may also be the mediator of reduced splanchnic blood flow.[15] Mild reductions in regional cerebral oxygen saturation in patients placed in TP were initially reported,[18] but others have recently shown only minimal net reductions in cerebral perfusion pressure and an increase in cerebral tissue oxygenation.[19,20]

Intraocular pressure (IOP) will increase, associated with hypertension, hypercarbia, position, and elevations in CVP.[21] It may be attenuated by general anesthesia in patients without ocular disease or it may be worsened in TP to a point of being contraindicated in those with intraocular hypertension. The intraocular pressure changes during gynecologic laparoscopic surgery in TP were lower when using propofol TIVA anesthesia compared to isoflurane, perhaps through propofol-induced inhibition of vasopressin release.[21] Posterior ischemic optic neuropathy has been reported after a long duration of TP during RALRP.[22] Others have also reported time- or CO_2-dependent increases in IOP, specifically during RALRP.[23]

6.2.4 Cardiovascular Effects

6.2.4.1 Background

Table 6.2 categorizes and summarizes the hemodynamic effects of CPT and posture.[24–38] TP for lower abdominal surgery causes significantly different effects upon the heart and circulation, which dictates

Table 6.2 Hemodynamic effects of capnoperitoneum (CPT) and posture

Ref.	Author–Year	Posture	CV risk	Surg	IAP	Monitor	MAP	CO	HR	SVR	MPAP	PVR	CVP	PCWP	SV	LVEDV	LVEF
24	Odeburg 1994	Supine	Healthy	Chole	12	PA	↑	↔	↔	↑	↑	↔	↑	↑		←	↔
25	Gannedahl 1996	Supine	Healthy	Chole	12	PA–TEE	↑	↔	↔	↑	↑	↔	↑	↑			↔
26	Fahy 1999	Lat	Healthy	Neph	15	TEE	↑		↔								↔
27	Cunningham 1993	r-TP	Healthy	Chole	15	TEE	↑		↔						→		
24	Odeburg 1994	r-TP	Healthy	Chole	12	PA	↑	→	↔	↑	↔	↔	→	→		→	↔
28	Dorsay 1995	r-TP	Healthy	Chole	15	TEE	↑		←						→	→	↔
25	Gannedahl 1996	r-TP	Healthy	Chole	12	PA–TEE	↑	↔	↔	↔	→		↑	→		←	
29	Joris 1998	r-TP	Healthy	Chole	14	PA	↔↑	↓↔	↔	↔↑	↑↑	↔↑	↑↑	↑↑			
24	Odeburg 1994	TP	Healthy	Chole	12	PA	↑	↔	↔	↔	←	↔	↑↑				
30	Hirvonen 1995	TP	Healthy	Hyst	14	PA	↑	→	→	↔	↑	↔	↑↑	↑↑		←	↔
25	Gannedahl 1996	TP	Healthy	Chole	12	PA–TEE	↑	↔	→	↑	↑				←	←	
31	Falabella 1907	TP	Healthy	RALRP	15	TEE	↑	↔	↔	↔			↑		←		
32	Meininger 1909	TP	Healthy	RALRP	12	TDCI	↑	→	↔	↑			↑				↔
33	Harris 1996	Supine	↑ risks	Colec	15	PA–TEE	↑	↔	↔	↑	↑	↔	↑	↔		↔	↔
34	Zollinger 1997	Supine	↑ risks	Chole	14	PA	↑	↔	↔	↑	←	↔	↑	↑	→		↔
35	Popescu 1906	Supine	↑ risks	Nissen	15	PA	↓↑		↔	←							↑→
36	Alfonsi 1906	Lat	↑ risks	AAA	14	TEE	↑	↔	←	↔					↑	↔	↑→
37	Safran 1993	r-TP	↑ risks	Multi	15	PA	↑	→	←	↑↑			←				→
34	Zollinger 1997	r-TP	↑ risks	Chole	14	PA	↑	↔	↔	←	←	↔	↑	↑			
38	Koivusalo 08	r-TP	↑ risks	Chole	10	PA	↔	↔	↔	↔	↔	↔	←	↔↑			
33	Harris 1996	TP	↑ risks	Colec	15	PA–TEE	↑	↔	↔	↑	↑↑		↑↑			←	↔

Lat, lateral; CV, cardiovascular; PA, pulmonary artery catheter; TEE, transesophageal echocardiography; Neph, nephrectomy; Hyst, hysterectomy; Intstn, intestinal; Chole, cholecystectomy; Colec, colectomy; AAA, abdominal aortic aneurysm; Nissen, Nissen fundoplication; Multi, multiple

a different anesthetic approach. Initially, most hemodynamic studies relied upon questionable PAP measurements (with high IAP and hydrostatic forces) but recent data from transesophageal echocardiography (TEE) are thought to be more reliable. Hemodynamic derangements arise from a complex interaction of direct pressure, posture, volume, and neurohumoral effects.[14,29,39,40]

6.2.4.2 Hemodynamic Changes

Increases in IAP (in supine patients; Table 6.2) consistently cause increases in MAP, SVR, and variable or no changes in CO and heart rate (HR). PA, PCWP, and CVP measurements all increase. SVR is highest during venous pooling in r-TP but mitigated during TP. IAP will cause a biphasic increase and then decrease in cardiac preload from splanchnic and caval compression, respectively. Administration of fluid would attenuate a decrease in blood pressure if in supine or in r-TP, but MAP typically rises consistently with higher SVR. TEE confirms an increase in end-diastolic volume (EDV) in the supine patient[41] but a decrease in EDV in r-TP.[27,28] EDV may be elevated in TP[25,33] with lessened SVR, but new data indicating diastolic dysfunction may cause a decrease in EDV and decrease in SV.[40] Such differences suggest that volume loading may not be indicated in TP.

SVR consistently increases because of resistance to aortic outflow across the diaphragm, and/or from immediate increases in vasopressin and/or norepinephrine[29] secondary to ICP elevations[15] from IAP. Such might explain the maintenance of CO, when it might otherwise be expected to fall. Renin–angiotensin is stimulated through reductions in renal blood flow (RBF) and glomerular filtration rate (GFR), either with r-TP or with IAP. Cardiac index (CI) in RALRP is stable[32,40] but stroke volume might be reduced with diastolic dysfunction.[40] Intermittent sequential pneumatic compression (ISPC) devices restore CO and lessen the increase in SVR, in r-TP patients.

6.2.4.3 Special Considerations with Cardiac Disease

Worsened valvular regurgitation after PPT and TP has been documented through TEE monitoring[26] and may be effectively treated with vasodilators. Most patients

seem to equilibrate over time and do not sustain complications.[34,37] With SVR increases of 65% and PVR increases of 90%,[42] there can be an increase in LV end-systolic area[36] attributed to increased afterload with systolic dysfunction. Right ventricular afterload also increases significantly, possibly as a result of both increased PVR and increased mechanical ventilation pressures, potentially leading to RV dysfunction with compression of the LV causing diastolic dysfunction. Myocardial wall stress of both ventricles can increase,[27] leading to concerns about increased oxygen demand, compromised intramyocardial coronary blood flow, and ischemia in susceptible patients. Heart rate is typically maintained or increased as a result of CO_2 absorption and catecholamine release.[29,42] An increase in volatile anesthesia or beta blockade to counteract increased MAP may be deleterious by virtue of their myocardial depressant effects.[33] Alternatively, increased filling, wall stress, and SVR might better be counteracted through the use of vasodilators and/or modulation of sympathetic activity through alpha-2 receptor agonists such as clonidine and dexmedetomidine[29,43] or through a phosphodiesterase inhibitor such as milrinone.

6.2.5 Pulmonary Effects

6.2.5.1 Lung Volumes

PPT and TP will significantly reduce total lung capacity (TLC) and total lung compliance,[44] and increase airway resistance. The diaphragm is shifted cephalad and FRC is reduced >50%, while the volume of the lung may reach its closing capacity (CC).[45] This causes atelectasis and shunt leading to oxygen desaturation and is overcome through the application of optimal PEEP, identified through spirometry and illustrated in Fig. 6.1. Clinically, one may be able to increase compliance from 15 mL/cmH$_2$O to as much as 40 mL/cmH$_2$O through such maneuvers. PEEP is not devoid of detrimental effects, however, and might reduce venous return and cause hypotension.

6.2.5.2 Hypercarbia and Hypoxia

Hypercarbia from CPT is generally overcome by increasing minute ventilation approximately 10–25%,[46,47] but complications of pneumothorax,

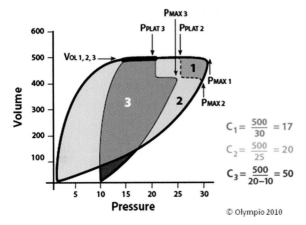

Fig. 6.1 Spirometry pressure–volume loops indicating no PEEP and no inspiratory pause in loop 1 (*blue*) with a resultant (dynamic) compliance of 17 mL/cm H_2O. The addition of an inspiratory pause may lead to a greater distribution of gas and a lower inspiratory plateau pressure ($P_{PLAT 2}$ of 25 cm H_2O), without the contribution of resistance to airflow. An improvement in (static) compliance to 20 mL/cm H_2O (loop 2, *orange*) is evident. If PEEP is added in loop 3 (*red*), the compliance might dramatically improve as the curve is shifted to the *right*, with lesser change in pressure ($P_{PLAT 3}$ – PEEP), thus improving compliance to 50 mL/cm H_2O

pneumomediastinum, pneumopericardium, and subcutaneous emphysema have all occurred.[48] Sudden or even gradual deterioration in oxygen saturation, peak inspiratory pressure, or development of hypercarbia must not be confused with the possibility of endobronchial intubation as the abdomen is inflated.[49] Although PPT typically leads to atelectasis and shunt with hypoxemia,[45,48] there is evidence that pO_2 may steadily increase over time[50] through recruitment of vascular perfusion to ventilated areas of the lung or reduction in flow (via compression) to previously atelectatic areas.

6.2.5.3 Ventilation Strategies

The optimal type of ventilation for PPT with or without TP has not been determined.[41] Newer modes of operative ventilatory strategies beyond VCV include PCV and adaptive support ventilation. Adjustment of the I:E ratio should be made to effect the greatest volume for the least amount of pressure, without creating auto-PEEP. PCV has not been shown to consistently improve compliance compared to VCV.[41] The retroperitoneal approach causes less peak inspiratory and plateau pressure and higher compliance than does the transperitoneal approach.

6.2.6 Lower Limb Circulation

PPT will enhance venous stasis and vascular resistance in the lower extremities in proportion to the IAP,[51] with evidence of an ischemia–reperfusion syndrome derived from elevations in plasma oxidative stress markers and reductions in total antioxidant status.[52] These effects are posture dependent occurring in r-TP, but not in TP. Nevertheless, massive PE has occurred during laparoscopic hysterectomy in TP.[53] IPSC devices reverse some of the physiological causes of ischemia/reperfusion.[54] If the pressure gradient from peritoneum to lower extremities (in r-TP) is neutralized, there is normalization of otherwise elevated SVR, associated with significant increases in CO,[55] but that study did not include a subgroup of TP patients. EAES clinical practice guidelines[14] recommend the IPSC device on all prolonged laparoscopic procedures, and in combination with low molecular weight heparin (LMWH), protection against DVT seems evident.[56]

Hydrostatic effects causing relative hypotension to the calves may be implicated in TP-dependent calf compartment syndrome and rhabdomyolysis after prolonged robotic cystoprostatectomy.[57] Other risk factors may include constant compression stockings, use of vasoactive drugs, hypovolemia, and hypertrophied calf muscles.

6.3   Special Monitoring Issues

6.3.1 Routine Monitoring

Routine monitoring includes a recent mandate for audible alarms for pulse oximetry and capnography so that a misconnection, hypoventilation, or oxygen desaturation would be more readily detectable.[58]

6.3.2 Peripheral Nerve Stimulation

The arms and legs in RALRP are inaccessible for monitoring the degree of neuromuscular blockade (NMB). Understanding the facial twitch is imperative to avoid direct muscle stimulation and subsequent overdosing of agents. Residual NMB in patients having critical respiratory events on admission to the PACU is highly likely.[59] The orbicularis oculi twitch response is most similar to the adductor pollicis in onset time and duration and may be preferred over the corrugator supercilii when monitoring on the face.

6.3.3 Hydrostatic Gradients, Blood Pressure, and CVP

For those robotic patients placed in extremes of positioning, the measuring device must be at or referenced to heart level. For example, the "beach-chair" position for orthopedic shoulder surgery has been of significant concern to anesthesiologists since Pohl and Cullen[60] reported four cases of catastrophic neurological outcomes in otherwise healthy patients. The Anesthesia Patient Safety Foundation (APSF) *Newsletter* published serial discussions on measurement and management of CBF and cerebral perfusion pressure (CPP).[60,61] Essentially, the complexities of "syphon" versus "waterfall" effects are not completely understood. Figure 6.2 emphasizes these postural hydrostatic effects. Understanding the difference between "referencing" a cuff or a transducer and "zeroing" a transducer is critical to having a sensible discussion on this issue. When monitoring BP, CVP, PAOP, or PAP with an arterial line in patients positioned in steep TP for RALUS, the transducer must be zeroed at the stopcock that is referenced horizontally to the right atrium (5 cm below the sternum at the forth intercostal space). One must then account for any negative hydrostatic gradients to the calf or positive gradients to the cranium. Similarly, a blood pressure cuff should be close to the heart level, on the biceps, and certainly not on the elevated calf or ankle. Experts suggest that the pressure

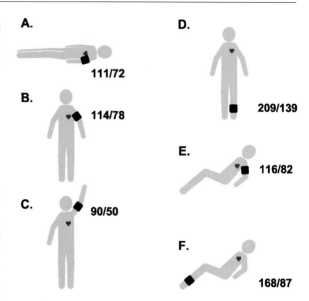

Fig. 6.2 Actual blood pressure readings of the author, taken in triplicate in various locations and body positions. Note similar readings in **A**, **B**, and **E** when the cuff is near heart level, despite posture, and note the decrease in pressure reading when the measurement site is above the heart in **C**. This reading is lower because of a negative hydrostatic gradient. Alternatively, when the pressure is measured below the heart in **D** and **F**, the reading may be dramatically higher, depending on the depth of the hydrostatic gradient. See text for details

reading be adjusted for hydrostatic gradient, according to the organ at greatest risk of hypoperfusion[61] (Fig. 6.3).

6.3.4 Pulse Oximetry

The continual measurement of oxygen saturation via pulse oximetry (SpO$_2$) is a standard of care.[58] The typical placement of a digital probe is not accessible

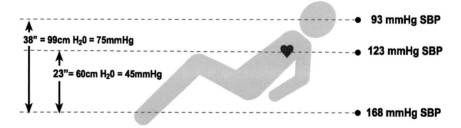

Fig. 6.3 Mathematical corrections of a systolic pressure of 123 mmHg measured at heart level. Since the brain is 15 in. above the heart (= 39 cm H$_2$O = 30 mmHg), the pressure is reduced to 93 mmHg. Similarly, the ankle reading is 23 in. below the heart and the pressure is increased by 45–168 mmHg. Generally, 1 vertical in. converts to 2 mmHg pressure change. Similarly 4 vertical cm converts to 3 mmHg

after positioning. Probes placed on the earlobe may read unreliably low,[62] while relatively new forehead reflectance pulse oximetry probes have also been contraindicated by the manufacturer for patients in TP (OxiMax MAX FAST, Nellcor/Tyco Healthcare). Although readings may well be obtained, they are more variable than concurrent digit-sensor recordings, and they read lower saturations.[63] A recommendation must be made for using conventional digit sensors in patients placed in TP with PPT.

6.3.5 Capnography and Pulmonary Function

The capnogram yields very useful information about resistance to exhalation from alterations in pulmonary mechanics, or from obstructive lung disease or bronchospasm during PPT. With expectations of particularly difficult ventilation, arterial cannulation should be considered for blood gas sampling. Caution is advised in the use of capnography to predict pCO_2 in the elderly patient and those with cardiopulmonary disease, since there is an increase in the $P(a\text{-}Et)CO_2$ difference in patients under PPT for Lap-C[46,64] secondary to an increase in dead space ventilation (increased V/Q) and/or a decrease in CO.

6.3.6 Renal Function

Assessments of renal function[65] include a BUN, creatinine (Cr), and calculation of GFR but these are not helpful in rapidly changing renal function. Cr is acutely decreased by intravenous volume dilution throughout all body compartments and may therefore slowly rise postoperatively when edema subsides. Intraoperative urine output is unreliable as an indicator of renal function, affected by salt/water balance, increases in antidiuretic hormone (ADH), endothelin, renin, and aldosterone associated with PPT, but it may actually reflect renal perfusion and volume status.[29,65,66] Reductions in RBF and GFR are reported in a majority of laparoscopic studies and are correlated with preoperative decreased renal function, or lower levels of hydration, r-TP, duration of PPT, and

higher IAP.[66] Renal blood flow and function typically return to normal after exsufflation.[66] Hypovolemia is suggested by the urine to plasma osmolarity ratio (U:Posm of >1.5, with urine >450 mOsm/L). With ATN, diluted urine may occur 24–48 h before Cr or BUN begins to rise. Intraoperative attenuation of renal hypoperfusion has been accomplished with nitroglycerine, clonidine,[29] dexmedetomidine,[43] dopamine, and epidural anesthesia.

6.4 Pre-anesthesia Assessment

The pre-anesthetic evaluation of the laparoscopic[3] and RALUS [67] patient specifically addresses potential problems with ICP, IOP, hemodynamics, ventilation, volume loading, and positioning. Since postoperative edema of the face, eyes, and larynx might delay extubation, necessitate re-intubation, or require insertion of oral or nasal airways, any known or suspected preoperative airway challenges will be magnified in the postoperative period. Compression of nerves is not always directly responsible for postoperative deficits, as preexisting susceptibilities have been described, particularly for ulnar neuropathy. Anesthesiologists should document these preexisting susceptibilities. Since IOP may rise during PPT and TP, glaucoma or visual problems may be a significant concern. Cervical spine disease and limited range of motion may be a factor if the patient is in the lateral position with flexion, causing lateral displacement of the cervical spine with potential stretch of the brachial plexus or exacerbation of spinal stenosis. Lateral flexion of the lumbar spine might exacerbate foraminal stenosis, back pain, or radiculopathy. Any calf pain, myopathies or use of statin drugs should be considered whenever the legs are elevated and compressed in leg holders.

Cardiac issues are common in the elderly urological patient. Those with new or unstable exertional angina or dyspnea should be evaluated with stress echocardiography to stratify risk and to optimize management with beta-blockers, nitrates, and/or aspirin preoperatively. Echo or stress testing in compromised patients[68] detects abnormalities in up to 71% and would lead the anesthesiologist to select optimal drug combinations in light of the SVR and PVR effects of PPT and TP. Those with drug-eluting coronary stents may need several days to discontinue thienopyridines[69] and should continue 81 mg aspirin according to a recent ASA practice alert.[70] The thienopyridine should be reinstituted as soon as possible after surgery. Murmurs require echocardiographic diagnosis since valvular dysfunction may profoundly alter hemodynamics under PPT and TP. Modern pacemakers or AICDs are complex and require specific interrogation of the battery, rate-responsive mode functions, and magnet effects.[71] The AICD function must be reactivated postoperatively.

Patients with severe COPD and/or reactive airways, and especially symptomatic obstructive sleep apnea (OSA), must be assessed for risk and counseled for postoperative recovery, CPAP, or ICU ventilation. OSA is predominantly associated with obesity and is caused by a decrease in pharyngeal muscle tone with soft tissue obstruction under sedation or during sleep. The syndrome leads to hypopnea, apnea, hypoxia, and hypercarbia with sympathetic activation, leading to hypertension, tachycardia, cardiac dysrhythmias, and congestive failure[72] Preoperative bronchodilator therapy may be indicated in those with COPD or reactive airways, and incentive spirometry could be helpful in all of these impairments to prevent postoperative atelectasis that might occur with splinting after renal procedures. Bowel preparations include magnesium citrate which will promote loss of intravascular/interstitial volume, causing hypovolemia in addition to NPO status, or previous intravenous dye studies that might further cause an osmotic diuresis.

6.5 Special Anesthesia Concerns

6.5.1 Airway Management

Although several studies describe the use of various laryngeal mask airway devices for spontaneous ventilation during laparoscopic surgery, these have typically been performed in short duration, outpatient surgery and/or cholecystectomy with the patient in r-TP. Endotracheal intubation would be considered standard management for robotic laparoscopic urologic surgery.

6.5.2 Neuromuscular Blockade

The advantage of NMB on respiratory mechanics during PPT is a controversial clinical issue, since investigators have reported using total intravenous anesthesia (TIVA) alone for laparoscopic surgery.[47] Most clinicians assume that deep NMB will soften the abdominal wall and increase intraperitoneal compliance, or increase pulmonary compliance. However, the use of NMB was shown to induce no change in PIP or IAP or ventilatory plateau pressure.[47,73] NMB did not significantly improve the pulmonary mechanics (increased pulmonary and chest wall compliance, or decreased pulmonary resistance) in patients undergoing Lap-C regardless of zero or high (10 cm H_2O) levels of PEEP.[47] Furthermore, the use of 1 MAC isoflurane/fentanyl without *any* NMB provided adequate surgical conditions in two-thirds of patients undergoing open radical prostatectomy.[74] Nevertheless, the use of neuromuscular blockade during robotic surgery would be considered routine.

6.5.3 Anesthetic Maintenance Drugs

Historically, numerous combinations of volatile and intravenous anesthesia have been described for laparoscopic surgery, with general emphasis upon the rate of emergence, the incidence of nausea and vomiting, the hemodynamic profiles, emergence delirium, postoperative pain, and the patient's satisfaction.[75] It is difficult to perceive significant clinical differences in outcome, with the lack of carefully controlled and numerous variables and myriad possibilities of combinations that exist. Choice of anesthetic agents is based upon preference, experience, hemodynamic and side-effect profiles, but specific adjuvants are discussed elsewhere in this chapter. TIVA without volatile agents is both possible and efficacious[75] and includes not only propofol but also midazolam, ketamine, and etomidate administered as infusions. The use of N_2O is controversial since it can diffuse into bowel with solubility much greater than nitrogen and also diffuses into a CPT. During laparoscopy, it cannot be appreciably detected by the surgeon,[76] and there seems to be no conclusive evidence against its use in laparoscopic surgery.[64]

6.5.4 Fluid Management

The perioperative inflammatory response and its effects upon the plasma–interstitial oncotic barrier may well be disrupted by indiscriminate amounts and types of intravenous fluid.[77] Hypervolemia increases perioperative risks of bowel dysfunction, anastomotic leakage, pulmonary edema, wound infection, and cardiovascular complications[78,79] in major abdominal surgery. Documented reductions in UOP with colloid fluid restriction do not cause acute renal failure.[79] Chappell et al.[77] emphasizes the use of crystalloid to replace urine output, actual deficits, and minimal insensible losses only and not presumed NPO deficits or ongoing third-space losses; judicious colloid use is recommended to replace intravascular blood loss (Table 6.3). Hypervolemic crystalloid therapy may worsen a shift (as much as 80%) into the interstitium that otherwise might be limited and caused by the surgical inflammation itself. Furthermore, 60% of colloid may also shift outward if given in excess of normovolemia and may trigger the release of atrial natriuretic peptide, a substance known to injure the endothelial glycocalyx causing a further cascade of immunological injury.[77] Intravenous fluids may need to be increased in TP patients prior to exsufflation and leveling the operating table, as sympathetic tone is removed. A reduction in volatile anesthetic or the elimination of an alpha-1 agonist sympathectomy, for example, may concurrently serve to restore the intravascular volume. Surgeons may request an induced diuresis in particular types of procedures.

6.5.5 Complications

The anesthesia provider may encounter a number of intraoperative complications that may be reduced, attenuated, or eliminated through proper preparation, monitoring, or intervention, and this subject is extensively reviewed by Joshi.[48] These include peripheral nerve injury, gas embolism, subcutaneous emphysema, peripheral and pulmonary edema, hypertension, sudden cardiovascular collapse, pneumothorax, and endobronchial intubation. A host of surgical complications are beyond the scope of this chapter. Subcutaneous emphysema is normally self-limited but may require

Table 6.3 A rational approach to perioperative fluid management

Current physiological insights into fluid management
- Blood volume after fasting is normal
- The extracellular deficit after usual fasting is low
- Insensible fluid loss is negligible
- A primarily fluid-consuming third space does not exist
- Crystalloid overload can induce fluid and protein shifts to the interstitium
- Crystalloids load the interstitial space 4:1
- Colloidal overload deteriorates the vascular barrier
- The endothelial glycocalyx is diminished by hypervolemia

Recommendations for fluid management
- *Optimizing* does not mean *maximizing* blood volume
- Maintain adequate circulation and oxygen delivery to tissues
- Abolish preoperative volume loading in normovolemic patients
- Abolish routine replacement of high insensible and third-space losses
- Replace urine output and insensible (0.5–1.0 mL/kg/h) losses with isotonic crystalloid
- Replace actual blood loss (and protein-rich fluid shifts, if any) with iso-oncotic colloid
- Replace all fluids in a timely, "as-needed" manner
- Use specific goal-directed therapy, not *restrictive* therapy

Chappell[77]

deflation of the abdomen and subsequently lower IAP should the gas traverse into the thorax, mediastinum, and cervical regions.[48] Sudden cardiovascular collapse may occur as the abdomen is inflated, induced by vagal stimulation,[80] but may also be caused by primary dysrhythmia, myocardial infarction, tension pneumothorax, severe respiratory acidosis, cardiac tamponade, anaphylaxis, or gas embolism.[48,81] The embolism of CO_2 gas is physically different from nitrogen, due to its higher solubility and easy elimination through ventilation, but cardiovascular collapse from sudden and massive CO_2 embolism would require similar aggressive intervention,[81] and the end-tidal CO_2 initially increases before decreasing.[48] The embolism typically occurs during the inflation of the abdomen through an open vessel that is subsequently collapsed after insufflation. Oxygen desaturation may be caused by the cephalad migration of the diaphragm causing endobronchial intubation.[49] Peripheral nerve injuries include the peroneal, femoral, and ulnar nerves. The former might be attenuated by carefully positioning the legs in stirrups and avoiding direct pressure on the common peroneal nerve, or avoiding tape compression across the thighs. Ulnar nerve compression is reduced by supination of the arms when tucked along the patient's side.[82] Brachial plexus injuries may be caused by shoulder braces, and these might be avoided by using tape across the torso to secure the patient. Blood loss is consistently minimal (mean 109–191 mL) for RALRP,[83,84] but may be far greater for radical cystectomy and nephrectomy depending upon the degree of anatomic abnormality, disruption by tumor, and/or vascular invasion.

6.6 The Specific Conduct of Anesthesia

6.6.1 Reported Methods

Very few published recommendations exist for the specific anesthesia management of RALUS.[67,85–89] Nishanian[85] recommended additional large-bore IV access; modification of ventilator settings to eliminate carbon dioxide load; consideration of an arterial line; caution using prolonged Trendelenburg in patients with history of stroke or cerebral aneurysm; silicone gel pads; and awake tucking of the arms to ensure comfort. Costello and Webb[87] described their management of 40 patients for RALRP: the use of fractionated heparin (enoxaparin) administered the evening before, and the evening of the surgery; thromboembolic deterrent (TED) stockings; large-bore intravenous access without CVP; intra-arterial cannulation of the radial artery; padding hands and arms; pulse oximeter probe on the earlobe; general anesthesia with midazolam/propofol induction, remifentanil/sevoflurane maintenance, and intravenous morphine for postoperative analgesia; subsequent lumbar epidural analgesia with oral clonidine to augment analgesia to provide better hemodynamic stability, to modulate the acute tolerance effects of remifentanil, and to lower intraocular pressure; dosing of the epidural at the end of the case with only local anesthesia, followed by catheter removal; a minimum 2 L of crystalloid and 1 L of colloid; and caution with the use of NSAIDs. Conacher et al.[67] minimize IAP to reduce its effect upon renal blood flow, GFR, and urine output, and used mannitol and/or furosemide to lower ICP and IOP or to induce diuresis

to flush the kidney in certain pyeloplasty procedures; concomitantly they routinely volume pre-loaded their patients to counteract the immediate effects of IAP but reduced fluid administration for those patients placed in TP; NSAID's were avoided in patients with borderline renal function; maintenance anesthesia included remifentanil and they placed central venous pressure lines but minimized radial pressure lines; analgesics included low-dose ketorolac and diamorphine, narcotics and only occasional PCA morphine, since it increased postoperative ileus (POI), nausea, and time to discharge; epidural analgesic techniques were discounted as unnecessary, except perhaps for cystectomy and ileal conduit, where the sympathetic blockade was observed to increase bowel activity thereby easing surgical manipulation and reducing POI. Phong and Koh[86] described post-extubation respiratory distress secondary to laryngeal edema from prolonged TP and IAP, in association with high ETT cuff pressure. They recommended the cuff leak test as a pre-extubation indicator of edema. They also described transient C5/6 brachial plexus neuropraxia with weakness only, ascribed to pressure from the shoulder brace. Gerges et al.[90] described the pharmacology of their anesthetics with multimodal techniques, incorporating oral and/or intravenous NSAIDS, acetaminophen, N-methyl-D-aspartate antagonists (ketamine), and alpha-2 agonists (clonidine and dexmedetomidine), added to short-acting volatile agents (sevoflurane and desflurane) and short-acting narcotics (remifentanil), or weak narcotics such as tramadol, to facilitate rapid emergence from anesthesia.

6.6.2 Local Anesthetics

Pain related to robotic-assisted laparoscopic urologic surgery may be visceral or somatic, secondary to the organ dissection, the trocar insertion sites, diaphragm stretch from PPT, and/or insufflant and residual insufflant chemical irritation.[46] Pre- or post-incisional injection of local anesthesia (LA) into the portal sites will reduce the incidence of postoperative pain, but a review of 24 studies of intraperitoneal local anesthesia showed only a mild indication of benefit when using 20 mL of 0.25 or 0.75% ropivacaine, each given twice during surgery.[91]

6.6.3 Neuraxial Blockade

6.6.3.1 Epidural Supplementation

Epidural analgesia with LA (LA-EA) provides superior postoperative analgesia compared to systemic opioids, particularly with patient ambulation.[92] IV-PCA was shown to have the highest risk of nausea and sedation, while EA had the highest risk of pruritus, urinary retention, and motor block. However, motor block and nausea were reduced with patient control of the epidural analgesia (PCEA). Specifically, thoracic epidural analgesia (TEA) is considered to be the most effective neuraxial technique for improving outcomes in pain, POI, stress response, catabolism, hypercoagulability, immune suppression, and cardiopulmonary complications.[92–94] Advantages over opioid PCA[94] are listed in Table 6.4. TEA (as opposed to LEA) also eliminates motor blockade, decreases dose requirements, improves sympathectomy of the bowel (reducing POI), and causes less urinary retention.[95] This elimination of narcotic side effects and early patient rehabilitation may be more significant than its analgesic effects.[94] Multimodal analgesia reduces POI,[96] and a Cochrane review demonstrated that TEA with LA alone shortens POI from 37 to 24 h compared to the use of IV or neuraxial narcotic agents.[97] Hypotension associated with TEA can be reversed by assuring normovolemia, reducing the basal infusion rate, temporarily suspending the

infusion, preventing excessive blockade, reducing the LA concentration, and by limiting parenteral narcotics. The duration of admission for RALUS may be the determining factor for consideration of LA-EA benefits.

Neuraxial analgesia may have beneficial effects on ventilation and lung compliance. During RALRP, in combination with GA,[98] TEA caused significantly lower peak inspiratory pressures and higher dynamic compliance with larger expiratory tidal volumes during surgery.

6.6.3.2 Neuraxial Alone

Although neuraxial anesthesia alone for laparoscopic procedures has been reported, there are no reports of such methods for robotic surgery, and such would not seem practical or safe in the event of patient movement or restlessness.

6.6.3.3 Subarachnoid Supplementation

Our practice has considered the use of adjunctive SAB in combination with GA, for the conduct of RALUS. In particular, we have utilized SAB (instead of TEA) out of convenience, expedition of care, and presumed benefits that would be analogous to TEA. Prolonged pre- and postoperative neuraxial blockade with CSE would presumably be more efficacious and more practical in

Table 6.4 Advantages (+) and disadvantages (−) of epidural analgesia vs. opioid patient-controlled analgesia

	Epidural analgesia (local anesthetic)	Opioid patient-controlled analgesia
Pain control		
At rest	+++	++
On mobilization	++	±
Side effects		
Hypotension	−	+
Postoperative ileus	++	−−
Nausea–vomiting	+	−−
Urinary retention	−−	−
Sedation	+	−
Reduction in postoperative morbidity		
Cardiovascular	+	−
Respiratory	+	−
Nurses' workload	+	+

Modified from Bonnet and Marret[94]

robotic cystectomy and nephrectomy than with robotic prostatectomy. The SAB is established prior to general anesthesia, for the primary purpose of providing a sympathectomy to overcome the physiological effects of relative hypervolemia and elevated SVR while in TP (specifically) with PPT. A secondary purpose is to provide a multimodal, narcotic-sparing anesthetic to reduce POI. We have also utilized this practice routinely in gynecologic RALS, with the intent of maintaining intestinal motility during the surgery, which the surgeon perceives as being helpful for laparoscopic visualization. Isobaric tetracaine with intrathecal fentanyl is typically used for the gynecologic patients, but we have used hyperbaric bupivacaine/epi without narcotics in the shortest (RALRP) cases, administered in the sitting position. Although we do not currently have data to defend these approaches, the literature supports the anti-inflammatory effects and metabolic stress reduction of neuraxial blockade, as a means to improve surgical recovery.[99] An outcome study in RALUS patients ought to test the effectiveness of multimodal, narcotic-sparing anesthesia with or without supplemental neuraxial blockade on bowel function and quality of recovery. Some report, however, that EA does not eliminate the shoulder pain from diaphragmatic irritation.[90]

6.6.3.4 Extended Release Epidural Morphine (EREM)

EREM is a significant alternative to TEA and is used at this institution[100] for orthopedic and gynecological patients admitted for at least 48 h postoperatively. The drug DepoDur® (Endo Pharmaceuticals) is administered as a single dose to the epidural space, with or without a single-dose SAB. EREM is released over 48 h and avoids the inconvenience and risk of epidural catheters, anticoagulation, and postoperative infusions; it provides excellent analgesia with visual analog scale (VAS) pain scores typically <2, using low-dose supplemental analgesics.[100] Our researchers believe that smaller doses (4–7.5 mg) are equally effective as the FDA-allowable 15 mg dosage and have a lower side-effect profile attenuated by stool softeners and nalbuphine. Such techniques are directly applicable to major RALUS procedures. Concerns over respiratory monitoring for EREM replace the concerns over hypotension and infusion management with narcotic-sparing LA-EA.

6.6.4 Pharmacologic Multimodal Analgesia

Pharmacologic multimodal analgesia (PMMA) has been evaluated as a discreet concept for greater than 16 years, and it serves to minimize the use of narcotic analgesics to avoid their complications of sedation, respiratory depression, nausea, vomiting, pruritus, POI, and urinary retention. PMMA refers to the adjunctive and continuous perioperative use of NSAIDS (e.g., ketorolac, ibuprofen, naproxen, diclofenac), selective cyclooxygenase-2 (COX-2) inhibitors (e.g., celecoxib, valdecoxib), and dexamethasone, ketamine, tramadol, dexmedetomidine, clonidine, acetaminophen, gabapentin, and pregabalin in various combinations. Neuraxial and local analgesia is also part of the PMMA concept but is separately considered above. The benefits of PMMA (only 30% reduction in postoperative narcotic requirement) are challenging to ascertain given various types of surgery and potentially adverse effects on coagulation, renal function, stroke, or coronary events.[101,102] However, White et al.[95] emphasize that most PMMA studies have compared only a single adjuvant in combination with morphine, and they found little to no data justifying specific treatments of post-RALUS pain.

Following a meta-analysis of NSAIDs, COX-2 inhibitors, and acetaminophen, Elia[102] determined that only NSAIDs resulted in a significantly combined reduction in pain scores, nausea/vomiting, and sedation. He also determined an association with new renal impairment in 1.7% of those on COX-2 inhibitors and an increase in surgical bleeding from 0.2 to 1.7% in those taking NSAIDs. Others have shown no significant increase in renal impairment from COX-2 inhibitors or NSAIDS.[103]

Ketamine (NMDA receptor antagonist) has shown similar reductions in morphine requirement but no reduction in the incidence of nausea and vomiting and questionably improved functional outcome.[92,104] Gabapentin showed no clinically significant reduction in pain score or PONV, and it increased the risk of sedation.[105] Liu[92] confirmed that only NSAIDs and ketamine demonstrated statistically significant reductions in pain scores, while only NSAIDs reduced the risk of opioid-related side effects (nausea, vomiting, and sedation). Future outcome research must focus on patient satisfaction, with pain being only one part of that outcome.

Acetazolamide has been shown to reduce the postoperative referred pain of laparoscopy secondary to the presumed actions of carbon dioxide in the acidification of the peritoneum.[106] Dexmedetomidine, like clonidine, is a specific alpha-2 adrenergic agonist that inhibits sympathetic activity and provides antinociceptive and sedative activity in animals[29] In humans, it is administered IV for sedation but may not alone provide significant amounts of analgesia without heavy sedative or even general anesthetic effects, and it is more effective for pain when given neuraxially. We use low-dose dexmedetomidine to attenuate the sympathetic response to PPT and TP in RALRP, but the cardiovascular and sympathetic effects of the drug are complicated and cause bradycardia or even cardiac arrest when other vagotonic drugs are administered.[107,108]

6.6.5 Promotility and Antiemesis

POI may be attributed to anastomotic leakage or pelvic hematoma, both of which may present with severe postoperative pain.[83] POI is recently reviewed by Gannon[96]: (1) metoclopramide has no advantage for motility, since it has no effect upon the colon and may cause sedation; (2) propranolol may help through inhibition of catecholamines; (3) neostigmine, despite its muscarinic effects, is ineffective; (4) NSAIDs and narcotic-sparing techniques are advantageous; (5) methylnaltrexone and alvimopan may be effective; and (6) lidocaine by infusion is recently advocated in laparoscopic colectomy. Effective antiemetic routines have been extensively reviewed,[109] but the incidence remains high at up to 30%.

6.6.6 Author's Preferences for Anesthetic Management

A second IV is typically placed in the external jugular to provide access, blood sampling, and avoidance of unrecognized infiltration of the arm. We do not routinely place intra-arterial catheters, except for longer duration radical cystectomy in which there is no intraoperative access to the radial artery. Hydrostatic issues for ICP and IOP are worrisome, but we do not administer mannitol or furosemide, and recent evidence suggests that cerebral perfusion pressure increases more than ICP in the TP.[19] We secure the patient with 3-in. tape over thin foam padding in a cross pattern over the chest and shoulders such that cephalad sliding of the patient is prevented by frictional posterior forces across the body and not by inferior axial resistance against the superior aspect of the shoulders. The arms are padded and tucked with the palms against the thigh, and thumbs anterior, to minimize pressure on the ulnar groove. We routinely use IPSC devices, as the evidence for improved physiology and circulation seems convincing. The depth of the ETT relative to the carina is determined during intubation to avoid endobronchial intubation and to avoid the opposite risk of herniation of the ETT cuff above the glottis if placed too shallowly. Our group has recently combined single-dose tetracaine spinal anesthesia with general anesthesia in a variety of RALUS procedures. We do this instead of TEA for simplicity and for the cardiovascular advantages of induced sympathectomy. Reduction of perioperative opioids is an added advantage, with reduced requirements for intraoperative volatile anesthesia, titrated through bispectral analysis. Patient comfort and wellness using supplemental neuraxial analgesia have not yet been measured in our practice. General anesthetic agents include isoflurane without N_2O or remifentanil. We desire low intraoperative fluid administration (<1,000 mL crystalloid) during PPT in TP for RALRP (without neuraxial blockade), recognizing the expected decline in UOP until the abdomen is deflated and table leveled, at which time an additional fluid bolus of approximately 1 L is administered. We have selectively used multimodal adjuncts and eliminated all narcotics in some cases, using acetaminophen or celecoxib premedicants, with intravenous dexmedetomidine, ketorolac, ketamine, and dexamethasone, but have not scientifically evaluated our outcomes. Hemodynamic stability is achieved with the alpha-2 agonists or subarachnoid block; alternatively hydralazine is selected for attenuation of the high SVR. Patients are routinely extubated at the conclusion of RALRP and nephrectomy but may require a period of postoperative intubation for laryngeal edema after prolonged cystectomy in TP.

References

1. Wu HL, Chan KH, Tsou MY, et al. Severe carbon dioxide retention during second laparoscopic surgery for urgent repair of an operative defect from the preceding laparoscopic surgery. *Acta Anaesthesiol Taiwan*. 2008;46:124–128.

2. Menes T, Spivak H. Laparoscopy: searching for the proper insufflation gas. *Surg Endosc*. 2000;14:1050–1056.

3. Henny CP, Hofland J. Laparoscopic surgery: pitfalls due to anesthesia, positioning, and pneumoperitoneum. *Surg Endosc*. 2005;19:1163–1171.

4. Mullett CE, Viale JP, Sagnard PE, et al. Pulmonary CO_2 elimination during surgical procedures using intra- or extraperitoneal CO_2 insufflation. *Anesth Analg*. 1993;76:622–626.

5. Streich B, Decailliot F, Perney C, et al. Increased carbon dioxide absorption during retroperitoneal laparoscopy. *Br J Anaesth*. 2003;91:793–796.

6. Minoli G, Terruzzi V, Spinzi GC, et al. The influence of carbon dioxide and nitrous oxide on pain during laparoscopy: a double-blind, controlled trial. *Gastrointest Endosc*. 1982;28:173–175.

7. Halverson A, Buchanan R, Jacobs L, et al. . Evaluation of mechanism of increased intracranial pressure with insufflation. *Surg Endosc*. 1998;12:266–269.

8. Bäcklund M, Kellokumpu I, Scheinin T, et al. Effect of temperature of insufflated CO_2 during and after prolonged laparoscopic surgery. *Surg Endosc*. 1998;12:1126–1130.

9. Makarov DV, Kainth D, Link RE, et al. Physiologic changes during helium insufflation in high-risk patients during laparoscopic renal procedures. *Urology*. 2007;70:35–37.

10. Schöb OM, Allen DC, Benzel E, et al. A comparison of the pathophysiologic effects of carbon dioxide, nitrous oxide, and helium pneumoperitoneum on intracranial pressure. *Am J Surg*. 1996;172:248–253.

11. Yau P, Watson DI, Lafullarde T, et al. Experimental study of effect of embolism of different laparoscopy insufflation gases. *J Laparoendosc Adv Surg Tech A*. 2000;10:211–216.

12. Catheline JM, Bihan H, Le Quang T, et al. Preoperative cardiac and pulmonary assessment in bariatric surgery. *Obes Surg*. 2008;18:271–277.

13. Gurusamy KS, Samraj K, Davidson BR. Abdominal lift for laparoscopic cholecystectomy. *Cochrane Database Syst Rev*. 2008;2:CD006574.

14. Neudecker J, Sauerland S, Neugebauer E, et al. The European Association for Endoscopic Surgery clinical practice guideline on the pneumoperitoneum for laparoscopic surgery. *Surg Endosc*. 2002;16:1121–1143.

15. Rosenthal RJ, Friedman RL, Chidambaram A, et al. Effects of hyperventilation and hypoventilation on $PaCO_2$ and intracranial pressure during acute elevations of intraabdominal pressure with CO_2 pneumoperitoneum: large animal observations. *J Am Coll Surg*. 1998;187:32–38.

16. Halverson AL, Barrett WL, Iglesias AR, et al. Decreased cerebrospinal fluid absorption during abdominal insufflation. *Surg Endosc*. 1999;13:797–80019.

17. Cooke SJ, Paterson-Brown S. Association between laparoscopic abdominal surgery and postoperative symptoms of raised intracranial pressure. *Surg Endosc*. 2001;15:723–725.

18. Lee JR, Lee PB, Do SH, et al. The effect of gynaecological laparoscopic surgery on cerebral oxygenation. *J Int Med Res*. 2006;34:531–536.

19. Kalmar AF, et al. Influence of steep Trendelenburg position and CO_2 pneumoperitoneum on cardiovascular, cerebrovascular, and respiratory homeostasis during robotic prostatectomy. *BJA*. 2010;104:433–439.

20. Park EY, et al. The effect of pneumoperitoneum in the steep Trendelenburg position on cerebral oxygenation. *Acta Anaesthesiol Scand*. 2009;53:895–899.

21. Mowafi HA, Al-Ghamdi A, Rushood A. Intraocular pressure changes during laparoscopy in patients anesthetized with propofol total intravenous anesthesia versus isoflurane inhaled anesthesia. *Anesth Analg*. 2003;97:471–474.

22. Weber ED, et al. Posterior ischemic optic neuropathy after minimally invasive prostatectomy. *J Neuro-ophthalmol*. 2007;27:285–287.

23. Awad H, et al. The effects of steep Trendelenburg positioning on intraocular pressure during robotic radical prostatectomy. *Anesth Analg*. 2009;109:473–478.

24. Odeberg S, Ljungqvist O, Svenberg T, et al. Haemodynamic effects of pneumoperitoneum and the influence of posture during anaesthesia for laparoscopic surgery. *Acta Anaesthesiol Scand*. 1994;38:276–283.

25. Gannedahl P, Odeberg S, Brodin LA, et al. Effects of posture and pneumoperitoneum during anaesthesia on the indices of left ventricular filling. *Acta Anaesthesiol Scand*. 1996;40:160–166.

26. Fahy BG, Hasnain JU, Flowers JL, et al. Transesophageal echocardiographic detection of gas embolism and cardiac valvular dysfunction during laparoscopic nephrectomy. *Anesth Analg*. 1999;88:500–504.

27. Cunningham AJ, Turner J, Rosenbaum S, et al. Transoesophageal echocardiographic assessment of haemodynamic function during laparoscopic cholecystectomy. *Br J Anaesth*. 1993;70:621–625.

28. Dorsay DA, Greene FL, Baysinger CL. Hemodynamic changes during laparoscopic cholecystectomy monitored with transesophageal echocardiography. *Surg Endosc*. 1995;9:128–134.

29. Joris JL, Chiche JD, Canivet JL, et al. Hemodynamic changes induced by laparoscopy and their endocrine correlates: effects of clonidine. *J Am Coll Cardiol*. 1998;32:1389–1396.

30. Hirvonen EA, Nuutinen LS, Kauko M. Hemodynamic changes due to Trendelenburg positioning and pneumoperitoneum during laparoscopic hysterectomy. *Acta Anaesthesiol Scand*. 1995;39:949–955.

31. Falabella A, Moore-Jeffries E, Sullivan MJ, et al. Cardiac function during steep Trendelenburg position and CO_2 pneumoperitoneum for robotic-assisted prostatectomy: a trans-oesophageal Doppler probe study. *Int J Med Robot*. 2007;3:312–315.

32. Meininger D, Westphal K, Bremerich DH, et al. Effects of posture and prolonged pneumoperitoneum on hemodynamic parameters during laparoscopy. *World J Surg*. 2008;32:1400–1405.

33. Harris SN, Ballantyne GH, Luther MA, et al. Alterations of cardiovascular performance during laparoscopic colectomy: a combined hemodynamic and echocardiographic analysis. *Anesth Analg.* 1996;83:482–487.

34. Zollinger A, Krayer S, Singer T, et al. Haemodynamic effects of pneumoperitoneum in elderly patients with an increased cardiac risk. *Eur J Anaesthesiol.* 1997;14: 266–275.

35. Popescu WM, Perrino AC Jr.. Critical cardiac decompensation during laparoscopic surgery. *J Am Soc Echocardiogr.* 2006;19(1074):e.

36. Alfonsi P, Vieillard-Baron A, Coggia M, et al. Cardiac function during intraperitoneal CO_2 insufflation for aortic surgery: a transesophageal echocardiographic study. *Anesth Analg.* 2006;102:1304 1310.

37. Safran D, Sgambati S, Orlando R III. Laparoscopy in high-risk cardiac patients. *Surg Gynecol Obstet.* 1993;176:548–554.

38. Koivusalo AM, Pere P, Valjus M, et al. Laparoscopic cholecystectomy with carbon dioxide pneumoperitoneum is safe even for high-risk patients. *Surg Endosc.* 2008;22:61–67.

39. O'Malley C, Cunningham AJ. Physiologic changes during laparoscopy. *Anesthesiol Clin N Am.* 2001;19:1–19.

40. Russo A, et al. Diastolic function: the influence of pneumoperitoneum and Trendelenburg positioning during laparoscopic hysterectomy. *Euro J Anaesthesiol.* 2009;26:923–927.

41. Balick-Weber CC, Nicolas P, Hedreville-Montout M, et al. Respiratory and haemodynamic effects of volume-controlled vs pressure-controlled ventilation during laparoscopy: a cross-over study with echocardiographic assessment. *Br J Anaesth.* 2007;99:429–435.

42. Joris JL, Noirot DP, Legrand MJ, et al. Hemodynamic changes during laparoscopic cholecystectomy. *Anesth Analg.* 1993;76:1067–1071.

43. Aho M, Scheinin M, Lehtinen AM, et al. Intramuscularly administered dexmedetomidine attenuates hemodynamic and stress hormone responses to gynecologic laparoscopy. *Anesth Analg.* 1992;75:932–939.

44. Lloréns J, Ballester M, Tusman G, et al. Adaptive support ventilation for gynaecological laparoscopic surgery in Trendelenburg position: bringing ICU modes of mechanical ventilation to the operating room. *Eur J Anaesthesiol.* 2009;26:135–139.

45. Andersson LE, Bååth M, Thörne A, et al. Effect of carbon dioxide pneumoperitoneum on development of atelectasis during anesthesia, examined by spiral computed tomography. *Anesthesiology.* 2005;102:293–299.

46. Joris JL. Anesthesia for laparoscopic surgery. In: Miller RD, ed. *Miller's Anesthesia.* 6th ed. Philadelphia, PA: Elsevier; 2005.

47. Maracajá-Neto LF, Verçosa N, Roncally AC, et al. Beneficial effects of high positive end-expiratory pressure in lung respiratory mechanics during laparoscopic surgery. *Acta Anaesthesiol Scand.* 2009;53:210–217.

48. Joshi GP. Complications of laparoscopy. *Anesthesiol Clin N Am.* 2001;19:89–105.

49. Lobato EB, Paige GB, Brown MM. Pneumoperitoneum as a risk factor for endobronchial intubation during laparoscopic gynecologic surgery. *Anesth Analg.* 1998;86: 301–303.

50. Andersson L, Lagerstrand L, Thörne A, et al. Effect of CO_2 pneumoperitoneum on ventilation-perfusion relationships during laparoscopic cholecystectomy. *Acta Anaesthesiol Scand.* 2002;46:552–560.

51. GüleçB, Oner K, Yigitler C, et al. Lower extremity venous changes in pneumoperitoneum during laparoscopic surgery. *ANZ J Surg.* 2006;76:904–906.

52. Glantzounis GK, Tsimaris I, Tselepis AD, et al. Alterations in plasma oxidative stress markers after laparoscopic operations of the upper and lower abdomen. *Angiology.* 2005;56:459–465.

53. Hsieh SW, Lan KM, Luk HN, et al. Massive pulmonary embolism presented as sudden cardiac arrest in the immediate postoperative period after laparoscopic hysterectomy. *J Clin Anesth.* 2003;15:545–548.

54. Bickel A, Drobot A, Aviram M, et al. Validation and reduction of the oxidative stress following laparoscopic operations: a prospective randomized controlled study. *Ann Surg.* 2007;246:31–35.

55. Bickel A, Arzomanov T, Ivry S, et al. Reversal of adverse hemodynamic effects of pneumoperitoneum by pressure equilibration. *Arch Surg.* 2004;139:1320–1325.

56. Lord RV, Ling JJ, Hugh TB, et al. . Incidence of deep vein thrombosis after laparoscopic vs minilaparotomy cholecystectomy. *Arch Surg.* 1998;133:967–973.

57. Galyon SW, Richards KA, Pettus JA, et al. Three limb compartment syndrome and rhabdomyolysis after robotic cystoprostatectomy. *J Clin Anesth.* 2009. In Press.

58. Basic Anesthetic Monitoring, Standards for (2010). Available at: http://www.asahq.org/For-Healthcare-Professionals/Standards-Guidelines-and-Statements.aspx. Accessed November 29, 2010.

59. Murphy GS, Szokol JW, Marymont JH. Residual neuromuscular blockade and critical respiratory events in the postanesthesia care unit. *Anesth Analg.* 2008;107: 130–137.

60. Cullen DJ, Kirby RR. Beach chair position may decrease cerebral perfusion: catastrophic outcomes have occurred. *APSF Newslett.* 2007;22(25):27.

61. Lanier WL. Cerebral perfusion: err on the side of caution. *APSF Newslett.* 2009;24(1):3–4.

62. Ludbrook G, Sutherland P. Erroneous pulse oximetry readings during robotic prostatectomy. *Anaesth Intensive Care.* 2007;35:144–145.

63. Casati A, Squicciarini G, Baciarello M, et al. Forehead reflectance oximetry: a clinical comparison with conventional digit sensors during laparotomic and laparoscopic abdominal surgery. *J Clin Monit Comput.* 2007;21: 271–276.

64. Cunningham AJ, Brull SJ. Laparoscopic cholecystectomy: anesthetic implications. *Anesth Analg.* 1993;76:1120–1133.

65. Moitra V, Diaz G, Sladen RN. Monitoring hepatic and renal function. *Anesthesiol Clin.* 2006;24:857–880.

66. Demyttenaere S, Feldman LS, Fried GM. Effect of pneumoperitoneum on renal perfusion and function: a systematic review. *Surg Endosc.* 2007;21:152–160.

67. Conacher ID, Soomro NA, Rix D. Anaesthesia for laparoscopic urological surgery. *Br J Anaesth.* 2004;93: 859–864.

68. American Society of Anesthesiologists Task Force on Preanesthesia Evaluation . Practice advisory for

preanesthesia evaluation: a report by the American Society of Anesthesiologists Task Force on Preanesthesia Evaluation. *Anesthesiology*. 2002;96:485–496.

69. Eisenberg MJ, Richard PR, Libersan D, et al. Safety of short-term discontinuation of antiplatelet therapy in patients with drug-eluting stents. *Circulation*. 2009;119:1634–1642.

70. American Society of Anesthesiologists Committee on Standards and Practice Parameters. Practice alert for the perioperative management of patients with coronary artery stents: a report by the American Society of Anesthesiologists Committee on Standards and Practice Parameters. *Anesthesiology*. 2009;110:22–23.

71. American Society of Anesthesiologists Task Force on Perioperative Management of Patients with Cardiac Rhythm Management Devices. Practice advisory for the perioperative management of patients with cardiac rhythm management devices: pacemakers and implantable cardioverter-defibrillators: a report by the American Society of Anesthesiologists Task Force on Perioperative Management of Patients with Cardiac Rhythm Management Devices. *Anesthesiology*. 2005;103:186–198.

72. Joshi GP. Are patients with obstructive sleep apnea syndrome suitable for ambulatory surgery? *ASA Newslett*. 2006;70:17–19.

73. Chassard D, Berrada K, Tournadre J, et al. The effects of neuromuscular block on peak airway pressure and abdominal elastance during pneumoperitoneum. *Anesth Analg*. 1996;82:525–527.

74. King M, Sujirattanawimol N, Danielson DR, et al. Requirements for muscle relaxants during radical retropubic prostatectomy. *Anesthesiology*. 2000;93:1392–1397.

75. Oikkonen M. Propofol vs isoflurane for gynaecological laparoscopy. *Acta Anaesthesiol Scand*. 1994;38:110–114.

76. Taylor E, Feinstein R, White PF, et al. Anesthesia for laparoscopic cholecystectomy. Is nitrous oxide contraindicated? *Anesthesiology*. 1992;76:541–543.

77. Chappell D, Jacob M, Hofmann-Kiefer K, et al. A rational approach to perioperative fluid management. *Anesthesiology*. 2008;109:723–740.

78. Nisanevich V, Felsenstein I, Almogy G, et al. Effect of intraoperative fluid management on outcome after intraabdominal surgery. *Anesthesiology*. 2005;103:25–32.

79. Brandstrup B, Tønnesen H, Beier-Holgersen R. Effects of intravenous fluid restriction on postoperative complications: comparison of two perioperative fluid regimens: a randomized assessor-blinded multicenter trial. *Ann Surg*. 2003;238:641–648.

80. Shifren JL, Adlestein L, Finkler NJ. Asystolic cardiac arrest: a rare complication of laparoscopy. *Obstet Gynecol*. 1992;79:840–841.

81. Brantley JCIII, Riley PM. Cardiovascular collapse during laparoscopy: a report of two cases. *Am J Obstet Gynecol*. 1988;159:735–747.

82. Prielipp RC, Morell RC, Walker FO, et al. Ulnar nerve pressure: influence of arm position and relationship to somatosensory evoked potentials. *Anesthesiology*. 1999;91:345–354.

83. Bhandari A, McIntire L, Kaul SA, et al. Perioperative complications of robotic radical prostatectomy after the learning curve. *J Urol*. 2005;174:915–918.

84. Farnham SB, Webster TM, Herrell SD, et al. Intraoperative blood loss and transfusion requirements for robotic-assisted radical prostatectomy versus radical retropubic prostatectomy. *Urology*. 2006;67:360–363.

85. Nishanian EV. Anesthesia for robotic surgery. In: Miller RD, ed. *Miller's Anesthesia*. 6th ed. Philadelphia, PA: Elsevier; 2005.

86. Phong SV, Koh LK. Anaesthesia for robotic-assisted radical prostatectomy: considerations for laparoscopy in the Trendelenburg position. *Anaesth Intensive Care*. 2007;35:281–285.

87. Costello TG, Webb P. Anaesthesia for robot-assisted anatomic prostatectomy. Experience at a single institution. *Anaesth Intensive Care*. 2006;34:787–792.

88. Malhotra V, Sudheendra V, Diwan S. Anesthesia and the renal and genitourinary system. In: Miller RD, ed. *Miller's Anesthesia*. 6th ed. Philadelphia, PA: Elsevier; 2005.

89. Danic MJ, Chow M, Alexander G, et al. Anesthesia considerations for robotic-assisted laparoscopic prostatectomy: a review of 1,500 cases. *J Robotic Surg*. 2007;1:119–123.

90. Gerges FJ, Kanazi GE, Jabbour-Khoury SI. Anesthesia for laparoscopy: a review. *J Clin Anesth*. 2006;18:67–78.

91. Labaille T, Mazoit JX, Paqueron X, et al. The clinical efficacy and pharmacokinetics of intraperitoneal ropivacaine for laparoscopic cholecystectomy. *Anesth Analg*. 2002;94:100–105.

92. Liu SS, Wu CL. The effect of analgesic technique on postoperative patient-reported outcomes including analgesia: a systematic review. *Anesth Analg*. 2007;105:789–808.

93. Block BM, Liu SS, Rowlingson AJ, et al. Efficacy of postoperative epidural analgesia: a meta-analysis. *JAMA*. 2003;290:2455–2463.

94. Bonnet F, Marret E. Influence of anaesthetic and analgesic techniques on outcome after surgery. *Br J Anaesth*. 2005;95:52–58.

95. White PF, Kehlet H, Neal JM. The role of the anesthesiologist in fast-track surgery: from multimodal analgesia to perioperative medical care. *Anesth Analg*. 2007;104:1380–1396.

96. Gannon RH. Current strategies for preventing or ameliorating postoperative ileus: a multimodal approach. *Am J Health Syst Pharm*. 2007;64(20 Suppl 13):S8–S12.

97. Jørgensen H, Wetterslev J, Møiniche S, et al. Epidural local anaesthetics versus opioid-based analgesic regimens on postoperative gastrointestinal paralysis, PONV and pain after abdominal surgery. *Cochrane Database Syst Rev*. 2000;4:CD001893.

98. Hong JY, Lee SJ, Rha KH, et al. Effects of thoracic epidural analgesia combined with general anesthesia on intraoperative ventilation/oxygenation and postoperative pulmonary complications in robot-assisted laparoscopic radical prostatectomy. *J Endourol*. 2009;23:1843–1849.

99. Holte K, Kehlet H. Epidural anaesthesia and analgesia – effects on surgical stress responses and implications for postoperative nutrition. *Clin Nutr*. 2002;21:199–206.

100. Nagle PC, Gernacher JC. Depodur® (extended release epidural morphine): A review of an old drug in a new vehicle. *Tech Reg Anesth*. 2007;11:9–18.

101. Kehlet H. Postoperative opioid sparing to hasten recovery: what are the issues? *Anesthesiology*. 2005;102: 1083–1085.

102. Elia N, Lysakowski C, Tramèr MR. Does multimodal analgesia with acetaminophen, nonsteroidal antiinflammatory drugs, or selective cyclooxygenase-2 inhibitors and patient-controlled analgesia morphine offer advantages over morphine alone? Meta-analyses of randomized trials. *Anesthesiology*. 2005;103:1296–1304.

103. Nussmeier NA, Whelton AA, Brown MT, et al. Complications of the COX-2 inhibitors parecoxib and valdecoxib after cardiac surgery. *N Engl J Med*. 2005;352:1081–1091.

104. Himmelseher S, Durieux ME. Ketamine for perioperative pain management. *Anesthesiology*. 2005;102:211–220.

105. Hurley RW, Cohen SP, Williams KA, et al. The analgesic effects of perioperative gabapentin on postoperative pain: a meta-analysis. *Reg Anesth Pain Med*. 2006;31: 237–247.

106. Woehlck HJ, Otterson M, Yun H, et al. Acetazolamide reduces referred postoperative pain after laparoscopic surgery with carbon dioxide insufflation. *Anesthesiology*. 2003;99:924–928.

107. Ingersoll-Weng E, Manecke GR Jr, Thistlethwaite PA. Dexmedetomidine and cardiac arrest. *Anesthesiology*. 2004;100:738–739.

108. Ebert TJ, Hall JE, Barney JA, et al. The effects of increasing plasma concentrations of dexmedetomidine in humans. *Anesthesiology*. 2000;93: 382–394.

109. Wilhelm SM, Dehoorne-Smith ML, Kale-Pradhan PB. Prevention of postoperative nausea and vomiting. *Ann Pharmacother*. 2007;41:68–78.

Chapter 7

The Development of a Robotic Urology Program in the UK

Harveer S. Dev, Nimish C. Shah, and David E. Neal

Abbreviations

LRP	Laparoscopic-assisted radical prostatectomy
NHS	National Health Service
NICE	National Institute for Clinical Excellence
OR	Operating room
PA	Patient-side assistant
QUALY	Quality-adjusted life years
RALP	Robotically assisted laparoscopic prostatectomy
RP	Radical prostatectomy
SCP	Surgical care practitioner
UK	United Kingdom
USA	Unites States of America
VUI	Vattikuti Urology Institute

7.1 History of Robotic Urology in the UK

The first recorded radical prostatectomy (RP) was performed in 1901, by the Frenchman Robert Proust.[1] In the early part of the twentieth century, surgeons reported mortality rates as high as 30%, and it took almost a century of developments from both sides of the Atlantic to significantly improve the morbidity and mortality associated with RP. The first use of minimally invasive surgery in urology came in 1991 when Schuessler and colleagues[2] performed the first

D.E. Neal (✉)
Department of Oncology, University of Cambridge,
Addenbrookes Hospital, Cambridge, UK
e-mail: den22@medschl.cam.ac.uk

laparoscopic RP (LRP); this procedure has also seen technical modifications in an effort to improve surgical outcomes. However, the technically demanding nature of laparoscopic surgery has meant that like the rest of the world, LRP has not gained popularity in the UK. The steep, and long, learning curve can be attributed to the fulcrum effect of the laparoscopic arms at the points of insertion, counter-intuitive movements of the instruments, a two-dimensional imaging system, and only four degrees of freedom at the instrument tips.

The introduction of robotics into urology began in 1989 when John Wickham (UK) described the use of a robotic system to assist in the transurethral resection of the prostate.[3] Around the same time, the National Aeronautics and Space Agency (NASA) began working with other American institutions on the concept of telepresent (i.e. remote) surgery. Although originally intended for use in war zones, the commercial potential of these prototypes was identified in the mid-1990s, leading to the development of minimally invasive master–slave robotic surgical systems. The most advanced of these in current clinical use is the da Vinci® series (Intuitive Surgical, Inc., Sunnyvale, CA, USA). The UK's early contributions to the development of robotic urology were to be its last, as these later innovations came entirely from the USA and mainland Europe. This hiatus may be attributed to the difficulties of funding such expensive programs within the UK's free National Health Service (see Section 7.4).

Frankfurt in Germany was home to the world's first robotically assisted laparoscopic prostatectomy (RALP) in May 2000, and the first case in the UK was performed at St Mary's Hospital, London, in August 2001.[4] The first structured robotic urology program

A.K. Hemal, M. Menon (eds.), *Robotics in Genitourinary Surgery*,
DOI 10.1007/978-1-84882-114-9_7, © Springer-Verlag London Limited 2011

was described by the Guy's and St. Thomas' robotics group in 2004, led by Mr. Prokar Dasgupta.[5]

This chapter describes how one of the earliest RALP services in the UK was established, as well as the current robotic training program. The difficulties in developing a robotics program within the NHS and the future of robotic urology in the UK will also be discussed.

7.2 Establishing a Robotics Program Within an NHS Foundation Trust Hospital

The decision to begin a robotics program within the USA is a relatively simpler exercise when compared to the UK. FDA approval of the da Vinci® in 2001 has provided plenty of time for innovators to lead and the more cautious to follow in the establishment of robotics programs across the USA. The system of health care within the UK, free at the point of delivery, means that spearheading such advancement is more challenging than in a system funded by private health insurance. Difficulties arise from more than simply financing such an endeavor; differences in health-care system infrastructure places even more emphasis on gaining managerial support, navigating local and regional levels of governance, attracting patients, and establishing a fully committed team. This section describes the process by which the Urology department of Addenbrooke's NHS Foundation Trust hospital (Cambridge, UK), led by Professor David Neal, began one of the UK's earliest robotics programs.

7.2.1 The Decision to Start a Robotics Program in the UK

For reasons discussed above, it is often fair to describe the UK as following closely in the shadow of America's technological superiority. For some, this itself may provide enough justification for the acquisition of a da Vinci®, based on successful reports emerging from the USA. However, differences in the health-care systems mean that the transition of a successful robotics program across the Atlantic cannot be guaranteed. The Addenbrooke's team had to consider

the risks and benefits of such a program within the NHS, as well as the feasibility of its implementation. Superseding any discussion by the Addenbrooke's team was the issue of how to ensure patient safety in a technology which has unfamiliar territory across the entire country.

By the middle of 2004, robotics programs in the USA were no more than 4 years old, but still evidence was emerging of superior operative outcomes such as reduced blood loss and faster recovery times postoperatively, when compared to RP.[6] As a regional cancer centre, the Addenbrooke's team already performing major surgery for urological cancers, together with surgeons and anesthetists with considerable experience in laparoscopic operations, provided an ideal setting to introduce the da Vinci® technology.

In 2004 Professor Neal began collaborating with experts in RALP from the USA. Establishing surgeon–mentor relationships during the process of developing the robotics program helped to identify and resolve any potential difficulties before they had arisen. This early contact also served to build the important relationship between surgeon and mentor.

Before selecting a specialist robotics team within the urology department, funding for the robotics program had to be secured.

7.2.2 Financing a Robotics Program

There were several issues which needed to be addressed when considering the financing of the robotics program. The costing of both hardware and the training program needed to be detailed, before seeking sources of funding.

The da Vinci® Surgical System costs around £1.3 million to install, with an annual servicing contract of £90,000. The disposable instruments add a real excess cost of around £1,400 over an open prostatectomy. Finally, any potential modifications to the operating room (OR) also needed to be considered.

Intuitive Surgical, Inc. provided guidance in terms of the ideal OR space and robot setup within this. An operating theatre within the existing theatre suite was identified, with adjacent storage area for the robotic system for its safe keeping. An outline of the robotic equipment (console and patient-side cart), operating table, anesthetic equipment, and operating instrument trolleys was traced using masking tape. Each operation typically involves 6–8 individuals, so assessing the logistics of their positions and movement during an operation was important in confirming the suitability of an OR.

The financial support necessary for the training program also had to be taken into account. The lead surgeon had to make several trips to the USA and Europe to visit highly experienced centers for RALP, accompanied on one occasion by the whole robotics team for their core training in the USA. In addition, a three-person mentoring team from the USA was then required to proctor the first five cases performed in the UK. Finally, administrative as well as marketing costs going into producing new patient information that explained the procedure also had to be considered.

Within the UK, hospitals with *Foundation Trust* status have a greater degree of financial independence compared to other more "centrally accountable" hospitals. Part of the financial assessment process at Addenbrooke's involved modeling various scenarios of different numbers of cases performed over the coming years. The population served by the Addenbrooke's hospital surpassed the critical population mass necessary to justify this investment. Eventually a competitive project grant was obtained for the value of £750 000, intended not only to purchase and maintain the robot but also for its scientific evaluation. The business case for acquiring the da Vinci® required setting various strategic objectives, which included satisfying the need for high-quality innovative services which meet local health priorities and the strengthening of the Trust's repertoire of specialist services.

The limited availability of NHS capital together with the high costs of acquiring this system provided a significant challenge to financing a robotics program. This was overcome by purchasing the asset through funds from the Mark Master Masons, and the Addenbrooke's Charitable Trust, which was subsequently donated to the Trust.

7.2.3 Establishing a Robotics Team

Great importance was placed on selecting the initial members of the dedicated robotics team. They needed to become self-sufficient in the entire RALP procedure from start to finish, which required inputs from multiple disciplines. Furthermore, a compromise had to be reached between training as many suitable individuals as possible and ensuring that the training of each member would not be compromised by the over-subscription of each role.

The surgical component of the robotics team consisted of the following:

Surgeons

i. Console: who possessed a large experience in open pelvic cancer, conferring great knowledge of pelvic anatomy and the process of prostatectomy.

ii. Patient-side assistant (PA): the primary (right-sided) PA had a substantial background in laparoscopy, including laparoscopic prostatectomy. The possession of basic laparoscopic skills in the robotics team is essential in the laparoscopic style setup of RALP. It is also important in ensuring that the PA can reach a minimum degree of competence from the very first case so as not to limit the progress of the operation.

Anesthetist

The urology anesthetist possessed an extensive background in laparoscopy anesthesia and was chosen based on this expertise. This would be particularly crucial in the earlier operations when operating times would be much longer.

Surgical care practitioner (SCP)

The role of a SCP incorporates more clinical responsibilities over and above that of a theatre nurse. The SCP was selected on the grounds of her extensive experience in operative urology, which would allow her to be trained initially as a secondary (left-sided) PA, before progressing onto the role of primary PA.

Theatre nurses

Senior theatre nurses from the urology team were chosen based on their extensive experience of working with the selected surgeons and anesthetist.

The surgical side of the robotics team would also need adequate administrative and managerial support. The surgical team met regularly with hospital management to discuss the timetable for training and any other operational requirements. Permission to begin the robotics program also involved formal registration of the project with the local Clinical Governance Committee, a hospital-based committee which oversees the safety and quality of care offered to patients.

Rigorous pre-operative, intraoperative, and postoperative data forms were designed to encompass all conceivable information pertaining to the surgery, allowing prospective data collection, which would be invaluable in assessing outcomes and comparisons with established centers. The project was also registered with the local research and ethics committee. The administrative task of documenting operative and post-operative outcomes was assigned to a team member from the very first operation, ensuring consistency in the data collected. This information would be used later during the review and integration stage (see Section 7.3).

The small size of the Addenbrooke's robotics team would allow each person not only to be present for every case but more importantly to implement their role and develop their own expertise. The entire team could become familiar with every step of the procedure, and by working together they could cohesively reduce operating time, improve efficiency, and maintain patient safety as the main priority. This small-sized team would also enable the fastest transition of skills from mentors to each individual and avoid dilution of any teaching experience. Team members could then train other hospital staff once they are completely comfortable with their own responsibilities. Finally, the small size and early establishment of the robotics team also helped to develop a sense of *team spirit*. Commitment to the success of the robotics program is perhaps the most important quality of the robotics team, which must be present in each member in abundance to overcome any technical and logistical difficulties they may encounter.

7.2.4 Training the First Robotics Team

Financial and logistical approval for the robotics program was eventually secured by the middle of 2005. For the previous year the entire robotics team was able to acquire theoretical knowledge of the RALP procedure and monitor procedural developments in the literature. The console surgeon had visited three robotic centers to observe the procedure and gain

familiarity with identifying tissue planes, as well as the novel perspective offered by the da Vinci® camera. The console surgeon and PAs also gained insight by reviewing videos of the RALP performed by highly experienced robotic units from the USA (led by Mani Menon). The primary PA was an accomplished laparoscopic surgeon performing upper tract laparoscopy and was fully trained up as a primary assistant for LRP.

In October 2005, the complete Addenbrooke's robotics team travelled to Hackensack University Medical Center (Hackensack, New Jersey, USA), an Intuitive Surgical, Inc. training centre, for 3 days of intensive training. On the first day the robotics team was taken through the fundamentals of the robot; setup of the robot, the proper use of the da Vinci® surgical system, and its full repertoire of EndoWrist® instruments. The basic principles of operating the instruments were described to the entire robotics team to improve general understanding of the RALP procedure for everyone involved.

The first afternoon was spent observing a live RALP procedure and discussing the details of patient positioning, port placement, surgical techniques, instrumentation applications, and anatomical references. The anesthetist gained valuable information from the host anesthetic team and hence developed an anesthetic recipe for safe patient setup, particularly as early experience typically resulted in longer anesthesia and operating times.

The following morning the patient operated upon the previous day was reviewed, and a further live RALP procedure was observed, gaining further information and experience of the procedure and equipment setup. In the afternoon the surgeons were taken to a dry lab, where they were able to practice using the robot and become familiar with the controls, both at the console and the patient side. Various exercises were performed to improve dexterity of handling the robotic instruments. This training also gave the console surgeon the opportunity to familiarize himself with clutching and motion-scaling controls which are also unique to the da Vinci®. Meanwhile, the rest of the robotics team performed dry runs on patient and robot setup, as well as mastering efficient draping and lens calibration.

On the third day these skills were transferred to the wet-lab setting, where the surgeons were able to spend the day operating on anesthetized pigs and gain an appreciation of manipulating tissue as guided by the 3D visual system, without the benefit of tactile feedback.

In training a new robotics team, there is an overwhelming emphasis placed on the short wet-lab experience on animal tissues, with widespread acceptance that completion implies proficiency to perform RALP safely on humans.[7] Unfortunately the complexity of this technology means that optimal use of the robotic controls cannot be achieved in such a short time. It was for this reason that a mentoring *team* was established, for the first five cases to be performed by the Addenbrooke's team in the UK.

7.2.5 The First Cases: A Mentor-Guided Approach

Dr. James Peabody, a senior staff member of the Vattikuti Urology Institute (VUI) at Henry Ford Health System (Detroit, Michigan, USA), served as the primary mentor for the Addenbrooke's robotics team. Working with Dr. Mani Menon, Dr. Peabody had helped to develop one of the earliest robotics programs in the USA and had an extensive experience of the RALP procedure. His interest in teaching robotic surgery also made Dr. Peabody an ideal mentor.

Professor Neal had previously visited the VUI to observe their preferred method of RALP. In addition, the mentors were fully informed of the robotic training the Addenbrooke's team had received. This was a critical part of the mentoring process ensuring that both teams were aware of each other's requirements.

In addition to the primary mentor, an experienced primary PA of the VUI team – Dr. Sanjeev Kaul – assisted in mentoring the PA for the first five cases performed at Addenbrooke's hospital. Given the importance of the role of the PAs in RALP, where the lead surgeon has no control of suction, retraction (using the three-arm da Vinci® system), and application of clips, it is imperative that the PAs are also given the undivided attention of a personal mentor. This also allowed Dr. Peabody to concentrate on mentoring the console surgeon. An experienced theatre nurse from the VUI also assisted the nursing team with preparing the robotic equipment for the first cases. Technical concerns regarding the robot itself were addressed by an

Intuitive Surgical, Inc. representative, who was present for the first 20 cases and immediately available by emergency contact thereafter.

Patients with localized prostate cancer were identified, vetted by the surgical team with a review of the histology and imaging at the multi-disciplinary meeting. The surgeons and mentors had previously agreed on the selection criteria for ideal patients for the first cases to reduce the complexity of the operation and the risk of complications. These included the following:

- Patients with low-risk disease (indicated by PSA < 10, clinically T2a or less and Gleason score ≤ 6)
- Prostate size < 80 g, without significant median lobe enlargement
- BMI < 30, without co-morbidities (especially COPD)
- No previous history of TURP, abdominal surgery, hormone, or radiotherapy. Previous appendicectomies or open inguinal hernia operations were acceptable

Patients were fully informed and counseled that the program of RALP at Addenbrooke's hospital was truly in its infancy, with an experienced mentor being present for the first five cases. All possible risk factors were discussed in obtaining patient consent, and patients were free to opt for traditional open surgery as was the norm at the time of RALP introduction. Furthermore, patients were informed that the surgeons could not claim any benefits in terms of their surgical outcome and recovery, compared to the then current practice of traditional open RP as they were truly the first cases to undergo the procedure.

The console trainee performed 40% of the first operation, 80% of the second, and was able to complete the third operation in its entirety. The console mentor continued to offer advice on surgical technique and the optimum use of robotic controls, improving the speed and efficacy of the operation in the fourth and fifth cases. The PA mentor was also directly involved in the first few cases, gradually transferring the responsibilities of assisting to the trainee in the safest manner possible.

The Addenbrooke's team members described a great benefit from the individual attention they received from their personal mentors. The presence of the same trainee at each position is also likely to offer a more efficient operating and learning experience than rotating training programs which have been previously described.[8]

Over the first five mentored cases, there was an improvement in setup and docking times. The operating time also showed a general decrease, from 300 min in the first case to 180 min in the fourth case. The Addenbrooke's team continued to maintain operative times below 240 min in the absence of the mentors, demonstrating a successful transfer of skills from mentors to trainees. Whilst this was an encouraging outcome, the Addenbrooke's team did not accept this as a sole indicator for success. It is commonly described that mastery of RALP is attained when the operating time falls below an arbitrarily set value (typically less than 3 h). However, the real indicators of success should incorporate several outcomes, most important of which are cancer control, gaining continence, erectile function, and reductions in complications.

Intraoperative capsular incisions occurred in the first two cases but were immediately corrected by the mentors. Similar transgressions in other difficult stages of the RALP were also corrected, avoiding adverse oncological and functional outcomes at this early phase of the learning curve. The mean age of the first five cases was 57.6 years (range 53–61 years). Nerve sparing was rated as excellent in four of the five first cases, and clear margins were reported for all five cases. Final histology correlated well with pre-operative biopsy results; all had adenocarcinoma of prostate Gleason score 3+3=6, two patients had pT2a, two patients had pT2c, and one patient had pT3a (focal extracapsular extension). Intraoperative blood loss showed a decreasing trend, remaining below 350 mL for all five cases, without any need for transfusion. Postoperatively, none of the patients had a urinary leak. The first four patients were all discharged within 24 h and the fifth patient on the second day after RALP.

At 40 months follow-up, all five patients remain free of biochemical recurrence (PSA < 0.02), four are fully continent and pad free, one patient uses one small pad per day. Three patients have erections sufficient for sexual intercourse with PDE5 inhibitors and the other two have failed to respond to PDE5 inhibitors and do not wish to pursue alternative treatments for their erectile dysfunction.

In terms of functional outcomes, the initial experiences of other robotics teams have been less successful compared to those seen at Addenbrooke's, though they all eventually improve as the teams mature.[7] This highlights the benefit of a mentor-guided approach when beginning a robotics program, ensuring safe and successful RALP whilst the robotics team gains experience.

7.3 Current Practice of RALP Within an NHS Foundation Trust Hospital: Development and Training

The Addenbrooke's team had reached an important milestone; the robotics team had been successfully established, and reports of positive outcomes were emerging from the first cases performed under the guidance of mentors. Nevertheless, difficulties lay ahead in developing the robotics program in a country where robotic urology was still in its infancy. The practicalities of arranging mentoring from international experts demanded conservative use of their time. The Addenbrooke's team would have to contend with these less than ideal conditions of developing their expertise, whilst still striving to achieve surgical outcomes comparable to the world's most experienced robotic centers. Finally, the team would have to establish a pragmatic training program which could bring the next generation of robotic surgeons to similarly high standards of practice and still maintain an absolute focus on patient safety. This section describes how Addenbrooke's RALP procedure evolved to what it is today and the training practices they currently employ.

7.3.1 Refining the Operative Technique

Like any other surgery, refining one's robotic technique requires a process of continual review: identifying suitable changes and integrating them into current practice. This review and integration process has taken place regularly as the robotics program at Addenbrooke's has matured.

The earliest example of this was with the VUI mentors, who were the first port of call for the first five cases, offering immediate technical advice and correcting any transgressions. A further 35 cases were closely monitored by Dr. Hervé Baumert, a highly experienced laparoscopic prostatectomy surgeon who had performed over 400 pure LRPs, with involvement at the Institut Mutualiste Montsouris (Paris). His presence offered another opportunity to develop the technique of the Addenbrooke's team.

In December 2006 after performing more than 70 cases, the Addenbrooke's team received additional mentoring by Dr. Ash Tewari of the Cornell Medical Centre (New York, USA), who had extensive experience in RALP. This process at such a late stage of the learning curve was essential in fine-tuning the technique which the Addenbrooke's team had developed. Upon mastering the fundamentals of the RALP procedure, the robotics team was able to further refine the operative technique with advancements reported in the literature.

The Vattikuti Institute Prostatectomy (VIP) has become the most popular method of RALP, incorporating principles taken from laparoscopic and open techniques.[9] Since its conception, numerous modifications have been made to the original technique, which the Addenbrooke's team have gradually incorporated into their practice. These modifications have been based on those described in the literature, as well as those observed in live robotic surgeries performed by experts at robotic symposia and international urological conferences.

The Addenbrooke's team have incorporated a posterior reconstruction suture prior to performing the vesicourethral anastomosis as described by Rocco et al.[10] with minor modifications. Using a single 3/0 poliglecaprone 25 (Monocryl) suture the free edge of Denonvilliers' fascia posterior to the bladder neck is opposed to the posterior aspect of the rhabdosphincter and posterior median raphe. The technique provides posterior support for the sphincteric mechanism and prevents caudal retraction of the urethra. The reconstruction also draws the bladder caudally into a supported position removing the tension on the vesicourethral anastomosis.

The Addenbrooke's team has been careful with neurovascular bundle preservation, ensuring an athermal dissection. The quality of nerve sparing is guided by the disease characteristics in terms of the presence of palpable disease, Gleason sum, and volume of disease on prostate biopsies. The preservation of the high lateral prostatic fascia (or "veil of Aphrodite") as described by Kaul et al.,[11] with its associated improvement in potency rates postoperatively, is reserved for patients with low-volume, low-risk disease, as this technique risks higher rates of positive margins.

The RALP procedure currently performed by the Addenbrooke's team is continuously evolving, incorporating new ideas as the evidence base develops, and pursuing each one only with the full support of every team member.

When initially learning the RALP procedure, the robotics team had used videos of recorded procedures to gain familiarity with the various steps of the surgery. In refining the operative technique, video recordings were used once again, this time to identify transgressions retrospectively for the first 50 cases, as has been described for open RP.[12] In this way one can, for example, correlate specific steps in surgical procedure with final pathology results, continence, and potency rates.

7.3.2 Perioperative Management

Patients who elect to undergo RALP as their definitive treatment for their localized carcinoma of prostate are reviewed pre-operatively in clinic by surgeons and the anesthetic team at least a week prior to surgery. All investigations including prostate biopsies and staging investigations are formally reviewed by independent pathologists and radiologists at a multidisciplinary team meeting to confirm diagnosis and planning of patient treatment. It is important to identify patients who would be deemed unsuitable for robotic prostatectomy, including those with significant respiratory disease, unable to tolerate steep head down position, body mass index greater than 35, and previous radiotherapy to the pelvis. Relative contraindications include ischemic heart disease, glaucoma, and previous major abdominal surgery. Patients are fully counseled regarding the RALP procedure, highlighting potential complications of the procedure, and advised on their post-operative recovery. They are reviewed by a urology nurse practitioner, who advises on pelvic floor exercises which patients are encouraged to commence pre-operatively. Patients are issued with printed information on all the above matters.

Patients are kept nil by mouth for 6 h prior to surgery. Pre-medication includes ranitidine (150 mg) on the night prior to surgery and on the morning of operation to avoid palatal ulcers, glycerine suppositories (two) on the morning of surgery to help evacuate the rectum, and anxiolytics as required. Thromboprophylaxis includes graduated compression stockings, pneumatic pressure boots intraoperatively, and low molecular weight heparin subcutaneously.

Patients are induced in the anesthetic room on the operating table with non-slip cushions. Arms are placed by the sides, with extensive padding to avoid neuropraxia; a chest strap over extensive padding allows additional support for the patient and the patient is secured in the lithotomy position (Fig. 7.1). The face is also carefully protected with padding to avoid inadvertent injury during surgery.

Following creation of the pneumoperitoneum and insertion of the ports as described for the three-arm system by the Vattikuti team (Fig. 7.2), the patient is positioned head down (by approximately 30°) and the robot is "docked in," ready for surgeons to begin the RALP.

All port sites are infiltrated with local anesthetic (levobupivacaine hydrochloride), and patients receive a bolus of morphine sulfate and a nonsteroidal anti-inflammatory (diclofenac sodium) intra-venously prior to waking. Patients are allowed oral fluids in the recovery room before being progressed onto a light diet later in the evening. They are encouraged to mobilize early, with an aim for discharging the next post-operative day.

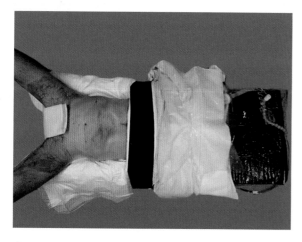

Fig. 7.1 Supine patient, padded and secured in the lithotomy position, ready to be prepped for RALP

7.3.3 Results and Learning Curves: A Personal Experience

When beginning any new surgical program, identifying appropriate performance indicators is one of the most challenging aspects of the evaluation process. The Addenbrooke's lead surgeon at the console was in the fortunate position of having expert mentors guiding him through an extensive series of cases, improving proficiency and efficiency as he ascended the learning curve. This was demonstrable in the low-positive margin rate and good functional outcomes recorded for the first cases. The next challenge facing the Addenbrooke's team was training the primary PA – Mr. Nimish Shah – to perform surgery at the console, under the tutorship of the lead surgeon who had comfortably mastered this role.

The primary PA was trained in an identical manner to that which had been used by the VUI mentoring team. The mentor would perform more challenging parts of the procedure and would guide the trainee through simpler stages. The responsibility would gradually increase over time until Mr. Shah was able to complete an entire RALP procedure independently. Despite the rapid ascent to independence, the original console surgeon still supervised Mr. Shah for several operations afterward, further refining his technique, as Ash Tewari had done in December 2007.

Mentoring of Mr. Shah was more easily facilitated with Professor Neal's presence as an "in-house" mentor, allowing Mr. Shah to gradually increase his responsibilities over time. Multiple contributors to any one surgery do however make documenting the progress of an individual surgeon more difficult. The Addenbrooke's team overcame this by recording the surgeon responsible for each *step* of the operation, as well as its duration. The operation was divided into nine surgical steps: bladder take down, opening the endopelvic fascia, ligation of the dorsal vein complex, dividing the bladder neck, dissection of the seminal vesicles, dividing the prostatic pedicles and sparing the neurovascular bundles, dissecting the apex of the prostate, clearance of lymph nodes, and anastomosis.

In doing so, the Addenbrooke's team was able to obtain operating times for Mr. Shah's independent contributions, producing the first accurate learning curve to be recorded for RALP. The trends in

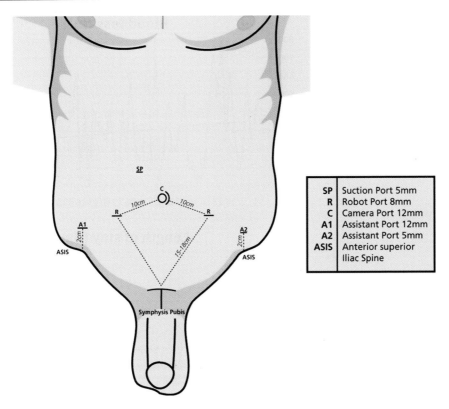

SP	Suction Port 5mm
R	Robot Port 8mm
C	Camera Port 12mm
A1	Assistant Port 12mm
A2	Assistant Port 5mm
ASIS	Anterior superior Iliac Spine

Fig. 7.2 Overhead view of port placement for performing RALP with a three-arm da Vinci® Surgical System

surgeries completed entirely by Mr. Shah are shown in Fig. 7.3.

As a group, the Addenbrooke's team has performed more than 420 cases, with a mean age of 62 years and a mean operating time of 180 min. The positive margin rate correlates with pathological stage, with 16% in pT2 and 36% in pT3. When drawing comparisons with American and European centers, one should note the low rate of PSA testing in the UK, resulting in the incidence of many more higher volume and higher grade cancers. Furthermore, the incidence of pT3 in the Addenbrooke's patient series has been 42%, indicating even higher stage cases in this center compared to American and European centers.

In terms of functional outcomes, 75% of men are potent sufficient for intercourse at 12 months, with 25% using no adjunctive treatment. Previously, 70% of patients were fully continent at 12 months, with a further 20% using up to one pad a day. Recent employment of the Rocco stitch in the last 100 patients led to 80% of patients being fully continent at 6 weeks and 94% at 10 months.

The Addenbrooke's team has been careful in counseling patients undergoing RALP, being clear during the early phase of introducing RALP that the program was in its infancy; and more recently, patients have been informed of the teams' outcome results from their own experiences. The Addenbrooke's team believe that careful presentation of outcome information and data, coupled with a more neutral approach with respect to discussion of radical versus conservative approaches, will result in lower rates of patient dissatisfaction, as has recently been reported.[13] In order for informed consent to be obtained, a frank and thorough discussion must take place, highlighting the likely outcomes for the patient based on the surgeon's own data, rather than the frequently quoted large studies in the literature with favorable outcomes. This is clearly not possible when establishing a new RALP program, thus necessitating a clear discussion with patients to ensure that

Fig. 7.3 Learning curve for
Mr. Shah's completed RALP
procedures (LOS, length of
stay)

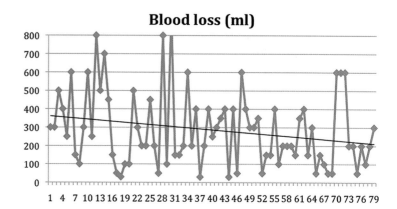

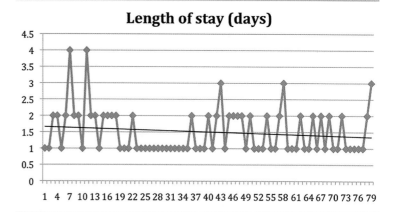

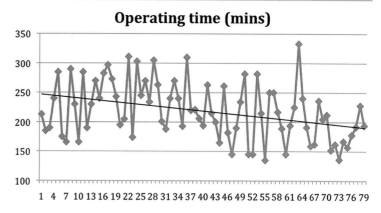

the experience of the team to date is clear, as has been
performed at Addenbrooke's hospital.

7.3.4 Training the Next Generation

Whilst RALP is still in its infancy, the USA has seen
a rapid expansion of robotic urology, with over 70%
of their prostatectomies currently being performed
robotically. This has meant that developing one's
expertise in robotics in the USA is relatively simple:
robotics has now become an essential part of many
urological training programs in the USA, and the abundance of da Vinci® robots allows trainees to gain
significant experience. Furthermore, the accessibility
of corporate support from Intuitive Surgical, Inc. and
the multiple regional and national courses and symposia provides the necessary infrastructure to build
successful robotics teams from scratch. In 2009 the

USA had more than 600 da Vinci® robots[14] compared to just 14 in the UK (1 per 500,000 population compared to 1 per 4,000,000). In addition to the UK's scarcity of da Vinci® robots, the dearth of training programs and corporate assistance in the UK also provides significant challenges to training their next generation of robotic surgeons.

The current practice of training robotic-naive surgeons in RALP in the UK is very much hospital specific. With so few da Vinci® robots in the UK, interest in training is particularly intense. Currently in Addenbrooke's hospital, robotic-naive consultant surgeons are given priority over training. The Addenbrooke's robotics group has developed their own structured training program, which is designed to impart expertise in the RALP procedure as efficiently as possible, whilst maintaining the same high standards in surgical outcomes that the original robotics team was able to report at the end of their learning curve. This has led to the Addenbrooke's team establishing guidelines, on operating times, for example, which ideally remain below 4 h in order to maintain similar standards. Whilst this can occasionally curtail the initial experience of a trainee, the Addenbrooke's team has deemed this the approach which maximizes patient safety.

Trainees first acquire the theoretical and observational knowledge of the RALP procedure, utilizing teaching videos and live procedures. They would then assist as a secondary (left-sided) PA for between 10 and 15 cases (establishing pneumoperitoneum and placement of laparoscopic ports), with the support of an experienced left-sided PA as is necessary. The trainee will then build up experience as a primary (right-sided) PA for around 20 cases (assisting with retraction, suction, placement of various haemostatic clips), receiving similar support from an experienced primary PA who will be actively involved in their first few cases to safely transfer their responsibilities. This allows the trainee to fully appreciate the roles of the primary and secondary (with a three-arm system) PA and identify any limitations before progressing onto the console.

At this point the trainee is reassessed to see whether they have developed an appreciation for handling the PA role, with further support offered if necessary. The trainee would then go on to participate in each of the nine surgical steps previously described, gradually gaining confidence and expertise at each stage.

From the learning curves the team could identify which stages would take longer to master and subsequently begin training at the relatively simpler stages. The order of surgical steps a trainee would follow (of increasing complexity, not the order of surgery) would be the following: bladder take down, opening the endopelvic fascia, ligation of the dorsal vein complex, dissection of the seminal vesicles, dividing the bladder neck, dissecting the apex of the prostate, clearance of lymph nodes, anastomosis, and nerve sparing. Once the individual steps are mastered, the trainee can begin completing several steps per operation until a degree of confidence and competence has been attained where the trainee can perform RALP independently, under close supervision. The Addenbrooke's team has found that it typically takes 30 cases for a previously experienced open prostatectomy consultant surgeon to reach this stage, using this training program.

Training of robotic-naive surgeons in UK hospitals with robotics programs is an entirely self-contained process. All trainees' experiences (practical and theoretical) must be acquired from that single robotics team who also has to continue to provide quality RALP during this training process. The Addenbrooke's team has successfully trained several consultants to perform RALP independently, in a safe and efficacious manner. Trainees benefit from the team's high throughput of cases, making training opportunities more frequent, as well as the permanent availability of the original robotics team to guide trainees at each role in RALP. The luxury of this setup overcomes the lack of corporate support or national training programs but highlights one of several difficulties of developing a robotics program in the UK health system, to be discussed in the next section.

7.4 The Difficulties of Developing a Robotics Program Within the NHS, and the Future...

It was over 60 years ago that a centrally funded health service, free at the point of delivery, was established in the UK. Since its launch, the NHS has grown to become one of the world's largest publically funded health services, receiving over £100 billion from taxations in 2010. Praise for the NHS and the egalitarianism upon which it is founded is abundant amongst both doctors and patients in the UK. Nevertheless, there is an increasing realization of the limitations that such a structure can impose. The following section describes the implications for developing robotics programs within the NHS and what this means for the future of robotic surgery in the UK.

7.4.1 Funding Robotic Surgery in the NHS

As outlined above (see Section 7.2.2) the costs for initiating a robotics program within a UK NHS hospital are particularly sizeable, requiring competitive research grants, bids for Trust funding, and generous charitable donations. Given the mechanism of financing the NHS, its market size, and the expansive definition encompassed by health and wellbeing (which the NHS seeks to maximize), public *demand* will always exceed the *supply* of health services. This forces the NHS to determine ethical frameworks for the allocation of resources amongst competing priorities in public health. With governments detailing those frameworks, NHS spending inevitably becomes politically, and subsequently publically, influenced.

Prostate cancer has received increasing attention from the NHS over the last few years, in an attempt to address public concern regarding inequities between spending on breast and prostate cancer. In part, this can be used as justification for supporting the funding of a robotic urology program within an NHS Foundation Trust hospital. However, complete support for establishing such a program would demand the endorsement of RALP by the National Institute for Clinical Excellence (NICE).

The role of NICE within the NHS was formalized in a 2004 white paper, which described how this independent body would serve to gather evidence in order to offer guidance on the provision of health services.[15] One of the types of guidelines that NICE offers are those for interventional procedures, where NICE presents its findings on both clinical and cost effectiveness of a particular treatment. In assessing cost effectiveness, NICE considers the increase in health (compared to current practice) which is likely to accrue from the increased expenditure, commonly expressing such a ratio in the form of cost per quality-adjusted life years (QUALYs).

Guidelines for LRP surgery have been issued, but the absence of interventional guidelines for RALP necessitates approval from individual NHS Trust's Clinical Governance Committees before a robotics program can begin. Furthermore, the absence of the gold-standard randomized controlled trials, for assessing differences between open RP, LRP, and/or RALP, prohibits the calculation of QUALYs by NICE. This will continue to force individual Trusts to make the final decision as to whether establishing a robotics program would be a cost-effective enterprise.

This high threshold for fiscal analysis absolves NICE from confronting the ethical decision of whether to fund a robotics program but still leaves individual NHS Foundation Trusts with the problem of whether this is an appropriate use of their resources. The end result is a more qualitative debate between a Trust board and surgical innovators, which ultimately determines whether the investment is made. The need for prudent financial planning, as well as a committed robotics team, will continue to make the decentralization of such decisions a risk for individual Trusts.

7.4.2 The Future of Robotic Urology in the UK

Addenbrooke's hospital has been privileged to see the development of a successful robotics program, but this result by no means guarantees the success of future programs to be established in the UK. Any decision to start a robotics program must not be taken lightly, and the future of robotic surgery in the UK will evidently be shaped by the strengths of individual Trusts across the nation.

As market demand for RALP increases with more public awareness of the technology, sales of da Vinci® surgical systems should also increase. This has the potential to earn UK hospitals additional corporate assistance for their robotics programs, in the form of increased financial support and the establishment of UK training centers. Increasing the expertise of robotic urology within the UK has the added benefit of creating local mentors. This will help save in costs when mentoring emerging robotics teams and may shorten the learning curve by providing access to mentors who are within more practical travelling distances.

Despite the possibility of increased patient interest in the UK, politicians and hospital Trusts alike should be vigilant of chasing changes in public opinion. The rapid uptake of RALP in the USA does not and *should not* serve as a guarantee for the future of robotic urology in the UK. Differences in the health systems and fundamentally in the cultures, of British and Americans, generate subtly different demands for their health-care providers. The future of robotic urology in the UK will have to be determined by the success of robotics programs being developed within the NHS over the coming years. A genuine benefit of RALP over traditional methods, which warrants the excess costs, first needs to be realized. Together with any international developments in the evidence base for RALP, this is the only realistic way of encouraging the central (government) support that is ultimately necessary to expand the robotics program throughout the nation. And such an expansion would be on the proviso that the critical population mass could be met in the areas surrounding each new robot (see Section 7.2.2). Without central support, robotic urology is likely to remain the domain of a few specialist centers across the UK.

Acknowledgments Special thanks to Ms Gillian Basnett, Dr. Vishal Patil, Miss Naomi Sharma, Mr. Edward Smith, and Mr. Jeremy Naylor for their assistance.

References

1. Proust R. Technique de la prostatectomie périnéale. *Ass Franc Urol.* 1901;5:361.
2. Schuessler W, Schulam P, Clayman R, Kavoussi L. Laparoscopic radical prostatectomy: initial short-term experience. *Urology.* 1997;50(6):854–857.
3. Davies BL, Hibberd RD, Coptcoat MJ, Wickham JE. A surgeon robot prostatectomy – a laboratory evaluation. *J Med Eng Technol.* 1989;13:273–277.
4. BBC News 2001. http://news.bbc.co.uk/1/hi/health/1481105.stm.
5. Dasgupta P, Hemal A, Rose K. Robotic urology in the UK: establishing a programme and emerging role. *BJU Int.* 2005;95(6):723–724.
6. Tewari A, Srivasatava A, Menon M. Members of the VIP team. A prospective comparison of radical retropubic and robot-assisted prostatectomy: experience in one institution. *BJU Int.* 2003;92(3):205–210.
7. Kaul S, Peabody J, Shah N, Neal D, Menon M. Establishing a robotic prostatectomy programme: the impact of mentoring using a structured approach. *BJU Int.* 2006;97(6): 1143–1144.
8. Mayer EK, Winkler MH, Aggarwal R, et al. Robotic prostatectomy: the first UK experience. *Int J Med Robot Comput Assist Surg.* 2006;2:321–328.
9. Menon M, Tewari A, Peabody J. The VIP team Vattikuti Institute Prostatectomy: technique. *J Urol.* 2003;169(6): 2289–2292.
10. Rocco B, Gregori A, Stener S, et al. Posterior reconstruction of the rhabdosphincter allows a rapid recovery of continence after transperitoneal videolaparoscopic radical prostatectomy. *Eur Urol.* 2007;51: 996–1003.
11. Kaul S, Bhandari A, Hemal A, Savera A, Shrivastava A, Menon M. Robotic radical prostatectomy with preservation of the prostatic fascia: a feasibility study. *Urology.* 2005;66(6):1261–1265.
12. Walsh PC, Marschke P, Ricker D, Burnett AL. Use of intraoperative video documentation to improve sexual function after radical retropubic prostatectomy. *Urology.* 2000;55(1):62–67.
13. Schroeck FR, Krupski TL, Sun L, et al. Satisfaction and regret after open retropubic or robot-assisted laparoscopic radical prostatectomy. *Eur Urol.* 2008;54(4): 785–793.
14. Intuitive Surgical, Inc. 2007. FAQs. http://www.intuitivesurgical.com/products/faq/index.aspx#19. Accessed June 1, 2009
15. Department of Health. 2004. Choosing health: making healthier choices easier. UK Government White Paper 264741.

Chapter 8

Robotic Urologic Surgery: How to Make an Effective Robotic Program

Arthur Caire, Michael N. Ferrandino, and David M. Albala

8.1 Introduction

In order for hospitals and physicians to remain competitive, continued training and the use of new technology are needed to keep up with the ever evolving health-care world. Robotic surgery is a perfect example of how technology has revolutionized the surgical field. From open to laparoscopic to robotic, surgical equipment has developed in order to improve precision and shorten recovery times. Robotic surgery was developed in part to manage the anatomical challenges of operating in the pelvis and allows for tremor filtering, movement scaling, improved ergonomics, better vision of the operative field, and increased range of motion.[1] The system is constantly advancing with a particular focus on improving tactile feedback[2]. Surgeons are regularly modifying procedures to improve functional outcomes.[3,4] Due to these advantages, robotic-assisted radical prostatectomy (RARP) has been on the forefront of the robotics movement. Minimally invasive surgery also has several clinical advantages including shorter hospital stay, decreased perioperative pain, and decreased blood loss[1,5,6].

Although the RARP was one of the first procedures to widely make use of this new technology, robotic surgery is not just limited to the urologist. It is an ever expanding practice in which many surgical fields are beginning to take advantage of this breakthrough technology. The number of surgical subspecialties that are currently taking advantage of this technology has grown substantially in the last 5 years. The robot has implemented itself in surgical practices ranging from gynecology to cardiac surgery to pediatrics as well as many others[7-9]. However, as with any new technology, robotic surgery is still very much in the developmental period and is ever expanding into the health-care market.

Although every hospital might like to have a robotics program, there are many requirements needed for a successful and self-sustaining program in the current health-care market. A thorough market analysis including competing entities and estimated surgical volume is necessary prior to purchasing a robot. Other issues to be addressed include determining whether you have the trained surgeons or the capability to recruit the appropriately trained surgeons to keep your robotics program afloat. An assessment of facilities and staff is also imperative prior to making this substantial investment. Ultimately, after a well thought-out analysis, a decision must be made as to whether the institution can support and maintain a robotics program. The goal of this chapter is to focus on the economic and developmental phase of starting a robotics program.

8.2 Market and Cost Analysis

The first step to establishing a successful robotics program is proper planning. Creating a robotics planning committee is a well-accepted initial action. The board should ideally consist of a multidisciplinary panel of hospital staff, for example, a hospital administrator, an

D.M. Albala (✉)
Division of Urologic Surgery, Department of Surgery, Duke Prostate Center, Duke University Medical Center, Durham, NC, USA
e-mail: dalbala@ampofny.com

A.K. Hemal, M. Menon (eds.), *Robotics in Genitourinary Surgery*,
DOI 10.1007/978-1-84882-114-9_8, © Springer-Verlag London Limited 2011

anesthesiologist, a surgeon, and a nursing administrator. By including a member from each group of the robotics team from the start, this will create the appropriate expectations and a smooth transition once the program begins. Subcommittees can then be created to evaluate specific tasks. For example, the market analysis should generally be performed by a subcommittee consisting of hospital administrators and surgeons.

A market analysis looks at two entities: (1) assessment of the health-care competition and (2) assessment of the patient population. For example, if a competing hospital has acquired a robotics program in the last several years, how has this affected your hospital? Also do you have a patient population that would find value in robotic surgery? Establishing a robotics program can have effects well outside your surgery department.

The impact of a robotics program can be evaluated in two ways. The first assessment includes an in-depth look at your surgical volume and personnel. Specifically looking at whether your institution has the appropriately trained surgeons to take advantage of the robot. If not, does your institution have surgeons interested in learning robotic surgery and undergoing the necessary training? If this is the case, the institution must take into account that an immature robotic surgeon will have certain limitations that may slow the initial development of the robotics program. A third scenario, which is the most ideal, is to recruit a mature robotic surgeon to become the director of robotic surgery at your institution. Having an experienced robotic surgeon will be a solid foundation for your program and will be essential to a smooth start to a robotics training program.

The second assessment should look at the overall impact of having a robotics program at your institution. Recent studies have shown that patients' interest in robotic surgery is growing[10]. Proper advertisement of your robotics program may generate patients for your institution by demonstrating the advanced technology offered at your facility. This is particularly important to assess if other hospitals in your area have established robotics programs. Evaluating a timeline of the start of their robotics program and comparing before and after patient volumes between your institutions will give you an idea of how their robotics program is affecting your hospital. If there are several robotics programs in your area, an assessment of whether there is an appropriate robotic surgical volume to sustain an additional program is necessary. Looking at your institution's current surgical volume and isolating procedures that could be performed robotically will provide an initial idea of the potential current robotic volume, although it must be remembered that this requires the appropriate surgical staff with the proper training.

To expand your patient volume, a marketing program should then be implemented for the benefit of the robotics program as well as the institution as a whole. Establishing a robotics program takes time and initial estimates should include a 5- and 10-year outlook as initial purchase of the robot is of substantial cost and will take time to pay itself off. Estimations of surgical volume alongside operating cost will then need to be calculated in order to assess if a robotics program is right for your institution. The market analysis is utterly important to the success of your future program as once you decide to establish a program, there are large start-up costs and cutting corners may hinder the opportunity to create a successful program.

8.3 Cost and Performance of a Urological Robotics Program

Due to the substantial cost associated with starting a robotics program, many groups have sought to evaluate the true cost of robotic surgery. Others have analyzed whether robotic surgery offers comparable outcomes. As with any new procedure, robotic surgery must be evaluated with evidence-based medicine and although the verdict is still out, preliminary reports have shown robotic surgery to be competitive from both an economic and an outcome standpoint. In the field of urology, the overwhelming majority of the current robotics caseload is the RARP. This is due to a combination of the high prevalence of prostate cancer and the specific benefits the robot can offer in the tight confines of prostate cancer surgery. Although other departments may also make use of the robot and other urologic procedures will be performed with the robot, the cost effectiveness of RARP remains one of the most well-studied and published procedures in robotic surgery.

In 2004, Lotan et al.[11] evaluated cost between open, laparoscopic, and robotic prostatectomies. They analyzed individual components of hospitalization, including operating room cost, surgical supplies, room and board, transfusion rates, medications, intravenous fluids, infusion pump costs, and professional fees between the three surgical methods. They assumed that the robot would last 7 years and be used for 300 cases per year. They found a nearly $1,800 difference in cost between radical retropubic prostatectomy (RRP) and RARP. The majority of this difference was related to the purchase and maintenance of the robot. Their analysis concluded that RARP needed significant decrease in both initial cost and maintenance to become cost competitive. Given an efficient surgeon and the appropriate surgical volume, this study no longer holds true. They assumed one case per day where it is not uncommon for three robotic procedures to be performed per day at our institution. This higher surgical volume allows the cost of the robot to be distributed over a larger case volume and therefore maintains cost competitiveness.

In 2005, Scales et al.[12] compared open and robotic prostatectomies head to head in a cost analysis. They divided cost into surgical or nonsurgical and evaluated cost between RRP and RARP. Surgical costs included anesthesia, operating room equipment, post-anesthesia care, and surgeon fee. Nonsurgical costs included hospital room and board and pharmacy costs. The initial cost of the robotic was included in the surgical costs by dividing the total cost of the robot by the amount of months in use. Their results were interesting as they showed that factors such as operative time and length of stay could skew cost competitiveness one way or another. Given a skilled surgeon who is able to generally perform a RARP in 90 min, the cost of a RARP and an RRP was equivalent. However, they found that once RARP went over 180 min, cost was increased due to the associated decrease in surgical volume. Their analysis demonstrates the importance of having a mature robotic surgeon for the foundation of your program as cost competitiveness relies not only on patient volume but also on surgical efficiency. Given the proper surgeon and a well-run efficient system, this article suggested RARP to be cost comparable to RRP.

Steinberg et al.[13] looked specifically at cost during the learning curve. They defined their learning curve as the time from adoption of RARP until a statistically significant nadir operative time was reached. Using their model, the learning curve range was between 24 and 360 cases at a cost from $95,000 to $1,365,000, respectively. Burgess et al.[14] showed operative charges to decrease 27% once the learning curve had been

overcome. As seen above the learning curve is highly variable and is dependent on your outcome measure. For example, Atug et al.[15] concluded that only 30 cases are needed to overcome the learning curve when using a positive surgical margin as the outcome measure. The above studies show that the learning curve can be highly variable based on your definition and put into perspective the cost saved by starting a robotics program with a mature robotic surgeon. In addition, there will be a robotics team learning curve associated with new equipment and procedures. These learning curve costs must be accounted for during the initial stages of the program.

Once the learning curve has lapsed, the RARP has shown competitive results compared to RRP. Smith et al.[16] analyzed 1,747 patients who underwent both RRP and RARP at their institution. From these cases, they isolated 200 consecutive RRPs and 200 consecutive RARPs. They then used surgical margin status as an outcome measure and concluded that in the hands of an experienced surgeon, patients undergoing RARP had a lower positive surgical margin rate. RARP has also shown higher short-term quality of life during the first 6 weeks postoperatively[17]. This study looked at 162 men undergoing both RRP and RARP for clinically localized prostate cancer.[17] Patients completed the SF-12 physical and mental health survey each week postoperatively for 6 weeks. They showed that the robotic group returned to baseline approximately 1.3 weeks earlier than did the open group. Although it is difficult to measure the value of an earlier return to baseline, this certainly offers an additional value to the robotic procedure. Not only has RARP been shown to have a quicker recovery time but also functional outcomes such as continence and potency have been competitive.

A more thorough review of the literature on the specifics of establishing a robotics program could also be useful during the planning process. The above studies give evidence that RARP has comparable outcomes once the learning curve has been overcome. Although one thing to remember is that each program and institution is unique and much of the data in the above studies are debatable because they are based on estimations and theoretical equations. In fact Gianino et al.[18] reviewed the current literature on the cost analysis of a robotic prostatectomy and concluded that due to statistical inconsistencies and assumptions, there is no valid evidence that RARP is more costly than

RRP. Therefore, the important aspect of reviewing the literature relies on learning principles and avoiding pitfalls. The above literature only looks at one procedure, although the learning curve undoubtedly applies to all robotic procedures. Further cost analysis studies are needed to properly assess other areas in robotic surgery. Although, the most important point to take into account is the cost of the learning curve from a financial and an outcomes standpoint. This will allow for a realistic view on the initial production of a robotics program.

8.4 Initial Purchasing and Maintenance Costs

The exact cost of establishing a robotics program is difficult to identify because each institution will negotiate its own pricing and service contract. Additionally, the surgical volume and reimbursement rates at each institution will offset the costs over differing time periods. Based on company estimates, the average purchase cost of a new da Vinci© platform is estimated at $1.33 million dollars. It is standard for the maintenance contract to begin in the second year, with costs ranging from $140 K to $160 K depending upon the type of platform and the particulars of the contract. Additionally, the per case disposable costs must be utilized to determine fiscal viability. On average, the estimated instrument and accessory cost per procedure is $1,800, ranging from $1,300 to $2,200. As previously stated, these are "ballpark" figures and will vary from institution to institution but can be used as estimates when considering purchase of a robotic system.

8.5 Robotic Surgical Procedures Currently Offered

The list of procedures being performed with robotic assistance is ever increasing. As more surgeons of all fields gain experience with robotic techniques, many previous open and laparoscopic procedures are being performed with robotic assistance. At our institution the primary fields utilizing the robot are urology and

Table 8.1 Robotic urological procedures

Urologic procedures
Radical prostatectomy
Radical/partial nephrectomy
Pyeloplasty
Nephroureterectomy
Radical/ partial cystectomy
Ureteral reimplantation
Bladder diverticulectomy
Simple prostatectomy
Sacrocolpopexy
Pelvic lymphadenectomy
Inguinal lymphadenectomy
Retroperitoneal lymphadenectomy

gynecology, but elsewhere, cardiac, general, otolaryngology, and pediatric surgical fields are exploring the usefulness and efficacy of robotic surgery. A complete list of surgical procedures described and performed with robotic assistance will potentially include all surgical procedures. Many of the commonly performed or described urologic procedures are listed in Table 8.1.

This list is clearly not exhaustive, even for the field of urology, and new applications for robotic surgery are constantly being described.

8.6 Facility Planning

8.6.1 Operating Room Requirements

Ideally an institution must have an operating room that can accommodate the robot, console, anesthesia cart, operating bed, nursing tables, and ancillary supplies necessary and still provide enough space to safely and efficiently navigate around the room. Optimally, the facility should have an operating room that is purely dedicated to robotic surgery. This will avoid the timely and arduous task of transferring the robotic between rooms. It will also avoid any damages that may occur during transport. The proper setup is essential to the development of an efficient operating room. The operating room must be well positioned and it is recommended to troubleshoot potential equipment malfunctions and have backup materials regularly accessible. A well thought-out operating room will save countless time during the initial cases when the robotics team is familiarizing themselves with the new equipment.

Having a sales representative available may also be beneficial during initial cases. This may seem like a daunting task although with proper planning, a recent study showed that a functional robotic surgical suite can be accomplished with dedicated engineers, trained surgical team members, a streamlined surgical setup, and efficient surgical technique[19].

8.6.2 The Robotics Team

Once the physical plant of the operating room is setup appropriately, the creation of a functioning robotics team is imperative to the success of the program. The ability of the operating room staff can make or break a program, therefore consistency of staff is necessary to avoid delays. The nursing staff are of particular importance, as they are needed to configure the appropriate instrumentation and troubleshoot any technical difficulties with the equipment during the procedure. A well-trained nursing staff allows the console surgeon to focus completely on the technical aspects of the procedure. Robotic surgery is unique in that the primary surgeon is not at the operating field, therefore the training and knowledge of the first assistant, as well as the nursing staff, plays a larger role in these procedures. Given the complexity of robotic procedures, it is often recommended to place an additional staff member in the room during initial cases. This will allow one staff member to focus on the machinery, while the other two focus on the patient.

8.6.3 Necessary Equipment

Guidelines regarding particular equipment necessary for a successful robotics procedure are difficult to provide as different instruments may be optimal for different procedures. Additionally, surgeon preference for one instrument over another will significantly affect what instruments are to be used.

Standard open should be available or open during the case, particularly early in the surgeon's experience. Though a rare occurrence, conversion to an open approach is more common early in a surgeon's learning curve and it is therefore recommended to have

this equipment readily available. As the operating surgeon gains experience and skill, this equipment will likely not be needed as rapidly but should however be available.

It is beneficial to have a standard set of nondisposable laparoscopic graspers and scissors at the beginning of robotic procedures. These will be useful for the bedside assistant during the operation but may also prove beneficial prior to docking of the robot, particularly in situations where adhesions limit insertion of secondary trocars. In addition to the standard laparoscopic instrumentation, a hot water bottle or thermos can prove invaluable to prevent fogging at the outset of the procedure and to clean the lens during the operation.

As mentioned above, the specific robotic tools will vary for different procedures and different surgeons. In general, a collection of various graspers (bipolar fenestrated, Maryland dissectors, and ProGrasp), a pair of needle drivers, and cutting instruments (monopolar scissors, hook) will suffice for the majority of urologic procedures. A full and growing catalog of available robotic instrumentation is available at Intuitive Surgical's Web site. It is recommended that the operating surgeon thoroughly review all previous descriptions, techniques, and instrumentation of any operation before attempting a new procedure.

8.6.4 Training Programs

Once you have established a robotics program, the focus shifts toward training. Properly training the next generation of robotics surgeons is a key aspect to maintaining a successful program. Although many residents are receiving more robotic experience during their core residency training, in a recent survey, only 38% of residents were satisfied with their laparoscopic training[20]. Robotic fellowship is currently available in many forms to aid in becoming a competent robotic surgeon. Although the term fellowship trained must be approached with caution as it is a broad term and can range from a 5 day program to a 2 year accredited fellowship. Ultimately, as robotic surgery continues to grow, it will be important to increase exposure in residency.

As with many surgical procedures, surgical volume and experience can be directly related and linked to outcomes and complications[21]. This is particularly important in robotics. The robotics training process is evolving alongside the increasing procedures and thus new training programs need to be established[22]. One limitation to robotics training is that due to the high cost of the robot, a training robot is not generally available. Hopefully, as equipment becomes more affordable, this will become common place as it has been shown that training in a nonclinical environment can carry over to the operating room[23,24]. Other concerns about training programs include whether having trainees involved from the start of the programs will affect the learning curve. Schroeck et al.[25] conducted a study to see how trainees affected the learning curve in RARP. They concluded that the trainees did not affect the learning curve and that outcomes were highly dependent on the skills of their mentor.

8.7 Research and Outcomes

Research efforts can be extremely beneficial in maintaining an effective and efficient robotics program. It is important to record outcome measures from the start, followed by regular internal reviews of your robotics program. This will assure quality control and diagnose any deficiencies in your program. An internal review should be carried out every year and ways to improve your program should be discussed throughout your robotics team. These internal reviews are particularly important during the first years of the program. By searching for and solving problems from the inside, this will avoid countless problems in years to come and lead to an efficiently run program. Published research can also be carried out to document the success of your program to the public. By conducting outcomes research, patients can study your literature and feel more confident about having a procedure at your institution.

Along with internal audits, yearly reviews, and review of published literature on outcomes, it is beneficial to create a database of all robotic procedures performed. Included in this database would ideally be pre-operative characteristics, intra-operative data (i.e., time required to complete particular steps, blood loss, and complications), and post-operative outcomes, both oncologic and functional. By doing this procedure over

and over again, week to week, overall improvements can be monitored. This data can then be monitored and provide rapid feedback on potentially necessary alterations in technique, such as wider excision in the case of an increasingly positive margin rate.

8.8 Establishing a Plan of Action – Is Robotics Program Sustainable at Your Institution?

After a well thought-out analysis, you have to ask whether a robotics program is right for your institution. If it is, then use the above information to formulate a well thought-out and detailed plan of action. Robotic surgery is here to stay and making the effort to create a sustainable program toward the beginning of the robotics movement will pay large dividends in the future.

References

1. Patel VR, Chammas MF Jr., Shah S. Robotic assisted laparoscopic radical prostatectomy: a review of the current state of affairs. *Int J Clin Pract*. 2007;61:309.
2. Grundfest WS, Culjat MO, King CH, et al. Development and testing of a tactile feedback system for robotic surgery. *Stud Health Technol Inform*. 2009;142:103.
3. Menon M, Shrivastava A, Bhandari M, et al. Vattikuti Institute Prostatectomy: technical modifications in 2009. *Eur Urol*. 2009;56:89.
4. Guru KA, Perlmutter AE, Sheldon MJ, et al. Apical margins after robot-assisted radical prostatectomy: does technique matter? *J Endourol*. 2009;23:123.
5. Menon M, Tewari A, Baize B, et al. Prospective comparison of radical retropubic prostatectomy and robot-assisted anatomic prostatectomy: the Vattikuti Urology Institute experience. *Urology*. 2002;60:864.
6. Ahlering TE, Woo D, Eichel L, et al. Robot-assisted versus open radical prostatectomy: a comparison of one surgeon's outcomes. *Urology*. 2004;63:819.
7. Hoekstra AV, Morgan JM, Lurain JR, et al. Robotic surgery in gynecologic oncology: impact on fellowship training. *Gynecol Oncol*. 2009;56:89.
8. Casale P. Robotic pediatric urology. *Curr Urol Rep*. 2009;10:115.
9. Morgan JA, Thornton BA, Peacock JC, et al. Does robotic technology make minimally invasive cardiac surgery too expensive? A hospital cost analysis of robotic and conventional techniques. *J Card Surg*. 2005;20:246.

10. Bultitude MF, Murphy D, Challacombe B, et al. Patient perception of robotic urology. *BJU Int*. 2009;103:285.

11. Lotan Y, Cadeddu JA, Gettman MT. The new economics of radical prostatectomy: cost comparison of open, laparoscopic and robot assisted techniques. *J Urol*. 2004;172:1431.

12. Scales CD Jr., Jones PJ, Eisenstein EL, et al. Local cost structures and the economics of robot assisted radical prostatectomy. *J Urol*. 2005;174:2323.

13. Steinberg PL, Merguerian PA, Bihrle W 3rd, et al. The cost of learning robotic-assisted prostatectomy. *Urology*. 2008;72:1068.

14. Burgess SV, Atug F, Castle EP, et al. Cost analysis of radical retropubic, perineal, and robotic prostatectomy. *J Endourol*. 2006;20:827.

15. Atug F, Castle EP, Srivastav SK, et al. Positive surgical margins in robotic-assisted radical prostatectomy: impact of learning curve on oncologic outcomes. *Eur Urol*. 2006;49:866.

16. Smith JA Jr., Chan RC, Chang SS, et al. A comparison of the incidence and location of positive surgical margins in robotic assisted laparoscopic radical prostatectomy and open retropubic radical prostatectomy. *J Urol*. 2007;178:2385.

17. Miller J, Smith A, Kouba E, et al. Prospective evaluation of short-term impact and recovery of health related quality of life in men undergoing robotic assisted laparoscopic radical prostatectomy versus open radical prostatectomy. *J Urol*. 2007;178:854.

18. Gianino MM, Galzerano M, Tizzani A, et al. Critical issues in current comparative and cost analyses between retropubic and robotic radical prostatectomy. *BJU Int*. 2008;101:2.

19. Coon TM. Integrating robotic technology into the operating room. *Am J Orthop*. 2009;38:7.

20. Duchene DA, Moinzadeh A, Gill IS, et al. Survey of residency training in laparoscopic and robotic surgery. *J Urol*. 2006;176:2158.

21. Klein EA, Bianco FJ, Serio AM, et al. Surgeon experience is strongly associated with biochemical recurrence after radical prostatectomy for all preoperative risk categories. *J Urol*. 2008;179:2212.

22. Amodeo A, Linares Quevedo A, Joseph JV, et al. Robotic laparoscopic surgery: cost and training. *Minerva Urol Nefrol*. 2009;61:121.

23. Sturm LP, Windsor JA, Cosman PH, et al. A systematic review of skills transfer after surgical simulation training. *Ann Surg*. 2008;248:166.

24. Tsuda S, Scott D, Doyle J, et al. Surgical skills training and simulation. *Curr Probl Surg*. 2009;46:271.

25. Schroeck FR, de Sousa CA, Kalman RA, et al. Trainees do not negatively impact the institutional learning curve for robotic prostatectomy as characterized by operative time, estimated blood loss, and positive surgical margin rate. *Urology*. 2008;71:597.

Chapter 9

Witnessing the Transition of Open to Robotic Surgery

John B. Malcolm, Michael D. Fabrizio, and Paul F. Schellhammer

9.1 Introduction

A paradigm shift has occurred in urologic surgery over the past 2 decades. Whereas the guiding principle of surgery – exposure – was formerly envisioned as a larger incision, it is now conceptualized as a video monitor, a laparoscope, and well-positioned trocars. In its infancy, basic diagnostic and extirpative laparoscopy demonstrated substantial clinical advantages over open surgery and introductory laparoscopic skills proved to be readily transferable. However, with more complex reconstructive laparoscopic procedures in urology, a steep learning curve has impeded widespread progress. In the context of this surgical transition, robotic technology is now playing a defining role, facilitating dissemination of increasingly complex laparoscopic procedures in urology.

9.2 A History of Robotic Technology

The first successful merger of robotic technology and surgery came with the Puma 560 robot. It was first used in 1985 to improve the precision of neurosurgical biopsies.[1] A few years later an automated system was developed for transurethral resection of the prostate in the first robotic urologic surgery.[2,3] Since then, a number of robotic surgical systems have been developed, with varying degrees of clinical application in urology.

J.B. Malcolm (✉)
Eastern Virginia Medical School/Urology of Virginia, Norfolk, VA, USA
e-mail: jbmalcol@sentara.com

Fixed path, or off-line, systems require no direct guidance from the surgeon. They are preprogrammed to execute precise movements within a space defined by preoperative imaging studies. Examples of fixed path systems include the Probot, which was designed in 1989 at the Imperial College in London for automated resection of the prostate,[2] and the PAKY device for percutaneous renal access (Fig. 9.1).[5] Off-line systems generally lack versatility and have not been widely utilized in urology.

Online systems are designed to mimic or replicate the surgeon's movements in real time in the surgical field. Online systems include endoscopic manipulators ("intern replacement" robotic systems), such as the Automated Endoscopic System for Optimal Positioning (AESOP; Intuitive Surgical, Inc., Sunnyvale, CA), and the more complex master–slave systems, such as the Zeus (Computer Motion, Inc., Goleta, CA) and da Vinci surgical robots (Intuitive Surgical, Inc., Sunnyvale, CA). Master–slave systems are composed of a control console and a mechanical device that performs directed tasks in the surgical field. The master–slave system has been the most versatile and clinically successful robotic platform. In 2000 and 2001, the FDA approved the da Vinci and Zeus surgical systems for use in laparoscopic surgery in humans. However, following the merger of Computer Motion and Intuitive Surgical in 2003, the Zeus became obsolete while the da Vinci Surgical System has become the pre-eminent robotic system in use today. The da Vinci's binocular optics provides 3D visualization, and the wristed instruments offer 7 degrees of freedom for precise maneuvering with tremor-free movement. The ergonomic console provides a comfortable working environment for the surgeon.[6] Although limitations include high start-up and maintenance costs, large size,

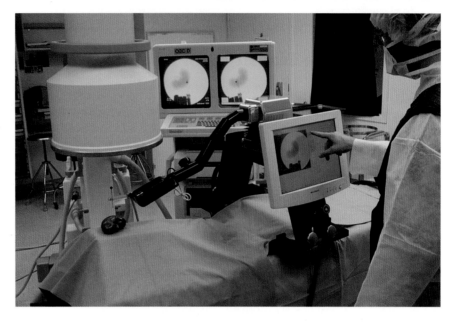

Fig. 9.1 Percutaneous access to the kidney (PAKY) device mounted to an operating room table with the injector positioned under a fluoroscopic C-arm. The PAKY is a fixed path robotic system with a passive arm allowing 6 degrees of freedom and an active injector for percutaneous renal access (*from* Kim and Schulam[4] with permission. Copyright © 2007 B.C., Decker Inc.)

and lack of haptic feedback, the da Vinci Surgical System is a tremendous technological achievement. Indeed, it has been the catalyst for the current robotic revolution in urologic surgery. Against the backdrop of widespread enthusiasm for, but limited success with, complex laparoscopic procedures in urology in the early twenty-first century, the da Vinci bridged a difficult technical divide and ushered in a new surgical era.

9.3 Robotic-Assisted Laparoscopic Radical Prostatectomy

The most commonly performed robotic procedure in urology today is the robotic-assisted radical prostatectomy (RAP). Robotic prostatectomy first came on the scene in 2000. Over the ensuing decade, RAP has rapidly grown in popularity, becoming a treatment of choice for patients and physicians alike. Over 60% of all radical prostatectomies performed in the United States in 2007 were performed with robotic assistance (Intuitive Surgical data, Sunnyvale, CA). At many centers, including our institution, RAP has replaced open radical prostatectomy (ORP) as the primary surgical treatment for localized prostate cancer.

The robotic prostatectomy was pioneered by Menon and colleagues at the Vattikuti Urology Institute in

an effort to bridge the difficult gap between open and laparoscopic prostatectomy. After laparoscopic nephrectomy demonstrated notable improvements in pain, blood loss, length of hospital stay, and convalescence compared to open nephrectomy,[7] efforts were made to extend similar benefits to radical prostatectomy. Laparoscopic radical prostatectomy (LRP) was reported by Clayman, Kavoussi, and Schuessler in 1997,[8] and the initial experience was discouraging. The challenges of working with 2D imaging and rigid instrumentation translated into prolonged operative times, increased perioperative complications, and outcomes that did not measure up to the time-tested and refined ORP. However, subsequent efforts by Guillonneau and Vallancian in France indicated that progress could be made toward a minimally invasive approach to radical prostatectomy. The Montsouris experience with LRP in 120 patients was published in 2000. This experience demonstrated the feasibility of the operation with evidence of oncologic efficacy and good functional outcomes in expert hands, albeit with prolonged operative times.[9] Although enthusiasm for LRP grew and favorable outcomes were reported,[9–12] the procedure was considered by many to be exceedingly difficult to master with a prohibitively prolonged and morbid learning curve. For surgeons with limited prior laparoscopic experience, the learning period for LRP could amount to 80–100 consecutive cases, extending over several years.[13]

In an effort to minimize the complications incurred during the learning curve, Fabrizio and colleagues at our institution utilized a mentored approach for the LRP. Dr. Ingolf Tuerk, having performed over 200 LRPs, was employed from March 2001 to August 2001 to mentor a fellowship trained laparoscopic surgeon (MDF) through the initial experience with LRP. We noted a significantly reduced learning curve with 30 mentored procedures but concluded that a minimum of 50 cases were required to produce consistent operative results.[14]

Similarly, Menon and colleagues initiated a mentored program for LRP at the Vattikuti Urology Institute under the mentorship of Drs. Guy Vallancien and Bertrand Guillonneau. They incorporated the da Vinci Surgical System into the program in hopes that the robotic platform might flatten the learning curve for a laparoscopic-naïve surgeon. Based on a preliminary analysis of this experience, the 3D visualization and wristed instrumentation of the robotic platform appeared to make laparoscopic prostatectomy accessible to an experienced open surgeon with no laparoscopic experience.[15] During the preliminary experience with 40 robotic prostatectomies, Menon and colleagues were able to achieve results that were similar to the "best-in-class" values for laparoscopic prostatectomy, including mean blood loss of 256 mL, 0% transfusion rate, 0% conversion rate, and 17% positive margin rate. Operative times diminished rapidly, with an overall mean time of 4.5 h and a trend toward accelerated operative efficiency. The relatively favorable learning curve for RAP would become a subject of considerable interest and a boon to broad incorporation or robotic assistance in urologic surgery.

9.3.1 RAP: The Learning Curve

Numerous authors have described the learning curve – or time required to achieve technical proficiency – for RAP. Because definitions of surgical proficiency or expertise may vary between surgeons, defining the learning curve may also be quite variable.[16] However, operative times, blood loss, and positive margin rates offer quantifiable benchmarks by which to evaluate the learning process with robotic prostatectomy.

Almost universally, acceptable operative times are readily achievable for the novice robotic prostatectomist, even if laparoscopically naïve. During the development phase of RAP at the Vattikuti Urology Institute, it took 18 cases for RAP operative times to become faster than LRP operative times.[15] Ahlering was able to achieve 4-h proficiency with robotic prostatectomy after 12 cases, with no prior laparoscopic experience and following a 1-day robotic training course.[13] While robotic prostatectomy was developed and pioneered at academic centers, Patel et al. demonstrated that robotic prostatectomy programs could also be developed at community hospitals, with a similarly favorable learning curve. Time to 4-h proficiency in their early experience was 20 cases. Operative times improved steadily, comparing favorably with LRP very early in the experience and ultimately comparing favorably with ORP, which remained the reference standard. The first 50 cases averaged just over 200 min and decreased to just over 100 min after 150 cases.[17]

Blood loss is consistently low during the learning curve for RAP. In point of fact, the reduced blood loss associated with robotic prostatectomy is one of the few undeniable advantages for robotic prostatectomy over ORP, and this advantage can be achieved with limited experience. Average blood loss early in the learning curve has been reported to range from 150 to 250 mL, and transfusions are uncommon.[13,15,17,18]

Positive margin rates during early experience with RAP have been variable – ranging from 13 to 45%.[13,15,17,19] Similar variability is seen in mature series of open, laparoscopic, and robotic prostatectomy and is not entirely attributable to the influence of the learning curve for RAP.[20,21]

9.3.2 RAP: Positive Margins and Oncologic Outcomes

The primary objective of radical prostatectomy is cancer control, and oncologic outcomes remain the critical measure for validation of any prostate cancer treatment. Because RAP is still a relatively new procedure, meaningful reports on biochemical-free survival, metastasis-free survival, and cancer-specific survival are limited. Therefore, the oncologic efficacy of RAP has been described largely in terms of positive margin rates.

Among early and mature robotic prostatectomy series reported in the literature, positive margin rates have varied widely from 2 to 59%.[22,23] Such variability reflects numerous biases, including lack of standardized analysis and reporting of pathologic specimens, heterogeneity of tumor grade and stage, and variability of surgeon experience and expertise. A consistent finding in the literature is a progressive reduction in positive margin rates with increasing surgeon experience. In the experience of Atug et al., positive margin rates decreased from 45, to 21, to 11% over the first 100 RAP cases analyzed as three consecutive groups of 33.[19] A similar trend was reported by Menon et al., with 7 and 4% positive margin rates for T2 disease in the first 200 and last 200 patients of a 2,766-patient series.[24] In the community setting, Patel et al. reported positive margin rates of 13% in the first 100 cases and 8% in the subsequent 100 cases.[17] Just as with ORP,[25] surgeon experience and technique appear to be a significant factor in positive margin rates following RAP. Nevertheless, positive margin rates equivalent to the best ORP experiences have been achieved with RAP.

A number of surgeons with significant experience with both open and robotic prostatectomy have compared margin rates between the two approaches in an effort to determine whether RAP is equivalent, inferior, or superior to ORP with respect to positive margin rates. Smith et al. compared margin rates between 200 consecutive ORPs and 200 RAPs, finding a significant advantage for RAP with 15% PSM vs. 35% for ORP.[26] Although critique of this report highlighted the fact that the two cohorts were not matched for preoperative positive margin risk factors, the statistically significant advantage for RAP remained when the comparison was limited to patients with pathologic T2 disease and Gleason 6 or less disease. Tewari et al. also found the positive margin rates were lower with RAP compared to ORP (9% vs. 23%).[27] In contrast, Ahlering found no significant difference in margin status in a comparative analysis of 60 RAPs and 60 ORPs (16.7% vs. 20%).[28] Although the available evidence is not definitive, it seems possible that with experience surgeons may be able to achieve better margin free rates with RAP than with ORP. In the final analysis, however, irrespective of surgical approach, margin rates will be most dependent on the pathologist's assessment – which may be subjective, preoperative risk factors – which are not modifiable, and surgeon technique –

which can always be improved upon with further experience.

9.3.3 RAP: Functional Outcomes

In experienced hands, RAP has been associated with excellent functional outcomes. From Menon's 12-month follow-up data on 1889 patients treated with robotic prostatectomy, 93% of patients were "socially dry" at 12 months, as defined by use of 1 pad or less per day, with a mean time to urinary control of 3 weeks.[24] Among patients with normal preoperative erectile function (SHIM score > 22), 82% reported successful sexual intercourse following robotic prostatectomy (44% required PDE5 therapy).[24] With a 500-case experience with robotic prostatectomy, Patel reported complete continence in 89 and 95% of patients at 3 and 6 months, respectively, and 12-month potency rates of 78% (with or without the use of PDE5 therapy).[29]

Functional outcomes have also been favorable with less robust experience. In Ahlering's first 45 robotic prostatectomies, 81% of patients reported being pad free at 3 months of follow-up. In Patel's first 200 cases, 82 and 98% of patients were pad-free at 3 and 12 months, respectively. In the early experience of Costello et al., 73% of patients used 0–1 pads at 3 months.[30] Erectile function outcomes have been more difficult to optimize early in the learning curve for RAP, and potency rates of 20–66% have been more typical for surgeons with less experience.[31–33]

Although numerous authors have reported excellent results with robotic prostatectomy, functional outcomes are indeed variable. They depend on many factors including surgeon experience, pretreatment urinary and sexual function, and means of evaluating and reporting functional outcomes. Numerous methodologies have been used to define functional outcomes after prostate cancer treatment. These have included retrospective, cross-sectional, and prospective studies based on chart review, interviews, and various questionnaires. As such, reported functional outcomes must be understood in the context of the metrics used to evaluate them. Direct comparisons of functional outcomes for open and robotic prostatectomy are problematic because outcomes analysis and reporting have not been standardized in the literature. A paucity of published studies is available with "apples to apples" comparisons of ORP and RAP functional outcomes. Tewari et al. reported a single institution experience with robotic and open prostatectomy and found that RAP allowed earlier return of urinary continence and potency than ORP.[27] At our center, we have used sequential UCLA-PCI questionnaires to prospectively evaluate 135 patients treated with open prostatectomy and 447 patients treated with robotic prostatectomy. In terms of return to baseline urinary function and sexual function, no statistically significant differences were observed between the two treatment groups.[34] Although RAP has replaced ORP as the surgical treatment of choice at our institution, we remain careful not to overstate the functional advantages of robotic prostatectomy relative to open prostatectomy.

9.3.4 RAP: Conclusions

From its infancy in 2000 until now, robotic prostatectomy has achieved mainstream status in a remarkably short period of time. It has proven to be a safe procedure with low rates of perioperative complications. Blood loss is lower than with open prostatectomy. The rise of robotic prostatectomy has fostered application of new clinical care pathways that facilitate earlier hospital discharge and catheter removal.[27,35,36] The da Vinci Surgical System has allowed urologists with or without prior laparoscopic expertise to perform a highly complex minimally invasive dissection, extirpation, and reconstruction, and the learning curve to 4-h proficiency has been relatively short in most reports. Positive margin rates have been comparable and long-term oncologic control will likely prove equivalent to open prostatectomy. Functional outcomes are variable and, as Menon writes, "robotic radical prostatectomy, like golf, is easy to learn, but difficult to master."[37]

The increased cost associated with robotic prostatectomy remains an unsolved problem. Cost analyses have suggested that because of reduced hospital expenses associated with shorter length of stay, RAP could be cost-effective for high-volume centers.[38] However, most centers with robotics programs do not maintain the 10–14 case per week volume needed to attain cost equivalence or cost benefit with ORP. Robotic prostatectomy has flourished in the United States despite increased costs, but cost concerns have limited the application of RAP in many countries.

With further limitations on resources, health-care policy may well have an impact on future utilization of robotic prostatectomy in the United States.

Nevertheless, the development of RAP has been a watershed event in the evolution of urologic surgery. The successes attributed to RAP have paved the way for the myriad applications of robotics in urology today, and RAP remains the introductory procedure for urologists endeavoring to develop robotic surgical skills.

9.4 Robotic-Assisted Laparoscopic Pyeloplasty

Open pyeloplasty has been the gold standard therapy for ureteropelvic junction (UPJ) obstruction with long-term success rates consistently exceeding 90%.[39,40] However, the open procedure may be associated with significant morbidity including pain, prolonged convalescence, flank bulge, and undesirable cosmesis. Efforts to reduce the morbidity associated with open pyeloplasty spawned the development of endoscopic treatments such as laser endopyelotomy or electrosurgical cutting balloon endopyelotomy. These treatments are well tolerated and are generally easy to perform with minimal morbidity, but long-term success rates are inferior to pyeloplasty. Conventional laparoscopic pyeloplasty achieves success rates comparable to open pyeloplasty and with less morbidity.[41–43] However, the laparoscopic reconstruction with intracorporeal suturing can be challenging. This technical challenge was a significant obstacle to widespread utilization of laparoscopic pyeloplasty. The da Vinci Surgical System has helped to overcome the challenges of intracorporeal suturing, and many urologists now prefer robotic pyeloplasty as the treatment of choice for high-grade UPJ obstruction.

The feasibility of robotic pyeloplasty was first demonstrated in a porcine model by Sung et al. in 1999.[44] Subsequent published case series indicated that the procedure translated well into clinical practice, with short-term outcomes comparable to conventional laparoscopic pyeloplasty.[45,46] Long-term outcomes are now available and, as anticipated, the results from robotic pyeloplasty are comparable to open and laparoscopic pyeloplasty, with long-term success rates exceeding 95%.[47,48]

Comparative studies of conventional laparoscopic and robotic pyeloplasty have not shown substantial advantages for one technique over the other. In a recent systematic review and meta-analysis of the available literature, robotic pyeloplasty was associated with a 10-min reduction in operative times and a 0.5-day reduction in hospital length of stay. Complication and success rates were equivalent.[49] Nevertheless, to our knowledge few urologists have favored conventional laparoscopic pyeloplasty after gaining experience with robotic pyeloplasty. To the contrary, even those experienced in laparoscopic pyeloplasty have appreciated the assistance of a robotic platform. In our experience, having performed over 175 laparoscopic prostatectomies and pyeloplasties before transitioning to robotic pyeloplasty, we have relished the benefits of the robotic platform – improved visibility, delicate tissue handling, improved ergonomics, and ease of the sutured anastomosis. Although these benefits are difficult to quantify and may not translate into demonstrably improved outcomes, we have no desire to return to conventional laparoscopic pyeloplasty now that the robotic platform is available.

The increased financial cost associated with robotic pyeloplasty remains the primary drawback to the transition from laparoscopic pyeloplasty.[50] The considerable inertia of market forces, novelty, patient and physician satisfaction have carried robotic pyeloplasty forward despite the increased cost. It is likely that ongoing technological advances, increased utilization, and decreased costs will continue to advance the application of robotic pyeloplasty.

9.5 Robotic-Assisted Laparoscopic Partial Nephrectomy

Momentum seems to be building for robotic partial nephrectomy (RPN). Partial nephrectomy (PN) has emerged as the preferred option for management of small renal masses, with improved renal functional outcomes and equivalent oncologic outcomes compared to radical nephrectomy (RN).[51,52] While laparoscopic partial nephrectomy (LPN) has advanced the management of small renal masses still further, it is a difficult procedure to master and has been associated with higher rates of postoperative complications, even in the most expert hands.[53] Because of the technical complexity of LPN, the procedure remains inaccessible to many urologists.

The first reports of RPN came from Gettman and colleagues at the Mayo Clinic and Stifelman and Taneja at New York University.[54,55] Initial reports demonstrated feasibility for certain well-selected candidates (anterior, small, exophytic tumors). However, neither of the initial reports made a particularly strong case for RPN. In comparison to a LPN cohort, Stifelman and Taneja found no advantages for RPN with respect to operative time, ischemia time, blood loss, hospital stay, change in creatinine, and change in hematocrit.[54] Both groups noted the disadvantages of increased cost and setup time for RPN. In addition, they noted that while LPN can be performed with one primary surgeon and an assistant, two experienced surgeons are needed for RPN; since the console surgeon is not scrubbed, the tableside "assistant" must be equipped to handle a conversion in the event of an emergency. Furthermore, renal hilar control is managed by the assistant, not the console surgeon.

Urologists have continued to pioneer RPN, and with growing experience some favorable outcomes are emerging. Bhayani's experience with 102 consecutive patients treated with LPN ($N = 62$) and then RPN ($N = 40$) demonstrated significantly reduced operative time (140 vs. 156 min), ischemia time (19 vs. 25 min), and length of stay for RPN (2.5 vs. 2.9 days).[56] Rogers et al. reported experience with RPN for more challenging renal hilar tumors, with favorable results.[57] In an unscientific but interesting comparison to the results of a far more experienced laparoscopic surgeon with LPN for renal hilar tumors,[58] Rogers et al. noted shorter mean warm ischemia time (29 vs. 36 min) with a similar mean tumor size (3.8 vs. 3.7 cm) during RPN. This comparison suggests that surgeons with more modest experience can utilize the robotic platform to extend the benefits of laparoscopic partial nephrectomy to patients with more challenging tumors. This finding has been reproducible.[59] Another development in RPN is the utilization of the fourth robotic arm, which gives the console surgeon more control and minimizes dependence on the bedside assistant for hilar control.[57,60]

Robotic-assisted laparoscopic partial nephrectomy is still in its infancy. However, the confidence engendered by a vast experience with robotic prosta-tectomy seems to have produced among urologists a willingness to undertake RPN on a scale that did not exist with conventional LPN. If it continues to safely expand the application of minimally invasive nephron-sparing surgery, RPN will likely become increasingly routine.

9.6 Robotic-Assisted Laparoscopic Radical Cystectomy

In 2009, open radical cystectomy (ORC) remains the gold standard treatment for invasive bladder cancer. It has been standardized to offer reproducible long-term oncologic results.[61] However, even in the best of hands, ORC is associated with substantial morbidity,[62] both because of the nature of the disease and because of the nature of the operation. Consequently, urologists have explored minimally invasive options to minimize the morbidity of radical cystectomy, while seeking to maintain the oncologic standards established by the open approach.

Laparoscopic radical cystectomy (LRC) has been shown to be feasible, and it has compared favorably to ORP, with less postoperative pain and faster recovery in some studies.[63] However, like laparoscopic prosta-tectomy, LRC is a technically challenging procedure and has not been widely adopted.

A number of small series of robotic radical cystec-tomy (RRC) have been reported. Oncologic outcomes have been limited by short follow-up. Perioperative advantages have not been uniformly pronounced; how-ever, some advantages over ORC have been suggested with respect to earlier return of bowel function and more rapid post-operative convalescence.[64,65] Rhee et al. compared 7 RRCs to 23 ORCs, noting longer operative times (638 vs. 507 min) but shorter hospi-tal stay (11 vs. 13 days) for the robotic cohort.[64] Wang et al. compared 33 RRCs and 21 ORCs, also noting longer operative times (390 vs. 300 min) and shorter hospital stay for robotic cystectomy (5 vs. 8 days).[65] Currently, the largest reported experience with RRC consists of 50 cases performed by Pruthi and Wallen with a mean follow-up of 13 months. Although patients were generally well selected for favorable oncologic outcomes, pathologic results were acceptable with no positive margins and mean lymph node count of 19.[66] Importantly, a learning curve analysis indicated that while operative times and blood loss improved with experience, lymph node counts and margin status were not compromised early in the series.[67]

Robotic radical cystectomy is an emerging min-imally invasive treatment for bladder cancer. It is gaining popularity. Its advocates are challenged to standardize and refine the operation in the context of a very unforgiving malignancy that has long challenged the best efforts of open surgeons. Further progress with robotic cystectomy appears almost a certainty, but a rapid transition away from open cystectomy is unlikely.

9.7 Expanding Application and the Future of Robotics in Urology

As urologists have gained familiarity with robotic-assisted surgery, primarily via robotic-assisted radical prostatectomy, its application has spread almost with-out bounds. At our institution, robotic assistance has been used in adult and pediatric urology; it has been used for prostatectomy, partial nephrectomy, pyelo-plasty, radical cystectomy, sacrocolpopexy, ureteral surgery, and ileal neovagina. Urologists have applied robotic technology for appendicovesicostomy, antire-flux surgery, adrenalectomy, vasovasostomy, donor nephrectomy, fistula repairs, ureteral reimplantation, and more. The robotic revolution has arrived, and the transition toward broader and better utilization of robotic technology in urology continues.

The next frontiers in minimally invasive surgery, natural orifice translumenal endoscopic surgery (NOTES) and laparoendoscopic single-site surgery (LESS), have generated considerable enthusiasm among urologists in recent years. Offering the advan-tages of improved cosmesis and reduced abdominal wall trauma, numerous LESS urologic surgeries have been successfully performed, including simple nephrectomy, donor nephrectomy, partial nephrec-tomy, pyeloplasty, sacrocolpopexy, and radical prostatectomy.[68] LESS is technically more challeng-ing than conventional laparoscopy and has benefited from the development of novel instrumentation such as multichannel ports and both bent and flexible laparoscopic graspers, scissors, and needle drivers. Indeed, robotic assistance has also shown utility in LESS surgery and will likely be an essential component of broader application of complex single-site surgery in urology. Kaouk et al. recently reported the initial Cleveland Clinic experience with robotic single-port surgery in humans.[69] Radical prostatectomy, dismembered pyeloplasty, and radical prostatectomy were successfully performed without complication. Difficulties encountered in this proof of principle series included clashing of the robotic arms, which could be improved upon with a lower profile robotic platform or flexible robotic arms. Nevertheless, the authors suggest that robotic assistance, even with the currently available platform, should make complex single-port surgery more accessible to most urologists.

Transvaginal and transgastric NOTES nephrectomy has been investigated in a porcine model at a number of centers.[70,71] Relying on flexible endoscopic and rigid laparoscopic instrumentation, the initial experience in animal models highlighted the need for improved instrumentation for better tissue visualization, maneuvering, and dissection. Subsequently, robotic technology has been utilized to push NOTES forward. In 2008, Box and colleagues reported the first experience with robotic-assisted NOTES nephrectomy in a porcine model. A da Vinci S robot was docked to transvaginal and transcolonic ports and the porcine nephrectomy was completed in 150 min with no intraoperative complications.[72] In the same year, Haber et al. reported robotic-assisted NOTES partial nephrectomy, pyeloplasty, and completion nephrectomy in a porcine model.[73] They noted that the currently available robotic platform significantly enhanced intracorporeal suturing in NOTES reconstructive surgery. However, they called for further innovations to the available robotic technology in order to support efforts toward clinical applications of reconstructive NOTES in urology. Future clinical application of NOTES in urology is likely to go hand in hand with innovation in robotic platforms and instrumentation.

One of the challenges for robotic technology innovators will be to miniaturize the currently available platforms. The da Vinci S, although more streamlined than the first generation da Vinci robot, is bulky. It occupies significant space over the surgical field and, in addition to crowding the working space of the bedside assistant, its bulkiness often results in camera and instrument collisions. This limitation has been particularly apparent in some of the early work with NOTES and robotic-assisted LESS. Although inventive port placement has allowed surgeons to work around this obstacle, miniaturization of the robotic platform would go a lot farther. Efforts to minimize the extracorporeal size and motion of the robotic platform are already underway. While not commercially available, the Laprotek system (EndoVia Inc., Hansen Medical, Inc., Mountain View, CA) has been designed with smaller robotic arms that are mounted to the rails of the operating table (Fig. 9.2). The intracorporeal portion of the robotic arm utilizes a curved guide tube that controls up and down movements, while the extracorporeal component moves in a single plane rather than in a cone (da Vinci System). This minimizes the external working space required by the robotic platform. Dachs and Peine have streamlined this concept further, proposing a robotic arm with extracorporeal movements confined to a line. Six degrees of freedom are provided by joints on the intracorporeal component of the robotic arm (Fig. 9.3).[74]

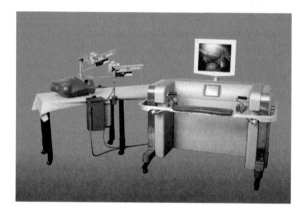

Fig. 9.2 Laprotek tool mounted to the operating table. The curved guide tube increases intracorporeal freedom of movement while confining extracorporeal movements to a single plane (*from* Dachs and Peine[74] with permission. Copyright © 2006 IEEE)

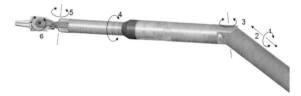

Fig. 9.3 Pictorial representation of a streamlined robotic arm allowing 6 df of movement intracorporeally, with extracorporeal movements confined to a single line (*from* Dachs and Peine[74] with permission. Copyright © 2006 IEEE)

In vivo microrobots have also been explored as a way to increase spatial freedom for robotic surgery. Rentschler and Oleynikov's group from the University of Nebraska has developed mobile and fixed-base cameras that can be deployed into the peritoneal cavity.[75] Similar prototypes supporting working instruments have also been considered. Although still early in conceptualization and development, in vivo microrobotic platforms could obviate the need for multiple incisions and access sites. Given the rapid rate of development in robotics technology in recent years, clinical application of deployable in vivo microrobots is not difficult to imagine in the near future.

9.8 Conclusions

The current decade has witnessed remarkable changes in the field of minimally invasive urologic surgery. Robotic-assisted surgery has moved from the fringes of medical science fiction to the mainstream of clinical urology, bringing with it an array of challenges, benefits, and opportunities. Urologists have embraced robotic technology and clinical ingenuity has flourished. The clinical benefits of this transition toward robotic surgery require continuous appraisal and valuation, as the cost of health care increasingly weighs in the balance against innovation. By most measures, robotic surgery in urology has been a profound success and the future holds even more promise.

References

1. Kwoh YS, Hou J, Jonckheere EA, et al. A robot with improved absolute positioning accuracy for CT guided stereotactic brain surgery. *IEEE Trans Biomed Eng.* 1988;35:153.
2. Davies BL, Hibberd RD, Coptcoat MJ, et al. A surgeon robot prostatectomy–a laboratory evaluation. *J Med Eng Technol.* 1989;13:273.
3. Ng WS, Davies BL, Timoney AG, et al. The use of ultrasound in automated prostatectomy. *Med Biol Eng Comput.* 1993;31:349.
4. Kim HL, Schulam P. Robotics: coming of age. In: Smith AD (ed) *Smith's textbook of endourology.* 2nd ed. Hamilton: BC Decker Inc.; 2007
5. Cadeddu JA, Stoianovici D, Chen RN, et al. Stereotactic mechanical percutaneous renal access. *J Endourol.* 1998;12:121.
6. Bagrodia A, Raman JD:. Ergonomics considerations of radical prostatectomy: physician perspective of open, laparoscopic, and robot-assisted techniques. *J Endourol.* 2009;23:627.
7. Dunn MD, Portis AJ, Shalhav AL, et al. Laparoscopic versus open radical nephrectomy: a 9-year experience. *J Urol.* 2000;164:1153.
8. Schuessler WW, Schulam PG, Clayman RV, et al. Laparoscopic radical prostatectomy: initial short-term experience. *Urology.* 1997;50:854.
9. Guillonneau B, Vallancien G:. Laparoscopic radical prostatectomy: the Montsouris technique. *J Urol.* 2000;163:1643.
10. Rassweiler J, Sentker L, Seemann O, et al. Laparoscopic radical prostatectomy with the Heilbronn technique: an analysis of the first 180 cases. *J Urol.* 2001;166:2101.
11. Olsson LE, Salomon L, Nadu A, et al. Prospective patient-reported continence after laparoscopic radical prostatectomy. *Urology.* 2001;58:570.
12. Turk I, Deger S, Winkelmann B, et al. Laparoscopic radical prostatectomy. Technical aspects and experience with 125 cases. *Eur Urol.* 2001;40:46.
13. Ahlering TE, Skarecky D, Lee D, et al. Successful transfer of open surgical skills to a laparoscopic environment using a robotic interface: initial experience with laparoscopic radical prostatectomy. *J Urol.* 2003;170:1738.
14. Fabrizio MD, Tuerk I, Schellhammer PF:. Laparoscopic radical prostatectomy: decreasing the learning curve using a mentor initiated approach. *J Urol.* 2003;169:2063.
15. Menon M, Shrivastava A, Tewari A, et al. Laparoscopic and robot assisted radical prostatectomy: establishment of a structured program and preliminary analysis of outcomes. *J Urol.* 2002;168:945.
16. Herrell SD, Smith JA Jr. Robotic-assisted laparoscopic prostatectomy: what is the learning curve? *Urology.* 2005;66:105.
17. Patel VR, Tully AS, Holmes R, et al. Robotic radical prostatectomy in the community setting–the learning curve and beyond: initial 200 cases. *J Urol.* 2005;174:269.
18. Hu JC, Nelson RA, Wilson TG, et al. Perioperative complications of laparoscopic and robotic assisted laparoscopic radical prostatectomy. *J Urol.* 2006;175:541.
19. Atug F, Castle EP, Srivastav SK, et al. Positive surgical margins in robotic-assisted radical prostatectomy: impact of learning curve on oncologic outcomes. *Eur Urol.* 2006;49:866.
20. Wieder JA, Soloway MS:. Incidence, etiology, location, prevention and treatment of positive surgical margins after radical prostatectomy for prostate cancer. *J Urol.* 1998;160:299.
21. Ficarra V, Cavalleri S, Novara G, et al. Evidence from robot-assisted laparoscopic radical prostatectomy: a systematic review. *Eur Urol.* 2007;51:45.
22. Menon M, Kaul S, Bhandari A, et al. Potency following robotic radical prostatectomy: a questionnaire based analysis of outcomes after conventional nerve sparing and prostatic fascia sparing techniques. *J Urol.* 2005;174:2291.
23. Sim HG, Yip SK, Lau WK, et al. Early experience with robot-assisted laparoscopic radical prostatectomy. *Asian J Surg.* 2004;27:321.

24. Badani KK, Kaul S, Menon M:. Evolution of robotic radical prostatectomy: assessment after 2766 procedures. *Cancer.* 2007;110:1951.

25. Eastham JA, Kattan MW, Riedel E, et al. Variations among individual surgeons in the rate of positive surgical margins in radical prostatectomy specimens. *J Urol.* 2003;170:2292.

26. Smith JA Jr, Chan RC, Chang SS, et al. A comparison of the incidence and location of positive surgical margins in robotic assisted laparoscopic radical prostatectomy and open retropubic radical prostatectomy. *J Urol.* 2007;178:2385.

27. Tewari A, Srivasatava A, Menon M:. A prospective comparison of radical retropubic and robot-assisted prostatectomy: experience in one institution. *BJU Int.* 2003;92:205.

28. Ahlering TE, Woo D, Eichel L, et al. Robot-assisted versus open radical prostatectomy: a comparison of one surgeon's outcomes. *Urology.* 2004;63:819.

29. Patel VR, Thaly R, Shah K:. Robotic radical prostatectomy: outcomes of 500 cases. *BJU Int.* 2007;99:1109.

30. Costello AJ, Haxhimolla H, Crowe H, et al. Installation of telerobotic surgery and initial experience with telerobotic radical prostatectomy. *BJU Int.* 2005;96:34.

31. Chien GW, Mikhail AA, Orvieto MA, et al. Modified clipless antegrade nerve preservation in robotic-assisted laparoscopic radical prostatectomy with validated sexual function evaluation. *Urology.* 2005;66:419.

32. Joseph JV, Rosenbaum R, Madeb R, et al. Robotic extraperitoneal radical prostatectomy: an alternative approach. *J Urol.* 2006;175:945.

33. Bentas W, Wolfram M, Jones J, et al. Robotic technology and the translation of open radical prostatectomy to laparoscopy: the early Frankfurt experience with robotic radical prostatectomy and one year follow-up. *Eur Urol.* 2003;44:175.

34. Malcolm JB, Fabrizio MD, Barone BB, et al. Quality of life after open or robotic prostatectomy, cryoablation or brachytherapy for localized prostate cancer. *J Urol.* 2010;183:1822.

35. Rocco B, Matei DV, Melegari S, et al. Robotic vs open prostatectomy in a laparoscopically naive centre: a matched-pair analysis. *BJU Int.* 2009;104:991.

36. Krambeck AE, DiMarco DS, Rangel LJ, et al. Radical prostatectomy for prostatic adenocarcinoma: a matched comparison of open retropubic and robot-assisted techniques. *BJU Int.* 2009;103:448.

37. Menon M, Shrivastava A, Kaul S, et al. Vattikuti Institute prostatectomy: contemporary technique and analysis of results. *Eur Urol.* 2007;51:648.

38. Scales CD Jr., Jones PJ, Eisenstein EL, et al. Local cost structures and the economics of robot assisted radical prostatectomy. *J Urol.* 2005;174:2323.

39. Lowe FC, Marshall FF:. Ureteropelvic junction obstruction in adults. *Urology.* 1984;23:331.

40. Persky L, Krause JR, Boltuch RL:. Initial complications and late results in dismembered pyeloplasty. *J Urol.* 1977;118:162.

41. Jarrett TW, Chan DY, Charambura TC, et al. Laparoscopic pyeloplasty: the first 100 cases. *J Urol.* 2002;167:1253.

42. Brooks JD, Kavoussi LR, Preminger GM, et al. Comparison of open and endourologic approaches to the obstructed ureteropelvic junction. *Urology.* 1995;46:791.

43. Chen RN, Moore RG, Kavoussi LR:. Laparoscopic pyeloplasty. Indications, technique, and long-term outcome. *Urol Clin North Am.* 1998;25:323.

44. Sung GT, Gill IS, Hsu TH:. Robotic-assisted laparoscopic pyeloplasty: a pilot study. *Urology.* 1999;53:1099.

45. Weise ES, Winfield HN:. Robotic computer-assisted pyeloplasty versus conventional laparoscopic pyeloplasty. *J Endourol.* 2006;20:813.

46. Gettman MT, Neururer R, Bartsch G, et al. Anderson-Hynes dismembered pyeloplasty performed using the da Vinci robotic system. *Urology.* 2002;60:509.

47. Mufarrij PW, Woods M, Shah OD, et al. Robotic dismembered pyeloplasty: a 6-year, multi-institutional experience. *J Urol.* 2008;180:1391.

48. Schwentner C, Pelzer A, Neururer R, et al. Robotic anderson-hynes pyeloplasty: 5-year experience of one centre. *BJU Int.* 2007;100:880.

49. Braga LH, Pace K, Demaria J, et al. Systematic review and meta-analysis of robotic-assisted versus conventional laparoscopic pyeloplasty for patients with ureteropelvic junction obstruction: effect on operative time, length of hospital stay, postoperative complications, and success rate. *Eur Urol.* 2009;56:848.

50. Bhayani SB, Link RE, Varkarakis JM, et al. Complete da Vinci versus laparoscopic pyeloplasty: cost analysis. *J Endourol.* 2005;19:327.

51. Huang WC, Levey AS, Serio AM, et al. Chronic kidney disease after nephrectomy in patients with renal cortical tumours: a retrospective cohort study. *Lancet Oncol.* 2006;7:735.

52. Fergany AF, Hafez KS, Novick AC:. Long-term results of nephron sparing surgery for localized renal cell carcinoma: 10-year followup. *J Urol.* 2000;163:442.

53. Gill IS, Kavoussi LR, Lane BR, et al. Comparison of 1,800 laparoscopic and open partial nephrectomies for single renal tumors. *J Urol.* 2007;178:41.

54. Caruso RP, Phillips CK, Kau E, et al. Robot assisted laparoscopic partial nephrectomy: initial experience. *J Urol.* 2006;176:36.

55. Gettman MT, Blute ML, Chow GK, et al. Robotic-assisted laparoscopic partial nephrectomy: technique and initial clinical experience with da Vinci robotic system. *Urology.* 2004;64:914.

56. Wang AJ, Bhayani SB. Robotic partial nephrectomy versus laparoscopic partial nephrectomy for renal cell carcinoma: single-surgeon analysis of >100 consecutive procedures. *Urology.* 2009;73:306.

57. Rogers CG, Metwalli A, Blatt AM, et al. Robotic partial nephrectomy for renal hilar tumors: a multi-institutional analysis. *J Urol.* 2008;180:2353.

58. Gill IS, Colombo JR Jr., Frank I, et al. Laparoscopic partial nephrectomy for hilar tumors. *J Urol.* 2005;174:850.

59. Deane LA, Lee HJ, Box GN, et al. Robotic versus standard laparoscopic partial/wedge nephrectomy: a comparison of intraoperative and perioperative results from a single institution. *J Endourol.* 2008;22:947.

60. Kaul S, Laungani R, Sarle R, et al. da Vinci-assisted robotic partial nephrectomy: technique and results at a mean of 15 months of follow-up. *Eur Urol*. 2007;51:186.

61. Herr H, Lee C, Chang S, et al. Standardization of radical cystectomy and pelvic lymph node dissection for bladder cancer: a collaborative group report. *J Urol*. 2004;171:1823.

62. Lowrance WT, Rumohr JA, Chang SS, et al. Contemporary open radical cystectomy: analysis of perioperative outcomes. *J Urol*. 2008;179:1313.

63. Basillote JB, Abdelshehid C, Ahlering TE, et al. Laparoscopic assisted radical cystectomy with ileal neobladder: a comparison with the open approach. *J Urol*. 2004;172:489.

64. Rhee JJ, Lebeau S, Smolkin M, et al. Radical cystectomy with ileal conduit diversion: early prospective evaluation of the impact of robotic assistance. *BJU Int*. 2006;98:1059.

65. Wang GJ, Barocas DA, Raman JD, et al. Robotic vs open radical cystectomy: prospective comparison of perioperative outcomes and pathological measures of early oncological efficacy. *BJU Int*. 2008;101:89.

66. Pruthi RS, Wallen EM:. Is robotic radical cystectomy an appropriate treatment for bladder cancer? Short-term oncologic and clinical follow-up in 50 consecutive patients. *Urology*. 2008;72:617.

67. Pruthi RS, Smith A, Wallen EM:. Evaluating the learning curve for robot-assisted laparoscopic radical cystectomy. *J Endourol*. 2008;22:2469.

68. Canes D, Desai MM, Aron M, et al. Transumbilical single-port surgery: evolution and current status. *Eur Urol*. 2008;54:1020.

69. Kaouk JH, Goel RK, Haber GP, et al. Robotic single-port transumbilical surgery in humans: initial report. *BJU Int*. 2009;103:366.

70. Gettman MT, Lotan Y, Napper CA, et al. Transvaginal laparoscopic nephrectomy: development and feasibility in the porcine model. *Urology*. 2002;59:446.

71. Matthes K, Yusuf TE, Willingham FF, et al. Feasibility of endoscopic transgastric distal pancreatectomy in a porcine animal model. *Gastrointest Endosc*. 2007; 66:762.

72. Box GN, Lee HJ, Santos RJ, et al. Rapid communication: robot-assisted NOTES nephrectomy: initial report. *J Endourol*. 2008;22:503.

73. Haber GP, Crouzet S, Kamoi K, et al. Robotic NOTES (Natural Orifice Translumenal Endoscopic Surgery) in reconstructive urology: initial laboratory experience. *Urology*. 2008;71:996.

74. Dachs GW 2nd, Peine WJ:. A novel surgical robot design: minimizing the operating envelope within the sterile field. *Conf Proc IEEE Eng Med Biol Soc*. 2006; 1:1505–1508.

75. Rentschler ME, Dumpert J, Platt SR, et al. Mobile in vivo camera robots provide sole visual feedback for abdominal exploration and cholecystectomy. *Surg Endosc*. 2006;20:135.

Chapter 10

Patient-Side Surgeons: The Unsung Heroes of Robotic Surgery

Phillip Mucksavage and Daniel D. Eun

There is much truth to the statement "The console surgeon is only as good as their assistant." As the only surgeon scrubbed during the procedure, the patient-side assistant is in large part responsible for the efficient and safe progression of the surgical procedure. We discuss the importance of a well-trained assistant and what is required in this demanding but often underappreciated position. Concepts in patient positioning, gaining access, port placement, docking, and basic operative principles are discussed. Important nuances such as parking in the sweet spot, "burping the ports," and assistant comfort are recommended. Troubleshooting and instructions on how to approach urgent and emergent scenarios are closely detailed and provided in a unique chart format.

10.1 Introduction

A dedicated team-based approach is critical for consistent success in the robotic operating room. Although often overlooked, the patient-side first assistant is central to this team. Due to the steep learning curve and highly specialized equipment, a skilled assistant is necessary to maximize efficiency and minimize complications.

10.2 Importance of the Assistant

There is much truth to the statement "The console surgeon is only as good as their assistant." As the only surgeon scrubbed during the procedure, the patient-side assistant is in large part responsible for the efficient and safe progression of the surgical procedure. It requires extensive knowledge of the robot, robotic instruments, and a plethora of laparoscopic equipment. The assistant must be familiar with the robot's limitations and constantly monitor the environment to prevent potential problems and delays. The assistant must be able to quickly identify the root cause and troubleshoot problems. An inexperienced or poorly trained assistant can severely disrupt the flow of the operation and potentially cause a major complication.

A firm understanding of the first assistant's role is a necessary step to gaining proficiency as a robotic console surgeon.[1] The ability to direct where and what the assistant should be doing at all times throughout a case is an essential part of learning how to perform the operation. Simply learning how to perform the console portion of the case is shortsighted and slows the console surgeon's progression on the learning curve. Therefore, programs dedicated to training robotic surgeons should incorporate intensive first-assistant experience as a cornerstone of the surgical training.[2,3]

10.3 Requirements of the Assistant

In addition to a keen knowledge of the robot, the patient-side first assistant must be skilled in positioning the patient, placing the ports properly,

D.D. Eun (✉)
Division of Urology, Penn Urology at Pennsylvania Hospital,
University of Pennsylvania, Philadelphia, PA, USA
e-mail: danieleun@hotmail.com

A.K. Hemal, M. Menon (eds.), *Robotics in Genitourinary Surgery*,
DOI 10.1007/978-1-84882-114-9_10, © Springer-Verlag London Limited 2011

docking, and managing the robot throughout the operation. Since robotic surgery is an extension of laparoscopic surgery, it requires the patient-side assistant to have a firm knowledge of basic laparoscopic principles. A thorough understanding of general safety issues and emergency scenarios should be mandated as part of the initial training protocol.[1,4] An excellent assistant should be familiar with an almost endless list of constantly changing laparoscopic tools. The job demands nimble two-handed assistance, requires keen eye–hand coordination, and expects one to manage multiple variables at once. Despite the industrious nature of the job, much of the effort goes unseen and can often seem thankless.

10.3.1 Patient Positioning, Gaining Access, and Port Placement

The patient-side assistant must understand the critical nature of proper patient positioning, port placement, and docking. Since the position of the patient in robotic surgery is often very different from open surgery, the assistant must understand optimal positioning concepts and provide sufficient padding and support for the patient. Improper position and padding can limit surgical access and hinder case progression. The association between poor positioning and neuromuscular–skeletal complications is well established.[5]

Attention to details in the initial setup and positioning of the ports cannot be overemphasized. Poor setup technique or mistakes in judgment here can subsequently lead to a multitude of technical problems. Access and trocar-related injuries are not an uncommon source of injury during laparoscopy that can often be avoided with proper technique and training.[6]

There are a number of different ways the abdomen can be accessed for robotic surgery. The techniques used by the primary surgeon are often based on previous training and comfort with laparoscopy. The two most common methods of establishing access are the Veress needle and Hassan port entry. Pneumoinsufflation technique using a Veress needle is well described in the literature.[7] The main advantages of the Veress needle are ease of use and quick access. In experienced hands, it is a safe and extremely reliable technique. However, due to the blind nature of its insertion, there is a small risk of inadvertent bowel or vascular injury.[8,9] The safest and most reliable point of intraperitoneal entry for the Veress needle is the periumbilical or left subcostal location. The surgeon must develop a feel for the needle as it passes through the fascia and recognize the characteristic "pop" of the needle point as it passes into the peritoneal cavity. The most reliable confirmatory tests of proper placement are achieved via two methods, the water drop test and opening pressure test. With the water drop test, a syringe with a small amount of saline is placed into the Veress needle, which should then quickly drop into the abdomen. Saline that does not drop immediately and quickly is suggestive that the needle is not intraperitoneal and should be repositioned. In this author's opinion, the rate of the saline drop is the most reliable indicator of proper Veress needle placement. Manually lifting up on the external abdominal wall during Veress needle placement can help with Veress needle access as it increases tension on the abdominal fascial layers as well as creating intraperitoneal negative pressures. After a satisfactory drop test, the gas should be attached and turned on at its highest flow, while keeping the needle completely steady. At this point, attention is focused on the initial pressures registered within the abdomen and should typically register at or below 4 mmHg. Intraperitoneal pressure should increase steadily and slowly, with flow rates over the Veress needle registering between 1.0 and 1.5 L/min. If the surgeon is unsuccessful in placing the Veress needle or is uncomfortable with the method, the Hassan technique can be employed.[10] With the Hassan technique, direct access is gained into the peritoneal cavity surgically. Advantages of the Hassan technique include direct visualization and can be preferable when attempting to access a hostile abdomen. Disadvantages of Hassan access include lengthier time for access and potential air leak issues once pneumo-peritoneum is established. Several methods exist for this type of access, but all are based on gaining direct surgical access into the peritoneal cavity under direct vision.[11,12] Although a point of controversy, Hassan entry is considered by some authors to be safer than the Veress needle. The technique, however, is useful for cases with especially difficult Veress placement and cases with hostile abdomens or for surgeons uncomfortable with the Veress needle. Using the Veress needle does provide some additional speed to establishing a pneumo-peritoneum, but is a "blind" procedure that relies on external clues to establish access into the abdomen. Unlike the Hassan technique, a camera port must be placed either blindly or with the use of a visually dilating port that allows the surgeon to observe entry through consecutive abdominal layers as access is gained into the peritoneum. With appropriate training, either method is acceptable and safe; however, each method's pros and cons should be understood.[13] Generally, the method of access obtained is surgeon specific and based on their comfort level with laparoscopy and each technique.

Once access to the peritoneum is gained and the camera port is placed, using a 30° angled-up camera can be useful to maximally visualize the anterior abdominal wall as other ports are subsequently placed. Improved visualization of the abdominal wall can provide superior abdominal wall transillumination, help avoid puncturing large abdominal wall blood vessels, and help in taking down difficult adhesions. During port placement, optimal visual conditions should be established by turning down room lights to augment abdominal wall transillumination. Ports should be strategically placed and spaced apart to minimize intra- and extracorporeal interference and instrument clashing. Poor choice in port site selection and/or suboptimal techniques can severely impede the operation. If the surgeon is unsure of an optimal port template, technique-related articles with illustrations regarding the proposed procedure should be referenced.

10.3.2 Principles of Docking, Sweet Spot, and Burping

Once the ports are placed, and attention is turned to docking the robot, it is important to drive and position the robot at an optimal distance and angle from the ports. This optimal distance is called the "sweet spot," and using the blue line and arrow on the camera arm can help determine how close to park the robot to the patient. Docking the robot is usually a coordinated effort between the patient-side assistant and the person driving the robot. Since the individual driving the robot often cannot see exactly where the robot needs to dock, it is the role of the scrubbed assistant to guide them in. Clear orientation as to which way to turn and how sharp to turn should be established prior to moving

the robot. Consistent directions from the assistant and practice as the driver also aid in creating a smoother and easier docking experience.

Once the robot is parked in the proper position and the arms are docked to the ports, it is essential to ensure that the robotic ports are inserted to the proper recommended depth. The abdominal fascia should be lined up with the wider grey line on the robotic ports. Failure to do so may result in ports pulling out inadvertently, especially when abdominal pressures run low. Once docked, the arms must be checked for possible areas of conflict. If the arms appear to have an external collision, the port should be readjusted while carefully stabilizing the port with one hand to prevent inadvertent port pullout during the process. Potential places where the robot can lean on the patient should be identified and adjusted before starting the case. As the camera and instruments are inserted and arms are directed toward the working area, the ports should be "burped" to minimize fascial torque being applied on the robotic port at the site of port insertion. Burping is achieved by grasping/stabilizing the port in one hand while clutching it with the other and essentially pulling up (toward ceiling) on the port. By minimizing the fascial torque being applied to the port, burping minimizes arm movement restrictions and abnormal feedback that the console surgeon may experience. Burping also may minimize potential for fascial tears resulting in air leakage and may result in less postoperative pain.

10.3.3 Being Comfortable

At this point the patient-side assistant is left alone as the console surgeon will begin the robotic portion of the procedure. To provide precise and high-quality tableside assistance for a prolonged period of time, the assistant must be comfortable. An ergonomically supportive chair with adjustable seat height, arm rests, and back support is recommended. This chair can be draped to maintain sterility. Prior to docking the robot, the operating table should be lowered to the lowest setting so that the assistant's arms are situated in a comfortable posture throughout the case. A dedicated monitor for the assistant should be placed in a comfortable location so that neck strain is minimized. The assistant should also have a clear line of sight to the real-time insufflation pressure values since air leaks and over-suctioning need to be readily identified. A Mayo stand to hold equipment that the assistant will need should be within arms length of the assistant. The assistant should remain spatially aware of the robotic arms to avoid getting hit by swift external movements and avoid injury and/or sterility issues. Remaining comfortable throughout the case is key to the success of the patient-side assistant, and its importance should not be overlooked.

10.4 Basic Rules and Principles During the Operation

During the course of the operation, the patient-side assistant is the eyes and ears of the console surgeon. There should be constant back and forth communication between the console surgeon and the first assistant, as the first assistant can add valuable input to the console surgeon's decision tree throughout the case. Moreover, the patient-side assistant should be encouraged to speak up and voice tableside concerns, providing valuable real-time feedback to the otherwise unaware console surgeon. For example, information that two robotic arms are externally clashing with each other would be very helpful to the console surgeon who may be struggling with movement limitations and unaware of this problem. Simple responses from the assistant, such as "needle out of the body" or "change to zero degree on console," keep the console surgeon and OR staff abreast of the current tableside events and should be mandated as protocol.

To be maximally efficient, the assistant should always be actively involved in the operation, maximizing exposure and retraction. The assistant should become comfortable using simultaneous two-handed retraction whenever two assistant ports are available. Dynamic two-handed triangulated traction of tissues to provide maximal tissue retraction is a key concept that is difficult to master but critical to maximize efficiency. It involves creating a three-dimensional field of view for the console surgeon by providing two opposite points of retraction at surgical site. This frees up both console surgeon's arms to freely dissect instead of employing one robotic arm for broad retraction. This is one major conceptual difference between conventional laparoscopic and robotic techniques. In difficult

situations with suboptimal exposure, additional fixed retraction can also be employed with an externally passed Keith needle. A Keith needle can be brought through the abdominal wall, attached to tissue that requires retraction, and brought out again and secured to the abdominal wall.

One of the most important roles of the assistant during the operation is providing a clear visual field for the console surgeon primarily with suction and retraction. As stated above, two-handed triangulation of tissues provides maximal tissue retraction and a three-dimensional surgical field for the operating surgeon. Suctioning is the second method to providing an adequate visual field. Clearing the field of excess blood, evacuating smoke from within the abdominal cavity, and revealing the source of small bleeders are an essential role of the assistant. Unlike open surgery, the use of suction must be in small bursts. Continuous suction will collapse the pneumo-peritoneum, and low pressures can exacerbate oozing from open venous vessels. Laparoscopic suction devices usually are equipped with irrigation that can aid in visualization. Irrigation can break up large blood clots and enable easier clot evacuation, while small bursts of irrigation can help expose an active bleeding point without compromising intra-abdominal pressures.

During the case, there must be constant attention paid to entry of instruments through all ports. Carelessness and lack of appropriate training can result in inadvertent tissue trauma and catastrophic consequences. Unrecognized injury such as bowel injuries can lead to delayed postoperative disasters. Instruments are often inserted through the assistant ports blindly, and the assistant must use extreme care to gently deliver the instrument in a safe angle while remaining attentive to tissue resistance. When placing an instrument through a port that is adjacent to the bowel, it is best to angle the instrument away from the bowel and toward the anterior abdominal wall. Sharp instruments, such as scissors, should ideally be inserted through more anteriorly placed ports that are further away from the bowel.

If there is any uncertainty during instrument insertion, the instrument should be withdrawn and the console surgeon should watch the instrument under direct vision. One should have a low threshold to stop the procedure and inspect for inadvertent bowel injury. In most instances, full-thickness bowel injuries can be repaired with an interrupted two-layered closure using

4-0 suture on a small tapered needle. Care should be taken not to close the bowel in a longitudinal fashion so as to avoid luminal narrowing.

Once the assistant understands the surgical steps and the console surgeon's needs, a flow of the case can be established. Movements become anticipated, and optimal suction and retraction are provided. Instruments required for the next step in the operation will be prepped earlier, and delays for instrument changes will be reduced. Failure to continuously utilize the assistant and to challenge the assistant to anticipate future steps can result in suboptimal assistance and slow surgical progression.

10.5 Urgent and Emergent Scenarios

The patient-side assistant should always be prepared for a crisis situation. It is recommended to discuss these potential situations and a plan of action prior to the procedure. The assistant should also mentally drill emergency maneuvers and techniques to minimize hesitation if an unfortunate situation unfolds. Preparation and calm, methodical thinking are keys to success in minimizing disasters.

Certain emergency supplies must be stocked in the robotic operating room and be immediately available. These include the laparoscopic Weck clip applicators, 5-mm titanium clip applicators, and vascular load staplers. The assistant surgeon should be familiar with their use. A 4-0 monofilament suture on small taper needles should be quickly available and cut to a 4 in. length for vascular repair if necessary. Other emergency options include the various flowable hemostatic agents such as Surgiflo (Ethicon) and Evicel (Ethicon) which can usually be quickly prepared on the back table with minimal preparation. Their use in conjunction with absorbable hemostatic fabrics such as Surgicel (Ethicon) can be very effective.

When faced with brisk bleeding, an expeditiously placed nontraumatic grasper on a bleeding vessel is the most simple and obvious maneuver that an assistant can do. Introduction of a compressive sponge such as a 4 × 18 Lap sponge (Medical Action Industries, Arden, NC) through a 12-mm port can quickly stabilize rapid bleeding by an experienced assistant and buy time to prepare for a coordinated attempt at repair.

If the abdomen needs to be opened quickly, the assistant should try to laparoscopically hold point pressure with a sponge on the bleeding source while the robot is quickly undocked and the robotic surgeon scrubs in. A cut-down incision can be made along the shaft of a port to rapidly enter the abdomen; however, caution must be made that once the intra-abdominal pressure is normalized to atmospheric pressure, a lacerated vessel can suddenly transform into a rapid bleeder.

10.6 Troubleshooting

In addition to providing assistants to the surgeon, a major role of the patient-side assistant is to constantly troubleshoot and adapt to the operation. As the only scrubbed surgeon, the patient-side assistant can provide immediate relief to common problems. Table 10.1 provides a list of common problems encountered during robotic surgeries and possible solutions. As more experience is gained, the assistant will develop a quick algorithm in diagnosing and fixing many of these commonly faced issues.

10.7 Summary

As the only surgeon scrubbed during most of the case, the patient-side assistant is largely responsible for the efficient and rapid progression of the procedure as well as the care and safety of the patient. In addition to assisting the console surgeon, the assistant must constantly identify and troubleshoot problems with the robot and patient. They are the first to respond to emergencies and must be able to quickly diagnose and manage each event. The patient-side surgeon is truly the unsung hero of robotic surgery. Sometimes spending hours in a darkened room, beaten up by the robotic arms in tight quarters, constantly cajoled by the console surgeon, the patient-side surgeons are rarely, if ever, congratulated with the type of respect or admiration the console surgeon receives. However, the assistant must remember that without them the case cannot be completed in an efficient and in some cases safe manner. Although the assistant is often overlooked and underappreciated, they command one of the most important jobs within the operating room.

Table 10.1 Common problems and solutions encountered by the patient-side assistant during robotic surgery

Problem	Possible causes	Solutions
Loss of pneumo-peritoneum	*Inflow problem*	
	Insufflation tube unplugged or not screwed on tight	Plug in or tighten insufflation tube
	Out of CO_2	Replace CO_2 container
	Line is kinked	Unwind tubing
	Port inflow valve open	Close port inflow valve
	Insufflation tube leak	Replace main line
	Leak problems – (Listen for leaks)	
	Port valve leak	Make sure all port valves closed
	Port site incision leak	Stitch port site or use towel clip
	Robotic port green seal leak	(1) Plug seal with finger to confirm seal leak location
		(2) Replace green seal
	Non-robotic port seal leak	(1) Plug seal with finger to confirm seal leak location
		(2) Replace reducer cap or port
	Suction issues	(1) Avoid over-suctioning by keeping eye on insufflation pressure
		(2) Make sure suction button not jammed on "on" position
Loss of suction	Suction tubing unplugged	Plug in suction tubing
	Suction motor/mechanism off	Turn on suction motor
	Suction tip clogged	Flush or replace suction tip
	Suction controller/tubing cracked	Replace component
	Vacuum generator failure or leak	Replace vacuum generator
	Charcoal filter clogged (Neptune device)	Replace Neptune filter
Port pullout	Camera port pullout	(1) Use translucent camera port to set proper shaft depth (fascia should be within ribbed area of port)
		(2) Use ribbed ports not smooth ports
		(3) Can switch to balloon port
		(4) Avoid complete loss of pneumo-peritoneum
		(5) Check for leaks or inflow issues
	Robotic port pullout	(1) Set to proper depth on robotic ports (thick dark line on the port)
		(2) Avoid complete loss of pneumo-peritoneum
		(3) Check for leaks or inflow issues
Robotic arm limitations (range of motion limited or "arm feels funny")	Robot parked too far/too close	Park robot within sweet spot
	Robot arms not set properly	Set robotic working arm elbows at 90°
	Robot arm–arm conflicts	Optimize robotic arm angles
	Robotic arm bumping assistant, patient, equipment, table	Reset arm or move obstruction
	Robotic arm not burped	Burp arm
	Robotic arm drape fasteners too snug	Loosen up arm drape
Incorrect needle count	Needle lost in abdomen	(1) Scan field immediately with minimal movement of field (more movement could hide the needle)
		(2) Obtain intraoperative KUB to confirm location in abdomen
		(3) Use C-arm to help locate needle

Table 10.1 (continued)

Problem	Possible causes	Solutions
Excess bleeding/loss of surgical field (nonemergency)	Suction clogged	(1) Flush or replace suction tip (2) Refer to *loss of suction* checklist above
	Low insufflation pressures	(1) Check for leaks (2) Refer to *loss of pneumo-peritoneum* checklist above (3) Compress/pack bleeder and allow pressures to recover (4) Increase insufflation pressure setting to 20 mmHg
Emergency situation	Emergency bleeding	(1) Attempt to grasp/compress vessel (2) Sponge via assistant port for compression and hold 5 min (3) Change arm to needle drivers and repair with 4-0 prolene (4) Consider stapler, clip applicator, or flowable hemostatic agent (5) Consider open conversion with rapid entry by cutting down directly on port (expect increased bleeding once exposed to atmospheric pressure)
	Crashing patient	(1) Desufflate and dedock immediately (2) Take out of Trendelenburg if air embolus (mill-wheel murmur) ruled out
	Air embolus (mill-wheel murmur)	(1) Turn to left lateral decubitus/Trendelenburg (2) Aspirate central line

References

1. Kumar R, Hemal AK. The 'scrubbed surgeon' in robotic surgery. *World J Urol*. 2006;24(2):144–147.
2. Menon M, et al. Laparoscopic and robot assisted radical prostatectomy: establishment of a structured program and preliminary analysis of outcomes. *J Urol*. 2002;168(3):945–949.
3. Lee DI, et al. Robotic laparoscopic radical prostatectomy with a single assistant. *Urology*. 2004;63(6):1172–1175.
4. Kaul SA, et al. Establishing a robotic prostatectomy programme: the impact of mentoring using a structured approach. *BJU Int*. 2006;97(6):1143–1144.
5. Winfree CJ, Kline DG. Intraoperative positioning nerve injuries. *Surg Neurol*. 2005;63(1):5–18.
6. Hemal AK, et al. Nuances in the optimum placement of ports in pelvic and upper urinary tract surgery using the da Vinci robot. *Urol Clin North Am*. 2004;31(4):683–692.
7. McKernan JB, Champion JK. Access techniques: Veress needle–initial blind trocar insertion versus open laparoscopy with the Hasson trocar. *Endosc Surg Allied Technol*. 1995;3(1):35–38.
8. Moberg AC, Montgomery A. Primary access-related complications with laparoscopy: comparison of blind and open techniques. *Surg Endosc*. 2005;19(9):1196–1199.
9. Molloy D, et al. Laparoscopic entry: a literature review and analysis of techniques and complications of primary port entry. *Aust N Z J Obstet Gynaecol*. 2002;42(3):246–254.
10. Gett RM, Joseph MG. A safe technique for the insertion of the Hasson cannula. *ANZ J Surg*. 2004;74(9):797–798.
11. Rosen DM, et al. Methods of creating pneumoperitoneum: a review of techniques and complications. *Obstet Gynecol Surv*. 1998;53(3):167–174.
12. Mayol J, et al. Risks of the minimal access approach for laparoscopic surgery: multivariate analysis of morbidity related to umbilical trocar insertion. *World J Surg*. 1997;21(5):529–533.
13. Catarci M, et al. Major and minor injuries during the creation of pneumoperitoneum. A multicenter study on 12,919 cases. *Surg Endosc*. 2001;15(6):566–569.

Part II
Training and Research

Chapter 11

Training in Robotic Urologic Surgery

David S. Wang and Howard N. Winfield

11.1 Introduction

Robotic surgery has become widespread in urology and is currently gaining abundant popularity among urologists. Virtually all major urologic procedures have been performed robotically assisted, including prostatectomy, pyeloplasty, cystectomy, nephrectomy, and partial nephrectomy.[1] At present, robot-assisted laparoscopic radical prostatectomy (RALP) is gaining widespread acceptance in the United States. Robotic radical prostatectomy was first described in 2001,[2,3] and since that time the number of robotic prostatectomies performed in the United States has grown rapidly. In 2008, more than 70,000 robotic prostatectomies were performed in the United States, accounting for over 50% of all radical prostatectomies[4] Currently, the da Vinci Surgical System (Intuitive Surgical, Sunnyvale, CA) is the only commercially available system available for performing RALP.

As robotic urologic surgery is emerging as an accepted standard of care, there is an increased recognition of the need to train resident physicians and practicing urologists on robotic urologic surgery. This chapter reviews the current state of robotic training in urology.

11.2 Learning Curve for Robotic Surgery

There is no accepted consensus definition of the term *learning curve* as it applies to robotic urologic surgery.

In general, it is the point at which the surgeon feels that he/she is comfortable performing a specific procedure on a regular basis. In actual practice, the learning curve of an operation refers to the point at which an operation is performed in a routine fashion in a reasonable operative time.

The learning curve for robotic urologic surgery appears to be shorter than that for traditional standard laparoscopy.[5] Robotic surgery affords the surgeon three-dimensional view and also removes the limitations of instrument movement which occur with traditional laparoscopy. Standard laparoscopic surgery requires the use of longer instruments which are limited to 4 degrees of freedom, whereas robotic surgery allows the surgeon to have 7 degrees of freedom.[6] Nonetheless, there are still difficulties inherent in training for robotic surgery.

For RALP the idea of the learning curve has been examined. Menon and colleagues[7] performed the first large-scale series of RALP in conjunction with two highly skilled laparoscopic surgeons with expertise in pure laparoscopic radical prostatectomy[8] and found that the learning curve for RALP based on OR time was 18 cases. Ahlering and colleagues[9] found that the learning curve for 4-h proficiency for RALP was 8–12 cases.

Zorn et al.[10] examined the learning curve for RALP by a fellowship-trained laparoscopic surgeon and found that the number of cases required to overcome the learning curve was 25–50 cases. In this study, a surgeon highly experienced in open RRP was involved with the first 25 cases, and it was felt that the involvement of a skilled open surgeon during the initial learning curve was critical.

On the other hand, Herrell and Smith[11] defined learning curve in a more stringent fashion, as the

D.S. Wang (✉)
Boston University Medical Center, Boston, MA, USA
e-mail: davids.wang@bmc.org

group had had extensive open surgical experience with prostatectomy prior to the initiation of RALP. The number of cases that were required to gain results comparable to that of open RRP was 150 cases, and the number of cases required until there was self-perception to a comparable degree of comfort by the surgeon was 250 cases.

Pruthi and colleagues examined the learning curve required for robot-assisted radical cystectomy[12] and found that when examining operative time, 20 cases were required to overcome the learning curve. Despite the longer operative time of surgery in the initial cases in this series, there were no differences observed in terms of oncologic parameters even in the earlier experience.

Most hospitals have a committee and/or process to determine if a surgeon is credentialed to perform robotic procedures. In the United States, most hospitals require that the urologist performing robotic surgery for the first time must attend a dedicated training course as well as have a proctor for the first three cases. Clearly, the training of the urologist prior to performing the first case is critical in determining the number of cases required to overcome the learning curve.

Ballantyne and Kelley[13] report on a very regimented credentialing process at Hackensack University Medical Center, a hospital with an extremely high robotic surgery volume. The credentialing process at this hospital is comprehensive and requires (1) board certification or board eligibility for the appropriate surgical board, (2) clinical privileges for the open and laparoscopic operations that will be performed telerobotically, (3) satisfactory completion of the Food and Drug Administration-mandated training course in the safe use of the robotic surgical system, (4) performance of telerobotic operations in animate models, (5) observation of clinical cases of telerobotic surgery by an expert surgeon, (6) acting as bedside assistant surgeon in telerobotic operations or supervision by a preceptor during the surgeon's initial operations, (7) observation by a proctor of the surgeon's initial clinical telerobotic operations, and (8) ongoing monitoring of surgical outcomes of telerobotic operations.

In summary, it appears that the number of robotic cases required to overcome the urologic surgeon's learning curve is highly variable. Also, the length of the learning curve depends on the surgeon's perception, the definition used for learning curve, the

operative time, and the surgeon's ability. Ultimately, however, the definition of the learning curve should depend on the overall outcome of the patient.

11.3 Robotic Training for Residents

Training in robotic urologic surgery to residents in training has been a challenging task. Traditional resident training in surgery was introduced by William Halsted from Johns Hopkins more than 100 years ago.[14] This type of training, where trainees learned to ultimately operate independently, often with various degrees of supervision, may not be as applicable to robotic surgery.[15]

In a survey of residency training in laparoscopic and robotic surgery from 2006, Duchene and colleagues[16] examined the status of residency training in laparoscopic and robotic surgery in the United States. It was found that robotic procedures were performed at 54% of institutions, primarily prostatectomy and pyeloplasty. When stratifying overall experience with laparoscopic and robotic surgery, only 38% of responders felt that their experience was satisfactory.

It is clear that learning robotic surgery (particularly RALP) requires advanced skills and significant experience, and thus teaching residents raises several concerns. For patients, having key steps of the operation performed by a resident physician may worsen the outcome. Also, there are concerns by hospitals that resident involvement may increase operative time and therefore cost.[17] Schroeck and colleagues[18] examined the effect of trainees on the learning curve for robotic prostatectomy in a large series of patients. Overall, there was no effect on EBL and positive surgical margins, although the operative times were higher in the resident trainees. In this training program, there was a highly structured teaching program where residents reviewed numerous videos of various cases prior to participating in RALP, and the procedure was divided into three portions. Each portion required at least 10 cases, or until proficiency was achieved.

In similar fashion, Rashid et al.[19] described a method of training residents on how to perform RALP. In this study, the operation was divided into five steps, including (1) bladder takedown, (2) endopelvic fascia incision and dorsal venous complex, (3) bladder neck and posterior dissection, (4) neurovascular bundles, and (5) vesico-urethral anastomosis. In this training paradigm, the resident was allowed to proceed to the next step once proficiency of the step was demonstrated on three separate occasions. Also, each procedure was recorded and reviewed with the attending physician following the completion of the operation. In this study there were no negative effects on patient outcome.

Thiel and colleagues[20] also tried to identify which factors affected operative time when involving residents with RALP in a training program. The operation was divided into nine different segments, and operative times were examined based on who was performing the operation and also on patient characteristics. The areas of significance identified were that there were the slowest decrease of operative times in performing the neurovascular bundle preservation and the bladder neck division, and operative times fluctuated the most with the vesico-urethral anastomosis. It was felt that resident involvement was possible in RALP cases even when the attending physician was still not completely over his/her own.

It is easier to teach robotic surgery than it is to teach traditional laparoscopic surgery. In one study by Stefanidis and colleagues,[21] robotic assistance greatly facilitated complex tasks such as intracorporeal suturing when compared with standard laparoscopy when evaluating notice surgeons. Also, the learning curve was shortened significantly. Nonetheless, even though robotics has facilitated laparoscopic surgery, significant hurdles exist in training urology residents on complex robotic urologic operations, including RALP. It is becoming increasingly apparent that intense training and relatively high numbers of cases are required. In addition, a formalized and regimented training program with close supervision by the attending physicians is necessary. In addition, the resident must be allowed to master individual steps before being able to perform the entire operation independently. Clearly the old adage "see one, do one, teach one" does not apply to robotic urologic surgery.

Recently Intuitive Surgical has released the new da Vinci Si robotic platform. This system allows a second console to be attached to the operative field, thus allowing the trained robotic surgeon to override the trainee's console and take over the controls. This would be synonymous with a driver's education training car where the instructor also has a steering wheel and breaks to prevent "an accident." Unfortunately the cost of this second console system is almost $500,000.

11.4 Robotic Training in Fellowship

Advanced laparoscopic and robotic training in the United States requires fellowship training following residency. In the United States, such programs are offered through the Endourological Society. In a recent survey of endourology fellowship programs,[22] respondents noted that in 73% of the programs the fellows performed more than 50 robotic procedures. The majority of fellows that receive training in advanced robotic techniques are comfortable performing robotic surgery at the completion of the fellowship. However, the demand for training surgeons advanced robotic surgery techniques does not appear to be met by the limited number of fellowship programs currently available in the United States.

11.5 Postgraduate Courses

For urologists that are already in practice, postgraduate training is necessary in order to become familiar with robotic techniques. Most postgraduate robotic training courses exist in 2- to 3-day didactic courses. In these courses, the participant first attends several didactic seminars prior to beginning robotic training, in which trainees become familiar with all working aspects of the robotic system.[15] This allows the course participant to become familiar with the basic concepts of robotics and also allows the opportunity to try and facilitate troubleshooting. It is during this time that the trainees review videos of the procedures and also have the opportunity to view live surgery.

It is during this course that the trainees also work with dry training on inanimate models, as it is necessary for trainees to become familiar with operating the robotic unit on an inanimate model. It has been shown that objective assessment of proficiency on a dry lab model can be measured in trainees using the da Vinci robot.[23] Moreover, practicing on an inanimate model can facilitate performing of robotic surgery,[24] but probably is not sufficient in and of itself.

During the short training course, attendees are given the opportunity to practice on live animal surgery, most commonly porcine surgery. This allows the surgeon to become familiar with docking the robot, become facile with manipulating the robot on real tissue, and becoming accustomed to the lack of tactile feedback. Moreover, it allows the surgeon to advance from an inanimate model to a live animal. Unfortunately, there are significant limitations of this animal training model. The porcine model does not really have a case equivalent to complex robotic urologic surgery, such as RALP. In addition, porcine anatomy is significantly different from human anatomy. Thus, the ability to perform robotic surgery in a porcine model does not necessarily translate over to the human model.

Performing robotic surgery (such as RALP) on a cadaver model is an effective method of simulating RALP on a patient. However, cadaveric robotic prostatectomy courses are increasingly rare, and the cost of running a cadaveric course is significant. When urologists were first performing robotic prostatectomy procedures, the company supplying the robot sponsored 2-day courses, which included a cadaveric lab. However, this is no longer the case and most urologists who now receive training in robotic prostatectomy do not participate in a cadaveric lab prior to performing robotic surgery on patients.

Completion of a 2-day course does not ensure that trainees will be qualified or comfortable performing robotic surgery. Indeed, in one study examining the effectiveness of a 2-day laparoscopic course in training urologists, only 54% of course participants performed any laparoscopic surgery at all 5 years from course completion.[25] Thus, although a 2–3-day postgraduate course is necessary prior to embarking upon robotic urologic surgery, it does not ensure that the trainee will be able to independently perform robotic surgery upon course completion.

11.6 Postgraduate Mini-Fellowship

McDougall and colleagues[26] have introduced a novel concept of a mini-fellowship program for RALP. In this new training paradigm, the participant attends an intensive 5-day training program. The 5-day course is limited to two participants per week and has a 1:2 faculty to attendee ratio. The course includes lectures, tutorials, videos, and laparoscopic and robot training in inanimate, animal, and cadaveric labs. In addition, numerous live cases are performed. If the participant wishes, a post-program proctoring experience is also offered.

The mini-fellowship program was highly effective in training urologists on how to perform RALP. Three years following the 5-day course, 86% of participants were performing RALP. In addition, it was found that those participants who were in a group practice were more likely to perform RALP than those in solo practice. In both the short and long term, most participants continued to perform RALP in their practice.

One major limitation of the 5-day course is the cost of the course. It is estimated that the course costs $10,000 per participant. The program was tuition free during the initial 3 years due to grant funding, and it is possible that participation in this program would have been less if the course were not tuition free. In addition, the course is limited to two participants per week. Finally, the intensive 5-day training program required an extensive commitment by the course faculty. Thus, the mini-residency appears to be effective in training urologists robotic surgery post-residency and allowing incorporation into urologic practice. However, limitations including cost and availability may limit this instructional paradigm to very select academic centers.

11.7 Simulators

In an effort to further decrease the learning curve of laparoscopic and robotic procedures, surgical simulators have emerged as an alternative training method for resident physicians and urologists already in practice. There are a variety of surgical simulators currently in existence, and a variety of these have been incorporated into urologic training.[27]

Such training alternatives range from simple pelvic trainers to advanced virtual reality simulators. Virtual reality simulators are already in use in other fields, such as aviation (flight simulators), the military, and in engineering (computer-aided design). In order for a virtual reality simulator to be considered worthwhile for teaching surgical skills to trainees, validation and reliability are required. Reliability refers to the required reproducibility and precision of the simulator whereas validity determines whether the simulator is appropriately teaching and evaluating what it is designed to do.[28] There are currently in existence virtual reality simulators which have been specifically designed for training in robotic surgery. The SEP robot system (Simsurgery, Oslo, Norway) is a virtual reality simulator which was developed to assist the trainee with tissue manipulation, dissection, and suturing skills. In one study, the SEP robot system was shown to enhance robotic suturing skills.[29] In another study it was found that practicing on the SEP robot allowed surgeons to decrease the learning curve, and it was felt that the SEP robot would be a useful adjunct to any training program.[30] The SEP robot has also been used in general surgery and felt to be useful for training purposes.[31]

Recently, the Mimic dV-Trainer (Mimic Technologies, Seattle, WA) has been introduced as a new virtual reality simulator which is based on the da Vinci system.[32] This system has been shown to have high validity as a virtual simulator for the da Vinci system in at least two studies.[32,33] In both studies, both trainees and experienced robotic surgeons felt that the Mimic dV-Trainer was useful for training and agreed into incorporating the simulator into a residency curriculum.

It is clear that virtual reality simulators are becoming more widespread in laparoscopic and robotic training. As such simulators are felt to be reliable and valid training tools, it is likely that all training programs will incorporate virtual reality simulators into their training curricula. Limitations at present include expense, availability, complexity, and realistic nature of simulators. Designing of robotic simulators requires collaboration between surgeons, engineers, and computer scientists. Sun et al.[34] offer an interesting article detailing how a robotic simulator is designed. In the future virtual reality simulators will become a major tool for training and evaluation of surgeons.

11.8 Conclusion

As robotic surgery has become widespread in urology, there is an increased need to train residents and practicing urologists on robotic surgery techniques. Significant challenges exist, but a number of training methods have been implemented to try and decrease the learning curve for robotic urologic surgery. It is likely in the future that robotic surgical simulators will become integral to robotic training.

References

1. Thiel DD, Winfield HN. Robotics in urology: past, present, and future. *J Endourol.* 2008;22(4):825–830.
2. Binder J, Kramer W. Robotically assisted laparoscopic radical prostatectomy. *BJU Int.* 2001;87:408–410.
3. Paticier G, Rietbergen JB, Guillonneau B, Fromont G, Menon M, Vallencien G. Robotically assisted laparoscopic radical prostatectomy: feasibility study in men. *Eur Urol.* 2001;40:70–74.
4. Intuitive Surgical Website. www.intuitivesurgical.com, 2008 statistics. Accessed 6/3/2009.
5. Blavier A, Gaudissart Q, Cadière GB, Nyssen AS. Comparison of learning curves and skill transfer between classical and robotic laparoscopy according to the viewing conditions: implications for training. *Am J Surg.* July, 2007;194(1):115–121.
6. Narula VK, Watson WC, Davis SS, et al. A computerized analysis of robotic versus laparoscopic task performance. *Surg Endosc.* December, 2007;21(12):2258–2261; [Epub May 24, 2007].
7. Menon M, Shrivastava A, Tewari A, et al. Laparoscopic and robot assisted radical prostatectomy: establishment of a structured program and preliminary analysis of outcomes. *J Urol.* September, 2002;168(3):945–949.
8. Guillonneau B, Vallancien G. Laparoscopic radical prostatectomy: the Montsouris technique. *J Urol.* June, 2000;163(6):1643–1649.
9. Ahlering TE, Skarecky D, Lee D, Clayman RV. Successful transfer of open surgical skills to a laparoscopic environment using a robotic interface: initial experience with laparoscopic radical prostatectomy. *J Urol.* November, 2003;170(5):1738–1741.
10. Zorn KC, Orvieto MA, Gong EM, et al. Robotic radical prostatectomy learning curve of a fellowship-trained laparoscopic surgeon. *J Endourol.* April, 2007;21(4):441–447.
11. Herrell SD, Smith JA Jr. Robotic-assisted laparoscopic prostatectomy: what is the learning curve? *Urology.* November, 2005;66(Suppl 5):105–107.
12. Pruthi RS, Smith A, Wallen EM. Evaluating the learning curve for robot-assisted laparoscopic radical cystectomy. *J Endourol.* November, 2008;22(11):2469–2474.
13. Ballantyne GH, Kelley WE Jr. Granting clinical privileges for telerobotic surgery. *Surg Laparosc Endosc Percutan Tech.* February, 2002;12(1):17–25.
14. Osborne MP. William Steward Halsted: his life and contributions to surgery. *Lancet Oncol.* 2007;8:256–265.
15. Guzzo TJ, Gonzalgo ML. Robotic surgical training of the urologic oncologist. *Urol Oncol.* March–April, 2009;27(2):214–217.
16. Duchene DA, Moinzadeh A, Gill IS, Clayman RV, Winfield HN. Survey of residency training in laparoscopic and

robotic surgery. *J Urol*. November, 2006;176(5):2158–2166.

17. Babineau TJ, Becker J, Gibbons G, et al. The "cost" of operative training for surgical residents. *Arch Surg*. April, 2004;139(4):366–369.

18. Schroeck FR, de Sousa CA, Kalman RA, et al. Trainees do not negatively impact the institutional learning curve for robotic prostatectomy as characterized by operative time, estimated blood loss, and positive surgical margin rate. *Urology*. April, 2008;71(4):597–601.

19. Rashid HH, Leung YY, Rashid MJ, Oleyourryk G, Valvo JR, Eichel L. Robotic surgical education: a systematic approach to training urology residents to perform robotic-assisted laparoscopic radical prostatectomy. *Urology*. July, 2006;68(1):75–79.

20. Thiel DD, Francis P, Heckman MG, Winfield HN. Prospective evaluation of factors affecting operating time in a residency/fellowship training program incorporating robot-assisted laparoscopic prostatectomy. *J Endourol*. June, 2008;22(6):1331–1338.

21. Stefanidis D, Wang F, Korndorffer JR Jr, Dunne JB, Scott DJ. Robotic assistance improves intracorporeal suturing performance and safety in the operating room while decreasing operator workload. *Surg Endosc*. February, 2010;24(2):377–382.

22. Yap SA, Ellison LM, Low RK. Current laparoscopy training in urology: a comparison of fellowships governed by the Society of Urologic Oncology and the Endourological Society. *J Endourol*. August, 2008;22(8):1755–1760.

23. Narazaki K, Oleynikov D, Stergiou N. Objective assessment of proficiency with bimanual inanimate tasks in robotic laparoscopy. *J Laparoendosc Adv Surg Tech A*. February, 2007;17(1):47–52.

24. Di Lorenzo N, Coscarella G, Faraci L, Konopacki D, Pietrantuono M, Gaspari AL. Robotic systems and surgical education. *JSLS*. January–March, 2005;9(1):3–12.

25. Colegrove PM, Winfield HN, Donovan JF Jr, See WA. Laparoscopic practice patterns among North American urologists 5 years after formal training. *J Urol*. March, 1999;161(3):881–886.

26. Gamboa AJ, Santos RT, Sargent ER, et al. Long-term impact of a robot assisted laparoscopic prostatectomy mini fellowship training program on postgraduate urological practice patterns. *J Urol*. February, 2009;181(2):778–782.

27. Wignall GR, Denstedt JD, Preminger GM, et al. Surgical simulation: a urological perspective. *J Urol*. May, 2008;179(5):1690–1699.

28. McDougall EM. Validation of surgical simulators. *J Endourol*. March, 2007;21(3):244–247.

29. Halvorsen FH, Elle OJ, Dalinin VV, et al. Virtual reality simulator training equals mechanical robotic training in improving robot-assisted basic suturing skills. *Surg Endosc*. October, 2006;20(10):1565–1569.

30. Balasundaram I, Aggarwal R, Darzi A. Short-phase training on a virtual reality simulator improves technical performance in tele-robotic surgery. *Int J Med Robot*. June, 2008;4(2):139–145.

31. Lin DW, Romanelli JR, Kuhn JN, Thompson RE, Bush RW, Seymour NE. Computer-based laparoscopic and robotic surgical simulators: performance characteristics and perceptions of new users. *Surg Endosc*. January, 2009;23(1):209–214.

32. Sethi AS, Peine WJ, Mohammadi Y, Sundaram CP. Validation of a novel virtual reality robotic simulator. *J Endourol*. March, 2009;23(3):503–508.

33. Kenney PA, Wszolek MF, Gould JJ, Libertino JA, Face MA. Content, and construct validity of dV-trainer, a novel virtual reality simulator for robotic surgery. *Urology*. June, 2009;73(6):1288–1292.

34. Sun LW, Van Meer F, Schmid J, Bailly Y, Thakre AA, Yeung CK. Advanced da Vinci Surgical System simulator for surgeon training and operation planning. *Int J Med Robot*. September, 2007;3(3):245–251.

Chapter 12

Animal Laboratory Training: Current Status and How Essential Is It?

Gyung Tak Sung and Yinghao Sun

For the successful transition of new technology into clinical practice, surgeons must continue to train concurrently with newly introduced technology for the benefit of both surgeons and future patients. Various training methods have been proposed to assimilate robotic-assisted technology for clinical applications. The methods of training may vary between utilizing inanimate models like bench models, pelvic trainers, and virtual reality simulators to animate models such as live animals, human cadavers, and animate cadavers. For decades, a live anesthetized animal has been utilized as a method of educating, developing, and refining complex surgical techniques. The ideal training model should be able to teach the surgical skills required, be easily accessible, cost-effective, and anatomically and physiologically akin to human patients. The potential advantages and disadvantages of the animal model for robotic training and comparison to other existing training models will be examined. Standardized robotic training curricula will be described. Several experimental studies will be reviewed in evaluating the da Vinci surgical system as regards refining and developing complex laparoscopic procedures.

12.1 Introduction

Modern-day surgeons face continuous challenges as technological advances, such as laparoscopy and robotic-assisted technology, are introduced into

existing practices.[1] In order for these advancements to be incorporated successfully, novel methods of learning must be employed to acquire necessary surgical skills that are inherently different from those previously known for traditional open surgery. Consequently, residents and surgeons suddenly find themselves in great need of continuous surgical training. Currently in urologic practice, minimally invasive surgery (MIS) primarily involves laparoscopic techniques which have become the "standard of care" for various urological procedures.[2]

As of now, laparoscopic surgery has some limitations, which include restricted range of motion, poor ergonomics of laparoscopic instruments, 2D image of operative field, reduced tactile feedback, and transfer of natural hand tremor to the instruments. The da Vinci robotic system (Intuitive Surgical, Valley View, CA) was introduced to overcome these limitations encountered in the standard laparoscopic surgery.[3] Robotic assistance offers several potential advantages over standard laparoscopy which includes improved ergonomics, 3D vision, articulated wrist instrumentation with 6 degrees of freedom, and telemanipulation capabilities. These advantages of the da Vinci allow advanced laparoscopic procedures to be more accessible to surgeons with no prior advanced laparoscopic training and allow them to develop and standardize a variety of complex laparoscopic procedures, thus expanding broader scope of laparoscopic surgical application.[4]

However, for successful incorporation of the new robotic-assisted technology into existing minimally invasive programs, a training program is required for both the novice and the skilled laparoscopic surgeon to optimize their performance. Therefore, acquiring new surgical skills to accommodate the innovative

G.T. Sung (✉)
Department of Urology, Dong-A University Hospital, Busan, South Korea
e-mail: Sunggt@dau.ac.kr

A.K. Hemal, M. Menon (eds.), *Robotics in Genitourinary Surgery*,
DOI 10.1007/978-1-84882-114-9_12, © Springer-Verlag London Limited 2011

technology is in a surgeon's best interest to attain best clinical results. To acquire surgical competency, the surgeon must be proficient in a combination of technical skills, decision-making, and team performance, as procedural development and instrument evaluation are very important aspects of surgical training.

Several training modalities for the clinical introduction of the da Vinci system have been implemented as robotic training opportunities continue to evolve with newer generations of the da Vinci robotic system.[5] These modalities are comprised of intensive operating experience during residency, postgraduate short courses, workshops or mini-apprenticeships, and full-time fellowship programs. Each training protocol incorporates animal models and surgical simulators as standardized and reproducible training methods to reduce and optimize the necessary learning curve. However, the learning curve associated with incorporation of robotic technology into a surgeon's armamentarium is not clearly defined. Therefore, various training models including both animate and inanimate models for robotic surgery training and education have been proposed.[6] The animate models include live animals, human cadavers or animate cadavers, and the inanimate models include bench and pelvic trainers. The ideal training model should be able to teach the surgical skills required, be easily accessible, economical, and anatomically and physiologically comparable to an anesthetized patient.

In this chapter, the potential advantages and disadvantages of the animal model for robotic training modality and comparison to other existing training models will be examined. Standardized robotic training curriculum offered at the centers of excellence will be presented. In addition, experimental studies will be described to emphasize how different animal models have been used to develop innovative robotic-assisted procedures with a review of the current literature.

12.2 Inanimate Models

Surgical skills laboratories are important components of curricula for surgical training. They provide trainees with a simulated environment with less stress, lower cost, and the opportunity to acquire technical skills that can be reproduced and receive immediate performance feedback. Bench models allow trainees to practice basic tasks such as moving beads around and passing a rope or dropping cotton peanuts into cylinders. The more commonly used inanimate models are pelvic trainers.[7] Trainees can practice various surgical skills such as cutting, clipping, grasping, positioning needles, intracorporeal suturing, and knot-tying, which should all be acquired prior to proceeding with animal or clinical procedures. Pelvic trainers allow trainees to develop hand–eye coordination and familiarize themselves with robotic instrumentations under 3D visualization. The use of commercially available inanimate simulators and mannequins allows trainees to practice port placement and actual surgical tasks. The main advantage of pelvic trainers is the ability to repeat specific reconstructive steps of a given surgery. For example, intracorporeal suturing and knot-tying can be performed to duplicate exact steps of dismembered pyeloplasty and vesicourethral anastomosis of the radical prostatectomy. In addition, the loss of tactile feedback can be offset by learning to use visual cues from 3D high resolution to guide instrument tip position and perform basic surgical maneuvers. In contrast, pelvic trainers have limited value in simulating dissection on humans. Advanced surgical skills, such as meticulous dissection, coagulation, and suturing, require more sophisticated animal or human cadaver models as it would develop higher psychomotor skills.[8]

12.3 Animate Models

A live anesthetized animal is the most realistic, non-patient environment that has been utilized for decades as a method of educating, developing, and refining complex surgical techniques.[9] In addition, animal models have been used in evaluating new instrumentations in both open and minimally invasive surgical approaches. Various minimally invasive training programs incorporate animal workshops as an important aspect in their systematic training curriculum.[10,11] Basic robotic surgical skills and dexterity should be acquired from dry labs and pelvic trainers before animal model training. Otherwise, beginning with an animal model would be a waste of time and financial resources.

In the animal lab, the surgeons have the opportunity to evaluate optimal port placement configuration and various robotic instrumentations specific for each procedures and learn surgical skills to improve operative techniques that can be transferred to the operating theater. Animals like pigs, dogs, sheep, and calves have similar anatomy and physiologic responses to humans. Also, the large animal model can be used to perform a complete robotic procedure. The physiologic responses to various surgical manipulations resemble to those seen in humans such as organ movements due to respiration, tissue resistance and reflection, vessel pulsations, and the possibility of bleeding when vessels are transected. The surgeon's anatomic awareness and confidence will be developed in concert with the ability to safely achieve exposure, identify, and control important structures. It is possible for the training director to create operative scenarios such as a vascular or bowel injury in order to train and evaluate how a trainee manages such complications.

Despite some anatomical differences in the urinary tracts of humans, the porcine model is the most often used for various urologic procedures in the kidney, ureter, bladder, and bowel.[12] They are most desirable when a trainer is teaching complex laparoscopic techniques before clinical application. The size of abdominal cavity and foregut anatomy in the porcine model are similar to those of humans. The porcine model allows the surgeon to establish transperitoneal pneumoperitoneum and a working space within the abdominal cavity, thereby allowing one to simulate different surgical situations.

It must be kept in mind that some of the anatomy may differ from humans. Retroperitoneum of the swine is a virtual space and is not surrounded by perirenal fat and Gerota's fascia. The ureter is thick, with a narrow lumen, and the prostate is indistinct. In contrast, the canine model is more often used for prostate surgery. The small and narrow pelvis in the canine model is an ideal environment to practice prostatectomy. The rat model facilitates and optimizes fine and delicate microsurgical techniques. Sometimes, calves are more ideal model for the kidney procedures since the size of the abdominal cavity and the kidney are quite comparable to humans. These animal models allow the simulation of the major steps of the procedure with similar surgical maneuvers, which can be considered suitable for training purposes. Performing procedures such as porcine nephrectomy, adrenalectomy, and cystectomy provide realistic environment where technical errors and complications such as bleedings, bowel injury, or

major vessel injury can arise without harming a human patient.[13]

In addition, trainees can experience robot-related incidents and malfunctions. Although 3D vision may compensate some of the precision and dexterity associated with tactile feedback, a number of situations can occur from lack of haptic feedback: such as inadvertent breaking of suture during knot-tying, instrument malfunction and breakage, and iatrogenic organ injury from instruments during instrument or camera exchange.[14] In addition, animal models allow trainees to work in a collaborative atmosphere, providing additional information regarding operative setup and intricacies of each surgical steps and thus reducing the learning curve.

Recently, Mehrabi et al. proposed an experimental training program to optimize the learning curve associated with the da Vinci system.[15] Four participants with different surgical experience were recruited in this study. The training scheme comprised of three different phases: initial evaluation of surgical performance using a porcine model, training of the participant using four standardized operations with a rat model, and final evaluation of the participant with four identical operations as in the initial phase by a porcine model. Procedures performed in the initial evaluation of surgical performance were standardized visceral and vascular operations (cholecystectomy, gastrostomy, anastomosis of the small intestine, and anastomosis of the aorta) in a porcine model. On the training phase with a rat model, the participants performed gastrostomy, anastomosis of the small and large intestines, and anastomosis of the aorta.

At the final evaluation stage, the operative durations have considerably decreased compared to the initial evaluation stage except in cholecystectomies. Also, complications were significantly less with improved operative proficiency in each procedure in the final evaluation phase, as compared with their counterparts in the initial evaluation phase. These improvements were documented at each phase of surgical experience. This study has demonstrated that a standardized training method using a small and large animal model allows a qualitative and quantitative evaluation of the surgical performance while shortening and optimizing the learning curve.

In another study, Hanly and coworkers reported successful multiservice laparoscopic surgical training program using the da Vinci surgical system.[16] A biphasic training program consisted of standardized da Vinci system training known as phase I, followed by self-guided learning in a porcine model known as phase II. A two day da Vinci course in phase I includes system basics, draping procedures, console and patient-side instructions, patient positioning, and port placement. Participants were trained in both inanimate model and an animal laboratory where they experienced various surgical movements and grip strength of each da Vinci instrument and practiced dissection and manipulation of tissues, ligation and transaction of vessels, intracorporeal suturing, and knot-tying, as well as system troubleshooting and emergency conversion procedures. Phase II of training is self-guided learning in a porcine model, where the surgeon will practice procedures that he is anticipating later in the clinical environment. Various intraoperative parameters were recorded including the da Vinci setup and operative times, the number of instrument and accessory port exchanges, and the complications. Twenty-three surgeons from seven surgical subspecialties participated in this program, and a total of 43 experimental procedures were performed in phase II of the training. The procedures performed include 10 cholecystectomies, 8 prostatectomies, 6 internal mammary artery take-down, 6 tubal anastomosis, 3 Nissen fundoplication, 2 bowel anastomosis, 2 pericardial window, 2 cystoureterostomy, 1 adrenalectomy, 1 cystostomy repair, 1 nephrectomy, and 1 pyeloplasty. The average number of procedures performed was 5.5 per surgeon. Significant reduction in the mean setup time of the da Vinci was documented from initial 45 min to 51% decrease on average by the third successive setup ($p < 0.0005$). Operative times decreased 39.0% by the third successive practice operation ($p < 0.0005$). Of the 43 cases performed, 10 operative complications were reported, and of the 10 intraoperative complications, 7 were considered robotic-related incidents. These robotic-related complications include system failure in one, frozen robotic arm in four, malfunctioning grasper in one, and robotic arm failure in one. Overall, the authors have demonstrated that the da Vinci is associated with increasing proficiency of learning, and preclinical animal model training was effective in developing surgical robotics skills.

As useful as animal labs are, there are some limitations. The psychological stress may not be as heightened as compared to the actual operating environment. Anesthesia time may be limited, and one may not be able to finish a complete procedure as initially planned. Also, ex vivo animal tissue or an organ can be used to teach procedure-specific surgical techniques. Their use is limited by variations from human anatomy and potential transmission of infectious disease. In addition, animal facilities are costly to establish and manage and require a housing facility on site with supporting staff. Furthermore, most institutions require ethics committee approval for use of animals in surgical training course, which adds to the administrative burden. Compounding the problem, animal activists and the general public at large are becoming quite sensitive to the use of the animals for surgical training and medical research.

12.4 Human Cadavers

The human cadaver has been used for centuries to teach human anatomy. They provide the benefit of high fidelity and an understanding of anatomy identical to the clinical situation. In addition, the cadaver requires no anesthesia and is not subjected to time constraints as normal physiological homeostasis has ceased. The establishment of pneumoperitoneum or retroperitoneum is feasible and simple. The position of the trocars in the cadaver is the same as it would be in a living patient. It provides the topography of all the different organs and structures with 3D images that are identical to those encountered with actual patients. Therefore, spatial perception of the anatomy is greatly enhanced. This is particularly important because the surgeons only have visual cues without any tactile feedback with the robotic surgery. Advanced procedures such as nephrectomy, radical prostatectomy, or pyeloplasty can be completely performed on cadavers. Those who have attended cadaver courses ranked highly in their understanding of surgical anatomy.[17,18] For a perfect understanding of the laparoscopic landmarks, cadaver lab provides critical training in terms of learning the surgical anatomy. In comparing porcine with cadaver models, trainees found cadavers to be superior.

However, the cadaver models have some disadvantages. First, the tissues do not bleed or respond normally. Despite the tissue dissection is easier with the clear surgical view, trainees cannot learn the principles of hemostasis. Second, surgical dissection of the defect tissue is not the same as real tissue and is quite different as is expected from a live human surgery.

Also, differences in tissue quality due to preservation techniques make this model less appealing. Third, a concern with the cadaver lab is that it is potentially dangerous due to the risk of disease transmission. In addition, human cadavers are not cost-efficient nor readily accessible and require appropriate facility and supporting staff. This is why both cadaver and porcine models are considered to be complementary steps in preclinical training.

12.5 Virtual Reality Simulators

Virtual reality simulators provide computer-simulated environment to practice surgical skills. Since robotic surgery and VR simulators use computer interfaces, both technologies will continue to grow and will undoubtedly provide a useful adjunct to minimally invasive surgical training.[19] In near future, VR simulators may replace other training media in specific applications as well as certify the surgeon's professional skills. The advantages, disadvantages, and challenges associated with this training model will be described in another chapter.

12.6 Standard Robotic Training Curriculum

Robotic surgery is a team approach with a main surgeon at the console, a surgical assistant at the bedside, and a scrub nurse. Each must understand the principles of laparoscopy and robotic technology as well as the functions of various laparoscopic and robotic instrumentations thoroughly. Important aspects of initial training prior to clinical application are proper patient positioning, trocar placement, robotic docking and setup, understanding the mechanism of various coagulation devices, potential thermal injuries, and their prevention and management. Familiarity with the mechanisms and instrumentations of the da Vinci robotic system and its operative setup is crucial to the smooth transition to the clinical application.

Currently, there are over 20 active training centers in the United States including the Intuitive Surgical corporate headquarters. In addition, there are several international training sites. Each training center has at least one da Vinci robotic system designated for training, research, and development. For proper training of the da Vinci robotic system, the Food and Drug Administration mandated two day courses for all users of the robot as taught by instructors from Intuitive Surgical. Intuitive Surgical offers three components of the da Vinci robotic system training: system training, procedure training, and clinical support. Pertinent topics covered in the system training include system preparation and management, inanimate labs, skills development with the da Vinci, and laboratory sessions. Procedure training covers case study review, clinical observation, laboratory sessions, surgical skills development, and surgeon-led training. Clinical support includes procedure map, surgeon proctoring, additional skills, laboratory session, and procedure dry run.

In the United States, East Carolina University (ECU) was selected as the initial training site.[20] Structured robotic surgical training curriculum was developed at ECU to optimize surgeon and team training. Surgical team usually consisted of two surgeons and two or three operating room nurses. Curriculum objectives for surgeons were to compare surgical robotic methods with prior training and clinical experiences and to understand and master surgical robotic technology. Team curriculum objectives were similar but focused more on operating room arrangement, sterile draping of the robot, instrument interfaces with the surgical cart, and device maintenance. Teams first underwent training in system troubleshooting that included electronic and mechanical problems as well as emergency shutdown maneuvers. After completion of system training, participants concentrated on specific procedure simulations. In the curriculum advancement levels, participants underwent didactic sessions, an inanimate laboratory, animal procedures, and fresh cadaver training before clinical observation.

12.7 Experimental Study

Since 1997, the Cleveland Clinic group has been investigating the experimental application of robotic-assisted surgery in urology. In a series of robotic-assisted laparoscopic urologic reconstructive and ablative studies, Sung and Gill have shown the feasibility and efficacy of performing pyeloplasty, nephrectomy, adrenalectomy, and bilateral extravesical ureteral reimplantation using the ZEUS system in a porcine model and a canine model.[21–23] These experimental studies have consistently demonstrated that robotic assistance provided accurate and reliable surgical performance with less surgeon fatigue and tremor when compared with standard laparoscopy. When the da Vinci system was newly introduced for the clinical evaluation, Sung and Gill have compared the da Vinci and ZEUS (V2 system) systems in performing various laparoscopic procedures in an acute porcine model.[24] The authors have demonstrated that the da Vinci system with EndoWrist technology was more intuitive with better dexterity and was associated with a shorter learning curve as compared to the ZEUS system. However, at the time of study, the ZEUS V2 system was not equipped with 3D visualization and extra wrist at the instruments tips.

Laparoscopic suturing is a technically demanding skill that requires overcoming a significant learning curve. In some cases, proficiency may never be achieved in a reasonable time because of limited case loads. The need for improving suturing ability has required development of animal models to evaluate new techniques. The main advantage of the robotic-assisted surgery is the ability to perform complex procedures, especially reconstructive surgery with less fatigue for the surgeon. In addition, any modification that reduces the learning curve in conventional laparoscopic technique to achieve proficiency would be of great benefit.

Hubert et al. used a porcine model to evaluate the feasibility of robotic-assisted pyeloplasty for ureteropelvic junction obstruction.[25] Eighteen pigs weighing 35–50 kg were used. Of the 18 procedures attempted, 14 pyeloplasties were performed successfully by transperitoneal approach. Due to unrelated robotic system technical problems, four could not be completed. In all cases, two absorbable 6/0 fine suture with close anastomosis were performed. The surgeons were able to perform various surgical steps with no particular difficulties, and the excellent anatomical results were confirmed without any leakage. The system installation time was significantly decreased from initial 45 min to 15 min at the end of the study. The surgeon reported no fatigue in five cases and moderate in nine cases, while the assistant surgeon reported none in 13 cases and moderate in one case. Also, the operative time decreased from initial 2 to less than 1 from seventh procedure. No complications were reported from these procedures.

In this study, it was successfully demonstrated that the robotic interface allows the surgeon to perform ergonomically at the console with wristed instrument tips under a 3D vision. For surgeons with limited laparoscopic experience, the robotic assistance will provide faster and easier learning. In addition, it would allow the surgeon to perform complex reconstructive techniques like tissue excision and spatulation, intracorporeal suturing, and knot-tying with no major difficulty. For seasoned laparoscopic surgeons, the robotic assistance will facilitate more complex reconstructive procedures with precision and reduced fatigue.

Recently, Passerotti and colleagues evaluated the quality of the ureteropelvic anastomosis and the learning curve associated with performing pyeloplasty using open, freehand, and robotic-assisted laparoscopic techniques in a porcine model by inexperienced surgeons.[26] Three inexperienced and one experienced surgeons were recruited in this study, and 57 swine weighing 30 kg were divided into three groups: open surgery (OS), freehand laparoscopy (LS), and robotic-assisted laparoscopy (RALS). Transperitoneal dismembered pyeloplasty was performed in all cases, and the anastomosis was evaluated for water tightness and patency using antegrade and retrograde urodynamic measurements immediately following surgery and 2 weeks postoperatively. Operated UPJ area was submitted for histology at 15 days postoperatively. Results showed that RALS had a shorter operative time and a shorter learning curve compared with LS. Urodynamic measurements for patency and water tightness of the UPJ with RALS were comparable to those in the OS group. Histological evaluation confirmed that there was less collagen III deposition around the operated UPJ in pigs that underwent RALS compared with LS and OS. These findings suggest that the robotic assistance had distinct advantages over freehand laparoscopy when the inexperienced surgeon is performing a pyeloplasty. This was the first study to directly evaluate the learning curve and the quality of the anastomosis associated with freehand and robotic-assisted laparoscopic suturing.

Laparoscopic bladder augmentation has not been performed widely due to its difficult technically demanding nature of extensive suturing; however, the use of robot-assisted laparoscopy may allow efficient suturing with less difficulty. Passerotti and coworkers described novel techniques of performing robot-assisted laparoscopic (RAL) bladder augmentation in a porcine model.[27] Of 10 pigs, 5 underwent intracorporeal anastomosis of ileal bladder augmentation and the other 5 underwent a freehand bowel anastomosis through one of the ports. The mean operative time was 6 h with a shorter learning curve. It was successfully demonstrated in this study that RAL bladder augmentation can be safely and efficiently performed with minimal complications. Minor technical modifications were necessary in reducing operative time and potential complications: placement of hitch stitches, extracorporeal irrigation of the isolated bowel loop, extracorporeal reconstruction of the bowel–bowel anastomosis, and keeping the bladder wall attachment intact to maintain bladder suspension.

Congenital obstructive uropathy, such as bladder outlet obstruction, can lead to devastating consequences in the kidney, leading to severe oligohydramnios, and cause fetal death. Although open fetal vesicostomy and percutaneous placement of a shunt into the bladder is an effective treatment, it is associated with a high fetal mortality and maternal morbidity. Therefore, as a promising alternative to traditional fetal treatments, sheep models are utilized to develop minimally accessing fetal surgery.

Ponsky et al. reported transuterine fetal vesicostomy by laparoscopic approach using a fetal sheep model.[28] However, performing freehand suturing in such restricted and mobile uterine space was quite a difficult task requiring advanced technical maneuvers, and consequently, only 4 of 10 lambs had a patent vesicostomy. More recently, Passerotti and colleagues used the da Vinci robotic system to evaluate the feasibility of performing fetal vesicostomy to overcome the technical limitations associated with standard laparoscopic techniques.[29] Fetal vesicostomy was performed after establishing bilateral hydronephrosis and distended bladder. However, in the first 10 fetuses, vesicostomy could not be completed laparoscopically, due to limited visualization and suboptimal port placement. But after specific modifications were made in the robot-assisted laparoscopic techniques including trocar placement and gas infusion, vesicostomy was successfully completed laparoscopically in the last eight fetuses in 2.5–4 h of operation. Subsequently, all of these fetuses had decompressed urinary tract system and a patent vesicostomy.

Schiff et al. evaluated the feasibility of performing robot-assisted urologic microsurgery in a rat model.[30] Hypothesis proposed that the advantages of the da Vinci surgical system would lead to the results as comparable or better than those of the conventional microsurgical techniques. A randomized prospective study comparing robotic microsurgical vasovasostomy and vasoepididymostomy to standard microsurgical vasovasostomy and vasoepididymostomy was conducted. In total of 24 adult male Wistar rats, the outcomes of robotic vs. standard microsurgical vasovasostomy and vasoepididymostomy were measured after 9 weeks postoperatively. Robotic vasovasostomy was shorter in the operative time compared to the conventional techniques (68.5 vs. 102.5 min, $p < 0.05$). However, there was no significant difference in the operative time between the robotic and the microsurgical vasoepididymostomy groups. Patency rates were excellent in both the robotic and the conventional groups (100 vs. 90%). Interestingly, the sperm granuloma rate was low in the robotic vasovasostomy group as 27% compare to 70% in the microsurgical vasovasostomy group. The sperm granuloma rate between the robotic and the microsurgical vasoepididymostomy was not significantly different (42 vs. 50%, $p = 0.37$). This is an interesting study that showed the da Vinci with improved stability and motion scaling during microsurgical suturing that helped to achieve excellent patency rates for vasovasostomy and vasoepididymostomy.

Various hemostatic methods have been evaluated during nerve-sparing robotic-assisted radical prostatectomy (RARP) to minimize collateral tissue injury, particularly to the cavernous nerves.[31] Examination of such techniques included ultrasonic shears, bipolar diathermy, laparoscopic clips, and bulldog clamps. Diathermy and ultrasonic shears can affect cavernous nerve with thermal injuries. Laparoscopic clips are usually larger than the periprostatic vessels and might tamper with dissection and perhaps dislodge as the dissection and tissue manipulation proceed.

Recently, several surgical lasers have been described that may potentially allow for precise tissue dissection with efficient hemostasis and minimal adjacent tissue damage. To evaluate feasibility of the laser energy for surgical precision, canine model was used in a pilot study by Gianduzzo and colleagues.[32] Ten dogs underwent laser-based RARP using the da Vinci S robotic system. The feasibility of laser dissection was initially assessed in the first five dogs to standardize the power settings and the procedure. The optimum laser settings determined for the KTP laser were 4–6 W for the bladder neck, common ejaculatory duct, and urethra and 2–4 W for the lateral pedicles, lateral prostatic fascia, and NVBs. The optimum Nd:YAG setting was 5 W. Pure laser RARP was then performed using predetermined laser generator settings in the later five dogs. The four-arm da Vinci S robotic system allowed the precise delivery of the laser and allowed to achieve narrow cutting widths. As a result, lower power setting was used for tissue dissection at 2–6 W rather than the 6 W that was used with handheld instruments in the previous study. For coagulating larger vessels, the neodymium-doped yttrium-aluminum-garnet laser at 5 W was employed. The EndoWrist technology of the laser instrument allowed the laser beam to be specifically targeted to optimize tissue cutting and vessel coagulation. The fourth arm allowed the main surgeon to be less dependent on the surgical assistant as well as providing optimal retraction of the tissue for dissection. Five dogs were euthanized immediately after RARP, and the other five were sacrificed after 72 h. All 10 procedures were successfully performed using only laser energy without any additional hemostasis. The mean excision time for prostate was 65 min. There were minimal changes in the intracavernosal pressure, the hemoglobin, and hematocrit levels postoperatively. Complications were anastomotic leakage in one and catheter-related problems in two. However, no complications were reported relating to the laser or postoperative hemorrhage.

Recently to further optimize MIS, the da Vinci system was employed in performing the transumbilical single-port laparoscopy. Haber et al. explored robotic natural orifice transluminal endoscopic surgery (R-NOTES) using a porcine model.[33] In each of the 10 female farm pigs, pyeloplasty, partial nephrectomy, and radical nephrectomy were performed. All 30 R-NOTES procedures were performed successfully without any complications. There were some modifications made in this study in order to optimize the surgical approach. Since the da Vinci is bulky, simultaneous umbilical and vaginal access was adapted that allowed a wide range of motion and avoiding clash of robotic instruments. To allow for larger instrument insertion, two standard ports were inserted through the same umbilical incision. Also, the ultrafine scaling option was used to minimize conflict between the laparoscope and the umbilical robotic instrument. Using a porcine model, they have demonstrated the potential for a less morbid and scarless surgery, incorporating

robotics into NOTES, thus enhancing intracorporeal suturing.

In another study, Hanly et al. reported their initial experience with a novel two-headed da Vinci surgical system in animal laboratory surgery.[34] This system has two collaborative modes that allow simultaneously to operate and actively swap control of the four robotic arms and allow them to share two of the robot's arms between two surgeons. The da Vinci mentoring console may facilitate surgeon collaboration during robotic surgery and improve the performance in surgical robotic cases, enhance resident education, and improve patient safety during robotic surgery. Recently, Intuitive Surgical has introduced the da Vinci Si HD model that is equipped with dual console capabilities for surgical training and education. Dual console capabilities feature built-in intercom to facilitate communication between surgeons and enable two surgeons to collaborate during a procedure for the da Vinci-enabled surgical assistance, such as exchanging control of the instrument arms and endoscope or facilitate teaching.

Now, possibility of telerobotic microsurgery from remote locations is possible using non-dedicated Internet lines. Sterbis et al. evaluated the validity of using the da Vinci system in urologic telesurgery and performed telerobotic nephrectomies on a porcine model using the public Internet.[35] Four right nephrectomies were performed telesurgically with resident surgeons operating at a console adjacent to the animal, while attending surgeons operated simultaneously on a second console of 1,300 and 2,400 miles from the operating room. This was the first report on collaborative transcontinental robotic telesurgery, with two separate consoles. Utilizing different parts of the same robot over non-dedicated Internet lines, the da Vinci system for a porcine nephrectomy model was innovative. Although the study acknowledges the several problems with telesurgery, such as liability, responsibility, and information security, its high rewarding potential for application into public health care is much anticipated.

12.8 Conclusion

For successful transition of new technology into clinical practices, surgeons must continue to train concurrently with the changing technology. Various methods have been proposed for training with the da Vinci surgical system. The method of training may vary between utilizing inanimate models like bench and pelvic trainers to animate models such as live animals, human cadavers, and animate cadavers. Utilization of these training models presents differing complications and shortcomings, especially in inanimate models. Nevertheless, the ideal training model should be able to teach the surgical skills required, be easily accessible, and be akin to an anesthetized patient. Ideal training strategy would be to learn basics of the da Vinci system and then train in both an inanimate model and an animal laboratory. Utilization of large animal models such as porcine or canine model, which display similar anatomy to humans, will be optimal in training and refining surgical skills, as well as developing new surgical procedures. Minimally invasive learning opportunities will evolve to incorporate animal training and advanced surgical simulators for optimal training and shorten the necessary learning curve.

Acknowledgments The authors would like to thank Ms. Seh-Rin Sung for her assistance in the preparation of this manuscript.

References

1. Hance J, Aggarwal R, Undre S, et al. Skills training in telerobotic surgery. *Int J Med Robotics Comput Assist Surg.* 2005;1(2):7–12.
2. Keeley FX, Eden CG, Tolley DA, et al. The British Association of Urological Surgeons: guidelines for training in laparoscopy. *BJU Int.* 2007;100(2):379–381.
3. Chitwood WR, Nifong LW, Elbeery JE, et al. Robotic mitral valve repair: trapezoidal resection and prosthetic annuloplasty with the da Vinci surgical system. *J Thorac Cardiovasc Surg.* 2000;120(6):1171–1172.
4. Thiel DD, Winfield HN. Robotics in urology: past, present and future. *J Endourol.* 2008;22(4):825–830.
5. McDougall EM, Corica FA, Chou DS, et al. Short-term impact of a robot-assisted laparoscopic prostatectomy 'mini-residency' experience on postgraduate urologists' practice patterns. *Int J Med Robotics Comput Assist Surg.* 2006;2:70–74.
6. Rashid HH, Leung YM, Rashid MJ, et al. Robotic surgical education: a systematic approach to training urology residents to perform robotic-assisted laparoscopic radical prostatectomy. *Urology.* 2006;68:75–79.
7. Cosman P, Hemli JM, Ellis AM, et al. Learning the surgical craft: a review of skills training options. *ANZ J Surg.* 2007;77:838–845.
8. van Velthoven RF, Hoffmann P. Methods for laparoscopic training using animal models. *Curr Urol Rep.* 2006;7(2):114–119.
9. Hammoud MM, Nuthalapaty FS, Goepfert AR, et al. To the point: medical education review of the role of simulators in surgical training. *Am J Obst Gynec.* 2008;199(34):338–343.
10. Vlaovic PD, Sargent ER, Boker JR, et al. Immediate impact of an intensive one-week laparoscopy training program on laparoscopic skills among postgraduate urologists. *JSLS.* 2008;12:1–8.
11. Belsley SJ, Byer A, Ballantyne GH, et al. 1st International Congress of the Minimally Invasive Robotic Association (MIRA), 7–10 December 2006, Innsbruck, Austria. Congress summary: MIRA and the future of surgical robotics. *Int J Med Robotics Comput Assist Surg.* 2006;2:98–103.
12. Pierorazio PM, Allaf ME. Minimally invasive surgical training: challenges and solutions. *Urol Oncol.* 2009;27(2):208–213.
13. Roberts KE, Bell RL, Duffy AJ. Evolution of surgical skills training. *World J Gastroenterol.* May 28, 2006;12(20):3219–3224.
14. Hanly EJ, Talamini MA. Robotic abdominal surgery. *Am J Surg.* 2004;188:19S–26S.
15. Mehrabi A, Yetimoglu CL, Nickkholgh A, et al. Development and evaluation of a training module for the clinical introduction of the da Vinci robotic system in visceral and vascular surgery. *Surg Endosc.* 2006;20:1376–1382.
16. Hanly EJ, Marohn MR, Bachman SL, et al. Multiservice laparoscopic surgical training using the da Vinci surgical system. *Amer J Surg.* 2004;187:309–315.
17. Cundiff GW, Weidner AC, Visco AG. Effectiveness of laparoscopic cadaveric dissection in enhancing resident comprehension of pelvic anatomy. *J Am Coll Surg.* 2001;291:492–495.
18. Lecuru F, Robin F, Taurelle R. Laparoscopic pelvic lymphadenectomy in an anatomical model: results of an experimental comparative trail. *J Obstet Gynecol Reprod Biol.* 1997;72:51–54.
19. Kunkler K. The role of medical simulation: an overview. *Int J Med Robot.* 2006;2:203–210.
20. Chitwood WR, Nifong LW, Chapman WH, et al. Robotic surgical training in an academic institution. *Ann Surg.* 2001;234(4):475–486.
21. Sung GT, Gill IS, Hsu TH. Robotic-assisted laparoscopic pyeloplasty: a pilot study. *Urology.* 1999;53(6):1099–1103.
22. Gill IS, Sung GT. Hsu et al. Robotic remote laparoscopic nephrectomy and adrenalectomy: the initial experience. *J Urol.* 2000;164(6):2082–2085.
23. Sung GT, Gill IS. Remote, robotic laparoscopic extravesical ureteral reimplantation with ureteral advancement technique. *Dialogues Pediatr Urol.* 2001;24:10.
24. Sung GT, Gill IS. Robotic laparoscopic surgery: a comparison of the da Vinci and ZEUS systems. *Urology.* 2001;58(6):893–898.
25. Hubert J, Feuillu B, Mangin P, et al. Laparoscopic computer-assisted pyeloplasty: the results of experimental surgery in pigs. *BJU Inter.* 2003;92:437–440.
26. Passerotti CC, Passerotti AM, Dall'Oglio MF, et al. Comparing the quality of the suture anastomosis and the learning curves associated with performing open,

freehand, and robotic-assisted laparoscopic pyeloplasty in a swine animal model. *J Am Coll Surg.* 2009;208: 576–586.

27. Passerotti CC, Nguyen HT, Lais A, et al. Robot-assisted laparoscopic ileal bladder augmentation: defining techniques and potential pitfalls. *J Endourol.* 2008;22(2): 355–360.

28. Ponsky LE, Cherullo EE, Banks KL, et al. Laparoscopic transuterine fetal vesicostomy: a feasibility study. *J Urol.* 2004;172:2391–2394.

29. Passerotti CC, Barnewolt C, Xuewu J, et al. In utero treatment for bladder outlet obstruction using robot assisted laparoscopic techniques. *J Urol.* 2008;180:1790–1794.

30. Schiff J, Li PS, Goldstein M. Robotic microsurgical vasovasostomy and vasoepididymostomy: a prospective randomized study in a rat model. *J Urol.* 2004;171: 1720–1725.

31. Gill IS, Ukimura O, Rubinstein M, et al. Lateral pedicle control during laparoscopic radical prostatectomy: refined technique. *Urology.* 2005;65(1):23–27.

32. Gianduzzo T, Colombo JR Jr, Haber GP, et al. Laser robotically assisted nerve-sparing radical prostatectomy: a pilot study of technical feasibility in the canine model. *BJU Inter.* 2008;102:598–602.

33. Haber GP, Crouzet S, Kamoi C, et al. Robotic NOTES (natural orifice translumenal endoscopic surgery) in reconstructive urology: initial laboratory experience. *Urology.* 2008;71:996–1000.

34. Hanly EJ, Miller BE, Kumar R, et al. Mentoring console improves collaboration and teaching in surgical robotics. *J Laparoendosc Adv Surg Tech A.* 2006;16(5):445–451.

35. Sterbis JR, Janly EJ, Herman BC, et al. Transcontinental telesurgical nephrectomy using the da Vinci robot in a porcine model. *Urology.* 2008;71:971–973.

Chapter 13

Training of Operating Room Technician and Nurses in Robotic Surgery

Stacey Dusik-Fenton and James O. Peabody

13.1 Introduction

Over the last several decades, there has been much technological advancement in the operating room. Laparoscopic surgery or minimally invasive surgery (MIS) was introduced over 20 years ago as an alternative to open surgery, and many surgical procedures can now be performed this way. However, some procedures have proven to be difficult to do in a pure laparoscopic environment. A new and increasingly common technological device is the master–slave robotic system. With a master–slave robot system, the surgeon controls the main operating instruments and the camera (operating the robot) from a remote console or workstation.[1] The most commonly used robotic system is the da Vinci Surgical System (Intuitive Surgical, Sunnyvale, CA). This robotic system provides the surgical team advantages such as 3D vision, magnification, wristed instrumentation, and tremor filtration for the robotic surgeon.[2] These advancements with the robotic system can overcome some of the drawbacks of laparoscopic surgery, in particular those related to suturing and working at difficult angles in smaller spaces. As the utilization of robots continues to evolve in the operating room and medical field, so will the role of the nurse and scrub technician.

During minimally invasive procedures, nurses must provide an increased amount and complexity of technical support. Nurses and technicians must seek opportunities to educate themselves about the technology, assess its impact, and determine how to best care for their patients with it.[3] While this increased knowledge is required for both laparoscopic and robotic surgeries, the complexity and novelty of the da Vinci system require a special educational effort. This knowledge will allow for educational and professional growth for the perioperative nurse and technician. A main role for nurses in the operating room is that of a patient advocate, and nurses must use this new technological knowledge and apply it to the overall care of their patient.

As of March 2009, there were 1,171 da Vinci robotic systems worldwide with 863 systems in the United States (Intuitive Surgical, Sunnyvale, CA). Over 140 hospitals own more than one da Vinci robotic systems, and one facility has five systems. Multiple robotic systems in a facility can increase the challenges and complexity of care for the perioperative nurse and technician. Multiple systems in an institution can increase the challenges because of a variety of instruments being used, different equipment, surgery services, and surgeons using the device. Nurses throughout the world are faced with the challenges, anxiety, and excitement of MIS, both laparoscopic and robotic, in the operating room.

13.2 Role of the Nurse and Technician

The primary role of the surgical nurse is to manage the environment in the operating room and to protect the patient within that environment.[4] A thorough understanding of the da Vinci system is critical for the perioperative nurse when caring for their patient. The nurse and technician must be able to prepare the robot,

J.O. Peabody (✉)
Department of Urology, Vattikuti Urology Institute, Henry Ford
Health System, Detroit, MI, USA
e-mail: jpeabod1@hfhs.org

A.K. Hemal, M. Menon (eds.), *Robotics in Genitourinary Surgery*,
DOI 10.1007/978-1-84882-114-9_13, © Springer-Verlag London Limited 2011

provide optimal patient care, and set up necessary instruments and supplies for every robot procedure. As well as preparing for successful robotic cases, the nurse and technician must be ready to troubleshoot any potential electrical or mechanical malfunctions with the robot. The team must also ready for potential conversions to laparoscopic or open cases. The perioperative nurse must function in a variety of roles ranging from patient advocate, educator, team leader, coordinator, and problem solver. With the help of an organized robotic team, the nurse and technician will develop individual roles yet continue to work together for a positive outcome for each patient undergoing a robotic-assisted laparoscopic procedure.

The perioperative nurse must function as an educator for both themselves and other team members. The lead nurse should keep aware of the new software installations and new hardware developed for the robot. The surgical team should communicate any problems with the function of the robot such as difficulty with the 3D vision or problems with the functioning of an instrument or robotic arm so that the field engineer can be promptly notified. Open communication with the company's field engineers enables the nurse and team members to be aware of these developments and help to troubleshoot any problems. Once nurses are confident in their knowledge base, they can begin to teach other team members and new team members so that all are aware of the robotic developments and new procedures. Nurses must seek opportunities to learn and educate others regarding new developments in the robotic field. These educational opportunities and resources may be found through the robotic company online, robotic courses, conferences for nurses and surgeons, journal articles, robotic texts, and via other robotic centers.

Team leader and coordinator are important aspects of the perioperative nurse's role. The nurse must work with the surgeon to coordinate and advocate for their patients. The perioperative nurse is the leader in the room. With this important role, the team will be coordinated, and all equipment and supplies will be readily available. All robotic procedures have the potential of conversion to laparoscopic or open surgery. As the coordinator, the nurse is aware and prepared for all emergencies. The nurse should have equipment and instruments available if any conversion is necessary. There are several emergency "backups" that are built into the robot. As the team leader, one must ensure

that the robot is always plugged into an electrical outlet, both the surgeon console and the patient-side cart. There is approximately 15 min of battery backup if there is a power failure in the medical facility. This backup allows the team enough time to safely remove the instruments and undock the robot. If the robot has been left unplugged, and the battery is empty, the robot will not function for the procedure to begin. It is important for the nurse to ensure and coordinate that the robot is always plugged into an electrical outlet, especially if the system has been moved around the operating room or from one room to another.

The da Vinci robot consists of three main components. These include the vision cart, patient-side cart, and the surgeon console (Fig. 13.1). The nurse and all team members in the operating room must be familiar with all three components. Preparation of the camera and scope, which is housed on the vision cart and draping of the robotic arms of the patient-side cart, must be completed for each robotic case. The operating room team must know how to connect, calibrate, and set up the three components of the robotic system.[3] There are potential mechanical and electrical malfunctions for each of the three components. Therefore, the nurse and operating team must be familiar with the system to properly troubleshoot all potential malfunctions. The operating team must also be familiar with the emergency procedures to remove the patient-side cart or robotic instruments from the patient.

Troubleshooting and problem-solving skills are important for the perioperative robotic nurse. Device failure with the robot may be mechanical or electrical.

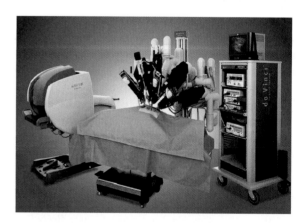

Fig. 13.1 Three components of the da Vinci robot – surgeon console, patient-side cart, and vision tower

The nurse and team members must be able to identify the issue with the robot and try to correct the problem. The correction phase will help avoid potential laparoscopic or open surgery conversions. The operating room should be equipped with sterilely packed scopes, extra light cables, camera, drapes, sterile adapters, light bulbs, and instruments for immediate use if there is a malfunction. Having these items set aside and ready can save valuable time during the procedure. Once the mechanical or electrical failure has been identified, the team members may correct the issue. Telephone communication with the field engineer of the company can also be of assistance during both the identification and the correction of the problem. Some problems can be corrected easily, occasionally by simply rebooting the system. According to *AORN*, "to prevent user error and rapidly recognize device failure, all healthcare team members must thoroughly understand robotic surgery and their role in the procedure."[5] Each team member must know their role for the team to function and avoidance of potential failures.

The role of the technician is that of an instrument engineer. With the assistance of the perioperative nurse, the technician coordinates the supplies and equipment necessary for the robotic surgery. The instruments, draping, calibration, and overall room preparation are completed in coordination between the technician and the nurse. The technician must also be aware of the differences in instrument use between the robotic surgeons, the differences between the three generations of da Vinci robots if they are all available in the same institution, and the variances between the instruments and the equipment. Educating other team members, troubleshooting and problem solving can be an important role of the technician. As a member of the dedicated team, the technician has an important role of the MIS team.

13.3 The Dedicated Operating Room Team

The hospital and health system must invest time and money into developing a successful robotic program. Initial setup costs for the hospital include the purchase of the robotic system, identifying and developing a lead surgeon and assistant surgeon, and purchase of instruments and supplies. A dedicated, committed, and a highly trained operating room team are also necessary for the program to be a success.

The costs for training operating room personal must be considered. The new team should attend the training sessions, preferably with the rest of the surgical team so that the group can begin to work together. The team must practice to learn how to drape, calibrate, and troubleshoot the system as well as learning the basic functions of the robot for things like optimal positioning of the robotic arms, instrument changes, and lens changes. If there is any confusion for the team members, this can lead to inefficient handling of the equipment, instruments, and supplies.[5] An inefficient team and robotic system use will increase operative time and decrease cost-efficiency while increasing inventory and maintenance costs.[5] Creating a dedicated operating room team may help to overcome these inefficiencies.

Together as a dedicated team, they will learn and understand the complexity of the robotic system as well as the robotic surgeon and the robotic procedures. Open communication and dedication among the members including the surgeon are vital for the team to be successful. This communication is not only among hospital team members but also with the company's field service engineer and customer service representative. The involvement of the service engineer and service representative will aid in the training and education of the team members. These individuals can provide information regarding the robotic system and assist in the troubleshooting process. As stated by Leach et al., the

> ...extent to which team members share the same understanding of operation, the major steps in the operation, and the critical points that might lead to surgical difficulties – and the OR environment – maintenance of a calm, positive working environment with expectations for respectful and supportive behaviors where "everyone matters" – influence surgical outcomes...[4]

A dedicated team that is training and communicating together and is working in a supportive environment facilitates in the establishment of a successful robotic program. The nurse and technician develop confidence in their roles and thus aid in the overall operating room efficiency. The efficiency is evident in room turnovers, room preparation, troubleshooting, patient care, and overall care of the complex robotic equipment. With an efficient and dedicated operating room team, the surgeons, hospital administration, management team, and patients will all benefit and notice a positive outcome. Positive patient results, decrease in operating room time, increase in productivity, and increase in staff satisfaction will be identified by all.

13.4 Robotic Room Preparation

When a hospital system makes the decision to purchase a robotic system, there are many factors that the administration, management, surgeon, and operating room team must appreciate and address. To begin, the type of robotic system and the generation of robotic system must be decided. Should the system be the high definition model, will there be 3D imaging system in the room for the assistants, what is the size and layout of the room, or are there other screens for assistant and visitors to view are a few other important questions that need to be addressed. The location of the system in the room and if the electrical outlets in the room can handle to voltage of the system are a few factors that must be thought through prior to the purchase of the system. Will the robotic system have a permanent "home" or will the system be moved throughout the operating room?

Once the type of system has been determined, it is beneficial for the hospital and operating room to have a permanent and stable room that will house the robot. If the robotic system must be moved from operating suites, there is a potential for damage to the system as well as injury to team members. The da Vinci robot consists of three components. These include the surgeon console, patient-side cart, and the vision tower. Each of these components requires its own electrical circuit and must be plugged in to maintain a constant charge on the battery. The battery backup is for emergency power failure and enables the surgeon to complete a portion of the surgery and the assistant to de-dock the robotic arms from the trocars. The system will not work if there is not sufficient life on the battery and may take up to 24 h for the battery to properly recharge. Failure to maintain the battery can cause surgery cancellations or require conversions to laparoscopic or open surgery. Due to a set length of the cables connecting the three components of the robotic system, the three components must be kept in close proximity to each other. This requires adequate

planning and developing of an organized robotic suite.

The assistant's ability to view either a 2D or a 3D screen is yet another factor to consider while preparing the robotic suite. Will the assistant be sitting or standing, will they be on the right side or the left side of the patient, will the assistant be able to communicate with the console surgeon, and where is the position of the patient in relation to the anaesthesia team. Once all components have been determined, the robotic room can be arranged and organized for a variety of robotic surgeries. The operating room's final arrangement must be beneficial for all those team members involved in the procedure, including the patient.

Once the room layout has been determined, the patient positioning equipment must be determined. There will be slight variances with patient positioning. This is related to the surgeon's preference and the type of surgery that will be performed. For the transperitoneal robotic-assisted prostatectomy, the patient is in a lithotomy position with extreme Trendelenburg position. The lithotomy position requires stirrups that will provide maximum support for the patient and adequate room for the robot. Due to the Trendelenburg position, the team must ensure that the patient is secured on the operating room table to prevent shift of position relative to the fixed robot during the procedure. The arms are tucked at the patient's side with ulnar nerve protectors around the hand and under the ulnar nerve (Fig. 13.2). The ulnar nerve protectors are taped

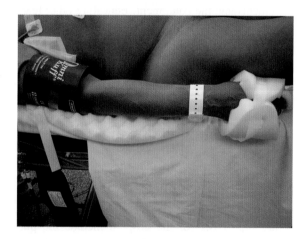

Fig. 13.2 Patient positioning of arms with ulnar nerve protectors for a robotic prostatectomy

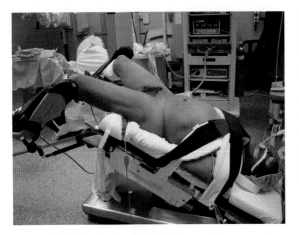

Fig. 13.3 Patient in lithotomy with *yellow* finn stirrups, secured with tape and safety straps and Trendelenburg position

and secured in an X configuration across the chest and taped to the operating room table. Safety straps are secured over the tape for an extra layer of security (Fig. 13.3). For robotic cystectomies or other pelvic robotic cases, the positioning is the same as the prostate. Robotic kidney cases have noticeable differences with positioning (Fig. 13.4). The patients are in a lateral decubitus position with operative side facing upward. An axillary roll is placed as well as a gel roll behind the patient to avoid potential rolling. The arm is placed in a Kranske arm holder, or pillows are placed between the two arms and secured with tape and rolled gauze dressing. The lower leg is flexed while upper leg is extended, with pillows between the two legs. Foam donuts are placed at the knee and ankle to protect from pressure points on the bed. The chest and legs are secured with tape and ulnar nerve protectors to secure patient to the bed. Once again, there are minor changes with surgeon preferences. Some surgeons prefer to use bean bags or gel pads between the patient and the

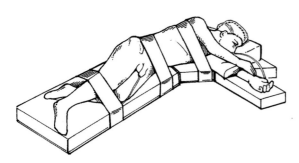

Fig. 13.4 Lateral robotic kidney position

bed. The ultimate goal for all the surgeries is to provide adequate security and protection for the patient while allowing access for the surgeon and the robot to perform the desired surgery.

For the operating room team, instrument trays and disposable products should be assessed, evaluated, and kept to a minimum for overall efficiency. The trays may be organized and based on laparoscopic instruments, robotic instruments, and open instruments. Each tray should have the minimum number of instruments that will be adequate to perform the surgery. If the tray has too many instruments, it will increase the turnover time for both central processing and room preparation. Similar to positioning, the trays will once again have slight variance depending on the robotic surgeon and surgery.

Efficiency in the operating room has a vested interest for all members of the operating room team as well as the surgeon, management, and hospital administration. Turnover time can be defined as "wheels out" to "wheels in." This definition is the time from when anaesthesia leaves the operating room with a patient until the time anaesthesia arrives at the room with the next patient. There are many factors that may affect the efficiency in the operating room, including instrument availability, operating room team, anaesthesia team, and team experience. Operating room efficiency improves with a dedicated team and with team experience.

13.5 Robotic Assistants

For the first time in the history of surgery the primary surgeon is not required to be by the bedside performing and assisting the surgery. This aspect puts phenomenal responsibility on the shoulders of the assistant in robotic surgery. The assistant surgeon may be a physician, a surgical assistant, or a registered nurse first assistant (RNFA). For robotic surgery with the da Vinci robotic system, the surgeon is operating from the console and the assistant is at the bedside. The surgeon then must rely on the assistant to provide direct hands on care to the patient. Communication among the members of the team is critical. The room should be arranged in such a way that it is easy for the team members to hear each other. During robotic surgery, the bedside assistant has a vital role in the overall care for the patient during the procedure.

The da Vinci robotic system used one robotic arm for the camera and may be equipped with two or three instrument arms. With three instrument arms (four-arm system), there is need for only one bedside assistant. Other surgeons may have the system with two instrument arms and may utilize either one or two bedside assistants. The main bedside assistant may assist from either the right side or the left side of the patient. This is dependent on a variety of factors. Factors include the surgeon training, experience and preference, assistant preference, the type of robotic surgery, and the operating room setup. For example, an assistant that is left handed may prefer to assist from the left side or visualization for the assistant might be optimal when the assistant is on the right side of the patient. It is beneficial for the console surgeon, bedside assistant, and the operating room team to identify these factors prior to the commencement of the robotic surgery.

The bedside assistant has a variety of roles and responsibilities. As mentioned before, the surgeon is at the robotic console and "unscrubbed" away from the patient's bedside. The assistant is the one at the bedside and must be prepared for potential emergencies such as conversions to laparoscopic or open surgery. The assistant should possess and develop expertise in laparoscopic skills such as gently grasping tissue to provide exposure, suctioning smoke, blood and other fluids, applying clips, and suture manipulation. As the laparoscopic skills and knowledge of the operative steps improve, the assistant is able to move in a coordinated fashion ("dance") with the robotic console surgeon. The assistant is able to anticipate the surgeon's next move and is prepared for each of the subsequent steps during the surgery. Robotic skills also are necessary for the bedside assistant to develop. The assistant aids in the placement of the ports, docking of the robotic arms, placement of the robotic instruments, and scope changes and maintenance. The console surgeon may assist in the port placement and wound closure, but the surgeon is dependent on the bedside assistant for all other manipulations of the robot.

A well-trained primary assistant may become an educator for others who are in training to become bedside assistants. The primary assistant must educate others and help train them with both their laparoscopic and robotic skill base. Teaching is a key role for the primary bedside assistant. Depending on the hospital setting, there are a variety of team members that may become the primary bedside assistant. Some hospital settings use other surgeons or retired surgeons as the assistant. In teaching facilities, residents and fellows are used as the primary assistant who then develop the skill base to become expert console surgeons. Other facilities utilize ancillary staff team members such as physician's assistants (PA), registered nurse first assistants (RNFA), or surgical technician first assistants. There are many benefits in the utilization of ancillary staff as the primary bedside assistants. These assistants are long-term staff members and do not rotate through the operating room in the manner that residents and fellows do. The ancillary staff may become part of the dedicated robotic team and aid in the development of OR efficiency and overall patient care.

13.6 Conclusion

A successful robotic surgery program is dependent on a well-trained, motivated, and involved team of perioperative nurses and technicians. Their strong involvement in the program will help the surgeons who are perfecting procedures and developing new ones. The team will do so by keeping the robotic equipment functioning at its capacity, by helping the flow of the operation through having the necessary instrumentation ready and available, by efficiently turning the room over between cases, by providing assistance at the patient side when called on to do so, and by serving in their role as patient advocate to make sure that the operating room environment is as safe as possible for their patient.

References

1. Thiel DD, Winfield HN. Robotics in urology: past, present, and future. *J Endourol.* 2008;22:825.
2. Palmer KJ, Lowe GJ, Coughlin GD, et al. Launching a successful robotic surgery program. *J Endourol.* 2008;22:819.
3. Francis P, Winfield HN. Medical robotics: the impact on perioperative nursing practice. *Urol Nurs.* 2006;26:99.
4. Leach LS, Myrtle RC, Weaver FA, et al. Assessing the performance of surgical teams. *Health Care Manage Rev.* 2009;34:29.
5. Francis P. Evolution of robotics in surgery and implementing a perioperative robotics nurse specialist role. *AORN J.* 2006;83:630.

Chapter 14

Impact of Virtual Reality Simulators in Training of Robotic Surgery

David A. Gilley and Chandru P. Sundaram

14.1 Overview of Simulation

The utilization of robotic surgery is increasing across surgical disciplines. This has created a need for training in robotic surgery for experienced and novice surgeons alike. Currently, this need is being met with participation in live surgery, animal labs, and skills labs with inanimate objects. Participation in live surgery increases risks for the patient due to the surgeon's inexperience. Animal models are expensive and are generally not available in volumes needed to acquire and maintain robotic surgery skills. The usefulness of training with inanimate objects is primarily limited to familiarization with the robotic console. This has left a large need for a safe, reproducible, cost-effective method to teach robotic surgery. This need is beginning to be filled by virtual reality simulation. Simulation alone has been used in many high-tech and specialized industries for years. Most notably the aerospace industry began developing simulators 70 years ago[1] and now utilizes simulation as an integral part of training programs.[2] Initially, these were crude mechanical representations of flight. Currently, these simulators are capable of recreating complex environments and reacting to user decisions. This is a safe, reproducible, and comparatively cheap environment in which one can learn a complex task. The defense industry also utilizes simulation for tank and submarine crews. Combat scenarios and strategies can be safely and repetitively practiced.

Simulation, in its broadest definition, has been used in surgery instruction for years. A basic example: a pig's foot with which to practice suturing. A simple model can provide trainees a basis for participation in live surgical procedures. In contrast to other industries, surgical simulation has certainly lagged behind. As surgical technology has changed the increased complexity has posed new problems for surgical education.[3] In the transition from open surgery to laparoscopic surgery, a multitude of new skills had to be learned and ultimately taught. This necessity to attain minimally invasive surgery skills in a safe and accurate way has made simulation important. Yet, its use as a core portion in training programs is not common.[4,5]

Laparoscopic simulators began simply as a box with instrument ports placed in them. Users could work with inanimate objects and complete simple tasks such as suturing and knot tying. These have evolved and gained wide acceptance as an important training tool.[6]

Box trainers certainly have established their value in the training of surgeons, but they are limited to relatively simple tasks. Taking a cue from the aerospace industry and advancing past the mechanical box trainers, virtual reality laparoscopic training systems have been developed.[7] The MIST-VR simulator was the first commercially successful virtual reality laparoscopic trainer and was able to demonstrate the value of simulation in live surgery.[1,8] Initially, these trainers were often limited to large medical centers with appropriate facilities and consisted of simplified tasks such as knot tying and placing rings on pegs.[9] More advanced trainers have been developed to simulate several urologic procedures including: TURP, cystoscopy, ureteroscopy, and PCNL. The value and validity of virtual reality training have been established by Seymour and colleagues.[8]

C.P. Sundaram (✉)
Department of Urology, Indiana University School of
Medicine, Indianapolis, IN, USA
e-mail: sundaram@iupui.edu

A.K. Hemal, M. Menon (eds.), *Robotics in Genitourinary Surgery*,
DOI 10.1007/978-1-84882-114-9_14, © Springer-Verlag London Limited 2011

14.2 Reliability and Validation

All simulators must be tested for their inherent reliability and validity. Basic simulators have inherent value in their ability to teach a basic task. The quality of a knot tied in a box trainer is easily assessed as are needle placement and handling. Their reliability and validity are easy to recognize and assess. The increasing surgical technology has demanded an associated increase in simulator capabilities. As simulators become more advanced and are used to teach more complex tasks and procedures, the tests used to evaluate the simulator must be more rigorous. As Mcdougall states,[3] complex simulators would need extensive testing to determine reliability and validity. By moving away from the basic mechanical simulators the testing must be rigorous.

Reliability is effectively the dependability of a simulator. The simulator must yield similar results under similar conditions each time it is used.[10] Reliability can be measured by comparing the performance on the first half of a test to that on the second half (split halves). Test–retest reliability is probably more practical for surgery simulation and involves the comparison of scores done at two separate points in time.

Validity in simulation means the device measures what it is supposed to measure.[10] There are several types of validity that are briefly outlined. Face validity is subjective and is attained by having an expert evaluate the simulation for its realism. For example, does it simulate what it is supposed to simulate?[3,10] Content validity is also subjective. It involves reviewing the simulation to ensure that it includes all of the appropriate steps as well as evaluating their level of cohesiveness. It is an evaluation of a simulators ability to realistically teach what it is intended to teach.[3,10]

Objective measures of validity include criterion and construct. Criterion validity is used to compare an old simulation method to a new method. Criterion validity has two subsets: concurrent and predictive. Concurrent validity is measured by having subjects complete a simulation and then perform a similar task with a different accepted model (i.e., cadaver, animal model). If the performance on the simulator and established model are correlated there is concurrent validity.[3,10] The other aspect of criterion validity is predictive validity. This is the ability of a simulator to reliably assess how the subject will do with the real task. Simply stated does good performance on the simulation relate to good performance in the operating room.[3] Construct validity is the ability of a simulator to distinguish from novice versus expert subjects. This is measured over time and continually updated.

14.3 Overview of Current Virtual Reality Robotic Simulators

To our knowledge three virtual reality simulators have been developed for robotic surgical training using the da Vinci Surgical system. All the systems continue to evolve and develop software to enhance their utility during training.

14.4 Mimic dV-Trainer

Mimic dV-Trainer is made by Mimic Technologies in Seattle, Washington, and represents a complete kinematic representation of the da Vinci Surgical system. It is a virtual reality simulator with a 3D visual interface provided by Mimic (Fig. 14.1). The interface has hand

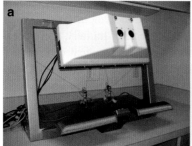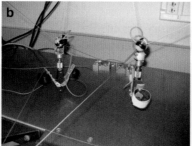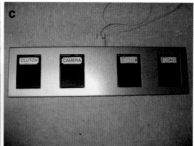

Fig. 14.1 **a** Mimic dV-Trainer interface console. **b** Mimic dV trainer hand controls. **c** Mimic dV trainer foot controls

controls that are very similar to the da Vinci surgery console. Mimic's software can be customized for a variety of tasks, including needle exchange, knot tying, and suturing.[11] Foot pedals representing those seen on the da Vinci system are also provided.

Training modules available on the dV-Trainer are for system training and skills training as seen below:

- System Training

    o Surgeon console awareness
    o EndoWrist manipulation
    o Camera and clutching
    o System assessment

- Skills Training

    o Needle exchange
    o Needle driving
    o Knot tying
    o Suturing

Face and content validity of the Mimic dV-Trainer have been established in a study by Sethi et al.[12] Twenty participants, including five experts, completed three virtual reality exercises. The exercises were selected based upon real drills used during our robotic training curriculum. They were a ring and cone, string walk, and letter board exercises. Virtual reality representations of the string walk and letter board were developed by Mimic specifically for this exercise. Face and content validity were established by a questionnaire in which the participants evaluated the system's realism, ease of use, and usefulness as a training tool. These questions revealed that participants thought that the virtual environment was overall realistic and easy to use, and the expert users all felt that it was useful as a training tool. Objective performance metrics were evaluated, and time to completion and time instruments were out of view. The performance of the novices was compared to the experienced group. The expert users were able to complete the tasks faster as well as have less time with instruments out of view. These differences were only statistically significant in one of the three exercises though.

In an unpublished follow up study we compared a group of 20 expert users to 20 novice users. Face and content validity were established with a postexercise questionnaire. All users rated the system well in categories of realism and ease of use. The expert

users unanimously rated the relevance of the system as very high, and all participants felt that it was a useful training tool. To establish construct validity time and performance metrics were logged and compared between the two groups. Expert users performed all tasks faster than the novice group. The expert group also demonstrated statistically significant differences in instrument collisions and economy of motion on certain exercises.

In a study by Kenney et al.,[13] experienced and novice surgeons completed four virtual tasks, two EndoWrist exercises (peg board and pick and place) and two needle-driving exercises (dots and numbers and suture sponge). A post-session questionnaire was completed by each user and established face and content validity of the dV-Trainer. Performance metrics including time to completion, instrument collisions, total motion, and others were recorded and analyzed. Construct validity was established by comparing the performance of experienced and novice users. Experienced users had statistically significant better performance in all measured metrics. Further studies will need to be completed to determine the two aspects of criterion validity.

14.5 Surgical SIM Robotic Surgery Simulator

The Surgical SIM RSS (SimSurgery AS, Oslo, Norway) distributed by Medical Education Technologies, Inc., Sarasota, Florida, in the United States uses the Surgical SIM VR system that can be used for other applications such as basic laparoscopy and transurethral resection of prostate. The system consists of a customized personal computer with a computer monitor. The controls can be changed to suit the appropriate training application. Centers that already possess a Surgical SIM VR system may be able to upgrade to the robotic simulator in a cost-effective manner.

It is a partial representation of the da Vinci controls. A 2D display on the monitor or an optional head mounted 3D display is available (Fig. 14.2). In a report by Lin and colleagues[14] participants at the 2006 Society of American Gastroesophageal Surgeons (SAGES) meeting were invited to complete suture

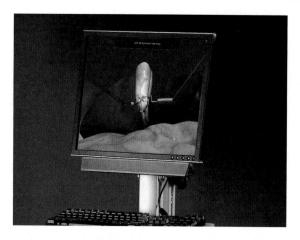

Fig. 14.2 METI robotic surgery simulator (RSS)

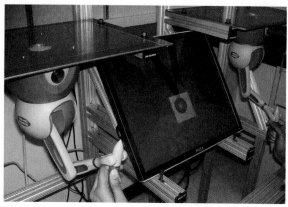

Fig. 14.3 RoSS robotic surgical simulator

placement and knot tying exercise on the METI robotic trainer. Users were stratified into expert or novice based upon their experience with robotic surgery. Task completion was higher in the expert group when compared to nonexpert users. The authors conclude that this difference is suggestive of construct validity.

14.6 RoSS System

Robotic Surgery Simulator (RoSS) is a new low-cost virtual reality training system developed by Roswell Park Cancer Institute and University at Buffalo and is being marketed by Simulated Surgical Systems LLC.[15] RoSS consists of a custom mock up of the DVSS master controls and console with two 6 degree of freedom input devices, stereo head mounted display, clutch and pedals, and custom-designed pinch device similar to the actual robot console (Fig. 14.3). The virtual reality simulation consists of lessons for robot-assisted operations, needle handling, catheter insertion and grasping, traversal stretching clipping of tissues, and needle capping. Advanced simulation modules consist of step by step tutorials for procedures such as prostatectomy and cystectomy. A preliminary study has demonstrated that RoSS helps in improvement of cognitive and visuomotor skills and familiarity with instruments. Validation studies are being planned.

Virtual reality simulation has great potential as a very advanced training tool. Currently, the hardware has been developed and is being refined. Most current

virtual models are simply representations of inanimate exercises used in basic robotic surgery training. The potential exists for incredibly advanced virtual environments in which to practice. There are several challenges where efforts are being focused.

Anatomic environments with accurate tissue structure and layering must be developed. The material properties of real tissue must be modeled to provide accurate deformation and interaction with the virtual instruments. These virtual tissues will deform, stretch, and tear like actual surgery.[15] Ultimately virtual reality simulators will be able to replicate entire operations in a safe environment. As more extensive models are developed an entire abdomen, complete with appropriate layers of tissue that deform, interact with virtual instruments, and respond to surgical tools (i.e. cautery) can be incorporated into simulations.

14.7 Incorporation of Virtual Reality Simulation in the Robotic Surgical Curriculum

Virtual reality simulation is only a part of a comprehensive surgical curriculum. The curriculum includes medical knowledge of the urologic conditions that can be treated with robotic surgery. The surgical aspects of the training consist of knowledge and skills related to the safe operation of the robotic surgical system and skills related to individual surgical procedures. Exercises using inanimate models help the trainee acquire several basic skills required for surgery: hand eye coordination, camera/laparoscope control, clutching, and efficient movement of instruments in the surgical field, intracorporeal suturing, pattern cutting, and dissection.

Robotic simulation has been incorporated into the teaching curriculum at our institution. Simulation can consist of training on the robotic system using inanimate or animal models or virtual reality simulators. We have established a weekend robotics course that allows our residents an opportunity to work with the full da Vinci robotic system. This training complements experience on the virtual reality simulator which is not fully developed. Until high-fidelity virtual reality simulators are developed with simulation of surgical procedures, the use of the da Vinci Surgical system in training labs continues to be required. Our skills training with inanimate models takes place on weekends when the operating room and the robotic system are not being used for surgeries. During the first session the participant is familiarized with the robotic system, including docking and undocking, trouble shooting, and trocar placement. Subsequent sessions include completion of five tasks modified and adapted from Albani and Lee[16] which are judged for time and accuracy. Each task is designed to utilize various aspects of the da Vinci system. A peg board is used for peg transition and requires camera repositioning and navigation, object transitioning, appropriate grasping force, and clutching. String walk is a piece of umbilical tape grasped at marked sites with alternating graspers. Letter board is the placement of letters and numbers on their appropriate place. Pattern cutting uses Potts scissors to cut out a circle from a piece of gauze. A suturing exercise involves needle driving and knot tying. Interrupted and running suturing is performed, followed by "running vesicourethral anastomosis" using a silicone model. Our residents find this curriculum very beneficial, as evidenced by very high participation and satisfaction rates.

We have started to incorporate the Mimic system into our robotics training curriculum. We have been able to develop virtual simulations of the same tasks that are performed during the weekend robotics course. Recently, Lerner et al.[17] were able to demonstrate that skills learned on a robotic simulator were able to be reliably transferred to the da Vinci system. Two groups were created. One group completed training tasks during five or six 1-h long sessions on the da Vinci system alone. The other group completed an initial session, to establish a baseline, and a final session on the full da Vinci with four sessions completed on the dV-Trainer in between. Three virtual exercises were performed on the dV-Trainer: a letter board, pick and place (rings picked up and placed over cones), ring walk (a ring is guided over a virtual tube), and a clutching cavity (users move the instruments across a virtual cavity using clutching and camera repositioning). Each individual group showed improvement in several performance metrics. Notably, the virtual reality group showed statistically significant improvement in performance on four of the five full da Vinci drills. This is certainly suggestive of concurrent validity.

The Mimic dV-Trainer continues to undergo development to enhance its usefulness. Though the hardware represents the controls of the da Vinci Surgical system, it requires further development to improve its durability, especially of the grippers. The simulation of force feedback is not a true representation of the da Vinci Surgical system. The software that has been validated so far includes basic exercises. However, further development of hardware and software is progressing and will correct the deficiencies in the early models.

14.8 Future Directions

Virtual reality robotic simulation could provide an opportunity to uncouple the da Vinci robot console from the robot itself. This would allow training to take place without requiring the usage of the entire da Vinci system reducing instrument degradation and cost. To reduce costs surgeons could use the console of the surgical system when not being used for surgery. This solution will eliminate the problems associated with hardware development in a simulator. Development can remain focused on software which is in early development. Development of simulation software required to fully realize the significant potential of simulation in robotic surgery includes procedure-specific simulation, troubleshooting and management of complications, and anatomical variations. Eventually, preoperative patient data and imaging details can be used to create patient-specific simulation where the surgeon can practice the entire surgery on a virtual patient before the actual surgery. Specific or critical parts of the operation can also be performed in the simulator as the surgeon becomes more experienced. Simulators can then be used as part of the certification or recertification process where not only knowledge is tested but so are the surgical skills. Assessing resident skills during their residency can also be accomplishment with objective assessment of their surgical skills on an annual basis along with their in-service examination. Simulators can also be used for patient education to assist them with selection of the appropriate treatment. Finally virtual reality simulators can be used during development and testing of new surgical instruments before being used on animal or human studies. The opportunities for virtual reality in robotic surgery are immense and extend from training and certification to patient education and instrument development.

References

1. Satava RM. Historical review of surgical simulation – a personal perspective. *World J Surg.* 2008;32(2):141–148.
2. Wignall GR, et al. Surgical simulation: a urological perspective. *J Urol.* 2008;179(5):1690–1699.
3. McDougall EM. Validation of surgical simulators. *J Endourol.* 2007;21(3):244–247.
4. Kapadia MR, et al. Current assessment and future directions of surgical skills laboratories. *J Surg Educ.* 2007;64(5):260–265.
5. Korndorffer JR Jr, Stefanidis D, Scott DJ. Laparoscopic skills laboratories: current assessment and a call for resident training standards. *Am J Surg.* 2006;191(1):17–22.
6. Fundamentals of Laparoscopic Surgery. July 6, 2009. Available at: http://www.flsprogram.org/index.php. Accessed July 6, 2009.
7. Satava RM. Virtual reality surgical simulator. The first steps. *Surg Endosc.* 1993;7(3):203–205.
8. Seymour NE, et al. Virtual reality training improves operating room performance: results of a randomized, double-blinded study. *Ann Surg.* 2002;236(4):458–463, discussion 463–464.
9. Hruby GW, et al. The EZ trainer: validation of a portable and inexpensive simulator for training basic laparoscopic skills. *J Urol.* 2008;179(2):662–666.
10. Gallagher AG, Ritter EM, Satava RM. Fundamental principles of validation, and reliability: rigorous science for the assessment of surgical education and training. *Surg Endosc.* 2003;17(10):1525–1529.
11. Mimic Technology. May 31, 2009. Available at: http://www.mimic.ws. Accessed May 31, 2009.
12. Sethi AS, et al. Validation of a novel virtual reality robotic simulator. *J Endourol.* 2009;23(3):503–508.
13. Kenney PA, et al. Face, content, and construct validity of dV-Trainer, a novel virtual reality simulator for robotic surgery. *Urology.* 2009;73(6):1288–1292.
14. Lin DW, et al. Computer-based laparoscopic and robotic surgical simulators: performance characteristics and perceptions of new users. *Surg Endosc.* 2009;23(1):209–214.
15. Baheti A, Kumar A, Srimathveeravalli G, Kesavadas T, Guru K RoSS: virtual reality robotic surgical simulator for the Da Vinci surgical simulator system, In Proc. of IEEE Haptics Symposium, 2008.
16. Albani JM, Lee DI. Virtual reality-assisted robotic surgery simulation. *J Endourol.* 2007;21(3):285–287.
17. Lerner MA, Ayalew M, Peine WJ, Sundaram CP. Does training on a virtual reality robotic simulator improve performance on the da Vinci surgical system? *J Endourol.* March, 2010;24(3):467–472.

Note: Mimic Technologies has been recently working with Intuitive Surgical to incorporate the simulation software into the daVinci Si surgical system's console.

Chapter 15

Training, Credentialing, and Hospital Privileging for Robotic Urological Surgery

Kevin C. Zorn and Gagan Gautam

Robotic surgery has undergone an evolution at an incredible rate in the last decade with robotic-assisted radical prostatectomy (RARP) now being the most commonly performed robotic procedure. More impressively, as a urologic community, we have witnessed a paradigm shift in that the robotic approach has now become the standard approach for radical prostatectomy in the majority of hospital centers. Despite this trend, the majority (>70%) of minimally invasive radical prostatectomies in the United States are being performed by low volume surgeons (<15 cases/year).[1] Although guidelines for the safe initiation of this technology are an overwhelming necessity, unfortunately no standardized credentialing system currently exists to assess competency and safety of the robotic surgeon. This is also the case for surgeon trainees who are Board certified only via oral examinations. The absence of an established training and credentialing protocol can result in undesirable complications – namely surgical and medicolegal. Above all, it can potentially compromise patient safety. Currently, various educational formats including residency, fellowship, "mini-residency," proctoring, teleproctoring, preceptoring, and simulation can provide the requisite training and evaluation for robotic urological surgeons. However, what is crucial is the establishment of a central credentialing authority which supervises these educational endeavors and formulates common guidelines for the safe initiation of a robotic program in any institution. Already implemented in the aviation milieu, simulation will become the means to ensure safe surgical training, objective credentialing and ongoing maintenance of skills. As we have sworn to the Hippocratic Oath, we must uphold our promise to "above all, do no harm".

15.1 Introduction

Robotic surgery has made rapid advances in the past decade, particularly in urology, and has now firmly established itself in most advanced centers around the world. Although the da Vinci® surgical system (Intuitive Surgical, Sunnyvale, CA) is also used for procedures on the kidney and the urinary bladder, it has found its greatest application in the surgical management of clinically localized prostate cancer. Robot-assisted radical prostatectomy (RARP) developed as a result of pioneering work performed by Binder,[2] Vallancien,[3] and Menon[4] and is now considered a frontline management modality for this condition. In the United States, 42 and 63% of all radical prostatectomies in 2006 and 2007, respectively, were performed with robot assistance. This number has continued to increase to over 85% for the years 2009–2010.[5] Approximately 18% (947/5223) of all US registered hospitals currently own a da Vinci robot. Although this may seem like a small proportion, it is impressive to note the rapid spread of this technology in that two new centers incorporate a robot every single week.[6] As of September 2010, the reported da Vinci Surgical System installed base was a total of 1,661 systems; 1,228 in the United States, 292 in Europe, and 141 in the rest of the world. (http://biz.yahoo.com/e/101020/isrg10-q.html FORM 10-Q).

K.C. Zorn (✉)
Department of Urology, Division of Robotic Surgery,
University of Montreal Medical Center, Montreal, QC, Canada
e-mail: kevin.zorn@gmail.com

A.K. Hemal, M. Menon (eds.), *Robotics in Genitourinary Surgery*,
DOI 10.1007/978-1-84882-114-9_15, © Springer-Verlag London Limited 2011

This explosive growth and adoption of robotic technology have resulted in an ever growing requirement for surgeons trained in robotic urological surgery (RUS). Unfortunately, due to the relatively recent introduction of this surgical approach, an overwhelming majority of current robotic surgeons have not been exposed to RUS during their residency and/or fellowship years. As such, it is imperative to establish set criteria for the training and credentialing of robotic surgeons to ensure the safe introduction of this technology while upholding patient safety.

15.2 Measuring the Robotic "Learning Curve" and Its Impact on Patient Care

Although a lack of long-term oncological data makes comparisons difficult, mid-term biochemical recurrence-free outcomes of RARP appear to be comparable between pure laparoscopic, robotic, and open radical prostatectomy series.[7–9] Similarly, in experienced hands, the incidence of positive surgical margins (PSM) has also been comparable between these modalities.[8–10] With regard to perioperative complication rates and functional outcomes (urinary continence and erectile function) after surgery, RARP has been able to match up to both open and laparoscopic radical prostatectomy.[8]

Like any other major surgical procedure, RARP is profoundly impacted by the experience of the surgeon. It has been demonstrated that the surgeon's learning curve (LC) influences all aspects of RARP outcomes, including the PSM rate.[11–13] Atug et al. compared PSM rates in the first 100 patients undergoing RARP in their institution by dividing them into three groups with equal number of patients in each group. The rates of PSM were significantly impacted by the team's prior surgical experience with the first group of 33 patients having a 45.4% positivity rate as compared to 21.2 and 11.7% for groups 2 and 3, respectively ($p = 0.0053$).[11] Vickers et al. evaluated the effect of surgeon experience on the rates of biochemical recurrence after RARP. They found that surgeons with a larger experience (>250 prior cases) had a significantly improved oncological outcome vis-a-vis their colleagues at the beginning of their LC (<10 prior

cases). At 5 years post-surgery, patients operated by the less experienced surgeons had a biochemical recurrence rate of 17.9% as compared to 10.7% for those treated by the more experienced ones ($p < 0.001$).[14] The same group subsequently demonstrated excellent 5-year cancer control rates (approaching 100%) for patients with organ-confined prostate cancer operated by experienced surgeons, thereby implying that most recurrences in such a situation reflect an inadequate surgical technique and may be a function of the LC rather than tumor biology.[15]

If operating time (OT) is used as the criterion, the LC of RARP has been estimated as 13–200 cases with a calculated OT improvement rate of 1–21 min per case.[6] In the same study by Steinberg et al., the cost of OT and anesthesia services during this RARP LC has been calculated to range from $95,000 to $1,365,000. However, several reports have demonstrated improvements in functional (urinary continence) and oncological (pT2-PSM rates) outcomes well beyond 250 cases, thereby implying that it may take a longer experience than is often assumed to reach a plateau on the RARP LC.[14–16]

A similar correlation between surgical experience and outcomes of radical prostatectomy (RP) can be inferred from studies which have evaluated the impact

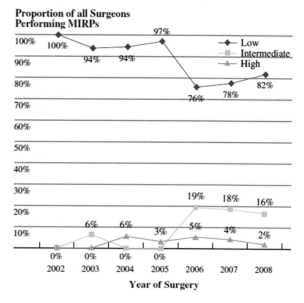

Fig. 15.1 Annual trends depicting the proportions of minimally invasive radical prostatectomy (MIRP) surgeons, stratified according to annual caseload tertiles: low (1–15 MIRP) vs. intermediate (16–63 MIRP) vs. high (63 MIRP). Permission for reprint by Springer, Lic No. 2562281240340

Table 15.1 Rates of in-hospital complications stratified according to surgeon's annual caseload[a]

Complications	Overall (%)	Annual caseload			χ^2 trend test
		Low (≤15 MIRP)	Intermediate (16–63 MIRP)	High (≥64 MIRP)	
Overall	243 (9.1)	127 (14.0)	69 (7.5)	47 (5.5)	<0.001
Miscellaneous medical	121 (4.5)	36 (7.0)	14 (3.5)	1 (2.9)	<0.001
Respiratory	85 (3.2)	42 (4.6)	29 (3.2)	14 (1.6)	<0.001
Miscellaneous surgical	63 (2.4)	36 (4.0)	14 (1.5)	13 (1.5)	<0.001
Genitourinary	30 (1.1)	15 (1.7)	9 (1.0)	6 (0.7)	0.2
Cardiac	18 (0.7)	4 (0.4)	5 (0.5)	9 (1.1)	0.2
Wound	12 (0.4)	4 (0.4)	2 (0.2)	6 (0.7)	0.3
Vascular	10 (0.4)	2 (0.2)	6 (0.7)	2 (0.2)	0.2
Transfusion rate	45 (1.7)	30 (3.5)	11 (1.0)	4 (0.5)	<0.001

Data are numbers with percentages in parentheses unless otherwise indicated.
[a]Beacuse more than one complication can occur, values add up to more than 100%.

of annual surgical volume on surgery outcomes.[17,18] Wilt et al., in a recent review, performed an analysis of databases from 1980 to 2007 and observed that for every 10 additional RP procedures performed annually in a hospital, the risk of surgery-related mortality and morbidity decreased by 13 and 1.21%, respectively. In fact, the relative risk (RR) of mortality was almost double in patients getting operated in low-volume (<22 cases per year) compared to high-volume (>50 cases per year) centers. Similarly teaching hospitals were found to have an 18% lower rate of surgery-related complications as compared to community hospitals.[17] In a recent population-based study of the 2002–2008 Florida Hospital Inpatient Datafile, Budäus et al. evaluated the temporal trends in RARP annual surgical caseload (AC), impact of RARP surgical experience and in-hospital complication and transfusion rates.[1] Between 2002 and 2005, 94–100% of surgeons were considered as low AC tertile (≤15 MIRP) vs. 76–82% between 2006 and 2008 (Fig. 15.1). For the same time periods, low AC tertile surgeons performed 46–100 and 27–32% of all MIRPs, respectively. Multivariable logistic regression models revealed 51 and 68% lower complication rates in patients operated on by surgeons of intermediate (17–76 MIRPs) and high SE (≥77 MIRPs) relative to surgeons of low SE (≤16 MIRPs) (Table 15.1). Similarly, transfusion rates were 80 and 83% lower for the same groups. This study is the first to indicate that high SE reduces MIRP complication and transfusion rates. Despite this observation, even in the most contemporary study year, most MIRP surgeons (82%) were in the low AC tertile and contributed to as many as 32% of all MIRPs.

Such an impact of the LC and surgical volume on oncological and functional outcomes stresses the importance of introducing mechanisms and guidelines by which the trainee surgeons can attain a sufficient level of skill without compromising on the safety of their initial patients.

15.3 Current Status of Robotic Urological Surgery Credentialing

Although several institutions have taken the initial steps toward establishing a credentialing system for robotic surgery, a majority of hospital centers have no safe measures for surgeon privileging. With no pathways in place, any qualified urologist may schedule a RARP with no verification of sufficient training or competence. A small number of centers have initiated specific credentialing guidelines (Table 15.2); however, they do not appear to be a universal consensus or consistency between the institutional requirements. As such, an overwhelming need currently exists for the creation of standardized guidelines applicable to all institutions, under the oversight of a centralized authority (such as the AUA or EUA) responsible for recommending and implementing training, certification, and credentialing in RUS.

At present, the responsibility of physician credentialing and granting privileges to perform surgeries is the responsibility of the individual institution. The chief of medical staff/medical staff offices/committees/operating room committee or other

Table 15.2 Guidelines for institutional robotic credentialing

	University of Iowa Hospitals and Clinics (UIHC)	University of Rochester Medical Center	University of Texas MD Anderson Cancer Center
Institutional implementation	October 2008	May 2005	January 2007
Proctor definition	– Proctor represents the medical staff and is responsible to the medical staff – Should be present and attentive throughout the entire robotic procedure, including port placement – Should hold hospital privileges in robotic-assisted surgery and have completed 10 robotic procedures	–	–
Proctor role	– Proctor provides objective evaluation of a physician's actual surgical competence (procedure performance and judgement)	–	–
Credentialing guidelines for robotic certification	*All physicians requesting privileges for robotic-assisted surgery must meet criteria 1, 2, and 3 or 4 and 5 or criteria 6, 7, and 8:* (1) Provide evidence of completing a hands-on training practicum in the use of robot of at least 8-h duration which includes 3 h of personal experience using the system on an animal model during this training (2) Provide evidence of observing at least two live clinical cases using the robotic surgical system (3) Provide evidence of performing two patient cases using the robotic surgical system that was proctored by a second surgeon who holds privileges in robotically assisted surgery or	*Provisional* Laparoscopic/robotic prostate surgery privileges are granted to initiate the process of credentialing in prostate robotic surgery. The following are criteria for granting provisional privileges: (1) Completion of an approved fellowship or preceptorship program (2) Completion of a laparoscopic prostate training course of at least 1-week duration which includes formal didactic sessions and laboratory sessions with cadavers, provided that the surgeon has prior experience in advanced laparoscopic surgery (greater than 12 laparoscopic cases per year). If the surgeon is not experienced, completion of an approved fellowship is required	*Provisional privileges:* 1. Initial privileging request is within the physician's department. Requests approved by the department chairman will be reviewed by MINTOS and forwarded to the credentials committee of the medical staff which will make a recommendation to ECMS and the president 2. To ensure patient safety and minimize the risks of complications, surgeons will initially be limited to a specific set of procedures and additionally should limit procedures to those they would normally and routinely be performing by other techniques

Table 15.2 (continued)

University of Iowa Hospitals and Clinics (UIHC)	University of Rochester Medical Center	University of Texas MD Anderson Cancer Center

(4) Provide evidence of completing a hands-on training practicum in the use of the da Vinci Surgical Platform of at least 8-h duration which includes 3 h of personal experience using the system on an animal model during this training
 	
(5) Provide evidence of performing two patient cases at UIHC using the robotic surgical system prior to August 1, 2004
 	
or
 	
(6) Provide evidence of completing a hands-on training practicum in the use of the robot of at least 8-h duration which includes 3 h of personal experience using the system on an animal model during this training
 	
(7) Provide evidence of prior privileges for robotically assisted surgery at another hospital
 	
(8) Provide evidence of performing two patient cases within the previous 12 months using the robotic surgical system
	(3) Established credentials to perform open prostate surgery
	
	To obtain *full robotic surgical privileges*, the surgeon must meet the following requirements:
	
	(1) Have hospital privileges to perform open prostatectomy
	
	(2) Have met requirements noted above for provisional privileges
	
	(3) Document six proctored cases in which the assistant is fully trained and experienced in laparoscopic/robotic surgery; six cases proctored by a urology colleague credentialed in open prostate surgery
	
	(4) Provide information on outcomes of 20 laparoscopic/robotic prostatectomy cases performed as primary surgeon showing acceptable cure and perioperative complication rates
	
	– Surgical outcomes data will be reviewed by the institutional robotic committee at regular intervals to evaluate safety and compare to published benchmarks
	
	– Surgeons must also perform a minimum of 12 cases per year to maintain privileges in laparoscopic/robotic surgery
	
	– Active participation in the endourological society with documentation of related CME activities must also maintained
		Full robotic privileges:
		
		1. Requests for robotic surgery privileging should be supported by documentation of training or experience in robotics. This training may take the form of prior experience in a formal training program (residency, fellowship, prior practice) or prior extensive laparoscopic/endoscopic experience:
		
		a. For faculty without extensive prior laparoscopic or endoscopic experience (defined in this situation as less than 12 cases per year):
		  i. Formal training/orientation by the company in dry and wet lab
		  ii. Attendance at an advanced postgraduate course, which includes "hands-on" exposure to equipment and techniques
		  iii. Fulfillment of proctorship of 10 pelvic cases with written proctor approval at the conclusion
		
		b. For faculty with extensive prior laparoscopic/endoscopic practice (12 or greater cases per year) and no/minimal robotic experience:
		  i. Formal training/orientation by the company
		  ii. Attendance of company technician or proctor in first three to five cases
		
		c. For new faculty with prior robotic experience:
		  i. Documentation of a minimum of 10 cases as primary, non-proctored surgeon

qualified individual or committee may formulate requirements for RUS credentialing. Credentialing for individual urologic procedures should ultimately involve the chief of the urology service or the clinical supervisor of the urologist.

15.4 Current Status of Robotic Urological Surgery Training

Training in RUS can be accomplished under various formats. At present, most US urology residency training programs incorporate basic laparoscopy and robotic skills into their curriculum.[19] Similarly, a majority of fellowship programs pertaining to endourology and uro-oncology have access to robotic training. A dilemma, however, exists for surgeons who completed their residency and/or fellowship at the time when RUS was unavailable. Although basic 1-day equipment training is offered by Intuitive Surgical, this is unlikely sufficient to attain the level of skill necessary for the safe and effective performance. Other processes are available to ensure that the "new" robotic surgeon has the requisite level of surgical competence to justifiably initiate this procedure. These include "mini-residency" training, use of simulators, proctoring, remote presence, or teleproctoring and preceptoring.

15.4.1 Residency and Fellowship

The establishment of a robotic training curriculum within the framework of a formal residency or fellowship training program has been the subject of recent attention. A systematic approach to training urology residents was presented in 2006 by the University of Minnesota group. The residents initially underwent da Vinci® certification followed by training in table-side assistance under the supervision of a second attending urologist. Subsequently, they were systematically guided through various steps of RARP in the following order – (a) bladder takedown, (b) endopelvic fascia and dorsal venous complex, (c) bladder neck and posterior dissection, (d) neurovascular bundles, and (e) urethral anastomosis. The proficiency in each step was assessed on a scale of 0–5 (very poor to outstanding). The resident was permitted to move to the next step only

after demonstrating a score of 3/5 on three consecutive occasions. Additionally, a digital recording of the procedure was reviewed with the attending urologist at the end of each procedure. This approach resulted in a steady improvement in analog scores and operative time over the course of 7 months. The authors thus demonstrated that a systematic approach to RUS training with frequent feedback resulted in an efficient and safe acquisition of robotic skills by the residents.[20] Such systematic and controlled trainee teaching has been shown not to negatively impact on patient care.[21]

RUS curriculum is also a part of postgraduate fellowships supervised by either the Endourology society (EUS) or the Society of Urologic Oncology (SUO). RUS training is also imparted within the purview of institutional minimally invasive urology or robotic urology fellowships which are not affiliated to a governing body. A recent survey reported that 73% of EUS fellows perform more than 50 procedures during their training period as compared to 43% of SUO fellows. The percentage of fellows going on to secure academic positions after completion of their training was similar, however, and varied between 44 and 100% from year to year.[22] Considering that a majority of these fellows are future mentors for the next generation of robotic surgeons, it is essential to take steps to ensure adequate exposure and comprehensive training during the course of these fellowship programs. While a large proportion of RUS is currently performed in the United States, the global urological community is also in the midst of devising strategies to ensure the adequate laparoscopic and robotic training within the purview of a residency/fellowship program.[23]

Nevertheless, the training of residents and fellows does pose unique challenges, and the foremost among these pertains ensuring the safety of the patient. Unlike open or laparoscopic surgery, where the mentor and trainee are both at the patient side and the mentor is able to provide "hands-on" training, only one of the two can be at the console in robotic surgery.[24] This may alter the perception of comfort and control in both the trainee and the mentor thereby making the learning process more difficult. The recent availability of the dual-console da Vinci Si® surgical system may help to overcome some of these actual and perceived difficulties in RUS training. It is reassuring, however, to note that trainees are able to implement the safe and efficient techniques of their mentors quite systematically and do not adversely impact the learning curve of an institution in terms of operative time, estimated blood loss, and positive surgical margins.[25]

15.4.2 Mini-Residency Training

In 2003, McDougall et al. established a comprehensive, 5-day mini-residency (M-R) program at the University of California Irvine and over the following year trained 21 urologists from four countries in the practical nuances of RARP.[26] All the participants had preliminary experience in laparoscopy, having performed 20–60 cases prior to attending the program. None had performed RARP earlier. The M-R included dry lab and animal/cadaver laboratory skills training and live demonstration in the operating room. Within 14 months of completion of the course, 95% of the participants were safely performing RARP at their respective institutions and 25% had started robotic pyeloplasty procedures. All the M-R participants were keen to recommend this program to their colleagues. Recently, an updated report assessing the long-term practice impact of the 5-day mini-residency course having a 1:2 faculty-to-attendee ratio was published by the same group.[27] The percent of participants performing RARP at 1, 2, and 3 years following the M-R was 78% (33 of 42), 78% (25 of 32), and 86% (18 of 21), respectively. Among the surgeons performing the procedure there was a progressive increase in the number of cases each year with increasing time since the mini-fellowship training. Furthermore, at 1, 2, and 3 years following M-R, 83, 84, and 90% of partnered attendees were performing RARP compared to only 67, 56, and 78% of solo attendees, respectively. The authors concluded that the intensive, dedicated 5-day educational course focused on RARP learning enabled most participants to successfully incorporate and maintain this procedure in clinical practice in the short and long term. Unfortunately, to the best of our knowledge, this is the only M-R program in North America. Duplication of such a curriculum at other medical centers poses its own unique challenges. Such a program relies on the commitment of expert faculty to serve as tutorial instructors and proctors, in addition to the availability of an animal and cadaveric skill training laboratory. Although this program was tuition free during the 3 years of this study due to grant funding, the UCI program was estimated to cost upward of $10,000 per attending surgeon when all components of the teaching strategies were considered. Thus, these financial and logistical challenges need to be overcome for establishment of similar programs worldwide. This undoubtedly would facilitate in the faster and more effective transfer of skills from the experts to the novice robotic surgeon.

15.4.3 Simulators

A simulator has been defined "as a device that enables the operator to reproduce or represent under test conditions phenomena likely to occur in actual performance."[28] Simulators are being used more frequently as educational tools based on the assumption that repetitive performance of a manual task leads to improvement and learning from failure reduces errors. Simulators are applied in varied skill-based professions like aviation and military training. While regulations are in place to ensure that airline pilots undergo annual flight simulator training and testing, no such rules apply to surgery which is arguably a profession dealing with similar risk situations.[29] Simulation's greatest attribute is that it permits individuals to err without jeopardizing patient welfare.

Simulators have been categorized as low fidelity, high fidelity, and virtual reality.[28] Low-fidelity simulators are ones that are not lifelike as in the laparoscopic box trainer. Although they do not duplicate the actual surgical environment and cannot be used to teach the entire procedure, they have the advantage of portability and economy and have been proven to improve surgical skills over time. Moreover, several studies have concluded that the efficacy of a low-fidelity system is equivalent to that of a high-fidelity simulator, especially when it is used to teach basic surgical skills to junior trainees.[30,31] High-fidelity simulators include animal models, cadavers, and commercially available models and can be used to confer training in more realistic environment. However, these carry their own set of disadvantages including cost, lack of ready availability, veterinary assistance, and anatomical variance from human organs (for animal models) and lack of bleeding and actual tissue compliance (for cadavers).[28] The recently developed third category of simulators incorporate the concept of virtual reality and can potentially provide a computer-derived realistic virtual operative field with tactile feedback on laparoscopic instruments.

To the best of our knowledge, the only commercially available robotic virtual reality simulators include the dV-Trainer (Mimic Technologies, Seatle WA) and the RoSS Robotic Surgical Simulator (Simulated Surgical Systems, Williamsville, NY) (Fig. 15.2). The initial version of the dV-Trainer developed in 2003, included a 520-MHz microprocessor and ran with the Windows XP software, offering a three-dimensional simulator-mounted stereoscopic eyepiece and emulates Intuitive Surgical's InSite Vision System. Kenney et al. recently studied the face, content, and construct validity of the dV-Trainer.[32] The system was accepted by the trainees as a realistic reproduction of the da Vinci® console and was recommended for inclusion in the residency training curriculum. More importantly, the dV-Trainer was able to differentiate between novice and expert surgeons with statistically significant differences recorded between the two groups in terms of total task time, total motion, instrument collisions, time instruments out of view, time instruments out of center of the visual field, number of dropped targets, number of successful targets, and number of unattempted targets. Thus it achieved construct validity in a wide variety of simulated scenarios

except suturing. This kind of simulation undoubtedly holds promise for the future and can potentially shorten the learning curve of future robotic surgeons without putting patients at any risk.[32] Over the last year, the second generation dV-Trainer was released which offered a more robust console design, increased training modules and performance evaluation. Similarly, collaboration with Intuitive Surgical has allowed the union of Mimic technology with the newest Da Vinci Si models. Future robot purchases will allow the simulation software to be integrated in the robot console to be used for training and clinical surgical cases. The RoSS surgical simulator, released in 2010, is a collaboration between the Center for Robotic Surgery at Roswell Park Cancer Institute and the University at Buffalo's School of Engineering and Applied Sciences. Similar to the aforementioned simulator, the RoSS is an independent, cost-effective (no consumables or disposables are required) device which provides a comprehensive curriculum to train for motor, and cognitive skills required to operate surgical robot. It also hosts a database of simulated surgical procedures for fellow or resident to follow, and recreate the surgical steps of an expert surgeon.

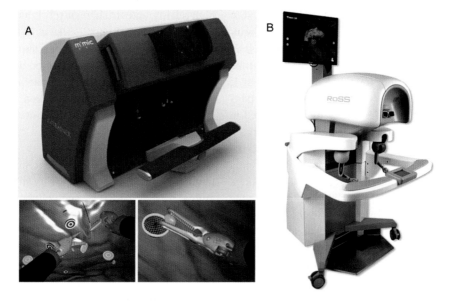

Fig. 15.2 Commercially available robotic virtual reality simulators include (**a**) the dv-Trainer by Mimic Technologies and (**b**) the RoSS robotic surgical simulator by Simulated Surgical Systems. Advantages of these systems include a safe, standalone, realistic cost-effective environment for trainees to acquire skills related to orientation, motor skills and procedure specific modules. They do not require an OR environment and there are no additive costs (i.e. disposables, models). Both surgical simulator system data management system can objectively measure and record training performance. As such, the user is provided teaching feedback with comprehensive performance evaluation and metrics history

In short, surgical simulation is an exciting area of surgical education. The future is bright as advancements in computing and graphical capabilities offer new innovations in simulator technology. Robotic tasks, not only with reconstructive skills but also with tissue dissection, are greatly needed. Simulators must continue to undergo rigorous validation studies to ensure that time spent by trainees on bench trainers and virtual reality simulators will translate into improved surgical skills in the operating room.[28]

15.4.4 Proctoring and Preceptoring

Proctoring is a process involving observation by another, preferably more experienced surgeon during the initial phase of the learning curve of a surgeon learner in order to assess his knowledge and skills in the use of a new equipment or technique. In RUS, a proctor can help to ensure that the new surgeon is able to establish a basic requisite level of competence during the steep phase of the learning curve. He/she reports the findings to the department head or the medical staff of the institution and provides recommendations based on his/her findings. These recommendations may result in the privileging of the surgeon learner in performing the particular procedure. The proctor may also recommend further training or preceptoring for the surgeon prior to privileging.

Preceptoring, on the other hand, is a form of training whereby an experienced surgeon scrubs in or supervises the procedure with the intention of guiding the surgeon learner and assisting him in the acquisition of new skills during the steep part of the learning curve. The preceptor provides feedback of the trainees' performance to the trainee himself and aims to transfer his/her skills to the surgeon learner by an active "hands-on" approach. In contrast to proctoring, in which the surgeon learner retains overall responsibility for the patient's care, a preceptor is the primary person responsible for the well-being of the patient and can readily take over a surgical procedure if the situation so demands.[33]

Both proctoring and preceptoring have an important role to play in the effective establishment of new procedures in all specialties, including RUS. While proctoring is invariably carried out in the surgeon learner's institution, preceptoring may be carried out

using various models. The preceptor and the surgeon learner may work together at the preceptor's or the surgeon learner's institution, or the transfer of skills may take place within the framework of a mini-fellowship/mini-residency.[34]

While proctors and preceptors have a crucial role in observing and certifying surgeon competence in RUS, the need for a governing body to lay down the standards for a surgeon to become a proctor or a preceptor cannot be overemphasized. At present there are no guidelines or authorities for certifying proctors in RUS. Currently, after performing only 20 such procedures, a surgeon is considered by Intuitive Surgical to be eligible to proctor other surgeons in RARP. This leads to a heterogeneous pool of robotic "experts" which is far from ideal for ensuring trainee competency.

For a complex RUS procedure, like RARP, an initial period of proctoring must be a prerequisite for granting privileges on the robot. However, there is a question surrounding the temporal relationship of this initial period of proctoring and granting of unrestricted robotic privileges. If the full privileges are granted beforehand and subsequently withdrawn based on a proctor's adverse report, the information has to be sent to the National Practitioners Data Bank (NPDB) and the state licensing board, potentially jeopardizing the surgeon's career. On the other hand, if the grant of unrestricted privileges is subject to a successful proctoring period, a subsequent decision not to grant privileges to a surgeon is not reportable to the NPDB or the licensing board and is professionally safer for the surgeon. Hence, a way to circumvent the problem is for the institutional credentialing committee to grant privileges to perform the initial RARP cases only under the observation of a proctor and withholding unrestricted privileges until the proctor's report is evaluated.[35]

Another caveat of proctoring a complex procedure is the medicolegal implication and liability that a proctor is subject to in case of a surgical mishap. While performing proctored (as opposed to preceptored) cases, the surgeon learner carries the overall responsibility for the patient's well-being and as such is liable for any malpractice occurring during the course of the treatment. A potential medicolegal implication arises for the proctor in the event of an emergency during the course of surgery that he/she is observing or if the proctor is witness to malpractice by the surgeon learner. While most proctoring guidelines, citing medical ethics and patient welfare, recommend intervention by the proctor in such a situation, the law takes a conflicting view and does not hold the proctor responsible for patient well-being in such a situation since the proctor is not involved in a physician–patient relationship. The proctor is clearly not liable if he/she chooses not to intervene in such a situation. This scenario has been legally tested, and the rulings have consistently been in the proctor's favor.[36]

However, the laws regarding proctor liability, once he/she has intervened and taken over a procedure in an emergent situation, are relatively unclear. Although this has not yet been tested in court, it is likely that such a situation will be within the purview of the state's Good Samaritan laws and would protect proctor intervention. Nevertheless, it has been recommended that a prior consent should be obtained from the patient and the role of the proctor should be clearly defined at the outset.[35] The institute credentialing committee also must clearly lay down proctoring guidelines and the roles of those participating in the surgical procedure.

15.5 Remote Presence Proctoring

The expanding horizons of telemedicine technology have influenced various aspects of medicine including direct physician–patient interaction. A mobile, remotely controlled audiovisual "robot" has been used for rounding on surgical patients with high levels of satisfaction and acceptance among postoperative patients.[37] A recent multi-institutional randomized control trial on robotic telerounding reported similar results. In this study, 270 postoperative urological patients were randomized to either a traditional bedside round or a robotic telerounding with a physician–patient video conference. The final analysis revealed similar morbidity, length of hospital stay, and patient satisfaction in the two arms. Moreover, there were no missed complications that could be attributed to substituting traditional rounds with robotic telerounds.[38]

Proctoring presents practical difficulties both for the surgeon learner and for the expert. It either involves the expert taking out time from his own practice and going to a learner's institution to observe or the learner bringing his patient to the proctor's institution. Both these scenarios have logistical, financial, and legal implications. With the help of telemedicine technology, an expert surgeon stationed remotely can observe, oversee, and even actively supervise a surgical procedure being conducted by a surgeon learner at his own institution. A mobile, remotely navigated, teleconferencing system with public internet connectivity was recently used for teleproctoring of medical students during anatomy cadaveric dissection classes and reportedly resulted in a high level of satisfaction among the medical students and the surgeon proctor alike.[39] A similar incorporation of this concept in teleproctoring endoscopic sinus surgery has resulted in increased convenience with no increase in complication rates within the purview of a residency training program. In this study, 83 procedures were performed via conventional proctoring and another 83 were supervised by the faculty via video teleconferencing (VTC) from a nearby room. Although, the time taken was slightly longer for the VTC proctored cases (3.87 min per side, $p < 0.024$), there was no compromise on patient safety and the residents had a positive learning experience with a sense of control in the operating suite.[40] With the expansion of robotic facilities worldwide, the application of this facility for proctoring RUS will enable expert robotic surgeons to easily proctor, optimizing outcomes and improving safety.

15.6 Credentialing and Privileging in Other Surgical Specialities

Several authors have addressed the issue of systematic and safe introduction of newer technology and skills in surgical practice.[41] Acquisition of new procedures and technology needs to be based on the level of evidence available in its support, the practice patterns of the surgeon, and the needs of the community.[34]

The American College of Surgeons has pioneered and implemented several steps for evaluating evidence pertaining to newer technologies and has introduced several courses for disseminating information and education among practicing surgeons.[42] Through the appointments of various national faculties, the division of education of the ACS has supported the development and implementation of several educational courses on emerging technologies and procedures. Establishment of a network of ACS-accredited education centers as well as accreditation of institutional surgical teams in newer technologies are some key areas that the division has recently been pursuing.[42,43]

The ACS has also suggested guidelines for the verification of individual surgeons in emerging technological procedures and equipment. These include criteria for assessing eligibility of surgeons for verification based on previous training and experience, education required for adequate understanding of the technological process, and the environment recommended for the appropriate use of the subject technology.[44,45]

Thus, similar procedure-specific and general guidelines have been deliberated and proposed by other surgical specialties (gynecology and general surgery) and organizations.

15.7 Conclusions and Current Recommendations

RUS is in the midst of rapid evolution and global expansion. Proper and effective guidelines for the safe introduction of these procedures are of upmost importance. A recently published consensus paper on training, credentialing, and proctoring RUS (specifically, RARP) by the Society of Urologic Robotic Surgeons (SURS) dealt with these considerations and presented suggested guidelines for the initiation and expansion of RUS in institutions (Table 15.3).[41]

Subsequently, further work is currently in progress to develop and outline guidelines for robotic surgery training, which will be presented to the AUA Educational Council for further deliberations and approval for 2011. The purpose of these proposed guidelines is to facilitate the credentialing of urologists seeking privileges after 2011 to perform RUS. Minimum training requirements for granting urologic privileges as well as a continuing monitoring process involving a peer review of the surgeon's volume, performance, and complications are some of the aspects that would be elaborated on in these proposed guidelines. Furthermore, individualized pathways based on residency/fellowship training or no formal training will be created as well as suggested requirements for privilege maintenance. More appropriate guidelines for robotic proctors and their medicolegal safety will also

Table 15.3 SURS committee recommendations for the safe implementation and credentialing of RUS, particularly RARP in an institution. (Reprinted with permission from Elsevier, license No. 2275071092928)

1. The establishment of a national/international, centralized, certification authority which would institute and uphold standards for safe introduction of RARP in an institutional credentialing committee setup

2. Credentialing of institutions and individuals to be based on these standard guidelines. The guidelines need to cover basic requirements with regards to training, certification courses, departmental staffing and infrastructure

3. Until residency programs provide an abundance of skilled robotic urologists (5–10 years), we recommend an increased number of regional centers to assist with preceptoring through mini-residency programs

4. The central certification authority, rather than the robotic industry, should assume responsible for identifying and promoting expert robotic surgeons. Only such designated experts, based on peer-support, submitted videos and case logs, should be permitted to serve as a proctor

5. The central certification authority will need to develop a standardized report for proctors to complete for each RUS which will need to be submitted to the institutional robotic committee for review

6. The first few (3–5) cases of the novice urologist will need to be proctored by an approved proctor, preferably by the same proctor for all cases. Individualized requirements may be necessary for those with laparoscopic vs. open radical prostatectomy experience and background. The proctors reports will then collectively be reviewed by the institutional departmental staff/credentialing committee prior to granting unrestricted, robotic privileges

7. Legal liability of the proctor/preceptor to be minimized by including the institutional legal counsel in the credentialing committee of the institution. He/she should be actively involved in the formulation of guidelines and their implementation

8. The institution should indemnify the proctor against any possible legal implications while performing proctoring services for RARP

9. Informed consent must be obtained from the patient with regards to the role of the proctor during the surgery and thereafter

10. The role of the proctor should be clearly defined by the institutional credentialing committee. Whether or not the proctor is expected to intervene in case of a possible intraoperative necessity should be clearly established and documented beforehand

11. A system of periodic review by the institutional robotic committee of the performance of the surgeon including case selection, surgical competence, management of complications and postoperative outcomes should be set in place. Continuance of robotic privileges should be subject to consistent performance in all these criteria. Failure to perform adequately should result in a recommendation for a refresher training or additional preceptoring prior to continuity of these privileges

be proposed. Like aviation science, the ultimate goal will be train and certify surgeons before (rather than during) clinical experience. Surgical simulation will be the educational vector to meet today's challenges of resident education (reduced resident work hours and increased utilization of new technology and minimally invasive equipment), and clinical work environment (increased medicolegal risk, increased awareness to outcomes and patient safety). In the very near future, we should expect to not only train urologists in a virtual reality environment with objective robotic measures, but also certify and ensure maintenance of skills on a periodic basis, particularly for low volume surgeons.

References

1. Budäus L, Sun M, Abdollah F, Zorn KC, Morgan M, Johal R, Liberman D, Thuret R, Isbarn H, Salomon G, Haese A, Montorsi F, Shariat SF, Perrotte P, Graefen M, Karakiewicz PI. Impact of Surgical Experience on In-Hospital Complication Rates in Patients Undergoing Minimally Invasive Prostatectomy: A Population-Based Study. *Ann Surg Oncol*. 2010; in press [DOI: 10.1245/s10434-010-1300-0].

2. Binder J, Kramer W. Robotically-assisted laparoscopic radical prostatectomy. *BJU Int*. 2001;87:408–410.

3. Pasticier G, Rietbergen JB, Guillonneau B, Fromont G, Menon M, Vallancien G. Robotically assisted laparoscopic radical prostatectomy: feasibility study in men. *Eur Urol*. 2001;40:70–74.

4. Menon M, Tewari A, Peabody J. Vattikuti Institute prostatectomy: technique. *J Urol*. 2003;169:2289–2292.

5. Intuitive Surgical web site. www.intuitivesurgical.com. Accessed August 15, 2009.

6. Steinberg PL, Merguerian PA, Bihrle W III, Seigne JD. The cost of learning robotic-assisted prostatectomy. *Urology*. 2008;72:1068–1072.

7. Badani KK, Kaul S, Menon M. Evolution of robotic radical prostatectomy: assessment after 2766 procedures. *Cancer*. 2007;110:1951–1958.

8. Hermann TR, Rabenalt R, Stolzenburg JJ, Liatsikos EN, Imkamp F, Tezval H, et al. Oncological and functional results of open, robot-assisted and laparoscopic radical prostatectomy: does surgical approach and surgical experience matter? *World J Urol*. 2007;25:149–160.

9. Boris RS, Kaul SA, Sarle RC, Stricker HJ. Radical prostatectomy: a single surgeon comparison of retropubic, perineal, and robotic approaches. *Can J Urol*. 2007;14: 3566–3570.

10. Patel VR, Thaly R, Shah K. Robotic radical prostatectomy: outcomes of 500 cases. *BJU Int*. 2007;99: 1109–1112.

11. Atug F, Castle EP, Srivastav SK, Burgess SV, Thomas R, Davis R. Positive margins in robotic-assisted radical prostatectomy: impact of learning curve on oncologic outcomes. *Eur Urol*. 2006;49:866–871.

12. Ahlering TE, Eichel L, Edwards RA, Lee DI, Skarecky DW. Robotic radical prostatectomy: a technique to reduce pt2 positive margins. *Urology*. 2004;64:1224–1228.

13. Zorn KC, Orvieto MA, Gong EM, Mikhail AA, Gofrit ON, Zagaja GP, et al. Robotic radical prostatectomy learning curve of a fellowship – trained laparoscopic surgeon. *J Endourol*. 2007;21:441–447.

14. Vickers AJ, Bianco FJ, Serio AM, et al. The surgical learning curve for prostate cancer control after radical prostatectomy. *J Natl Cancer Inst*. 2007;99:1171–1177.

15. Vickers AJ, Bianco FJ, Gonen M, et al. Excellent rates of cancer control for patients with organ-confined disease treated by the most experienced surgeons suggest that the primary reason such patients recur is inadequate surgical technique. *Eur Urol*. 2008;53:960–966.

16. Zorn KC, Wille MA, Thong AE, et al. Continued improvement of perioperative, pathological and continence outcomes during 700 robot assisted radical prostatectomies. *Can J Urol*. 2009;16:4742–4749.

17. Wilt TJ, Shamliyan TA, Taylor BC, MacDonald R, Kane RL. Association between hospital and surgeon radical prostatectomy volume and patient outcomes: a systematic review. *J Urol*. 2008;180:820–829.

18. Nuttall M, Van der Meulen J, Phillips N, Sharpin C, Gillatt D, McIntosh G, et al. A systematic review and critique of the literature relating hospital or surgeon volume to health outcomes for 3 urological cancer procedures. *J Urol*. 2004;172:2145–2152.

19. Duchene DA, Moinzadeh A, Gill IS, Clayman RV, Winfield HN. Survey of residency training in laparoscopic and robotic surgery. *J Urol*. 2006;176:2158–2166.

20. Rashid HH, Leung YY, Rashid MJ, Oleyourryk G, Valvo JR, Eichel L. Robotic surgical education: a systematic approach to training urology residents to perform robotic-assisted laparoscopic radical prostatectomy. *Urology*. 2006;68:75–79.

21. Schroeck FR, de Sousa CA, Kalman RA, Kalia MS, Pierre SA, Halebilan GE, Sun L, Moul JW, Albala DM. Trainees do not negatively impact the institutional learning curve for robotic prostatectomy as characterized by operative time, estimated blood loss and positive surgical margin rate. *Urology*. 2008;71:597–601.

22. Yap SA, Ellison LM, Low RK. Current laparoscopy training in urology: a comparison of fellowships governed by the society of urologic oncology and the endourological society. *J Endourol*. 2008;22:1755–1760.

23. Gautam G. The current three-year postgraduate program in urology is insufficient to train a urologist. *Indian J Urol*. 2008;24:336–338.

24. Guzzo TJ, Gonzalgo ML. Robotic surgical training of the urologic oncologist. *Urol Oncol*. 2009;27:214–217.

25. Schroeck FR, de Sousa CA, Kalman RA, Kalia MS, Pierre SA, Haleblian GE, et al. Trainees do not negatively impact the institutional learning curve for robotic prostatectomy as characterized by operative time, estimated blood loss, and positive surgical margin rate. *Urology*. 2008;71: 597–601.

26. McDougall EM, Corica FA, Chou DS, Abdelshehid CS, Uribe CA, Stoliar G, et al. Short-term impact

of a robot-assisted laparoscopic prostatectomy 'mini-residency' experience on postgraduate urologists' practice patterns. *Int J Med Robotics Comput Assist Surg*. 2006;2: 70–74.

27. Gamboa AJ, Santos RT, Sargent ER, Louie MK, Box GN, Sohn KH, et al. Long-term impact of a robot assisted laparoscopic prostatectomy mini fellowship training program on postgraduate urological practice patterns. *J Urol*. 2009;181:778–782.

28. Wignall GR, Denstedt JD, Preminger GM, Cadeddu JA, Pearle MS, Sweet RM, et al. Surgical simulation: a urological perspective. *J Urol*. 1699;2008(179): 1690–1699.

29. Satava RM. Accomplishments and challenges of surgical simulation. *Surg Endosc*. 2001;15:232–241.

30. Matsumoto ED, Hamstra SJ, Radomski SB, Cusimano MD. The effect of bench model fidelity on endourological skills: a randomized controlled study. *J Urol*. 2002;167: 1243–1247.

31. Grober ED, Hamstra SJ, Wanzel KR, Reznick RK, Matsumoto ED, Sidhu RS, et al. The educational impact of bench model fidelity on the acquisition of technical skill: the use of clinically relevant outcome measures. *Ann Surg*. 2004;240:374–381.

32. Kenney PA, Wszolek MF, Gould JJ, Libertino JA, Moinzadeh A. Face, content, and construct validity of dv-trainer, a novel virtual reality simulator for robotic surgery. *Urology*. 2009;73:1288–1292.

33. Sachdeva AK, Russell TR. Safe introduction of new procedures and emerging technologies in surgery: education, credentialing and privileging. *Surg Clin N Am*. 2007;87: 853–866.

34. Sachdeva AK. Acquiring skills in new procedures and technology: the challenge and the opportunity. *Arch Surg*. 2005;140:387–389.

35. Livingston EH, Harwell JD. The medicolegal aspects of proctoring. *Am J Surg*. 2002;184:26–30.

36. Sachdeva AK, Blair PG. Enhancing patient safety through educational interventions. In: Manuel BM, Nora PF, eds. *Surgical Patient Safety: Essential Information for Surgeons in Today's Environment*. Chicago, IL: American College of Surgeons; 2004:Chapt 14.

37. Ellison LM, Pinto PA, Kim F, Ong AM, Patriciu A, Stoianovici D, et al. Telerounding and patient satisfaction after surgery. *J Am Coll Surg*. 2004;199:523–530.

38. Ellison LM, Nguyen M, Fabrizio MD, Soh A, Permpongkosol S, Kavoussi LR. Postoperative robotic telerounding: a multicenter randomized assessment of patient outcomes and satisfaction. *Arch Surg*. 2007;142:1177–1181.

39. Smith CD, Skandalakis JE. Remote presence proctoring by using a wireless remote-control videoconferencing system. *Surg Innov*. 2005;12:139–143.

40. Burgess LPA, Syms MJ, Holtel MR, Birkmire-Peters DP, Johnson RE, Ramsey MJ. Telemedicine: teleproctored endoscopic sinus surgery. *Laryngoscope*. 2002;112: 216–219.

41. Zorn KC, Gautam G, Shalhav AL, Clayman RV, Ahlering TE, Albala DM, et al. and The Society of Urologic Robotic Surgeons. Training, credentialing, proctoring and medicolegal risks of robotic urological surgery: recommendations of the society of urologic robotic surgeons. *J Urol*. 2009;182:1126–1132.

42. Sachdeva AK. Invited commentary: educational interventions to address the core competencies in surgery. *Surgery*. 2004;135:43–47.

43. Sachdeva AK. Acquisition and maintenance of surgical competence. *Semin Vasc Surg*. 2002;15:182–190.

44. Verification by the American College of Surgeons for the use of emerging technologies. *Bull Am Coll Surg*. 1998;83:34–40.

45. Statements on emerging surgical technologies and the evaluation of credentials. American college of surgeons. *Surg Endosc*. 1995;9:207–213.

Chapter 16

Research in Urologic Oncology in an Era of Minimally Invasive Surgery

Ralph W. deVere White, Kirk A. Keegan, and Karim Chamie

16.1 Introduction

Urologists have a rich and proud tradition of innovation and research, leading to significant advances within the discipline of urologic oncology and the field of urology. Most prominently, Huggins et al. evaluated the effect of androgens on advanced prostate cancer in 1941, and they were subsequently awarded the Nobel Prize in 1966 for their landmark insight into the impact of hormones on neoplastic cells.[1] Further milestones such as the elucidation of PSA as a marker for prostate cancer by Murphy,[2] the discovery of human chorionic gonadotropin (hCG) and alpha fetoprotein (AFP) as biomarkers for testicular cancer by Lange,[3] the role of Bacillus Calmette-Guerin (BCG) treatment for superficial bladder cancer by Morales,[4] and the molecular underpinnings of renal cancer by Linehan[5] were led by urologists with a focus on research in urologic oncology. Procedural advances by such open surgical pioneers as Walsh,[6] Novick,[7] and Skinner[8,9] demonstrated that effective oncologic control can be maintained with a view toward the preservation of function. The explosion of minimally invasive surgery, and its natural marriage with urologic oncology, has been led by groundbreaking and creative surgeons such as Clayman,[10] Gill,[11] and Menon.[12] Basic science and clinical research in urology clearly has a storied past. It is our job to ensure that the future is equally illustrious.

16.2 The Surgeon Scientist

However, as has been eloquently argued by Dr. Paul Lange,[13] the role of the surgeon scientist in urology may be tenuous. The reasons cited are multifactorial. The length of the urologic residency, especially when combined with subspecialty fellowship, is particularly long. Many medical students today graduate with considerable debt. For some, this may preclude a budding interest in academic medicine, given the inequities between private practice and academic salaries. Furthermore, the advent of capitated and managed care health plans place additional time and efficiency constraints on already busy clinicians. Finally, it is no longer sufficient to publish data on a natural history description of a disease process. Rather, the explosion of molecular biology and the "-omics" has ushered in an age where the reductionist training of Ph.D.s and post-doctoral fellows is favored over the systems-based learning of the typical medical student or urologic resident. With this in mind, it is not surprising that an increasing number of research grants are being awarded to Ph.D.s rather than surgeon scientists and an increasingly small proportion of federally funded grants are awarded to principal investigators who are urologists.[10]

16.3 Challenges

Prosperity requires the recognition and specific identification of current challenges and the subsequent implementation of appropriate corrective action. The challenges for research in urologic oncology in an era

R.W. deVere White (✉)
UC Davis Cancer Center, Sacramento, CA, USA
e-mail: ralph.devere-white@ucdmc.ucdavis.edu

A.K. Hemal, M. Menon (eds.), *Robotics in Genitourinary Surgery*,
DOI 10.1007/978-1-84882-114-9_16, © Springer-Verlag London Limited 2011

of minimally invasive surgery are focused along three fronts: challenges posed to the discipline of urologic oncology itself, potential threats to minimally invasive urology, and the hurdles created by current and future health policy changes.

The previously stated challenges that face the surgeon scientist are particularly germane to the urologic oncologist. The relatively long duration of residency and fellowship training, a diminished role of research within residency training, high debt burden, increased clinical demands of junior faculty, and the need to hone still-developing surgical skills after fellowship are barriers to the development of a fledgling research career for young urologic oncologists. As stated previously, many more basic scientists are now competing for a static amount of research dollars. As a result, urologic oncologists will need to embrace an emerging role as "clinician scientists." By this, we mean the urologist who not only understands basic science but is also a leader focused on collaborative endeavors with clinical and basic science colleagues generating correlative research projects. This collaborative cross-talk is at the root of "team science" (Fig. 16.1).

If urologic oncologists do not assume a leadership position in this paradigm of team science, we are at risk of losing influence in the care of our patients to medical oncologists. The dedicated subspecialty of genitourinary medical oncology is relatively nascent. However,

the discipline has made great strides in recent years, with a majority of recent Prostate Cancer Foundation grants and NIH dollars going to medical oncologists rather than to urologic oncologists. In certain fields within urology, in particular, infertility and stone disease, urologists have been able to maintain control of the full course of treatment, from diagnosis to medical treatment to surgical therapy to follow-up management. As Lange[3] and Clayman[14] have argued, "Who is best equipped to manage the patient but the physician who diagnoses, treats, and manages the patient postoperatively?" While this may resonate with urologists, it may not with patients who harbor urological cancers. Furthermore, this cycle of diagnosis, treatment, and management is being eroded in urologic oncology, largely because medical oncologists have seized the opportunity. This is particularly true with regard to systemic treatment of castration-resistant prostate cancer, a domain previously controlled by urologists. If we are not leading in the realms of research innovation and design of clinical trials, do we deserve to lead in determining the direction of therapy?

Disconcertingly, urologists have a history of relinquishing their leadership role in certain urologic diseases, namely renal transplant to general surgery, female incontinence surgery to urogynecology, and percutaneous renal access to interventional radiology. The concern with this historical precedent is

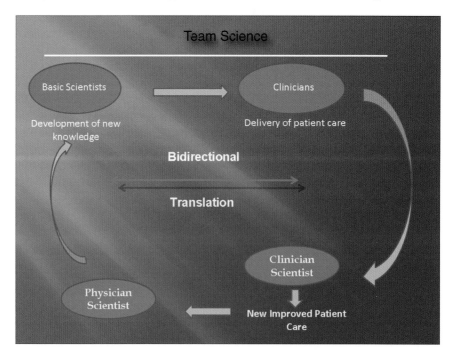

Fig. 16.1 Team science

the challenge it poses to minimally invasive urologic oncology. There has been an incredibly rapid adoption of robotic-assisted laparoscopic procedures in urologic oncology, particularly with regard to prostate cancer,[15] while there has been a much slower adoption of minimally invasive surgery for renal disease.[16] There is no doubt that these extirpative procedures will become increasingly minimally invasive, possibly to the point of being purely ablative. Minimally invasive urologic oncologists stand to lose influence regarding the management of their patients with small renal masses or localized prostate cancer to interventional radiologists performing high-intensity focused ultrasound, radio frequency ablation, or cryotherapy. Urologic oncologists may need to retool themselves to provide the diagnostic and procedural skills to avoid relinquishing the management role for these disease states.

The final challenge facing the discipline of minimally invasive urologic oncology is one that the entire health-care system faces, impending public policy changes. We are likely perched on the brink of significant health-care reform. It is important to realize that the health-care system can go bankrupt (Fig. 16.2) and that hospitals can fail. Health-care industry groups have noted that up to 50% of short-term acute care hospitals in the United States do not make a profit from patient care.[17] In California alone, at least 17 hospitals

have closed in the last 5 years.[18] The federal government has long dictated how our research dollars are allocated, with largely flat NIH congressional appropriations over 6 of the last 7 years[19] (Fig. 16.3). While it has not come to health-care rationing in this country, it is possible that the federal government may dictate how patients are cared for, by virtue of what it will pay for. Each marginal health-care dollar spent represents an opportunity cost to the system, i.e., what we spend for one treatment limits our ability to pay for other treatments. Therefore, in an era of 1.5 million dollar robotic consoles that demonstrate only oncologic equivalency, urologic oncologists must maintain leadership positions that advocate for continued minimally invasive treatment and research that will allow the essential advances in the field.

16.4 Corrective Action

Strengthening the role of research in urologic oncology needs to begin at the medical school and residency level. Urology often attracts the best and brightest of the medical school class. These students and residents should be identified and mentored early in their training. Unfortunately, a significant proportion of urologic

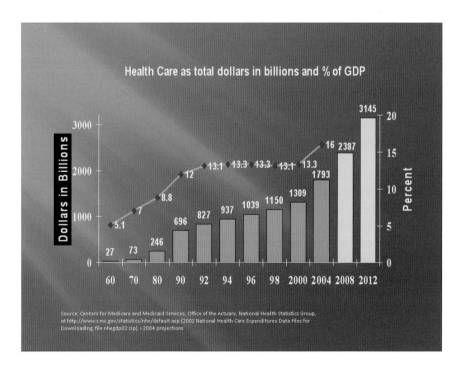

Fig. 16.2 Congressional appropriations for National Institutes of Health

Fig. 16.3 Costs of health care

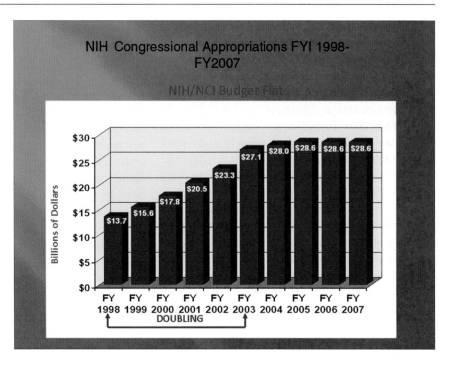

residency programs have restructured to a 5-year format reducing the residency research experience and shifting the burden to fellowship training.

Therefore, we should support standardized fellowship training in urologic oncology. This will be led and organized by the Society of Urologic Oncology (SUO). It is important to realize that the production of fellowship-trained urologic oncologists will benefit not only the membership of the SUO but rather all urologists. As has been addressed by Buscarini and Stein,[20] Olumi and DeWolf,[21] and authors from Memorial Sloan-Kettering,[22] the training of urologic oncologists should focus on a multidisciplinary approach, with incorporation of coursework and clinical activities in hematology/oncology and radiation oncology. We should strive for minimum training criteria, standardized course work, and exams. With regard to research, training should place emphasis on medical and grant writing, biostatistics, as well as design and management of clinical trials.

Not only should resident and fellow training address the cognitive aspects of urologic oncology, but it must address the burgeoning technical demands. Due to expanding clinical loads, a shortened work week, decreasing overall surgical volumes, increased complexity of patient cases, a more rigorous medicolegal environment, and an explosion of complex minimally

invasive procedures with a substantial learning curve, the era of "see one, do one, teach one" is appropriately over. Clearly, part of our strategy should be an integration of urologic oncology and minimally invasive urology. The tenets of surgical resection hold, regardless of the size of the incision. It is clear that surgery, and perhaps particularly urologic surgery, is moving in a more minimally invasive direction, a shift we should all support. To meet these increasing demands, we may have to turn to alternative and creative means of preparing future minimally invasive urologic oncologists. While data have been conflicting,[23,24] virtual reality and intensive surgical simulation may be our best means to achieve the necessary technical proficiency balanced against expanding clinical demands.

As we work toward codifying the training necessary to become successful urologic oncologists and clinician scientists, we must increase our support of those residents and fellows who are entering that critical "establishment phase"[10] of their careers. A report by the American Academy of Orthopedic Surgeons[25] notes several barriers to the development of a thriving clinician scientist: few successful mentors and role models, lack of a fostering clinical environment, educational debt, institutional emphasis on primary care, diminished financial support for training and education, and peer pressure to assume greater clinical responsibilities. New and aspiring urologic oncologists face these same hurdles. As a discipline, we need to work toward promoting young urologic oncologists with salary support and mentoring during these critical formative years. Astellas Rising Star awards, institutional matching grants, and the AUA Career Development awards are creative means to address these issues. We will need to continue to foster these measures to support rising clinician scientists.

As we train and mentor our future urologic oncologists in this era of expanding minimally invasive surgery, it is imperative to foster improved coordination and relationships with our colleagues in minimally invasive urology, endourology, and medical oncology. Nowhere is this more beneficial than the realm of clinical trials. As we have discussed, team science (Fig. 16.1) is not support of the weak by the strong, but a mutually beneficial collaboration and bidirectional exchange of ideas and knowledge culminating in the integration of clinical research with patient care. In the future, the number of purely basic science-oriented physician scientists likely will be few. However, as trained urologic oncologists, we should all strive to be legitimate members of a team of clinician scientists. This leadership role should drive the development and management of meaningful clinical trials and correlative science, which can and must involve the community physician, as well as the academic.

The drive to create substantive clinical trials necessitates the adoption of solid evidence-based medicine. The growing influence of outcomes or health services research represents a natural and expected progression between basic science, translational, and clinical research. The role of health services research in urology, and health care in general, will likely become increasingly important in light of future health policy changes. It is paramount for urologic oncologists to be drivers in this arena in order that we remain in leadership positions within the field. While it will be important to develop good evidence-based medicine, perhaps more importantly, we will need to incorporate these data into practice. We must avoid the sins of our past (e.g., poor utilization of neoadjuvant chemotherapy in bladder cancer or cystectomy without extended node dissection) in order to optimize quality patient care. Urologic oncologists should be leading the investigation and dissemination of this information. Emerging fields such as molecular epidemiology hold promise as a translational discipline between basic science and health services research. It is also very important to realize that the increased role played by medical oncologists in treating patients with urologic malignancies is due to their laurel of involvement in clinical research. It is up to urologists to match this effort. The SUO is committed through both their fellowship program and the recently initiated clinical trials consortium to help urologic oncologists meet these demands.

16.5 Conclusion

The field of urology has an impressive history of successful researchers and thought leaders whose discoveries were based upon groundbreaking research. The challenges of medicine in the modern era will make it difficult for many to pursue a pure surgeon scientist track. However, the role of the clinician scientist in urology has never been more important. If we neglect research, urologists will lose influence in how our patients are treated because we will lose leadership positions within the medical community and increasingly decisions will be directed by medical oncologists or bureaucrats. If this occurs, ultimately, our specialty will become less attractive to the best and brightest medical students and residents. A continued focus on comprehensive and cohesive resident and fellow training, solid mentoring and support of junior faculty, as well as collaborative clinical research will allow the future of urologic oncology to remain bright.

References

1. Huggins C, Stevens RE, Hodges CV. Studies on prostate cancer. II. The effects of castration on advanced carcinoma of the prostate gland. *Arch Sur*. 1941;43:209–223.
2. Murphy GP. The current and potential status of screening for prostate cancer in asymptomatic populations. *Prog Clin Biol Res*. 1989;303:19–25.
3. Lange PH, McIntire KR, Waldmann TA, et al. Serum alpha fetoprotein and human chorionic gonadotropin in the diagnosis and management of nonseminomatous germ-cell testicular cancer. *NEJM*. 1976;295:1237–1240.
4. Morales J, Eidinger D, Bruce AW. Intracavitary Bacillus Calmette-Guerin in the treatment of superficial bladder cancer. *J Urol*. 1976;116:180–183.
5. Linehan WM, Gnarra JR, Lerman MI, et al. Genetic basis of renal cell cancer. *Imp Adv Onc*. 1993:47–70.

6. Walsh PC, Lepor H, Eggleston JC. Radical prostatectomy with preservation of sexual function: anatomical and pathological considerations. *Prostate*. 1983;4:473–485.

7. Novick AC, Stewart BH, Stratton RA, et al. Partial nephrectomy in the treatment of renal adenocarcinoma. *J Urol*. 1977;118:932–936.

8. Skinner DG, Boyd SD, Lieskovsky G. Clinical experience with Kock continent ileal reservoir for urinary diversion. *J Urol*. 1984;132:1101–1107.

9. Doerr A, Skinner EC, Skinner DG. Preservation of ejaculation through modification of retroperitoneal lymph node dissection in low stage testis cancer. *J Urol*. 1993;149:1472–1474.

10. Clayman RV, Kavoussi LR, Soper NJ, et al. Laparoscopic nephrectomy: initial case report. *J Urol*. 1991;146: 278–282.

11. Gill IS, Canes D, Aron M, et al. Single port transumbilical (E-NOTES) donor nephrectomy. *J Urol*. 2008;2:637–641.

12. Menon M, Shrivastava A, Bhandari M, et al. Vattikuti Institute Prostatectomy: Technical Modifications in 2009. *Eur Urol*. July, 2009;56(1):89–96.

13. Lange PH. Whitmore lecture: genitourinary oncology and its surgeon scientists: triumphant past, but does it have a future? *Urol Oncol*. 2007;25:2–10.

14. Clayman RV. Pursuit of a paradigm for professional progress. *J Urol*. 2007;177:425.

15. Intuitive Surgical Statistics, http://www.intuitivesurgical.com. Accessed June 2009.

16. Miller DC, Taub DA, Dunn RC, et al. Laparoscopy for renal cell carcinoma: diffusion versus regionalization? *J Urol*. 2006;176:1102–1106.

17. The Alvarez and Marsal Healthcare Industry Group. Hospital Insolvency: The Looming Crisis. March 2008, http://www.alvarezandmarsal.com. Accessed June 2008.

18. California Hospital Association Statistics, June 2008.

19. National Institute of Health Congressional Appropriations, fiscal years 2000–2009. http://officeofbudget.od.nih.gov. Accessed June 2008.

20. Buscarini M, Stein JP. Training the urologic oncologist of the future: where are the challenges? *Urol Oncol*. 2009;27:193–198.

21. Olumi AF, DeWolf WC. The hybrid of basic science and clinical training for the urologic oncologist: necessity or waste? *Urol Oncol*. 2009;27:205–207.

22. Thompson RH, Eastham JA, Scardino PT, et al. Critical elements in fellowship training. *Urol Oncol*. 2009;27: 199–204.

23. Champion H, Gallagher A. Simulation in surgery: a good idea whose time has come. *Br J Surg*. 2003;90:767–768.

24. Seymour N, Gallagher A, Roman S, et al. Virtual reality training improves operating room performance: results of a randomized double-blinded study. *Ann Surg*. 2002;236:458–464.

25. Brand RA, Hannafin JA. The environment of the successful clinician scientist. *Clin Orthop Relat Res*. 2006;449: 67–71.

Chapter 17

Databases and Data Management for Robotic Surgery

Charles-Henry Rochat and Usha Seshadri-Kreaden

17.1 Motivation

As with any new technology, the importance of tracking surgical experience through the collection of clinical data within a given specialty and particular operation is critical to its success. Clinical data provide evidence for the scientific community through peer-reviewed publications. It enables collaboration among surgeons, supports expanding clinical indications, and provides ongoing quality control of patient outcomes. The information gained from the ongoing quality control of clinical outcomes may have significant impact for a particular operation, leading to refinements in operative techniques. This may in turn lead to improved patient outcomes – an obvious benefit for everyone concerned.

The US Food and Drug Administration approved most of the clinical indications for robotic surgery after the conduct of successful clinical trials.[1] These trials were a mix of prospective and retrospective studies. In both circumstances, clinical data were consistently collected from multiple institutions in order to provide evidence of feasibility, efficacy, and safety of the operation in question. Conduct of these multicenter trials was made possible through the collection of data using a standardized methodology. In this chapter we will discuss the fundamental elements that make this possible and reproducible for various operations of interest.

17.2 Form Design

When designing a data collection tool, the information to be collected is generally dictated by a prospectively designed protocol. While this represents the ideal scenario, it is not always the case. There are instances when the researcher's goal is to monitor outcomes and perform quality control outside the context of a clinical trial. In the absence of a formal protocol, it is important to design a *data collection sheet* or *form* that effectively captures the endpoints of interest for a given operation.

An ideal form is one that is easy to use and captures pertinent data without overburdening the research staff.[2] This is often seen as a laborious and unattractive pursuit as investigators are often anxious to get the trial underway or to simply start the process of data collection. Before starting a trial or a data collection effort, it is imperative that careful thought be given to design of the data collection tools. Failure to do this can result in the following problems:

- An "over-collection" of data may result where much of the data collected ends up not being used.
- The quality of the data recorded may be compromised.
- Clear definitions of the precise data that are required may be unclear.
- Data may not be recorded in a manner that lends itself to statistical analysis.

There are two possibilities that one may encounter; there is the extreme case of too much data being collected and at the other end of the spectrum, insufficient data being collected such that one is unable to draw meaningful conclusions from the data.

C.-H. Rochat (✉)
Robot-Assisted Laparoscopic Surgery Center, Clinic Generale
Beaulieu, Geneva, Switzerland
e-mail: rochat@deckpoint.ch

A.K. Hemal, M. Menon (eds.), *Robotics in Genitourinary Surgery*,
DOI 10.1007/978-1-84882-114-9_17, © Springer-Verlag London Limited 2011

In the case of collecting too much data, the process may be so over burdensome that it becomes difficult for participating centers to follow. This can result in a slowdown in the recruitment of cases, as well as non-compliance in data collection and loss of motivation on the part of the investigators.

As for the case of collecting an insufficient amount of data, one may have failed to overlook critical variables required for an effective analysis. This omission may cause the investigator to have to go back and make modifications to the form while the study is ongoing or even after the initial recruitment and data-gathering period. This lack of sufficient information in a data collection form can be corrected so as to minimize the impact of the study. Effective form design coupled with a well-designed data management system is the only way to ensure that your intended analysis can be performed at the end of your study – with full compliance across all of your sites.

17.3 Selection of Variables

The selection of clinical variables pertaining to a study is done in close collaboration with the investigators involved in the particular operation. When collecting clinical information, the manner in which questions are asked must be objective and free from ambiguity. Investigators and researchers involved with a study seek a simplistic means to answer key clinical questions. Hence the answers should be in the form of binary options (yes, no) or chosen from list of options. In responding to the clinical questions, one should minimize the ability to answer in free form or open-ended answers. This information, while of academic interest, does not lend itself to a quantitative (standardized) method for analysis.

Before developing a database, data collection forms are designed to capture clinical information in the natural course corresponding to the patient's care (preoperative, operative, pathologic, postoperative, long-term follow-up). At each time-point, the particular clinical information matches one to one with questions that would be asked of the patient's condition. The information is captured in an objective manner, with minimal chance for interpretation. When there are validated questionnaires in use, the questions are used in the database in the same manner as their hard copy counterpart. In such instances, it may be advisable to create separate data entry screens for each questionnaire.

17.4 Data Collection Tool Development

To provide an illustrative discussion of the development of data collection tools for the study of prostate cancer, we will explore what was done in a study of robotic radical prostatectomy cases. We will discuss the development of data collection tools for studying prostate cancer in a longitudinal manner. One should realize that this may apply to any operation for that matter and the same principles would apply.

We modeled the evaluation of a patient with prostate cancer taking place in phases of the evaluation:

A *preoperative assessment form* providing baseline information was used to capture the patient's demographic information, medical history, and current state of disease – with key measures of clinical stage, Gleason pattern, preoperative PSA, and the number of positive biopsies.

Next, an *intra-operative form* was used to capture data pertaining to

- techniques used during the operation (intraperitoneal, extraperitoneal, VIP,[3] etc.);
- whether or not a nerve-sparing procedure was done;
- preoperative urinary continence of the patient;
- duration of the intervention;
- various operative characteristics such as the estimated blood loss, need for transfusion, length of ICU stay, and length of hospital stay.

A *pathologic assessment form* was used to describe the current pathology status (including but not limited to)

- pathologic stage;
- pathologic Gleason score;
- seminal vesicle involvement;
- capsular invasion;
- size of the prostate gland;
- the presence or absence of a positive surgical margin;
- whether or not the positive margin was focal or extensive in nature;
- the definition of what is meant by a focal margin;
- the anatomic location of the positive surgical margin.

A *postoperative follow-up form* captured data within 30 days of the operation and included information on the incidence of complications. This follow-up form also captured longer term oncologic outcomes as measured by PSA recurrence at preset time-points, treatment with hormonal therapy, radiation or chemotherapy, and functional outcome measurements of continence and potency at prescribed time intervals.

Measures of the return to continence and potency have been studied using additional validated standard questionnaires. These questionnaires include the Sexual Health Inventory for Men (http://www.erectilefunction.org) (SHIM) or the International Index of Erectile Function Questionnaire[4] (IIEF), and International Consultation on Incontinence Modular Questionnaire[5] (ICIQ). This mode of data gathering often has poor compliance with respect to actually being completed. Furthermore, results may vary depending on who completes the survey (patient, spouse, or partner). Experience to date demonstrates that continence at a particular time-point may be better determined by posing the simple question "When did you become free from the use of pads?"[6] Furthermore, potency may be measured more precisely based on measuring the number of days to successful erection and/or experiencing an erection strong enough for penetration.[7]

In the evaluation of continence and potency, the time at which follow-up information is collected is critical in monitoring and reporting outcomes. Consistency across patients and compliance with respect to office visits are crucial for successful data collection and the minimization of missing data.

17.5 Database Considerations

Prior to selecting what database to use, a careful needs analysis should be undertaken. A series of key questions should be posed. These include the following: Who is the end user? What tasks will they perform? Who will be responsible for database modifications (schema, logic, and user interface)? What are the hardware requirements if you choose to run the system yourself? The choice of database will depend largely on the needs analysis performed.

Database tools for data management, analysis, and reporting range from the familiar (and simple) spreadsheet to the more robust and capable RDBMS (relational database management system). A further consideration is whether to own (and build out) your own IT infrastructure on premise – software, servers, storage, backups, security, or subscribe to one of the many Internet-based services that have become more prevalent in recent years.

Regardless of approach taken, accounting for the total cost in ownership (TCO), along with the requisite responsibilities that you, your clinical staff, and IT group will have in managing the database, and resulting data will have to be considered in selecting your data collection and management tool set.

Familiar personal or workgroup databases such as Microsoft Access and Filemaker can handle the task of managing data into the tens of thousands of records, but tend to be problematic to set up for scalable multiuser operation and secure accessibility over the Internet. Enterprise-grade database platforms from vendors such as Oracle (Oracle, MySQL), IBM (DB2), and Microsoft (SQLServer) are all more than capable of powering the most sophisticated clinical applications and data volumes – although the costs associated with purchasing software, developing the data collection application, setting up the infrastructure (servers, etc.), and managing these systems can be prohibitive for most small-scale studies.

Considerations for choosing a database can be affected by your end goals. Your options will differ if the goal is to manage data for a publication and/or monitor patient outcomes long term, as opposed to conducting a multicenter trial intended for a regulatory submission.

The requirements for databases used to support regulatory submissions are high. One of the most stringent requirements for regulatory submissions is the mandate to provide a complete audit trail on database changes. The Code of Federal Regulations Part 21 Section 11[8] requires controls for closed systems with respect to electronic records. What this means is full traceability of changes within a validated database used to house clinical data in support a regulatory submission. This level of traceability is often not required when the goal of data collection is to solely monitor outcomes and to publish results in peer review journal.

Table 17.1 lists features to consider in a database tool depending on whether it is to be used solely as

Table 17.1 Database Requirements

	Peer-reviewed publication	Regulatory submission
Operating under prospectively defined protocol	●	●
Import and export to a statistical analysis tool	●	●
Cross-form and cross-variable edit checks	●	●
Flexibility of platform	●	●
Need to collaborate with multiple investigators and different institutions	●	●
Need for multiple investigators to view data	●	
21 CFR Part 11 compliance		●
Electronic signatures		●

Dots denote the potential requirements depending on the purpose of the database.

a repository for publications or for the purpose of a regulatory submission.

17.6 Cloud Computing

In the case of robotic surgery, there has been an increasing interest and need for collaboration across multiple investigators in different institutions around the globe. Beyond multiuser capabilities, the ability to access the database securely over the Internet became crucial to the success of our study.

Accessing applications over the Internet is not a new concept – it has gone through various incarnations from the early days of the Internet when it was referred to as application services from application service providers (ASPs), more recently known as Software as a Service (SaaS) and now culminating in the all-encompassing term *cloud computing*. The IT analyst firm Gartner defines cloud computing as "a style of computing where scalable and elastic IT capabilities are provided as a service to multiple customers using Internet technologies."[9]

What this typically translates to is that you subscribe to a service for your computing needs, and only pay for the use of your applications as you need them. Scalability, reliability, security, and expansion are all handled automatically for you. You get to concentrate on your task at hand – definition of database, application, and the use of your application. Once your needs have been satisfied, you can discontinue use of these services or scale back your subscription to better manage costs.

What is new with cloud computing is that major vendors like Google, Microsoft, Amazon.com, Intuit, and Salesforce.com are all offering enterprise-scale online technologies that provide an alternative to traditional premise-based RDBMS systems. This can considerably reduce the complexity and cost of developing and maintaining your clinical trial data collection system.

What this also means for the end user is that their database is accessible from any computer that has Internet access. Gone are the days when you had to be in the office or lab to enter data. Other advantages are that they allow the user to update data once and share this information with multiple investigators simultaneously. Many of these cloud computing services provide robust analytics and reporting engines for real-time review and analysis of data.

Careful consideration relating to security and privacy of data is required when providing access to any system over the Internet (whether the database is premise based or provided by utilizing a cloud computing vendor). All of the major cloud computing providers have well-documented privacy policies, and their data security policies and systems are equal to (or better) than what is found in the largest institutions and governmental agencies.

It should be noted that these services are likely not fully compliant with 21 CFR Part 11, but they can be brought into compliance with some customization and process documentation work. Such systems are currently ideal for research purposes when the level of documentation is less rigorous than that of a submission to a governmental agency. As with any system or technology selection, be sure to match your choice to your key requirements.

17.7 Private Clouds

While cloud computing encompasses the current movement of large-scale applications and infrastructure available as a service over the Internet, it is typically thought of as being provided by the major

Fig. 17.1 Intra-operative characteristics

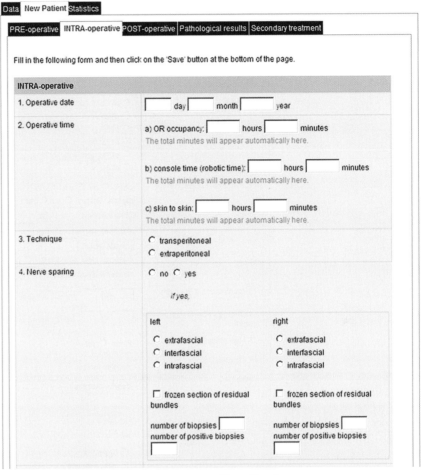

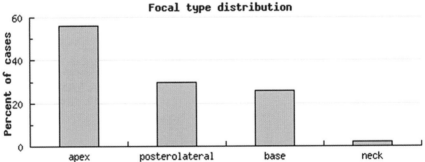

web vendors such as Google, Amazon, and Salesforce. But what happens when a third party leverages these cloud computing services to provide an application for their institution or limited set of users? Such a setup has recently been referred to as a *private cloud*.

An example of a private cloud is a web-based system for clinical data management that was recently developed by the Geneva Foundation for Medical Education and Research (GFMER).[10] GFMER is a nonprofit organization supported by numerous affiliates (including the Department of Health of the Canton of Geneva, Department of Social Affairs of the City of Geneva, the Faculty of Medicine, Geneva University, and the World Health Organization). This foundation embarked on the development of a web-based database for research in gynecologic and urologic surgery for use by its affiliates.

Fig. 17.2 Pathological results

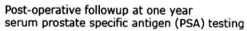

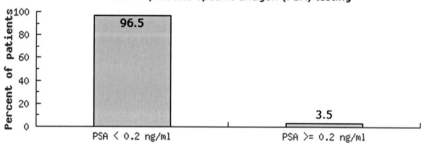

The GFMER efforts have resulted in the participation of five international centers collectively known as the European Group of Robotic Urology (EGRU) involved with performing robotic-assisted prostatectomy with a total of over 1,200 cases logged in the online system to date (http://www.gfmer.ch/Formation_Fr/Chirurgie_laparoscopique_robotisee.htm). The web-based nature of this tool has allowed for real-time data monitoring and statistical analysis while facilitating collaboration between colleagues at different institutions.

Examples of data entry screens for the intra-operative and pathological evaluations are seen in Figs. 17.1 and 17.2. The figures demonstrate the level of detail of data collection that can be captured using this tool. The majority of variables and their values are given in the form of drop-down menus or check boxes with very little need for written descriptions. This ultimately makes the export and subsequent analysis straightforward. This web-based tool allows for some rudimentary graphs, which assist in tracking progress and data trends.

The database developed by GFMER represents one type of private cloud solution that can be used to track robotic prostatectomy outcomes. Other premise-based solutions include ones that are specific to *electronic data capture systems* including but not limited to *Phase Forward* and *Open Clinica*.[11] Many of these existing systems are more complex to set up and run for the single institutional user and are not as cost-effective unless being considered for a multicenter trial for the purpose of a regulatory submission.

17.8 Conclusion

In summary, the careful selection of clinical variables needed for analysis of outcomes is paramount to creating an effective data collection form. Look to segment your data collection according to the natural course of patient treatment – for example, preoperative, intra-operative, postoperative. The structure of the forms will dictate the architectural design of the database. Your selection of database will likely be driven by the long-term needs of your study, taking into consideration the total cost of ownership (TCO).

It is difficult to predict how the use of web-based tools will affect individual researchers in the future; however, with the increasing need for multi-institutional collaboration across the globe this option of data management is proving to be ideal.

References

1. FDA clearances for the da Vinci Surgical System. http://www.accessdata.fda.gov/scripts/cdrh/cfdocs/cfPMN/pmn.cfm
2. Pocock SJ. *Clinical Trial: A Practical Approach.* New York, NY and Chichester: Wiley; 1983.
3. Menon M, Tewari A. Vattikuti Institute Prostatectomy Team. Robotic radical prostatectomy and the Vattikuti Urology Institute technique: an interim analysis of results and technical points. *Urology.* April 2003;61(4 Suppl 1):15–20.
4. Bristol Urological Institute. "International Index of Erectile Function Questionnaire". URL: http://www.iciq.net. Updated 2010. Accessed July, 2009
5. International Index of Erectile Function (IIEF) Questionnaire. http://www.urologyspecialists.net/print/iief.html. Updated February 2010. Accessed June, 2009
6. Rodriguez E Jr, Skarecky DW, Ahlering TE. Post-robotic prostatectomy urinary continence: characterization of perfect continence versus occasional dribbling in pad-free men. *Urology.* 2006;67(4):785–788. Epub 2006 March 29. Accessed 2006.
7. Ahlering TE, Eichel L, Skarecky D. Early potency outcomes with cautery-free neurovascular bundle preservation with robotic laparoscopic radical prostatectomy. *J Endourol.* 2005;19(6):715–718.
8. Code of Federal Regulations, Title 21 – Food & Drugs Good Clinical Practice Part 11. Available at: http://www.accessdata.fda.gov/scripts/cdrh/cfdocs/cfcfr/CFRSearch.cfm?CFRPart=11. Published April 1st, 2008. Accessed June, 2009
9. Gartners Newsroom. "*Gartner Says Cloud Computing Will Be as Influential as E-business.*" Available at: http://www.gartner.com/it/page.jsp?id=707508. Published June, 2008. Accessed June, 2009
10. Geneva Foundation for Medical Education and Research. Available at: http://www.gfmer.ch. Accessed July, 2009
11. Solution Providers: Electronic Document Management Systems. Available at: http://www.21cfrpart11.com/pages/sol_prov/edms.htm. Updated 2009. Accessed July, 2009

Chapter 18

The Role of Scientific Journals in Disseminating New Technology

Barry B. McGuire and John M. Fitzpatrick

Scientific journals have been at the heart of medical technological advancements and remain an integral role in distributing information. The path of discovery in many of the commonly used technologies has really been quite interesting. Advancements in laparoscopy have been astonishing since the first clinical laparoscopic nephrectomy in 1991 by Clayman et al. Observing the application of laparoscopy to new and innovative ways is fascinating with tangents such as robotics, laparoscopic-augmented reality images, and natural orifice surgery. This chapter walks you through the scientific journals' progressive description of these old and new technologies from case reporting to randomized controlled trials to illustrate the important role they play in disseminating information.

18.1 Introduction

Scientific journals have retained a central role in the clinical arena for so long due to the combination of demand for knowledge and speed at which new technologies come to the market. Scientific journals can be traced back to the middle of the seventeenth century and continue to provide an up-to-date, comprehensive archive for knowledge in a discipline and facilitate the generation and flow of information. Since the dawn of surgery, different techniques have been employed to aid the surgeon perform their required duties. Early innovative surgical advancements have included Asian

tribes lighting a mix of saltpeter and sulfur placed onto wounds as a form of cautery, Dakota Indians using the quill of a feather attached to an animal bladder to suck out purulent material, and the discovery of needles from the Stone Age which were used in the suturing of cuts. Ambroise Pare, a sixteenth-century French surgeon, stated that there were five reasons to perform surgery: "To eliminate that which is superfluous, restore that which has been dislocated, separate that which has been united, join that which has been divided and repair the defects of nature." Much has happened in the development of surgical techniques and technologies since these past times where only the most basic of tools were available to the physician. In the last century there has been such technological advancements that we as physicians are continuously presented with new cutting edge tools that may, or indeed may not, benefit our patients.

18.2 Appraisal of New Technology

As surgeons we are continuously faced with new technologies and need to appraise them. There is a natural curiosity when faced with a new device coupled with the desire to do what is best for our patients. Despite temptation, we must remember that a methodical and scientific approach to new technology must be applied as if it were a new pharmaceutical agent we would administer to a patient. In addition, newer technologies often seem more expensive and a rigorous health economic analysis must be performed focusing not only on consumables used intra-operatively but also on previously overlooked issues such as economic productivity of the patient and how this is altered by the

J.M. Fitzpatrick (✉)
Department of Surgery, Mater Misericordiae University Hospital, Dublin, Ireland
e-mail: jfitzpatrick@mater.ie

A.K. Hemal, M. Menon (eds.), *Robotics in Genitourinary Surgery*,
DOI 10.1007/978-1-84882-114-9_18, © Springer-Verlag London Limited 2011

intervention. Unfortunately, properly conducted randomized control trials are often lacking as the thrill of a new technology is embraced hastily. New pharmaceutical agents are subjected to rigorous levels of scrutiny from phase I trials to clinical practice. Logically one would not blindly try a new medication on a patient without knowing it has been tested rigorously and likewise one should not use an instrument that has not had the same standards applied to it. For example, the Mersilene sling was utilized for the surgical treatment of urinary stress incontinence in the early 1990s[1] and following some long-term data it became apparent that there was an unacceptably high erosion rate associated with it.[2] It could be argued that if rigorous pre-clinical trials were carried in similar stepwise fashion as the pharmaceuticals, then there would not have been so many subjected to the complication of urethral erosion. On the other hand, in situations where important information pertaining to the use of new technologies affects our patients, be it good or bad, it is important to have a peer-reviewed forum for discussion so that as professional we can openly discuss the pros and cons in a non-threatening manner without fear of reproach. Quite often, in the media, a new technology will be brought to open attention due to its perceived futuristic clinical application and in turn it is perceived publicly that the medical community is slow to embrace new ideas. However, despite all pressures and eagerness to be at the cutting edge, one must strictly adhere to the law of clinical science and progress all new technologies from infancy to randomized controlled blinded trials.

18.3 Regulating New Technologies

The regulation of new technologies varies from country to country. In the United States, the Food and Drug Administration (FDA) controls all new technologies that have a clinical application. Its centre for devices and radiological health is responsible for regulating firms that manufacture, repackage, re-label, and/or import medical devices sold in the United States Devices are classified into class I, II, and III. Regulatory control increases from class I to III with class I devices exempt from pre-market approval and most class III devices requiring pre-market approval. In the United Kingdom, The National Institute for Health and Clinical Excellence (NICE) is

an independent organization responsible for providing national guidance on promoting good health and preventing and treating ill-health in the UK. NICE, similar to FDA, independently assesses new technologies that come into clinical use, albeit non-legislatively. Another excellent source of validation and scientific appraisal is the Cochrane Database. The Cochrane library contains high-quality independent evidence to inform healthcare decision making. It includes reliable evidence from systematic reviews and clinical trials. Cochrane reviews publish combined results of the world's literature on topics and are truly a very valuable tool for appraisal of new technologies that should be present in every clinician's armamentarium.

18.4 Scientific Journals at the Hub of Disseminating New Technologies

To look at the role of scientific journals in disseminating new technologies, we must look at the landmark technologies which have come to be used in everyday urology throughout the world. It is easier for us to analyze a new technology when there is a gold standard to compare to, e.g., TURP, open radical prostatectomy. This gives us the opportunity to evaluate new equipment and technology comparing all parameters, not just clinical. It is difficult to know which technology is the best one for our patients bearing in mind our sacrosanct Hippocratic oath of "doing no harm." It is in this very arena that scientific journals play the absolutely essential role of not only disseminating new technologies but also following them through properly conducted trials assessing their real value.

Three common urological operations that are performed are TURP, nephrectomy, and radical prostatectomy, all of which have a constant flow of new technologies and have established gold standards to which they can be compared to.

18.5 Transurethral Resection of the Prostate

Since the first transurethral resection of the prostate (TURP) was performed by Guyon at the Necker Hospital in Paris in 1901, we have seen a myriad of new technologies come and go. TURP remains the most common surgical intervention for LUTS secondary to BPH as it provides excellent short- and long-term results, as assessed by urodynamics and patient symptom scores.[3] It remains the "gold standard" despite the morbidity such as blood loss, fluid absorption, and retrograde ejaculation. Morbidities have stimulated the development of new technologies and have introduced many different modalities of treating benign prostatic hypertrophy with the aim of reducing length of stay and blood loss. Numerous energy delivery systems have been used, including interstitial, contact and side-firing lasers, microwaves, high-intensity focused ultrasound, and direct heating of the prostate with interstitial needles. Whereas the standard TURP would necessitate a 2–3 day inpatient stay, newer techniques can be undertaken as day-case procedures and incur minimal blood loss.

Examples of promising alternatives to TURP, albeit at different points of maturation, include Holmium laser enucleation of the prostate (HoLEP) and The GreenLight[TM] laser. Holmium laser enucleation of the prostate (HoLEP) as proposed by Fraundorfer and Gilling[4] results in the excision of the prostatic adenoma with minimal blood loss and complications. The irrigation fluid used does not have to be nonionic, as no electrical currents are used; fluid absorption is therefore less of a problem and will not result in the TUR syndrome. Sufficient data prove HoLEP's durability for most prostate sizes at longterm follow-up; KTP laser vaporization needs further evaluation to define the re-operation rate.[5] The clinical results of GreenLight[TM] prostate vaporization are equivalent to those following transurethral resection of the prostate, with reduced operative risks, even for the high-risk patient.[6] However, despite promising early results, there appears to be some reluctance in adopting new technologies due to feared complications associated, e.g., prolonged catheterization or dysuria. Also, none of these novel technologies achieve equivalent urodynamic improvements to those after TURP.[3]

Another alternative technique is transurethral microwave therapy techniques and is an effective alternative to TURP in certain circumstances. However, a Cochrane review of TUMT versus TURP reports that TURP provides greater symptom score and urinary flow improvements and reduces the need for subsequent BPH treatments compared to TUMT.[7] Small sample sizes and differences in study design limit comparison between devices with different designs and energy levels. The effects of symptom duration, patient characteristics, or prostate volume on treatment response are unknown. There are many promising alternatives to TURP and increasing the number of quality prospective randomized controlled trials with adequate follow-up is mandatory to tailor each technique to the right patient.

18.6 Laparoscopic Radical Nephrectomy

There is an increasing incidence of all stages of kidney cancer in the last two decades.[8] Surgical excision remains the primary treatment for localized RCC and the technique and technology has come a long way since open radical nephrectomy was first popularized by Robson in 1969.[9] Percutaneous removal of the kidney began in 1988 when Weinberg and Smith attempted to remove a porcine kidney by means of a single tract, percutaneous retroperitoneal approach.[10] Unfortunately this was complicated by a colonic injury, and the project was abandoned. Subsequently, Ikari et al.[11] reported a single clinical case in which they attempted to remove a non-functional kidney by a single-tract, percutaneous retroperitoneal approach. After first embolizing the renal artery, they used myriad grasping forceps to avulse bits of renal parenchymal tissue, which were then delivered through the nephrostomy tract. Much of the kidney was removed but postoperative sonography of the flank showed that about 17 g of kidney tissue remained in place. With the quest for reducing morbidity and cost through reduced length of stay and peering enviously at other specialities utilizing minimal access surgery, the first real case report of a laparoscopic nephrectomy was reported in 1991 in the *Journal of Urology* by Ralph Clayman[12] 6 years after Prof. Erich Mühe of Böblingen, Germany, performed the first laparoscopic cholecystectomy.[13] It was a 190 g right kidney extracted through an 11-mm port. From then multiple series[14] were reported which progressed to multiple randomized controlled trials comparing open versus laparoscopic nephrectomy.[15,16] It illustrates the role of scientific journals in disseminating new technologies, as a variety of international publications that quickly came to light after the first report was published illustrate how it became a popular method of nephrectomy. Publishing on a

new subject such as laparoscopic nephrectomy in scientific journals by surgeons allows us to validate new
technologies through initial case reports, series, editorials, and comparison trials as demonstrated. Such is
the success of laparoscopic nephrectomy that it has
become an acceptable first-line surgical method of
removing the kidney with acknowledged low morbidity and shorter hospital stay and recovery.[17] Indeed,
renal surgery including simple nephrectomy, radical nephrectomy, donor nephrectomy, partial nephrectomy, and nephroureterectomy has now become the
most frequent laparoscopic procedure performed by
urologists. It has only been through the sharing of
information through scientific journals that pushing
the boundaries of keyhole surgery has been allowed.
It is demonstrated time and time again that laparoscopic nephrectomy has a reduced pain level, faster
convalescence, and excellent cosmetic results.[17] There
are acceptable oncological outcome reports for laparoscopic radical nephrectomy[18] and the management of
small renal tumors using laparoscopic nephrectomy is
gradually approaching the new standard of care.[17,19]
Such is the popularity of this procedure that laparoscopic nephrectomy is replacing open nephrectomy
in certain centers with the rapid expansion of this
specialty.

18.7 Applying Technology in New and Innovative Ways

With the popularity of laparoscopic nephrectomy and
the excellent established results both in reduced morbidity and oncological parameters, it was obvious that
this would spill over into the domain of the pelvic urologist. Retropubic radical prostatectomy (RRP) using
the nerve sparing technique popularized by Walsh in
1983 has long been the gold standard[20] with established and expected objectives – "The triad of per-
fection": oncological control, continence, and potency.
Laparoscopic prostatectomy was first described in
1997[21] quite soon after reports from multiple other
institutions surfaced.[22–24] As the technique was published and attempted by other international institutions,
it is interesting to see a different outcome which
occurred compared to laparoscopic nephrectomy. With

laparoscopic nephrectomy we observed a natural stepwise progression to usage with good quality publications and research to back this up as an appropriate
method to operating, from case report to randomized
controlled trial. However, in relation to laparoscopic
radical prostatectomy, publications began discussing
the many reservations they had with the procedure,
such as length of operating time and the long arduous learning curve. It is considered a technically very
challenging operation[25] as even in strict mentoring circumstances, at least 50 cases must be performed,[25]
the learning curve for operating time and blood loss
can take at least 100–150 cases, complication and
continence rates 150–200 cases, and potency up to
700 cases.[26] These learning curves are likely to be
shorter when surgeons are taught in departments with
a high throughput of cases; however both surgeons and
patients need to be aware of them. Laparoscopic radical prostatectomy needs to be learned within an immersion teaching program and even then, a large surgical
volume is needed to maintain clinical outcomes at the
highest level. Outside of tertiary or quaternary referral
centers, most do not have this level of throughput to
support or justify this slow learning curve.

More recently, technological advancements in
robotics have enabled the development of robotic-
assisted laparoscopic radical prostatectomy as a possible alternative to conventional laparoscopic radical
prostatectomy[27] and its timing could not have been
more perfect. It was with reluctance that the ever
enthusiastic minimally invasive surgeon was embracing the laparoscopic radical prostatectomy. The robotic
prostatectomy changed that however and quickly.
Surgeons untrained in laparoscopic technology have
embraced robotic prostatectomy, reporting success
comparable to pure laparoscopic and open prostatectomy approaches. Surgeons experienced in open
prostatectomy made a smooth transition to robotic
prostatectomy, while pure laparoscopic radical prostatectomy remains beyond their reach. The number of
cases taken to perform a robotic prostatectomy in 4 h,
or the 4-h learning curve, has been estimated at 15–30
cases for experienced surgeons. This number increases
to 60–100 cases for surgeons switching from open
to pure laparoscopic radical prostatectomy. It would
appear that there is a real niche for the robot with
prostatectomy; however, a randomized controlled trial
is eagerly awaited.

18.8 Exciting New Technologies Surfacing in Scientific Journals: Augmented Reality Images

With the advent of minimally invasive surgery the surgeon has been forced to learn to operate with little or no tactile feedback. As more and more surgeries are performed laparoscopically now, the surgeon depends on quality pre-operative imaging. There is no ability to see what is beyond the displayed image and a technology that could combine pre- and intra-operative images together could lend itself to enhance the surgeons' ability and protect the patient. A tool that assists in identifying structures that lie beyond the image displayed, e.g., vessels, nerves, organs, would be of assistance to those learning the skill of laparoscopic operating or indeed difficult dissection such as adhesions. "Augmented reality" is a novel technology which combines the preoperative and/or intraoperative radiologic images onto the visualized surgical field in a real-time manner and is used as a tool to assist in dissection.[28–30] For example, real-time virtual sonography combines real-time ultrasound with a pre-operative MRI or CT[31,32] and enhances the ultrasonographic image in front of the user. This technology has already been used for laparoscopic partial nephrectomy and laparoscopic radical prostatectomy,[31] where the computerized digital images are projected and superimposed in a three-dimensional image in real-time endoscopic image. Another modality in which this technology is useful for is in cryoablation of renal tumors. The shape of the target lesion may become distorted by the ice ball and augmented imaging using ultrasound, which better images the ice ball compared to computed tomography, allows real-time ablation zone imaging for better precision. As we have seen in all aspects of technological development in surgery, all advancements come from a basic idea, performed in an environment most likely for success, and from there more complex and challenging obstacles are overcome, in the confidence that it has been successful at the most basic level. Augmented reality is no different and has been used in the field of neurosurgery for over 10 years now. It is easier to use in this setting as the brain is confined within steady bony confines of the skull and the image does not move at all, therefore fusing preoperative images with

needle direction is possible.[28] Unfortunately within the abdomen there is considerable movement and there can be considerable variation between the preoperative image and that which is in front of the surgeon which is now the biggest hurdle to the application of this technology to a different environment such as the abdomen.[33] We are still in the early stages of the development of this exciting new technology and eagerly await the progression from case reports to real clinical use and hopefully randomized controlled trials.

18.9 Natural Orifice Surgery

Another good example of the role scientific journals play in disseminating new technologies can be observed through the history of natural orifice surgery. The growth of this specialized technique can clearly be seen to gather momentum from the very first description to its successful application to a human model. Needless to say that as a specialty this would not have developed without the publishing of successes with laparoscopic surgery and the thoughtful application of this technology to go one step further. Anthony Kalloo of Johns Hopkins University in Baltimore and Venkat Rao and Nageshwar Reddy of the Asian Institute of Gastroenterology in Hyderabad, India, are credited with conceiving natural orifice abdominal surgery. Interestingly, the first described natural orifice surgery was a hybrid, laparoscopic small non-functioning tuberculous nephrectomy removed through a posterior colpotomy in 1993[34] and since then there has been great interest and development in natural orifice translumenal endoscopic surgery (NOTES) due to perceived reduced morbidity and improved cosmesis. Clearly a chain reaction of interest was created following this publication and similar hybrid models of laparoscopic nephrectomy and transvaginal extraction of intact nephrectomy specimens in 10 patients were subsequently reported by Gill and colleagues.[35] Although the specialty began as a hybrid model, by publishing this material in peer–reviewed, high-powered journals, the world stage looked upon NOTES as a possible alternative to standard operative techniques. Experiments continued; however, the technique was heavily criticized due the cumbersome and difficult nature of the instruments. There appeared to be a waning interest in the specialty until 2004 when a publication by Kalloo and colleagues described access to the peritoneal cavity for a liver biopsy with transgastric peritoneoscopy in a porcine model also.[36] There were no immediate postoperative complications and following this report there was an explosion of cross-specialty studies performed, e.g., appendectomy[37] and cholecystectomy.[38] With all of this interest and publishing of results, there was marked enthusiasm for NOTES as a technique and enough interest spurred the Natural Orifice Surgery Consortium for Assessment and Research (NOSCAR)[39] which gathered to discuss any potential future to NOTES. A white paper was generated during this meeting which recommended that additional studies were to be performed under the watchful eye of NOSCAR.[39,40] It is apparent that as a specialty those who were enthusiastic about it realized that a careful approach was needed prior to embracing it and that the technical limitations represented the most significant barrier to its safe application in humans.[39,41] In response to, and in accordance with, the recommendations of NOSCAR, additional animal experiments were performed transvaginally, transgastrically, and transvesically in instrumentation and equipment was refined. NOTES procedures in humans that have successfully been performed to date include transgastric, transvaginal, and transvesical peritoneoscopy, transgastric cholecystectomy, appendectomy, liver biopsy and tubal ligation, and transvaginal appendectomy.[42-45]

The progression of NOTES in urology surgery has also been interesting. The initial experiments in animals have been met with good success with multiple centers reporting success with NOTES nephrectomy. Mathes reported transgastric nephrectomy in 2007 using a dual-chamber gastroscope, Clayman in 2007[46] performed a transvaginal nephrectomy in a pig removing the kidney through the vagina, and in 2008 Crouzet[47] reported bilateral transgastric and transvesical renal cryoablation in a porcine model. The response to criticism of the poor instrumentation led to a publication by Box where they placed ports through the umbilicus, the vagina, and the colon and successfully completed a nephrectomy without complications.[48] In 2009 the world's first transvaginal NOTES nephrectomy on a 57-year-old female with a non-functioning kidney was performed in the Cleveland clinic.[49]

18.10 Summary

Some of the incredible technological advancements in urological surgery over the last 100 years led to the rise of the scientific journal. The journals have been the hub at the centre of each development disseminating both positive and negative attributes in an open forum for discussion. The environment encouraged openness and competitiveness which pushed the technological advancements and standards higher and higher, without which we would not be able to offer our patients such vast options in their treatment.

References

1. Guner H, Yildiz A, Erdem A, Erdem M, Tiftik Z, Yildirim M. Surgical treatment of urinary stress incontinence by a suburethral sling procedure using a Mersilene mesh graft. *Gynecol Obstet Invest*. 1994;37:52–55.
2. Wohlrab KJ, Erekson EA, Myers DL. Postoperative erosions of the Mersilene suburethral sling mesh for antiincontinence surgery. *Int Urogynecol J Pelvic Floor Dysfunct*. 2009;20:417–420.
3. Gordon NS. Day-case holmium laser enucleation of the prostate for gland volumes of ml: early experience. *BJU Int*. 2003;92:330.
4. Fraundorfer MR, Gilling PJ. Holmium:YAG laser enucleation of the prostate combined with mechanical morcellation: preliminary results. *Eur Urol*. 1998;33:69–72.
5. Naspro R, Bachmann A, Gilling P, et al. A review of the recent evidence (2006–2008) for 532-nm photoselective laser vaporisation and holmium laser enucleation of the prostate. *Eur Urol*. 2009;55:1345–1357.
6. Van Cleynenbreugel B, Srirangam SJ, Van Poppel H. High-performance system GreenLight laser: indications and outcomes. *Curr Opin Urol*. 2009;19:33–37.
7. Hoffman RM, Monga M, Elliot SP, Macdonald R, Wilt TJ. Microwave thermotherapy for benign prostatic hyperplasia. *Cochrane Database Syst Rev*. 2007:CD004135.
8. Hock LM, Lynch J, Balaji KC. Increasing incidence of all stages of kidney cancer in the last 2 decades in the United States: an analysis of surveillance, epidemiology and end results program data. *J Urol*. 2002;167:57–60.
9. Robson CJ, Churchill BM, Anderson W. The results of radical nephrectomy for renal cell carcinoma. *J Urol*. 1969;101:297–301.
10. Weinberg JJ, Smith AD. Percutaneous resection of the kidney: preliminary report. *J Endourol*. 1988;2:355–361.
11. Ikari O, Netto NJ, Palma PC, D'Ancona CA. Percutaneous nephrectomy in nonfunctioning kidneys: a preliminary report. *J Urol*. 1990;144:966–968.
12. Clayman RV, Kavoussi LR, Soper NJ, et al. Laparoscopic nephrectomy: initial case report. *J Urol*. 1991;146:278–282.
13. Reynolds W Jr. The first laparoscopic cholecystectomy. *JSLS*. 2001;5:89–94.

14. Pisani E, Austoni E, Trinchieri A, et al. Urological laparoscopy: our preliminary results. *Arch Ital Urol Androl*. 1993;65:687–694.

15. Andersen MH, Mathisen L, Veenstra M, et al. Quality of life after randomization to laparoscopic versus open living donor nephrectomy: long-term follow-up. *Transplantation*. 2007;84:64–69.

16. Burgess NA, Koo BC, Calvert RC, Hindmarsh A, Donaldson PJ, Rhodes M. Randomized trial of laparoscopic v open nephrectomy. *J Endourol*. 2007;21:610–613.

17. Hemal AK, Kumar A, Kumar R, Wadhwa P, Seth A, Gupta NP. Laparoscopic versus open radical nephrectomy for large renal tumors: a long-term prospective comparison. *J Urol*. 2007;177:862–866.

18. Dunn MD, McDougall EM, Clayman RV. Laparoscopic radical nephrectomy. *J Endourol*. 2000;14:849–855.

19. Eskicorapci SY, Teber D, Schulze M, Ates M, Stock C, Rassweiler JJ. Laparoscopic radical nephrectomy: the new gold standard surgical treatment for localized renal cell carcinoma. *ScientificWorldJournal*. 2007;7:825–836.

20. Walsh PC, Lepor H, Eggleston JC. Radical prostatectomy with preservation of sexual function: anatomical and pathological considerations. *Prostate*. 1983;4:473–485.

21. Schuessler WW, Schulam PG, Clayman RV, Kavoussi LR. Laparoscopic radical prostatectomy: initial short-term experience. *Urology*. 1997;50:854–857.

22. Guillonneau B, Cathelineau X, Barret E, Rozet F, Vallancien G. Laparoscopic radical prostatectomy. Preliminary evaluation after 28 interventions. *Presse Med*. 1998;27:1570–1574.

23. Guillonneau B, Cathelineau X, Barret E, Rozet F, Vallancien G. Laparoscopic radical prostatectomy: technical and early oncological assessment of 40 operations. *Eur Urol*. 1999;36:14–20.

24. Guillonneau B, Vallancien G. Laparoscopic radical prostatectomy: initial experience and preliminary assessment after 65 operations. *Prostate*. 1999;39:71–75.

25. Fabrizio MD, Tuerk I, Schellhammer PF. Laparoscopic radical prostatectomy: decreasing the learning curve using a mentor initiated approach. *J Urol*. 2003;169:2063–2065.

26. Eden CG, Neill MG, Louie-Johnsun MW. The first 1000 cases of laparoscopic radical prostatectomy in the UK: evidence of multiple 'learning curves'. *BJU Int*. 2009;103:1224–1230.

27. Menon M, Hemal AK. Vattikuti Institute Prostatectomy: a technique of robotic radical prostatectomy: experience in more than 1000 cases. *J Endourol*. 2004;18:611–619.

28. Iseki H, Masutani Y, Iwahara M, et al. Volumegraph (overlaid three-dimensional image-guided navigation). Clinical application of augmented reality in neurosurgery. *Stereotact Funct Neurosurg*. 1997;68:18–24.

29. Marescaux J, Rubino F, Arenas M, Mutter D, Soler L. Augmented-reality-assisted laparoscopic adrenalectomy. *JAMA*. 2004;292:2214–2215.

30. Sato Y, Nakamoto M, Tamaki Y, et al. Image guidance of breast cancer surgery using 3-D ultrasound images and augmented reality visualization. *IEEE Trans Med Imaging*. 1998;17:681–693.

31. Ukimura O, Gill IS. Imaging-assisted endoscopic surgery: Cleveland Clinic experience. *J Endourol*. 2008;22:803–810.

32. Ukimura O, Mitterberger M, Okihara K, et al. Real-time virtual ultrasonographic radiofrequency ablation of renal cell carcinoma. *BJU Int*. 2008;101:707–711.

33. Ukimura O, Gill IS. Image-fusion, augmented reality, and predictive surgical navigation. *Urol Clin North Am*. 2009;36:115–123, vii.

34. Breda G, Silvestre P, Giunta A, Xausa D, Tamai A, Gherardi L. Laparoscopic nephrectomy with vaginal delivery of the intact kidney. *Eur Urol*. 1993;24:116–117.

35. Gill IS, Cherullo EE, Meraney AM, Borsuk F, Murphy DP, Falcone T. Vaginal extraction of the intact specimen following laparoscopic radical nephrectomy. *J Urol*. 2002;167:238–241.

36. Kalloo AN, Singh VK, Jagannath SB, et al. Flexible transgastric peritoneoscopy: a novel approach to diagnostic and therapeutic interventions in the peritoneal cavity. *Gastrointest Endosc*. 2004;60:114–117.

37. Sumiyama K, Gostout CJ, Rajan E, et al. Pilot study of the porcine uterine horn as an in vivo appendicitis model for development of endoscopic transgastric appendectomy. *Gastrointest Endosc*. 2006;64:808–812.

38. Pai RD, Fong DG, Bundga ME, Odze RD, Rattner DW, Thompson CC. Transcolonic endoscopic cholecystectomy: a NOTES survival study in a porcine model (with video). *Gastrointest Endosc*. 2006;64:428–434.

39. Rattner D, Kalloo A. ASGE/SAGES working group on natural orifice translumenal endoscopic surgery. October 2005. *Surg Endosc*. 2006;20:329–333.

40. White WM, Haber GP, Doerr MJ, Gettman M. Natural orifice translumenal endoscopic surgery. *Urol Clin North Am*. 2009;36:147–155, vii.

41. Rattner D. Introduction to NOTES white paper. *Surg Endosc*. 2006;20:185.

42. Gettman MT, Blute ML. Transvesical peritoneoscopy: initial clinical evaluation of the bladder as a portal for natural orifice translumenal endoscopic surgery. *Mayo Clin Proc*. 2007;82:843–845.

43. Hazey JW, Narula VK, Renton DB, et al. Natural-orifice transgastric endoscopic peritoneoscopy in humans: initial clinical trial. *Surg Endosc*. 2008;22:16–20.

44. Marescaux J, Dallemagne B, Perretta S, Wattiez A, Mutter D, Coumaros D. Surgery without scars: report of transluminal cholecystectomy in a human being. *Arch Surg*. 2007;142:823–826.

45. Tsin DA, Colombero LT, Lambeck J, Manolas P. Minilaparoscopy-assisted natural orifice surgery. *JSLS*. 2007;11:24–29.

46. Clayman RV, Box GN, Abraham JB, et al. Rapid communication: transvaginal single-port NOTES nephrectomy: initial laboratory experience. *J Endourol*. 2007;21:640–644.

47. Crouzet S, Haber GP, Kamoi K, et al. Natural orifice translumenal endoscopic surgery (NOTES) renal cryoablation in a porcine model. *BJU Int*. 2008;102:1715–1718.

48. Box GN, Lee HJ, Santos RJ, et al. Rapid communication: robot-assisted NOTES nephrectomy: initial report. *J Endourol*. 2008;22:503–506.

49. Kaouk JH, White WM, Goel RK, et al. NOTES transvaginal nephrectomy: first human experience. *Urology*. 2009;74:5–8.

Chapter 19

Predicting Robotic Utilization in Urologic Disease: An Epidemiology-Based Model

Jed-Sian Cheng and Gabriel P. Haas

19.1 Introduction

Robotic surgery is a new minimally invasive approach readily endorsed by patients, surgeons, and institutions alike. As with so many new technologies, the concept started out slowly with only a few selected medical applications, but as it became increasingly popular, there has been an explosion of indications (Table 19.1).

At the same time, rapid technological advances in the field of robotic surgery have made the equipment increasingly user-friendly, and this has further resulted in the willingness to cultivate new applications. For some surgeries, it is on the horizon of new applications; for others it has already become the "standard of care." Robotic surgery can not only replace traditional open or laparoscopic operations, but its many advantages may provide the opportunity for some patients to benefit from surgery when they would have chosen nonsurgical interventions in the past. Where is robotic surgery going? What new, expanded applications await us in the future? There are solid data for utilization trends between 2002 and the present for US and international da Vinci installations (Fig. 19.1). But can we predict the utilization of robotic surgery 5, 10, or more years into the future? The answers to these questions are important information for institutions, investors, and manufacturers alike. They may guide health-care policy, reimbursement, and even educational need assessment.

The answer to these questions requires the development of accurate models to predict future robotic utilization based upon population trends, disease epidemiology, and clinical management trends.

19.2 Overview of Epidemiology

Epidemiology is the study of the causation, spread, and patterns of a specific disease in relation to the demography of a defined population. It may be cancer, infection, social habit, or any medical condition.

Incidence is defined as the number of new cases of disease *detected over a period of time*. Prevalence is the number of cases at a given time. The prevalence is a *snapshot in time* that includes detected and undetected diseases. The detection rate is how many cases that are in the population are detected by screening or other methods. The detection rate will predict how many prevalent cases become detected. A low detection rate leaves a large proportion of cases undetected. A new and improved method of detection may change the estimate dramatically.

Multiple studies have shown that the prevalence of prostate cancer is high[1,2] and much higher than newly diagnosed cases. Therefore, incidence depends on both the existence of a condition and the intensity of the efforts to diagnose it. This is a very important issue to consider in the case of prostate cancer, incidental renal masses, pelvic floor dysfunction, and many other medical conditions, because the more intensive the efforts to diagnose it, the more cases will come to light, and the more likely that patients will be offered treatment.

Sometimes the prevalence is not known, and the model must rely on incidence only. For example,

G.P. Haas (✉)
Astellas Pharma Global Development, Inc., Deerfield, IL, USA
e-mail: gabsihaas@aol.com

A.K. Hemal, M. Menon (eds.), *Robotics in Genitourinary Surgery*,
DOI 10.1007/978-1-84882-114-9_19, © Springer-Verlag London Limited 2011

Table 19.1 A list of attempted surgical procedures using the da Vinci robot (obtained from Intuitive Surgical, Inc.)

Urology	Gynecology	Cardiothoracic	General
Prostatectomy	Hysterectomy	Mitral valve repair and replacement	Gastric bypass
Nephrectomy	Myomectomy	Single vessel beating heart bypass	Nissen fundoplication
Partial nephrectomy	Sacral colpopexy	Multi-Vessle beating heart bypass	Heller myotomy
Pyeloplasty	Pelvic lymphadenectomy	Single vessel arrested heart bypass	Gastrectomy
Cystectomy	Tubal reanastomosis	Multi-Vessel arrested heart bypass	Colon resection
Donor nephrectomy	Vaginal prolapse repair	IMA harvesting	Thyroidectomy
Ureterolithotomy	Dermoid cyst	Coronary Anastomosis	Arteriovenous fistula
Pelvic lymphadenectomy	Endometrial ablation	Atrial septum aneurysm	Toupet
Adrenalectomy	Oophorocystectomy	Atrial septal defect repair	Pancreatectomy
Cystocele repair	Oophoroectomy	Tricuspid valve repair	Adrenalectomy
Excision of renal cyst	Ovarian cystectomy	Thrombectomy	Hemi-colectomy
Lymphadenectomy	Ovarian transposition	Thymectomy	Sigmoidectomy
Testicular resection	Salpingectomy	Esophagectomy	Splenectomy
Renal cyst decortication	Salpingo-oophrectomy	Percardial window	Pyloroplasty
Uretetro transplant	Colposuspension (Burch)	Lobectomy	Gastroplasty
Nephropexy	Tubal Ligation	Pneumonectomy	Appendectomy
Ureterectomy	Tubalplasty	Pacemaker lead implantation	Intra-rectal surgery
Rectocele repair		Mediastinal resectioin	Bowel resection
Varicocele		Pulmonary wedge resection	Lumbar sympathectomy
Ureteroplasty			Liver resection
Ureteral implantation			Cholecystectomy
Vaso-vasostomy			Hernia repair

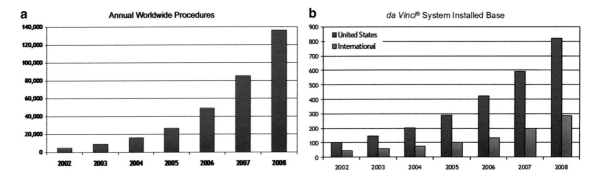

Fig. 19.1 **a** Number of annual da Vinci procedures worldwide. **b** Number of da Vinci robots installed annually in the United States and internationally. Obtained from Intuitive Surgical, Inc.

Creutzfeldt–Jakob disease has a long latent period and is not actively screened in populations. Sometimes the incidence and prevalence numbers may be similar. In diseases like pyelonephritis, almost all patients will present for treatment and few, if any, undetected cases are left in the population. Finally, for some diseases it is important to define what context the intervention should be investigated. For example, estimating pelvic slings for female urinary incontinence: is it placed in a proportion of *all* women with incontinence (prevalence), or women with *new* incontinence (incidence), or women *who fail medical therapy* for incontinence

(a different incidence)? It is important to understand the specifics in the definitions.

19.3 Description of the Model

Predicting the future can be a complex task. Using methods that are based on researched numbers and known clinical practice of a given disease will result in more reliable projections. Therefore, a model was created based on this premise and should result in an educated estimate of future trends.

The key to making a good functional model is to create a conceptually easy to understand, yet adaptable, scheme. There is also a need to make the model dynamic enough to account for changes in gathered data or practice. Our model is illustrated by the flow diagram below. The model begins with a more general population and becomes more specific in each step (Fig. 19.2).

First, a population needs to be defined. Then information of that population can be gathered from published statistics, internal data, or data that may need to be researched. Ideally the prevalence of the disease of interest needs to be known. This will help in estimating potential if all cases were to be known. In general, the population being evaluated is usually patients with newly detected disease. Although incidence is a function of detection rate, we list detection rate as a distinct entity. This is to remind us that method of detection plays a significant role in predicting cases.

Once the incidence, prevalence, and detection rate are defined, one must look at the staging or severity of the disease. This is important as low-stage or low-severity disease may be treated differently than high-stage or high-severity disease. Determine which stage(s) are relevant to the intervention. In the flow diagram, the intervention of interest is surgery.

Not all disease that *can be* treated surgically *will be* surgically treated. It is important to determine what proportion of surgical candidates actually chooses surgery. Note that these numbers may be population dependent. More elderly and sickly patients may not be treated with surgery. Some cultures are averse to surgery. Populations with poor medical follow-up may choose surgery for easier management.

After assembling these statistics, an estimate can be calculated. Understand that assumptions are made at every step. Sometimes it is possible to compare the predictions with actual numbers. Calculations were based on known numbers from previous years, and see if the estimate approximates the *actual* cases and surgeries. If they do not, then the assumptions at each step need to be examined.

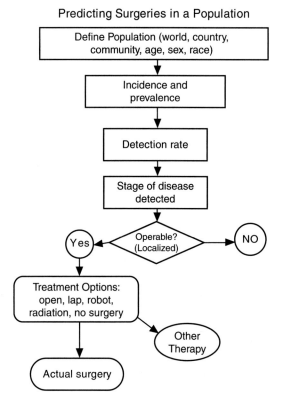

Fig. 19.2 Predicting surgeries in a population. General scheme for surgical disease

19.3.1 Variables

Projections can change due to a number of factors. These influences have been added to the flow diagram below (Fig. 19.3). The dotted lines and boxes illustrate the variables that may affect the projection at the particular data point. There may be more factors that influence a model that may not be illustrated here.

19.3.2 Changes in Population Trends

The projections are calculated by projected population change, and most of the examples use the US population, which expects growth. However, populations can change dramatically. This may be a result of war, famine, or plague. During times of war, the proportions of the population may change. Often, there are less young men, and the female population comprises a larger percentage of the total. Migration may also be a significant factor as some diseases are associated with certain races. A disease epidemic will change the population composition dramatically.

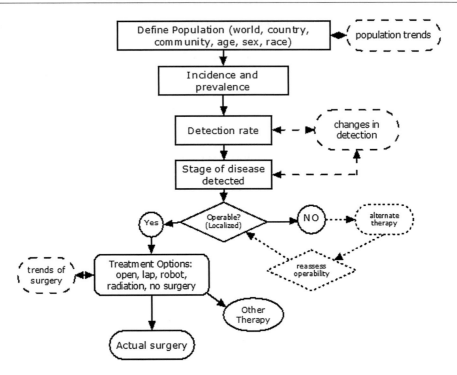

Fig. 19.3 Predicting surgeries in a population. General scheme for surgical disease including variables affecting estimates

19.3.3 Changes in Incidence or Progression

For some diseases, there are interventions that may change incidence or disease progression. Interventions such as folic acid for prevention of neural tube defects have immediate results while others have delayed results. Currently there are a number of studies attempting to prevent prostate cancer: the Prostate Cancer Prevention Trial (PCPT) and Reduction by Dutasteride of Prostate Cancer Events (REDUCE).[3] Moreover, the Reduction by Dutasteride of Clinical Progression Events in Expectant Management (REDEEM)[3] for prostate cancer attempts to evaluate if dutasteride therapy can slow the progression of low-grade, low-risk, localized prostate cancer.

19.3.4 Changes in Detection

The method of detection will greatly affect the incidence of the disease. The more sensitive the process,

the more disease cases will be detected. A good example is prostate cancer. There is a large population of undetected disease based on autopsy studies.[2] With the usage of PSA, there was a tremendous spike in prostate cancer incidence. This phenomenon was not due to an increase in prostate cancer prevalence but an increase in the detection (or incidence) of prostate cancer. The incidence has since leveled off.

If a new assay were to be developed for prostate cancer that had a better sensitivity and specificity, an increase in incidence is expected. If new guidelines were to be made to decrease the PSA threshold, then we would expect the incidence of prostate cancer to increase. By lowering the PSA threshold, we would be increasing the sensitivity. This is because more men would undergo prostate biopsy, but more clinically insignificant prostate cancers would be detected. Thus, changing the PSA threshold may affect the stage of disease at the time of detection. Therefore a fine balance exists between the benefit of detecting significant disease and the cost and risks of a negative or insignificant cancer on biopsy.

19.3.5 Therapies That Make Inoperable Patients Operable

This leads to the part of the flow diagram that shows patients that are not operable that then become operable. Not all patients are operable. Generally, metastatic cancer is considered not operable. Depending on the cancer, currently many patients are treated with radiation and/or chemotherapy to allow the shrinkage of the tumor or metastases. The tumor may then be "downstaged" and the patient deemed resectable and appropriate for surgery.

19.3.6 Treatment Trends or Changes in Paradigms

In 2009, two large studies offered differing conclusions in the benefit of prostate cancer treatment.[4] This brings into question whether prostate cancer is being overtreated. This is a perfect example of treatment trends and paradigms shift. Currently, there is a trend toward watchful waiting/expectant management.[7] This means that there are less men diagnosed with prostate cancer, who choose to have surgery. At the same time, those men who do choose surgery are increasingly using the robot-assisted laparoscopic prostatectomy as the mode for prostatectomy.[8]

19.3.7 Price and Popularity

Another significant factor that affects treatment choices is cost to the patient. Can the patient afford the surgery or medications? Does the surgery save the patient money in the long run? In a country where most people do not have health insurance, a generic drug that treats the disease is preferred. If a population is well insured, then the newest brand name drug that treats the disease and has the least side effects is often chosen.

On the other side, how procedures are reimbursed by insurance may influence the treatment decision. The choice between treatments of equal efficacy is often driven by reimbursement. While the cost to an insured patient may be the same, insurance companies and government may use reimbursement as an incentive to drive preference for one treatment over another.

Since an open, laparoscopic, or robotic prostatectomy results in the same cancer control,[9,10] why would a patient choose one over the others? Patient preference and cosmetic results may drive decisions for treatment. Patients generally do not want to stay in the hospital. The most commonly asked question is, "When will I go home?" or "How long will I stay in the hospital?" In the case of robotic surgery, there is a clear cosmetic advantage and length of stay advantage.[11]

19.4 Examples of Its Application

19.4.1 Prostate Cancer

The robot-assisted laparoscopic prostatectomy (RALP) is one of the new standards of treating prostate cancer. Although the treatment modalities of prostate cancer are established, the proportions of surgical treatment compared to other treatments are still variable. Using this model, a projection will be demonstrated for the year 2020. We do not attempt to project any further into the future, since we believe that knowledge is ever increasing and that treatments are ever improving. Even now, there are clinical trials using 5-α-reductase inhibitors to prevent prostate cancer.[3]

19.4.1.1 Epidemiology

The prevalence of prostate cancer is high. About one in three to one in four men have prostate cancer based on autopsy studies.[1,2] The incidence of prostate cancer is trending down but had previously seen a large spike in the 1990s during the start of the PSA screening era. Although incidence is trending down, the current incidence is still much higher than before the development of PSA screening.

However, current methods of prostate screening do not identify all the cases in the population. Therefore the annual incidence of prostate cancer may potentially increase due to screening methods. However, a debate continues to rage as to the screening and treating of prostate cancer.[12,5,6]

19.4.1.2 Treatments and Trends

Numerous treatment options have been shown to be effective in treating prostate cancer. They include observation/expectant management, androgen deprivation, radiation, cryosurgery, prostatectomy, and others. The natural course of prostate cancer generally affects individuals 10 years after initial diagnosis. Therefore the current treatment trend is to be more conservative with older patients with multiple comorbidities by using expectant management or androgen deprivation. Conversely, younger patients with higher Gleason scores are treated aggressively with prostatectomy.

19.4.1.3 Sample Calculation

An example is calculated assuming that the current methods for prostate cancer screening are unchanged (Fig. 19.4). First with a more basic calculation for RALP and then a more elaborate calculation will be shown in an attempt to be more specific. In addition, current trends and variables will be discussed.

We begin by looking at the US census for population data. According to the census data, a projected 168 million men will make up the 2020 population.[13] Then we researched the prostate cancer incidence according to *Cancer Statistics* 2009 which states that an estimated 158.2 men per 100,000 men will be diagnosed with prostate cancer. The detection rate of the total number of men with prostate cancer in year 2020 is estimated at 266,184 (population × incidence).

Moreover, the number of localized disease in prostate cancer is >90%. This means that almost all prostate cancer patients are potential surgical candidates. According to Miller et al. 31.4% of all prostate diagnoses have prostate surgery for treatment. Taking 31.4% of all prostate cancer diagnoses projected in 2020 results in about 91,000 prostatectomies. The diagram below illustrates the steps for our calculations.

Now reality may not be as simple as the calculation above. We know that male population in the United States is aging. The incidence of prostate cancer by age is different. A proportionally larger older population will exist in 2020, as Fig. 19.5 illustrates. Using the same model, age and age-specific incidence can be adjusted for. Age-specific incidence was

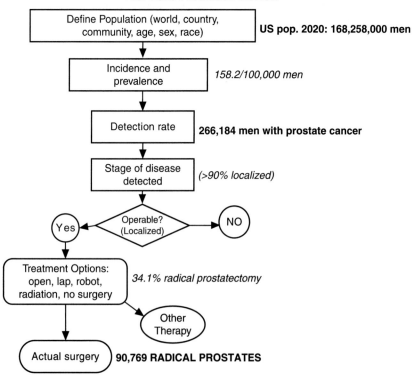

Fig. 19.4 Year 2020 estimate for radical prostatectomies: a basic calculation is illustrated using current published data

Aging Male Population

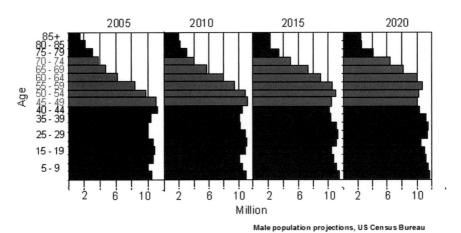

Male population projections, US Census Bureau

Fig. 19.5 The aging male population in the United States. The *red highlighted* age group is the portion of the population most likely to be screened and diagnosed with prostate cancer

obtained through the SEER database which reported data by age intervals. Again the US census database was queried, but now with 5-year age intervals identified.

The age-specific prostate cancer incidence by 5-year intervals as reported by the SEER study[14] is calculated. The estimated age-specific cases are then combined to give the overall cancer incidence for a given year. Again the 34.1% surgery rate for prostate cancer is used. The recalculation is summarized in Fig. 19.6.

As expected, the 2020 estimate is higher than the simple calculation: about 105,000 radical prostatectomies. However, adjusting for age does not always result in increasing numbers. In a population where age proportions are not equal or a disease that affects different age groups, adjusting for age results in more accurate numbers.

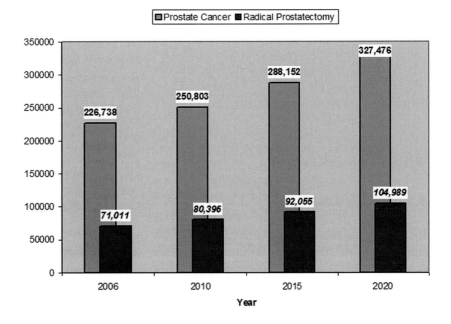

Fig. 19.6 Year 2020 estimate for radical prostatectomies: revised for age adjustment

19.4.1.4 Variables

The variables that can affect the prostate cancer prediction are many. One such example is the discovery of a carcinogen that is modifiable to reduce incidence and prevalence. A similar scenario would be the introduction of a carcinogen to the population that increases incidence and prevalence of prostate cancer. As mentioned above, currently there are trials for the prevention of prostate cancer. If successful, prevention programs may be started on patients with significant risk of prostate cancer resulting in decreased incidence and prevalence. A better prostate cancer screen is continually being developed. The goal is to develop a screen that detects prostate cancer accurately and find more of the prevalent cases and increase incidence. Moreover, prognostic factors are continually elucidated and may guide changes in management: surgical, nonsurgical, or even observation. New treatments are always being developed to increase efficacy and/or decrease morbidity. Potentially, a breakthrough new surgery or medication may be developed that completely changes the management of prostate cancer.

19.4.1.5 Summary

Presently, only a proportion of prostatectomies are done with the robot. We believe that the robot will follow the path of the laparoscopic surgery. As the laparoscopic appendectomy is now the surgery of choice for appendicitis, RALP will become the new surgery of choice for prostatectomies.

In this estimate, only prostate cancer cases were included. Cases for prostatectomy for benign diseases were not accounted for. RALP may become popular for patients requiring an open prostatectomy.

19.4.2 Renal Cell Cancer

19.4.2.1 Epidemiology

The incidence of renal tumors has increased since the new development of the CT scanner. Rarely do patients present with the classic flank pain, hematuria, and palpable mass. Most of the renal tumors discovered today are incidentally found on imaging. Hence, 75% of renal tumors are found at an early stage.[15] The prevalence of renal cell is higher than we used to think. Now that more renal tumors are detected, urologists are left to decide the optimum therapy.

19.4.2.2 Treatment and Trends

The classic answer is excision of the tumor since it has shown to be a significant prognostic factor in survival.[16] Recently, large proportion of renal tumors is detected incidentally by CT scan. Most of these are small, and many of them are currently being followed by serial imaging without intervention unless the tumor size increases dramatically. Moreover, these smaller tumors are candidates for radiofrequency ablation or cryoablation for treatment. However, these treatments cannot confirm eradication of cancer like a partial or total nephrectomy. Small tumors located in upper or lower poles are more amenable to partial nephrectomy. Partial nephrectomies are also indicated for solitary kidneys or patients with poor renal function in an attempt to prevent the need for dialysis. Partial nephrectomy has become a more popular surgical option since the procedure results in the retention of some renal function along with removal of the tumor and a tissue diagnosis.

19.4.2.3 Sample Calculation

After reviewing the literature and available databases, a simple calculation was performed to predict the number of resectable renal cancer cases in the year 2020 (Fig. 19.7). Population information was obtained from the US census database. The incidence is based on 2000–2005 SEER database calculations.[14] Assuming that the incidence of renal tumors does not change, the calculated new cases in 2020 is 44,380. According to Hock et al.[15], the 25% of newly detected renal tumor patients had distal metastases. That leaves 75% with surgically resectable disease. Using those numbers, we conclude that there are potentially more than 30,000 nephrectomies in 2020.

19.4.2.4 Variables

Currently there are no prevention programs and few great exposure modifications for renal cancer. An

Predicting Nephrectomies in 2020 (Total and Partial)

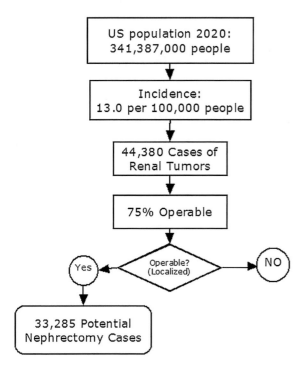

Fig. 19.7 Simple prediction of potential nephrectomy cases in 2020. The numbers used were obtained from multiple sources, and references can be found in the text

important variable for renal tumors is screening. Most cases are found incidentally, and the prevalence is most likely much greater than currently reported. If a screening protocol or test was developed, an increase in incidence is likely.

Another key variable is treatment modality and efficacy. Some patients with small tumors or poor surgical candidates may choose to observe their tumors or undergo cryoablation or radiofrequency ablation and therefore reduce the total surgical intervention. Surgery is still the gold standard, and ablation therapies are just starting to have long-term data regarding efficacy. Moreover, observation of small renal tumors is becoming an increasingly accepted practice.

Currently, the most successfully treated histologic type is clear cell. All other histologic types have poor response to current drug regimens. Therefore a new medical therapy can change the face of renal cancer.

19.4.2.5 Summary

If the robot technology becomes readily available, most of the projected cases can be done as robot total or partial nephrectomies. On the other hand, there are patients with large tumor burden that still requires resection of primary tumor and patients with solitary metastases that are still deemed resectable and thus increasing total surgical cases.

The robot has distinct advantage in performing partial nephrectomies due to the precise motion and control.[17] This is also true for more difficult radical nephrectomies. With more small incidental renal tumors detected, the trend has been to preserve renal function by performing partial nephrectomies. We believe that the more partial nephrectomies will be performed as robot technology is incorporated.

19.4.3 Bladder Cancer

19.4.3.1 Epidemiology

The incidence of bladder cancer has been increasing steadily over the last decade or so. Men are more likely to have bladder cancer than women, as seen by a four to one ratio of men to women with bladder cancer. The incidence increases in people older than 65 years and has a poorer prognosis. This may be the result of comorbidities or more advanced stage at detection. Interestingly, very few bladder cancers are found on autopsy, and hence most cases will eventually become symptomatic.

19.4.3.2 Treatment and Trends

Bladder cancer has a broad spectrum of treatments. Less invasive approaches include transurethral resection of bladder tumor (TURBT), *Bacille Calmette-Guerin* (BCG), and other bladder-sparing techniques. Those treatments are reserved for less invasive disease, but a cystectomy is indicated for invasive disease. Cisplatin and gemcitabine chemotherapy is indicated for metastatic or advanced locally invasive disease. Although bladder preservation is ideal, muscle invasive disease is best treated with a cystectomy. In this section, a prediction for potential robot-assisted cystectomies is calculated.

19.4.3.3 Sample Calculation

The US census projects that about 341 million people will live in the United States in the year 2020.[13] According to Cancer Statistics 2009 from the American Cancer Society, the incidence of bladder cancer is 48.2 per 100,000. This results in over 164,000 cases of bladder cancer. Of these cases, the 12-month cystectomy rate is 69 per 1,000 bladder cancer patients based on the SEER database.[18] This means that about 11,000 patients will undergo a radical cystectomy for bladder malignancy in the year 2020 (Fig. 19.8).

19.4.3.4 Variables

A number of carcinogens have been identified for bladder cancer. These include cigarette smoking, aniline dyes, and other industrial chemicals. As carcinogens

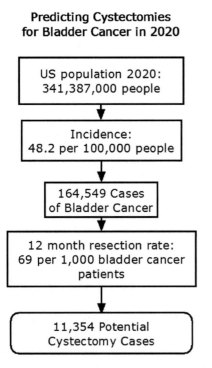

Predicting Cystectomies for Bladder Cancer in 2020

US population 2020: 341,387,000 people

↓

Incidence: 48.2 per 100,000 people

↓

164,549 Cases of Bladder Cancer

↓

12 month resection rate: 69 per 1,000 bladder cancer patients

↓

11,354 Potential Cystectomy Cases

Fig. 19.8 Simple prediction of potential cystectomy cases in 2020. The numbers used were obtained from multiple sources, and references can be found in the text

are identified and exposures minimized, the incidence and prevalence of bladder cancer would decrease. Almost all bladder cancers become symptomatic, and current screening is only done on patients with hematuria. No random screening or more advanced testing is currently recommended. A new bladder cancer screen may affect the incidence of bladder cancer. Prevention in bladder cancer is limited to smoking cessation and exposure modification. An active prevention program may change the prevalence of bladder cancer. New treatments may be developed to increase efficacy and/or decrease morbidity of bladder cancer. If a breakthrough new surgery or medication is developed that can treat muscle invasive bladder cancer and is bladder sparing, it could potentially make the cystectomy a rare procedure.

19.4.3.5 Summary

Robotic approach for cystectomy is an emerging procedure. Many urologists are receiving training for robotic cystectomy, and at large cancer centers the robotic cystectomy with diversion will be soon readily available.

19.4.4 Female Pelvic Dysfunction

19.4.4.1 Epidemiology

Female urinary incontinence is a well-known social and urologic problem that is associated with increased age. Depending on the definition, the prevalence can be as high as 50% in women older than 50 years or as low as 2.5% in women younger than 65 years.[19] Of these women, a fraction will have pelvic organ prolapse that will require surgery with an urethropexy and/or a colpopexy. In these cases, the robot has distinct advantage in reducing incision size and hospital stay. The robot used for female pelvic surgery is a more attractive option for both patients and surgeons.

19.4.4.2 Treatment and Trends

Depending on the type of incontinence, there are many new therapies available. For urge incontinence, the main treatments are medical and/or sacral neurostim-ulation. The treatment of stress urinary incontinence is surgery. The development of the pubovaginal sling has recently changed the management of stress inconti-nence. The procedure is short, and results are effective for a majority of patients. Pelvic surgery with ure-thropexy and/or a colpopexy is used in patients with significant pelvic organ prolapse.

19.4.4.3 Sample Calculation

The populations most studied for incontinence are females 65 and older, and therefore these statistics will be used to illustrate this model (Fig. 19.9). It is esti-mated that there will be about 30 million women 65 years or older in the year 2020.[13] Using the defini-tion of "SEVERE INCONTINENCE," daily leakage of urine "most or all of the time" approximately 10% of women 65 or older would be surgical candidates.[20] This amounts to about 3 million women.

Only a proportion of these women would likely undergo surgery. Looking at reported Medicare data,[20]

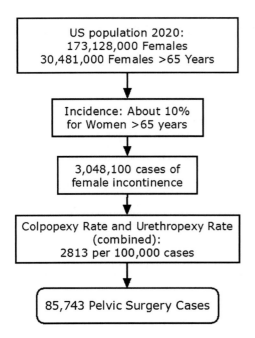

Predicting Female Pelvic Surgeries for Incontinence in 2020

US population 2020:
173,128,000 Females
30,481,000 Females >65 Years

↓

Incidence: About 10%
for Women >65 years

↓

3,048,100 cases of
female incontinence

↓

Colpopexy Rate and Urethropexy Rate
(combined):
2813 per 100,000 cases

↓

85,743 Pelvic Surgery Cases

Fig. 19.9 Adapted model for predicting female pelvic surgeries for incontinence in year 2020. The numbers used were obtained from multiple sources, and references can be found in the text

about 2,813 per 100,000 diagnoses of incontinence undergo urethropexy and/or colpopexy.

This calculation results in over 85,000 potential robotic pelvic operations for incontinence. This is likely an underestimation of likely total cases. The nature of the disease, variable age range, and clin-ical definition of incontinence introduce uncertainty. Furthermore, as the procedure becomes more accepted and more widely available, there may be an influx of patients seeking surgical treatment with the robot.

19.4.4.4 Variables

The screening for urinary incontinence is currently not a routine practice and is dependent on patients request for help. If a national screening campaign were to be introduced, the incidence of urinary incontinence would be dramatically increased. Some incontinence risk factors such as obesity and pelvic trauma at child-birth may be preventable and modifiable. Since such a large portion of the population has incontinence, sur-gical treatments are being redefined and the robot will play an increasing role.

19.4.4.5 Summary

The creation of the surgical robot has revolution-ized minimally invasive pelvic surgery. The ability to achieve great visibility and instrument accuracy dur-ing surgery has made procedures like the urethropexy and the colpopexy a less morbid procedure. As incon-tinence treatments are being refined, the use of robot-assisted surgery for traditionally open surgeries will become the norm.

19.5 Conclusion

The presence of the robot is ever increasing. More hos-pitals are offering robot-assisted surgery. More surgical residents are trained to use the robot. We believe that almost all cases that can be done by the robot will be done by the robot. Since the laparoscopic era, over 80–90% of cholecystectomies are done laparoscopically.[21] Achieving similar numbers with the robot is realistic. Moreover there are more surgeries still in the early phases of robot use. As more uses are discovered and current uses established, the robot will be a standard of surgical care.

In this chapter, a method for estimating cases was illustrated. It is a model that is conceptually easy to understand and adaptable to many different diseases and scenarios. Built into the flow diagram are factors to consider that may alter the projection. The estimation method may be simplistic or detailed depending on the desired accuracy.

This model attempts to include as many assumptions as possible to account for diverse clinical situations. No projection model is perfect, but we believe that using this method we can generate reliable and realistic results. The method is applicable for any given population, any given disease, and any given treatment modality.

References

1. Haas GP, Delongchamps NB, Jones RF, et al. Needle biopsies on autopsy prostates: sensitivity of cancer detection based on true prevalence. *J Natl Cancer Inst*. October 3, 2007;99(19):1484–1489.
2. Sakr WA, Grignon DJ, Haas GP, et al. Epidemiology of high grade prostatic intraepithelial neoplasia. *Pathol Res Pract*. September 1995;191(9):838–841.
3. Andriole GL. Overview of pivotal studies for prostate cancer risk reduction, past and present. *Urology*. May 2009;73(5 Suppl):S36–S43.
4. Van den Bergh RC, Roemeling S, Roobol MJ, et al. Outcomes of men with screen-detected prostate cancer eligible for active surveillance who were managed expectantly. *Eur Urol*. January 2009;55(1):1–8. Epub 2008 Sep 17.
5. Schröder FH, Hugosson J, Roobol MJ, et al. ERSPC investigators. Screening and prostate-cancer mortality in a randomized European study. *N Engl J Med*. March 26, 2009;360(13):1320–1328.
6. Andriole GL, Crawford ED, Grubb RL 3rd, et al. PLCO project team. Mortality results from a randomized prostate-cancer screening trial. *N Engl J Med*. March 26, 2009;360(13):1310–1319.
7. Miller DC, Gruber SB, Hollenbeck BK, Montie JE, Wei JT. Incidence of initial local therapy among men with lower-risk prostate cancer in the United States. *J Natl Cancer Inst*. August 16, 2006;98(16):1134–1141.
8. Kawachi MH. Counterpoint: robot-assisted laparoscopic prostatectomy: perhaps the surgical gold standard for prostate cancer care. *J Natl Compr Canc Netw*. August 2007;5(7):689–692.
9. Krambeck AE, DiMarco DS, Rangel LJ, et al. Radical prostatectomy for prostatic adenocarcinoma: a matched comparison of open retropubic and robot-assisted techniques. *BJU Int*. February 2009;103(4):448–453.
10. Drouin SJ, Vaessen C, Hupertan V, et al. Comparison of mid-term carcinologic control obtained after open, laparoscopic, and robot-assisted radical prostatectomy for localized prostate cancer. *World J Urol*. October 2009;27(5):599–605. Epub 2009 May 7.
11. Hakimi AA, Feder M, Ghavamian R. Minimally invasive approaches to prostate cancer: a review of the current literature. *Urol J*. Summer 2007;4(3):130–137.
12. Barry MJ. Screening for prostate cancer – the controversy that refuses to die. *N Engl J Med*. March 26, 2009;360(13):1351–1354.
13. National Population Projections Released 2008. US Census Bureau Population Division Web Site. http://www.census.gov/population/www/projections/summarytables.html. Accessed July 8, 2009.
14. Surveillance, Epidemiology, and End Result (SEER) Program. Cancer Statistics.US National Institutes of Health Web Site. http://seer.cancer.gov/canques/incidents.html. Accessed July 8, 2009
15. Hock LM, Lynch J, Balaji KC. Increasing incidence of all stages of kidney cancer in the last 2 decades in the United States: an analysis of surveillance, epidemiology and end results program data. *J Urol*. January 2002;167(1):57–60.
16. Motzer RJ, Mazumdar M, Bacik J, Berg W, Amsterdam A, Ferrara J. Survival and prognostic stratification of 670 patients with advanced renal cell carcinoma. *J Clin Oncol*. August 1999;17(8):2530–2540.
17. Talamini MA, Chapman S, Horgan S, Melvin WS. Academic robotics group. A prospective analysis of 211 robotic-assisted surgical procedures. *Surg Endosc*. October 2003;17(10):1521–1524.
18. Konety BR, Joyce GF, Wise M. Bladder and upper tract urothelial cancer. *J Urol*. May 2007;177(5):1636–1645.
19. Thom D. Variation in estimates of urinary incontinence prevalence in the community: effects of differences in definition, population characteristics, and study type. *J Am Geriatr Soc*. April 1998;46(4):473–480.
20. Thom DH, Nygaard IE, Calhoun EA. Urologic diseases in America project: urinary incontinence in women-national trends in hospitalizations, office visits, treatment and economic impact. *J Urol*. April 2005;173(4):1295–1301.
21. McAneny D. Open cholecystectomy. *Surg Clin North Am*. December 2008;88(6):1273–1294, ix.

Part III
The Prostate

Chapter 20

Development of the Vattikuti Institute Prostatectomy: Historical Perspective and Technical Nuances

Piyush K. Agarwal, Sanjeev A. Kaul, and Mani Menon

Time Line for Radical Prostatectomy.

1867	Bilroth attempts perineal prostatectomy
1891	Goodfellow attempts transurethral perineal prostatectomy
1901	Proust performs radical perineal prostatectomy
1904–1905	Young performs radical perineal prostatectomy
1947	Millin performs radical retropubic prostatectomy
1983	Walsh performs "nerve-sparing" radical prostatectomy, based on Donker's anatomical dissections
1991	Schuessler and colleagues perform first laparoscopic radical prostatectomy
1997–1998	Guillonneau and Vallancien describe the "Montsouris" technique
2000	Binder and Kramer, Abbou, Rassweiler, and Vallancien perform "robotic" prostatectomy
2000–2001	Menon establishes first robotic urology program in the world, describes the VIP technique of robotic prostatectomy
2003–2010	Modifications of VIP including extended nerve sparing (2003), avoidance of Foley catheter (2008), primary hypogastric node dissection (2008), anastomosis with barbed wound closure device (2010)
May 2010	Over 300,000 robotic radical prostatectomies done worldwide

P.K. Agarwal (✉)
Vattikuti Urology Institute, Henry Ford Hospital, Detroit, MI, USA
e-mail: pagarwal1@hfhs.org

20.1 Introduction

This chapter will describe the evolution of the robotic radical and will highlight key publications and steps in that process that took place at the Vattikuti Urology Institute at the Henry Ford Hospital in Detroit, Michigan.

20.2 Historical Perspective (See Timeline)

Radical prostatectomy was a morbid procedure marred by blood loss, poor visualization, impotence, and high rates of incontinence. Perineal prostatectomy improved upon an abdominal approach, but did not allow for sampling of lymph nodes and potency was still difficult to reliably establish. In 1982, however, Walsh and Donker described the anatomic retropubic approach.

Since then, open radical retropubic prostatectomy has been the standard of care for prostate cancer.[1] However, the beauty of modern medicine is the constant drive for improvements and refinements to well-established techniques and dogma. It is unclear where minimally invasive, specifically laparoscopic prostatectomy was attempted first. To our knowledge, the first publication was from Schuessler and colleagues in the United States. They reported on the initial feasibility and efficacy of laparoscopic-assisted radical prostatectomy.[2] Schuessler demonstrated no advantage over open surgery in terms of tumor removal, continence, potency, length of stay, cosmetic result, and convalescence and suggested that the procedure not be performed.

A.K. Hemal, M. Menon (eds.), *Robotics in Genitourinary Surgery*, 219
DOI 10.1007/978-1-84882-114-9_20, © Springer-Verlag London Limited 2011

In 1997–1998, the brilliant French laparoscopic surgeon, Richard Gaston from Bordeaux was performing a laparoscopic procedure to remove a cyst of the seminal vesicle (personal communication). He had approached the seminal vesicle through the peritoneal cul-de-sac. At the end of the procedure, he found that he had an excellent view of the area of the verumontanum of the prostate. In an "aha" moment, Gaston reasoned that the prostate may be removed with a similar approach. He then embarked on doing just so, but did not present or publish these results. The young French urologist, Bertrand Guillonneau of Paris, heard about these procedures. Encouraged by his visionary chairman, Professor Guy Vallancien, at the Institut Mutualiste Montsouris, Guillonneau visited Gaston at Bordeaux and witnessed the procedure first hand. Guillonneau and Vallancien applied their technical virtuosity to streamlining Gaston's technique. Their approach, the Montsouris technique, rapidly became the gold standard for laparoscopic prostatectomy.[3] Many other surgeons such as Abbou from Paris, Rassweiler from Germany, and Bollens from Belgium started to work independently in the field and published their own modifications of the Guillonneau/Vallancian laparoscopic prostatectomy.

In 1999, Mani Menon obtained philanthropic funding from the Vattikuti Foundation for the specific purpose of developing minimally invasive techniques for radical prostatectomy. In June 2000, Menon traveled to Paris to observe the laparoscopic radical prostatectomy program at Montsouris. Impressed by the results, Menon arranged for a formal collaboration with the French surgeons to visit Detroit for an extended period and help establish a laparoscopic radical prostatectomy program there. By happenstance, Vallancien had leased a da Vinci robot and was determining the feasibility of performing robotic prostatectomy. Although Vallancien was able to complete the operation, he saw no added value for the robot in terms of time, bleeding, or ease of surgery.[4]

Menon was fascinated by the robot. By self-admission, he was a neophyte laparoscopic surgeon. As one with extensive training in open surgery, Menon found standard laparoscopy restricting with its two-dimensional images, counterintuitive movements, rigid instruments, limited degrees of motion,[5] and ergonomic difficulties.[6] Further, he found that even Guillonneau and Vallancien found it difficult to duplicate their Parisian results in the Michigan patients.

The Detroit patients were on average 40 pounds heavier and 4 in. taller than their French counterparts, and that appeared to make a difference. Meanwhile, the da Vinci robot surgical system received Food and Drug Administration (FDA) approval for abdominal surgery in November of 2000. It was leased and integrated into the minimally invasive prostatectomy program in Detroit, and the first robotic prostatectomy was attempted by Vallancien on November 29, 2000, with Menon providing enthusiastic, but, sadly, inexpert assistance.

At the time the da Vinci robot was incorporated into Henry Ford Hospital's structured program, no published reports of its use in radical prostatectomy were available. The first cases were performed by Binder and Kramer, although they did not report it immediately.[7] They performed a minilaparotomy, inserted the robotic ports under direct vision, closed the incision, and proceeded with the prostatectomy. Several small case series were published shortly after. The first "pure" robot-assisted radical prostatectomy was reported by Abbou and colleagues in 2000.[8] Small case series were then reported by Pasticier et al.[4] (five cases) and Rassweiler et al.[9] (six cases). In the United States, the first robot-assisted radical prostatectomy may have been performed at Henrico Hospital in Virginia, although details were never reported. This case was followed in a short period of time by a series of cases performed by Menon at the Henry Ford Hospital.[10] The procedure has evolved over the years to what is now known as the Vattikuti Institute Prostatectomy (VIP) procedure. We chronicle this process.

20.3 Comparison with Open and Laparoscopic Radical Prostatectomy

The Vattikuti Urology Institute's minimally invasive radical prostatectomy program started in October 2000 with laparoscopic radical prostatectomy but quickly moved to a robotic radical prostatectomy program in March 2001. The outcomes of robotic-assisted prostatectomy were compared separately to that of open radical prostatectomy[11] and laparoscopic radical prostatectomy.[10] In general, robotic-assisted prostatectomy was superior to open radical prostatectomy in terms

Table 20.1 Odds ratio for important outcomes for laparoscopic, robotic, and radical prostatectomies performed at the Vattikuti Urology Institute in 2004

Variables	Open radical prostatectomy (reference values)	Laparoscopic radical prostatectomy (odds ratio)	Robotic prostatectomy (odds ratio)
Operating room time	163 min	1.51[a]	0.91[b]
Estimated blood loss	910 mL	0.42[a]	0.10[a]
Positive margins	23%	1	1
Complications	15%	0.67[a]	0.33[a,b]
Catheterization time	15.8 d	0.50[a]	0.44[a]
Hospital stay >24 h	100%	0.35[a]	0.07[a,b]
Postoperative pain score (0–10)	7	0.45[a]	0.45[a]
Median time to continence	160 d	1	0.28[a,b]
Median time to erection	440 d	NA[c]	0.4[a]
Median time to intercourse	>700 d	NA[c]	0.5[a]
Detectable prostate-specific antigen	15%	1	0.5

The reference values were those from conventional radical prostatectomy; odds ratio was the ratio of the observed to the reference value. Abbreviation: NA, not available
[a]$p < 0.05$ compared with radical retropubic prostatectomy
[b]$p < 0.05$ compared with laparoscopic radical prostatectomy
[c]Most patients undergoing laparoscopic radical prostatectomy were not sexually active at baseline

of estimated blood loss, postoperative pain score, hospital stay, and percentage discharged within 24 h. In comparison to laparoscopic radical prostatectomy, no key difference was noted except for less blood loss in the robotic-assisted group. Using open radical prostatectomy at our institution as a standard, we compared the outcomes of laparoscopic prostatectomy and robotic-assisted prostatectomy performed at our institution (Table 20.1). The odds ratios for operating room time, estimated blood loss, complications, catheterization time, hospital stay greater than 24 h, median time to continence, and prostate-specific antigen (PSA) recurrence are lowest for the robotic-assisted group. Laparoscopic radical prostatectomy had lower odds ratios than open surgery for all parameters except for operating room time.

20.4 Outcomes After First 1,100 Cases

By 2004, over 1,100 robotic radical prostatectomies were performed. The operating time (calculated from placement of Veress needle to wound closure) ranged from 70 to 160 min with the actual console (robotic) time being approximately 90–100 min. Blood loss ranged from 50 to 250 mL and no patient required intraoperative blood transfusion. Over 95% of patients were discharged within 24 h. In terms of urinary continence (defined as the use of no pads or liners), an analysis of 200 VIPs through a third-party telephone survey during the initial 400 VIPs performed revealed a 50% return of continence at 44 days compared to 160 days in a cohort of 100 open radical prostatectomies ($p < 0.05$). For erectile function in the same groups of patients, there was a 50% return of erections at a mean of 180 days in the VIP cohort compared to 440 days in the open cohort ($p < 0.05$) although 42 and 65% were using sildenafil at the time of analysis.[11]

20.5 Nerve Preservation

Postoperative impairment of potency has traditionally been one of the complications of radical prostatectomy. Even in the hands of the most skilled of surgeons, postoperative potency overall can range from 13[12] to 86%.[13,14] Erectile function can also vary with the age of the patient, preoperative potency, operative skill of the surgeon, and the stage of the lesion. Although we initially performed nerve preservation in a standard fashion by assuming the neurovascular bundles travel along the dorsolateral aspect of the prostate bilaterally, we learned later with cadaveric dissections and magnified intraoperative photos that the traditional understanding of the pathway of the bundles is overly simplified. Instead, a large pelvic plexus is located over the surface of the rectum with cross-communicating fibers and its important branches are located lateral and posterior to the seminal vesicles.[15] As a result, it is important to avoid electrocautery and traction lateral to the seminal vesicles. In addition, since the space containing the neurovascular bundles is larger near the base of the prostate than it is at the apex, it may be easier to perform nerve sparing in an antegrade fashion as opposed to a retrograde approach.

Although these maneuvers enhanced standard nerve sparing, we continued to search how we could maximize nerve preservation. Subsequent anatomic studies have shown that the branches of the neurovascular plexus travel more anteriorly near the apex.[16,17] In addition, Kiyoshima and colleagues demonstrated that varying amounts of adipose tissue exist between the prostatic fascia and prostatic capsule and that in patients with adipose tissue, distinct neurovascular bundles are not seen and instead a neurovascular

plexus is seen along the anterolateral surface of the prostatic fascia.[18] We postulated that high anterior release of the prostatic fascia off the prostatic capsule would allow preservation of the neurovascular plexus and its anterior branches and, therefore, maximize nerve preservation in comparison to a standard nerve-sparing procedure (Fig. 20.1).

Therefore, we evaluated the feasibility of prostatic fascia nerve sparing relying on the magnification of the robotic da Vinci system to distinguish the prostatic capsule from the prostatic fascia.[19] This new preserved veil of neurovascular tissue was termed the "veil of Aphrodite" out of deference to the Greek Goddess of Love. In our early studies, we performed this nerve-sparing procedure in 15 patients undergoing robotic cystectomy for bladder cancer where inadvertent entry into the prostatic capsule would be of no ill consequence and then in 6 impotent men with low D'Amico risk prostate cancer undergoing VIP procedure. We

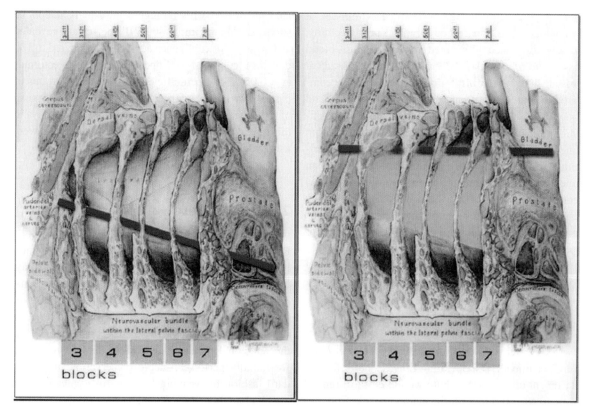

A   B

Fig. 20.1 **a** Plane of dissection for standard nerve sparing. **b** Plane of dissection for "veil of Aphrodite." *Yellow area* depicts prostatic fascia, which is preserved

determined that the technique was feasible and onco-logically safe with no positive margins seen in the region of the veil.

20.6 Outcomes with the "Veil of Aphrodite" Nerve-Sparing Technique

After our initial feasibility study, we prospectively compared potency outcomes in 35 men undergoing bilateral prostatic fascia nerve sparing with 23 men undergoing standard bilateral nerve sparing in patients with localized prostate cancer and normal baseline erectile function (defined as Sexual Health Inventory for Men [SHIM] score greater than 21 without use of medications). All patients were encouraged to use phosphodiesterase-5 inhibitors (PDE5-I) within 4 weeks of surgery. At 12 months, 74% (17 of 23) of the standard nerve-sparing group and 97% (34 of 35) of the prostatic fascia-sparing group achieved erections firm enough for intercourse ($p = 0.002$). Normal erections, defined as SHIM >21, were lower in both groups with 26% (6 of 23) in the standard group and 86% (30 of 35) in the prostatic fascia-sparing group ($p < 0.0001$) with or without the use of phosphodiesterase-5 inhibitors (PDE5-I). Restricting this latter analysis to patients with normal erections without the use of PDE5-I found that 17% (4 of 23) of the standard patients and 51% (18 of 35) of the prostatic fascia-sparing patients had normal erections ($p < 0.0001$) (Fig. 20.2).[20]

In 2007, after performing more than 2,600 procedures, approximately 42% of patients underwent standard nerve sparing, 25% of patients underwent unilateral "veil" nerve sparing, and 33% of patients underwent bilateral "veil" nerve sparing. In patients with no preoperative erectile dysfunction, defined by SHIM >21, successful intercourse was reported in 70% of patients at 12 months and 100% of patients at 48 months in those undergoing bilateral "veil" nerve-sparing surgery. However, only half of these patients were able to do so without medication.[21] Stratified by preoperative erectile dysfunction as none, mild, and moderate, postoperative return to baseline erectile function and to intercourse was better in the patients undergoing a "veil" nerve-sparing procedure compared to patients undergoing a standard nerve-sparing procedure (Fig. 20.3).

20.7 Progression to the "Super Veil" Nerve-Sparing Technique

The "veil of Aphrodite" or prostate fascia-sparing technique has also been adopted by open surgeons and termed "interfascial dissection"[22] or "high anterior release."[23] Encouraged by our early results and the acceptance of our technique by other robotic and non-robotic prostate cancer surgeons, we sought to see if we could improve upon the "veil" nerve-sparing technique. Although we preserve the tissue lateral to

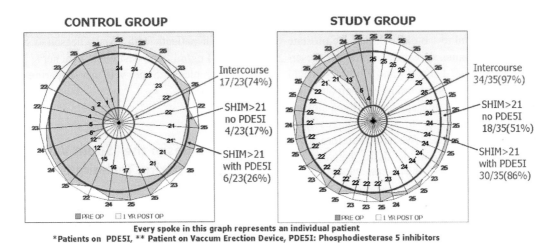

Fig. 20.2 Radar graph shows preoperative and postoperative SHIM scores in each patient (spokes) and ability of procedure to preserve sexual function. Extent of *blue areas* correlates with postoperative loss of potency

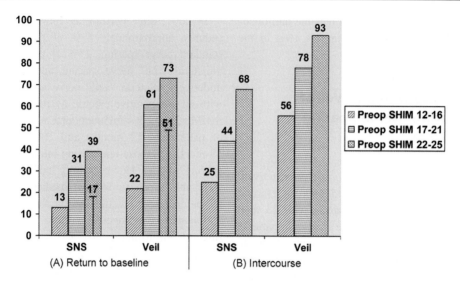

Fig. 20.3 Postoperative return of potency in patients with various levels of preoperative erectile dysfunction (The *line* inside the *bars* represents the percentage of patients not receiving postoperative phosphodiesterase-5 inhibitors)

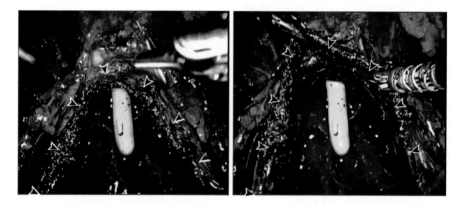

Fig. 20.4 Tissue preserved during "Super veil" nerve-sparing technique. *Arrowheads* correspond to preserved "Super veil" and "veil" tissues

11 o'clock and lateral to 1 o'clock during the prostate fascia-sparing technique, we wondered whether preservation of the tissue medial to 11 and 1 o'clock would enhance erectile function. A study has demonstrated that up to 21–28% of prostate nerve tissue lies on its anterior surface with up to 10% of nerves lying between 11 and 1 o'clock.[24] We have therefore advocated additional sparing of the tissue between the 11 and 1 o'clock regions during the "veil" procedure called the "Super veil" procedure. The "Super veil" procedure is more difficult than the "veil" procedure as the tissue on the anterior surface of the prostate is more fibromuscular than the lateral prostatic fascia and so precise separation from the prostatic capsule is challenging. Therefore, this procedure is only

performed in patients with focal Gleason 6 disease with PSA <4 ng/mL who desire maximal nerve preservation. A completed "Super veil" nerve sparing can be seen in Fig. 20.4.[25]

20.8 Outcomes of the "Super Veil" Nerve-Sparing Technique

We analyzed 171 consecutive patients that underwent the "Super veil" nerve-sparing technique who had preoperative SHIM scores >17, focal Gleason 6 adenocarcinoma of the prostate, and serum PSA <4 ng/mL.[25] We asked them to complete a postoperative SHIM

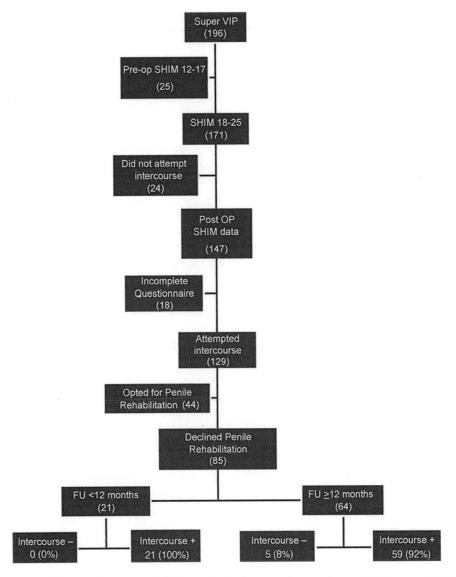

Fig. 20.5 Flowchart for "Super veil" patients. SHIM, sexual health inventory for men; Super VIP, "Super veil" Vattikuti Institute Prostatectomy; Pre-op, preoperative; Post OP, postoperative; FU, follow-up

questionnaire. We excluded 86 patients: 24 (14%) that did not attempt intercourse, 18 (11%) that failed to return questionnaires, and 44 (26%) that opted for immediate penile rehabilitation (using intracavernosal injection therapy or vacuum erection device) (Fig. 20.5). The remaining 85 patients attempted sexual intercourse of which 74 had used PDE5-I and 13 were current users. At a median follow-up of 18 months, 94% (80 of 85) of these patients had erections firm enough for penetration with a median SHIM score

of 18. The oncologic outcomes were sound for this procedure as only one patient had a positive margin with final pathology demonstrating a Gleason 7, pT3a adenocarcinoma of the prostate. To date, no patient has had a biochemical recurrence (Table 20.2).

In summary, we have progressed from standard nerve sparing to "veil" nerve sparing and now to "Super veil" nerve sparing. Although a rigorous comparison between "veil" and "Super veil" nerve sparing has not been performed, a comparison of consecutive

Table 20.2 Postoperative sexual health inventory for men (SHIM) scores in 85 men undergoing "Super veil" nerve sparing

No. of patients	214	85		
No. able to penetrate (%)	209 (98%)	80 (94%) median follow-up, weeks	156	78
Preoperative SHIM score, median	25	25		
Postoperative SHIM score, median	19	18		

SHIM, sexual health inventory for men

cases demonstrates that return of erectile function is similar with both procedures but tends to occur earlier in the "Super veil" group. However, the "Super veil" nerve-sparing technique is only performed in patients with minimal and low-risk disease. The type of nerve sparing performed in a patient is tailored to their biopsy results and therefore we perform all nerve-sparing techniques as well as wide resections when appropriate.

20.9 Optimization of Urinary Continence Through Precise Apical Dissection

The magnification of the apex afforded by the robotic procedure allows precise dissection. The technique is described in detail below but we routinely spare the puboprostatic ligaments. In addition, the dorsal venous complex is carely exposed. In our initial experience, it was routinely ligated. But it often compromised dissection near the apex and we have found that transecting it expeditiously with cautery can control bleeding and allow for more precise visualization of the apex. It can be subsequently ligated after the urethra and apex are exposed. The urethra is then divided distal to the prosatic apex with the use of articulated scissors. An important detail is leaving the periurethral connective tissue untouched during apical dissection. We do *not* pass the Maryland forceps behind the urethroprostatic junction. While this does help in identifying the junction, it also may disrupt the supporting tissues. In any event, the time to return of continence is greatly improved by avoiding extra dissection.

20.10 Anastomosis Using a Barbed Wound Closure Device: the Knotless Anastomosis

We initially only performed a single running anastomosis as a modification of the technique described by van Velthoven and colleagues.[26] Although traditionally the anastomosis has been commonly performed using a monofilament suture (3-0 polyglecaprone on a RB-1 needle), the monofilament suture has a tendency to slip, leading the surgeon to retighten the anastomosis with every throw and revisit each throw several times throughout the anastomosis to assure integrity. Assistants have been used to hold the suture in place between throws but this requires experienced assistants performing delicate retraction. Hem-o-lok and Lapra-Ty clips have been used to secure the posterior layer of the anastomosis; however, these are associated with erosion into the bladder and subsequent bladder neck contractures (Blumenthal et al.[27]), irritative voiding symptoms (Tunnard and Biyani[28]), and stone formation (Tugcu et al.[29]).

The V-Loc barbed wound closure device suture (Covidien, Mansfield, MA) is a unidirectional, self-anchoring barbed suture composed of absorbable copolymer of glycolic acid and trimethylene carbonate (polyglyconate) (Fig. 20.6). It received FDA approval for soft tissue approximation in January 2010. Almost immediately, we initiated a prospective study to evaluate the feasibility and safety of the barbed wound closure device for urethrovesical anastomosis in VIP (Kaul et al.[30]). The approach we used is a slight modification of the van Velthoven approach. We used a 3-0 polyglyconate wound closure device fashioned into a double-armed stitch (Fig. 20.7) rather than a conventional monofilament suture. The anastomosis itself proceeds similarly to the van Velthoven technique (Figs. 20.8, 20.9, and 20.10). Conventional monofilament suture and technique is shown in Fig. 20.11.

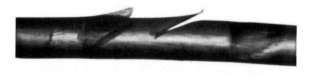

© Copyright 2008 Angiotech Pharmaceuticals, Inc.

Fig. 20.6 Magnified view of self-anchoring barbed suture

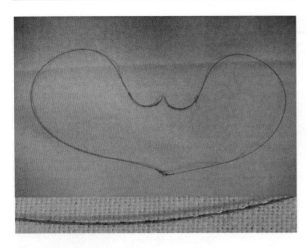

Fig. 20.7 Double armed self-anchoring barbed suture

We pass the needle of each wound closure device (suture) through the loop of a second device extracorporeally to make a single, double-armed suture with roughly 6 in. of suture on each side of the knot, for a total of 10–11″ of barbs. The left-side end is used first to approximate the posterior plate of the anastomosis with three throws in the bladder (outside-in) and two throws in the urethra (inside-out) starting roughly at the 3 or 4 o'clock position and proceeding clockwise. In the past, assistants maintained tension on the suture with each throw by "following" the console surgeon; however, since the barbs lock into the tissues with each throw, no assistance or "following" is required. The

suture is continued clockwise until about the 9 o'clock position where the suture is now passed back outside the bladder (inside-out) with a Connell stitch. Now the suture is run to the 12 o'clock position outside-in on the urethra and inside-out on the bladder. The right-side needle is now used from the 4 o'clock position outside-in on the urethra and inside-out on the bladder and the suture is run in a counterclockwise fashion until the right-sided suture is reached at 12 o'clock. With each throw, the suture is cinched tight by the console surgeon. The barbs hold the suture in place, essentially "locking" each throw. The two unidirectional barb sutures prevent slippage, obviate the need for "following" by the assistant, and minimize revisiting of the throws by the surgeon to confirm that the anastomosis has not loosened. Upon completion of the anastomosis, the needles are cut without the need for tying a knot.

As of May 2010, 128 patients have undergone anastomosis using the barbed wound closure device. All anastomoses were completed by the console surgeon independently, without any assistance whatsoever from the patient-side assistant. Specifically, the assistant or surgeon did not provide traction on the suture during anastomosis. The median time for anastomosis was 11 min (IQR, 9–15) including the time for bladder neck reconstruction, with 45% performed in less than 10 min. Median time for posterior reconstruction was 4 min (IQR, 3–6). At a mean follow-up of 4 months no patients had intraoperative or cystogram detected

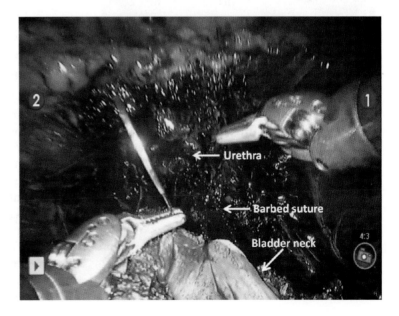

Fig. 20.8 Posterior anastomosis using the double-armed self-anchoring barbed suture

Fig. 20.9 Anterior anastomosis using the double-armed self-anchoring barbed suture

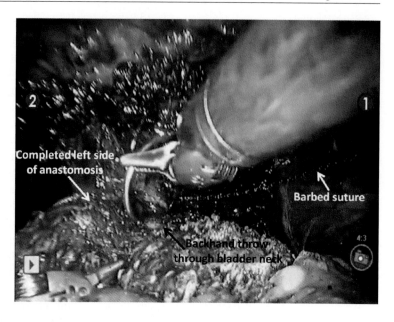

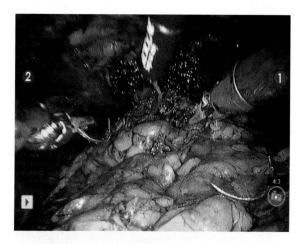

Fig. 20.10 Completed anastomosis using the double-armed self-anchoring barbed suture with cutting of the needles. Note that the anastomosis does not need to be tied

is instilled to check for leakage. In the absence of leakage, the balloon is inflated to 30 mL. In the initial 1,100 cases, a drain was routinely placed but now is rarely placed. Recently, a number of patients have undergone the VIP procedure with placement of a percutaneous suprapubic tube (PST) which will be described later. Although a Foley catheter is also placed in the urethra, it is removed the subsequent day prior to discharge.

20.11 Initial Outcomes with Single-Layer Running Urethrovesical Anastomosis

urinary leaks and there were no episodes of urinary retention after removal of catheter or urethral strictures. Mean duration of catheterization was 7.1 days. Table 20.3 depicts a comparative analysis of perioperative outcomes in patients undergoing anastomosis with monofilament and barbed suture, respectively (Kaul 2010).

We have recently performed a double-layer running anastomosis that will be described below. A new Foley catheter is inserted and approximately 250 mL

We initially reported an analysis on 120 consecutive patients performed by a single surgeon in 2004. The mean (range) time for completion of the anastomosis was 13 (5–34) min. All patients underwent a cystogram at 4 days and if no leak was noted, the catheter was removed. A mild leak was seen in 24 patients who had to wait 7 days to have their catheters removed. Urinary retention requiring recatheterization only occurred in two patients. An analysis at 3 months consisting of a self-reported mailed questionnaire revealed that 96% used no liners/pads and the remaining 4% used a single

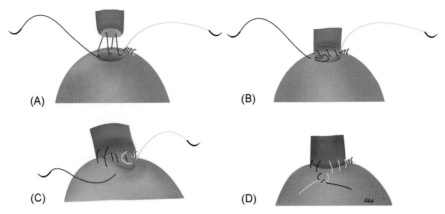

Fig. 20.11 Urethrovesical anastomosis. **a** Posterior wall with anti-clockwise dyed monocryl arm of suture. **b** Change of direction of needle passage at transition of anterior and posterior walls. **c** Clockwise stitches with undyed monocryl arm of suture. **d** Completion of anastomosis

Table 20.3 Comparison of perioperative outcomes in the two groups

Characteristic	Monofilament suture group ($n = 36$)	Barbed suture group ($n = 36$)	p value
Operative characteristic			
Operative time, min (SD)	166.5 (37.4)	146.5 (32.8)	0.146
Console time, min (SD)	130.0 (35.6)	118.7 (32.4)	0.135
Dual layer anastomosis time, min (SD)	*21.8 (6.5)*	*15.9 (5.1)*	*0.003*
Bladder neck reconstruction, n (%)	*1 (2.8)*	*7 (20.0)*	*0.001*
Estimated blood loss, mL (SD)	149.3 (55.9)	139.7 (82.8)	0.280
Duration of catherization, days (SD)	7.25 (1.5)	7.21 (1.0)	1.000
Adverse events			
Cystogram leak[a], n (%)	1 (2.8)	0 (0.0)	1.000
Anastomotic leak[b], n (%)	3 (8.3)	0 (0.0)	0.330
Urethral tear[c], n (%)	0 (0.0)	1 (2.8)	0.357
Urinary retention, n (%)	0 (0.0)	0 (0.0)	1.000
Anastomotic stricture, n (%)	0 (0.0)	0 (0.0)	1.000

SD, standard deviation; UVA, urethrovesical anastomosis
[a]Grade I (minor extraperitoneal) leak. Catheter removed on postoperative day 10
[b]Two patients required additional figure of 8 stitch. Cystogram showed on contrast extravasation
[c]Anastomosis completed with same suture. UVA watertight intraoperatively and on cystogram

security liner.[31] An updated analysis published in 2007 after performing greater than 2,600 robotic prostatectomies revealed that early urinary continence (defined stringently as 0 pads/24 h) was 25% at 1 day, 50% at 4 weeks, and 90% at 3 months. Total urinary continence was achieved in 84% after 12 months. Although 16% did not achieve total continence, 8% only used a liner for security. True incontinence was seen in 3.2% using 1 pad/day, 4% using 2–3 pads/day, and total incontinence in 0.8% (Table 20.4).[21]

Table 20.4 Rates of incontinence after 2,600 robotic prostatectomies

Return of continence in 12 months	%
No urinary leak (total control)	84
Liner for security (stress incontinence about	8
1 pad/day (occasional stress incontinence)	3.2
2–3 pads/day (frequent stress incontinence)	4
Total incontinence	0.8

20.12 Double-Layer Urethrovesical Anastomosis

Some reports have suggested that posterior and anterior reconstruction may improve early continence after catheter removal. Rocco and colleagues have described rapid return of urinary continence (0–1 pads in a 24 h period) within 30 days (83.8% vs. 32.3%) of laparoscopic radical prostatectomy modified by reconstruction of the posterior rhabdosphincter compared to patients without reconstruction.[32] Tewari and associates have described improvements in urinary continence by adding lateral and anterior reconstruction to preserve the puboprostatic collar. They have demonstrated continence of 29% at 1 week, 62% at 6 weeks, and 88% at 12 weeks.[33] Encouraged by these results, we incorporated posterior and anterior reconstruction suggested by the above groups into a double-layer anastomosis technique (described below) and in a pilot study, we observed encouraging initial results with early continence of 69% at 1 day, 77% at 7 days, and 83% at 30 days.[34]

The double-layer anastomosis technique requires two separate 3-0 double-armed monofilament sutures. The first suture is passed through the posterior rhabdosphincter and the posterior layer of Denonvilliers' fascia from the 5 o'clock position to the 8 o'clock position to begin the external layer and then set aside. The urethrovesical anastomosis or internal layer is now performed using a separate, second suture as the standard single-layer urethrovesical anastomosis. After completion of the urethrovesical anastomosis, we resume the external layer by completing the lateral and anterior reconstruction by approximating the puboprostatic ligaments to the midline bladder tissue and anterior pubovesical collar (Fig. 20.12).

20.13 Outcomes of the Double-Layer Urethrovesical Anastomosis

Although we were pleased with the results of the pilot study, we sought to determine the difference in early continence between the two techniques in a randomized controlled trial. Patients were randomized to a single-layer (35 patients) or a double-layer

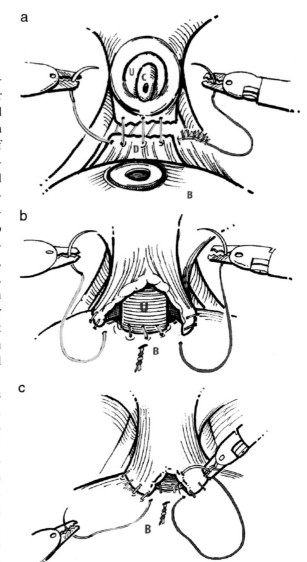

Fig. 20.12 Surgical technique. **a** Posterior external layer approximating Denonvilliers' fascia and posterior rhabdosphincter. Following reconstruction between 5 and 8 o'clock positions formal urethrovesical anastomosis (or internal layer) is begun. **b** After completion of urethrovesical anastomosis lateral aspects of external layer are completed in stepwise fashion from 8 to 11 o'clock position on *left side* and from 5 to 1 o'clock position on *right side*. **c** Anterior pubovesical collar reconstruction is completed approximating puboprostatic ligaments to midline anterior bladder tissue. *B*, bladder; *U*, urethra; *C*, Foley catheter; *D*, Denonvilliers' fascia

(43 patients) technique and patients and data collectors were blinded to technique. Early continence was defined as the proportion of patients using 0–1 pads in a 24-h period and was assessed at 1, 2, 7, and 31

days after catheter removal. At these time points, continence was 20 and 21%, 26 and 26%, 34 and 35%, and 63 and 77% for single layer and double layer, respectively. These differences were not statistically significant. Analysis with a more stringent definition of continence (0 urinary pads/24 h) and mean and median urinary loss also resulted in no statistically significant differences between the techniques.[34]

We confirmed the same excellent early continence rates as described by Rocco et al. and Tewari et al. However, we achieved similar results without reconstruction. Longer follow-up at 12 months continues to show no difference between the two groups (91 and 91% continence, respectively). We did note, however, a decreased incidence of cystographic leaks with the double-layer technique as compared to the single-layer technique (3.4% vs. 8.8%, $p < 0.05$). We postulate that it allows for better hemostasis behind the bladder, thereby potentially reducing the incidence of pelvic hematomas and subsequent cystographic leaks. This allows catheter-less VIP (described below).

20.14 Percutaneous Suprapubic Tube (PST) Drainage

Most patients after radical prostatectomy complain about catheter discomfort. One study showed that 19% of patients had moderate bother from the incision but 46% of patients had severe bother from the urethral catheter after radical retropubic prostatectomy.[35] Tewari et al. have successfully used a modified suprapubic tube with an extension that stents the urethrovesical anastomosis in 10 patients and found a decrease in penile pain but not in bladder spasms after robotic prostatectomy.[36] We investigated the feasibility and early results of a standard PST without a urethral catheter beyond 24 h after VIP.[37]

In 2008, we offered PST drainage to patients with waist circumference <45 in. After completion of the urethrovesical anastomosis, its integrity is checked with intravesical instillation of 250 mL of sterile saline. Under robotic visualization, a 14 Fr PST is placed through the anterior abdominal wall and held above the bladder. The bedside assistant places a 2-0 nonabsorbable polypropylene suture on a straight needle

through the skin adjacent to the PST which is grasped by the console surgeon. The suture is passed through the full thickness of the bladder wall with a horizontal mattress suture and then advanced back through the anterior abdominal wall. The PST is then advanced into the bladder wall through the limbs of the horizontal mattress suture as they are pulled up by the bedside assistant to maintain tension on the anterior bladder wall (Fig. 20.13). Upon extraction of the specimen and release of pneumoperitoneum, the external suture is tied to the skin over a sterile plastic button to cinch the bladder to the anterior abdominal wall (Fig. 20.14).

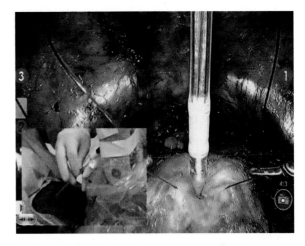

Fig. 20.13 Placement of percutaneous suprapubic tube. *Inset:* simultaneous view from outside the patient

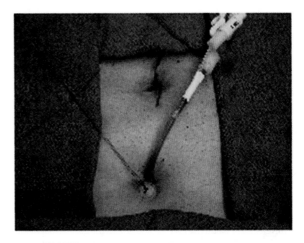

Fig. 20.14 Final external appearance of percutaneous suprapubic tube

20.15 Outcomes of Percutaneous Suprapubic Tube (PST) Drainage

The PST was drained to gravity until postoperative day 5 when it was clamped and patients were encouraged to void per urethra, measuring any postvoid residuals.[37] After 48 h of voiding with residuals less than 30 mL, the PST was removed. We assessed catheter discomfort in the initial 202 patients undergoing this procedure using a visual analog scale (0 = no discomfort and 10 = agonizing discomfort) on postoperative days 2 and 6. This was compared to scores from a control group (50 patients) that underwent similar VIP procedure but with a urethral catheter. The median score went from 4 (interquartile range (IQR): 2–5) on postoperative day 2 to 2 (IQR: 1–3) on postoperative day 6 in patients with urethral catheters. Four patients (8%) required anticholinergic medication for bladder pain and median duration of catheterization was 7 days. Three patients (6%) required recatheterization because of retention. For patients with PST, the median score went from 2 (IQR: 1–3) on postoperative day 2 to 0 (IQR: 0–1) on postoperative day 6. This was statistically significant when compared to patients with a urethral catheter ($p < 0.001$) (Fig. 20.15). One patient (0.5%) required anticholinergic medication and median duration of catheterization was 7.6 days. Five patients (2.5%) required urethral catheterization for retention after PST was removed. At 90 days, continence defined as 0 pad/24 h and 0–1 pads/24 h was 64 and 82% for urethral catheter patients and 67 and 90% for PST patients, respectively ($p > 0.2$ for all time points).[37] At a mean follow-up of 9 months, one patient had a urethral dilation, one patient required urethrotomy, and two patients had urinary tract infections.[25]

20.16 Isolated Internal Iliac Node Dissection for Low-Risk Prostate Cancer

Although most surgeons, including us, would agree to perform a complete and extended node dissection consisting of external iliac, obturator, and internal iliac regions for high-risk aggressive prostate cancer, many debate the type of dissection to perform in low-risk prostate cancer. Some surgeons advocate omitting the dissection entirely[38] or performing a limited dissection of the external iliac region.[39] However, when nodes are positive, they usually localize to the internal iliac lymph nodes. Schumacher and colleagues demonstrated that 70% of all lymph node-positive patients had positive internal iliac lymph nodes either alone (21%) or in combination with other positive lymph nodes (49%). Conversely, lymph node-positive disease localized only to the external iliac lymph nodes and obturator fossa occurred in only 4% of the patients.[40]

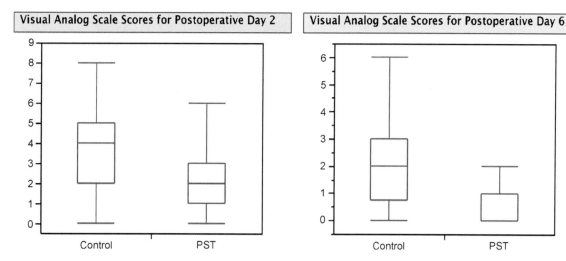

Fig. 20.15 Catheter discomfort assessed by visual analog scale scores

This is consistent with pre-PSA reports localizing positive lymph nodes to the internal iliac lymph nodes in up to two-thirds of patients.[41] We asked ourselves why perform a limited external iliac node dissection instead of an internal iliac node dissection in low-risk disease? Because it is easier?

We modified our node dissection for 90 patients with low-risk prostate cancer defined as primary Gleason score of 3 on biopsy (3+3 or 3+4), T1c, PSA < 10 ng/mL, and 0–1% predicted probability of nodal metastasis (based on 2007 Partin Tables[42]). In these patients, a limited internal iliac node dissection was performed (described as a zone 2 nodal dissection by Mattei et al.[43]). The technique is described in detail elsewhere[25] but after dropping the bladder, the superior vesical artery is traced back to the internal iliac artery. Dissection proceeds distal to the superior vesical artery which protects the ureter which lies beneath the artery. The tissue below the obturator nerve and along the lateral pelvic wall is dissected to clear the obturator fossa and then tissue from the fossa to the lateral surface of the bladder is also removed. A completed node dissection exposes several vessels (Fig. 20.16).

20.17 Outcomes for Isolated Internal Iliac Node Dissection for Low-Risk Prostate Cancer

We compared 1,006 patients that underwent a limited zone 1 dissection (external iliac and obturator regions), 90 patients that underwent a limited zone 2 dissection (internal iliac) as described above, and 55 patients that underwent an extended zone 1 and 2 node dissection (all three regions). The number of nodes retrieved on average was 6.4, 5.5, and 12.3, respectively (see Table 20.5). The total number of patients with positive nodes retrieved among all patients was 5 (0.5%) in zone 1, 6 (6.7%) in zone 2, and 6 (10.9%) in zones 1 and 2. However, five of six patients undergoing zones 1 and 2 dissection with positive nodes had positive nodes only in the internal iliac region. Also, the observed probability of nodal metastasis was higher in patients with a zone 2 dissection than would be expected, suggesting that dissection in this zone has a greater positive nodal yield. When comparing patients that underwent a zone 2 dissection only with patients that underwent a zone 1 dissection only, the incidence

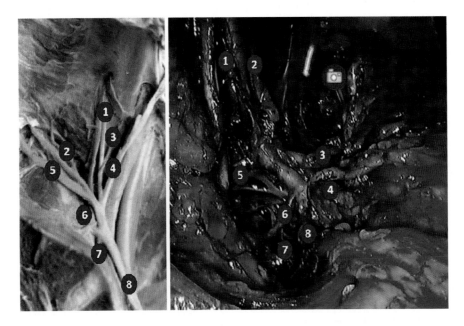

Fig. 20.16 Completed internal iliac/obturator lymphadenectomy on the *left side* compared with cadaveric dissection: (*1*) obturator artery; (*2*) internal pudendal artery; (*3*) inferior vesical artery; (*4*) superior vesical artery; (*5*) inferior gluteal artery; (*6*) superior gluteal artery; (*7*) lateral sacral artery; (*8*) internal iliac artery

Table 20.5 Lymph node metastases by type of lymph node dissection

	Zone 1 (external iliac/obturator) (extended)	Zone 2 (internal iliac)	Zones 1 and 2
No. of patients	1,006	90	55
Preoperative PSA level, ng/dL (SD)	6.1 (2.9)	5.1 (1.8)	7.4
(4.3) biopsy Gleason score (SD)	6.6 (0.8)	6.2 (0.9)	7.5
(0.8) cT1, no. (%)	755 (75%)	90 (100%)	41
(25%) No. of nodes removed	6.4	5.5	12.3
Positive lymph nodes, no. (%)	5 (0.5%)	6 (6.7%)	6
(10.9%) Partin 2007 prediction	0–1%	N/A	4–11%

cT1, Clinical T1 stage; PSA, prostate-specific antigen

of positive nodes was 13.7 times higher (6.7% vs. 0.5%). A caveat is that the average PSA and Gleason score was lower in the zone 2 group compared to the zone 1 group (5.1 vs. 6.1 ng/mL and 6.2 vs. 6.6 ng/mL, respectively). Although addition of zone 1 to the zone 2 dissection would increase the yield of positive nodes in 0.5% patients, we think that the marginal yield does not justify an extended dissection in patients with low-risk disease. However, if node dissection is to be performed, according to our data, positive nodal yield is best in a zone 2 template of dissection.

20.18 Biochemical Recurrence and Oncologic Outcomes

We have performed two large analyses of our oncologic outcomes after the VIP procedure. In one analysis, we looked at 1,142 patients with a minimum follow-up of 12 months (range: 12–66 months) who were seen on follow-up at our institution. With median follow-up of 36 months, 26 patients (2.3%) had a biochemical recurrence with predicted 5-year biochemical

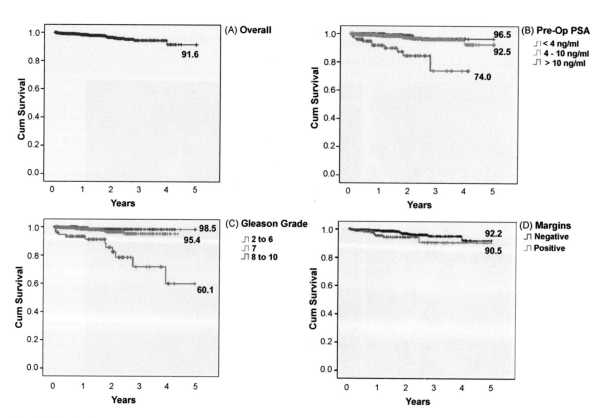

Fig. 20.17 Biochemical recurrence-free survival in 1,142 patients

recurrence rate of 8.4%. This result is further stratified by preoperative PSA, Gleason grade, and margin status (Fig. 20.17).[21] On multivariate analysis, only preoperative PSA and pathologic Gleason score were independent predictors of biochemical recurrence. Biopsy Gleason score, tumor volume, and margin status were not predictive. Biochemical recurrence correlated well with pathologic Gleason score with 5-year rates of 1.5% for Gleason 6, 4.6% for Gleason 7, and 39.9% for Gleason 8 and 9 disease.

A subsequent analysis looked at 2,766 consecutive patients with median follow-up of 22 months (mean follow-up of 25.8 months).[44] Table 20.6 summarizes preoperative and postoperative data for the patients. Overall, 22% of patients had palpable disease and 42.4% of patients had a Gleason score ≥ 7. Ninety-five patients (7.3%) had a biochemical recurrence and 5-year actuarial biochemical recurrence-free survival (BRFS) rate was 84%. These rates were 84.2% for organ-confined disease and 66.3% for extracapsular extension. The BRFS rates based on pathologic Gleason grade were 87.5% for Gleason 6, 79.7% for Gleason 7, and 52.8% for Gleason 8–10. On multivariate analysis, only preoperative PSA, pathologic Gleason score, and pathologic stage were independent predictors of biochemical recurrence. Adjuvant therapy consisting of radiation and/or hormonal therapy was given in 33 patients (2.5% of the cohort).[44]

20.19 Effect of the Learning Curve

In 2007, we directly compared the effect of the learning curve after 2,766 cases by comparing the outcomes of the first 200 cases with the outcomes of the last 200 cases (Table 20.7).[44] It can be seen that with increased experience, patients with more aggressive disease were operated on based on higher preoperative Gleason biopsy scores and postoperative pathologic stages and pathologic Gleason scores in the last 200 patients when compared to the initial 200 patients. Other significant differences are that more patients with prior abdominal surgery (45% vs. 20%, $p < 0.05$) underwent VIP, and mean console times improved (97 vs. 121 min,

Table 20.6 Preoperative, perioperative, and pathologic parameters in 2,766 robotic prostatectomies

Parameters	Overall (three surgeons)
Mean age (range), years	60.2 (39–80)
Mean PSA (range), ng/mL	6.43 (0.1–77.2)
<2.5	152 (6.8)
2.5–4	294 (13.3)
4.1–10	1,527 (69.2)
>10	236 (10.7)
No. in each clinical stage (%)	
T1a	4 (0.3)
T1b	0 (0)
T1c	1,713 (77.3)
T2a	407 (18.4)
T2b	80 (3.6)
T3	6 (0.4)
No. of each biopsy Gleason score (%)	
5	7 (0.3)
6	1,263 (57.2)
7	768 (34.7)
8	131 (5.9)
9–10	41 (1.8)
No. in each D'Amico risk group (%)	
Low	1,492 (69.1)
Intermediate	491 (22.7)
High	177
Mean BMI (range), kg/m^2	27.6 (19–44)
No. with prior abdominal surgery (%)	637 (30.1)
Surgical time, min	
Mean (range)	154 (71–387)
Median	148
Console time, min	
Mean (range)	116 (45–331)
Median	111
Estimated blood loss	
Mean (range)	142 (10–1,350)
Median	100
No. of postoperative blood transfusions	41 (1.5)
Mean no. of units transfused (range)	2.6 (2–8)
No. in each pathologic stage (%)	
T2a	344 (15.5)
T2b	879 (39.8)
T2c	497 (22.4)
T3a	372 (16.9)
T3b	112 (5.1)
T4	6 (0.3)
No. with each pathologic Gleason score (%)	
5	23 (1)
6	764 (34.6)
7	1,185 (53.6)
8	113 (5.1)
9	122 (5.5)

Table 20.6 (continued)

Parameters	Overall (three surgeons)
Mean prostate weight (range)	49.91 (13–220)
Mean tumor volume (range) (%)	17.2 (1–90)
Mean hospital stay (range)	1.14 (0–35)
Mean duration of catheterization (range)	10 (4–36)
No. of cystograms with no evidence of leakage (%)	1,951 (88.3)
No. of complications	
Clavien I	221 (8)
Clavien II	102 (3.7)
Clavien III	13 (0.5)
Clavien IV	2 (0.01)
Clavien V	1 (<0.01)
No. of PSA recurrences (%)	95 (7.27)
No. of positive surgical margins	
pT2 (%)	170 (13.0)
pT3 (%)	169 (35)
No. of conversions (%)	2 (0.1)
No. aborted (%)	8 (0.3)
No. of positive lymph nodes (%)	20 (9.0)

$p < 0.05$) as comfort with the procedure increased. Finally, positive surgical margins also improved for organ-confined disease (4% vs. 7%, $p < 0.05$). At the time of this publication, we have performed over 4,000 VIPs and the procedure has evolved over time with different techniques performed in certain clinical situations as highlighted above. The description of the current technique is below.

20.20 Steps of the Vattikuti Institute Prostatectomy (VIP) Procedure

Using the knowledge we gained from our anatomic and operative study of the anatomy of the neurovascular plexus, we embarked upon a higher degree of nerve sparing.

Our approach is unique and combines a transperitoneal approach with extraperitoneal techniques of dissection as learned from open surgery. The procedure has undergone several improvements and technical refinements over the years. For details beyond the limits of this chapter, refer to the complete description with figures in 2007[21] with newer modifications described in 2009.[25] We will highlight some salient points and include some images from these manuscripts.

20.21 Basics

The procedure is performed with the patient's arms tucked to prevent a brachial plexus injury and in Trendelenburg position. The legs are separated and placed in low lithotomy position and the robot is brought into position over the patient's abdomen between his legs. A Veress needle is used to gain pneumoperitoneum and then 5–6 trocars are placed as shown in Fig. 20.18. Normally a left- and right-side bedside assistant is employed during the case. We attempt to minimize the number of robotic instruments used and often employ a monopolar hook, a bipolar Maryland dissector, two needle drivers, and cold scissors. Intravenous fluids are limited to 600–800 mL during the case so as to minimize the production of urine during the procedure that can obscure the view and require copious suctioning. The initial part of the surgery begins with a 30° lens angled upward.

20.22 Release of Bowel

With the patient in deep Trendelenburg, the small bowel falls away from the pelvis. The sigmoid colon (on the left side) and the cecum (on the right side), however, can be adherent to the posterior and lateral peritoneum. In these situations, the large bowel has to be mobilized in order to facilitate pelvic lymphadenectomy.

20.23 Bladder Mobilization

After adequate mobilization of the large bowel, the extraperitoneal space is entered by making an inverted U-shaped incision on the anterior peritoneum superior to the dome of the bladder and lateral to the medial umbilical ligaments. The incision is made medial to the internal inguinal ring bilaterally and the only structure of concern that passes through the vertical limb of these peritoneal incisions is the vas deferens. The vasa can be either preserved or transected at this point. The vertical limbs are then deepened inferiorly until the pubic bone is seen bilaterally. The incisions are then joined anteriorly and the urachus is released to drop the bladder off the anterior abdominal wall.

Table 20.7 Comparison of first and last 200 patients in a cohort of 2,766 patients

Parameter	First 200 cases	Last 200 cases	p value
Mean age (range), years	59.9 (40–72)	60 (44–80)	NS
Mean PSA (in ng/mL) (range)	6.4 (0.6–41)	6.14 (0.87–27.5)	NS
No. with clinical stage (%)	1 (0.5)	0	<0.05
T1b	NA	0	
T1c	98 (49)	133 (66.5)	
T2a	20 (10)	57 (28.5)	
T2b	78 (39)	8 (4)	
T3	3 (1.5)	1 (0.5)	
No. with a biopsy Gleason score (%)			
5	0	0	<0.01
6	132 (66)	76 (38)	
7	56 (28)	98 (49)	
8	8 (4)	19 (9.5)	
9–10	4 (2)	7 (3.5)	
Mean BMI (range), kg/m^2	27.7 (19–38)	28.17 (20–40)	NS
No. with prior abdominal surgery (%)	40 (20)	90 (45)	<0.05
Surgical time, min			
Mean (range)	160 (71–315)	131 (83–242)	<0.05
Median	NA	135	
Console time, min			
Mean (range)	121 (53–280)	97 (40–204)	<0.05
Median	119	96	
Estimated blood loss			
Mean (range)	153 (25–750)	133 (50–250)	NS
Median	NA	100	
No. with each pathologic stage (%)			
T2a	30 (15)	19 (9.5)	<0.05
T2b	144 (72)	0 (0)	
T2c	0	105 (52.5)	
T3a	14 (7)	60 (30)	
T3b	12 (6)	15 (7.5)	
T4	0	1 (0.5)	
No. with each pathologic Gleason score (%)			
5	1 (0.5)	2 (1)	<0.01
6	86 (43)	60 (30)	
7	80 (40)	108 (54)	
8	16 (8)	15 (7.5)	
9	5 (2.5)	7 (3.5)	
Cannot be assessed	NA	8 (4)	
Mean prostate weight (range)	43 (11–117)	45.58 (80.18)	NS
Mean tumor volume (range) (%)	20.3 (1–80)	23 (1–100)	NS
Mean hospital stay (range)	1.2 (<1–5)	1.09 (1–5)	NS
Mean duration of catheterization (range)	7 (1–18)	8.1 (5–36)	NS
No. of cystograms with no leakage (%)	176 (88)	183 (91.5)	NS
No. of PSA recurrences (%)	8	0 (at 3 months of follow-up)	NA
No. of positive surgical margins			
pT2 (%)	12 (7.0)	5 (4)	<0.05
No. of conversions (%)	0 (0)	0 (0)	NA
No. aborted (%)	1 (0.5)	1 (0.5)	NS
No. of positive lymph nodes (%)	2 (1.0)	1 (0.5)	NS

NS, not significant; PSA, prostate-specific antigen; NA, not available; BMI, body mass index

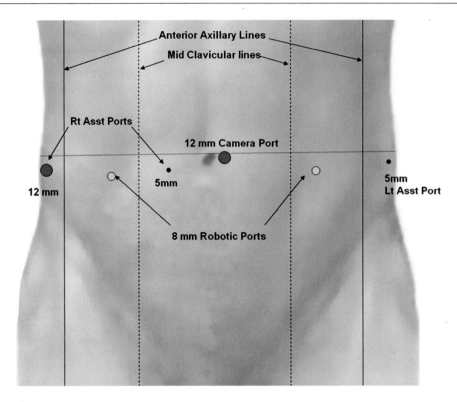

Fig. 20.18 Port placement

20.24 Division of the Bladder Neck

In the past we would open the endopelvic fascia and ligate the dorsal venous complex. We now minimize dissection near the apex and proceed directly to the bladder neck. This allows for precise suturing of the dorsal venous complex after the urethra is divided. At this point, the 30° lens is pointed downward. The right assistant places the anterior bladder wall on traction in the midline. The dissection is performed laterally as the prostatovesical junction is easier to identify. Once the bladder neck is divided anteriorly in the midline, the Foley catheter balloon is deflated and the catheter is pulled upward from the incision and grasped by the assistant and placed on traction, thereby retracting the prostate upward. The posterior bladder neck is now divided.

20.25 Incision of Denonvilliers' Fascia and Dissection of Vas Deferens and Seminal Vesicles

Dissection is now continued underneath the prostate until the anterior layer of Denonvilliers' fascia is identified. Through this thin layer, the vas deferens and the seminal vesicles can be identified. The left assistant places the prostate base on upward traction to facilitate the dissection. Care is taken to carefully dissect these structures and their accompanying blood vessels. In cases where preservation of potency is desired and disease is low risk and/or minimal, the tips of the seminal vesicles may be intentionally preserved provided that intraoperative frozen sections of the margins are normal. However, the tips can be resected using clips or fine bipolar coagulation only as the neurovascular bundles are near this location. With the seminal vesicles now retracting upward, the posterior layer of Denonvilliers' fascia is opened sharply down to perirectal fat as shown in Fig. 20.19. As a result, the dissection posterior to the prostate is essentially done at the end of this step.

20.26 Nerve Sparing

The nerve-sparing technique has evolved over time and based on preoperative characteristics, some patients may be candidates for prostatic fascia-sparing ("veil of Aphrodite" or "Super veil of Aphrodite") techniques. We have discussed these approaches above along with

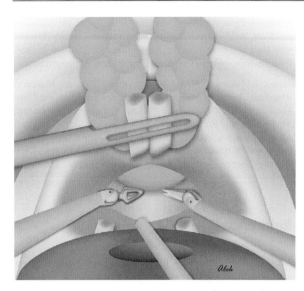

Fig. 20.19 Posterior dissection

Table 20.8 What is the Vattikuti Institute Prostatectomy?

Year	Technique	Benefit
2001	Initial approach to bladder neck	↓ Operating time
2002	Running anastomosis	↓ Leak, strictures
2002	Avoid monopolar cautery after seminal vesical transaction	Not evident
2003	"Veil" nerve-sparing technique	Decreased ED
2004	Anterior traction on bladder to identify bladder neck	Easier transference of skill
2004	Delayed ligation of the dorsal venous complex	More precise urethral transaction, ↓ Apical margins
2004	Not opening the endopelvic fascia	Not evident
2005	Fully athermal nerve-sparing technique	Not evident
2007	Double-layer anastomosis	Unchanged continence; ↓ urinary leak
2008	Percutaneous suprapubic tube	↓ Patient discomfort
2008	Primary hypogastric node dissection for low-intermediate risk disease	Increased node positivity
2010	Barbed anastomotic suture	↓ Anastomotic time

outcomes and associated figures. In patients who are not candidates for the "veil" or "Super veil" nerve sparing, standard nerve sparing is performed. The prostatic pedicles divided between Hem-o-lok (Weck) clips and individual vessels are ligated using bipolar electrocautery.

20.27   Apical Dissection and Division of the Urethra

Using the hook monopolar electrocautery, the puboprostatic ligaments and dorsal venous complex are divided. A 0° lens can be used at this point if visualization is difficult with the 30° downward lens. If the dorsal venous complex bleeds excessively after division, a suture is placed now. Usually, however, the apical dissection can be completed and the stitch through the complex can be placed later. Now the urethra and apical junction are easily seen. The urethra is intentionally kept thick and scissors are used to transect the urethra with care to transect beyond a posterior lip of the apex of the prostate. Frozen sections can easily be obtained if necessary. The posterior striated sphincter/rectourethralis muscle is carefully divided with attention to the fact that the rectum is clearly separated from this area. The prostate is now placed in a specimen back and placed out of the pelvis. The preserved neurovascular and periurethral tissues are inspected for hemostasis.

20.28   Bilateral Pelvic Lymphadenectomy

This is an additional part of the operation that has evolved. We have recently appreciated that the internal iliac nodal basin is the primary landing zone for lymph node metastases from prostate cancer. Therefore, we now routinely perform an internal iliac lymphadenectomy. This was discussed earlier; however, an extended or standard external iliac lymphadenectomy can also be performed at this point.

20.29   Running Urethrovesical Anastomosis

This has been described above in detail along with accompanying images. Although our randomized controlled trial demonstrates no improvement in early continence with the double-layer anastomosis over the single-layer anastomosis, we still perform the double layer at times, especially when anastomotic leak or pelvic hematoma is anticipated. The anastomosis can be performed with a 30° lens directed downward but often is easier with a 0° lens. It is a running anastomosis that approximates mucosa to mucosa and is completed with a single intracorporeal knot.

20.30 Postoperative Care

Patients are discharged within 24 h of surgery. Initially, patients were returning in 4–7 days for office cystogram and catheter removal in the event of no contrast extravasation. However, recently, cystograms are not being routinely performed unless a patient required extensive bladder neck repair or the anastomosis was not noted to be watertight at the time of surgery. If extravasation is noted, the cystogram is repeated in 7 days and the catheter is maintained.

20.31 Summary

Below is a brief summary of technical modifications evaluated during the evolution of the current procedure. During this evolution, suggestions made by our team influenced the development of specific instrumentation for the Intuitive Surgical da Vinci system including the Prograsp, monopolar scissors, hook, and the bipolar.

20.32 Conclusion

Our goal in developing robotic prostatectomy was not to replace open radical prostatectomy, but to build upon and improve it. Immediately, we saw a 90% decrease in blood loss and transfusions. The luxury of working in a bloodless (at least relatively) field allowed us to concentrate on the reconstructive rather than the extirpative aspect of the operation. Simultaneously, this has allowed us to concentrate on the functional aspects of prostate cancer surgery. As evolved, the Vattikuti Institute Prostatectomy procedure is much different from its open counterpart of 2000. In our hands, this approach has significantly decreased blood loss and complications and improved the temporal return of continence and erectile function.

Acknowledgments We would like to recognize the following residents, fellows, and staff of the Vattikuti Urology Institute who have contributed to the development of Vattikuti Institute Prostatectomy over the years and shaped it to its present form.

James O Peabody, Hans Stricker, Craig Rogers, Mahendra Bhandari, Ashok K. Hemal, Ashutosh Tewari, Khurshid Guru, Melissa Fisher, Nikhil Shah, Richard Sarle, Ketan Badani, Michael Fumo, Ronald Boris, Daniel Eun, Rajesh Laungani, Alok Shrivastava, Akshay Bhandari, Ram Dasari, James Brown, Ramgopal Satyanarayana, Sameer Siddiqui, Katherine Rhee, Ronney Abazza, Spencer Krane, Fred Muhletaler, and Nilesh Patil.

References

1. Walsh PC, Donker PJ. Impotence following radical prostatectomy: insight into etiology and prevention. *J Urol.* 1982;128(3):492–497.
2. Schuessler WW, Schulam PG, et al. Laparoscopic radical prostatectomy: initial short-term experience. *Urology.* 1997;50(6):854–857.
3. Guillonneau B, Vallancien G. Laparoscopic radical prostatectomy: the Montsouris experience. *J Urol.* 2000;163(2):418–422.
4. Pasticier G, Rietbergen JB, et al. Robotically assisted laparoscopic radical prostatectomy: feasibility study in men. *Eur Urol.* 2001;40(1):70–74.
5. Menon M, Tewari A, et al. Vattikuti institute prostatectomy, a technique of robotic radical prostatectomy for management of localized carcinoma of the prostate: experience of over 1100 cases. *Urol Clin North Am.* 2004;31(4): 701–717.
6. Hemal AK, Srinivas M, et al. Ergonomic problems associated with laparoscopy. *J Endourol.* 2001;15(5):499–503.
7. Binder J, Kramer W. Robotically-assisted laparoscopic radical prostatectomy. *BJU Int.* 2001;87(4):408–410.
8. Abbou CC, Hoznek A, et al. Remote laparoscopic radical prostatectomy carried out with a robot. Report of a case. *Prog Urol.* 2000;10(4):520–523.
9. Rassweiler J, Frede T, et al. Telesurgical laparoscopic radical prostatectomy. Initial experience. *Eur Urol.* 2001;40(1):75–83.
10. Menon M, Shrivastava A, et al. Laparoscopic and robot assisted radical prostatectomy: establishment of a structured program and preliminary analysis of outcomes. *J Urol.* 2002;168(3):945–949.
11. Tewari A, Srivasatava A, et al. A prospective comparison of radical retropubic and robot-assisted prostatectomy: experience in one institution. *BJU Int.* 2003;92(3):205–210.
12. Schover LR, Fouladi RT, et al. Defining sexual outcomes after treatment for localized prostate carcinoma. *Cancer.* 2002;95(8):1773–1785.
13. Walsh PC. Radical prostatectomy, preservation of sexual function, cancer control. The controversy. *Urol Clin North Am.* 1987;14(4):663–673.
14. Walsh PC, Marschke P, et al. Patient-reported urinary continence and sexual function after anatomic radical prostatectomy. *Urology.* 2000;55(1):58–61.

15. Tewari A, Peabody JO, et al. An operative and anatomic study to help in nerve sparing during laparoscopic and robotic radical prostatectomy. *Eur Urol*. 2003;43(5): 444–454.

16. Takenaka A, Murakami G, et al. Variation in course of cavernous nerve with special reference to details of topographic relationships near prostatic apex: histologic study using male cadavers. *Urology*. 2005;65(1):136–142.

17. Costello AJ, Brooks M, et al. Anatomical studies of the neurovascular bundle and cavernosal nerves. *BJU Int*. 2004;94(7):1071–1076.

18. Kiyoshima K, Yokomizo A, et al. Anatomical features of periprostatic tissue and its surroundings: a histological analysis of 79 radical retropubic prostatectomy specimens. *Jpn J Clin Oncol*. 2004;34(8):463–468.

19. Kaul S, Bhandari A, et al. Robotic radical prostatectomy with preservation of the prostatic fascia: a feasibility study. *Urology*. 2005;66(6):1261–1265.

20. Menon M, Kaul S, et al. Potency following robotic radical prostatectomy: a questionnaire based analysis of outcomes after conventional nerve sparing and prostatic fascia sparing techniques. *J Urol*. 2005;174(6):2291–2296, discussion 2296.

21. Menon M, Shrivastava A, et al. Vattikuti institute prostatectomy: contemporary technique and analysis of results. *Eur Urol*. 2007;51(3):648–657, discussion 657–648.

22. Graefen M, Walz J, et al. Open retropubic nerve-sparing radical prostatectomy. *Eur Urol*. 2006;49(1):38–48.

23. Nielsen ME, Schaeffer EM, et al. High anterior release of the levator fascia improves sexual function following open radical retropubic prostatectomy. *J Urol*. 2008;180(6):2557–2564, discussion 2564.

24. Eichelberg C, Erbersdobler A, et al. Nerve distribution along the prostatic capsule. *Eur Urol*. 2007;51(1):105–110, discussion 110–101.

25. Menon M, Shrivastava A, et al. Vattikuti institute prostatectomy: technical modifications in 2009. *Eur Urol*. 2009;56(1):89–96.

26. Van Velthoven RF, Ahlering TE, et al. Technique for laparoscopic running urethrovesical anastomosis: the single knot method. *Urology*. 2003;61(4):699–702.

27. Blumenthal KB, Sutherland DE, Wagner KR, et al. Bladder neck contractures related to the use of Hem-o-lok clips in robot-assisted laparoscopic radical prostatectomy. *Urology*. 2008;72:158–161.

28. Tunnard GJ, Biyani CS. An unusual complication of a Hemo-Lok clip following laparoscopic radical prostatectomy. *J Laparoendosc Adv Surg Tech A*. 2009;19:649–651.

29. Tugcu V, Polat H, Ozbay B, et al. Stone formation from intravesical Hem-o-lok clip migration after laparoscopic radical prostatectomy. *J Endourol*. 2009;23:1111–1113.

30. Kaul S, Sammon J, Bhandari A, Peabody J, Rogers CG, Menon M. A novel method of urethrovesical anastomosis during robot-assisted radical prostatectomy using a unidirectional barbed wound closure device: feasibility study and early outcomes in 51 patients. *J Endourol*. November, 2010;24(11):1789–1793.

31. Menon M, Hemal AK, et al. The technique of apical dissection of the prostate and urethrovesical anastomosis in robotic radical prostatectomy. *BJU Int*. 2004;93(6): 715–719.

32. Rocco B, Gregori A, et al. Posterior reconstruction of the rhabdosphincter allows a rapid recovery of continence after transperitoneal videolaparoscopic radical prostatectomy. *Eur Urol*. 2007;51(4):996–1003.

33. Tewari AK, Bigelow K, et al. Anatomic restoration technique of continence mechanism and preservation of puboprostatic collar: a novel modification to achieve early urinary continence in men undergoing robotic prostatectomy. *Urology*. 2007;69(4):726–731.

34. Menon M, Muhletaler F, et al. Assessment of early continence after reconstruction of the periprostatic tissues in patients undergoing computer assisted (robotic) prostatectomy: results of a 2 group parallel randomized controlled trial. *J Urol*. 2008;180(3):1018–1023.

35. Lepor H, Nieder AM, et al. Early removal of urinary catheter after radical retropubic prostatectomy is both feasible and desirable. *Urology*. 2001;58(3):425–429.

36. Tewari A, Rao S, et al. Catheter-less robotic radical prostatectomy using a custom-made synchronous anastomotic splint and vesical urinary diversion device: report of the initial series and perioperative outcomes. *BJU Int*. 2008;102(8):1000–1004.

37. Krane LS, Bhandari M, et al. Impact of percutaneous suprapubic tube drainage on patient discomfort after radical prostatectomy. *Eur Urol*. 2009;56(2):325–330.

38. Bishoff JT, Reyes A, et al. Pelvic lymphadenectomy can be omitted in selected patients with carcinoma of the prostate: development of a system of patient selection. *Urology*. 1995;45(2):270–274.

39. Clark T, Parekh DJ, et al. Randomized prospective evaluation of extended versus limited lymph node dissection in patients with clinically localized prostate cancer. *J Urol*. 2003;169(1):145–147, discussion 147–148.

40. Schumacher MC, Burkhard FC, et al. Good outcome for patients with few lymph node metastases after radical retropubic prostatectomy. *Eur Urol*. 2008;54(2): 344–352.

41. McDowell GC 2nd, Johnson JW, et al. Pelvic lymphadenectomy for staging clinically localized prostate cancer. Indications, complications, and results in 217 cases. *Urology*. 1990;35(6):476–482.

42. Makarov DV, Trock BJ, et al. Updated nomogram to predict pathologic stage of prostate cancer given prostate-specific antigen level, clinical stage, and biopsy gleason score (Partin tables) based on cases from 2000 to 2005. *Urology*. 2007;69:1095–1101.

43. Mattei A, Fuechsel FG, et al. The template of the primary lymphatic landing sites of the prostate should be revisited: results of a multimodality mapping study. *Eur Urol*. 2008;53(1):118–125.

44. Badani KK, Kaul S, et al. Evolution of robotic radical prostatectomy: assessment after 2766 procedures. *Cancer*. 2007;110(9):1951–1958.

Chapter 21

Transferring Knowledge of Anatomical Dissection from the Laboratory to the Patient: An Australian Perspective

Ben Challacombe and Anthony J. Costello

The surgical treatment of localized prostate cancer with nerve-sparing radical prostatectomy (RP) has undergone a substantial improvement in outcomes in recent years due to new insights into the anatomy of the prostate and the adjacent tissues. Minimally invasive approaches to RP have served to focus surgeons on these anatomical landmarks, and interest in the precise anatomy of the neurovascular bundle (NVB) has increased since the advent of telerobotic laparoscopic prostatectomy, where the magnification using the da Vinci's optical system may allow easier recognition and preservation of these nerves. This has served to "raise the bar" with regards to oncological efficacy, urinary incontinence, and erectile dysfunction, the three primary outcomes following RP. In this chapter we look at the intricate anatomy of the neurovascular bundle as revealed by recent cadaveric dissections and differential immunohistochemical staining and focus on the translation of our anatomical dissections into clinical practice.

21.1 Introduction

The ancient science of human anatomy has allowed a progressive understanding of the structure and function of the organs and connective tissues of the human body over thousands of years. Anatomical dissections have been performed since Egyptian times followed by the masterful dissections of Hippocrates and Galen, and even today anatomy remains one of the cornerstones of a doctor's education. Since the times of the British anatomist and surgeon John Hunter in the 1760s, surgeons have based their operative surgical knowledge of human anatomy primarily on cadaveric dissection.

The intimate understanding of the peri-prostatic neurovascular bundles and sphincter mechanisms has only relatively recently begun to be fully understood. The major long-term morbidity from radical prostatectomy (RP) remains sexual dysfunction, despite many advances in surgical techniques, as incontinence is now increasingly well maintained or corrected with slings and artificial sphincters. The ability of urological surgeons to perform potentially nerve-sparing radical prostatectomy was highlighted by the seminal fetal and neonatal studies of Walsh and Donker in the 1970s[1] and subsequently investigated in the clinical outcomes of men on whom these new techniques were attempted.[2] By tracing the autonomic innervation of the corpora cavernosa, Walsh and Donker proposed and later showed that erectile dysfunction occurred secondary to injury of these nerves (termed the cavernosal nerves). These nerves were identified branching from the pelvic plexus (formed by the union of the sympathetic hypogastric nerve and the parasympathetic pelvic splanchnic nerves) and running as a plexus of small nerves within a prominent NVB on the posterolateral border of the prostate, before piercing the urogenital diaphragm and descending along the lateral aspect of the urethra. Detailed histological studies performed in Australia and by Walsh's group have also revealed the cross-sectional profile of the NVB and shown it to run through leaves of the lateral pelvic fascia.[3,4]

B. Challacombe (✉)
Division of Surgery, Department of Urology, The Royal Melbourne Hospital, University of Melbourne, Melbourne, Australia
e-mail: benchallacombe@doctors.net.uk

Respecting and observing these anatomical details during robotic radical prostatectomy can result in improved postoperative functional outcomes, as well as reliable oncological control. The development of 'nerve-sparing' RP has led to improved potency rates, with studies reporting the recovery of erectile function in 16–76% of men in whom both neurovascular bundles (NVBs) were preserved and 0–56% in those with one NVB preserved.[5]

21.2 Preliminary Anatomical Dissection of the Neurovascular Region of the Prostate

21.2.1 Background to the Study

Deliberate bilateral excision of the cavernosal nerves during prostate surgery to achieve adequate cancer resection margins results in erectile dysfunction in almost all men.[6] For men with intentional unilateral or bilateral cavernosal nerve resection, nerve reconstruction using an interposition sural nerve graft was previously proposed as a means of restoring neurological control of erectile function. Studies assessing the ability of sural nerve grafts to enhance cavernosal nerve regeneration were conducted in both rats and humans.[7–9] Despite some promising preliminary data in these models, we viewed this technique with a degree of skepticism. Criticism of the technique in humans focused on the ability to accurately interpose the sural nerve graft into the appropriate area of the neurovascular bundle. The debate surrounding this technique stimulated our team at the Royal Melbourne Hospital to conduct detailed anatomical studies to describe the anatomy of the NVB and outline potential technical difficulties in sural nerve grafting.

21.2.2 Dissection Protocols

The pelves of 12 fixed male human adult cadavers (age at death 56–74 years) were dissected in detail. The NVB was dissected bilaterally in each cadaver and its anatomy and relationship to surrounding pelvic

structures documented photographically. The dissection sequence varied with two different approaches adopted, with four cadaver specimens hemi-sected and eight prepared by en bloc pelvic resection. The branches of the pelvic plexus were meticulously dissected under magnification ($\times 6$). The constituents of the NVB were traced to their target organs, with the findings documented and the relationship of the NVB to surrounding pelvic structures recorded.[10]

The en bloc dissection sequence enabled the pelvic plexus to be dissected in full and exposed the additional branches innervating the bladder, seminal vesicles, anterolateral prostate, and levator ani musculature. The cavernosal nerves were traced to the corpora cavernosa.

In all 24 (12 pairs) dissections, the plexus of nerves running within the NVB branch from the postero-inferior aspect of the pelvic plexus was found to be 0.5–2 cm inferior to the level of the tip of the seminal vesicle (Fig. 21.1). The number of macroscopic nerves present varied, with 6–16 noted. On branching from the pelvic plexus these nerves are spread significantly, with up to 3 cm separating the anterior- and posterior-most nerves. Generally, most of the NVB descends posteriorly to the seminal vesicle. The nerves converge en route to the mid-prostatic level, forming a denser NVB, only to diverge once again when approaching the prostatic apex. These micro-dissections of the NVB have confirmed the course of the cavernosal nerves in the posterolateral groove between the prostate and rectum.

21.2.3 Discussion of NVB Anatomy

The nerves of the NVB are intimately associated with vessels branching from the inferior vesical vein and artery. As these vessels course distally toward the prostatic apex numerous terminal branches are given off which, in most cases, mimic the course of the nerves. The nerves running in the NVB innervate the corpora cavernosa, rectum, prostate, and levator ani musculature. The nerves innervating the posterior aspect of the prostate are intimately associated with capsular arteries and veins of the prostate. These structures penetrate the prostatic capsule along its base, mid-portion, and apex. The cavernosal nerves and several small vessels pierce the urogenital diaphragm posterolateral to the

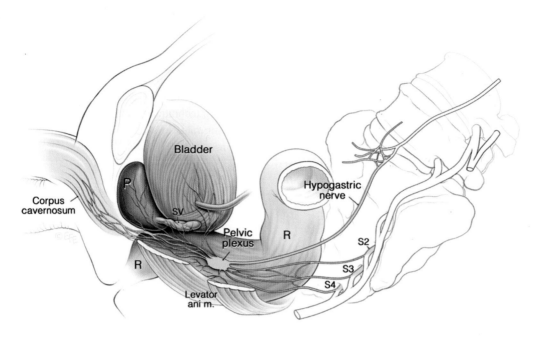

Fig. 21.1 Schematic diagram of the autonomic nerves of the pelvis. Adapted from images courtesy of Department of Anatomy, The University of Melbourne

prostatic apex. At this level the clearly visible cavernosal nerves divide into numerous small branches that descend along the posterolateral aspect of the membranous urethra, before penetrating the posterior aspect of corpora cavernosa.

What was particularly significant about this work was the discovery and description of distinct fascial compartments within the neurovascular bundle itself. The constituents of the NVB were seen to be organized into three functional compartments. The neurovascular

supply to the rectum is generally in the posterior and posterolateral section of the NVB, running within the leaves of Denonvilliers' and pararectal fasciae. The levator ani neurovascular supply is in the lateral section of the NVB, descending along and within the lateral pelvic fascia. The cavernosal nerves and the prostatic neurovascular supply descend along the posterolateral surface of the prostate, with the prostatic neurovascular supply most anterior (Fig. 21.2). The functional organization of the NVB is not absolute and is less

Fig. 21.2 The fascial compartments of the NVB. RNV, neurovascular supply to the rectum; DF, Denonvilliers' fascia; PF, pararectal fascia; LPF, lateral pelvic fascia; LANV, neurovascular supply to levator ani; PNV, neurovascular supply to the prostate; CN, cavernosal nerves. Adapted from images courtesy of Department of Anatomy, The University of Melbourne

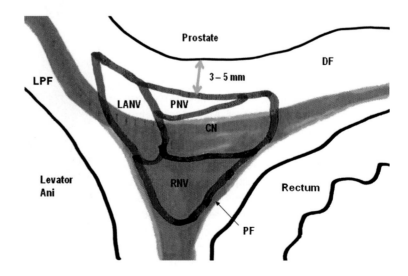

pronounced proximally at the levels of the seminal vesicles and the prostatic base. In addition to the nerves descending within the NVB, a scattering of nerves extends from the medial margin of the NVB to the prostatic midline.

Prior to this study and when assessing previous publications it was apparent that the terms NVB and cavernosal nerve were often used synonymously[11]; such reference is no longer appropriate. This study also illustrated significant difficulty in placing the proposed sural nerve grafts for enhancing erectile function after RP; as having identified the large proximal NVB, to which severed proximal nerves should the nerve graft be anastomosed was difficult to answer.

21.3 Autonomic Immunohistochemical Staining

21.3.1 Background to the Study

In the new millennium surgeons have continued to refine their techniques in an attempt to minimize the morbidity of radical prostatectomy. In the era of robotic-assisted radical prostatectomy the exact positioning of the physiologically active cavernous nerves and the concept of a well-defined neurovascular bundle posterolateral to the prostate have been challenged by several investigations. Some authors have located nerve fibers on the anterolateral aspect of the prostate, outside of the neurovascular bundle.[11,12] These authors speculate that a proportion of these anteriorly placed nerves are parasympathetic in nature and as a result contribute fibers to the pro-erectile cavernous nerves. Despite a lack of hard evidence relating to the actual function of these nerves, some institutions have developed nerve-sparing techniques aimed at preserving these structures.[13,14] This new nerve-sparing approach, dubbed the 'Veil of Aphrodite' technique by Menon's group in Detroit or curtain dissection, releases the lateral prostatic fascia high on the anterolateral margins of the prostate above the midpoint of the prostate. The Veil approach was named after Aphrodite, the Greek goddess of love. Aphrodite's urological relevance extends to her mythological origins. She was born of the foaming water off Cyprus when Cronus cut off Uranus' testicles and threw them over his shoulder into the sea. Early reports from

some centers have indicated improved postoperative potency using this technique.[14,15] However, there is little anatomical evidence to justify this approach, given that the higher placed nerves are potentially destined to innervate the prostatic stroma and not the cavernosal tissue of the penis. It is also a more technically demanding technique that may increase positive surgical margin rates in all but highly experienced robotic surgeons.

21.3.2 Experimental Techniques

As a result of this lack of concordance between anatomy and surgical technique, we designed a further investigation primarily focused on characterizing the position and functionality of the autonomic nerves on the anterolateral aspects of the prostate, with the hope of optimizing postoperative potency rates and providing justification for the different nerve-sparing approaches. To achieve this we needed to differentially stain parasympathetic and sympathetic nerves running along the prostate.

Four blocks of pelvic tissue were serially histologically sectioned from the prostatic base proximally, to the apex distally (Fig. 21.3). The blocks of tissue were from the pelves of two embalmed cadavers and two fresh cadavers, which had been hemi-sectioned. The hemi-sected pelvic blocks were then divided into 4 mm

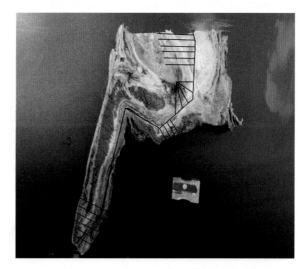

Fig. 21.3 Sectioning technique for hemi-pelves. Stylized representation of sectioning process. *Lines* indicate sites of sectioning (4 mm approx.). Courtesy of Emma Clarebrough, Department of Anatomy, The University of Melbourne

Fig. 21.4 Method of sector analysis. Adapted from images courtesy of Department of Anatomy, The University of Melbourne

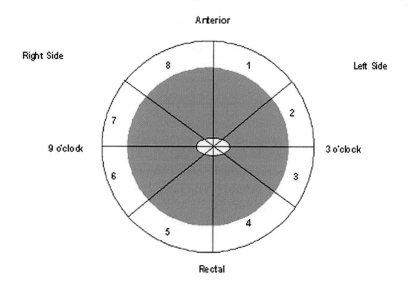

sections and embedded into paraffin for histological analysis.

To localize the parasympathetic nerves an antibody directed against neuronal nitric oxide synthase (bNOS) was used. bNOS is a 150 kDa protein that is found in peripheral parasympathetic nerves and catalyzes the formation of nitrous oxide (NO).[16] Nitric oxide is released by parasympathetics and is a potent vasodilator, implicated in the physiology of the male erection. To localize the sympathetic nerves we used a primary antibody directed against tyrosine hydroxylase (TH). TH is the rate-limiting enzyme in the synthetic pathway of catecholamines including noradrenaline (NA), which is a neurotransmitter found in peripheral sympathetic nerves and their associated ganglia.

In addition to the standard H&E staining to identify somatic nerves, slides were stained with these immunohistochemical (IHC) stains – using tyrosine hydroxylase (sympathetics) and nNOS (parasympathetics). Each slide was analyzed according to nerve fiber number, type (somatic, parasympathetic, or sympathetic), and position relative to the prostate. The analysis subdivided and allocated nerves as they were observed, to a particular region as shown in Fig. 21.4.

21.3.3 Results

At the prostatic base parasympathetic nerves accounted for 43.3% of all nerve fibers present. This proportion increased slightly to 45.5% at the prostatic apex. Of particular note is the observation that parasympathetic nerves found above the 3–9 o'clock level accounted for only 4, 5, and 6.8% of the total number of nerves at the base, mid-prostate, and apical regions, respectively.

The proportion of nerves characterized as sympathetic remained relatively constant, staying within the range of 38.7–39.1%. Sympathetic nerves found above the 3–9 o'clock level represented approximately 15% of the total number of nerves at any given prostatic level.

Somatic nerves corresponded to 18, 16.5, and 15.5% of the total nerve fibers at the base, mid-prostate, and apex, respectively. Somatic nerves found above 3–9 o'clock level were about 7.5% of the total nerves at each level of the prostate. Interestingly a little over a quarter (27.4, 26.5, and 29.6%) of all the nerve fibers identified was found on the anterior half of the prostate, above the 3–9 o'clock level.

21.3.4 Parasympathetic Nerve Fiber Distribution

At the prostatic base parasympathetic nerves accounted for only 14.3% of the nerves located on the anterior aspect of the prostate. However, these nerves correspond to only 9% (Table 21.1) of the total number of parasympathetic nerves found at the base. A significant proportion of the parasympathetic

Table 21.1 Functional nerve distribution in anterior sectors: as a percentage of all nerve fibers in sectors 1, 2, 7, and 8

	Parasympathetic	Sympathetic	Somatic
Prostate base	14.3	55.7	30
Prostate mid-gland	18.8	53	28.2
Prostate apex	23.1	52.3	18.6

nerves at the base were localized to the region of the neurovascular bundle (sectors 4 and 5). At this level 69.4% of the parasympathetic nerves were found within the anatomically defined NVB (Table 21.1).

Likewise at the mid-prostate 65.3% of the parasympathetic nerves were found inside the NVB. Only 11.1% of parasympathetics at this level were found above the 3–9 o'clock junction, which as a proportion of the total nerves at this level represents 18.8% of those nerves found on the anterior aspects of the prostate.

Apically, 57% of all parasympathetic fibers were found within the region of the NVB, with 15% found above the 3–9 o'clock level. Importantly, the proportion of parasympathetic nerves found within the posterolateral NVB dropped slightly from the base to the apex.

The fascial architecture of the posterolaterally located neurovascular bundle (NVB) was also analyzed and in 18 of the 32 slides examined the neurovascular bundle exhibited a fascial architecture with three separate compartments as previously described.[10] Figure 21.5 illustrates the compartmental architecture found within the neurovascular bundle on a slide. Three compartments containing nerves and blood vessels can be clearly seen, the most medial of which conveyed a significant proportion of the parasympathetic nerve fibers. This indicates that the cavernous nerves probably remain within a distinct

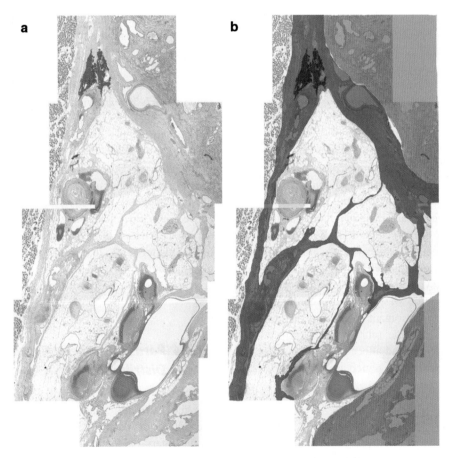

Fig. 21.5 Compartmental architecture of the NVB (mid-prostate). **a** *Left*: H&E slide showing compartmental NVB architecture. **b** *Right overlay*: prostate (*green*), fascial bands (*blue*), nerves (*yellow*), pararectal tissue (*grey*), levator ani musculature (*spotted pink*). Courtesy of Emma Clarebrough, Department of Anatomy, The University of Melbourne

structural compartment and the higher parasympathetic nerves do not contribute to the pro-erectile innervation of the penis.

21.3.5 Discussion of Immunhistochemical Staining

In the differential nerve staining study autonomic nerve fibers were found occupying positions on the anterolateral aspect of the prostate between the prostate and lateral prostatic fascia. At the mid-prostatic level autonomic nerves accounted for 83.5% of all nerve fibers. Autonomic fibers found above 3–9 o'clock accounted for only 19% of all nerves at the same level. In studies of operatively resected prostates both Eichelberg et al.[3] and Kiyoshima et al.[4] also identified nerves placed anteriorly and anterolaterally to the prostate further confirming their existence. These authors speculated that a proportion of these nerves were parasympathetic in nature and as a result contributed fibers to the pro-erectile fibers of the cavernous nerves and therefore attempts should be made to spare these fibers. Without investigation into the function of these higher placed nerves and in the absence of entire anatomical blocks of tissue to determine their course, the speculation by these authors remained unsubstantiated.

This immunohistochemical investigation revealed that at the mid-prostate only 18.8% of the nerves found on the anterior aspect of the prostate were parasympathetic in nature, with the vast majority of parasympathetics (68%) found in the traditional NVB region, posterolateral to the prostate. The anteriorly placed parasympathetic nerve fibers are likely to be destined for innervation of the prostatic stroma and not the copra cavernosum of the penis. This observation is supported by two pieces of evidence.

First, the total number of visible nerve fibers was smaller at the prostatic apex as compared to the base. This decrease in the number of fibers has been reported by some authors[11,12,17] and may be related to a significant proportion of nerves penetrating the prostate to provide innervation to the gland itself. In the fresh cadavers included in this study, 134 nerve fibers were located at the base as opposed to 115 at the apex. Of these, the absolute number of parasympathetic nerves found on the anterior half of the prostate at the apex

was only eight – further supporting this hypothesis of nerves entering the prostate as they course along it.

Second, fascial architecture of the neurovascular bundle (NVB) itself supports the view that prostatic innervation is the role of these anterior nerve fibers. In our earlier work with 12 micro-dissected cadavers we showed distinct compartments within the neurovascular bundle, each supplying separate structures.[10] A similar compartmental structure of the NVB was again confirmed in this study.

Figure 21.6 clearly illustrates this anatomy, showing the neural elements in the other compartments innervating levator ani (LA), rectum (Rec), and the prostatic stroma (P).

Interestingly, the majority of the nerve fibers found on the anterolateral regions examined were sympathetic in nature. The tendency for sympathetics to be found at these locations is due to three reasons. First, the sympathetic nerves contribute significant innervation to the prostatic stroma. Second, they also are responsible for innervation to the vascular structures in the region and as such may extend outside the typical neurovascular bundle, which is predominantly parasympathetic. Finally, the external urethral sphincter (EUS) – located immediately distal to prostatic apex – receives input from the autonomic sympathetic nerves.[17,18] The sympathetics may course over the anterior aspects of the prostate to provide innervation to the anterior EUS.

Apically the absolute number of the parasympathetic fibers above the 3–9 o'clock junction increased

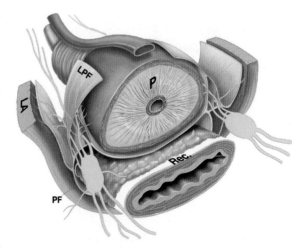

Fig. 21.6 Schematic diagram of peri-prostatic innervation. Adapted from images courtesy of Department of Anatomy, The University of Melbourne

slightly. This is consistent with studies that show the cavernous nerves ascending to assume a higher position distal to the apex.[4,19,20] Takenaka et al.[19] claimed the cavernous nerves assume a higher 2–10 o'clock position at the apex. Our investigation did not confirm these findings; however, careful dissection and ligation of the dorsal venous complex is recommended to preserve the neural anatomy.

Several authors have reported the use of the 'Veil of Aphrodite' technique (Fig. 21.7) as a nerve-sparing method.[13,14,21] As previously discussed this technique releases the lateral prostatic fascia from a higher position, therefore preserving the nerves found on the more anterior aspects of the prostate. In one series Menon et al. reported potency rates at 12 months postoperatively of 90%[15] using this method. The question that remains is the following: Are these results a function of surgical skill and careful patient selection or are they representative of the actual functional anatomy in the region? The results of our investigation point toward the former as the true source of these superior outcomes. This inference is in light of the fact that the majority of parasympathetic nerves are located in the posterolateral regions of the prostate, enclosed in the predominant pro-erectile neurovascular bundle. Consequently, from an anatomical perspective, the functionally relevant parasympathetic nerves

are spared during standard nerve-sparing procedures. Those that are spared using the Veil technique are probably destined for innervation of the prostatic stroma itself and are not implicated in the physiology of erections.

21.4 Discussion

The neuroanatomy of the male pelvis is as complex as it is important. Much of the complexity relevant to the urological surgeon centers on the course of the pro-erectile parasympathetic fibers also known as the cavernous nerves. Injury to these structures is directly linked to iatrogenic impotence in the post-radical prostatectomy setting.

We have characterized the autonomic nerves, including the cavernous nerves, in the peri-prostatic region. The existence of ventrally placed peri-prostatic nerves has been previously documented in cadaveric and fetal dissections[13,19] and we have in this investigation again shown that autonomic nerve fibers do exist on the anterior aspects of the prostate, above the 3–9 o'clock level. Only a small minority of these fibers, however, correspond to the pro-erectile parasympathetic cavernous nerves, with the majority of parasympathetic nerves in the posterolateral region of the prostate. Many of these nerves are localized into a neurovascular bundle which exhibits a distinct compartmental structure, with the cavernous nerves occupying the most posterior of the compartments. These findings suggest that the nerves found higher in the lateral prostatic fascia may be responsible for innervation to prostatic stroma itself and not the cavernous tissue of the penis. In effect we have found little anatomical justification for the 'Veil of Aphrodite' technique of nerve sparing, despite reports of improved potency outcomes.

These observations, yielded from immunohistochemical analysis, illustrate that the function and location nerves vary to those purported in the literature. When placed into the context of nerve-sparing radical prostatectomies, these results require us to question the pro-erectile nature of the anteriorly placed nerves and have significant implication on the methodology employed in pelvic surgery. Recognition of this anatomy is essential to optimize the functional outcomes and oncological outcomes from nerve-sparing radical prostatectomies. Tewari et al.[22] characterized

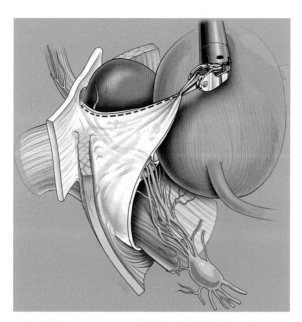

Fig. 21.7 Veil of Aphrodite nerve-sparing technique. Courtesy of Department of Anatomy, The University of Melbourne

these nerves in a similar fashion, referring to a tri-zonal neural architecture. They dissected the pelvic plexus in 12 male adult cadavers and by comparing their findings with intra-operative robotic-assisted laparoscopic radical prostatectomy (RARP) videotapes of 200 cases, they produced a three-dimensional model of the relevant neural pathways. They observed that 'the predominant neurovascular bundle carries impulses to the cavernosal tissue. . . and is located posterolateral to the prostate, as described by Walsh.' These findings support the standard technique of nerve-sparing radical prostatectomy.

Urologists have increasingly been focusing on improving the clarity of their vision of the anatomy during radical prostatectomy and reducing the thermal energy applied to the prostate. This has been stimulated by the minimally invasive techniques that have served to 'raise the bar' for all approaches generally and has increased the functional outcomes expected by our patients, whichever technique they choose. We believe it likely that the high or Veil-type dissection technique contributes to better potency outcomes because of the early release of the fascia, which assists in preserving the more inferiorly placed cavernous nerves. The rationale for this high release might be less traction, less thermal energy damage, and better vascular preservation, rather than preservation of any functional ventrally placed nerves.

The term 'trifecta' has been used to describe the three key goals of radical prostatectomy: oncological control, urinary continence, and potency.[23] One must be careful not to sacrifice one element of this trifecta to achieve another. In appropriate patients, the positive surgical margin (PSM) rate does not appear to be adversely affected by nerve-sparing radical prostatectomy using the standard technique.[24] Because the 'Veil' technique approaches the prostatic capsule much more intimately, some concern exists about the impact this technique may have on PSMs.[25] Menon et al.[22] have acknowledged this concern in their publications on this technique and have maintained a PSM rate of 5% in their 'Veil' series.

21.5 Future Directions

Criticisms of our immunohistochemical analysis of the peri-prostatic nerves include the small number of cadavers dissected and stained and hence further specimens are being dissected to verify and improve the validity of these findings. The observation that parasympathetic nerves may swing upward from posterior to a more anterior distribution along the sphincter urethrae and at the penile hilum and pubic arch en route to join the dorsal sensory nerves needs further clarification. It is possible that the high anterior release may do more as one approaches the apex to preserve those nerves rising anteriorly at this level than it does for any anterior placed nerves at the level of the prostatic base. In this setting a nerve-sparing technique that starts posterolaterally and sweeps anteriorly at the apex might prove to be the optimal anatomically based technique.

Kaiho's group have electrically stimulated ventral peri-prostatic nerves during RP in 12 patients and assessed changes in pressure at the middle of the urethra using an inserted balloon catheter to detect increases in cavernosal pressure.[26] This is a further attempt to prove physiological function of ventrally placed nerves and they observed evoked urethral pressure responses in all patients. A similar study was performed by Takenaka with simultaneous intracavernous and intraurethral pressure measurement and they concluded that distribution of cavernous nerves was wider than anticipated.[27] However, artificial electrical stimulation of peri-prostatic nerves is perhaps too crude an analytical technique to rely on for precise anatomical proof of function. The same group has also investigated the use of multiphoton microscopy to provide intra-operative guidance during RP in a rat model. This technique provides high-resolution images without necessitating any extrinsic labeling agent and with minimal phototoxic effect on tissues. Tissue was excited with a femtosecond pulsed titanium/sapphire laser and nerves detected by their auto-fluorescence.[28] Although promising this technique cannot delineate different types of nerve or their function.

An alternative approach to understanding pelvic neuroanatomy is to trace the cavernous nerves from the penis backward using nerve-specific dyes. We have begun work focusing on real-time visualization, using UV light, of pelvic nerves in a rat model using fluorescent nerve tracers to illustrate the course of the pro-erectile cavernous nerves retrogradely from penis to spinal level. This technique appears to have negligible neural toxicity and avoids the difficulty of tracing nerves anterogradely when they are within a large neurovascular bundle. In clinical use this technique could potentially lead to an individualized approach to nerve sparing in RP as the fluorescent-stained nerves would directly guide the surgeon intra-operatively reducing errors due to patient variability.

21.6 Conclusions

The rationale for nerve-sparing radical prostatectomy as a technique to maximize erectile function must have a sound anatomical foundation. Though nerves have been demonstrated in the lateral prostatic fascia, our anatomical micro-dissections have suggested that these nerves innervate the prostate, not the cavernosal spaces. This work therefore does not support an anatomical basis for why the 'Veil' technique should produce vastly superior potency results. The only clinical data to support this technique has emerged from a nonrandomized single-center series and a randomized trial investigating this issue is unlikely to recruit due to strongly held perceptions of both patients and clinicians. Further work to characterize the nerves of the NVB at the apex of the prostate and beyond into the cavernosal tissue continues in our anatomy department.

These high fascial release techniques described, although attractive to maximize potential ventral nerve sparing, are likely to risk increasing positive surgical margins in inexperienced hands. It is not clear if centers with less experience would note any deterioration in their PSMs if they adopted the 'Veil' technique. We have found no anatomical evidence to perform this additional technique as part of an already demanding procedure as we feel that it may actually worsen outcomes in all but the most experienced centers. We recommend an anatomically proven 'standard' nerve-sparing technique which has excellent outcomes without risking the added and unnecessary complexity of the high fascial release.[29]

Acknowledgments We thank Dr. Matthew Brooks and Dr. Owen Cole for their initial anatomical dissections; Dr. Ben Namdarian, Mr. Ben Dowdle, and Miss Emma Clarebrough for the immunohistochemical analyses; and Dr. Declan Murphy for help with the discussion.

References

1. Walsh PC, Donker PJ. Impotence following radical prostatectomy: insight into etiology and prevention. *J Urol.* 1982;128:492.
2. Walsh P, Lepor H, Eggleston J. Radical prostatectomy with preservation of sexual function: anatomical and pathological considerations. *Prostate.* 1983;4:473.
3. Kourambas J, Angus DG, Hosking P, Chou ST. A histological study of denonvilliers' fascia and its relationship to the neurovascular bundle. *Br J Urol.* 1998;82:408.
4. Lepor H, Gregerman M, Crosby R, et al. Precise location of the autonomic nerves from the pelvic plexus to the corpora cavernosa: a detailed anatomical study of the male pelvis. *J Urol.* 1985;133:207–213.
5. Walsh PC, Mostwin JL. Radical prostatectomy and cystoprostatectomy with preservation of potency. Results using a new nerve-sparing technique. *Br J Urol.* 1984;56:694–697.
6. Quinlan DM, Epstein JI, Carter BS, et al. Sexual function following radical prostatectomy with wide unilateral excision of the neurovascular bundle. *J Urol.* 1991; 145:998.
7. Quinlan DM, Nelson RJ, Walsh PC. Cavernous nerve grafts restore erectile function in denervated rats. *J Urol.* 1991;145:380–383.
8. Burgers JK, Nelson RJ, Quinlan DM, et al. Nerve growth factor, nerve grafts and amniotic membrane grafts restore erectile function in rats. *J Urol.* 1991;146:463–468.
9. Kim ED, Nath R, Slawin KM, et al. Bilateral nerve graft during radical retropubic prostatectomy: extended follow-up. *Urology.* 2001;58:983–987.
10. Costello AJ, Brooks M, Cole OJ. Anatomical studies of the neurovascular bundle and cavernosal nerves. *BJU Int.* 2004;94:1071.
12. Eichelberg C, Erbersdobler A, Michl U, et al. Nerve distribution along the prostatic capsule. *Eur Urol.* 2007;51: 105–111.
11. Kiyoshima K, Yokomizo A, Yoshida T, et al. Anatomical features of periprostatic tissue and its surroundings: a histological analysis of 79 radical retropubic prostatectomy specimens. *Jpn J Clin Oncol.* 2004;34:463.
13. Lunacek A, Schwentner C, Fritsch H, et al. Anatomical retropubic prostatectomy: 'curtain dissection' of the neurovascular bundle. *BJU Int.* 2005;95:1226–1231.
14. Menon M, Shrivastava A, Jaul S, et al. Vattikuti institute prostatectomy: contemporary technique and analysis of results. *Eur Urol.* 2007;51:648–658.
15. Menon M, Kaul S, Bhandari A, et al. Potency following robotic radical prostatectomy: a questionnaire based analysis of outcomes after conventional nerve sparing and prostatic fascia sparing techniques. *J Urol.* 2005; 174:2291–2296.
16. Stanarius A, Uckert S, Machtens S. Immunocytochemical distribution of nitric oxide synthase in the human corpus cavernosum: an electron microscopical study using the tyramide signal amplification technique. *Urol Res.* 2001;29:168–172.
17. Yucel S, Erdogru T, Baykara M. Recent neuroanatomical studies on the neurovascular bundle of the prostate and

cavernosal nerves: clinical reflections on radical prostate-ctomy. *Asian J Androl*. 2005;7:339–349.

18. Walz J, Greaten M, Huland H. Basic principles of anatomy for the optimal surgical treatment of prostate cancer. *World J Urol*. 2007;25:31–38.

19. Takenaka A, Murakami G, Matsubara A. Variation in course of cavernous nerve with special reference to details of topographic relationships near prostatic apex: histo-logical study using male cadavers. *Urology*. 2005;65(1):136–142.

20. Paick J, Donatucci C, Lue T. Anatomy of cavernous nerves distal to prostate: microdissection study in adult male cadavers. *Urology*. 1993;42:145–149.

21. Kaul S, Bhandari A, Hemal A, et al. Robotic radical prostatectomy with preservation of the prostatic fascia: a feasibility study. *Urology*. 2005;66:1261–1265.

22. Tewari A, Takenaka A, Mtui E, et al. The proximal neurovascular plate and the tri-zonal neural architecture around the prostate gland: importance in the athermal robotic technique of nerve-sparing prostatectomy. *BJU Int*. 2006;98:314–323.

23. Bianco FJ Jr, Scardino PT, Eastham JA. Radical prostatec-tomy: long-term cancer control and recovery of sexual and urinary function ("trifecta"). *Urology*. 2005;66(S5):83–94.

24. Ward JF, Zincke H, Bergstralh EJ, et al. The impact of surgical approach (nerve bundle preservation versus wide local excision) on surgical margins and biochemical recur-rence following radical prostatectomy. *J Urol*. 2004;172:1328–1332.

25. Goldstraw MA, Dasgupta P, Anderson C, Patil K, Kirby R. Does robotically assisted radical prostatectomy result in better preservation of erectile function? *BJU Int*. 2006;98:721–722.

26. Kaiho Y, Nakagawa H, Saito H, et al. Nerves at the ventral prostatic capsule contribute to erectile function: initial electrophysiological assessment in humans.

27. Takenaka A, Tewari A, Hara R, et al. Pelvic autonomic nerve mapping around the prostate by intraoperative elec-trical stimulation with simultaneous measurement of intra-cavernous and intraurethral pressure. *J Urol*. 2007;177:225–229.

28. Yadav R, Mukherjee S, Hermen M, et al. Multiphoton microscopy of prostate and periprostatic neural tis-sue: a promising imaging technique for improving nerve-sparing prostatectomy. *J Endourol*. 2009;23:861–867.

29. Murphy DG, Kerger M, Crowe H, et al. Operative details and oncological and functional outcome of robotic-assisted laparoscopic radical prostatectomy: 400 cases with a minimum of 12 months follow-up. *Eur Urol*. 2008;55:148–155.

Chapter 22

Robot-Assisted Radical Prostatectomy: A Prostate Surgeon's Perspective

Cole Davis, Matthew R. Cooperberg, and Peter R. Carroll

22.1 Introduction

The availability and promulgation of robotic technology has resulted in a paradigm shift in the use of radical prostatectomy. Historically radical prostatectomy was performed using an open approach, usually the retropubic approach and rarely using a laparoscopic approach. However, robotic-assisted radical prostatectomy (RARP)[1] has swept across the United States at an extremely rapid rate, accounting for approximately 75% of cases performed in 2008. While the early adopters and promoters of RARP were laparoendoscopic specialists, the robotic-assisted approach is becoming the procedure of choice for urologic oncologists as well. In addition, residents are being trained in the use of such technology. The actual costs, benefits, and risks of robotic as compared to open radical prostatectomy remain somewhat controversial. Often lost in such debate is the role of radical prostatectomy, by whatever approach, in the management of prostate cancer, given the considerable stage/grade migration that has occurred because of widespread PSA testing and the mounting concerns regarding prostate cancer over detection and treatment.

Annual prostate cancer mortality in the United States has been declining steadily and substantially over the past 15 years, from a peak of nearly 40,000 in 1994 to a projection of 27,360 in 2009.[2] The explanations for this encouraging trend are controversial, but are almost certainly multifactorial, reflecting advances in both screening and treatment timing and type. This favorable trend is offset, however, by the fact that the number of deaths annually is far exceeded by the number of new diagnoses – 192,280 in 2009.[2] The natural history of prostate cancer, in many cases, may be protracted and/or indolent even in the absence of treatment.[3] Essentially all available treatments may have adverse side effects including declines in health-related quality of life (HRQOL).[4]

22.2 Radical Prostatectomy in Perspective

Radical prostatectomy has been shown in a large, well-controlled randomized trial to offer improved prostate cancer survival compared to watchful waiting.[5] Declines in HRQOL, risks of incontinence, and erectile dysfunction after surgery were offset by progressive local symptoms in the observation arm, with little difference in overall subjective well-being between both groups.[6] Randomized trials comparing prostatectomy to other active treatments, on the other hand, have not been completed successfully, and most retrospective comparative studies have been performed with biochemical endpoints and have been confounded by issues of patient selection, case-mix adjustment, and variation in definition of recurrence.[7] A recent systematic review of the literature concluded that no conclusions may be drawn regarding the benefit of any local treatment approach over another for most patients.[4]

In the absence of clear guidelines or evidence, great variation has been noted in the use of radical prostatectomy,[8] as well as other treatments for prostate cancer.[9]

P.R. Carroll (✉)
Department of Urology, UCSF-Helen Diller Family
Comprehensive Cancer Center, University of California,
San Francisco, CA, USA
e-mail: pcarroll@urology.ucsf.edu

A.K. Hemal, M. Menon (eds.), *Robotics in Genitourinary Surgery*,
DOI 10.1007/978-1-84882-114-9_22, © Springer-Verlag London Limited 2011

Radical prostatectomy is the most common treatment for localized prostate cancer, particularly among those with low-risk disease[10]; with increasing risk, use of prostatectomy falls in favor of radiation and androgen deprivation therapy.[11] Increasingly, active surveillance in lieu of immediate treatment, including radial prostatectomy, may be considered for those men with low-risk disease.[10,12] Conversely, recent series have reported favorable outcomes for men with high-risk prostate cancer, suggesting that prostatectomy might have a greater role in this setting.[13–15] Other studies have demonstrated additional benefit to adjuvant radiation or androgen deprivation therapy,[16,17] suggesting that multimodal therapy including prostatectomy may be an increasingly important strategy for those with high risk disease as defined by serum PSA, T stage, and cancer grade.

As alluded to in the introduction, a significant paradigm shift in the technique of radical prostatectomy has occurred. The open technique of radical prostatectomy was refined considerably over the past 25 years. Many have emphasized the importance of a clear understanding of the pelvic anatomy surrounding the prostate and meticulous surgical technique to ensure urinary control and sexual function while avoiding incomplete cancer excision. Clear visualization with magnification, appropriate lighting, and fine instruments are required for the achievement of good outcomes. The use of fixed retraction, a limited incision followed by complete dorsal vein control, and anatomic nerve-sparing technique are hallmarks of the modern retropubic radical prostatectomy.[18,19] A high standard has been set over many years of outcomes analysis at centers of excellence with high-volume, advanced open surgeons. In our series at UCSF, we have seen a 5-year survival rate of 97% and very low perioperative morbidity associated with open radical retropubic prostatectomy (rectal injury 0.018%, ureteral injury 0.018%, hospital stay 1.8 days with 37% leaving in day 1, median blood loss of 400 cc, and transfusion rate of 1%). This with a patient cohort composed of 67% intermediate and high-risk patients.

After being introduced in 2002, the use of robotic-assisted laparoscopic prostatectomy has grown at an exponential rate with 10% of prostatectomies performed robotically in 2004 growing to near 80% by 2008. Several factors have influenced the dramatic dissemination of this technology leading to patient and hospital demand. Ultimately surgeon preference driven by postoperative outcomes and costs should be the primary factors influencing surgical technique in a health-care system already overburdened with costs and unacceptable variability in outcomes, quality, safety, and access. Unfortunately, definitive oncologic outcomes often require many years of follow-up. Therefore, in order for new techniques and technology to progress at a reasonable pace, surgeons may rely on surrogate oncologic outcomes, as well the documentation of cost, perioperative morbidity and HRQOL endpoints, and their own experience to draw conclusions on a new technique's value. To this end, we incorporated robotic-assisted laparoscopic prostatectomy at UCSF in 2005 and have accumulated a large and rapidly growing experience to date. Robotic technology has improved and refined our ability to identify important anatomic details through magnification, very limited blood loss, and perhaps a refined approach to the neurovascular pedicles. Experienced open surgeons are already quite familiar with pelvic anatomy and the necessary steps to ensure cancer control and preservation of sexual and urinary function. Studies evaluating surrogate oncologic endpoints as well as surgical morbidity have largely shown at least equivalence with the historical, gold standard, open radical retropubic approach. The wide variation in results of these studies must be interpreted with caution due to the heavy influence of selection bias. Some have shown that patients who underwent a robotic – assisted radical prostatectomy had higher levels of regret compared to those who underwent an open approach, suggesting that patients' expectations for an improved outcome with the use of new technology may be higher.[20] A recent review of case series evaluating comparative data between surgical approaches for radical prostatectomy indicated an overall advantage to the robotic approach.[21] Operative time has been a major factor influencing the open surgeon's consideration for implementation of a laparoscopic or robotic-assisted program. However, the comprehensive review found that operative times for open RP, robotic RP, and laparoscopic RP have become similar with weighted means of 147, 164, and 227 min, respectively.[21]

Surgical learning curves exist for all procedures, and radical prostatectomy is no exception. The learning curve for open techniques has been described by several authors including Catalona et al. as requiring greater than 100 cases to acquire baseline proficiency.[22] The shift from open to laparoscopic radical prostatectomy requires a completely new skill set for the open surgeon due to its decreased range of motion, two-dimensional vision, and reduced haptic feedback.[23] It has been estimated that laparoscopic radical prostatectomy requires 50–100 cases before the learning curve begins to level.[24] While some insist robotic-assisted laparoscopic prostatectomy requires similar effort for proficiency, considerable debate exists as to the number of cases needed. The robotic interface to laparoscopic surgery provides a much more comfortable environment for an experienced open surgeon to work within. Magnified vision with loupes is replicated and potentially improved by the robotic camera; the disorientation is reduced as are the range of motion problems encountered during the learning curve of laparoscopic techniques. A large portion of the open prostatectomy learning curve involves acquiring a detailed understanding of the anatomic relationships associated with good nerve-sparing technique and interpretation of tissue planes to ensure negative margin status. This observation has led several high-volume experienced surgeons to conclude that a much shorter learning curve is may be required for mastery of the robotic approach if a firm base of open experience has previously been achieved. Alternatively, Herrell and Smith have stated that surgeons advanced in open radical retropubic prostatectomy are likely to hold higher standards for their performance and thus prolonging the learning curve required to achieve results similar to large open series.[25] If a 4-h operative time is considered an indicator of proficiency for robotic RP, then Zorn et al. found that 120 cases were required to consistently achieve this goal.[26] On the other hand, Ahlering et al. reported a decrease in 4-h operative time and 150 mL blood loss after just 12 robotic-assisted laparoscopic prostatectomy cases (though a positive margin rate of 35%) in the hands of an experienced open surgeon.[27] However, experience counts and all surgeons, whether open, laparoscopic, or robotic, need to be committed to having the necessary volume, environment, and commitment to life-long surgical learning that will best ensure good outcomes for their patients.

Ultimately oncologic outcomes must be the primary concern of any urologist performing prostatectomy by any approach available. Evaluation of the large, multi-institutional community, and university-based CaPSURE database revealed a positive surgical margin after radical prostatectomy for localized disease is an independent predictor of recurrence.[28] Data from another large international database indicated 10-year freedom from recurrence drops from approximately 80 to 40% with a positive surgical margin.[29] Relatively long-term oncologic outcomes data are still lacking for robotic RP, but given the predictive ability of positive surgical margins, the oncologic efficacy debate regarding surgical approach becomes a debate, to some degree, on surgical margins. Review of our institutional database has supported the use of the robotic approach. Characteristics of both our open RP and robotic-assisted RP patient cohorts have similar clinical and pathologic stage and grade. No significant difference has been seen in positive surgical margin rate between open RP (16%) and robotic RP (18%) ($p < 0.01$) (Table 22.1). More importantly, the biochemical-free survival has shown no significant difference between open RP (94%) and robotic RP (91%) at 3-year follow-up incorporating our entire robotic RP series (Fig. 22.1). Length of stay, estimated blood loss, and transfusion rates have all shown advantages for the robotic approach (Table 22.1). It is recognized that the benefits, although statistically significant, may lack the clinical significance that might be seen elsewhere, given the very positive experience documented with the open technique at UCSF. The risk of bladder neck contracture, although low with the open technique, appears to be reduced with the robotic approach. Comprehensive reviews of outcomes comparing open RP, laparoscopic RP, and robotic RP reveal an advantage with the robotic approach when evaluating estimated blood loss, complication rate, and positive margin rate while requiring similar operative time.[21,25] Several reports have described the equivalence of positive margin rates for laparoscopic/robotic prostatectomy vs. open prostatectomy.[27,30–34] Smith and colleagues reported positive margin rates of 24.1%

Table 22.1 Comparison of open and robotic-assisted radical prostatectomy

Characteristic	Open (mean, SD)	Robotic (mean, SD)	p value
Length of stay	1.8 (1.21)	1.6 (1.04)	<0.01
Blood loss	509 (375)	215 (160)	<0.01
Positive margins	16%	18%	<0.01
Bladder neck contracture	3%	1%	0.02

Fig. 22.1 PSA relapse-free or second treatment-free survival for contemporary men undergoing open ($N = 687$) or robotic-assisted ($N = 403$) radical prostatectomy with adequate follow-up ($p = 0.14$)

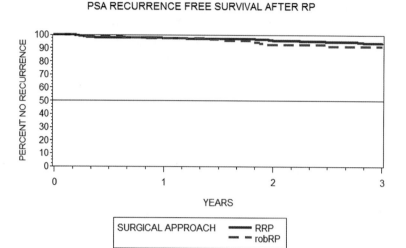

PSA RECURRENCE FREE SURVIVAL AFTER RP

for open prostatectomy compared to 9.4% for robotic-assisted prostatectomy in pT2 patients and 60 vs. 50% in the open vs. robotic groups, respectively, for pT3 patients.[35] Additionally, the review data reveal a mean positive margin rate of 12.5, 19.6, and 23.5% for robotic RP, laparoscopic RP, and open RP, respectively, although the open series had more pT3 patients.[21] The apparent equivalence or even advantage in positive margin rate with the use of robotic assistance seems to hold true even with decreased robotic experience in the hands of experienced open and laparoscopic surgeons as evidenced by Trabulsi et al. Their study found an 18% positive margin rate in 150 laparoscopic RPs, followed by a 6% rate in their first 50 robotic RPs. The difference remained significant even when considering only pT2 disease.[36] Obviously, positive margin rates are affected not only by technique but also by patient selection. Low positive margin rates are seen most often in those with low-grade, low-volume disease, a patient population that may be equally good candidates for surveillance in lieu of immediate treatment. Alternatively, avoiding surgery in those with higher risk disease because of concerns about positive margins may deny this group of patients treatment, which may be associated with improved outcomes as compared to the initial use of other therapeutic modalities as alluded previously.

A report by Hu et al. has called into question the oncologic efficacy of robotic-assisted laparoscopic prostatectomy. The authors reported a statistically significant decrease in the length of stay for patients undergoing the robotic-assisted and laparoscopic approaches as compared to the open approach, but a significant increase in the requirement for salvage therapy was seen in the robotic group (27.8 vs. 9.1%) as well as a significant increase in postoperative anastomotic strictures.[37] This difference became insignificant when evaluating the results of high-volume robotic and laparoscopic surgeons. Studies have also shown equivalence in hospital stay length and recovery time for robotic and open approaches.[38] High variability is seen in the rates of continence and potency with consistently high rates being reported from high-volume surgeons within high-volume centers (continence 95%, potency 65–85%), and very few prospective studies evaluating HRQOL comparing open vs. laparoscopic vs. robotic prostatectomy have been reported.

There is little debate as to the cost in-effectiveness of a robotic prostatectomy program when compared directly to a stable or growing open radical prostatectomy practice. With high purchase prices, costly maintenance contracts, slightly longer operative times, similar hospital stays, and fixed reimbursement, conversion to a robotic prostatectomy program can be costly. In a meta-analysis using models based on the literature and local costs, Lotan and colleagues found a US $1,726 per-case cost advantage of open radical retropubic prostatectomy over the robotic approach. This advantage remained US $1,155 even after discounting the original purchase price of the robot.[39,40] Actual costs rather than models were used in a more recent study that found the open retropubic approach to be less expensive (US $2,315) per case than the robotic approach. This cost difference was generated primarily by the surgical supply cost since purchase and maintenance costs of the robot were excluded.[41] However, such costs can be offset by potentially improved outcomes, shorter hospital stay, earlier return to work, improved HRQOL, and less preoperative morbidity.

22.3 Summary

Radial prostatectomy is an important and effective treatment modality for a very large number of men with prostate cancer. Its use, whether done open or with robotic assistance, will be refined in the coming years, given the current emphasis on comparative effectiveness. Cancer control, urinary function, and sexual function after prostatectomy are more dependent on surgeon training and technical expertise than approach. The use of robot assistance for laparoscopic prostatectomy has enabled high-volume open surgeons to translate their experience and expertise into precisely executed laparoscopic steps without the prohibitively long learning curve required for standard laparoscopic radical prostatectomy.

References

1. Castle EP, Lee D. Nomenclature of robotic procedures in urology. *J Endourol*. 2008;22: 1467.
2. Jemal A, Siegel R, Ward E, et al. Cancer statistics, 2009. *CA Cancer J Clin*. 2009;54(4):225.
3. Albertsen PC, Hanley JA, Fine J. 20-Year outcomes following conservative management of clinically localized prostate cancer. *JAMA*. 2005;293: 2095.
4. Wilt TJ, MacDonald R, Rutks I, et al. Systematic review: comparative effectiveness and harms of treatments for clinically localized prostate cancer. *Ann Intern Med*. 2008;148: 435.
5. Bill-Axelson A, Holmberg L, Filen F, et al. Radical prostatectomy versus watchful waiting in localized prostate cancer: the Scandinavian prostate cancer group-4 randomized trial. *J Natl Cancer Inst*. 2008;100: 1144.
6. Steineck G, Helgesen F, Adolfsson J, et al. Quality of life after radical prostatectomy or watchful waiting. *N Engl J Med*. 2002;347: 790.
7. Cookson MS, Aus G, Burnett AL, et al. Variation in the definition of biochemical recurrence in patients treated for localized prostate cancer: the American urological association prostate guidelines for localized prostate cancer update panel report and recommendations for a standard in the reporting of surgical outcomes. *J Urol*. 2007;177: 540.
8. Cooper MM, Birkmeyer JD, Bronner KK, et al. *The Quality of Medical Care in the United States: A Report on the Medicare Program*. Hanover, NH: The Center for the Evaluative Clinical Sciences, Dartmouth Medical School; 1999.
9. Shahinian VB, Kuo YF, Freeman JL, et al. Determinants of androgen deprivation therapy use for prostate cancer: role of the urologist. *J Natl Cancer Inst*. 2006;98: 839.
10. Cooperberg MR, Broering JM, Kantoff PW, et al. Contemporary trends in low risk prostate cancer: risk assessment and treatment. *J Urol*. 2007;178: S14.
11. Cooperberg MR, Cowan J, Broering JM, et al. High-risk prostate cancer in the United States, 1990–2007. *World J Urol*. 2008;26: 211.
12. Dall'Era MA, Cooperberg MR, Chan JM, et al. Active surveillance for early-stage prostate cancer: review of the current literature. *Cancer*. 2008;112: 1650.
13. Yossepowitch O, Eastham JA. Radical prostatectomy for high-risk prostate cancer. *World J Urol*. 2008;26: 219.
14. Ward JF, Slezak JM, Blute ML, et al. Radical prostatectomy for clinically advanced (cT3) prostate cancer since the advent of prostate-specific antigen testing: 15-year outcome. *BJU Int*. 2005;95: 751.
15. Berglund RK, Jones JS, Ulchaker JC, et al. Radical prostatectomy as primary treatment modality for locally advanced prostate cancer: a prospective analysis. *Urology*. 2006;67: 1253.
16. Thompson IM, Tangen CM, Paradelo J, et al. Adjuvant radiotherapy for pathological T3N0M0 prostate cancer significantly reduces risk of metastases and improves survival: long-term follow-up of a randomized clinical trial. *J Urol*. 2009;181: 956.
17. Messing EM, Manola J, Yao J, et al. Immediate versus deferred androgen deprivation treatment in patients with node-positive prostate cancer after radical prostatectomy and pelvic lymphadenectomy. *Lancet Oncol*. 2006;7: 47.
18. Walsh PC. Anatomic radical prostatectomy: evolution of the surgical technique. *J Urol*. 1998;160: 2418.
19. Nielsen ME, Schaeffer EM, Marschke P, Walsh PC. High anterior release of the levator fascia improves sexual function following open radical retropubic prostatectomy. *J Urol*. 2008;180(6):2557.
20. Schroeck FR, Krupski TL, Sun L, et al. Satisfaction and regret after open retropubic or robot-assisted laparoscopic radical prostatectomy. *Eur Urol*. 2008;54: 785.
21. Berryhill R, Jhaveri J, Yadav R, et al. Robotic prostatectomy: a review of outcomes compared with laparoscopic and open approaches. *Urology*. 2008;72: 15.
22. Catalona WS, Carvalhal GF, Mager DE, Smith DS. Potency, continence and complication rates in 1,870 consecutive strategies for radical prostatectomy. *J Urol*. 1999;162(2):433.
23. Ficarra V, Cavalleri S, Novara G, Aragona M, Artibani W. Evidence from robot-assisted laparoscopic prostatectomy: a systematic review. *Eur Urol*. 2007;51: 45.
24. Guillonneau B, Vallancien G. Laparoscopic radical prostatectomy: the Montsouris experience. *J Urol*. 2000;163(2):418.
25. Herrell SD, Smith JA Jr. Robotic-assisted laparoscopic prostatectomy: what is the learning curve? *Urology*. 2005;66: 105.

26. Zorn KC, Orvieto MA, Gong EM, et al. Robotic radical prostatectomy learning curve of a fellowship-trained laparoscopic surgeon. *J Endourol*. 2007;21: 441.

27. Ahlering TE, Woo D, Eichel L, Lee DI, Edwards R, Skarecky DW. Robot-assisted versus open radical prostatectomy: a comparison of one surgeon's outcomes. *Urology*. 2004;63(5):819.

28. Grossfeld GD, Chang JJ, Broering JM, Miller DP, Yu J, Flanders SC, et al. Impact of positive surgical margins on prostate cancer recurrence and the use of secondary cancer treatment: data from the CaPSURE database. *J Urol*. 2000;163: 1171.

29. Karakiewicz PI, Eastham JA, Graefen M, et al. Prognostic impact of positive surgical margins in surgically treated prostate cancer: multi-institutional assessment of 5831 patients. *Urology*. 2005;66: 2292.

30. Ghavamian R, Knoll A, Boczko J, Melman A. Comparison of operative and functional outcomes of laparoscopic radical prostatectomy and radical retropubic prostatectomy: single surgeon experience. *Urology*. 2006;67(6):1241.

31. Fromont G, Guillonneau B, Validire P, Vallancien G. Laparoscopic radical prostatectomy, preliminary pathologic evaluation. *Urology*. 2002;60(4):661.

32. Roumeguere T, Bollens R, Vanden Bossche M, Rochet D, Bialek D, Hoffman P, et al. Radical prostatectomy: a prospective comparison of oncological and functional results between open and laparoscopic approaches. *World J Urol*. 2003;20(6):360.

33. Menon M, Tewari A, Baize B, Guillonneau B, Vallancien G. Prospective comparison of radical retropubic prostatectomy and robot-assisted anatomic prostatectomy: the Vattikuti Urology Institute experience. *Urology*. 2002;60(5):864.

34. Tewari A, Srivasatava A, Menon M. Members of the VIP team. A prospective comparison of radical retropubic and robot-assisted prostatectomy: experience in one institution. *BJU Int*. 2003;92(3):205.

35. Smith JA Jr, Chan RC, Chang SS, et al. A comparison of the incidence and location of positive surgical margins in robotic assisted laparoscopic radical prostatectomy and open retropubic radical prostatectomy. *J Urol*. 2007;178(6):2385.

36. Trabulsi EJ, Linden. RA, Bomella LG, McGinnis DE, Strup SE, Lallas CD. The addition of robotic surgery to an established laparoscopic radical prostatectomy program: effect on positive surgical margins. *Can J Urol*. 2008;15(2):3994.

37. Hu JC, Wang Q, Pashos CL, Lipsitz SR, Keating NL. Utilization and outcomes of minimally invasive radical prostatectomy. *J Clin Oncol*. 2008;26(14): 2278.

38. Nelson B, Kaufman M, Broughton G, Cookson MS, Chang SS, Herrell SD, et al. Comparison of length of hospital stay between radical retropubic prostatectomy and robotic assisted laparoscopic prostatectomy. *J Urol*. 2007;177(3):929.

39. Lotan Y. Economics of robotics in urology. *Cur Opin Urol*. 2010;20: 92.

40. Lotan Y, Cadeddu JA, Gettman MT. The new economics of radical prostatectomy: cost comparison of open, laparoscopic, and robot assisted techniques. *J Urol*. 2004;172(4pt1):1431.

41. Bolenz C, Gupta A, Hotze T, et al. Cost comparison of robotic, laparoscopic, and open radical prostatectomy for prostate cancer. *Eur Urol*. 2009; doi:10.1016/j.eururo.2009.11.008.

Chapter 23

Cautery-Free Technique of Robot-Assisted Radical Prostatectomy: Impact on Nerve Preservation and Long-Term Outcome on Recovery of Sexual Function

David S. Finley, Anthony J. Costello, and Thomas E. Ahlering

In this chapter we discuss cavernous neuroanatomy, mechanisms of nerve injury, and strategies to minimize damage including the emerging use of local hypothermia. We summarize our surgical technique for cautery-free robotic prostatectomy with an emphasis on neurovascular bundle dissection and report on potency outcomes.

23.1 Introduction

The anatomic basis for erectile function and the technique for nerve-sparing radical retropubic prostatectomy were first described by Lepor and Walsh in 1983.[1] While early emphasis was placed on proper anatomic dissection of the neurovascular bundle (NVB), more recently, however, the avoidance of "trauma" has developed as an important yet incompletely understood factor. Accumulating evidence suggests that trauma to the NVB is multifactorial. While direct injury to the NVB can occur by traction (stretching) or mechanical damage, other mechanisms occur, such as thermal injury and inflammation. In this chapter we will examine anatomic principles of the cavernous nerve preservation, athermal techniques for nerve preservation during robot-assisted radical prostatectomy (RARP), nerve injury, and potency outcomes.

D.S. Finley (✉)
UCLA Department of Urology, Clark Urology Center,
Los Angeles, CA, USA
e-mail: dfinley@mednet.ucla.edu

23.2 Cavernous Neuroanatomy

Walsh and Donker[2] described the tortuous path of the parasympathetic nerves that run from the pelvic plexus past the seminal vesicles and then along the posterolateral aspect of the prostate between the true capsule and the lateral prostatic fascia (the supralevator pathway); the nerves continue on just posterior and lateral to the urethra where they pierce the urogenital diaphragm and continue on below the pubic bone (the so-called infra-levator pathway) where there are delicate neural interconnections at the penile hilum between the cavernous and dorsal nerves, Fig. 23.1.[3,4] Recently, much attention has been paid to the network of nerves that surround the prostate and seminal vesicles. Tewari et al.[5] described this lattice work of interconnecting nerves as a hammock, which they believe are crucial to potency. Takenaka and associates[6] performed precise gross and histologic dissections of male cadavers defining the cranial and caudal paths of the cavernous nerves. Their group determined that, in most individuals, the traditional NVBs contain few parasympathetic nerve components proximal to the prostato-vesical junction. Instead, parasympathetic nerve branches configured in a "spray-like" distribution were found approaching the dorso-lateral prostate at least 2 cm below the prostato-vesical junction. Of note, in some individuals, they noted the cavernous nerves appeared to be located deep to the traditional NVB. Such a finding may account for the rare patient who retains sexual function following non-nerve-sparing surgery. In a corollary paper, Takenaka et al.[7] identified the presence of pelvic autonomic ganglion cells, which lack the capacity for regeneration and hence may contribute to recovery of potency.

A.K. Hemal, M. Menon (eds.), *Robotics in Genitourinary Surgery*,
DOI 10.1007/978-1-84882-114-9_23, © Springer-Verlag London Limited 2011

Fig. 23.1 Supralevator and infra-levator neural pathways of the cavernous nerves (reproduced with courtesy of Elsevier)

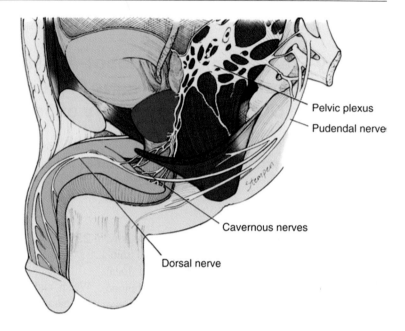

Pelvic plexus

Pudendal nerve

Cavernous nerves

Dorsal nerve

Ganglion cells were found throughout the surfaces of the pelvic viscera including the pelvic plexus, the seminal vesicles, the levator ani muscle, the bladder, the prostate as well as the NVB. The number and distribution of these ganglia varied tremendously between specimens, suggesting an explanation for variability in patient susceptibility or resistance to impotence.

Interestingly, similar studies by Tewari and colleagues have also shown that the pelvic plexus is located on the lateral wall of the rectum.[8,9] The midpoint of the plexus (proximal neurovascular plate) was found to correspond approximately to the tip of the seminal vesicle. These authors, like Takenaka, also reported the presence of multiple autonomic ganglia in the vicinity of the cavernous nerves. Both authors described interconnections between the left and right cavernous nerves along the anterior rectal wall within Denonvilliers' fascia. Unlike Takenaka, however, Tewari and associates noted cavernous branches of the pelvic plexus coalescing to form a more traditional "bundle" that runs within a triangular area (the neurovascular triangle) between the inner and outer layers of the periprostatic fascia and Denonvilliers' fascia. The inner layer of periprostatic fascia (prostatic fascia) forms the medial vertical wall of this triangle; the outer layer of periprostatic fascia (lateral pelvic fascia) forms the lateral wall, and the posterior wall of this triangle is formed by the anterior layer of Denonvilliers' fascia. This triangular space is

wide near the base of the prostate and becomes narrower near the apex. Menon contends that additional nerves important for sexual function exist within the periprostatic fascia that covers the lateral and anterior surface of the prostate (aptly named the Veil of Aphrodite; see Section 23.8).[10] The authors acknowledge they have not traced these nerves to the corpora cavernosa. They also hypothesize that because the plane of dissection is away from the cavernosal nerves, other factors such as decreased traction, avoidance of thermal injury, and preservation of extra blood supply may also play a role in preservation of nerve function.

In 2005, Costello and associates reported a detailed description of the plexus of nerves running within the NVB based upon a series of elegant microdissections in human cadavers.[11] They found multiple nerve branches (6–16 in number) that emanated from the pelvic plexus and spread significantly, with up to 3 cm separating the anterior and posterior nerve fibers, much like the findings of Takenaka and associates. Importantly, they found in all 24 dissections, the NVB ran 0.5–2 cm inferior to the tip of the seminal vesicle. Similar to Menon, Costello noted that the NVB courses along the posterolateral border of the prostate within the bounds of lateral pelvic fascia, the pararectal fascia, and Denonvilliers' fascia (Fig. 23.2). However, in distinction to Menon and associates, they feel that the nerves located within the Veil of Aphrodite innervate the prostate only. They also noted branches to the

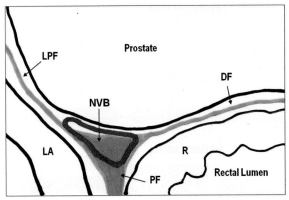

Fig. 23.2 Position of the NVB and its relationship to the prostate (P), rectum (R), and fascial layers. The widening Denonvilliers' fascia (DF) laterally fuses with the lateral pelvic fascia (LPF) and pararectal fascia (PF). The posterior and lateral divisions of the NVB run within these fibrous leaves

levator ani and anterior rectum. Similar to Takenaka, Costello found that the nerves converge at the mid-prostate, forming a more condensed bundle, and then diverge again when approaching the prostatic apex, where they divide into numerous small branches that descend along the posterolateral aspect of the membranous urethra before penetrating the corpora cavernosa. Figure 23.3 demonstrates the functional organization of the NVB according to their findings.

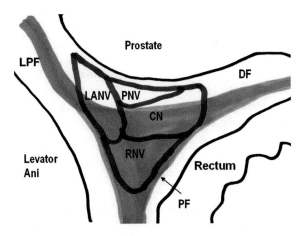

Fig. 23.3 Functional organization of the NVB: RNV, neurovascular supply to the rectum; DF, Denonvilliers' fascia; PF, pararectal fascia; LPF, lateral pelvic fascia; LANV, neurovascular supply to levator ani; PNV, neurovascular supply to the prostate; CN, cavernosal nerves

23.3 Classification of Nerve Injury

Injury to peripheral nerves (as opposed to central or spinal cord injuries) was initially classified by Sir Herbert Seddon in 1943 (Fig. 23.4).[12] According to his classification, three categories of severity occur: (1) *Neurapraxia*: a mild compression, blunt impact, or stretch injury to the nerve with no structural damage. A concussion-like state results in a transient conduction block from which full recovery is likely to occur; recuperation may take hours to weeks; (2) *Axonotmesis*: a moderately severe injury, which results in axonal disruption and Wallerian degeneration; the nerve can regenerate or regrow from the point of injury to the end organ at approximately 1 in./month – recovery takes 8–24 months; (3) *Neurotmesis*: occurs after severe injury or laceration that transects the nerve completely with no capacity for regrowth. A neuroma or scar may form resulting in a permanent injury with a potential for only partial recovery. During radical prostatectomy, injury to the pelvic nerves and neurovascular bundles (i.e., wide excision, partial excision, transection, or incision of the NVB) occurs according to this mechanism along a spectrum of nerve injury.

23.4 Thermal Injury

The use of thermal energy on or near the nerves is a major mechanism of damage leading to delayed or impaired recovery of potency. An increase in temperature of just 4–41°C can produce neural injury.[13–15] At 45–55°C, coagulation occurs.[16] As temperatures continue to rise beyond that point, cell death occurs, with denaturation occurring at 57–60°C and protein coagulation at 65°C.[17] Donzelli and associates have shown that both monopolar and bipolar cautery cause primarily thermal injury to nearby neural tissue.[18]

Importantly, the use of thermal energy can have effects beyond the site of cautery. Mandhani and colleagues measured temperature changes at the NVB during RARP with monopolar and bipolar cautery.[19] The average temperature rise with monopolar and bipolar cautery at the NVB during distant (>1 cm from the NVB) anterior black neck incision was 43.6 and 38.8°C, respectively, after approximately 60 s

Fig. 23.4 Classification of nerve injury according to Seddon[12]

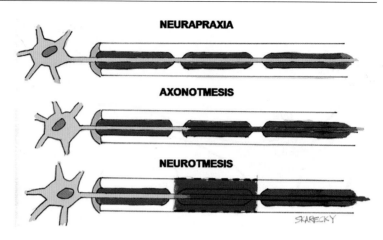

of cautery. During NVB dissection itself using both cautery modalities, the mean temperatures within the NVB measured within 1 cm of the cautery rose to 53.6 and 60.9°C, respectively. The average time for the temperature to return to baseline with each modality was 3.4 and 6.4 s, respectively.

A landmark paper by Ong and associates described the effects of electrocautery and thermal injury on cavernous nerves performed in a canine model.[20] In this study, monopolar electrocautery, bipolar electrocautery, and harmonic shears were compared to standard suture ligatures for unilateral NVB dissection. The contralateral bundle was not dissected and acted as an internal control. Upon cavernous nerve stimulation, only the energy-free (suture ligature) group maintained similar-to-baseline intracavernosal pressure responses immediately after dissection and 2 weeks later. The other modalities using electrical energy, heat, or both all resulted in a >95% decrease in cavernosal pressures. Histologic studies comparing the individual groups confirmed an increased amount of inflammation associated with the use of heat and/or electrocautery. Because of these findings, transection of the vascular pedicles should be accomplished without thermal energy, unless thermoprotective simultaneous cold irrigation is being used.

Currently we are investigating the use of judicious point monopolar cautery with concurrent cold, 4°C, irrigation (see Section 23.6) to minimize collateral thermal injury. When cautery is used we generally use the lowest effective power setting: 10 W at the endopelvic fascia and 35 W at PVP. We find that point cautery using a single blade of the monopolar scissors is most efficient and precise.

23.5 Inflammatory Damage

Following primary injury (direct mechanical trauma of dissection, traction, and thermal energy) to the NVB and other sensitive tissues there is undoubtedly a secondary wave of inflammatory damage that ensues possibly leading to additional delays in functional recovery of the erectile nerves. The inflammatory cascade includes activation of coagulation factors, pro-inflammatory cytokine formation, hypoxia, microcirculatory impairment from endothelial damage, acidosis, free radical production, and apoptosis.[21] Neutrophil and macrophage infiltration with subsequent release of proteolytic enzymes further contribute to tissue destruction.[22,23]

23.6 Hypothermia

Theoretically, this secondary inflammatory cascade might be blocked (or at least mitigated) with the use of local tissue hypothermia. Application of hypothermia pre-emptively (before dissection starts) should prepare tissues for imminent damage by lowering their metabolic rate and oxygen demands. With sufficient temperature reduction, the cell enters into a quiescent state of low energy utilization. When injury ensues, energy reserves are available for repair without going into anaerobic metabolism. As a result, less lactate formation occurs, protein synthesis is preserved, and most importantly, the inflammatory cascade is blunted. With less pro-inflammatory molecules and free radical species generated, the risk of apoptotic cell death is reduced. Tissue damage from leukocyte infiltration is further reduced because cooling also blocks adhesion molecule transcription and inhibits neutrophil adherence.[24]

The use of local tissue hypothermia for injury is well established. Everyone is familiar with applying an ice pack to an injured extremity. Icing is well known to greatly reduce pain and edema after closed soft tissue injury.[25,26] There is objective proof of this therapeutic effect; Schaser and coworkers quantified this effect by assessing microvascular permeability after controlled striated muscle injury in rats with or without superficial cold therapy for 20 min.[27] The cold-therapy group was found to have significantly decreased interstitial fluorescent-labeled albumin levels compared to sham animals. In addition, cold therapy was found to preserve microcapillary density and reduce leukocyte adhesion, chemotaxis, and myonecrosis. Kelly and colleagues showed that regional hypothermia to 4°C protected against ischemic peripheral nerve injury after prolonged application of a tourniquet to the hind limb in rats.[28]

Hypothermia has been demonstrated to have a dramatic protective impact in numerous experimental injury models of the central and peripheral nervous systems. The use of mild to moderate hypothermia (i.e., 33–28°C) has been shown to be effective in shielding neurons from damage. In a rabbit model of spinal cord ischemia, Isaka and colleagues applied trans-vertebral cold packs and infused cold saline into a cross-clamped aorta to produce spinal cord cooling.[29] A modest reduction in spinal cord temperature of just 4.3°C completely prevented paraplegia compared to complete paraplegia in all of the control rabbits. Sun and coworkers studied the effects of hypothermia on protecting guinea pig optic nerves from stretch injury to the optic nerve.[30] Significant axonal ultra structural changes occurred under room temperature conditions. In contrast, optic nerves that were maintained under moderate hypothermia (32°C) for 2 h showed no difference compared with sham-operated animals.

A large body of clinical data exist demonstrating the value of hypothermia for ischemic events such as anoxic brain injury, cardiac arrest, and prevention of spinal cord injury during thoracic–aortic aneurysm repair.[31–33] Cambria and coworkers reported among patients undergoing thoracic–aortic aneurysm a 3% rate of spinal cord injury in 61 patients treated with hypothermia induced by continuous epidural infusion of 4°C saline compared with 23% in 55 matched controls ($p < 0.001$).[34]

We have implemented two strategies to accomplish local hypothermia. The first uses a cooling balloon in the rectum which effectively cools the NVBs and surrounding structures (i.e., urethra).[35] The second technique utilizes adjunctive cold irrigation by the laparoscopic assistant. Previous studies have shown that irrigation may not only protect against thermal energy but also minimize inflammatory damage. Donzelli et al. demonstrated the thermoprotective effects of simultaneous room temperature irrigation during bipolar cautery to protect rat sciatic nerves.[18] With room temperature normal saline irrigation, they found simultaneous irrigation significantly reduced the temperature response to cautery. Blinded review of the cauterized nerves found preservation of myelin and axons. Rats that received irrigation showed enhanced functional recovery and less paresis according to the Sciatic Functional Index score. During nerve-sparing RARP, we use copious cold irrigation simultaneously with minimal cautery to lower target tissue temperatures and minimize collateral thermal injury. In addition to cold irrigation, we also use an endorectal cooling balloon to lower tissue temperatures.

23.7 Preoperative Planning

Careful preoperative evaluation of potency is a key factor in tracking patient outcomes and expectations after surgery. It is impossible and inappropriate to evaluate the presence of preoperative sexual function by asking the patient, "Are you potent?" It is mandatory to have a quantitative assessment of potency, and it should be acquired in an unbiased manner via validated questionnaire. There are a number of validated questionnaires that assess sexual function. We prefer the International Index of Erectile Function (IIEF) to reliably assess preoperative sexual function. It has been our experience that men are more likely to complete shorter forms such as the abbreviated 5-item questionnaire known as IIEF-5 (see Appendix), also identified as Sexual Health Inventory for Men (SHIM). An IIEF-5 score of 22–25 is considered normal; 17–21 mild; 12–16 mild to moderate; 8–11 moderate, and 1–7 severe dysfunction.

It is recognized that age, especially over age 65, has a deleterious effect on return of sexual function. Lastly, medical conditions (diabetes, coronary artery disease, and hyperlipidemia) and associated medications (e.g., anti-hypertensives) can have a significant negative impact on return of sexual function. It is very important to evaluate and decide preoperatively which patients are candidates for bilateral vs. unilateral nerve preservation based on factors that assess risk for extra-capsular extension. From a clinical basis, most surgeons assess risk based on the clinical T stage, Gleason score, the number of cores, and the volume of disease on prostate needle biopsy. Some surgeons will assess risk of extra-capsular extension based on endorectal magnetic resonance imaging.[36,37] It is also necessary for surgeons to know their own pattern of positive margin locations in order to guide and counsel patients. The important point, however, is that it is indeed a risk assessment. With adequate risk assessment, patients can and should play a most definitive role in the decision process of sparing or excising a NVB. We recommend wide excision with abnormal digital findings and/or higher volume disease (>30–40% cores involvement) and higher grade disease (Gleason score 4 + 3 and higher).

23.8 Neurovascular Bundle Dissection

As discussed previously, a major mechanism of neurapraxic injury is traction. In this regard, there are two primary schools of thought existing with regard to the direction of NVB dissection and minimization of nerve traction. The technique as described by Walsh is considered retrograde as the prostate is freed initially at the apex and carried back toward the bladder. In this technique one first releases the superficial levator fascia at the bladder neck to release the bundle laterally, making it easier to free the NVB posteriorly at the apex.[38] Once the medial border of the NVB is identified at the apex, the dissection is carried posteriorly toward the rectum. The NVB is then dissected, beginning at the apex and moving toward the base. Walsh notes that if unilateral wide excision is planned, the contralateral NVB should be freed from the prostate at the apex to avoid traction injury. The counter-school favors antegrade dissection of the NVB during laparoscopic or robotic-assisted radical prostatectomy. Some believe an antegrade approach has several advantages. First, geometrically speaking, the use of long straight instruments makes the antegrade approach more practical because it is easier to see (especially with a 30° lens). This technique also allows for dissection in an intuitive, straightforward direction toward the penis, as compared to trying to see around the prostate and dissect back toward the bladder. In addition, this dissection may be accomplished with less traction on the NVBs. When contemplating forces associated with traction during the antegrade approach, we believe there is less risk of traction injury when the prostate is dissected off of the NVB rather than dissecting the NVB off of the prostate.

Patel combines an antegrade and a retrograde approach. After controlling the pedicles with clips, he initiates the separation of the nerve in the mid-prostate and dissects antegrade to the apex and retrograde to the PVP. Patel developed this hybrid technique to more clearly separate the NVB from the PVP. He notes this separation permits precise clipping of the PVP without concern for inadvertent injury to the NVB, which he believes is not necessarily the case with a pure antegrade approach.[39]

Our technique begins with division of the PVP (see Section 23.11). The transition between the PVP and NVB is reliably identified when after transecting the last vessels in the PVP the prostate suddenly springs or releases forward. On the right side, we use the fourth arm as a fixed retractor to gently hold up on the prostate. An interfascial dissection is done in antegrade fashion sharply with scissors. The assistant uses the suction irrigator to hold the rectum down with minimal lateral traction on the NVB. Bleeders are left alone, sutured, or controlled with point monopolar cautery with simultaneous hypothermic irrigation. As the dissection is carried toward the urethra, the prostate is continually regrasped with the left hand (PK dissector) to "see around the corner." On the left side, the assistant holds the prostate with a grasper just superolateral to the seminal vesicle and gently pulls the prostate out of the pelvis toward the camera and medially. The antegrade approach also facilitates the difficult task of separating the NVB from the urethra until last, when the prostate is completely mobilized. Near the apex, an important maneuver which can facilitate release of the NVB is to switch the scissors to the left for dissection of the left NVB (or to the right for left-handed surgeons). This allows the surgeon to avoid crossing instruments.

23.9 Irrigation

Another important instrument in terms of exposure and keeping the field clear is the suction irrigator. During dissection of the NVB, the assistant uses a grasper to retract the prostate upward, out of the pelvis, and medially. The suction irrigator is used to gently retract the rectum and NVB laterally, which accentuates the proper plane of dissection between the bundle and the prostatic capsule. If the side holes on the suction irrigator are pointed at this plane, irrigation can be applied toward the area of dissection without obstructing or losing exposure. Since January 2008 we have been using 4°C sterile water irrigation. Copious cold irrigation is used during the nerve dissection not only to improve visualization, but also to promote local hypothermia of the neurovascular bundle (and urethra), minimize collateral thermal spread (if cautery is used), and reduce inflammation.[35] We prefer the Davol X-stream irrigation pump (Davol Inc, Cranston, RI), which can be used on gravity, low-power, or high-power settings. We also favor a re-usable 5 mm/33 cm suction tip with side holes or a 5 mm/46 cm suction tip for larger patients.

23.10 Anatomic Factors Affecting Operative Technique

23.10.1 High Anterior Release and the Veil of Aphrodite

Menon's technique emphasizes the presence of accessory nerves located in the anterior prostatic fascia which may be important for potency. In their approach, the lateral prostatic fascia is incised anteriorly – the so-called high anterior release (HAR) or Veil of Aphrodite. In 2005, Kaul et al. reported on outcomes with this technique. A total of 154 consecutive men underwent RARP with antegrade NVB preservation and Veil of Aphrodite modification.[40] The dissection for the Veil of Aphrodite begins by entering the intrafascial plane between the prostatic fascia and the capsule, starting infero-laterally near the PVP and carried up to the apex. The authors note that at the conclusion of the dissection, an intact "Veil" of periprostatic tissue should extend from the pubo-urethral ligament to the bladder neck. Among men with an average age of 57.4 and preoperative SHIM of >21, at 12 months 96% were having intercourse (defined as an answer of ≥ 2 to question 2 of the SHIM), 69% had "normal erections," and 20.6% achieved a median post-operative SHIM of 22. Of note, oncologic efficacy was not compromised with this technique – positive surgical margin rates among patients with pT2 disease was 5%, mostly at the apex, but none within the region of the Veil of Aphrodite.

Walsh's group has also recently described a modification to their interfascial NVB dissection technique which includes a release of the levator fascia much higher on the prostate (more medial and anterior at the apex) than they previously did.[41] In this report, the authors compared outcomes of 93 pre-potent men (IIEF-5 22–25) who underwent bilateral nerve sparing with HAR and 74 patients who underwent standard nerve-sparing radical prostatectomy. Post-operative potency was defined, with or without PDE5 inhibitors, as a IIEF-5 of ≥ 16 and/or a response of "most times or almost always" to the question "In the last 4 weeks, when you attempted sexual intercourse, how often was it satisfactory to you?" Return to baseline was defined as an IIEF-5 of ≥ 22. Of note, overall median age was 53 (range 49–57). Patients who underwent unilateral or bilateral nerve sparing with HAR achieved a 90.9% potency rate compared with 76.8% for patients who did not ($p = 0.03$); 69.7% of men in this HAR group returned to baseline potency status, compared with 54% ($p = 0.07$). The authors suggest that improved potency with this technique occurs due to decreased traction injury as there was no apparent improvement in outcomes when the HAR was unilateral or bilateral.

Anatomically, there is little evidence to support the notion that HAR release preserves more autonomic nerve fibers important for erections. Using intraoperative electrical stimulation nerve mapping during radical prostatectomy, Takenaka and colleagues found that stimulation at the base of the putative NVB (where the more anterior fibers would be running) increased intraurethral pressures rather than intracavernous pressures.[42] Nerve stimulation at the rectal wall

1 cm posterolateral to the putative NVB resulted in increased intracavernous pressure. This finding was substantiated clinically by the previously described study by Kaul et al. who found improved continence rates with the Veil of Aphrodite technique (97% required no pads at 12 months).[40]

Finally, similar controversy exists regarding the presence of nerve tissue responsible for erectile function adjacent to the lateral edge of the seminal vesicle (SV). In our experience, it is difficult to anatomically picture how cavernosal nerves could course along the length of the SVs and then traverse the prostatic vascular pedicle and not be transected in conjunction with the vascular pedicle. We agree with the findings of Costello and associates that these nerves innervate the SVs, bladder neck, and prostate.[11]

23.11 Controlling the Prostatic Vascular Pedicle

The vascular pedicle to the prostate, in our opinion, is the most important factor to successful nerve preservation with the antegrade approach. There are multiple reasons, including the fact that the vascular pedicle is a reliable and easy to identify landmark; it always enters the prostate laterally at the base and is a very sturdy complex that requires sharp transection. Transection of the vascular pedicle is optimized when accomplished with minimal bleeding, and there is growing evidence of the crucial role of no – or minimal – thermal energy in this process. These vessels can be controlled with 5 mm laparoscopic Hem-o-lok clips, temporarily occluded with a vascular bulldog clamp and oversewn later, or cut through cold with point monopolar cautery with concurrent hypothermic irrigation. More recently, we have been controlling the pedicle with an innovative technique adapted from Bhayani: a monocryl suture with a pre-formed loop in the end to create a slipknot. The suture is passed deep and then superficial. The needle is passed through the loop and pulled up. A Hem-o-lok clip is then applied to the suture and cinched down until tight, locking the tension on the suture.

After the vascular pedicle has been transected, identification of the plane between the prostatic capsule and the NVB is reliably simple to identify and enter. At this point, when the last of the PVP vessels are divided

the prostate springs forward and the texture of the tissue dramatically changes, allowing gentle sweeping of the NVB off of the prostatic capsule. As the sweeping process continues toward the apex, smaller but sturdy vessels that enter the prostatic capsule and resist the gentle sweeping are essentially always encountered. These vessels should be transected in order to avoid entering the prostatic capsule and potentially creating a positive surgical margin.

The prostatic vascular pedicle requires cautery, clips, bulldogs, or suture ligation for control. To avoid cavernosal nerve injury while transecting the prostatic vascular pedicle and dissecting the NVB, it is advisable to avoid electrical and/or thermal injury unless thermoprotective simultaneous cold irrigation is being used. Commercially available non-absorbable polymer vascular clips are an option, but the disadvantages are the potential for inadvertently clipping some of the NVB over clips slipping off or migrating into the anastomosis. Many surgeons favor the use of 5 mm Hem-o-lok clips (Weck Closure Systems, Research Triangle Park, NC). The clips can be applied with a standard 5 or 10 mm laparoscopic applier or with a robotic applier. Vessels or tissue packets ranging from 1 to 16 mm can be clipped.

In 2005, both Gill and associates and our group advocated the use of a temporary vascular clamp (bulldog clamp) to occlude the vascular pedicle of the prostate.[43,44] In this technique, the prostate is retracted upward and a straight or curved bulldog clamp (30 mm) is placed on the pedicle approximately 10 mm from the prostate. Cold scissors are used to divide the pedicle. When the PVP is completely divided, the prostate is more mobile and an obvious change occurs signifying the transition to the NVB. Once the nerve sparing is completed, the bulldog clamps are removed, and the pedicles are precisely ligated with absorbable 4-0 suture (i.e., polyglycolic acid) on an RB-1 needle.

23.12 Potency Outcomes with Cautery-Free Technique

Our own potency data with CFT have demonstrated significant improvements compared with early patients in which cautery was used. Previously, we reported

Table 23.1 Potency outcomes over time with cautery vs. cautery-free technique

	3 months	9 months	15 months	24 months
Cautery				
Number of patients	36	34	37	38
All NS	3/36 (8.3%)	5/34 (14.7%)	16/37 (43.2%)	24/38(63.2%)
Bilateral NS	3/26 (11.5%)	4/24 (16.7%)	12/27 (44.4%)	19/28 (67.9%)
Unilateral NS	0/10 (0%)	1/10 (10%)	4/10 (40%)	5/10 (50%)
Cauteryfree				
Number of patients	160	159	96	52
All NS	53/139 (38.1%)	60/86 (69.8%)	51/60 (87%)	46/50 (92.0%)
Bilateral NS	46/120 (38.3%)	51/70 (72.8%)	43/48 (89.6%)	36/38 (94.7%)
Unilateral NS	7/19 (36.8%)	9/16 (56.3%)	8/12 (66.7%)	10/12 (83.3%)

on a select group of men <66 years of age with IIEF scores of 22–25 (to minimize non-surgical factors) who underwent nerve-sparing cautery-free RARP.[45] Group 1 ($N = 23$) had preservation of the NVB with CFT whereas group 2 ($N = 36$) had traditional dissection using bipolar cautery. Data were collected prospectively via validated questionnaires; potency was defined as an erection adequate for vaginal penetration. At 3 months, 43% in the CFT group reported potency vs. just 8.3% in the bipolar-cautery group ($P = 0.003$). In addition, only 18% of those having CFT reported zero penile fullness compared with 68% in the bipolar-cautery group ($P = 0.01$). With subsequent long-term follow-up, at 3, 9, 15, and 24 months only 3 of 36 (8.3%), 5 of 34 (14.7%), 16 of 37 (43.2%), and 24/38 (63.2%) in the cautery group were potent.[46,47] At 24 months their average IIEF-5 was 18.4 and erectile firmness was 75–100% of baseline. The cautery-free group, however, at each time point fared significantly better, with potency rates of 38.1, 69.8, 87, and 92%, respectively (Table 23.1).

Gill's group reported 1-year potency outcomes of an athermal bulldog antegrade NVB-sparing technique and compared the potency data with patients undergoing a thermal-based NVB-sparing technique.[48] The cohort consisted of 76 patients, 22 who had undergone nerve-sparing LRP using a harmonic scalpel and 54 who had undergone nerve-sparing LRP using an energy-free technique. Sexual intercourse ability was defined as the ability to achieve erections sufficient for vaginal penetration with or without the use of phosphodiesterase-5 inhibitors. At 3, 6, 12, and 18 months, 9, 14, 36, and 64% of men were potent in the cautery group vs. 20, 42 ($p = 0.02$), 70 ($p = 0.04$), and 75% in the athermal group. In patients with preoperative SHIM ≥ 22 ($n = 7$ cautery vs. $n = 16$ athermal),

potency rates at 3, 6, 12, and 18 months were 14, 29, 71, and 86% vs. 50, 73, 88, and 83%, respectively ($p=$ non-significant). In this group of men, the mean overall SHIM score at 18 months was 16.6 (69% of baseline) in the cautery group vs. 18.3 (77% of baseline). Erectile function recovered about 6 months faster in patients undergoing energy-free technique. From these data it is evident that patients who underwent athermal technique had superior potency outcomes.

Fagin reported a single surgeon series comparing thermal to athermal techniques.[49] He divided a consecutive series of 400 patients into three groups: group 1 used selective bipolar cautery, group 2 used an athermal technique with Weck clips and posterior NVB dissection ("clip and peel"), and group 3 used an athermal technique with a high anterior/posterior dissection of the NVB. Inclusion criteria were age less than 66, preoperative SHIM score of greater than 14, and bilateral nerve sparing. Potency was evaluated by post-operative SHIM score and erections capable of intercourse were defined as the ability to achieve vaginal penetration. Although sample size was not reported, at 3 months, erections capable of intercourse were achieved by 14% of the men in series 1, 24% of the men in series 2, and 71% of the men in series 3. SHIM scores in each group were 5, 5, and 20, respectively.

23.13 Effect of Unilateral Wide Excision on Potency

Excision of one of the NVBs may be necessary in efforts to control cancer. Walsh et al.[50] and Kundu et al.[51] both reported their experience with unilateral nerve-sparing (UNS) surgery. In 1987, Walsh et al.

reported that 69% of men potent before RP who had unilateral wide excision were potent after RP, compared to 85% who had bilateral NS (BNS). Kundu et al. reported a similar trend in overall potency rates at 18 months, of 53 and 76% after UNS and BNS RP, respectively. A unifying theme among these reports is that doubling the volume of nerve tissue improved potency rates only by about 15–20%. We sought to better understand this disproportionality by evaluating the effect of reducing the volume of cavernous nervous tissue on the time to recovery and overall recovery of sexual function after robotic-assisted RARP by analyzing the return of potency after unilateral wide excision of one NVB vs. preserving both NVBs.[52] We define UNS as preservation of one NVB using a standard interfascial technique on one side and wide excision of the entire NVB on the other side, defined as excision included all tissue from the midline of the rectum from the bladder neck to the urogenital diaphragm. In this chapter, we analyzed a highly selected group of men who were aged ≤65 years and had "normal" preoperative sexual function, i.e., International Index of Erectile Function-5 (IIEF-5) scores of ≥22 to insulate the analysis from non-surgical factors (i.e., patient-related variables) that could adversely affect the recovery of potency. We performed this analysis for two different groups of consecutive patients – cautery and CFT.

We found the mean 2-year IIEF-5 score for potent men in group 1 was 19.0 (11–25) the mean UNS and BNS IIEF-5 scores were statistically equal, at 19.6 (15.7–23.5) and 18.9 (16.6–21.0), respectively ($P = 0.72$). The qualitative results were similar in group 2; the overall IIEF-5 score was 21.2 (16–25) and for UNS and BNS in the CFT group, the mean IIEF-5 score was 22.0 (20.2–23.8) and 21.0 (19.8–22.1), respectively ($P = 0.37$). We also assessed patient-reported "fullness of erections" (vs. preoperative levels) for potent men at 2 years in both groups, with similar findings to the IIEF-5 scores. In group 1, there was no significant difference between the UNS and BNS groups, with percentage fullness (95% CI) of 85.0 (73.0–97.0%) and 79.4 (70.7–88.1%), respectively ($P = 0.53$). Similarly, the mean fullness at 2 years between UNS and BNS in group 2 was not statistically different, at 90.0 (82.8–97.2%) vs. 91.4 (86.3–96.5%), respectively ($P = 0.37$). Thus, when comparing potency with a single NVB vs. two (i.e., essentially doubling of nervous input), there was only a 35% improvement in group 1 and a 15% improvement in group 2. Similar findings with

open and laparoscopic techniques have been reported by others, with ratios of 1.1–1.43.[53–55] Importantly, we found that patients in both groups reported comparable quality of erections at 24 months, whether one or two NVBs were spared, as measured by IIEF-5 scores or an assessment of erectile fullness. Of note, the absolute difference in IIEF-5 score and erectile fullness between UNS and BNS was negligible for both group 1 and 2 (about 1 point and 1.5–5%, respectively). This observation suggests that the remaining NVB will either compensate functionally or cross over somehow (i.e., anatomically or biochemically) to provide similar erectile quality to both corpora as with two NVBs. Analysis of our recovery of potency time lines favors a cross-over mechanism. This information implies that there is significant redundancy in this system. These findings should raise questions about the logic of "maximally" sparing nerves, especially with regard to risking a PSM.

23.14 Conclusion

With a progressive understanding of the neuroanatomy of the male pelvis efforts to preserve the cavernosal nerves during radical prostatectomy have been met with increased success. Great care should be taken to avoid electrocautery, excessive heat application, and traction in the vicinity of the cavernous nerves. Our results using a cautery-free technique seem to promote the return of erectile function. Novel therapies to hasten the recovery of erectile function following RARP, including local hypothermia, are forthcoming.

References

1. Walsh PC, Lepor H, Eggleston JC. Radical prostatectomy with preservation of sexual function: anatomical and pathological considerations. *Prostate*. 1983;4:473.
2. Walsh PC, Donker PJ. Impotence following radical prostatectomy: insight into etiology and prevention. *J Urol*. 1982;128:492.
3. Breza J, Aboseif SR, Orvis BR, Lue TF, Tanagho EA. Detailed anatomy of penile neurovascular structures: surgical significance. *J Urol*. 1989;141:437.
4. Yucel S, Baskin LS. Identification of communicating branches among the dorsal, perineal and cavernous nerves of the penis. *J Urol*. 2003;170:153.

5. Tewari A, Takenaka A, Mtui E, Horninger W, Peschel R, Bartsch G, et al. The proximal neurovascular plate and the tri-zonal neural architecture around the prostate gland: importance in the athermal robotic technique of nerve-sparing prostatectomy. *BJU Int.* 2006;98:314.

6. Takenaka A, Leung RA, Fujisawa M, Tewari AK. Anatomy of autonomic nerve component in the male pelvis: the new concept from a perspective for robotic nerve sparing radical prostatectomy. *World J Urol.* 2006;24(2):136–143.

7. Takenaka A, Kawada M, Murakami G, et al. Interindividual variation in distribution of extramural ganglion cells in the male pelvis: a semi-quantitative and immunohistochemical study concerning nerve-sparing pelvic surgery. *Eur Urol.* 2005;48:46.

8. Tewari A, Peabody JO, Fischer M, et al. An operative and anatomic study to help in nerve sparing during laparoscopic and robotic radical prostatectomy. *Eur Urol.* 2003;43:444.

9. Tewari A, El-Hakim A, Horninger W, et al. Nerve-sparing during robotic radical prostatectomy: use of computer modeling and anatomic data to establish critical steps and maneuvers. *Curr Urol Rep.* 2005;6:126.

10. Savera AT, Kaul S, Badani K, Stark AT, Shah NL, Menon M. Robotic radical prostatectomy with the "Veil of Aphrodite" technique: histologic evidence of enhanced nerve sparing. *Eur Urol.* 2006;49(6):1065–1073; discussion 1073–4.

11. Costello AJ, Brooks M, Cole OJ. Anatomical studies of the neurovascular bundle and cavernosal nerves. *BJU Int.* 2004;94:1071.

12. Seddon HJ. Three types of nerve injury. *Brain.* 1943;66:237–288.

13. Wondergem J, Haveman J, Rusman V, Sminia P, VanDijk JD. Effects of local hyperthermia on the motor function of the rat sciatic nerve. *Int J Radiat Biol.* 1988;53:429–438.

14. Hoogeveen JF, Troost D, Wondergem J, van der Kracht AH, Haveman J. Hyperthermic injury versus crush injury in the rat sciatic nerve: a comparative functional, histopathological and morphological study. *J Neurol Sci.* 1992;108: 55–64.

15. Xu D, Pollock M. Experimental nerve thermal injury. *Brain.* 1994;117:375–384.

16. Smith TL, Smith JM. Electrosurgery in otolaryngology-head and neck surgery: principles, advances, and complications. *Laryngoscope.* 2001;11:769.

17. Lantis JC, Durville FM, Connolly R, Schwaitzberg SD. Comparison of coagulation modalities in surgery. *Laparosc Adv Surg Tech.* 1998;8:381.

18. Donzelli J, Leonetti JP, Wurster RD, Lee JM, Young MR. Neuroprotection due to irrigation during bipolar cautery. *Arch Otolaryngol Head Neck Surg.* 2000;126:149.

19. Mandhani A, Dorsey PJ Jr, Ramanathan R, et al. Real time monitoring of temperature changes in neurovascular bundles during robotic radical prostatectomy: thermal map for nerve-sparing radical prostatectomy. *J Endourol.* 2008;22(10):2313.

20. Ong AM, Su LM, Varkarakis I, et al. Nerve sparing radical prostatectomy: effects of hemostatic energy sources on the recovery of cavernous nerve function in a canine model. *J Urol.* 2004;172:1318.

21. Ni Choileain N, Redmond HP. The immunological consequences of injury. *Surgeon.* 2006;4(1):23–31.

22. Osborn L. Leukocyte adhesion to endothelium in inflammation. *Cell.* 1990;62(1):3–6.

23. Weiss SJ. Tissue destruction by neutrophils. *N Engl J Med.* 1989;320(6):365–376.

24. Westermann S, Vollmar B, Thorlacius H, Menger MD. Surface cooling inhibits tumor necrosis factor-alpha-induced microvascular perfusion failure, leukocyte adhesion, and apoptosis in the striated muscle. *Surgery.* 1999;126(5):881–889.

25. Deal DN, Tipton J, Rosencrance E, Curl WW, Smith TL. Ice reduces edema. *J Bone Joint Surg Am.* 2002;84(9):1573–1578.

26. Laing DR, Dalley DR, Kirk JA. Ice therapy in soft tissue injury. *N Z Med J.* 1973;78:155–158.

27. Schaser KD, Disch AC, Stover JF, Laufer A, Bail HJ, Mittlmeier T. Prolonged superficial local cryotherapy attenuates microcirculatory impairment, regional inflammation, and muscle necrosis after closed soft tissue injury in rats. *Am J Sports Med.* 2007;35:93.

28. Kelly C, Creagh T, Grace PA, Bouchier-Hayes D. Regional hypothermia protects against tourniquet neuropathy. *Eur J Vasc Surg.* 1992;6:288–292.

29. Isaka M, Kumagai H, Sugawara Y, Okada K, Orihashi K, Ohtaki M, et al. Cold spinoplegia and transvertebral cooling pad reduce spinal cord injury during thoracoabdominal aortic surgery. *J Vasc Surg.* 2006;43:1257–1262.

30. Sun X, Tang W, Zheng L. Ultrastructural observation of effect of moderate hypothermia on axonal damage in an animal model of diffuse axonal injury. *Chin J Traumatol.* 2002;5:355–360.

31. Hypothermia after Cardiac Arrest Study Group. Mild therapeutic hypothermia to improve the neurologic outcome after cardiac arrest. *N Engl J Med.* 2002;346: 549–556.

32. Nolan JP, Morley PT, Vanden Hoek TL, Hickey RW and ALS Task Force. Therapeutic hypothermia after cardiac arrest. An advisory statement by the Advanced Life Support Task Force of the International Liaison Committee on Resuscitation. *Resuscitation.* 2003;57:231–235.

33. Celik T, Iyisoy A, Yuksel UC, Celik M, Jata B. Chill therapy in the patients with resuscitated cardiac arrest: a new weapon in the battle against anoxic brain injury. *Int J Cardiol.* 2010;138(3):300–302.

34. Cambria RP, Davison JK. Regional hypothermia for prevention of spinal cord ischemic complications after thoracoabdominal aortic surgery: experience with epidural cooling. *Semin Thorac Cardiovasc Surg.* 1998;10(1): 61–65.

35. Finley DS, Osann K, Skarecky D, Ahlering TE. Hypothermic nerve-sparing radical prostatectomy: rationale, feasibility, and effect on early continence. *Urology.* 2009;73(4):691–696; Epub Febraury 28, 2009.

36. Torricelli P, Barberini A, Cinquantini F, Sighinolfi M, Cesinaro AM. 3-T MRI with phased array coil in local staging of prostatic cancer. *Acad Radiol.* 2008;15(9): 1118–1125.

37. Nishimoto K, Nakashima J, Hashiguchi A, et al. Prediction of extraprostatic extension by prostate specific antigen velocity, endorectal MRI, and biopsy Gleason score in clinically localized prostate cancer. *Int J Urol.* 2008;15(6): 520–523.

38. Walsh PC, Partin AW. Ch. 97, anatomic radical retropubic prostatectomy. In: Wein AJ, *Campbell-Walsh Urology*, 9th ed. Saunders: Philadelphia, PA; 2007.

39. Patel VR. Da Vinci Prostatectomy with the 4th Arm, March 2008 World Robotic Urology Symposium (WRUS) Full-Length Procedure, Intuitive Surgical Video. 2008

40. Kaul S, Savera A, Badani K, Fumo M, Bhandari A, Menon M. Functional outcomes and oncological efficacy of Vattikuti Institute prostatectomy with Veil of Aphrodite nerve-sparing: an analysis of 154 consecutive patients. *BJU Int*. 2006;97(3):467–472.

41. Nielsen ME, Schaeffer EM, Marschke P, Walsh PC. High anterior release of the levator fascia improves sexual function following open radical prostatectomy. *J Urol*. 2008;180:2557–2564.

42. Takenaka A, Tewari A, Hara R, et al. Pelvic autonomic nerve mapping around the prostate by intraoperative electrical stimulation with simultaneous measurement of intracavernous and intraurethral pressure. *J Urol*. 2007;177(1):225–229.

43. Gill IS, Ukimura O, Rubinstein. M. Lateral pedicle control during laparoscopic radical prostatectomy: refined technique. *Urology*. 2005;65:23–27.

44. Ahlering TE, Eichel L, Chou D, Skarecky DW. Feasibility study for robotic radical prostatectomy cautery-free neurovascular bundle preservation. *Urology*. 2005;65(5):994–997.

45. Ahlering TE, Eichel L, Skarecky D. Rapid communication: early potency outcomes with cautery-free neurovascular bundle preservation with robotic laparoscopic radical prostatectomy. *J Endourol*. 2005;19(6):715–718.

46. Ahlering TE, Skarecky D, Borin J. Impact of cautery versus cautery-free preservation of neurovascular bundles on early return of potency. *J Endourol*. 2006;20(8):586–589.

47. Ahlering TE, Eichel L, Skarecky D. Evaluation of long-term thermal injury using cautery during nerve sparing robotic prostatectomy. *Urology*. 2008;72(6):1371–1374.

48. Gill IS, Ukimura O. Thermal energy-free laparoscopic nerve-sparing radical prostatectomy: one-year potency outcomes. *Urology*. 2007;70(2):309–314.

49. DaFagin R. Vinci prostatectomy: athermal nerve sparing and effect of the technique on erectile recovery and negative margins. *J Robotic Surg*. 2007;1:139–143.

50. Walsh PC, Epstein JI, Lowe FC. Potency following radical prostatectomy with wide unilateral excision of one neurovascular bundle. *J Urol*. 1987;138:823.

51. Kundu SD, Roehl KA, Eggener SE, Antenor JA, Han M, Catalona WJ. Potency, continence and complications in 3,477 consecutive radical retropubic prostatectomies. *J Urol*. 2004;172:2227.

52. Finley DS, Rodriguez E Jr, Skarecky DW, Ahlering TE. Quantitative and qualitative analysis of the recovery of potency after radical prostatectomy: effect of unilateral vs bilateral nerve sparing. *BJU Int*. 2009;104(10):1484–1489.

53. Catalona WJ, Bigg SW. Nerve-sparing radical prostatectomy: evaluation of results after 250 patients. *J Urol*. 1990;143:538.

54. Michl U, Friedrich MG, Graefen M, Haese A, Heinzer H, Huland H. Prediction of sexual function after nerve-sparing radical retropubic prostatectomy. *J Urol*. 2006;176:227.

55. Katz R, Salomon L, Hoznek A, de la Taille A, Vordos D, Cicco A, et al. Patient reported sexual function following laparoscopic radical prostatectomy. *J Urol*. 2002;168:2078.

Chapter 24

Current Concepts in Cavernosal Neural Anatomy and Imaging and Their Implications for Nerve-Sparing Radical Prostatectomy

Gerald Y. Tan, Sonal Grover, Atsushi Takenaka, Prasanna Sooriakumaran, and Ashutosh K. Tewari

24.1 Introduction

Over the past 2 decades, widespread prostate-specific antigen screening has resulted in a downward stage migration of prostate cancer, with most patients being diagnosed nowadays at a younger age with early organ-confined disease.[1-3] With radical prostatectomy delivering better survival outcomes,[4,5] preservation of sexual function has become an increasing priority for patients deliberating upon surgery as first-line treatment. Despite advances in surgical technique and technologies, return of erectile function sufficient for sexual intercourse at a year after surgery varies from 15 to 87% in contemporary series of radical prostatectomy.[6-8] For younger men, postprostatectomy erectile dysfunction (PPED) significantly affects their sense of masculinity and their daily interactions with women.[9,10] Patient age, clinical and pathologic stage of cancer, preoperative potency status, and aggressiveness of nerve sparing are the most significant factors for recovery of potency after surgery.[11-13] Other reported variables include surgeon experience and surgical volume, intraoperative neurovascular bundle injury, penile ischemia and subsequent fibrosis, and veno-occlusive disease for successful return of sexual function following surgery.[14,15]

Much of the progress achieved in the past 2 decades in improving potency outcomes after radical prostatectomy has been wrought through an improved appreciation of the anatomic basis of the nerves responsible for erection. Diminished innervation of the corpora cavernosal tissue prevents the release of nitrous oxide from NANC nerves; decreases the production of cyclic nucleotides within the vascular smooth muscle; and causes impairment of vascular engorgement. Vascular injury, namely arterial insufficiency and veno-occlusive leakage, has also been proposed as possible etiologies for PPED, although the evidence for this is still early.[16-18] Recent advances in the anatomical course of these cavernosal nerves have led to various innovative techniques for improving nerve-sparing radical prostatectomy (nsRP). In addition, developments in fiber optic imaging technologies have led urologists to explore their potential for improved visualization of the erectogenic neural scaffold during nsRP.

24.2 Anatomic Basis of Erectogenic Nerve Preservation

24.2.1 Neurovascular Bundles and Cavernosal Nerves

The autonomic neural system is directly responsible for penile erection. The inferior hypogastric plexus (IHP) is responsible for the mechanisms of erection, ejaculation, and urinary continence. The IHP contains sympathetic and parasympathetic components. The sympathetic fibers arise from the T11–L2 ganglia, while the parasympathetic fibers originate from the ventral rami of S3 and S4. The IHP is a dense network of neural fibers located within a fibro-fatty,

A.K. Tewari (✉)
Lefrak Center of Robotic Surgery and Prostate Cancer Institute, Brady Foundation Department of Urology, Weill Medical College of Cornell University, New York, NY, USA
e-mail: ashtewarimd@gmail.com

A.K. Hemal, M. Menon (eds.), *Robotics in Genitourinary Surgery*,
DOI 10.1007/978-1-84882-114-9_24, © Springer-Verlag London Limited 2011

Fig. 24.1 Cross section of adult prostate demonstrating the posterolaterally situated neurovascular bundle running between the layers of the lateral pelvic fascia – the levator fascia lies lateral and the prostatic fascia lies medial to the bundle (© Brady Urological Institute)

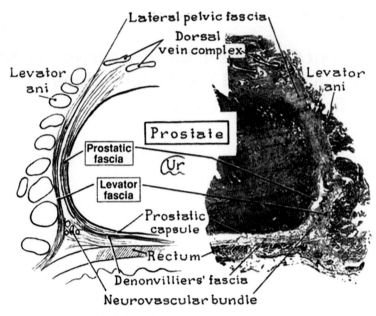

sub-peritoneal plate between the urinary bladder and rectum.[19]

Walsh and Donker[20] first detailed the anatomy of the nerves supplying the corpora cavernosal in male stillborns. Subsequent cadaveric and intraoperative studies by Walsh and colleagues[21,22] demonstrated that the neurovascular bundles (NVB) run posteriolateral to the prostate between two layers of lateral pelvic fascia – the prostatic fascia medially and levator fascia laterally (Fig. 24.1). These neurovascular bundles consist of (1) the cavernosal nerves (CN) directly responsible for erectile function, which originate from the most inferior portion of the IHP; (2) the arterial branches from the inferior vesical artery; and (3) venous vessels. The majority of these cavernous nerve fibers, approximately 6 mm wide, then run caudally at the 3 and 9 o'clock position of the membranous urethra beneath the striated sphincter at the prostatic apex (Fig. 24.2).

24.2.2 Anatomic Variants of Cavernosal Nerves

Recent studies have reported variants to the course of cavernosal nerves previously described by Walsh. Costello et al.[23] demonstrated that the NVBs in male cadavers descend posteriorly to the seminal vesicles, converging at the mid-prostatic level and then diverging on approaching the prostatic apex into indistinguishable fibers. Takenaka[24] highlighted the lattice-like distribution of the NVB on the lateral surface of the prostate, demonstrating that the NVB is more a network of multiple fine dispersed nerves than a distinct structure. Kiyoshima et al.[25] further reported that these dispersed nerve fibers are located between the prostate capsule and the lateral pelvic fascia. Eichelberg et al.[26] also found that only 46–66% of all nerves were found in the classical posterolateral location as described by Walsh, while 21–29% were found on the anteriolateral surface of the prostate.

24.2.3 Trizonal Hammock Concept

Tewari and colleagues[27,28] proposed that the periprostatic nerves consistently fell into three broad surgically identifiable zones: the proximal neurovascular plate (PNP), the predominant neurovascular bundle (PNB), and the accessory neural pathways (ANP) (Fig. 24.3). The predominant neurovascular bundles are usually located in a posteriolateral groove on the side of the prostate. Significant variations in the location, shape, course, and composition of this

Fig. 24.2 a Cross section of membranous urethra just distal to the prostatic apex, demonstrating the relationship of the neurovascular bundle to the striated urethral sphincter and the perineal body. **b** Lateral view of the neurovascular bundle, tracing its course from the pelvic plexus through the layers of the lateral pelvic fascia distally to lie lateral to the membranous urethra (© Brady Urological Institute)

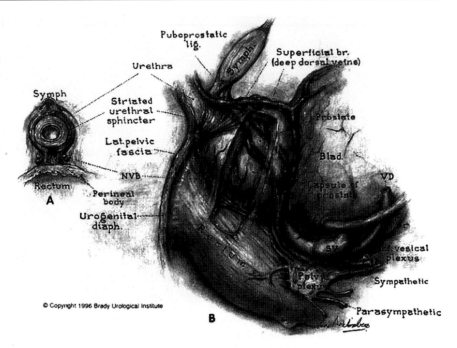

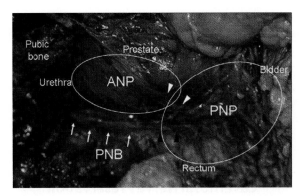

Fig. 24.3 Gross anatomy photograph (*right*) showing the proximal neurovascular plate (PNP) and predominant neurovascular bundle (PNB)

bundle occur. They can be widespread on the rectum, Denonvilliers' fascia, and lateral prostatic fascia or they can be circumscribed on the posterolateral groove enclosed in the triangular space. The PNB is closely related to the prostatic pedicle and prostatic fascia, and its branches can sometimes be intermingled with the lateral pedicles of the prostate (Fig. 24.4). Correlating their anatomic findings from cadaveric dissections to intraoperative video footage and final histology slides, Tewari's group observed accessory neural pathways in several locations around the prostate: specifically, between the prostatic and lateral prostatic fascia, posterior to the prostate and in the layers of Denonvilliers'

fascia, in several planes between the layers of periprostatic fascia, and even in the outer layers of the prostatic capsule. The superficial layer of Denonvilliers fascia has cross-communicating fibers between the left and right neurovascular bundles. Distally, these bundles coalesce to form a retro-apical plexus. In up to 35% of cases, this distal plexus penetrates the rectourethralis muscle (Fig. 24.5). Being the final exit pathway for the cavernous and retro-apical nerves, these delicate structures may easily be damaged during urethral transection and anastomosis. Tewari observed that the overall architecture of these delicate erectogenic nerves coursing around the prostatic capsule is similar to suspension of a weight in a hammock (Fig. 24.6), and that nerve preservation should not be considered a discrete technical maneuver, but rather an overarching surgical priority to be pursued at all stages of this complex procedure for achieving optimal outcomes.[28]

24.2.4 Fascial Planes Surrounding the Prostate Capsule

Correlating their intraoperative observations during robotic-assisted radical prostatectomy with histological specimens, Tewari and Menon recognized that

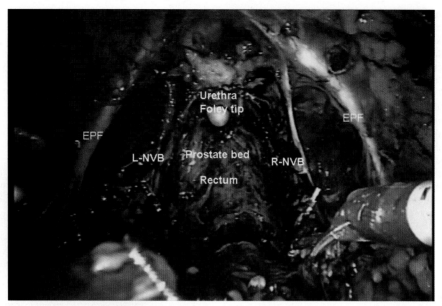

Fig. 24.4 View of the neurovascular bundles (NVBs) in the prostatic fossa after removal of the prostate gland. Note that the NVBs are closely related to the prostatic pedicle and prostatic fascia, and its branches can sometimes be intermingled with the lateral pedicles of the prostate

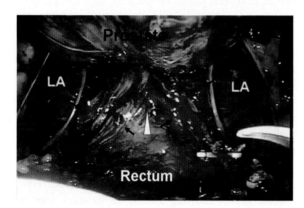

Fig. 24.5 Retro-apical region of prostate has a rich plexus of nerves formed by cross-communicating fibers between the *left* and *right* neurovascular bundles and fibers (LA, Levator ani, *Black arrows*, neural tissue)

numerous nerve bundles are present in the different layers of fascia enveloping the prostate[29] (Figs. 24.7 and 24.8). The lateral pelvic fascia (LPF) – a multilayered fascial covering – surrounds the prostatic capsule. The medial, well-defined component of the LPF is known as the prostatic fascia and directly wraps around the prostate capsule. The laterally defined part of LPF is the levator fascia, which lies on the levator muscles. Interposed between the prostatic fascia and the levator fascia are the periprostatic venous plexus and the

neurovascular tissue that travel distally to supply the sphincter, urethra, and cavernous tissue. These neural fibers can travel close to the vessels or occasionally, independently, on the surface of prostate or laterally on the rectum.

24.3 Techniques for Optimizing Cavernosal Nerve Preservation

24.3.1 Techniques for Retropubic Radical Prostatectomy

Based on their anatomic elucidations of the neurovascular bundles, Walsh[31] proposed the following technical considerations to avoid inadvertent NVB injury during open retropubic radical prostatectomy: (1) Securing venous backbleeding on the anterior prostate after ligation and division of the dorsal venous complex – this should be achieved with a V-shaped running suture instead of apposing the edges toward the midline, as the latter causes medial displacement of the NVB at the apex, making accurate dissection difficult; (2) transecting the membranous urethra only at the lateral edges while refraining from blind dissection

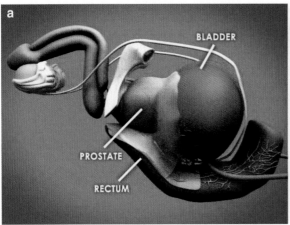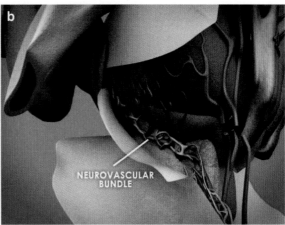

Fig. 24.6 **a** Graphical representation of the pelvic anatomy encountered by surgeons during robotic-assisted radical prostatectomy. **b** Close-up pictorial representation of the delicate scaffold of erectogenic nerves that run in the fascial planes around the prostatic capsule

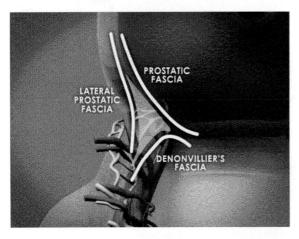

Fig. 24.7 Graphical representation of the neurovascular triangle, which is a potential avascular space bounded posteriorly by the Denonvilliers' fascia, laterally by the levator fascia, and medially by prostatic capsule covered by prostatic fascia

to the NVBs on the anterolateral prostate prior to apical dissection and division of the deep venous complex.

24.3.2 Periprostatic Planes of Fascial Dissection

Deviating from Walsh's technique of leaving prostatic fascia on the prostatectomy specimen, Menon and colleagues[35] from the Vattikuti Urology Institute adopted an aggressive nerve-sparing approach during robotic-assisted radical prostatectomy called the "veil of Aphrodite" technique, wherein the lateral pelvic fascia is dissected down to the glistening prostatic capsule surface and the veil of periprostatic tissue teased away in a relatively avascular plane (Fig. 24.9). In their cohort of 154 men, 96% reported return of potency (either with or without medical assistance) at 12 months follow-up, with a positive margin rate of 5%.[36] Adopting this aggressive intrafascial approach of dissection down to the shiny prostatic capsule for laparoscopic radical prostatectomy, Stolzenburg[37] also reported return of potency in 89.7% of their patients aged less than 55 years at 12 months following surgery, with margin positivity rates of 4.5% in pT2 and 29.4% in pT3 disease. Interestingly, Walsh's group[38] also adopted this approach in performing *high anterior release of the levator fascia* during bilateral nerve-sparing retropubic RP and reported similar sexual function outcomes without compromise of surgical margins.

of the prostatic apex; (3) releasing the superficial layer of the lateral pelvic fascia, which facilitates dissection of the posteriolateral groove between the prostate and the rectum posteriorly and augments intraoperative appreciation of the NVBs; (4) avoiding excessive traction on the NVBs during the posteriolateral dissection by gently rolling the prostate side to side; and (5) careful dissection of the seminal vesicles to avoid injury to distal branches of the inferior hypogastric plexus.

Alternative approaches to preservation of the NVBs described by Ruckle and Zincke,[32] Scardino,[33] and Klein[34] involve incising the lateral pelvic fascia medial

Fig. 24.8 Microscopic images of the nerves in the lateral pelvic fascia (*brown structures*) (note the small nerves posterior and anterolateral to the prostate): **a** low magnification; **b** medium magnification; **c** high magnification (© Elsevier Inc.[29])

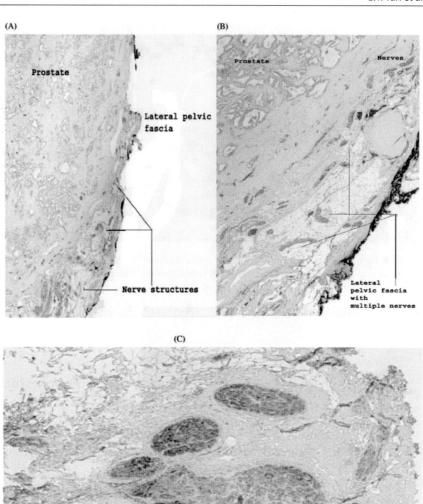

24.3.3 Trizonal Risk-Stratified Nerve-Sparing Approach

Based on their anatomic findings of the trizonal distribution of the erectogenic neural lattice, Tewari et al. propose the following technical modifications for optimizing nerve preservation (Table 24.1).[28]

To balance the competing goals of optimizing potency preservation with avoiding positive surgical margins, Tewari's group also employed a risk-stratified approach toward aggressiveness of nerve sparing according to the patient's likelihood of ipsilateral extraprostatic extension of cancer, which involves varying degrees of preservation of the nerve fibers in the periprostatic fascial planes (Figs. 24.10 and 24.11). In their cohort of potent men who met criteria for aggressive bilateral Grade 1 nerve sparing (PSA <10 ng/dL, clinical stage ≤T2, primary Gleason grade <4, cancer volume <5% in all cores, and absence of cues suggestive of extraprostatic extension on endorectal MRI and during surgery), 95% of these hitherto

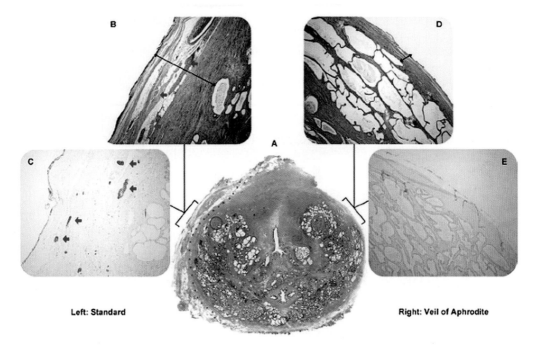

Left: Standard   **Right: Veil of Aphrodite**

Fig. 24.9 **a** H&E of whole mount radical prostatectomy specimen demonstrating Walsh's conventional nerve-sparing technique on *left* and "veil of Aphrodite" technique on the right. Note the presence of tumor (*red circle*) and the lateral pelvic fascia on the *left* and absence of LPF external to the prostatic capsule on the *right*. **b**, **c** H&E of the lateral pelvic fascia, demonstrating nerve bundles and extended margin to the capsule. **d**, **e** Absence of LPF and close proximity of margin to the capsule (© Elsevier Inc.[35])

Table 24.1 Technical maneuvers for athermal trizonal nerve-sparing robotic prostatectomy

Zone 1	Preservation of primary neurovascular plate (PNP)
	• Athermal dissection when opening endopelvic fascia around the proximal prostate
	• Perform bladder neck incision from the midline
	• Avoiding PNP injury during athermal seminal vesicle dissection from medial avascular plane outward using clips to control pedicles
Zone 2	Preservation of predominant neurovascular bundles (PNB)
	• Athermal dissection of seminal vesicles and neurovascular structures
	• Use of clips for controlling lateral pedicles
	• Risk-stratified approach to nerve sparing based on patient's likelihood of extracapsular extension of cancer (Fig. 24.8)
Zone 3	Preservation of accessory neural pathways
	• Athermal posterior and apical dissection to preserve peri-apical and retro-apical neural cross-fibers

potent men had partial erections with and without use of PDE5 inhibitors and 86% had erection sufficient for penetrative intercourse at a mean follow-up of 26 weeks.[39]

24.3.4 Alternatives to Electrocautery

Collateral thermal injury to the neurovascular bundles during radical prostatectomy is a well-recognized phenomenon. Tissue coagulation is achieved with temperatures above 45°C; tissue denaturation ensues at 57–60°C and protein coagulation at temperatures above 65°C[40]. Ong and colleagues[41] elegantly demonstrated a decrease in erectile function following application of thermal energy to the neurovascular bundles in a canine model. In their series of robotic-assisted radical prostatectomies, Ahlering et al.[42] reported that avoidance of thermal energy results in nearly a fivefold improvement in early return of sexual function, and that thermal injury induces a pronounced but mostly recoverable injury after 2 years from time of surgery. Recently, Tewari's group[43] also reported that bipolar cautery during robotic-assisted radical prostatectomy causes significantly higher and more persistent rise in temperature to tissues within 1 cm of its use, compared to monoploar cautery applied at the same distance, challenging the widely held belief that bipolar cautery causes less collateral tissue damage. Using a porcine

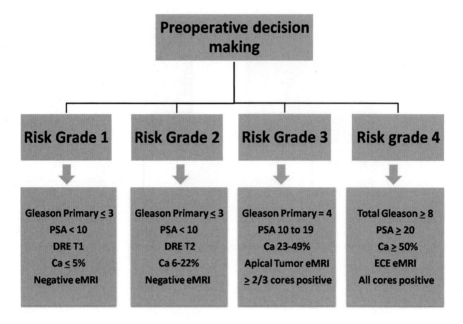

Fig. 24.10 Risk-stratified algorithm for nerve-sparing athermal nerve-sparing robotic radical prostatectomy

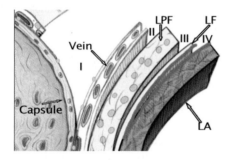

Fig. 24.11 Layers of fascia enveloping prostatic capsule, demonstrating the planes of dissection for differing grades (I–IV) of nerve sparing. *Grade 1* – incision of the Denonvilliers' and LPF is taken just outside the prostatic capsule. *Grade 2* – incision through the Denonvilliers' (leaving deeper layers on the rectum) and LPF is taken just outside the layer of veins of the prostate capsule, preserving most large neural trunks and ganglions. *Grade 3* – incision taken through the outer compartment of LPF, excising all layers of Denonvilliers' fascia. *Grade 4* – wide excision of the LPF and Denonvilliers' fascia containing the majority of the periprostatic neurovascular tissue

model, Khan et al.[44] also demonstrated that the lateral prostatic pedicles serve as a heat sink during bladder neck transection using cautery, protecting the NVBs from thermal injury.

Various alternatives to thermal energy have been explored. Ahlering and colleagues[45] reported their experience placing laparoscopic bulldog clamps on the lateral pedicles 1 cm from the prostate, followed by division of the lateral pedicles with cold scissors. After mobilization of the neurovascular bundle off the prostatic capsule, FloSeal™ was applied along its entire length and the NVB covered with a dry 1 × 4 cm sheet of Gelfoam™. The bulldog clamps were sequentially withdrawn following completion of prostatectomy and 3-0 figure-of-eight sutures used for hemostasis of bleeding from the lateral pedicles. Shalhav's group[46] also reported 47% of patients returning to baseline potency at 1 month after robotic prostatectomy using an antegrade dissection of the neurovascular bundle that avoided the use of clips or monopolar cautery.

Gill and colleagues[47,48] from the Cleveland Clinic adopted an energy-free technique of lateral pedicle ligation during laparoscopic radical prostatectomy, wherein the lateral prostatic pedicles were first controlled with atraumatic bulldog clamps, then divided using cold scissors and the NVBs preserved with blunt and sharp dissection. Hemostasis was then secured with superficial suturing of the transected pedicle. Using real-time Doppler transrectal ultrasound guidance, they demonstrated that application of bulldog clamps on the lateral pedicles did not impair blood flow through the NVBs throughout this maneuver. More recently, these investigators reported their preliminary experience comparing the KTP laser against ultrasonic shears and athermal cold Endoshear[TM] scissors dissection of the lateral pelvic fascia during laparoscopic unilateral NVB mobilization in a canine radical prostatectomy model.[49] Measuring peak intracavernosal pressure upon cavernous nerve stimulation both acutely and at 1 month follow-up in 36 dogs, they found that the KTP laser was comparable to the athermal technique, and superior to the ultrasonic shears, for preserving cavernous nerve function. In addition, intraoperative thermography revealed less collateral thermal spread from the KTP laser than from the ultrasonic shears. These animal studies suggest laser energy as a less traumatic alternative for periprostatic fascial dissection, and their feasibility in human trials is awaited.

24.3.5 Nerve Reconstruction and Regeneration

Quinlan and Walsh first reported successful return of erectile function in rats using interposition cavernous nerve grafts after iatrogenic denervation.[50] Kim and Scardino[51,52] subsequently reported excellent results using bilateral sural interposition nerve grafts (SNG) in 23 erstwhile potent patients with aggressive cancer undergoing non-nerve-sparing retropubic radical prostatectomy with deliberate wide NVB resection, compared to a control group of 12 men undergoing similar surgery who did not have SNG. Of the patients receiving bilateral SNG, 26% had spontaneous medically unassisted erections sufficient for penetrative intercourse; 26% reported spontaneous erections insufficient for intercourse; and 43% had intercourse with sildenafil. The greatest return of potency occurred at 18 months follow-up, although none of the patients reported erections before 5 months. This technique was subsequently adapted by other investigators for laparoscopic-and robotic-assisted radical prostatectomy with similar encouraging results.[53,54] However, a randomized phase II trial involving a cohort of 107 men undergoing unilateral nerve-sparing radical prostatectomy failed to demonstrate any additional improvement of potency with unilateral sural nerve grafting at 2 years following surgery.[55]

Tewari and colleagues[56] proposed an alternative approach of nerve advancement during robotic prostatectomy, wherein they performed end-to-end reconstruction after partial resection of the neurovascular bundle in clinically high-risk patients with MRI evidence of extracapsular extension of disease, most of whom had pT3 disease at final histology. In these patients, athermal partial resection of the NVBs was performed outside the lateral pelvic fascia, and the proximal and distal ends of the severed NVB then mobilized and approximated without tension using 6-0 polypropylene interrupted sutures. At a median of 20 months follow-up, five of these seven patients reported recovery erections with or without phosphodiesterase inhibitors and a median SHIM score of 18.

Atala and colleagues[57] reported significant recovery of erectile function in adult male Sprague-Dawley rats with bilateral cavernous nerve excision, using acellular nerve matrices processed from donor rat corporal nerves for interposition nerve grafting. Subsequent electromyography of the acellular nerve grafts at 3 months after surgery demonstrated adequate intracavernosal pressures, confirming their feasibility as an alternative to autologous nerve grafts in aiding recovery of cavernosal nerve function. Other innovative approaches currently being explored in animal models include use of embryonic stem cells[58] and growth factors[59] to augment cavernous nerve regeneration.

24.4 Advances in Cavernosal Neural Imaging

In recent years, significant efforts have been made to improve real-time identification and preservation of the cavernosal nerves during radical prostatectomy. Optical magnification of the operative field with surgical loupes has been demonstrated to improve earlier return of potency and lower rate of positive surgical margins following retropubic radical prostatectomy.[60,61] Intraoperative nerve stimulation and tumescence monitoring using the CaverMap[TM] has been reported to help improve potency outcomes, although its specificity for accurate NVB identification has remained weak with considerable background variables contributing to penile tumescence.[62–64] In their experience with real-time power Doppler transrectal ultrasonography imaging of the neurovascular bundles

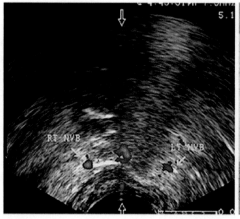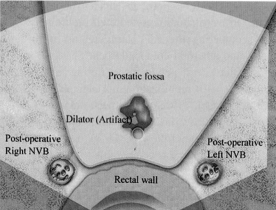

Fig. 24.12 Neurovascular bundles seen with power Doppler ultrasonography after bilateral nerve-sparing laparoscopic radical prostatectomy. A urethral dilator (typical ultrasound reflector, hyperechoic) and irrigation fluid (water-echo-texture, hypoechoic) are used as imaging contrasts to identify the NVBs on the surface of relatively hyperechoic periprostatic tissues (© Elsevier Inc.[65])

during laparoscopic radical prostatectomy, Ukimura and Gill reported that real-time TRUS helped the surgeon identify the anatomic course of the NVB, measure the number of visible vessels, and quantify arterial blood flow resistive index in the NVB[65] (Fig. 24.12). However, the variability of NVB imaging with positioning of the ultrasound probe, insufficient resolution for defining microscopic structures, and operator dependency of this approach have not resulted in this technique being adopted by other centers.

In contrast, promising advances have been made in fiber optic-based imaging technologies for visualizing biologic structures at a cellular and microscopic level, and we review some of these potential applications for identifying cavernosal nerves.

24.5 Optical Coherence Tomography

Optical coherence tomography (OCT) was first developed in 1991 as an imaging modality to visualize tissue microstructures.[66] Similar to B-mode ultrasonography but using near-infrared light instead of acoustic waves, OCT works by focusing an optical beam into the tissue and then measuring the time delay of reflected light from the internal microstructure at different depths by interferometry. A two-dimensional cross-sectional view of the cellular structures is then obtained by analyzing the intensity of backscattered light at different transverse positions as the optical beam is scanned across the tissue. Notable features of OCT for its use as a real-time intraoperative imaging tool are (1) its compact size and portability; (2) its compatibility with existing surgical platforms such as handheld probes, laparoscopes, and needles; (3) its ability to operate without tissue contact, avoiding visual obstruction of the operative field; (4) delivery of localized, high-resolution images of the area of interest, without requiring a distal imaging transducer; and (5) its relative affordability given the prevalent use of this technology in telecommunications industry. Nonetheless, image resolution is limited by signal attenuation with increasing tissue depth, with useful information only obtainable at depths of less than 1 mm.

Using the Niris[TM] OCT system and an 8 Fr handheld probe (Imalux Corporation, Cleveland, OH), Fried and Rais-Bahrami[67] from Johns Hopkins performed real-time in vivo imaging of the cavenosal nerves and periprostatic tissue in male Sprague-Dawley rats (Fig. 24.13). These nerves appeared as relatively intense, linear structures distinct from the underlying prostatic stroma and glands and correlated well with images obtained at final histopathology. However, poorer tissue discrimination between nerves and underlying prostate was reported by these same investigators on using OCT to image fresh ex vivo human radical prostatectomy specimens.[68] The thicker capsule and dense stroma of human prostates, as well as the abundance of blood vessels and fat found alongside the neurovascular bundles in human specimens,

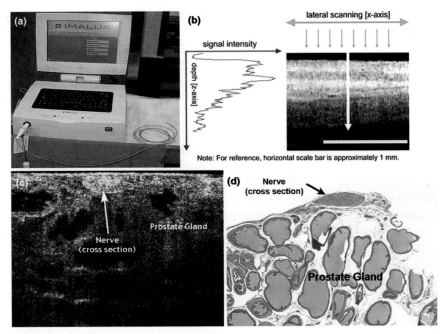

Fig. 24.13 **a** Imalux Niris™ Optical Coherence tomography imaging system. **b** Illustration of two-dimensional image creation based on scatter. **c** OCT imaging. **d** Histologic (hematoxylin–eosin) correlation of rat cavernous nerve in cross section (© Elsevier Inc.[68])

resulted in significant loss of signal contrast. Similar results were reported by Aron and colleagues[69] from the Cleveland Clinic, who demonstrated the feasibility of deploying the 8 Fr Niris probe through a 5-mm laparoscopic port for real-time in vivo imaging of the NVBs during laparoscopic- and robotic-assisted radical prostatectomy. More recently, Patel and colleagues[70] examined the use of OCT for predicting margin positivity on 100 ex vivo radical prostatectomy specimens. On correlation with final histopathology, they reported sensitivity, specificity, and negative predictive value of 70, 84, and 96%, respectively, for predicting final margin positivity, suggesting it may have an intraoperative role in helping surgeons identify true negative margins around the NVBs and avoiding overzealous dissection to optimize nerve preservation.

24.6 Spectroscopy

Alternative imaging modalities using reflected light include elastic scattering spectroscopy, Raman spectroscopy, and coherent anti-Raman spectroscopy (CARS). *Elastic scattering spectroscopy* (also known as diffuse reflective spectrometry) detects photons that are reflected and scattered by cell and tissue constituents. Capturing signals of reflected light at the same wavelength as emitted source, elastic spectroscopy detects differences in wavelength intensity. It does not yield anatomic images, but may be useful in distinguishing tissue constituents. As such, its clinical use to date has been limited to imaging of bladder urothelium via a cystoscope to distinguish malignant from benign tissue.[71] *Raman spectroscopy* operates on a similar principle to elastic scattering, except that it depends upon molecule-specific inelastic scattering of photons to analyze cellular constituents. Crow and colleagues reported an accuracy of 86% in distinguishing malignant from benign/inflammatory snap-frozen prostate samples collected during transurethral resection of prostate.[72]

24.7 Fluorescent Imaging

Fluorescent imaging technologies capture light emitted from target tissues in response to photons absorbed by specific target constituents and/or markers.[73] Two broad strategies employing this optical phenomenon for imaging and diagnosis have been (1) *exogenous fluorescence techniques,* which rely on introduction of fluorescent markers or labels into target tissue to visualize specific structures or distinguish between healthy and diseased targets and (2) *endogenous fluorescence techniques,* wherein specific tissue constituents emit characteristic their own autofluorescence upon photon excitation. In the latter approach, normally endogenous molecules such as collagen, elastin, amino acids, and other cellular proteins display autofluorescence and have been used to provide information on cellular interactions (e.g., nicotinamide adenine dinucleotide) and connective tissue integrity in normal and cancerous host tissue. Its primary limitations are the bulky footprints occupied by attendant equipment and complex software required for image processing.

24.8 Exogenous Fluoroscopy

This approach involves the administration of small molecules into the target tissue by a variety of routes, either systemically or location specific. The inherent advantages with this modality are its potential for specific identification of altered cellular/tissue architecture when conjugated to specific biomarkers, avoiding confounding signals generated by neighboring autofluorescent tissue. Comparing five different fluorophores administered via penile injection in male Sprague-Dawley rats, Davila and colleagues[74] demonstrated successful retrograde uptake of Fluoro-Gold in the NVBs and major pelvic ganglion of the rats after 3 days. More recently, Boyette and colleagues[75] successfully demonstrated in vivo fluorescent imaging of the rat cavernosal nerves at 40 μm resolution using the Cellvizio® fibroptic confocal microscope (Mauna Kea Technologies, Cambridge, MA, USA) following injection of the fluorescent retrograde nerve tracer CTb-488 (Fig. 24.14). As well as demonstrating the absence of tissue toxicity/mutagenicity caused by these fluorophores, Boyette's group reported no compromise in cavernous nerve function following fluorophore administration on subsequent intracavernosal pressure manometry with electrical stimulation of the cavernosal nerves. These studies highlight the potential for using fiber optic confocal fluorescent microscopy as an intraoperative imaging tool for identifying the cavernosal nerves during radical prostatectomy.

24.9 Endogenous Autofluorescence

Nobel laureate Maria Goeppert-Mayer first proposed in 1931 that absorption of two low-energy photons can cause sufficient excitation of electrons to emit a fluorescence normally produced by the absorption of a single high-energy photon.[76] This optical phenomenon, known as two-photon or multi-photon excitation, was later developed as an imaging technology in the form of *multiphoton nonlinear microscopy* (MPM) by Denk and Webb from Cornell University in the 1990s.[77] Since then, MPM has been used extensively to image cellular and subcellular processes, offering increased depth of tissue imaging (500–600 μm), higher spatial resolution, less phototoxicity and photobleaching, and minimal background fluorescence compared to confocal microscopy.[78]

Yadav and colleagues[79] recently reported their initial experience with ex vivo imaging of cavernosal nerves in a Sprague-Dawley rat model using multiphoton microscopy in combination with second harmonic generation. They demonstrated good correlation between MPM images of neural and prostate tissue with those obtained at final histopathology and also highlighted the capability of using this modality for high-resolution "optical sectioning" of tissue at various depths (Figs. 24.15 and 24.16). *Coherent anti-Raman Spectroscopy (CARS),* a new type of multiphoton microscopy, has also generated significant interest. This third-order nonlinear optical imaging modality operates by generating two spatially and temporally overlapping pulsed laser beams (a pump beam and a Stokes beam) with different wavelengths.[80] The difference in wavelengths, when tuned to match a certain molecular vibration energy level, significantly enhances the CARS signal to produce vibrational contrast. Huff and Cheng[81] successfully demonstrated in vivo CARS imaging of the sciatic nerve in mice. Using a wavelength difference of 2,840 cm^{-1}, the peak frequency of CARS band for symmetric CH_2 stretch vibration, a large E-CARS signal was observed from the myelinated axons in the sciatic nerve as well as the surrounding fat cells (Fig. 24.17). Further combination of CARS with second harmonic generation (SHG) facilitated high signal-to-background ratio, three-dimensional spatial resolution images of the nerves and surrounding tissue without the need for exogenous fluorophore labeling. However, the primary drawback of CARS remains its limited depth of penetration at ~100 μm.

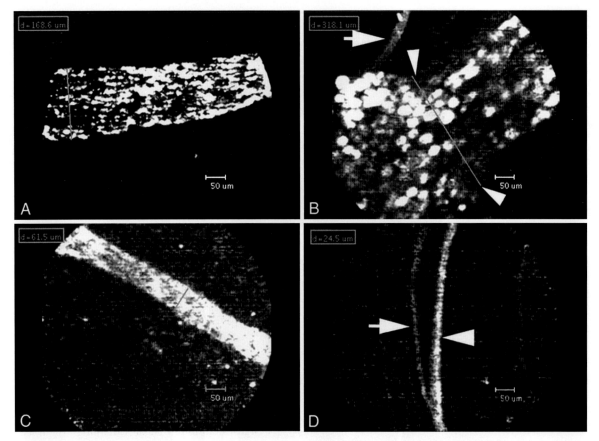

Fig. 24.14 Variation in rat cavernosal nerve (CN) appearance and thickness was noted during sequence acquisition 9 days after CTb-488 injection. **a** Sharply granular appearing CN with distinct parts of nerve containing no fluorescent signal (diameter 186.6 m). **b** Junction of CN with MPG (*arrowheads*) (diameter 318.1 m) and accessory nerve branching from MPG (*arrow*). **c** Evenly distributed bright fluorescent nerve image (diameter 61.5 μm). **d** Accessory nerve branching into larger (*arrowhead*) (diameter 24.5 μm) and smaller (*arrow*) (diameter 10.0 μm) bundles. Scale bar represents 50 μm (© Elsevier Inc.[75])

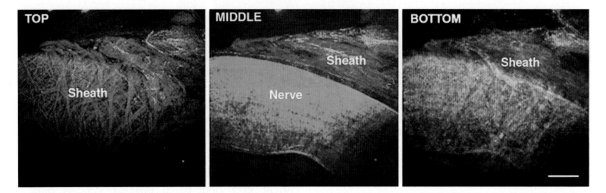

Fig. 24.15 High-magnification (×20) multiphoton microscopy image of rat femoral nerve. Seen are the second harmonic generation signal from the fibrocollagenous sheath (*red*) and autofluorescence (*green*) from the nerve, presumably coming from the axoplasm and the cytoplasm of Schwann cells. Note how the sheath wraps around the nerve bundle at different optical depths. Scale bar: 100 μm

Fig. 24.16
Low-magnification (×4) multiphoton microscopy image of rat cavernous nerve. A single optical section from the middle of the tissue is shown. Second harmonic generation signal is from the fibrocollagenous sheath (*red*) and autofluorescence (*green*) is from the nerve. Scale bar: 500 μm

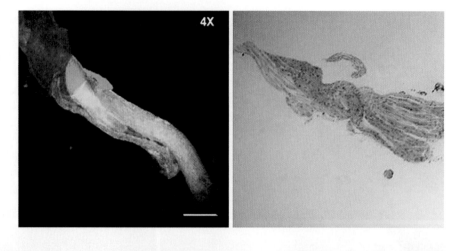

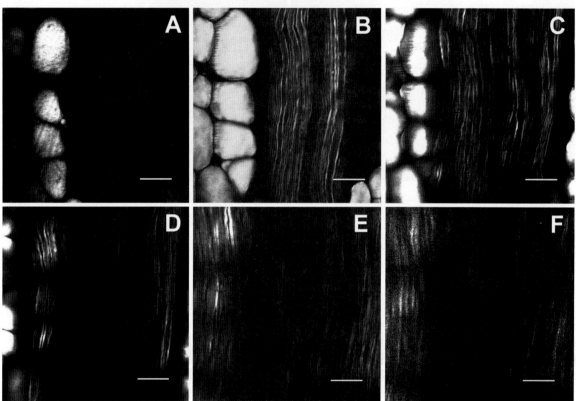

Fig. 24.17 E-CARS images of sciatic nerve at increasing depth (**a**) 0, (**b**) 10, (**c**) 20, (**d**) 30, (**e**) 40, and (**f**) 50 μm. The dark contrast along the axons in the *left-hand side* of (**d**), (**e**), and (**f**) is due to defocusing of excitation beams and scattering of E-CARS signals by adipocytes right beneath the axons. Bar = 20 μm (© The Royal Microscopical Society[81])

24.10 Conclusion

Better appreciation of the variable and often invisible anatomical course of the cavernosal nerves continues to engender innovations in surgical technique to optimize their preservation. Nonetheless, most current fiber optic-based imaging systems remain limited by image attenuation with increasing tissue depth and their sizable footprint. Exciting frontiers of research that include efforts in stem cell neural regeneration, development of specific fluorophores and biomarkers, and performing radical prostatectomy under hypothermic conditions may provide much needed breakthroughs to improving potency outcomes following radical prostatectomy in this current age of improved life expectancy and heightened patient expectations.[58,82]

References

1. Schröder FH, Hugosson J, Roobol MJ, et al. Screening and prostate-cancer mortality in a randomized European study. *N Engl J Med*. 2009;360:1320–1328.

2. Jemal A, Siegel R, Ward E, et al. Cancer statistics, 2009. *CA Cancer J Clin*. 2009;59:225–249.

3. Quinn M, Babb P. Patterns and trends in prostate cancer incidence, survival, prevalence and mortality. Part 1: international comparisons. *BJU Int*. 2002;90:162–173.

4. Bill-Axelson A, Holmberg L, Ruutu M, et al. Radical prostatectomy versus watchful waiting in early prostate cancer. *N Engl J Med*. 2005;352(19):1977–1984.

5. Tewari A, Johnsson CC, Devine G, et al. Long-term survival probability in men with clinically localized prostate cancer: a case-control, propensity modeling study stratified by race, age, treatment and co-morbidities. *J Urol*. 2004;171:1513–1519.

6. Zippe C, Nandipati K, Agarwal A, Raina R. Sexual dysfunction after pelvic surgery. *Int J Impot Res*. 2006;18:1–18.

7. Berryhill R Jr, Jhaveri J, Yadav R, et al. Robotic prostatectomy: a review of outcomes compared with laparoscopic and open approaches. *Urology*. 2008;72:15–23.

8. Ficarra V, Novara G, Artibani W, et al. Retropubic, laparoscopic and robot-assisted radical prostatectomy: a systematic review and cumulative analysis of comparative studies. *Eur Urol*. 2009;55:1037–1063.

9. Penson DF, Feng Z, Kuniyuki A, McClerran D, Albertsen PC, Deapen D, et al. General quality of life 2 years following treatment for prostate cancer: what influences outcomes? Results from the prostate cancer outcomes study. *J Clin Oncol*. 2003;21:1147–1154.

10. Kirschner-Hermanns R, Jakse G. Quality of life following radical prostatectomy. *Crit Rev Oncol Hematol*. 2002;43:141–151.

11. Quinlan DM, Epstein JI, Carter BS, Walsh PC. Sexual function following radical prostatectomy: influence of preservation of neurovascular bundles. *J Urol*. 1991;145:998–1002.

12. Rabbani F, Stapleton AM, Kattan MW, Wheeler TM, Scardino PT. Factors predicting recovery of erections after radical prostatectomy. *J Urol*. 2000;164(6):1929–1934.

13. Dubbelman YD, Dohle GR, Schroder FH. Sexual function before and after radical retropubic prostatectomy: a systematic review of prognostic indicators for a successful outcome. *Eur Urol*. 2006;50:711–720.

14. McCullough AR. Rehabilitation of erectile function following radical prostatectomy. *Asian J Androl*. 2008;10(1):61–74.

15. Bianco F, Kattan M, Eastham J, Scardino P, Mulhall JP. Surgeon and surgical volume as predictors of erectile function outcomes following radical prostatectomy. *J Sex Med*. 2004;1:33.

16. Kim ED, Blackburn D, McVary KT. Post-radical prostatectomy penile blood flow: assessment with color Doppler ultrasound. *J Urol*. 1994;152:2276–2279.

17. Mulhall JP, Slovick R, Hotaling J, et al. Erectile dysfunction after radical prostatectomy: haemodynamic profiles and their correlation with the recovery of erectile function. *J Urol*. 2002;167:1371–1375.

18. Kawanishi Y, Lee KS, Kimura K, Kojima K, Yamamoto A, Numata A. Effect of radical retropubic prostatectomy on erectile function, evaluated before and after surgery using color Doppler ultrasonography and nocturnal penile tumescence monitoring. *BJU Int*. 2001;88:244–247.

19. Walz J, Graefen M, Huland H. Basic principles of anatomy for optimal surgical management of prostate cancer. *World J Urol*. 2007;25:31–38.

20. Walsh PC, Donker PJ. Impotence following radical prostatectomy: insight into etiology and prevention. *J Urol*. 1982;128:492–497.

21. Lepor H, Gregerman M, Crosby R, Mostofi FK, Walsh PC. Precise localization of the autonomic nerves from the pelvic plexus to the corpora cavernosa: a detailed anatomical study of the adult male pelvis. *J Urol*. 1985;133:207–212.

22. Walsh PC. Anatomic radical prostatectomy: evolution of surgical technique. *J Urol*. 1998;160:2418–2424.

23. Costello AJ, Brooks M, Cole OJ. Anatomical studies of the neurovascular bundle and cavernosal nerves. *BJU Int*. 2004;94:1071–1076.

24. Takenaka A, Murakami G, Matsubara A, et al. Variation in course of cavernous nerve with special reference to details of topographic relationships near prostatic apex: histologic study using male cadavers. *Urology*. 2005;65:136–142.

25. Kiyoshima K, Yokomizo A, Yoshida T, et al. Anatomic features of periprostatic tissue and its surroundings: a histological analysis of 79 radical retropubic prostatectomy specimens. *Jpn J Clin Oncol*. 2004;34:463–468.

26. Eichelberg C, Erbersdobler A, Michl U, Schlomm T, Salomon G, Graefen M, et al. Nerve distribution along the prostatic capsule. *Eur Urol*. 2007;51(1):105–111.

27. Tewari A, Takenaka A, Mtui E, et al. The proximal neurovascular plate and the tri-zonal neural architecture around the prostate gland: importance in the athermal robotic technique of nerve-sparing prostatectomy. *BJU Int*. 2006;98:318–323.

28. Tewari A, Tan GY, Dorsey PJ Jr, et al. Optimizing erectogenic outcomes during athermal robotic prostatectomy: a risk-stratified tri-zonal approach. *Urol Times* (Clinical Edition). 2008;3:s4–s12.

29. Tewari A, Peabody JO, Fischer M, et al. An operative and anatomic study to help in nerve-sparing during laparoscopic and robotic radical prostatectomy. *Eur Urol*. 2003;43:444–454.

30. Tewari AK, Patel ND, Leung RA, et al. Visual cues as a surro gate for tactile feedback during robotic-assisted laparoscopic prostatectomy: posterolateral margin rates in 1340 consecutive patients. *BJU Int*. 2010;106(4):528–536.

31. Walsh PC. Anatomic radical retropubic prostatectomy. In: Walsh PC, Retik AB, Vaughan ED Jr, Wein AJ, eds. *Campbell's Urology*, Volume 4, Chapter 90. 8th edn. WB Saunders Co: Philadelphia, PA; 2002: p3107–p3129.
32. Ruckle HC, Zincke H. Potency sparing radical retropubic prostatectomy: a simplified anatomical approach. *J Urol.* 1995;153:1875–1877.
33. Goad JR, Scardino PT. Modifications in the technique of radical prostatectomy to minimize blood loss. *Atlas Urol Clin North Am.* 1994;3:65–80.
34. Klein EA, Kupelian PA, Tuason L, Levin HS. Initial dissection of the lateral fascia reduces the positive margin rate in radical prostatectomy. *Urology.* 1998;51: 766–773.
35. Savera AT, Kaul S, Badani K, Stark AT, Shah NL, Menon M. Robotic radical prostatectomy with the "veil of aphrodite" technique: histologic evidence of enhanced nerve sparing. *Eur Urol.* 2006;49:1065–1074.
36. Kaul S, Savera A, Badani K, Fumo M, Bhandari A, Menon M. Functional outcomes and oncological efficacy of Vattikuti Institute prostatectomy with Veil of Aphrodite nerve-sparing: an analysis of 154 consecutive patients. *BJU Int.* 2006;97:467–472.
37. Stolzenburg JU, Rabenalt R, Do M, et al. Intrafascial nerve-sparing endoscopic extraperitoneal radical prostatectomy. *Eur Urol.* 2008;53:931–940.
38. Nielsen ME, Schaeffer EM, Marschke P, Walsh PC. High anterior release of the levator fascia improves sexual function following open radical retropubic prostatectomy. *J Urol.* 2008;180:2557–2564.
39. Dorsey P Jr, Tan G, Jhaveri J, et al. Early return of potency and orgasmic function during aggressive bilateral intrafascial nerve-sparing during trizonal athermal robotic prostatectomy: a prospective cohort study. *(Abstract) CUAJ.* 2009;3(3 Suppl 1):S11 (POD-3.03).
40. Lantis JC, Durville FM, Connolly R, Schwaitzberg SD. Comparison of coagulation modalities in surgery. *J Laparoendosc Adv Surg Tech.* 1998;8: 381–394.
41. Ong AM, Su LM, Varkarakis I, et al. Nerve sparing radical prostatectomy: effects of hemostatic energy sources on the recovery of cavernous nerve function in a canine model. *J Urol.* 2004;172:1318–1322.
42. Ahlering TE, Rodriquez E, Skarecky DW. Overcoming obstacles: nerve-sparing issues in radical prostatectomy. *J Endourol.* 2008;22:745–749.
43. Mandhani A, Dorsey PJ Jr, Ramanathan R, et al. Real time monitoring of temperature changes in neurovascular bundles during robotic radical prostatectomy: thermal map for nerve-sparing radical prostatectomy. *J Endourol.* 2008;22:2313–2317.
44. Khan F, Rodriguez E, Finley DS, Skarecky DW, Ahlering TE. Spread of thermal energy and heat sinks: implications for nerve-sparing robotic prostatectomy. *J Endourol.* 2007;21:1195–1198.
45. Ahlering TE, Eichel L, Chou D, Skarecky DW. Feasibility study for robotic radical prostatectomy cautery-free neurovascular bundle preservation. *Urology.* 2005;65:994–997.
46. Chien GW, Mikhail AA, Orvieto MA, et al. Modified clipless antegrade nerve preservation in robotic-assisted laparoscopic radical prostatectomy with validated sexual function evaluation. *Urology.* 2005;66: 419–423.
47. Gill IS, Ukimura O, Rubinstein M, et al. Lateral pedicle control during laparoscopic radical prostatectomy: refined technique. *Urology.* 2005;65:23–27.
48. Haber G, Aron M, Ukimura O, Gill IS. Energy-free nerve-sparing laparoscopic radical prostatectomy: the bulldog technique. *BJU Int.* 2008;102:1766–1769.
49. Gianduzzo TRJ, Colombo JR Jr, Haber GP, et al. KTP laser nerve sparing radical prostatectomy: comparison of ultrasonic and cold scissor dissection on cavernous nerve function. *J Urol.* 2009;181:2760–2766.
50. Quinlan DM, Nelson RJ, Walsh PC. Cavernous nerve grafts restore erectile function in denervated rats. *J Urol.* 1991;145:380–383.
51. Kim ED, Scardino PT, Hampel O, et al. Interposition of sural nerve restores function of cavernous nerves resected during radical prostatectomy. *J Urol.* 1999;161: 188–192.
52. Kim ED, Nath R, Slawin K, Kadmon D, Miles BJ, Scardino PT. Bilateral nerve grafting during radical retropubic prostatectomy: extended follow-up. *Urology.* 2001;58: 983–987.
53. Turk IA, Deger S, Morgan WR, Davis JW, Schelhammer PF, Loening SA. Sural nerve graft during laparoscopic radical prostatectomy: initial experience. *Urol Oncol.* 2002;7:191–194.
54. Kaouk JH, Desai MM, Abreu SC, Papay F, Gill IS. Robotic assisted laparoscopic sural nerve grafting during radical prostatectomy: initial experience. *J Urol.* 2003;170: 909–912.
55. Davis JW, Chang DW, Chevray P, et al. Randomized phase II trial evaluation of erectile function after attempted unilateral cavernous nerve-sparing retropubic radical prostatectomy with versus without unilateral sural nerve grafting for clinically localized prostate cancer. *Eur Urol.* 2009;55:1135–1144.
56. Martinez-Salamanca JI, Rao S, Ramanathan R, et al. Nerve advancement with end-to-end reconstruction after partial neurovascular bundle resection: a feasibility study. *J Endourol.* 2007;21:830–835.
57. Conolly SS, Yoo JJ, Abouheba M, Soker S, McDougal WS, Atala A. Cavernous nerve regeneration using acellular nerve grafts. *World J Urol.* 2008;26:333–339.
58. Bochinski D, Lin GT, Nunes L, et al. The effect of neural embryonic stem cell therapy is a rat model of cavernosal nerve injury. *BJU Int.* 2004;94:904–909.
59. Hsieh PS, Bochinski DJ, Lin GT, et al. The effect of vascular endothelial growth factor and brain-derived neurotrophic factor on cavernosal nerve regeneration in a nerve-crush rat model. *BJU Int.* 2003;92:470–475.
60. Chuang MS, O-Connor RC, Laven BA, Orvieto MA, Brendler CB. Early release of the neurovascular bundles and optical loupe magnification lead to improved and earlier return of potency following radical retropubic prostatectomy. *J Urol.* 2005;173: 537–539.

61. Magera JS, Inman BA, Slezak JM, Bagniewski SM, Sebo TJ, Myers RP. Increased optical magnification from 2.5× to 4.3× with technical modification lowers the positive margin rate in open radical retropubic prostatectomy. *J Urol*. 2008;179:130–135.

62. Klotz L, Herschorn S. Early experience with intraoperative cavernous nerve stimulation with penile tumescence monitoring to improve nerve sparing during radical prostatectomy. *Urology*. 1998;52:537–542.

63. Walsh PC, Marschke P, Catalona WJ, Lepor H, Martin S, Myers RP, et al. Efficacy of first-generation cavermap to verify location and function of cavernous nerves during radical prostatectomy: a multi-institutional evaluation by experienced surgeons. *Urology*. 2001;57:491–494.

64. Holzbeierlein J, Peterson M, Smith JA Jr. Variability of results of cavernous nerve stimulation during radical prostatectomy. *J Urol*. 2001;165:108–110.

65. Ukimura O, Gill IS, Desai MM, et al. Real-time transrectal ultrasonography during laparoscopic radical prostatectomy. *J Urol*. 2004;172:112–118.

66. Huang D, Swanson EA, Lin CP, et al. Optical coherence tomography. *Science*. 1991;254:1178–1181.

67. Fried NM, Rias-Bahrami S, Lagoda GA, et al. Imaging the cavernous nerves in the rat prostate using optical coherence tomography. *Lasers Surg Med*. 2007;39:36–41.

68. Rias-Bahrami S, Levinson AW, Fried NM, et al. Optical coherence tomography of cavernous nerves: a step toward real-time intraoperative imaging during nerve-sparing radical prostatectomy. *Urology*. 2008;72:198–204.

69. Aron M, Kaouk JH, Hegarty NJ, et al. Preliminary experience with the Niris™ optical coherence tomography system during laparoscopic and robotic prostatectomy. *J Endourol*. 2007;21:814–818.

70. Dangle PP, Shah KK, Kaffenberger B, Patel VR. The use of high resolution optical coherence tomography to evaluate robotic radical prostatectomy specimens. *Int Braz J Urol*. 2009;35:344–353.

71. Mourant JR, Bigio IJ, Boyer J, et al. Spectroscopic diagnosis of bladder cancer with elastic light scattering. *Lasers Surg Med*. 1995;17:350–357.

72. Crow P, Molckovsky A, Stone J, et al. Assessment of fibreoptic near-infrared raman spectroscopy for diagnosis of bladder and prostate cancer. *Urology*. 2005;65: 1126–1130.

73. Tuttle JB, Steers WD. Fibreoptic imaging for urologic surgery. *Curr Urol Rep*. 2009;10:60–64.

74. Davila HH, Mamcarz M, Nadelhaft I, et al. Visualization of the neurovascular bundles and major pelvic ganglion with fluorescent tracers after penile injection in the rat. *BJU Int*. 2007;101:1048–1051.

75. Boyette LB, Reardon MA, Mirelman AJ, et al. Fiberoptic imaging of the cavernous nerve in vivo. *J Urol*. 2007;178:2694–2700.

76. Dunn KW, Young PA. Principles of multiphoton microscopy. *Nephron Exp Nephrol*. 2006;103:e33–e40.

77. Denk W, Strickler J, Webb W. Two-photon laser scanning microscope. *Science*. 1990;248:73–76.

78. Benninger RK, Hao M, Piston DW. Multi-photon imaging of dynamic processes in living cells and tissues. *Rev Physiol Biochem Pharmacol*. 2008;160:71–92.

79. Yadav R, Mukherjee S, Hermen M, et al. Multiphoton microscopy of prostate and periprostatic neural tissue: a promising imaging technique for improving nerve-sparing prostatectomy. *J Endourol*. 2009;23:861–867.

80. Cheng JX, Xie XS. Coherent anti-stokes Raman scattering microscopy: instrumentation, theory, applications. *J Phys Chem*. 2004;108:827–840.

81. Huff TB, Cheng J-X. In vivo coherent anti-stokes raman scattering imaging of sciatic nerve tissue. *J Microsc*. 2007;225:175–182.

82. Finley DS, Osann K, Skarecky D, Ahlering TE. Hypothermic nerve-sparing radical prostatectomy: rationale, feasibility, and effect on early continence. *Urology*. 2009;73:691–696.

Chapter 25

Robot-Assisted Radical Prostatectomy for Large Glands and Median Lobe

Ugur Boylu and Raju Thomas

25.1 Introduction

With the introduction of robotic surgery, robotic-assisted radical prostatectomy (RARP) is rapidly becoming the preferred surgical approach for management of localized prostate cancer. In 2005, approximately 35,000 RARPs were performed in the United States[1]; this number is estimated to exceed 60,000 in 2009.[2] However, with increasing numbers of RARPs, the robotic surgeon can expect to be confronted with various challenging scenarios given the variation of anatomy from patient to patient, such as large-sized prostates and varying sizes and configurations of median lobes.

25.2 Embryology of the Prostate

The prostate gland develops as multiple endodermal outgrowths of the urogenital sinus. Between the 11th and 16th week of gestation these simple tubular outgrowths develop in five distinct groups. These prostatic ducts branch multiple times and result in a complex system that meets the mesenchymal cells around this segment of the urogenital sinus. The muscular stroma is markedly developed by the 22nd week. Five lobes are eventually formed from the five groups of epithelial buds: anterior, posterior, median, and two lateral lobes.[3] Although these lobes are widely separated

initially, they later converge without any dividing septa. The tubules of the posterior lobe extend posterior to the developing median and lateral lobes and form the posterior aspect of the gland. According to Glenister,[4] the epithelium covering verumontanum has a composite origin from a mixture of endodermal urogenital sinus cells, mesodermal mesonephric or Wolffian cells, and paramesonephric or Mullerian cells. The median lobe is developed from the upper limit of the mixed epithelium covering the verumontanum. Therefore, the median lobe of the prostate behaves differently from the rest of the prostate in disease and under experimental conditions.

25.3 RARP for Median Lobe

Not all patients have a clinically discernable median lobe. The estimates of a clinically significant median lobe encountered during surgical procedures vary between 8 and 18%.[5,6] Obviously, the larger the median lobe, the greater the challenge and increase in variables, such as operative time, size of bladder neck requiring reconstruction, injury to the ureteral orifices, and level of frustration, especially to the relatively novice robotic surgeon.

Although the presence of a large median lobe is discovered at the time of surgery, the diagnosis can be made preoperatively. A large median lobe can be diagnosed based on the patient's voiding history and voiding pattern, such as urinary intermittency, and can also be visualized on preoperative abdominal and even transrectal ultrasound as a protruding smooth mass from the bladder neck. Additionally, cystoscopy may help in diagnosis of a large median lobe preoperatively.

R. Thomas (✉)
Department of Urology, Center for Minimally Invasive and Robotic Surgery, Tulane University School of Medicine, New Orleans, LA, USA
e-mail: rthomas@tulane.edu

A.K. Hemal, M. Menon (eds.), *Robotics in Genitourinary Surgery*,
DOI 10.1007/978-1-84882-114-9_25, © Springer-Verlag London Limited 2011

However, the necessity of such preoperative interventions to determine the existence of a large median lobe prior to RARP is debatable. Although the presence of a large median lobe does not necessitate a change in surgical approach for the experienced robotic surgeon, it may be challenging for the initial cases of one's robotic learning curve. Therefore, during the early phases of the learning curve for RARP, we suggest appropriate patient selection, and if the patient's voiding history is suspicious for the presence of a median lobe, appropriate preoperative workup, such as performing a preoperative abdominal or transrectal ultrasound or cystoscopy, is highly recommended. Presence of a known median lobe should be cause for appropriate patient counseling regarding the challenges that may be encountered intraoperatively.

The main concerns regarding the existence of a large median lobe during RARP is the possibility of ureteral injury during dissection of the median lobe/bladder neck and risk of ureteral obstruction during urethrovesical anastomosis.[7] Additionally, in an attempt to remove the complete median lobe, a wide excision of the trigone results in a large bladder neck defect and leaves the ureteral orifices closer to the bladder neck's resected margins.[8]

25.3.1 Literature Review

Several studies have evaluated the impact of encountering a median lobe on the outcomes of RARP. Jenkins et al.[5] published a retrospective review of 29 patients (8%) with median lobe in a series of 345 patients undergoing RARP. In all patients, the existence of a large median lobe was found at surgery. A comparison of surgical, clinical, and pathologic outcomes between these patients and 29 consecutive patients without a median lobe was performed. The authors found the presence of a median lobe did not increase operative time required for bladder neck dissection or urethrovesical anastomosis. Additionally, there was no difference in surgical margin status and time to continence between patients with median lobe and control group. Meeks et al.[6] reported the impact of prostatic median lobe on RARP. Of the 154 patients, 29 (18%) were found to have large median lobes. Contrary to the previous study, the authors reported greater operative time because of increased dissection requirements

around the posterior bladder neck and seminal vesicles in patients with median lobes. Moreover, estimated blood loss and hospital stay were significantly greater in men with large median lobes.

25.3.2 Surgical Technique

Trocar placements and the steps for proceeding with a routine RARP are unchanged until the presence of a median lobe is suspected. During dissection at the anterior bladder neck, deviation of the Foley catheter to one side and significant intravesicular prostatic extension are the hallmarks of the presence of a large median lobe. Traction on the Foley catheter should better delineate the presence of a median lobe. Once the median lobe has been identified, either preoperatively or intraoperatively, the robotic surgeon needs to make adjustments to appropriately and safely handle the median lobe. If the median lobe is relatively small, approximate total volume of 5–10 cc, then this may not be very challenging and no significant adjustments need to be made. In this case, we recommend that the surgeon score the mucosa at the very top end or the caudal end of the median lobe close to the bladder neck (Fig. 25.1), peel the mucosa off the median lobe, dissect out the median lobe, and then evaluate if this would pose a significant technical challenge in proceeding with the prostatectomy. If the median lobe visually obstructs the surgical field of dissection, the recommended option is to excise only the median lobe to be sent off as a separate specimen. Due to its known embryological origin the median lobe is usually benign.

If the median lobe is of significant volume and a challenge for intraoperative dissection, the recommendation is as follows: As mentioned above, the mucosa is scored, then peeled off the median lobe, and then lateral dissections are carried out to free up the median lobe, hopefully in its entirety. If possible, a 30° down lens is placed to see if the ureteral orifices can be identified. Every effort should be made to identify the ureteral orifices, so as to protect them. Intraoperative administration of indigo carmine or methylene blue may also be useful in the identification of the orifices, thus avoiding any possible injury. The optics of the robotic camera can be affected by either of these dyes staining the tissue and impairing vision by darkening

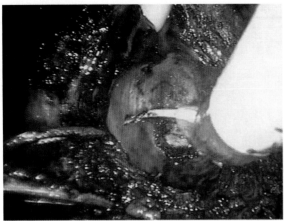

Fig. 25.1 The mucosa of the median lobe is scored and cut, as distally as possible, with scissors

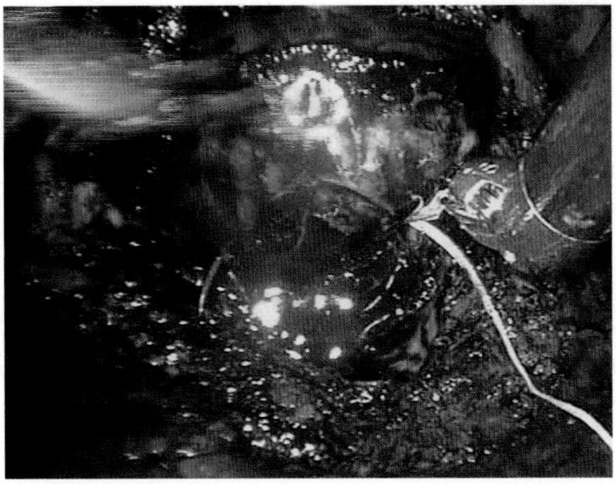

Fig. 25.2 2-0 polyglactin sutures on a CT-1 needle being placed for traction of the median lobe

the operative field during the procedure.[8] Other techniques used to avoid injury to the orifices include extra upward traction on the Foley balloon, use of a 30° down lens, and increasing magnification. If the median lobe is of a significant size, it might obscure the identification of the ureteral orifices. In these cases, extreme caution should be exercised to prevent trauma to the trigone and ureteral orifices. With this caution in mind, several techniques may be employed to manipulate the median lobe out of the operative field, from left to right or from right to left, so as to adequately visualize the operative field as one proceeds with the remaining portion of the RARP.

After the median lobe has been completely dissected free of the mucosa and of the trigonal area, the recommended means of retracting this off the operative field would be as follows:

1. If the surgeon has the 4-arm robot, the 4th arm can be used to retract the median lobe as needed, be it from left to right, right to left, or from the inferior to the superior aspect, to expose the appropriate surgical plane, to proceed with the prostatectomy.
2. If this option is not available or impossible, we recommend using 2-0 or 1-0 polyglactin sutures on a CT-1 needle for traction (Fig. 25.2). This large needle can adequately affix a firm suture or sutures to the median lobe so as to promote adequate traction, either by the 4th arm of the robot or by the assistant, on either side, using grasping forceps to retract the median lobe away from the surgical field. Often,

depending on the size of the median lobe, more than one traction suture may be needed.

Once the median lobe has been adequately retracted away or excised, further dissection is continued as per the surgeon's preference whether it is to move toward the posterior bladder neck and the ampullae of the vas or to move laterally so as to drop the pedicles before further developing the plane between the bladder and the prostate.

25.3.3 Management of the Ureteral Orifices

An important aspect of performing a safe robotic prostatectomy (or for any radical prostatectomy) is to adequately locate and ensure that the ureteral orifices or ureter is not compromised or traumatized in any way during the dissection underneath the significant median lobe.

One recommendation we have followed successfully, after the median lobe and/or the prostate is removed off the field, is to identify the ureteral orifices as follows:

1. A 30° down lens may be required for this maneuver. We highly recommend a 5 Fr infant feeding tube be used instead of the usual ureteral catheters, since the infant feeding tubes are softer, less traumatic,

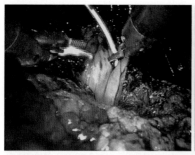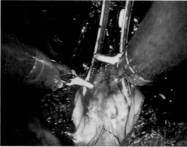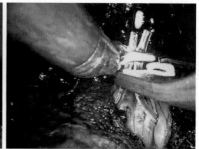

Fig. 25.3 a Right ureteral orifice being catheterized with 5 Fr infant feeding tube. **b** Both infant feeding tubes in place. **c** The distal ends are clipped together with Hem-o-lok clips

and more rounded at the tips. The valve end of the infant feeding tube is cut and removed prior to inserting it into the laparoscopic trocars. We recommend both orifices to be individually catheterized and that the two distal ends be clipped with Hem-o-lok clips, so as to ensure its presence in the orifice without being extruded or pushed into the bladder by ureteral peristalsis (Fig. 25.3).

2. If the robotic surgeon is comfortable with the distance of the orifices from the resected margins, intravenous indigo carmine or methylene blue with efflux of blue-tinged urine may be adequate.

In any case, we recommend the orifices be clearly identified prior to closure of the bladder neck or prior to the urethrovesical anastomosis in the presence of a significant median lobe.

If the ureteral orifices are relatively close to the excised margin we recommend that the infant feeding tubes be left in as the posterior bladder neck is very carefully rolled over the mucosa to make the ureteral orifices roll into the bladder during closure of the posterior aspect of the bladder or with the urethrovesical anastomosis. Once the anastomosis is approximately 70% completed and the subsequent sutures are away from the posterior aspect of the bladder, we recommend that the infant feeding tube be removed prior to completion of the urethrovesical anastomosis. As a cautionary note, we recommend careful monitoring of the urine output postoperatively to ensure there is no inadvertent pressure on the ureteral orifices.

In case of any question or concerns, or if the patient does have any unexpected postoperative discomfort, an ultrasound or other appropriate imaging, such as CT scan, is recommended to ensure the absence of

silent hydronephrosis secondary to edema around the ureteral orifices. Further management, if hydronephrosis is encountered, will include measures such as percutaneous placement of nephrostomy tube or a gentle attempt to percutaneously place ureteral stents. Careful clinical correlation with objective findings, prior to any postoperative invasive procedures, is highly recommended.

In conclusion, if at all possible, it is important to make a preoperative diagnosis of not only the presence, but also the size of the median lobe. Once the median lobe is encountered, adequate traction should delineate the operative field and thus protect the ureteral orifices.

25.4 RARP for Large Prostate

RARP in patients with a massive prostate gland that fills the pelvic outlet is a technical challenge, as compared to performing prostatectomy on smaller glands. The difficulty in performing RARP in patients with larger-sized prostates concerns the smaller working space of the pelvis, which reduces the ability to manipulate, retract, and rotate the gland. Additionally, a large prostate displaces the neurovascular bundles posteriorly.[9] There is no definition as to what constitutes a large prostate, in the radical prostatectomy literature. Previous studies have used values 70–80 g to define a large prostate.[10–15] Published open and laparoscopic prostatectomy series have demonstrated an inverse relationship between prostate volume and both extraprostatic extension and positive surgical margins.[10–13]

El-Hakim et al.[16] reported their athermal RARP technique in 30 men with prostates larger than 75 g. The mean operative time was 193 min and mean estimated blood loss was 208 mL. All surgical margins were found to be negative. The authors concluded that although RARP for patients with large prostates is challenging, the robotic approach does not compromise oncologic control. Zorn et al.[15] reported a series of 375 men undergoing RARP. The patients were divided into four groups as less than 30 g ($n = 20$), 30–50 g ($n = 201$), 50–80 g ($n = 123$), and larger than 80 g ($n = 31$). The authors found no significant difference in operative time, estimated blood loss, hospital stay, length of Foley catheterization, and complication rates. The positive surgical margin rates were significantly different among the groups, demonstrating a trend of increase in surgical margin positivity with lower prostate volumes. Yadav et al.[14] studied 700 RARP procedures. The authors compared surgical and oncologic outcomes among small prostate (<40 cc, $n = 217$), intermediate size (40–70 cc, $n = 375$), and large prostate (>70 cc, $n = 108$) groups. Cumulatively, 14.6% had extraprostatic extension and 8.6% had positive surgical margins on final pathology. The authors, however, found greater incidence of extraprostatic extension in the small prostate group (16.7%) compared to the larger prostate (7.3%) group and concluded that small prostates have a higher cancer density and, therefore, a greater incidence of extraprostatic extension. Msezane et al.[17] performed a multivariate analysis in a series of 709 men who underwent RARP and found an inverse relationship between prostate volume and extraprostatic extension and positive surgical margins. The authors concluded that prostate volume is an independent predictor of both extraprostatic extension and positive surgical margins. While the aforementioned studies were performed transperitoneally, Boczko et al.[18] evaluated the effects of prostate size on treatment outcomes after extraperitoneal RARP. In this study, patients with prostate weight <75 g ($n = 319$) were compared with those having glands ≥75 g ($n = 36$). The authors found a large prostate volume is associated with an increase in postoperative urinary complications. A significantly higher percentage of cases of urinary tract infection (1.5% vs. 8.3%) and urinary retention after catheter removal (<1% vs. 13%) occurred in patients with larger prostates. The 6-month continence rate was significantly lower (84% vs. 97%) in the large prostate group.

25.4.1 Technical Modifications for Large Prostates

As with patients with large median lobes, traction sutures may have to be deployed so that the assistant (or 4th arm) can retract the prostate appropriately to visualize the prostatic pedicles and the rectum. In these cases, the traction sutures are placed laterally and posteriorly. Despite these efforts, management of large and wide-based prostates is challenging and will require patience and increased operative time. An additional challenge facing the robotic surgeon in this clinical situation is the probability of additional robotic instrument-induced bleeding, because of lack of adequate space between the prostate gland, the pubic bones, and the pelvic sidewall.

Preoperative assessment of the prostate size is crucial to prevent any complications or frustrations during RARP. Adequate patient counseling regarding outcomes, based on published literature as mentioned above, is important.

25.4.2 Management of the Large Bladder Neck

It is possible that after RARP for patients with large median lobe or a large prostate gland, the resulting bladder neck will be larger than is normally expected.

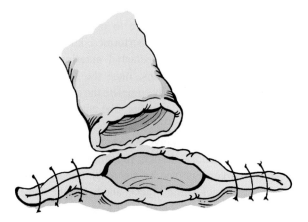

Fig. 25.4 Fish-mouth closure: Anterior view of large open bladder neck (BN); sutures from 3 and 9 o'clock positions are run medially, decreasing the BN size

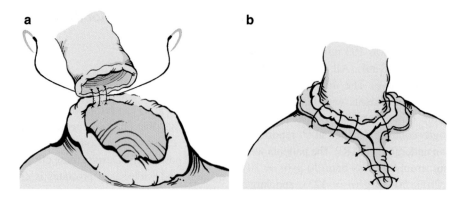

Fig. 25.5 **a** Anterior view showing start of vesico-urethral anastomosis in standard fashion. **b** The residual large bladder neck is closed anteriorly (tennis racket closure)

Most urethro-vesical anastomosis factors in a bladder neck that is much larger than the urethral margin, with the robotic surgeon making appropriate adjustments to take wider "suture-bites" on the bladder side as compared to the urethral side. Occasionally, if this maneuver is insufficient, the residual bladder is closed anteriorly.

However, if the bladder neck defect is too large, then the two following techniques are suggested:

a. *Fish-mouth closure*: In this technique, sutures are taken at 3 and 9 o'clock on the bladder neck and run medially until the bladder neck is of a sufficient size to meet the surgeon's comfort level (Fig. 25.4). Once this has been accomplished, the remainder of the vesico-urethral anastomosis is continued in a usual manner. Caution should be exercised to safeguard the ureteral orifices.

b. *Anterior tennis racket technique*: With this technique, recommendations are to proceed with the anastomosis as is usually performed, knowing that there will still be a substantial anterior bladder defect (Fig. 25.5a). Thus, once the anastomotic sutures circumferentially complete the anastomosis, these sutures are tied together. The anterior bladder neck defect is then closed in a side-to-side manner using 2-0 or 3-0 polyglactin sutures (Fig. 25.5b) similar to bladder closures for other surgical procedures when the bladder has to be opened. This closure mimics a tennis racket and hence the name.

In summary, RARP for patients with larger prostates appears to have similar surgical outcomes when compared to smaller prostates. Although there is no randomized prospective study, all retrospective studies demonstrated lesser incidence of positive surgical margins with the increasing prostate volume, though increased operative time should be allocated. Challenges will be encountered in these patients because of limited operating space between the large prostate gland and the pelvic sidewall.

References

1. Badani KK, Kaul S, Menon M. Evolution of robotic radical prostatectomy: assessment after 2766 procedures. *Cancer.* 2007;110:1951.
2. Pruthi RS, Wallen EM. Current status of robotic prostatectomy: promises fulfilled. *J Urol.* 2009;181:2420.
3. Tanagho EA, Nguyen HT. Embryology of the genitourinary system. In: Tanagho EA, McAninch JW, eds. *Smith's General Urology.* 17th ed. New York, NY: McGraw-Hill Professional; 2007:17–29.
4. Glenister TW. The development of the utricle and of the so-called 'middle' or 'median' lobe of the human prostate. *J Anat.* 1962;96:443.
5. Jenkins LC, Nogueira M, Wilding GE, Tan W, Kim HL, Mohler JL, et al. Median lobe in robot-assisted radical prostatectomy: evaluation and management. *Urology.* 2008;71:810.
6. Meeks JJ, Zhao L, Greco KA, Macejko A, Nadler RB. Impact of prostate median lobe anatomy on robotic-assisted laparoscopic prostatectomy. *Urology.* 2009;73:323.
7. Sarle R, Tewari A, Hemal AK, Menon M. Robotic-assisted anatomic radical prostatectomy: technical difficulties due to a large median lobe. *Urol Int.* 2005;74:92.
8. Rehman J, Chughtai B, Guru K, Shabsigh R, Samadi DB. Management of an enlarged median lobe with ureteral orifices at the margin of bladder neck during robotic-assisted laparoscopic prostatectomy. *Can J Urol.* 2009;16:4490.

9. Myers RP. Practical surgical anatomy for radical prostatectomy. *Urol Clin North Am*. 2001;28:473.
10. Chang CM, Moon D, Gianduzzo TR, Eden CG. The impact
of prostate size in laparoscopic radical prostatectomy. *Eur
Urol*. 2005;48:285.
11. Freedland SJ, Isaacs WB, Platz EA, Terris MK, Aronson
WJ, Amling CL, et al. Prostate size and risk of high-grade,
advanced prostate cancer and biochemical progression after
radical prostatectomy: a search database study. *J Clin
Oncol*. 2005;23:7546.
12. Frota R, Turna B, Santos BM, Lin YC, Gill IS, Aron
M. The effect of prostate weight on the outcomes of
laparoscopic radical prostatectomy. *BJU Int*. 2008;101:
589.
13. Hsu EI, Hong EK, Lepor H. Influence of body weight and
prostate volume on intraoperative, perioperative, and postoperative outcomes after radical retropubic prostatectomy.
Urology. 2003;61:601.
14. Yadav R, Tu JJ, Jhaveri J, Leung RA, Rao S, Tewari
AK. Prostate volume and the incidence of extraprostatic
extension: is there a relation? *J Endourol*. 2009;23:383.
15. Zorn KC, Orvieto MA, Mikhail AA, Gofrit ON, Lin S,
Schaeffer AJ, et al. Effect of prostate weight on operative and postoperative outcomes of robotic-assisted laparoscopic prostatectomy. *Urology*. 2007;69:300.
16. El-Hakim A, Leung RA, Richstone L, Kim TS, Te AE,
Tewari A. Athermal robotic technique of prostatectomy in
patients with large prostate glands (>75 g): technique and
initial results. *BJU Int*. 2006;98:47.
17. Msezane LP, Gofrit ON, Lin S, Shalhav AL, Zagaja GP,
Zorn KC. Prostate weight: an independent predictor for
positive surgical margins during robotic-assisted laparoscopic radical prostatectomy. *Can J Urol*. 2007;14:3697.
18. Boczko J, Erturk E, Golijanin D, Madeb R, Patel H,
Joseph JV. Impact of prostate size in robot-assisted radical
prostatectomy. *J Endourol*. 2007;21:184.

Chapter 26

Extraperitoneal Robot-Assisted Radical Prostatectomy: Simulating the Gold Standard

Ahmed Ghazi and Jean Joseph

26.1 Introduction

While open prostatectomy is routinely performed in the extraperitoneal space, the newer methods of laparoscopic radical prostatectomy (LRP) and robot-assisted radical prostatectomy (RARP) are instead more commonly performed transabdominally. The familiar laparoscopic transperitoneal anatomy and larger working area have made it the preferred approach for the majority of surgeons performing these procedures laparoscopically or using robot assistance. Herein the procedure and the arguments for the extraperitoneal robot-assisted radical prostatectomy technique, which has been my preferred approach in nearly 2,000 cases, are presented.

26.1.1 Robot-Assisted Radical Prostatectomy Procedure

26.1.1.1 Access

Extraperitoneal access is the first step in all procedures. The initial access is obtained via a 2–3 cm periumbilical incision to expose the posterior rectus sheath. A 1 cm incision is made in the anterior sheath, bringing the rectus muscle fibers into view. This incision should be very superficial to avoid bleeding which

may result from incising the muscle fibers. Using a small clamp, the muscle fibers are retracted laterally allowing visualization of the posterior sheath. Once the latter is visualized, a balloon dilator is inserted over the posterior sheath, down to the retropubic space of Retzius. With the scope inserted through the balloon, the retroperitoneal space is created under direct vision. The epigastric vessels can be visualized, with care taken not to dissect them off of the lower aspect of the rectus muscle belly. This can lead to bleeding compromising visualization. The external iliac vessels can be easily visualized and care taken not to compress them or tearing the epigastric vessels from their takeoff point. Once the space has been created the balloon dilator is removed. If more space is needed a long beveled trocar can be used to bluntly push the peritoneum cephalad. A fan retractor or laparoscopic clamp can be used to push the peritoneum off the anterior abdominal wall. This step is necessary to facilitate placement of the assistant trocars. Extreme caution is advised at this stage to avoid entering the peritoneal cavity. This can be a significant challenge in patients with prior lower abdominal surgeries, such as a herniorrhaphy or appendectomy. Entering the peritoneal cavity decreases the extraperitoneal space due to bulging of the peritoneum. The procedure can still be carried out extraperitoneally as discussed below.

26.1.1.2 Port Placement

Four to five additional ports are placed under direct vision, with enough space left between the robotic trocars, to avoid instrument collision. Care should be taken not to place the assistant ports too lateral. This can lead to decreased ability to reach the pelvis, or

J. Joseph (✉)
Section of Laparoscopic and Robotic Surgery, University of Rochester Medical Center, Rochester, NY
e-mail: jean_joseph@urmc.rochester.edu

A.K. Hemal, M. Menon (eds.), *Robotics in Genitourinary Surgery*,
DOI 10.1007/978-1-84882-114-9_26, © Springer-Verlag London Limited 2011

work area, due to restriction from the pelvic brim. Both a 3-arm and a 4-arm robot can be used with this approach, with enough space available for one or two assistant ports.

26.1.1.3 Endopelvic Fascia

Once the extraperitoneal space is developed, access to the endopelvic fascia is immediate. The bladder dissection or "takedown" step is eliminated with the extraperitoneal approach. The endopelvic fascia is incised freeing the prostate from its lateral attachments. Accessory vessels, if present, are identified and preserved. Puboprostatic ligaments are trimmed to further facilitate mobilization of the prostatic apex.

26.1.1.4 Dorsal Vein Ligation

The groove between the urethra and dorsal vein can often be identified with lateral retraction of the prostate apex. A 2-0 vicryl suture ligature is used to ligate the dorsal vein. We do not routinely ligate the branches of Santorini's plexus, but this can be done to help minimize bleeding during the bladder neck dissection.

26.1.1.5 Bladder Neck Dissection

Using a Prograsp in the 4th arm, or a fan retractor if a 3-arm unit is used, tension is placed on the bladder to help visualize the bladder neck. Blunt dissection and cautery are used to facilitate visualization of the bladder neck fibers. These are pushed cephalad, with care taken not to enter the prostate capsule. Once the longitudinal urethral fibers are identified, the bladder neck is transected sharply. Cautery is used selectively to control bleeding from the bladder neck. Upon entering the anterior aspect of the bladder, the trigonal ridge is identified, prior to transecting the posterior bladder neck.

26.1.1.6 Seminal Vesicle Dissection

Following the bladder neck transection, the longitudinal muscular fibers overlying the seminal vesicles can be visualized. They are incised transversely in the

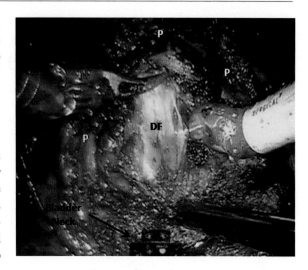

Fig. 26.1 Division of the posterior Denonvilliers' fascia (seminal vesicle fascia) for identification of the vasa deferens and seminal vesicles; DF, Denonvilliers' fascia

midline bringing the ampullae into view (Fig. 26.1). The ampullae are clipped and retracted anteriorly using the 4th arm, or a grasper, to assist in visualizing the seminal vesicles. The artery to the vas can be seen coursing between the seminal vesicles and ampullae. The ampullae and artery to the vas are clipped en bloc.

26.1.1.7 Posterior Prostate Dissection

Retracting the ampullae anteriorly allows visualization of Denonvilliers' fascia (Fig. 26.2). The latter is incised exposing the perirectal fat. Using blunt dissection, the prostate is freed from the anterior rectal wall. Care should be taken to avoid injuring the rectum, particularly in patients with conditions causing significant periprostatic inflammation, where the rectal wall is adherent to the posterior prostate. An assistant's finger or a rectal bougie can be helpful in delineating the tissue planes and avoid a rectal injury. The rectal wall should be inspected immediately if an injury is suspected.

26.1.1.8 Neurovascular Bundle Dissection

We perform a cautery-free technique using clips to control all vessels entering the prostate. The ampulla from the contralateral side being dissected is used

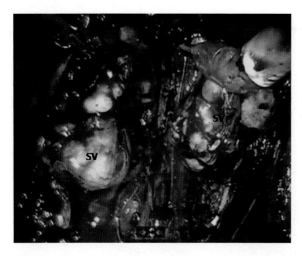

Fig. 26.2 Complete dissection of both seminal vesicles and vas deferens

to place traction on the prostate. The prostate capsule is exposed bluntly. Vessels and surrounding neural tissues coursing behind the prostate are pushed posteriorly. Once the main neurovascular trunks are identified, vessels entering the prostate are clipped (Fig. 26.3). We perform an interfascial dissection in nerve-sparing cases. Once the main vessels entering the base of the prostate are controlled, the remainder of the dissection is carried out bluntly, pushing the neurovascular bundle posteriorly. In non-nerve-sparing cases, the pelvic fascia is incised next to levator ani. The bundles and investing fascia are left attached

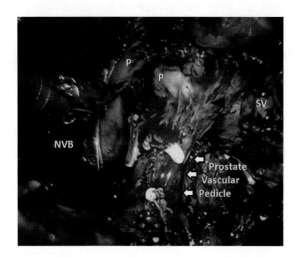

Fig. 26.3 Plane for nerve-sparing dissection along the lateral border of the prostate (indicated by the *black arrowhead*); P, prostate; SV, seminal vesicle; NVB, neurovascular bundle

to the prostate when a wide resection is performed. Figure 26.4a demonstrates a completely resected bundle on the right side, versus the left where the bundle has been preserved. A bilateral neurovascular bundle preservation is shown in Fig. 26.4b. We do not perform or recommend an intrafascial dissection due to the increased risk of positive surgical margin.

26.1.1.9 Apical Dissection

The previously ligated dorsal vein is transected, identifying the urethra (Fig. 26.5a). When a very broad dorsal vein is present, it can also be transected with subsequent oversewing using a 2-0 vicryl on an SH or RB needle. The previously placed suture can at times become loose during the apical dissection, due to traction on the prostate. Increasing the intra-abdominal pressure to 20 mmHg helps achieve hemostasis before the vein stump is oversewn. The contour of the prostate should be followed during this step, to avoid transecting the prostate apex. This dissection is carried out in a caudal direction, to limit this risk.

The Foley catheter is inserted through the prostate to allow visualization of the anterior urethra. We prefer transecting this sharply to avoid ischemic mucosal trauma to the urethra (Fig. 26.5b). This also helps prevent cautery damage to the adjacent neurovascular bundles. Once the prostate is freed, it is placed in an endocatch bag and pulled near the tip of one of the assistant's trocar.

26.1.1.10 Vesicourethral Anastomosis

Prior to starting the anastomosis, Denonvilliers' fascia is sewn to the posterior urethra (Figs. 26.6, 26.7a). This step helps approximate the bladder to the urethra, in preparation for the vesicourethral anastomosis.

The anastomosis is completed using two separate (2-0 vicryl, RB 1 needle) sutures. The first suture is placed at the 5 o'clock position in the urethra and anastomosed to its corresponding position at the bladder neck (Fig. 26.7b). This is carried out in a counterclockwise direction to the 11 o'clock position. The second suture is done in the opposite direction from the 5 to 11 o'clock (Fig. 26.7c). The Foley catheter is used to help identify the urethral lumen. We routinely decrease the pressure in the retroperitoneal space to 8–10 mmHg to

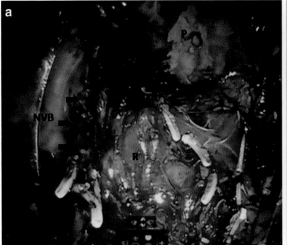
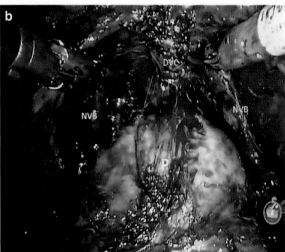

Fig. 26.4 Operative view of a bilateral and unilateral nerve-preserving dissection prior to apical dissection. **a** Unilateral nerve-sparing dissection (left nerve-preserving technique and right non-nerve-preserving technique). **b** Bilateral nerve-sparing dissection. Note the use of fewer clips during preservation of the nerve; NVB, neurovascular bundle; R, rectum; P, prostate; DVC, dorsal venous complex

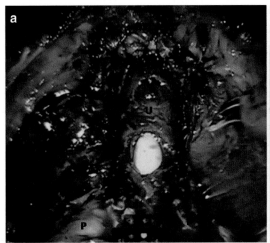
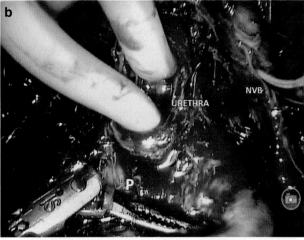

Fig. 26.5 Division of the urethra following dissection and ligation of the dorsal venous complex. **a** Division of the anterior lip of the urethra, revealing the Foley catheter. **b** Division of the posterior lip of the urethra; NVB, neurovascular bundle; U, urethra; P, prostate; DVC, dorsal venous complex

facilitate approximation between the bladder and urethra. A 20 Fr 30 cc Foley catheter is placed into the bladder, prior to tying the anterior anastomotic suture.

26.1.1.11 Specimen Retrieval and Closure

Once the robot is disconnected from the patient, the specimen bag is passed through the midline trocar. A 19 Fr Blake drain is placed in the space of Retzius.

The working and assistant trocars are removed under direct vision, ensuring hemostasis from these sites. The anterior rectus sheath is incised according to specimen size and subsequently closed. No other fascial closure is necessary using the extraperitoneal approach. When trapped intra-abdominal air is suspected, a small opening in the posterior rectus sheath and peritoneum is recommended to evacuate the air, for improved patient comfort postoperatively.

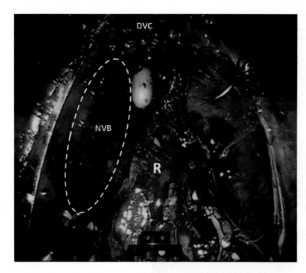

Fig. 26.6 Operative view following removal of the prostate with preservation of the left neurovascular bundle. *Dotted circle* delineating the preserved bundle; R, rectum; NVB, neurovascular bundle; DVC, dorsal venous complex

26.1.1.12 Postoperative Care

Patients are generally discharged home on postoperative day 1 or when they tolerate oral nutrition and do not require intravenous analgesia. A Jackson–Pratt drain placed after surgery is removed prior to discharge if output is less than 30 cc in an 8-h period. The drain is otherwise removed as an outpatient when the output meets such criteria. Foley catheter removal is done 7–10 days postoperatively as an outpatient.

26.1.2 Comparing to the Gold Standard

Unlike open prostatectomy which is generally performed by accessing the space of Retzius, in a completely extraperitoneal fashion, to date there is no uniform way of performing a laparoscopic or robot-assisted radical prostatectomy. Most of these procedures are performed transperitoneally, connecting the abdominal cavity with the space of Retzius. In the extraperitoneal approach, the peritoneum serves as a natural retractor keeping the bowel away from the operative field. In transperitoneal procedures, a steep Trendelenburg position may be required to achieve this task. This can lead to ventilation difficulties and anesthetic complications in patients with compromised respiratory function.

A number of advantages and disadvantages to these two approaches have been described in the literature.[1,2] Several studies have compared the transperitoneal and extraperitoneal laparoscopic/robotic approaches.[3] Patients with prior abdominal surgeries were found to be best suited for the extraperitoneal approach to avoid potential lysis of adhesions and associated bowel complications.

With the transperitoneal approach, the removal of the natural peritoneal barrier places blood from the operative site and potential urine leak from the vesicourethral anastomosis in direct contact with the bowel which can lead to postoperative ileus. The dissipation of blood into the abdominal cavity does not allow small bleeders to potentially tamponade. Access to the intra-abdominal cavity is useful in the setting of lymphatic fluid leakage. The peritoneal surface allows prompt resorption of lymphatic fluid. With meticulous clipping, such lymphatic fluid leak can be avoided. This step is generally fast, since the pelvic vessels are often already exposed with the balloon dilation step.

As with pure laparoscopic prostatectomy, increased experience with robotic procedures has led many centers to adopt an extraperitoneal approach. Following the description of the extraperitoneal approach by Raboy et al.[4] and Bollens et al.[5] who presented the first case report and the first case series of extraperitoneal radical prostatectomy, a number of centers have performed these procedures with several having experience well above a thousand.[6] Gettman and Abbou reported their first four cases with this approach using robotic assistance.[7] In 2006, we published one of the larger robotic series using the extraperitoneal approach.[8] Whether a pure laparoscopic or robot assistance is used, the rationale for the extraperitoneal approach has been the avoidance of the peritoneal cavity and potential complications, similar to the well-accepted open radical prostatectomy technique.

26.1.3 The False Arguments Against the Extraperitoneal Approach

26.1.3.1 The Anastomosis

Critics of the extraperitoneal approach often cite tension at the vesicourethral anastomosis, due to the bladder or urachal attachments to the abdominal wall.

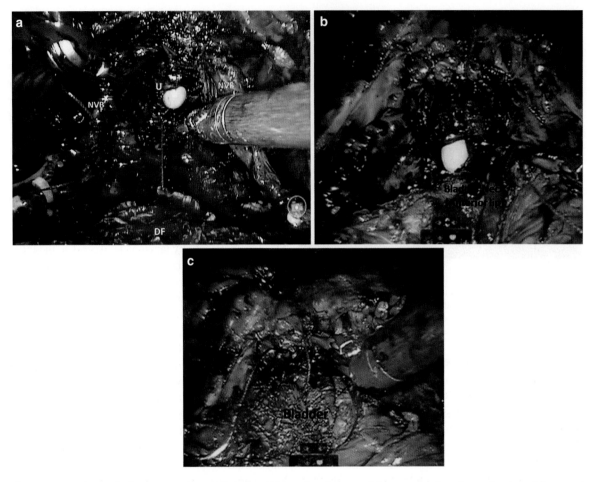

Fig. 26.7 Urethro-vesical anastomosis. **a** Dorsal suture, approximating severed ends of the Denonvilliers' fascia at the posterior bladder neck and urethral stump. **b** Completing the dorsal aspect of the anastomosis. **c** Approximation of the ventral aspect of the anastomosis before applying tension on the running suture

We have found no difficulty approximating the bladder to the urethra. Our recommendation is to decrease the pneumopreperitoneum insufflation pressure to 8–10 mmHg and to have the assistant suction to collapse the space. This allows the bladder to easily approximate to the urethra with the first knot, which is the most difficult. Subsequent suture placement approximating the bladder neck to the urethra is generally easier. We prefer not to move the patient, or change the incline of the table, while the robot is docked. A more commonly used alternative is the application of perineal pressure which leads to protrusion of the urethral stump, facilitating suture placement in difficult cases. As for open radical retropubic prostatectomy, once the gas is evacuated from the retroperitoneal space, or the retractors are removed, the bladder neck remains approximated to the urethra with no undue tension.

26.1.3.2 The Working Space

The extraperitoneal approach has been reported to be more difficult due to a smaller working space. When properly developed, with no peritoneal rent, the space is quite large and non-limiting. A peritoneal rent, however, can significantly collapse the space making visualization difficult. In such setting a fan retractor can be used to retract the bladder cephalad. A steeper Trendelenburg may be required to keep the intra-abdominal contents and peritoneum cephalad. A

5 mm trocar can also be placed in the peritoneal cavity to help evacuate trapped intraperitoneal air. These steps eliminate the need to convert to a transperitoneal laparoscopic procedure.

Faster port placement following intra-abdominal insufflation has been reported with the transperitoneal approach. In the setting of prior abdominal surgery, however, longer operative time may be associated with lysis of adhesions, while the extraperitoneal approach would allow expeditious access to the space of Retzius. The extraperitoneal method is most advantageous in patients with prior abdominal operations. Over a third of my patients have had prior abdominal surgeries, including bowel resection, liver transplant, and others. In my experience with both approaches, I have had faster surgery time due to a shorter time interval between skin incision and endopelvic fascia incision. Intra-abdominal dissection or bladder takedown steps are not necessary.

Besides rapid access to the target organ, another advantage worth mentioning is the rapid completion of wound closure. With the posterior rectus sheath, and peritoneum intact, this approach eliminates the need for fascia closure. Only the fascial opening for retrieval of the specimen requires closure. In my series of extraperitoneal cases, I have not experienced either bowel or omental adhesions when the procedure is completed extraperitoneally. Entering the abdominal cavity requires meticulous fascial closure to eliminate such risks.

Unifying the peritoneal cavity with the space of Retzius can lead to bowel adhesions to the operative site. Not only can this potentially complicate subsequent laparoscopic or open intra-abdominal interventions, it potentially places the bowel in the path of radiation should adjuvant radiation become necessary.

Developing the working space is nearly impossible in patients with prior laparoscopic extraperitoneal mesh hernia repair. This is the main indication that I use to perform a transperitoneal procedure. Besides the previous dissection of the extraperitoneal space, the mesh causes significant inflammatory reaction obliterating the space, causing troublesome peritoneal rents. In such settings it is best to proceed immediately to a transperitoneal route.

26.1.3.3 The Extended Node Dissection

Open prostatectomists with decades of experience and large series of open radical prostatectomists have yet to show conclusive evidence that an extended lymph node dissection provides therapeutic benefit. This argument persists for both laparoscopic and robotic surgeons. Critics of the extraperitoneal approach have cited the inability to perform an extended lymph node dissection. Proper retraction and a downward angled scope can easily permit cephalad dissection up the common iliac node chain (Fig. 26.8a) and further to allow a

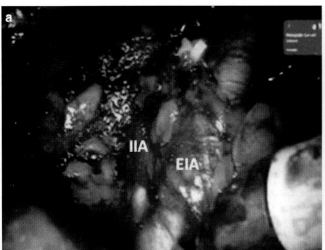
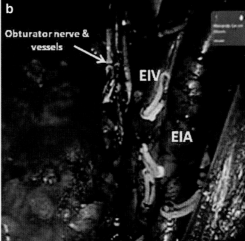

Fig. 26.8 a Cephalad limit of an extended lymph node dissection at the bifurcation of the iliac arteries, using a downward angled scope. EIA, external iliac artery; IIA, internal iliac artery. **b** An extended lymph node dissection performed using an extraperitoneal approach. EIA, external iliac artery; EIV, external iliac vein

thorough and extended node dissection. Similar to open retropubic radical prostatectomy, an extended lymph node dissection can be performed using an extraperitoneal approach (Fig. 26.8b). As mentioned above, the absence of the resorptive peritoneal surface is associated with a higher risk of lymphocele, which is not a trivial drawback. Meticulous clipping of all lymphatic channels is necessary to mitigate such risks. A lymphocele collection is possible in both approaches, but it is much less likely during intraperitoneal surgery. For patients undergoing an extended lymph node dissection, a transperitoneal route helps minimize the risk of lymphocele.

26.2 Conclusions

The extraperitoneal approach is increasingly preferred at a number of centers, once they have overcome the perceived limitations discussed above. Avoiding the abdominal cavity furthers the goals of minimal invasiveness and best duplicates the gold standard open radical retropubic prostatectomy.

References

1. Cathelineau X, Cahill D, Widmer H, Rozet F, Baumert H, Vallancien G. Transperitoneal or extraperitoneal approach for laparoscopic radical prostatectomy: a false debate over a real challenge. *J Urol.* 2004;171:714.
2. Erdogru T, Teber D, Frede T, et al. Comparison of transperitoneal and extraperitoneal laparoscopic radical prostatectomy using match-pair analysis. *Eur Urol.* 2004;46:312.
3. Madi R, Daignault S, Wood DP. Extraperitoneal v intraperitoneal robotic prostatectomy: analysis of operative outcomes. *J Endol.* 2007;21:1553.
4. Raboy A, Ferzli G, Albert P. Initial experience with extraperitoneal endoscopic radical retropubic radical prostatectomy. *Urology.* 1997;50:849.
5. Bollens R, Vanden BM, Roumeguere T. Extraperitoneal laparoscopic radical prostatectomy. Results after 50 cases. *Eur Urol.* 2001;40:65.
6. Stolzenburg JU, McNeill A, Liatsikos EN. Nerve sparing endoscopic extraperitoneal radical prostatectomy. *BJU Int.* 2008;101:909.
7. Gettman MT, Hoznek A, Salomon L, Katz R, Borkowski T, Antiphon P. Laparoscopic radical prostatectomy:description of the extraperitoneal approach using the da Vinci robotic system. *J Urol.* 2003;170:416.
8. Joseph JV, Rosenbaum R, Madeb R, Erturk E, Patel HR. Robotic extraperitoneal radical prostatectomy: an alternative approach. *J Urol.* 2006;175:945.

Chapter 27

The Retrograde Extraperitoneal Approach: Robotic Retrograde Extraperitoneal Laparoscopic Prostatectomy (RRELP)

Charles-Henry Rochat and Pierre Dubernard

27.1 Introduction

It is possible with the da Vinci robot to reproduce exactly the surgical protocol of an open retropubic prostatectomy and to give to the patient all the advantages of mini-invasive surgery.

Nowadays there is no longer a debate when it comes to defining the best way to approach a laparoscopic prostatectomy either in conventional laparoscopy or robotic: intraperitoneal or extraperitoneal. It is the operator's experience that is critical whatever the technique. However, we have to admit that in a majority of high-volume robotic centers, the transperitoneal approach is performed most of the time, which is mainly due to the larger and easier accessible working space than in an extraperitoneal approach. The extraperitoneal approach is recommended in particular to patients with a history of prior abdominal surgery and therefore it should be known in detail.[1–4] In addition it is the only approach that replicates exactly the surgical protocol of open retropubic prostatectomy, which is still the standard operation in many countries.

In this chapter we will develop the aspects of the extraperitoneal prostatectomy and the step-by-step description. This description is based on the experience gained over the past 10 years by the authors and particularly by Pierre Dubernard, who was the first to perform a retrograde extraperitoneal laparoscopic prostatectomy.[5] He joined our team at the robotic centre of the Clinique Générale Beaulieu in Geneva in 2003 in order to adjust his technique to the da Vinci robot. The principle of the retrograde extraperitoneal laparoscopic prostatectomy is the retrograde prostato-semino-rectal cleavage up to the bladder neck, and the key of the of the procedure is the initial approach of the apexo-ureteral junction with ascending dissection of the erectile neurovascular bundles (ENVB).The dissection is facilitated by the use of the 30° lens.

All patients requiring a radical prostatectomy can benefit from a robotic extraperitoneal prostatectomy,[3,6] except those needing an extended lymph node dissection, patients with an indication of salvage prostatectomy after radiotherapy for whom primary access to the rectum through the Douglas is more secure, and patients who had a preperitoneal hernia repair with mesh surgery and a possibly difficult dissection of the Bogros space. Conversely we think that a transabdominal approach is not appropriate for patients with a history of heavy abdominal surgery (peritonitis, occlusion, iterative abdominal surgery) or patients with an associated inguinal hernia where an extraperitoneal approach would be better suited. For obese patients with a high BMI, the extraperitoneal approach has the advantage of the support of the abdominal content by the peritoneum, and the light Trendelenburg position is easier to bear from an anesthesiologic point of view.

27.2 Indication and Preoperative Preparation

There is no difference in the preoperative preparation between a retrograde extraperitoneal robotic prostatectomy and a transabdominal robotic prostatectomy.[7] We recommend waiting at least 6 weeks after the diagnostic biopsies so that the periprostatic inflammatory reactions are resorbed. A preoperative injection of

C.-H. Rochat (✉)
Robot-Assisted Laproscopic Surgery Center, Clinic Generale Beaulieu, Geneva, Switzerland
e-mail: rochat@deckpoint.ch

A.K. Hemal, M. Menon (eds.), *Robotics in Genitourinary Surgery*,
DOI 10.1007/978-1-84882-114-9_27, © Springer-Verlag London Limited 2011

low molecular weight heparin is not a standard procedure but every patient is given a preoperative enema. Antibiotics are given at the time of induction and for as long as the patient keeps the catheter (at our institution the catheter is kept for an average 6 days).

27.3 Operative Setup

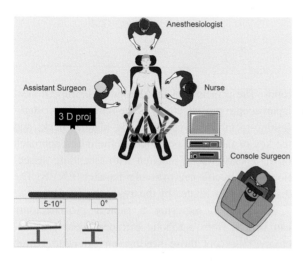

Fig. 27.1 The extraperitoneal approach does not require extended Trendelenburg

27.4 Patient Positioning

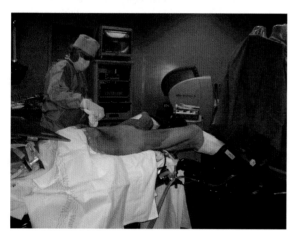

Fig. 27.2 Supine position, legs on supports with pneumatic compressing socks. Table in slight Trendelenburg (note the tray table above the head of the patient)

The operation is performed under general anesthesia and standard monitoring with one or two venous approaches connected by the extenders, protected at arm and hand level and with non-invasive control of arterial pressure via a wristband.

The patient is positioned supine with the arms at the sides of his body and is placed on a gel mattress.

The legs are spread to the sides on a leg support allowing the access of the robot. Compression socks are routinely used. After the patient has been draped, an 18 Fr Foley catheter is inserted. It should be sufficiently flexible so that it can be manipulated using forceps in order to mobilize the prostate upward, backward, and laterally in an atraumatic fashion during the dissection of the apex and the retrograde, prostato-semino-rectal cleavage up to the bladder neck, then during the final section of the bladder neck and the subsequent antegrade vesico-prostatic cleavage.

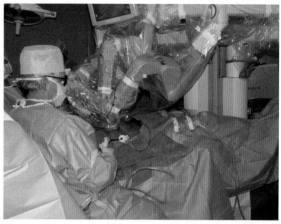

Fig. 27.3 The assistant surgeon is seated at the right side of the patient

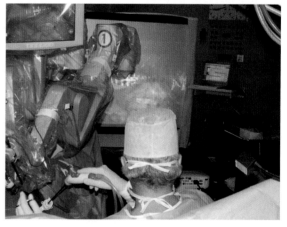

Fig. 27.4 The assistant surgeon wears 3D goggles to view the screen

27.5 Instrumentation List

1. Exposure of the retroperitoneal space:

   • Round preperitoneal distention balloon and inflation bulb (OMS-PDB1000 Auto-Suture)

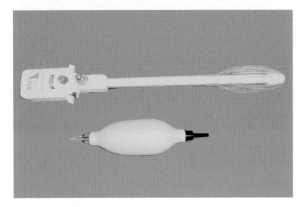

Fig. 27.5   Round preperitoneal distention balloon

   • 12 mm Endopath Xcel bladeless trocar with stability sleeve (B12LT)

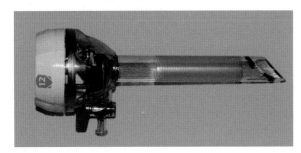

Fig. 27.6   Endopath Xcel bladeless trocar

   • 12 mm VerSastep trocar (Tyco, Norwalk, CO) (×2)
   • 5 mm trocar (×2)

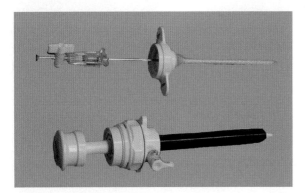

Fig. 27.7   VerSastep trocar

2. Robotic procedure:

   • Robotic trocars da Vinci (×2–3)

Table 27.1   Console surgeon instrumentation (see Fig. 27.1)

Right arm (yellow)	Left arm (green)	Fourth arm (red)	First arm
• Monopolar scissors • Large needle driver (cutting needle holder)	• Cadière forceps	• Maryland bipolar forceps or plasmakinetic • Large needle driver	• 0° 12 mm endoscope • 30° 12 mm endoscope

3. Assistant tools:

   • Long Johan forceps
   • Standard Johan forceps
   • Babcock forceps
   • Laparoscopic scissors
   • Suction device
   • Endoclips:

      ○ Hem-o-lok Wecks ML + L
      ○ Aesculap Challenger

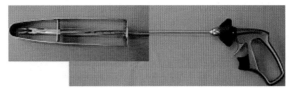

Fig. 27.8   Aesculap Challenger

4. Suture material:

   • Monocryl 3/0 UR 6
   • Vicryl 1 CT-2
   • Vicryl 2-0 JB
   • Ethibond 1 CP 1
   • Stapler Vista 3 M

5. Miscellaneous items:

   • Gyrus® Plasmakinetic generator
   • Electric lancet generator
   • Endobag

27.6 Step-by-Step Technique

Table 27.2 Operative technique step by step

1	Exposure, trocars placement, and robot docking
2	Initial approach to the erectile neurovascular bundle
3	Division of the Santorini plexus and exposure of the anterior hemi-circumference of the urethra
4	Lateral and posterior dissection of the apico-urethral junction
5	Retrograde prostato-semino-rectal cleavage
6	Final section of the bladder neck and latero-vesical prostatic pedicles
7	Vesicourethral anastomosis
8	Lymphadenectomy
9	Closure and drainage

1. Exposure, trocars placement, and robot docking

A transverse incision 2 cm under the umbilicus, slightly on the right side, and 25 mm long is made. The preparation of the subcutaneous incision of the anterior sheet of the right rectus muscle and smooth dissection with the Mayo scissors is carried out in order to lateralize the muscle. Langenbeck retractor keeps the muscle on the side and a dilatation balloon is introduced and pushed until placed below the pubic bone. A conventional laparoscopic 30° lens is introduced in the dilatation balloon and the balloon is inflated.

Hand pressure on the abdomen and lateral movement on the balloon allow a larger dissection of the peritoneum. The dilatation trocar is then exchanged to a 12 mm trocar and under vision we introduce the additional robotic and assistant trocars. All the operating trocars are inserted under direct visual

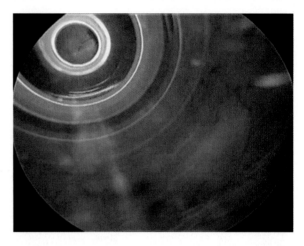

Fig. 27.10 Exposure of the extraperitoneal space, vision through the dilatation balloon

control to avoid the risk of visceral or vascular damage. The use of Johan or bipolar forceps helps to complete the dissection especially to clear the peritoneum laterally to the epigastric vessels. Peritoneal detachment is performed below the epigastric vessels, above the spermatic cord, and above the iliopsoas muscles and then laterally and upward to the anterior abdominal wall.

This stage is performed with caution, carefully avoiding tearing the peritoneum, particularly as it may be hampered by an inguinal hernia, fibrous sequelae resulting from an appendectomy or low lying expansion of the line of Douglas – these will be freed or sectioned.

This detachment should be continued extensively up to the anterior superior iliac spine in order to introduce a 12 mm Versastep trocar, external to the epigastric vessels, on both sides.

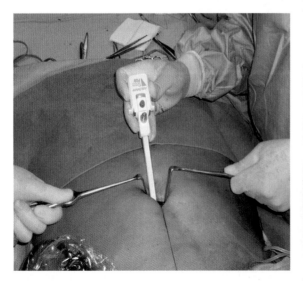

Fig. 27.9 Introduction of the dilatation balloon

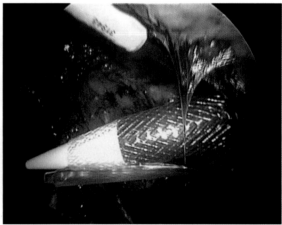

Fig. 27.11 Introduction of the 12 mm trocar through the VerSastep sheet

These Versastep trocars are placed around two fingers medially to the anterior superior iliac spine. The principle of the Versastep is to use the Verrès needle through an extensible sheet which allows for a very precise puncture of the abdominal wall. The 30° camera can also be introduced in the Versastep trocar to finalize the preparation of the space.

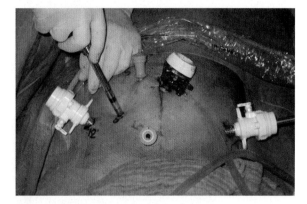

Fig. 27.12 30° camera and conventional laparoscope from the left controlling the trocars placement in the opposite side (patient head up)

The robot trocars are inserted at a distance of 16–18 cm from the pubic bone and one hand-wide from the camera trocar and the robot is docked. For the fourth arm, the robotic instrument trocar will be inserted directly in the Versastep trocar on the left side.[8] An additional 5 mm trocar is inserted between the camera trocar and the right robot instrument trocar. The surgeon console is ready to start the procedure and the patient-side assistant stays on the right side of the patient and is seated on a chair covered with sterile sheets. He uses a long tip suction device through the right Versastep trocar and a Johan forceps through the 5 mm trocar.

2. Initial approach to the ENVB

For the procedure we use monopolar scissors on the first arm, a Cadière forceps on the second arm, and a bipolar or plasmakinetic forceps on the third arm (during the surgery the tools can be exchanged between the second and the third arms depending on the exposure in the field). The cautery is set to 40 W on both instruments.

The 30° camera down is used and we start by removing the fatty tissue covering the anterior surface of the prostate. The endopelvic fascia is then incised with the scissors on both sides avoiding the use of electrocautery. The puboprostatic ligaments are partially incised. We identify the upper third of the lateral side of the prostate and we open transversally the periprostatic fascia. With sharp and smooth dissection we push away the neurovascular bundles starting at the level of the apex and moving backward.

Visualization of the neurovascular bundles is facilitated through the use of the 30° camera and the mobilization of the lateral wall of the prostate, which is reclined toward the central line. Cleavage continues in the front, at the level of the capsule, along the length of the posterior external aspect of the inferior pole of the apex, to the apico-urethral junction, which is exposed by holding the musculo-sphincteral sleeve forward.

Dissection up to this level, which preserves the muscular fibers of the striated sphincter, will also facilitate the subsequent section of the posterior semi-circumference of the urethra and the retrograde prostate-rectal cleavage in an optimal way, while also reducing the risk of positive apical surgical margins.

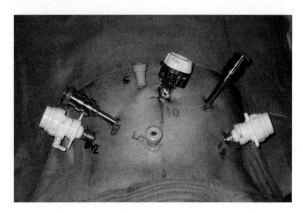

Fig. 27.13 Final trocars position (patient head up)

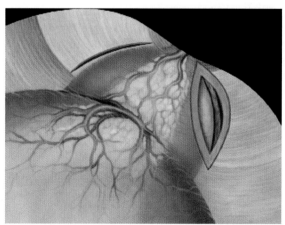

Fig. 27.14 Incision of the endopelvic fascia and initial approach to the ENVB

During the nerve-sparing portion of the procedure we do not use any form of electrocautery. Small 2 mm clips are used to secure small perforating vessels. Once the neurovascular bundles are well identified and pushed away from the prostate we move to the next step, division of the Santorini and the urethra.

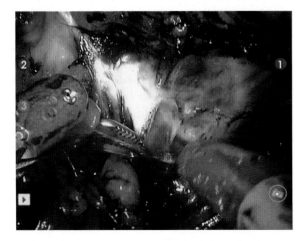

Fig. 27.15 Incision of the endopelvic fascia and initial approach to the ENVB with curvated cissors

3. Division of the Santorini plexus and exposure of the anterior hemi-circumference of the urethra

A Babcock forceps is introduced through the 5 mm trocar and grasps the Santorini plexus. With the scissors we complete the incision of the puboprostatic ligaments and we recline the periureteral sphincteric muscle fibers. The tools are changed for two Endowrist® needle drivers and a Vicryl 2/0 JB 14 cm is introduced by the assistant. An X point secures the Santorini plexus. Another similar suture is placed in the middle of the prostate to control the backflow. At this time of the procedure the assistant plays a very important role to expose symmetrically the apex by placing on both sides the Johan forceps and the tip of the suction device. With the monopolar scissors the console surgeon cuts through the Santorini and through the anterior part of the urethra leaving a security margin of 2–4 mm from the apex. This stage can be performed in various ways and thus adapted to the individual anatomic situation:

• While Santorini's plexus is easily pediculized, it is grasped using Babcock forceps and then sectioned with the scissors up to the urethra before being secured and subsequently tied.

• After this initial dissection and tying, Santorini's plexus can then be grasped with forceps and sectioned using scissors up to the latero-prostatic pillars on both sides of the urethra.

The anterior and lateral faces of the urethra will be dissected after the sectioning of the Müller ligaments; the thickness of which differs from case to case.

This approach facilitates access to the anterio-inferior side of the apical poles, which extend under the urethra and taper at the end.

We recommend a cold section with a minimum of cautery to avoid thermal damage to the sphincter and to the nerves.

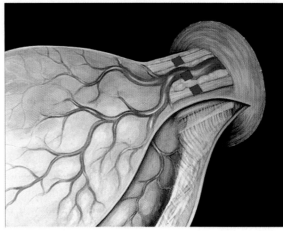

Fig. 27.16 Schematic view of the lateral aspect of the Santorini plexus

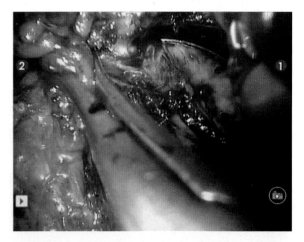

Fig. 27.17 Exposure of the Santorini plexus with Babcock forceps

4. Lateral and posterior dissection of the apico-urethral junction

This is the critical stage of the technique, which aims to reduce the apical margin risks as much as possible and preserve the sphincteric and erectile structures.

Once the anterior half of the urethra has been divided the Foley catheter is grasped with the robot forceps and the apico-urethral junction is exposed. The 30° camera down allows for perfect vision in this critical step of the operation. The neurovascular bundles are pushed laterally and fibers of the Denonvilliers' fascia are incised first on the right side until we can enter the inter-prostatorectal plan as we proceed in open surgery. This allows for perfect visualization of the posterior part of the apex of the prostate as it tapers under the urethra and the expansion of Denonvilliers' fascia to the recto-urethral muscle. These are well individualized and cleaved at the anterior face of the rectum at the rear and at the posterior semi-circumference of the urethra at the front.

The apical poles are reclined gradually upward, backward, and inward, which perfectly exposes the apico-urethral junction at the front, Denonvilliers' fascia internally, the anterior wall of the rectum at the rear, the sphincteral sleeve below, and the erectile neurovascular bundle externally. We complete then the posterior division of the urethra under perfect visual control.

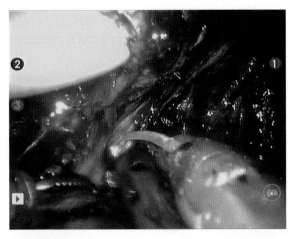

Fig. 27.20 Athermal dissection of the apico-urethral junction

5. Retrograde prostato-semino-rectal cleavage

The prostate is raised by pulling the Foley catheter upward and backward. The neurovascular bundles are easily identified and perforating vessels are secured with 2 mm clips. We continue the retrograde cleavage by pulling the prostate backward and lateralizing the neurovascular bundles. Once we are at the level of the base of the prostate we open again the Denonvilliers' fascia and we grasp the vas deferens. The two vas are

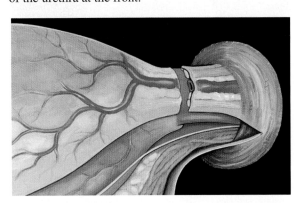

Fig. 27.18 Section of the Santorini plexus

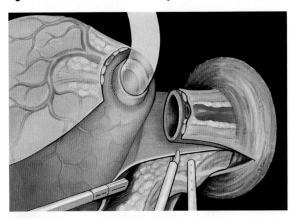

Fig. 27.19 Dissection of the apico-urethral junction

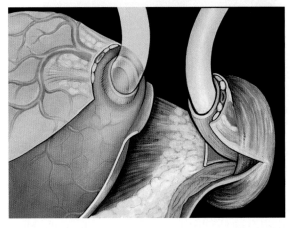

Fig. 27.21 Initiation of retrograde prostato-semino-rectal cleavage

then cut and cauterized without clipping the proximal end. The seminal vesicles are dissected and the small pedicles are clipped. If the dissection is easy and free of adhesion, we completely remove the vesicles, and if it is not the case we leave the tip in place in order to avoid further damage to the neurovascular bundles. We try to extend this retrograde dissection nearly to the level of the trigone. In small-volume prostates care should be taken not to injure the ureters. The latero-prostatic pedicles are clipped and sectioned as far backward as possible.

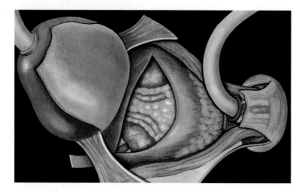

Fig. 27.22 Completed retrograde prostato-semino-rectal cleavage with exposure of the seminal vesicles

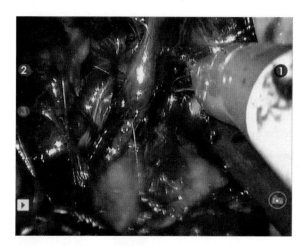

Fig. 27.23 Retrograde prostato-semino-rectal cleavage (the left ENVB is lateralized)

6. Final section of the bladder neck and latero-vesical prostatic pedicles

The last step of the prostatectomy is the bladder neck dissection which is done in an antegrade manner. The bladder catheter is pushed away from the bladder neck and the prostate is elevated with the Cadière forceps grasping the ligature placed at the beginning of the procedure in the middle of the prostate. As we

did to expose the apex, again the patient-side assistant will expose the bladder neck with a suction device and the Johan forceps on both sides of the Foley catheter. Once prepared the division of the bladder neck is not done immediately. We first divided the vesical prostatic pedicles after having clipped them with median size Hem-o-lok clip. By pulling the prostate and the bladder in an opposite side, the pedicles are kept under tension which allows to control and separate them easily. The bladder neck is then divided. We try to keep a small bladder neck at distance of the ureteric orifices which should always be identified. The last attachments of the prostate are divided and the prostatectomy is completed. The prostate is inspected in order to check the integrity of the capsule and the apex, then the prostate is put on the prepared space, laterally to one of the Versastep trocars.

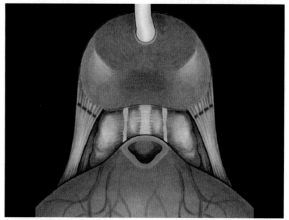

Fig. 27.24 Final section of the bladder neck and latero-vesical prostatic pedicles

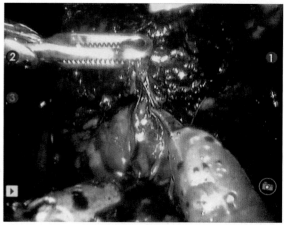

Fig. 27.25 Final section of the bladder neck

7. Vesicourethral anastomosis

After having controlled the hemostasis of the dissection field we perform the anastomosis without specific posterior reconstruction. The vesicourethral anastomosis is done with two half running sutures with 3/0 Monocryl. Special attention should be paid to keep the running suture under tension to avoid any posterior leakage. A new 18 Fr Foley catheter is inserted and its position is controlled before knotting the suture. The balloon is inflated and the bladder is filled with 200 ml of saline to check if the suture is watertight and also in order to rinse the bladder of eventual clots.

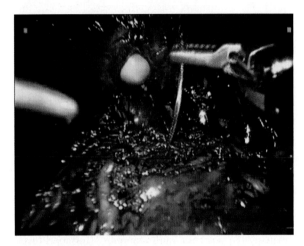

Fig. 27.26 Running suture for the vesicoureteral anastomosis

8. Lymphadenectomy

If a lymphadenectomy has been planned we do it at the end of the prostatectomy. Most of the time it is performed in a traditional way by clearing the nodes in the obturator fossa. The obturator nerve is free of all lymphatic tissue, as the external iliaca vein up to its crossing with the hypogastric artery. The lymphostasis is assured by mini-clips or by bipolar cautery. The lymph nodes are then extracted through the 12 mm trocar.

9. Closure and drainage

After undocking the robot, the prostate is placed in an endobag inserted through the camera trocar, under vision of the lens placed in one of the 12 mm Versastep trocars. The prostate is extracted after having enlarged the abdominal wall incision. A suction drain is placed. The anterior sheet of the rectus muscle is closed with a running suture. The other orifices are only closed with skin staples.

27.7 Postoperative Management

The pneumatic compression socks are applied two to three times a day for a few days and the patient is put under low molecular weight heparin from the sixth postoperative hour. The patient is fed progressively from day 1 and rapidly fully mobilized. The suction drain is removed between day 2 and day 3 even if it is still draining lymph. The catheter is removed on day 6 after a cystogram. A prophylactic antibiotic therapy is given as long as the patient keeps the catheter. We give corticoids for 3 days starting at the induction in order to decrease the inflammation and perioperative edemas. In our country, patients are not usually discharged with a catheter, so the hospitalization time is approximately 1 week.

27.8 Data Management

We have developed since 2005 through the European Group of Robotic Urology an Internet database (see Chapter 17). This allows us to record and to analyze all of the clinical, surgical, pathological, and functional outcomes. We think that it is a mandatory step for quality control, improving surgical technique and outcomes, and to compare our results with other institutions, thereby ultimately benefitting our patients.

27.9 Special Considerations

Extraperitoneal prostatectomy and combined hernia repair:

It is not infrequent that patients scheduled for prostatectomy present with concomitant inguinal hernia.[9] The extraperitoneal approach allows for an easy dissection of the hernia.

If the patient has an indirect hernia, the suture of the hedge hernia's ring with a running suture as in the Nyhus procedure is possible. But in the case of a large direct hernia, a mesh prosthesis is more advisable. The combined repair of an inguinal hernia during a laparoscopic prostatectomy is feasible and safe provided the mesh is not exposed to the bowel. In this case, the extraperitoneal prostatectomy should be preferred.

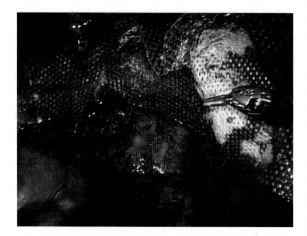

Fig. 27.27 Bilateral hernia mesh repair associated with a radical extraperitoneal prostatectomy

27.10 Steps to Avoiding Complications

During the extraperitoneal procedure, some air can enter and inflate the peritoneal cavity which will reduce the working space.[10] In this case, a Verrès needle can be inserted in the left hypochondrium in order to decrease the abdominal pressure.

27.11 Discussion

After having described the purely technical aspects of this operation, some fundamental questions still need to be emphasized:

1. Why a robotic approach?

If one is still not convinced, the answer is obviously given by the 3D magnification of the anatomic structures. The precision and the advantages of minimally invasive surgery will not be discussed further in this section.

2. Why an extraperitoneal approach?

Reasons for this choice:

First, why a transperitoneal route when this route is almost never used via open surgery and as there is

no truly valid reason for using it, not even for primary access to the seminal vesicles, which does not appear to be an essential preliminary phase of the operation?

The prostate's location in the subperitoneal space means that an intraperitoneal approach requires successive and unnecessary invasions of the peritoneal cavity, which is a source of iatrogenic risk.

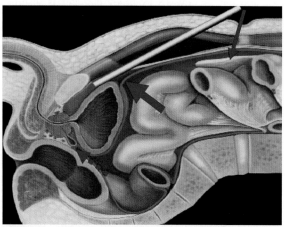

Fig. 27.28 The extraperitoneal approach prevents intraabdominal complications

Urologists have a long experience with endoscopy, but many have still a limited experience of laparoscopic surgery and robotics. Intraperitoneal laparoscopy is more widely used in visceral surgery, particularly in the field of gynecology, especially as insertion of ports is simpler and more rapid than via the extraperitoneal route. When a difficult technique has been laboriously acquired, it is not very easy to change one's habits.

The technique of extraperitoneal exposure of the surgical field with insertion of ports is relatively more difficult. However, once this technique has been mastered, it allows exact and more accurate reproduction of the conventional open operation by visualizing the already identified and recognized landmarks.[11]

The initial creation of the extraperitoneal space requires the use of the 30° camera and conventional laparoscope and a dilatation balloon to ensure correct conduct of the peritoneal detachment and to reduce bleeding and the risk of peritoneal tears. It is not suitable to perform it by blind and traumatic movements of an index finger or laparoscope holder sheath. The dilatation trocar is replaced by 12 mm and the preparation is extended under complete vision with the conventional laparoscope. The heavy da Vinci endoscope is only inserted at the time of docking.

The extraperitoneal approach allows for immediate access on the Retzius and Bogros spaces.

A rational choice:

Preserving the peritoneal barrier facilitates a conversion if necessary, protects the intraperitoneal viscerae, and reduces iatrogenic risks (intra-operative intestinal lesions, fistulae, uroperitoneum, transient ileus) and postoperative scapular pain which guarantee a higher level of comfort following the intervention.[12–14]

It avoids the uncertain medium-term or long-term outcome of intestinal loops that accumulate in the bottom of an exposed pelvis (risks of intestinal obstruction and furthermore operative difficulties in the case of subsequent intra-abdominal operations, more particularly in case of adjuvant radiotherapy). In the literature the oncological and functional outcomes of trans- or extraperitoneal laparoscopic robotic prostatectomies are similar.[1, 2, 13, 15, 16]

3.

Table 27.3 Advantages of the extraperitoneal approach

History of heavy abdominal surgery
Prevention of intra-abdominal complications
Obese patient
Better ventilation (light Trendelenburg)
Less abdominal pain and sub-ileus
Associated inguinal hernia repair
Interest of reproducing the classic RP

4. Why a systematic fore-oblique vision?

In spite of the reduction of the visual field, the 30° camera allows an exceptional lateral approach to the apexo-ureteral crossroad and is absolutely essential for the retrograde dissection. It is the key of the extraperitoneal and retrograde technique.

5. Why a retrograde dissection?

First, why perform antegrade prostatic dissection, which does not particularly facilitate identification and dissection of the neurovascular bundles, while in the great majority of open prostatectomies, this dissection is performed via a retrograde approach after initial dissection of the apex and section of the urethra?

The anatomic landmarks are imprecise at the base of the prostate, and initial antegrade, vesico-prostatic dissection proves more dangerous as it carries the danger of following the wrong path at the base of the prostate, along the adenomectomy planes (1) or in the trigone (2), but also mainly because laterally there is the risk of capsular perforation (3) and perforation of the vascular laminae (4) hidden by the latero-prostatic pedicles.

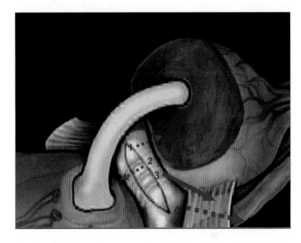

Fig. 27.29 Risk of wrong path at the base of the prostate while performing an antegrade dissection

Furthermore, the apex, in close contact with the fragile anterior wall of the rectum, is at the junction of the surgical and, in particular, oncologic risks, associated with the frequency of tumor locations, with the absence of the capsule at its level and thus the margins, but also functional risks due to the contiguity of the sphincteral and erectile structures. It would therefore appear preferable to start the dissection at the apex right at the beginning of the intervention under the best circumstances for accuracy and surgical precision and then continue the retrograde ascending cleavage path culminating with the final section of the bladder neck when the base of the prostate has been completely freed in a retrograde manner and the erectile neurovascular laminae have first been displaced sufficiently backward and externally under permanent visual control, during their ascending dissection.

27.12 Conclusion

The retrograde robotic extraperitoneal laparoscopic prostatectomy (RRELP) is a logical operation which recreates the conditions of open surgery but minimizes the risks of abdominal complications. Supporters of a transabdominal approach should also have good knowledge of the extraperitoneal technique because it can be more adapted to patients with anticipated abdominal adhesions.[15] The lack of popularity of this approach is mainly related to the particular dissection of the extraperitoneal space. From experience we realize that the extraperitoneal approach is convenient and perfectly safe, the aim of this chapter is then to guide the reader through a step-by-step approach.

Acknowledgments The authors acknowledgments Nicole Walch for the drawings and Thierry Vedrenne for the technical assistance.

References

1. Atug F, Thomas R. Transperitoneal versus extraperitoneal robotic-assisted radical prostatectomy: which one? *Minerva Urol Nefrol.* 2007;59(2):143–147.
2. Atug F, et al. Transperitoneal versus extraperitoneal robotic-assisted radical prostatectomy: is one better than the other? *Urology.* 2006;68(5):1077–1081.
3. Boczko J, Joseph JV. Robot-assisted extraperitoneal radical prostatectomy in a patient with a pelvic kidney. *Urology.* 2006;68(5):p. 1122 e3–4.
4. Joseph JV, et al. Robotic extraperitoneal radical prostatectomy: an alternative approach. *J Urol.* 2006;175(3 Pt 1):945–950. discussion 951.
5. Dubernard P, Benchetrit S, Hamza T, Van Box Som P. Radical prostatectomy by simplified extra-peritoneal laparoscopic technique. *J Urol.* 2002;167 (Suppl 4):180. abstract no.724.
6. Boczko J, Erturk E, Joseph JV. Is there a proper pelvic size for an extraperitoneal robot-assisted radical prostatectomy? *J Endourol.* 2007;21(11):1353–1356.
7. Rochat C-H, Sauvain J. Robotic radical prostatectomy: transperitoneal access. John H, Wiklund P, eds. *Robotic Urology.* Berlin: Springer; 2008.
8. Clayman RV. Use of fourth arm in da Vinci robot-assisted extraperitoneal laparoscopic prostatectomy: novel technique. *J Urol.* 2006;175(5):1750.
9. Finley DS, Rodriguez E Jr, Ahlering TE. Combined inguinal hernia repair with prosthetic mesh during transperitoneal robot assisted laparoscopic radical prostatectomy: a 4-year experience. *Urology.* 2007;178 (4):1296–1300.
10. Bivalacqua TJ, et al. Intraperitoneal effects of extraperitoneal laparoscopic radical prostatectomy. *Urology.* 2008;72(2):273–277.
11. Rassweiler J, Hruza M, Teber D, Su LM. Laparoscopic and robotic assisted radical prostatectomy: critical analysis of the results. *Eur Urol.* 2006;49:612–624.
12. John H, Schmid DM, Fehr JL. Extraperitoneal radical prostatectomy da Vinci. *Actas Urol Esp.* 2007;31(6):580–586.
13. Madeb R, et al. Patient-reported validated functional outcome after extraperitoneal robotic-assisted nerve-sparing radical prostatectomy. *JSLS.* 2007;11(3):315–320.
14. Stolzenburg JU, Rabenalt R, Do M, et al. Endoscopic extraperitoneal radical prostatectomy: the University of Leipzig experience of 1300 cases. *World J Urol.* 2007;25:45–51.
15. Capello SA, et al. Randomized comparison of extraperitoneal and transperitoneal access for robot-assisted radical prostatectomy. *J Endourol.* 2007;21(10):1199–1202.
16. Lee YS, et al. Comparison of extraperitoneal and transperitoneal robot-assisted radical prostatectomy in prostate cancer: a single surgeon's experience. *Korean J Urol.* 2009;50(3):251–255.

Chapter 28

Technical Modifications for Robotic Prostatectomy

Kenneth J. Palmer, Rafael E. Coelho, Sanket Chauhan, and Vipul R. Patel

28.1 Introduction

Robotic radical prostatectomy is a procedure that has evolved considerably in the last 10 years as the main treatment for prostate cancer. Published literature currently describes in detail the procedure and outcomes. However, as widespread as it may be, we believe that certain technical modifications have greatly improved our technique hence improving early and medium-term outcomes. These include placement of the suspension stitch, athermal dissection of the seminal vesicles, athermal early retrograde release of the neurovascular bundle, and the modified posterior reconstruction of the rhabdosphincter for recovery of early continence.

Since, the first report of RRP in 1905 by Young the prostate has represented a difficult surgical challenge. These technical challenges (location in pelvis and significant blood supply) led to increased surgical morbidity life threatening for the patient. Over the subsequent decades the procedure has been refined significantly into one that is less harmful to the patient and provides improved quality of life. However, it is still associated with a high perioperative morbidity which led to the search for less invasive options.

The need for continuous improvement resulted in less invasive approaches that offered decreased blood loss and perioperative pain, shorter hospital stay, and faster convalescence with a more rapid return to normal activity while maintaining oncologic efficacy. The

addition of robotic technology to the armamentarium of urologists is one such example.

Robotic technology was introduced to overcome these limitations and aids the surgeon to transition from open surgery to the minimally invasive arena. The interface was created to enhance technique and reduce learning curve by providing 3D-vision, wristed instrumentation with seven degrees of freedom of motion, lack of tremor, and a comfortable seated position making it ideal for a technically challenging reconstructive procedure. This technology has the potential to provide significant surgical advantages especially in challenging areas of a patient's anatomy and with in difficult-to-remove structures, like the pelvis.

28.2 Periurethral Suspension Stitch

Originally described by Walsh[1] as a means to decrease blood loss during division of the DVC or prevent damage to the striated sphincter, the use of pubourethral suspension stitches or the application of sutures anchoring the vesicourethral anastomosis to the ligated dorsal vein complex (DVC) also helps in improving early urinary continence rates after RRP.[2] The maneuver consists in passing a suture through the DVC and then through the periostium of the pubic symphysis, in a reverse direction. The suture is tied, suspending the DVC. This maneuver can help to control the venous bleeding and provides a recapitulation of the puboprostatic ligaments, supporting the striated sphincter. These technical variations showed a significant effect on the earlier recovery of urinary continence without compromising oncological outcomes.[2,3]

K.J. Palmer (✉)
Department of Urology, College of Medicine, University of
Central Florida, Florida, USA
e-mail: kenneth.palmer@flhosp.org

A.K. Hemal, M. Menon (eds.), *Robotics in Genitourinary Surgery*,
DOI 10.1007/978-1-84882-114-9_28, © Springer-Verlag London Limited 2011

28.2.1 Surgical Technique

The anterior peritoneum is incised to enter the retropubic space of Retzius. The endopelvic fascia is opened immediately lateral to the reflection of the puboprostatic ligaments bilaterally and the elevator muscle fibers are pushed off the prostate until the dorsal vein complex (DVC) and urethra are visualized. The DVC is ligated using a 12 in. monofilament polyglytone suture on a CT-1 needle.

We analyzed our data of 331 consecutive patients who underwent RALP. Ninety-four of these patients underwent RALP without the placement of suspension stitch (group 1) and 237 patients underwent RALP with the application of the suspension stitch (group 2), as described below. The only difference between the groups with and without suspension stitch was the placement of the pubo-periurethral stitch after the ligation of the DVC (Fig. 28.1a). In the suspension group a periurethral retropubic stitch was placed using another 12 in. monofilament polyglytone suture on a CT-1 needle. The stitch was placed holding the needle two-thirds the way back in a 90° position and passed from

right to left between the urethra and DVC (Fig. 28.1b) and then through the periostium on the pubic bone (Fig. 28.1c). The stitch was passed again through the DVC (Fig. 28.1d) and then through the pubic bone (Fig. 28.1e), in a figure of eight, and then tied with a mild amount of tension (Fig. 28.1f). The DVC was typically divided later during the operation, prior to the apical dissection of the prostate and division of the urethra.

We received the questionnaires (EPIC) from all the 94 patients evaluated in group 1 and all the 237 patients in group 2. In group 1 the continence rate at <1, 3, 6, and 12 months postoperatively was 33 and 83%, 94.7 and 95.7%, respectively. In group 2 the continence rate at <1, 3, 6, and 12 months postoperatively was 40 and 92.8%, 97.9 and 97.9%, respectively. The suspension technique resulted in significantly greater continence rates at 3 months after RALP ($p = 0.013$), although the rates at 6 and 12 months were not significantly affected (Table 28.1).

The interval to recovery of continence was statistically and significantly lower in the suspension group (median = 6 weeks/mean = 7,338 weeks; 95%

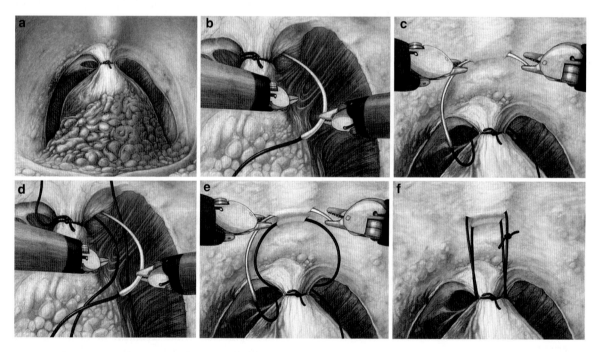

Fig. 28.1 **a** Endopelvic fascia has been opened and DVC ligated. **b** CT1 needle held at 90° passed from *right* to *left* between the urethra and DVC. **c** Stitch placed through the periostium on the posterior aspect of the pubis. **d** Second pass through the DVC. **e** Second pass through periostium on posterior aspect of pubis. **f** Final stitch tied

Table 28.1 Continence rates at <1, 3, 6, and 12 months of follow-up with and without the suspension stitch

Follow-up time (months)	Without suspension stitch ($N = 94$)	With suspension stitch ($N = 237$)	p value
1	31 (33.0%)	95 (40.0%)	0.282
3	78 (83.0%)	220 (92.8%)	0.013
6	89 (94.7%)	232 (97.9%)	0.237
12	90 (95.7%)	232 (97.9%)	0.479

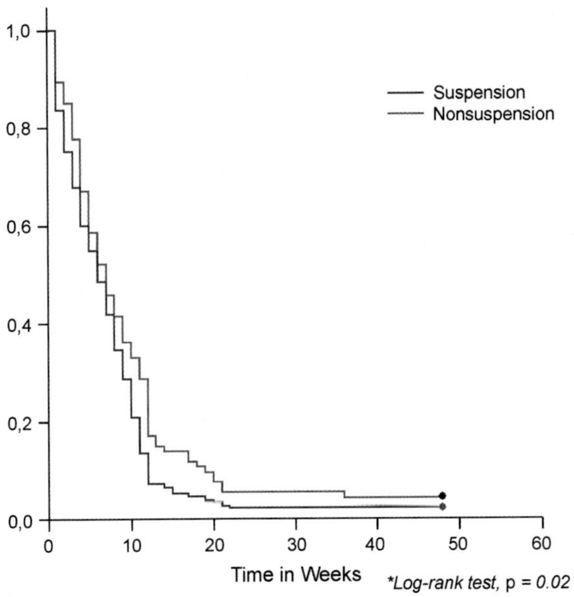

Fig. 28.2 Kaplan–Meier curves showing the urinary incontinence probability after RALP with and without the placement of the suspension

CI: 6,387–8,288) than in the non-suspension group (median = 7 weeks/mean = 9,585 weeks; 95% CI: 7,558–11,612) (log-rank test, $P = 0.002$) (Fig. 28.2).

28.2.2 Comments

Our results showed a higher recovery of complete urinary continence at 3 months after the RALP with the placement of the suspension stitch. Positive margin rate was unaffected. Complete removal of the cancer is still the primary endpoint of the RALP and any modifications of the surgical technique must not compromise the oncological outcome.

The exact mechanism of the early recovery of continence using the suspension stitch is unclear. We believe that the suspension of the periurethral complex can provide better vision, urethral length, and additional anterior support to the striated sphincter, stabilizing the posterior urethra in its anatomical position in the pelvic floor. This stabilization aids in the preservation of urethral length during the dissection of the prostatic apex facilitating the vesicourethral anastomosis and preventing descent and destabilization of the continence mechanism.

Furthermore, we believe that the suspension stitch helps to control the venous bleeding from the DVC and enables the surgeon to visualize more clearly the plane between the anterior prostatic apex and the DVC, as emphasized by Walsh previously.

28.3 Modified Posterior Reconstruction of the Rhabdosphincter

We have previously described our technique for RALP.[4] After extraction of the specimen, posterior reconstruction is performed prior to beginning the vesicourethral anastomosis. This is performed according to the two-layer reconstruction described by Rocco et al. with some minor technical modifications.[3]

28.3.1 Surgical Technique

The reconstruction is carried out utilizing a continuous suture of two 3-0 monocryl sutures (RB1 needles) of different colors that are tied together with each individual length being 12 cm. Ten knots are placed when tying the sutures together to provide a bolster.

The free edge of the remaining Denonvilliers' fascia is identified following prostatectomy. It is located anterior to the rectum just caudal to the bladder and seminal vesicle dissection. This edge is approximated to the posterior aspect of the rhabdosphincter and the posterior median raphe using one arm of the

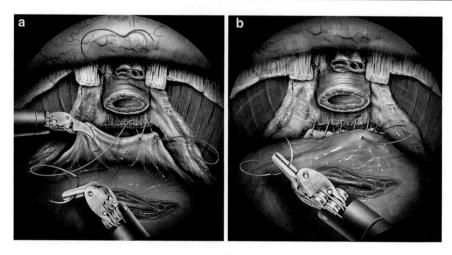

Fig. 28.3 **a** Posterior reconstruction. First plane: Attaching Denonvilliers' fascia to the rhabdosphincter. **b** Posterior reconstruction. Second plane: The posterior bladder neck is sutured to the reconstructed rhabdosphincter

continuous monocryl suture. Typically four bites of Denonvilliers' fascia and the rhabdosphincter/posterior median raphe are taken; the edges are approximated in a tension-free manner and the suture tied (Fig. 28.3a).

We have further modified our technique from its early description. At present, we incorporate the posterior bladder neck in the second layer. This is commenced with the other arm of the monocryl suture approximating the posterior bladder neck to the initial reconstructed layer of posterior rhabdosphincter and Denonvilliers' fascia (Fig. 28.3b). The running suture takes the posterior rhabdosphincter/Denonvilliers' complex, and incorporates the posterior bladder neck preparing for a tension-free anastomosis. A continuous modified van Velthoven vesicourethral anastomosis[5] is then performed with a running suture.

Care must be taken to avoid potential complications, such as damage to the neurovascular bundles, urethra, and/or ureters during the placement of reconstruction sutures. Careful identification of target anatomy and accurate suture placement is of the utmost importance for prevention.

28.3.2 Comments

We have recently incorporated the technique during RALP. Our complete 'early continence' rate (defined by use of no pads) of 58% at 1 week is encouraging. If the definition of continent is broadened to that of Rocco et al.[6,7] (0 or 1 pad per day) the rate is 72%. We felt there was a learning curve of approximately 20 cases to perform this modification optimally. During this time we learned precise identification of the target anatomy and the technical refinements to both the reconstruction and the subsequent vesicourethral anastomosis.

28.4 Athermal Seminal Vesicle Dissection

The anatomy and location of the seminal vesicles (SVs) warrant an athermal and careful dissection due to their proximity to the hypogastric plexus and cavernous nerves. We have developed a simple technique for dissection and liberation of the SVs without trauma.

28.4.1 Surgical Technique

After dissection of the posterior bladder neck, the vas deferens is identified. The fourth arm is used to grasp and elevate first the left vas deferens. Blunt dissection starts on the medial surface developing an avascular plane between vas deferens and the SV. Once the SV is identified, the fourth arm is used for upward and lateral traction to continue dissection until the tip is reached. Once this occurs, a 10 mm hemolock clip is placed on the vas deferens increasing exposure of the tip of the SV being able to place a following clip on the vascular supply entering the tip. Dissection is then continued until the base of the SV is reached. Important to point out is that no thermal energy is used during this step of the procedure due to the proximity of neurostructures (hypogastric plexus and cavernous nerves) to the tip of the SVs. Dissection of the right SV is carried out in a similar manner.

28.4.2 Comments

Our experience encompasses over 3,000 cases during which we have continuously modified our technique. The SVs constitute an essential part of the nerve-sparing procedure due to the proximity of the cavernous nerves and hypogastric plexus to the tip of the SVs. As we previously mentioned advantages of this technique include an athermal dissection and precise placement of clips as to avoid inadvertent injury to these vital neurostructures. Once performed dissection of the posterior plane (separation of rectum from prostate) can be carried out safely preparing for the nerve-sparing part of the procedure.

28.5 Athermal Early Retrograde Release of the Neurovascular Bundles

Precise identification and delineation of the neurovascular bundle during nerve-sparing radical prostatectomy is a challenging but critical component of the operation. The neurovascular bundle can be damaged at various locations along its path and by various methods of injury. Damage can occur via transection, ligation, thermal injury, or excessive traction. Common points of injury include at the prostatic pedicles, seminal vesicles, during the apical dissection, and inadvertent inclusion of the neurovascular bundle during the vesicourethral anastomosis.[8]

Different operative techniques present various unique challenges during nerve-sparing radical prostatectomy. In open radical prostatectomy the levator fascia is opened and the neurovascular bundle is released from the prostate beginning at the apex and moving toward the base of the gland. The neurovascular bundle is released from the prostate prior to controlling the vascular pedicles. Challenges of the open retropubic technique include obtaining adequate hemostasis and visualization to allow the surgeon to perform such an intricate dissection.

The standard approach to nerve sparing with laparoscopic or robotic radical prostatectomy is antegrade. Here the prostatic pedicle is controlled and divided and then the neurovascular bundle is released from the prostate beginning at the base and moving toward the apex of the gland. Advantages of the laparoscopic approach include improved visualization with magnified vision and improved hemostasis secondary to the pneumoperitoneum. With the antegrade approach, however, the neurovascular bundle risks inadvertent injury during control of the vascular pedicle prior to precise delineation of the path of the neurovascular bundle. Hence the need for a technique which can overcome these limitations is required.

Based upon our experience with both the open and standard laparoscopic approaches we developed a hybrid technique for nerve preservation during RALP. Our approach to RALP is an antegrade prostatectomy; however, prior to controlling the vascular pedicles we release the neurovascular bundle from the prostate beginning at the apex and extending back toward the base of the gland.

28.5.1 Surgical Technique

Our approach to RALP has been described previously in detail.[9] Here we will focus solely on the key step of neurovascular bundle preservation. Our approach is based upon the philosophy of minimal traction, use of no thermal energy, and early release of the neurovascular bundle with precise identification of its location at the base of the gland prior to ligating the prostatic pedicle.

Prior to approaching the neurovascular bundle the bladder neck has been divided, the seminal vesicles have been dissected athermally, and the posterior dissection has been performed. A complete posterior dissection is critical to successful nerve sparing. It is essential to maximally release the prostate from the

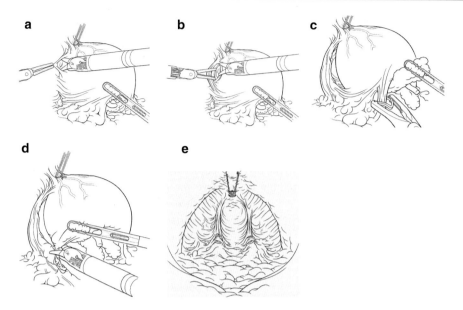

Fig. 28.4 **a** Dissection of fascial layers at midportion of the prostate until the plane between neurovascular bundle and prostate is reached. **b** Complete dissection of interfascial plane connecting to the posterior plane (already dissected). **c** Vascular control of the prostatic pedicle is achieved using 10 mm hem-o-lock® clips. **d** Retrograde release of the neurovascular bundle and complete section of the prostatic pedicle. **e** Bilateral nerve preservation

rectum all the way to the apex and laterally to the bundles. The prostate is then rotated laterally by the assistant to aid with identification of the lateral fascial attachments. Early release of neurovascular bundle is then performed.

The levator fascia is incised along the lateral aspect of the prostate. At the level of the apex and midportion of the prostate the avascular plane between the levator fascia and prostatic fascia is developed (Fig. 28.4a). The plane is continued posteriorly between the neurovascular bundle and the prostatic fascia as an interfascial nerve-sparing dissection (Fig. 28.4b). The neurovascular bundle is stabilized with plasma kinetic forceps and the prostate is gently stroked medially away from the bundle. The dissection continues posteriorly to meet the plane of the posterior dissection between the prostate and rectum. The prostate is then stroked medially off of the bundle back to the base of the gland in a retrograde manner. No thermal energy is used during dissection of the bundle or ligation of the pedicle. The path of the bundle has been clearly delineated prior to controlling the prostatic vascular pedicle. The pedicle is then controlled with a 10 mm hemolock clip above the level of the already released bundle (Fig. 28.4c). This technique allows complete neurovascular bundle sparing without the use of any thermal energy or trauma.

The neurovascular bundle is then released distally to the level of the pelvic floor to avoid damaging it during the apical dissection or vesicourethral anastomosis (Fig. 28.4d). The procedure is repeated on the contralateral side. Final appearance of the neurovascular bundles after bilateral nerve sparing resembles train tracks (Fig. 28.4e).

28.5.2 Comments

Our experience with RALP is now over 3,000 cases and we have continually refined our technique to improve patient outcomes. We have found this technique to be both reliable and reproducible and is mainly a hybrid utilizing advantages of both conventional open and laparoscopic techniques. The major advantage is precise delineation of the course of the neurovascular bundle prior to controlling the pedicle. This allows the vascular pedicle to be ligated while avoiding inadvertent injury to the bundle. The pneumoperitoneum, magnified vision, and wristed instrumentation of robotics allow this intricate step of the dissection to be performed.

28.6 Conclusions

Radical prostatectomy remains today the gold standard for the treatment of organ-confined prostate cancer. Robotic prostatectomy has evolved to challenge the former offering comparable and in some instances improved outcomes regarding continence, potency, and oncologic control with the modifications herein described. However, experience is a crucial factor in these outcomes and only the availability of long-term outcomes will determine its true validity.

References

1. Walsh PC. Anatomical radical prostatectomy: evolution of the surgical technique. *J Urol.* 1998;160:2418–2424.
2. Noguchi M, Kakuma T, Suekane S, Nakashima O, Mohamed ER, Matsuoka K. A randomized clinical trial of suspension technique for improving early recovery of urinary continence after radical retropubic prostatectomy. *BJU Int.* 2008 Sep;102(8):958–963.
3. Campenni MA, Harmon JD, Ginsberg PC, Harkaway RC. Improved continence after radical retropubic prostatectomy using two pubo-urethral suspension stitches. *Urol Int.* 2002;68:109–112.
4. Patel VR, Shah K, Thaly R, Lavery H. Robotic-assisted laparoscopic radical prostatectomy: the Ohio State University technique. *J Robot Surg.* 2007;1:51–60.
5. van Velthoven RF, Ahlering TE, Peltier A, Skarecky DW, Clayman RV. Technique for laparoscopic running urethrovesical anastomosis: the single knot method. *Urology.* 2003;61:699.
6. Rocco F, Carmignani L, Acquati P, et al. Early continence recovery after open radical prostatectomy with restoration of the posterior aspect of the rhabdosphincter. *Eur Urol.* 2007;52:376–383.
7. Rocco B, Gregori A, Stener S, et al. Posterior reconstruction of the rhabdosphincter allows a rapid recovery of continence after transperitoneal videolaparoscopic radical prostatectomy. *Eur Urol.* 2007;51:996–1003.
8. Dubble men YD, Dohle GR, Schroder FH. Sexual function before and after radical retropubic prostatectomy: a systematic review of prognostic indicators for a successful outcome. *Eur Urol.* 2006;50(4):711–718.
9. Patel VR, Shah KK, Rahul K. Thaly hugh lavery. Robotic-assisted laparoscopic radical prostatectomy: the Ohio state university technique. *J Robot Surg.* 2007;1:51–59.

Chapter 29

Robotic Radical Prostatectomy: Cancer Control and Implications of Margin Positivity

Mark H. Katz, Kevin C. Zorn, and Arieh L. Shalhav

Abbreviations

BMI   Body mass index
BRFS   Biochemical recurrence-free survival
DVC   Dorsal venous complex
LRP   Laparoscopic radical prostatectomy
NVB   Neurovascular bundle
ORP   Open radical prostatectomy
PSM   Positive surgical margin
RARP   Robot-assisted radical prostatectomy
RT   Radiation therapy
SWOG   Southwest Oncology Group

Current robot-assisted radical prostatectomy (RARP) data suggest comparable and, perhaps, improved pathologic outcomes when compared with laparoscopic and open techniques. In mature RARP series, overall positive surgical margin (PSM) rates have ranged between 9 and 19%. Independent risk factors for PSMs include lower surgeon case volume, pathologic stage and Gleason sum, lower prostate weight, higher pre-operative PSA level, and PSA density. Other possible prognostic indicators include biopsy Gleason sum, body mass index, and neurovascular bundle preservation. Various surgical techniques and tailoring nerve preservation based on disease severity appear to improve cancer control during RARP. The most common locations for PSMs during RARP are posterolateral and apical, but location and number do not appear to impact recurrence. An extensive PSM, however, does appear to be an adverse

prognostic finding. Short- and mid-term biochemical recurrence-free survival appears equivalent for robotic, laparoscopic, and open radical prostatectomy. Unfortunately, the RARP data are too immature to estimate cancer-specific and overall survival. Based on level 1 evidence from open radical prostatectomy literature, adjuvant radiation therapy (RT) for locally advanced disease and/or PSMs significantly improves biochemical recurrence-free, metastasis-free, and overall survival compared to observation. PSMs predict an improved response to RT. These findings should be applicable to RARP patients as well.

29.1 Introduction

Since its introduction in 2001, robot-assisted radical prostatectomy (RARP) has evolved into a highly effective treatment option for localized prostate cancer. Favorable marketing combined with a plethora of studies demonstrating a relatively short safety learning curve and impressive perioperative outcomes has favored a rapid dissemination of RARP. Limited to academic centers for the initial 2–3 years, RARP has since expanded into the community setting. In less than a decade, we have witnessed a paradigm shift in the surgical treatment of prostate cancer such that in 2008, over 80% of radical prostatectomies in the United States were performed robotically.[1]

As with all new technology, careful study of outcomes and safety were critically assessed prior to its adoption. Initial research focused on procedure feasibility, technical variations, and perioperative outcomes.[2] Such early evaluation was instrumental in refining surgical techniques and establishing RARP as a safe and effective surgical modality. Several

A.L. Shalhav (✉)
University of Chicago Medical Center, Chicago, IL, USA
e-mail: ashalhav@surgery.bsd.uchicago.edu

A.K. Hemal, M. Menon (eds.), *Robotics in Genitourinary Surgery*,
DOI 10.1007/978-1-84882-114-9_29, © Springer-Verlag London Limited 2011

short-term endpoints such as blood loss, pain control, and hospital stay were consistently improved with RARP when compared to open radical prostatectomy (ORP).[3] Subsequent research evaluated the role of learning curve for surgeons transitioning from open or laparoscopic surgery to RARP.[4,5] Although results from these studies varied tremendously, they consistently demonstrated the ability of surgeons to learn and continue to improve the procedure. Current intermediate RARP follow-up demonstrates that urinary and sexual function outcomes are equivalent or improved when compared with ORP.[6]

Intuitively, early studies lacked oncologic outcomes including biochemical recurrence, cancer-specific survival, and overall survival. Positive surgical margin (PSM) rates, an oncologic surrogate, were reported in early series.[7,8] As such, without sufficient data on cancer control, there was still reluctance by many experts to consider RARP a standard of care for localized prostate cancer.

With almost a decade of RARP experience, large series with meaningful oncologic data have finally emerged. The following chapter will comprehensively review the cancer control data for RARP. In particular, PSMs in both organ-confined and locally advanced disease will be summarized as well as the more recent data on biochemical recurrence and survival. Appropriate patient selection and surgical techniques to optimize cancer control will also be addressed. When appropriate, comparisons will be made with historical and contemporary studies of ORP and laparoscopic radical prostatectomy (LRP). Finally, the impact and role of adjuvant radiation therapy (RT) after radical prostatectomy will be outlined.

29.2 Definitions of Positive Surgical Margins

Although seemingly simple and straightforward, the definition of a PSM can be quite variable from study to study. As such, caution must be taken when comparing outcomes among series with different definitions of a PSM. In most series, a PSM is defined as the presence of tumor at the inked margin of a resected specimen.[9,10]

A PSM results from incision across malignant cells that are extracapsular in pT3 disease or from inadvertent capsular incision into tumor in organ-confined prostate cancer. Artifact from tissue handling may also result in a PSM, and the type of pathologic processing may impact the detection of PSMs. Whole mount sectioning is less likely to overlook a PSM when compared with the more common step sectioning techniques. It has been well described that a PSM is an independent predictor of disease recurrence after ORP[11] and RARP.[12] However, controversy exists over the relative significance of capsular incision compared with PSMs in extracapsular disease (pT2 vs. pT3 PSMs). Furthermore, the extent, location, and number of PSMs may have an independent effect on disease recurrence. These issues are discussed in detail below.

29.3 Positive Surgical Margins with RARP

Several important factors must be considered before comparing PSM rates among reported series. Most importantly, patient clinical and pathological characteristics should be similar across studies or else a selection bias exists in favor of one group. At a minimum, pre-operative PSA, Gleason score, number and percentage of tumor in biopsy cores, as well as clinical and pathological stage, should be similar in order to make fair comparisons. Other factors undoubtedly also play a role such as experience of the surgeon and body mass index (BMI).

Early in its evolution, RARP raised concerns due to the lack of tactile feedback possibly contributing to an increase in PSMs. However, RARP was developing as a new technique, with large tertiary centers performing cases in the infancy of their experience. Thus, early series reporting PSM rates should be interpreted with caution, especially when comparing results to mature ORP series. As experience with RARP has grown over the past 5 years, larger series have demonstrated improved PSM rates comparable to, if not better than, data from the ORP literature.

29.3.1 Early RARP PSM Outcomes

The earliest case series of RARP originate from two centers in Germany and one in France.[13–15] They included ≤10 patients and reported PSM rates as high

Table 29.1 Positive surgical margins in early RARP series

Series	N	Overall (%)	pT2 (%)	pT3/T4 (%)
Menon et al.[7]	30	26	–	–
Menon et al.[2]	100	15	11	40
Bentas et al.[18]	40	30	8	67
Ahlering et al.[19]	First 50	36	27	53
	Next 90	17	5	46
Patel et al.[16]	200	11	6	26
Mikhail et al.[17]	100	16	10	42

as 30%. Meanwhile, in the United States, Dr. Menon and colleagues were pioneering and standardizing the RARP procedure. In 2002, Menon et al. performed a non-randomized, prospective study comparing 30 consecutive ORP cases and 30 initial RARPs.[7] Pre-operative parameters were comparable between groups with the exception mean PSA being significantly higher in the RARP cohort (9.9 vs. 8.4 ng/ml). Overall PSM rates were 29 and 26% for ORP and RARP, respectively. Of note, surgeons performing ORP had extensive experience (collectively over 2,500 cases) as opposed to the robotic surgeon performing his first 30 RARP cases. Even after acknowledging all the limitations of this small study, this early experience demonstrated comparable PSM rates between the open and robotic techniques and, perhaps, encouraged other centers to embark on RARP programs.

In 2003, the same group from Henry Ford reported the results of their first 100 patients undergoing RARP between 2001 and 2002.[2] Fifteen percent had PSMs, of which 10% were focal (<1 mm length) and 5% were established (>1 mm length). Pathologic T2 and pT3 PSM rates were 11 and 40%, respectively. Pre-operatively, this was a relatively low-risk cohort, with 70% of patients having biopsy Gleason ≤ 6 pathology, 81% with clinical stage T1c, and an overall mean pre-operative PSA of 7.2 ng/ml. However, on final pathology, 15% of patients had pT3 disease and 18% demonstrated Gleason ≤ 8. Compared with their previous study of 30 RARP cases,[7] PSM rates decreased from 26 to 15% after the addition of only 70 cases, highlighting the importance of surgical experience in improving outcomes.

Following the lead of the group from Henry Ford, other centers began publishing their initial RARP series. In 2005, Patel et al. reported on their first 200 cases and found an overall PSM rate of 10.5%.[16] The pT2 and pT3 PSM rates were 5.7 and 26%, respectively. There was a non-significant trend toward a decreased incidence of PSMs when comparing the first 100 (13%) and second 100 (8%) cases. This was

a higher risk cohort than the Menon et al. series,[2] as 52% of patients had a biopsy Gleason sum ≥ 7 and 22% had extracapsular disease. Additional early RARP series of 40–140 cases, including one from Germany, demonstrated overall PSM rates between 16 and 36%.[17–19]

Table 29.1 summarizes the PSM data for the above early RARP series. Taken together, the initial RARP experience demonstrated encouraging results. Larger, more mature, series were needed to demonstrate improved outcomes and to analyze risk factors and technical aspects associated with PSMs.

29.3.2 Experienced RARP PSM Outcomes

Several academic centers have published large RARP series, allowing for comparison with earlier experiences and with the ORP literature. Henry Ford Hospital reported the largest series known to date of 2,766 RARPs over a 6-year period.[20] The overall, pT2 and pT3 PSM rates were 19, 13, and 35%, respectively. Other large series have been published, including 1,500 patients by Patel et al.[21] The overall PSM rate was 9% and an impressive 4% for organ-confined (pT2) disease. From the University of Chicago, 945 patients underwent RARP, demonstrating an overall and pT2 PSM rate of 18 and 13%, respectively.[22] Murphy et al. from Australia reported an overall PSM rate of 19%, with pT2 and pT3 PSM rates of 10 and 42%, respectively, in a cohort of 400 RARP patients.[23]

Table 29.2 summarizes the PSM data for the above large RARP series. At first glance, there does not appear to be a significant improvement in outcomes when comparing the early, smaller series to the more recent, larger studies. Selection bias in favor of the early studies undoubtedly plays a role in this finding, as more challenging and higher risk cases are included in the larger series. Thus, to better assess the impact

Table 29.2 Positive surgical margins in large RARP series

Series	N	Overall (%)	pT2 (%)	pT3/T4 (%)
Badani et al.[20]	2,766	19	13	35
	First 200	–	7	–
	Last 200	–	4	–
Patel et al.[21]	1,500	9	4	33
Wiltz et al.[22]	945	18	13	40
Murphy et al.[23]	400	19	10	42

of surgeon experience on PSM rates, comparing a subset of early cases to more recent cases may be most appropriate. In the above Henry Ford series,[20] when comparing their first and last 200 cases, pT2 margin rates significantly decreased from 7 to 4%, suggesting that surgical experience can improve outcomes. This is despite the fact that the last 200 patients were higher risk with regard to Gleason score and pathologic stage. In addition, whole mount sectioning was introduced after the first 200 cases, making it more likely to identify all PSMs.

29.4 Risk Factors for Positive Surgical Margins

Surgical experience plays a significant role in decreasing PSMs.[24,25] Data from Ahlering et al.[19] and Badani et al.[20] clearly demonstrate a reduction in PSM rate over time despite applying broader inclusion criteria for RARP. Moreover, in a multivariate analysis of 216 RARP cases by Ornstein et al. increasing case volume was an independent predictor of decreasing PSMs ($p = 0.025$), particularly in men with pT3 disease.[26] With increasing experience, multiple factors likely contribute to decreasing PSMs including improved appreciation of pelvic anatomy, better control of the da Vinci™ system, and technical modifications that evolve over time. Furthermore, the role of the robotic team and the bedside assistant becomes more refined to facilitate surgical dissection. Other PSM risk factors noted by Ornstein et al. on multivariate analysis were pathological stage (pT3 vs. pT2), PSA density (>0.15 ng/ml/g), pathological Gleason score, and performing a nerve-sparing procedure. The impact of nerve preservation was greatest in pT3 disease, with 40% of patients undergoing nerve-sparing having PSMs compared with only 22% that had wide excision. This finding underscores the importance of identifying patients at high risk for adverse pathology and subsequently tailoring the surgical dissection

appropriately. Simply stated, those patients at high risk for extracapsular disease should not undergo aggressive nerve preservation at the cost of compromising cancer control. Another study confirmed a 3.5-fold increased risk of PSMs with extra-prostatic disease (pT3 + pT4) compared with organ-confined cancer.[27]

Shikanov et al. from the University of Chicago examined the effect of biopsy Gleason score on adverse pathologic outcomes.[28] In a high-risk cohort of 70 patients with biopsy Gleason scores of ≥8 undergoing RARP, the overall PSM rate was 24% (6% for pT2 and 42% for pT3). Over 50% of the patients had extraprostatic disease and 13% had positive lymph nodes, underscoring the high-risk nature of this group. There was no comparative low-risk group in this study, but previous series from the same institution have reported lower overall PSM rates between 16 and 18%,[17,22] further suggesting the negative effect of higher Gleason scores.

Zorn et al. at the University of Chicago further examined the impact of aggressive nerve preservation on PSMs.[29] Between 2003 and 2005, 300 consecutive RARPs were performed with selective interfascial nerve preservation at the discretion of the surgeon (i.e., plane closest to the prostate capsule). The overall, pT2, and pT3 PSM rates were 20, 15, and 52%, respectively. The most common location for a PSM was posterolateral (54%), and pT3 PSMs occurred significantly more often in the posterolateral location when ipsilateral interfascial nerve preservation was performed vs. wide excision (73 vs. 33%, $p = 0.05$). Thus, the plane of dissection closest to the prostate capsule may increase the risk of PSMs, especially for extracapsular disease.

There have been several retrospective studies examining the effect of BMI on perioperative outcomes of RARP.[17,22,30–33] Wiltz et al. reviewed 945 RARPs performed at a single institution and stratified patients by BMI into three groups (<25 kg/m², 25 to < 30 kg/m², and ≥30 kg/m²). They found no significant difference in overall, organ-confined, and pT3 PSM rates among the groups.[22] Another study by Ahlering et al. also found no difference in PSM rates for obese patients.[30] However, in a cohort of 140 RARPs, Castle et al. did observe a significantly higher PSM rate in obese (26.1%) vs. non-obese (13.1%) patients.[32] Herman et al. also demonstrated higher rates of PSMs in overweight and obese men.[33] Thus, there is still no consensus on obesity as an independent risk factor for PSMs, especially since multiple confounding variables likely exist. In particular, PSA levels are often lower as BMI increases, contributing to a delay in the diagnosis of prostate cancer and the subsequent identification of more aggressive disease at the time of surgery. As such, robotic surgeons should take extra precautions when performing RARP in obese patients.

The effect of prostate weight on PSMs has been well studied in ORP and LRP.[34–36] With both open and laparoscopic techniques, larger prostate weights correlated with fewer PSMs. More recently, studies have confirmed the same findings with RARP.[21,37] In their analysis of 1,500 RARPs, Patel et al. identified an inverse relationship between prostate weight and incidence of PSMs. For prostate volumes < 50, 50–99 g, and ≥ 100 g, positive margin rates were 14.3, 9.4, and 5.9%, respectively. Similarly, Zorn et al. identified lower prostate weight as a risk factor for overall and pT2 PSMs. For prostates <30 g, the pT2 PSM rate was 12.5% compared to only 7.7% for prostates ≥80 g. There was a similar trend with pT3 disease, but the relatively small number of pT3 cancers in each prostate weight group precluded statistical significance. The etiology of this inverse relationship between prostate weight and PSMs is likely multifactorial, including difficulty with identifying surgical planes and a higher density of disease in smaller glands. Results of the above studies should be interpreted with caution as the number of cases in each prostate weight group, especially at the extremes, was relatively small. Furthermore, prostate weight was calculated from the surgical specimen, which may not correlate well with pre-operative ultrasound measurements.

29.5 Comparison of PSM Outcomes Among RARP, ORP, and LRP Series

Comparing PSM rates among different radical prostatectomy approaches has significant limitations. This is particularly true when evaluating data across multiple institutions where patient characteristics, inclusion/exclusion criteria, and surgical experience vary tremendously. Comparison of contemporary results to historical ORP controls, which included men from the pre-PSA era, may be biased by the Will Rogers phenomenon.[38] Although no randomized, prospective trials are available, several single-institution retrospective series and one prospective study have compared the different surgical techniques. Menon et al., in a non-randomized prospective study, compared 30 RARPs to 30 ORPs.[7] Both groups had comparable pre-operative parameters, and overall PSM rates were similar at 29 and 26% for the ORP and RARP cohorts, respectively. This is despite the fact that the RARP cases were very early in the "learning curve" while the surgeons had extensive experience with ORP. A follow-up study at the same institution of 100 ORPs and 200 RARPs demonstrated fewer PSMs in the RARP cohort (23% ORP vs. 9% RARP).[39] A more recent study compared the initial 120 RARPs to a historical cohort of 240 ORPs.[27] The groups were well matched except for a higher incidence of extracapsular disease in the ORP patients. The rate of PSMs was similar in both groups (22% RARP vs. 25% ORP) even when stratified by pathologic stage. Other studies have also demonstrated no significant differences in PSM rates between RARP and ORP.[6,40] Comparing 200 RARPs and 200 ORPs, Smith et al. observed significantly lower overall (15 vs. 35%) and pT2 PSMs (9.4 vs. 24.1%) in the RARP group.[41] These findings should be interpreted with caution because the ORP cohort was higher risk based on pre-operative PSA, clinical stage, and biopsy Gleason score. Another small study found improved overall and organ-confined surgical margin rates with RARP when compared with ORP.[42] Conversely, one small series found a significantly higher rate of PSMs in RARP patients (50% RARP vs. 20% ORP).[43] This was, however, an analysis of the first 30 robotic cases performed by an experienced open surgeon. Furthermore, only 6.7% in the ORP cohort underwent nerve preservation vs. 53% in the RARP group, highlighting the potential impact of tailoring the dissection to optimize outcomes.

The PSM rates between LRP, ORP, and RARP have also been compared. Drouin et al. analyzed 239 patients who underwent ORP ($n = 83$), LRP ($n = 85$), and RARP ($n = 71$) and found no significant difference in overall, pT2, and pT3 PSM rates among the different techniques.[44] Similar to other reports, the ORP cohort was higher risk based on PSA, clinical stage, and biopsy Gleason score. Another study comparing 133 consecutive RARP cases with 133 well-matched LRP cases demonstrated equivalent PSM rates.[45] Finally, in a meta-analysis of 19 studies and 3,893 patients comparing ORP to either LRP or RARP, there was no difference in the risk of overall and stage-specific PSMs among the three techniques.[46] Table 29.3 summarizes the studies comparing PSM rates between ORP and RARP.

In summary, with limited retrospective data, PSM rates appear comparable between ORP, LRP, and RARP. Although three of the above series did demonstrate improved outcomes with RARP, the limitations of these studies are too significant to draw any firm conclusions. Importantly, patients undergoing ORP often had more adverse clinical characteristics. The large discrepancy in PSMs among series suggests that surgeon experience and patient characteristics play a significant role in outcomes, and larger, prospective studies are necessary to identify the true impact of surgical modality on PSMs. In the meantime, it seems as though proper patient selection and surgeon ability are more important than the type of technique utilized.

29.6 Location, Number, and Size of Positive Surgical Margins

It remains unclear whether the location of PSMs impacts cancer recurrence or progression. Analyzing 215 ORP cases, Watson et al. did not find the site of margin involvement to be an independent predictor of progression.[47] Conversely, Salomon et al. reported that a PSM at the apex yielded the worst prognosis of all locations, with only 54.5% 3-year biochemical-free progression.[48] Eastham et al. reviewed the results of 2,442 ORPs and also observed that margin location impacted the rate of biochemical recurrence.[49] In this study, however, the posterolateral location was associated with an increased risk for recurrence. Other ORP studies have shown a PSM at the prostate base or bladder neck to confer the highest likelihood of biochemical recurrence.[50–52] In the only known study in the RARP literature examining the impact of margin location, Shikanov et al. reported that the site of margin positivity was not an independent predictor of biochemical recurrence.[12]

Regardless of the impact on progression, identifying the most common locations for PSMs is important because it targets portions of the procedure requiring technical improvement. During retropubic ORP, the majority of studies report the apex as the most common site for PSMs.[39,45,9,53] Several factors contribute to the apex being a problematic location with the retropubic approach. Prostate cancer commonly occurs at the apex, and extracapsular extension is thought to commonly occur in this location via the perineural spaces.[54] Furthermore, attempts to preserve urinary continence by dividing the urethra close to the apex may contribute to an increase in PSMs. Finally, the confines of the pelvis coupled with bleeding from the DVC may hinder visualization

Table 29.3 Studies comparing positive surgical margin rates between RARP and ORP[a]

Series	N	Overall (%)	pT2 (%)	pT3/pT4 (%)
Menon et al.[7]	30 RARP	26	–	–
	30 ORP	29	–	–
Tewari et al.[39]	200 RARP	9 ($p < 0.05$)	–	–
	100 ORP	23	–	–
Smith et al.[41]	200 RARP	15 ($p < 0.001$)	9.4 ($p < 0.001$)	50
	200 ORP	35	24.1	60
Laurila et al.[40]	88 RARP	13	10	38
	84 ORP	14	15	9
White et al.[42]	50 RARP	22 ($p = 0.007$)	19.1	67
	50 ORP	36	34	67
Ou et al.[43]	30 RARP	50 ($p < 0.05$)	13.3	86.7 ($p < 0.05$)
	30 ORP	20	0	40
Rocco et al.[27]	120 RARP	22	15	34
	240 ORP	25	17	42
Ficarra et al.[6]	103 RARP	34	12	–
	105 RRP	30	12	–

[a]Only significant ($p < 0.05$) p-values are listed.

and increase the risk of apical PSMs. Not all ORP series describe the apex as the most prevalent site for PSMs. A large study from Memorial Sloan Kettering Cancer Center found the posterolateral and apical locations to be the first and second most common sites, respectively.[49]

In comparison with ORP, RARP benefits from improved visualization and less bleeding, particularly at the apex. The main drawback of RARP is the lack of tactile feedback. As a result of these differences, the location of PSMs has been somewhat dissimilar between ORP and RARP. Patel et al., in a review of 1,500 RARPs, identified the posterolateral location to be the most common site, accounting for 37% of all PSMs.[21] In contrast, Smith et al. found the apex to be the most prevalent site in both ORP and RARP.[41] In their series, 52% of RARP PSMs were located at the apex, followed by 24% posteriorly. In the largest study examining PSM location during RARP, Shikanov et al. found the posterolateral region to be the most common site for overall, organ-confined, and pT3 cancers.[12] Forty-five percent of all PSMs were located posterolaterally, followed by 29% at the apex. Thus, it seems as though the posterolateral location may be the most common site for PSMs after RARP, but additional studies are necessary to confirm this finding. Certainly from a technical standpoint, the lack of tactile feedback and the antegrade dissection in RARP vs. the retrograde approach in ORP may increase the chances of a capsular incision during posterior dissection and neurovascular bundle (NVB) preservation. Furthermore, the improved visualization and hemostasis beneath the pubic symphysis may help to decrease PSMs at the apex.

When compared with a single location, multifocal positive margins have also been shown to confer a worse prognosis in some ORP studies,[52,55] but other open series have not validated these findings.[56,57] In a large RARP study of almost 1,400 patients by Shikanov et al., margin multifocality was not an independent predictor of recurrence ($p = 0.3$).[12] This finding may imply that a single PSM is enough of a negative prognostic factor and that additional positive sites do not have a cumulative effect. However, the median follow-up was only 12 months and there were a small absolute number of recurrences, suggesting that the results may change as the data mature.

The extent of PSMs may also play a role in oncologic outcomes after RARP. Indeed, not all PSMs are equivalent, as some are focal, typically defined as <1 mm in length, while larger ones are considered extensive.[12] Another study defined a focal PSM as one only visible on a single step section and only involving one gland.[47] PSMs due to iatrogenic capsular incision are sometimes considered equivocal. Intuitively, larger, more extensive PSMs should have a more significant impact on recurrence. However, only a few studies have investigated the extent of PSMs. Watson et al. retrospectively reviewed 215 ORP cases and identified 73 PSMs, of which 66% were considered extensive.[47] On multivariate analysis, the extent of PSM was not an independent predictor of biochemical recurrence ($p = 0.122$). Ochiai et al. reviewed the outcomes of 117 men who underwent ORP with a PSM between 1991 and 1999.[58] Patients with seminal vesicle invasion or lymph node metastasis and those who received neoadjuvant or adjuvant therapy were excluded. They stratified the extent of PSMs into ≤ 1 mm, 1.1–3 mm, and > 3 mm and found that a PSM > 3 mm was an independent predictor of recurrence. In the RARP literature, only one study from the University of Chicago has assessed the impact of PSM length on biochemical recurrence.[12] A retrospective review of 1,398 RARP cases identified 243 (17%) PSMs, of which 161 were available for secondary review and margin length measurement (<1 mm, 1–3 mm, >3 mm). With a median follow-up of 12 months, the length of PSM proved to be an independent predictor of biochemical recurrence. Interestingly, outcomes for patients with negative margins were similar to those with PSMs < 1 mm, suggesting that very small PSMs may be false positives or that, with relatively short follow-up, microscopic residual disease has not yet translated into recurrence. Taken together, the above studies suggest that the extent of PSMs likely has prognostic significance. This is especially important given the findings from a recent RARP study demonstrating that the incidence of extensive PSMs decreases with increasing surgeon experience.[59] Longer follow-up and additional studies are necessary to confirm these findings.

29.7 Impact of PSMs on Oncologic Outcomes

Large retrospective studies with sufficient follow-up have demonstrated that ORP is an effective treatment option for clinically localized prostate cancer.[53,60,61] Roehl et al. reviewed 3,478 consecutive ORP cases performed by a single surgeon over a 20-year period.[60] With a mean follow-up of 65 months, 5- and 10-year estimated biochemical recurrence-free survival (BRFS) was 80 and 68%, respectively. PSA, clinical stage, Gleason sum, pathological stage, and era of treatment (before 1991) were independently associated with cancer progression. Only 49 men (2%) died of prostate cancer, yielding an actuarial 10-year cancer-specific survival rate of 97%. Since this study included patients dating back to 1983, a significant proportion of cases were from the pre-PSA era, resulting in more advanced disease for that subset men. In a similar study of 2,402 patients treated with ORP between 1982 and 1999, 5-, 10-, and 15-year BRFS was 84, 74, and 66%, respectively.[61] At a mean follow-up of 6.3 years, actuarial cancer-specific survival at 10 and 15 years was 96 and 90%, respectively. Similar to the study by Roehl et al., a large subset of patients treated in the pre-PSA era had more advanced disease. Another large study of 5,679 patients from the Mayo Clinic with a median follow-up of 76 months demonstrated slightly lower 5- (76%) and 10-year (63%) BRFS.[53] Taken together, the above studies demonstrate robust long-term outcomes with ORP for clinically organ-confined disease. Caution must be taken when comparing these outcomes to more recent LRP and RARP series that only include patients from the PSA era, as significant down-staging and down-grading of disease has occurred.

The LRP technique was pioneered in the late 1990s and further refined by the start of the new millennium. Several large, retrospective studies have assessed mid-term oncologic outcomes. Touijer et al. studied 1,564 consecutive patients who underwent LRP for clinically organ-confined disease.[62] Disease progression was defined as a PSA $\geq$ 0.1 ng/ml with a confirmatory rise or the initiation of secondary therapy. The overall 5- and 8-year BRFS was 78 and 71%, respectively. Higher risk (based on Kattan nomogram) and higher pathologic stage patients demonstrated lower BRFS. Defining relapse as a PSA of $\geq$ 0.2 ng/ml, Pavlovich et al. reviewed the results of 528 LRPs performed between 2001 and 2005 at a single institution.[63] With a mean follow-up of 13 months, overall 3-year BRFS was 94.5% (98% for organ-confined and 79% for pT3 and/or N1 disease). Pathological Gleason sum and stage were the only independent predictors of recurrence. The presence of a PSM trended toward, but did not attain, statistical significance. Importantly, this study represented a screening-detected patient population from the United States with less aggressive clinical features than the Touijer et al. study based primarily in France. Differences in patient characteristics, definition of biochemical recurrence, and length of follow-up may explain the discrepancy in outcomes between the two series.

In the largest published robotic series, Badani et al. reported on 2,766 patients who underwent RARP between 2000 and 2006.[20] Mean follow-up was 26 months (median 22 months) and biochemical recurrence was defined as a PSA of $\geq$ 0.2 ng/ml. Ninety-five patients (7.3%) had a PSA recurrence, and the 5-year BRFS was 84%. Pre-operative PSA, pathologic Gleason sum, and pathologic stage were independent predictors of disease recurrence. Nine patients died during the entire study period, two as a result of prostate cancer. Other large RARP series with shorter follow-up have also reported oncologic outcomes. Shikanov et al. reviewed 1,398 men who underwent RARP, and with a median follow-up of 12 months, 4% of patients experienced biochemical recurrence (PSA $\geq$ 0.1 on two occasions).[12] In addition to pre-operative PSA, pathological stage, and pathological Gleason sum being prognostic for PSA recurrence, the presence of a PSM and the length of the PSM were also both independent predictors of biochemical relapse. Eleven percent of patients with a PSM compared with only 3% with negative margins experienced recurrence. Longer follow-up is necessary to better assess cancer control in this cohort. With a median follow-up of 22 months, Murphy et al. assessed the oncologic outcomes in their first 400 RARP cases.[23] Fifty-three patients (13%) experienced biochemical recurrence, and the 5-year BRFS was 74%. Patients with PSMs were more likely to experience PSA relapse than those with negative margins ($p = 0.0001$).

In the only known study comparing cancer control outcomes among ORP, LRP, and RARP at a single institution, Drouin et al. reviewed the results of 239 men (83 ORP, 85 LRP, 71 RARP) who underwent radical prostatectomy between 2000 and 2004.[44] Overall mean follow-up was 50 months and was shortest for RARP (41 months) and longest for ORP (58 months). Patients undergoing ORP were highest risk based on PSA, clinical stage, and biopsy Gleason sum. The overall 5-year PSA-free survival was 88%, and when stratified by surgical technique, there was no significant difference in BRFS. Another matched

Table 29.4 Oncologic outcomes for large ORP, LRP, and RARP studies

Series	Technique	N	Mean F/U (months)	Recurrence definition	5-Year BRFS (%)	10-Year BRFS (%)
Roehl et al.[60]	ORP	3,478	65	PSA > 0.2 ng/ml	80	68
Han et al.[61]	ORP	2,402	76	PSA ≥ 0.2 ng/ml	84	74
Ward et al.[53]	ORP	5,679	76[c]	PSA ≥ 0.4 ng/ml	76	63
Touijer et al.[62]	LRP	1,564	18	PSA ≥ 0.1 ng/ml	78	71[a]
Pavlovich et al.[63]	LRP	528	13	PSA ≥ 0.2 ng/ml	95[b]	–
Badani et al.[20]	RARP	2,766	26	PSA ≥ 0.2 ng/ml	84	–
Krambeck et a.[64]	ORP	294	16	PSA > 0.4 ng/ml	92[b]	–
	RARP	588			92[b]	–
Murphy et al.[23]	RARP	400	22[c]	PSA ≥ 0.2 ng/ml	74	–
Drouin et al.[44]	ORP	83	50	PSA > 0.2 ng/ml	88	–
	LRP	85			88	–
	RARP	71			90	–

[a]8-Year BRFS.
[b]3-Year BRFS.
[c]Median follow-up.

cohort study comparing RARP and ORP at a single institution also found no significant difference in 3-year BRFS (92% RARP, 92% ORP).[64] Table 29.4 summarizes the oncologic outcomes of ORP, LRP, and RARP studies.

Based on the above studies, short- and mid-term oncologic outcomes appear similar among the various surgical techniques for radical prostatectomy. However, in the above retrospective studies, differences in patient characteristics, definition of biochemical recurrence, surgical experience, and length of follow-up make it difficult to directly compare outcomes. Due to the significantly longer follow-up, ORP remains the gold standard for clinically localized prostate cancer, but as the RARP studies continue to mature, oncologic equivalence between the two techniques will hopefully be established.

29.8 Adjuvant Radiation for Locally Advanced Disease and/or Positive Surgical Margins

The decision of whether or not to institute adjuvant therapy after radical prostatectomy is multifactorial and includes patient age, pathological findings (including surgical margin status), functional status (urinary control and sexual function), and patient preference. As described previously, the presence of a PSM is an independent risk factor for prostate cancer recurrence, suggesting that adjuvant RT may play a role

in this setting. Unfortunately, there are no studies in the RARP literature addressing the role of adjuvant RT. However, to date, there have been three randomized controlled trials evaluating adjuvant RT for locally advanced disease (pT3/pT4) and/or PSMs after ORP. Initiated in 1992, Bolla et al. performed a randomized clinical trial (EORTC 22911) to assess the impact of immediate adjuvant RT (60 Gy) on cancer control for patients with PSMs or pT3 disease[65]; 503 patients were randomized to immediate RT and 502 to a wait-and-see policy until local failure. At a median follow-up of 5 years, BRFS, clinical progression-free survival, and loco-regional control were significantly improved in the irradiated group, and 5-year BRFS was 74 vs. 53% in the RT and wait-and-see cohorts, respectively (p < 0.0001). This improvement was noted for all subgroups, including patients with organ-confined disease and PSMs. No significant differences were observed for cancer-specific or overall survival. Adverse effects were more prevalent in the irradiated group, but severe toxicities were rare in both cohorts. Although the study was randomized and prospective, limitations included the inclusion of patients with detectable PSA levels after surgery and variations in indication and type of salvage therapy in the observation group. After central pathological review of over 50% of the cases, a repeat analysis of the data revealed that patients with PSMs benefited most from adjuvant RT.[66]

Southwest Oncology Group (SWOG) 8794 was a similar randomized trial but with a primary endpoint of metastasis-free survival.[67] Between 1988 and 1997, 425 patients with extra-prostatic extension, seminal vesicle invasion, or PSMs were randomized after ORP to immediate RT (60–64 Gy) or observation. Similar to EORTC 22911, an undetectable PSA was not required for study eligibility. There were no significant differences between groups in metastasis-free or overall survival at a median follow-up of 10.6 years. However, PSA relapse (median BRFS 10.3 years vs. 3.1 years, $p < 0.001$) and disease recurrence were significantly improved with immediate RT. Adverse effects were more common with RT (24% RT vs. 12% observation). An updated analysis with over 12 years of follow-up was published in 2009 and metastasis-free and overall survival were significantly improved with adjuvant RT.[68]

More recently, a German study randomized 192 men to observation and 193 to immediate post-operative RT (60 Gy).[69] All patients had pT3N0 disease after ORP, with or without PSMs. Importantly, unlike in the above two studies, patients with a detectable PSA after ORP were excluded. At a median follow-up of 54 months, 5-year BRFS was significantly improved in the immediate RT group (72 vs. 54%, $p = 0.0015$). The number of events was too few and the follow-up too short to assess metastasis-free and overall survival. Among other variables, a PSM predicted an increased effect of the RT. Minor adverse effects were greater with RT, but grade 3 or 4 toxicity was rare in both cohorts.

The above three clinical trials clearly demonstrate a significantly improved BRFS with adjuvant RT after ORP vs. a wait-and-see approach for locally advanced disease and/or PSMs. The recently updated analysis of SWOG 8794 also demonstrates improved metastasis-free and overall survival with immediate post-operative RT. Although none of the trials included RARP patients, the results should be applicable to all patients fitting the study criteria regardless of surgical technique. One caveat is that many of the patients in the above studies were treated in the pre- or early-PSA era when prostate cancer was diagnosed at more advanced stages. Furthermore, there is no evidence to support improved outcomes with adjuvant RT compared with salvage RT initiated relatively early after PSA-only relapse. A large, multi-institutional, retrospective study of 1,540 men who underwent post-prostatectomy salvage RT (median 65 Gy) after biochemical recurrence demonstrated encouraging results.[70] At a median follow-up of 53 months after RT, overall 6-year progression-free probability was 32%, and outcomes

were better when treatment was initiated at a PSA level ≤ 0.50 ng/ml (48% disease-free at 6 years). Other variables predicting a durable response to salvage RT included longer PSA doubling time, lower prostatectomy Gleason score, PSMs, and no lymph node metastasis. Based on this study, a nomogram was constructed to predict outcomes after salvage RT. Thus, for patients with biochemical recurrence after radical prostatectomy, salvage RT can provide long-term disease control and is potentially curative in a subset of patients, especially those who receive treatment when PSA levels are still low. The impact of adjunctive hormonal therapy is presently under investigation, and a randomized clinical trial investigating the timing (adjuvant vs. salvage) of post-operative RT is currently underway. The bottom line is that the decision to begin adjuvant or salvage RT is complex and should be done on a case-by-case basis.

29.9 Surgical Techniques to Improve Cancer Control

Regardless of technique, surgeons performing radical prostatectomy strive to achieve what has been coined "the trifecta"—cancer control, urinary continence, and preservation of erectile function. There is no doubt that the most important component of "the trifecta" is cancer control and, from a technical standpoint, achieving negative surgical margins is paramount. Oftentimes, the desire to maximize functional outcomes can jeopardize surgical margins, particularly during the apical and posterolateral dissection where the preservation of tissue can improve urinary and sexual function. Thus, optimizing surgical margin rates is multifactorial and includes appropriate patient selection, tailoring surgery based on risk factors for adverse pathology, and surgical techniques during various steps of the procedure. Increasing surgical experience has been shown to improve surgical margin rates, likely due to a combination of the above factors. Previous sections of this chapter have discussed the various clinical and pathological characteristics associated with PSMs. As such, this section will focus on surgical techniques to minimize PSMs.

Since the introduction of NVB preservation techniques, it has been hypothesized that nerve-sparing radical prostatectomy may increase PSMs and the subsequent risk of biochemical recurrence. However, previous large ORP series have shown that a nerve-sparing approach is not an independent risk factor for PSMs. In a retrospective review of 7,268 men who underwent ORP at a single institution, Ward et al. found a significantly higher PSM rate for wide excision (42%) than for nerve-sparing (34%).[53] After controlling for disease severity, nerve preservation was not an independent risk factor for PSMs. A similar study from the University of Miami resulted in the same conclusion.[55] Thus, based on the ORP literature, it seems as though tumor biology dictates the likelihood of PSMs and not the wide resection or preservation of the NVB. With significantly improved visualization, robotic surgeons have been able to further stratify the extent of nerve preservation. No longer just an all or nothing phenomenon, the concept of partially sparing nerves based on disease severity has emerged. Zorn et al. implemented a protocol to select side-specific extent of nerve preservation based on pre-operative disease characteristics (PSA, clinical stage, biopsy Gleason score, percent of positive biopsy cores, greatest percent positive core).[71] Three levels of nerve-sparing were implemented: interfascial for lowest-risk, partial extrafascial for intermediate-risk, and wide excision for highest risk candidates. The extrafascial dissection leaves a thin layer of tissue and blood vessels on the capsule of the prostate and is made possible by the improved magnification with the da Vinci™ system. When comparing 150 RARPs performed with the above protocol to 245 cases of non-selective interfascial nerve preservation, the authors found significantly lower overall (12.6 vs. 20.4%, $p = 0.04$) and posterolateral margin rates (37 vs. 70%, $p = 0.04$) with the tailoring approach. At 12 months, potency was reported in 67% of men undergoing partial extrafascial nerve preservation. Although these findings need confirmation, the extrafascial plane seems to offer acceptable functional outcomes while significantly improving cancer control in select intermediate-risk patients. To facilitate the tailoring of NVB preservation, a 12-core biopsy with mapping of the locations sampled (e.g., apex, mid-gland, base) should be standard of care. Larger glands may require more cores sampled to adequately map the prostate. In the future, endorectal magnetic resonance imaging may also prove beneficial in assisting with a tailored surgical approach.

Along with the posterolateral location, the apex is another area with high rates of PSMs. Several studies have described surgical techniques to decrease apical PSMs during RARP. Ahlering et al. reported their apical dissection modification and a coinciding reduction in organ-confined PSMs from 27 to 5%.[19] Removing all of the peri-prostatic fat overlying the apex, dividing the pubo-prostatic ligaments, and stapling the DVC were the new techniques implemented. One caveat is that increasing surgical experience may have also contributed to the improved outcomes. Guru et al. compared suture ligation of the DVC followed by apical dissection to cold incision of the DVC and apical dissection.[72] They found a significantly lower apical PSM rate with the cold incision technique (2 vs. 8%, $p = 0.02$). Menon and colleagues reported a similar improvement in organ-confined apical PSMs when suture ligation of the DVC was performed after prostate removal instead of before apical dissection.[73]

The competing interest of maximizing functional outcomes without compromising cancer control during RARP is always a dilemma for the surgeon. The take-home message is, regardless of which technical modifications are implemented, cancer control should always take precedence.

29.10 Conclusions

Radical prostatectomy has evolved over the last three decades into a precise, sophisticated procedure with minimal mortality and excellent surgical outcomes. Since its incorporation, robotic technology has quickly demonstrated that it can duplicate and improve on standard laparoscopy. Current RARP data suggest that comparable and possibly improved pathological and functional results can be obtained with robotic assistance in experienced hands, while providing the urologist a more ergonomic surgical platform.

In experienced RARP series, overall PSM rates have ranged between 9 and 19%, which are comparable to the gold-standard ORP. Independent risk factors for PSMs include lower surgeon case volume, pathologic stage and Gleason sum, lower prostate weight, pre-operative PSA level, and PSA density. Some evidence also suggests that biopsy Gleason score and BMI may be risk factors. Similarly, NVB preservation appears to be a risk factor for PSMs; however, it is difficult to control for confounding variables such as surgical technique and disease severity. Finally, tailoring nerve preservation based on disease severity and certain surgical techniques, particularly at the apex, may improve cancer control during RARP. Regardless of technique, cancer control should never be compromised during attempts to maximize functional outcomes.

The most common locations for PSMs during RARP are posterolateral and apical. The PSM location and number (single vs. multifocal) do not appear to impact recurrence. An extensive PSM, however, does appear to be an independent predictor of PSA relapse. Conversely, very small PSMs may not significantly impact cancer control.

Short- and mid-term BRFS appear equivalent for RARP, LRP, and ORP. Unfortunately, the RARP data are too immature to estimate cancer-specific and overall survival. Based on level 1 evidence from ORP literature, adjuvant RT for locally advanced disease and/or PSMs significantly improves biochemical recurrence-free, metastasis-free, and overall survival compared to observation. PSMs predict an improved response to RT. Salvage RT, initiated in a timely fashion when PSA levels are low, can also provide durable outcomes. These findings should be applicable to RARP patients as well. The decision to pursue post-operative RT (adjuvant or salvage) is, however, complex and includes consideration of the added survival benefit vs. adverse effects from the radiation. The optimal timing of when to deliver additional RT is still unknown and awaits the results of randomized clinical trials.

RARP has already become, by far, the most common surgical approach performed for prostate cancer and de facto the gold standard. Functional outcomes mature in 2 years after a radical prostatectomy and currently show at least equal, if not superior, results compared to ORP. Cancer control outcomes mature in 10–15 years, and we believe that when longer term data become available, RARP will officially become the gold standard for the surgical management of prostate cancer.

References

1. Zorn KC, Wille MA, Thong AE, et al. Continued improvement of perioperative, pathological and continence outcomes during 700 robot-assisted radical prostatectomies. *Can J Urol.* 2009;16:4742–4749.
2. Menon M, Shrivastava A, Sarle R, et al. Vattikuti Institute prostatectomy: a single-team experience of 100 cases. *J Endourol.* 2003;17:785–790.
3. Tewari A, Shrivastava A, Menon M. A prospective comparison of radical retropubic and robot-assisted prostatectomy: experience in one institution. *BJU Int.* 2003;92:205–210.
4. Herrell SD, Smith JA Jr. Robotic-assisted laparoscopic prostatectomy: what is the learning curve? *Urology.* 2005;66 (5 suppl):105–107.
5. Samadi D, Levinson A, Hakimi A, et al. From proficiency to expert, when does the learning curve for robotic-assisted prostatectomies plateau? The Columbia University experience. *World J Urol.* 2007;25:105–110.
6. Ficarra V, Novara G, Fracalanza S, et al. A prospective, non-randomized trial comparing robot-assisted laparoscopic and retropubic radical prostatectomy in one European institution. *BJU Int.* 2009;104:534–539.
7. Menon M, Tewari A, Baize B, et al. Prospective comparison of radical retropubic prostatectomy and robot-assisted anatomic prostatectomy: the Vattikuti urology institute experience. *Urology.* 2002;60:864–868.
8. Ahlering TE, Skarecky D, Lee D, et al. Successful transfer of open surgical skills to a laparoscopic environment using a robotic interface: initial experience with laparoscopic radical prostatectomy. *J Urol.* 2003;170:1738–1741.
9. Wieder JA, Soloway MS. Incidence, etiology, location, prevention and treatment of positive surgical margins after radical prostatectomy for prostate cancer. *J Urol.* 1998;160:299–315.
10. Epstein JI. Incidence and significance of positive margins in radical prostatectomy specimens. *Urol Clin North Am.* 1996;23:651–663.
11. Chang SS, Cookson MS. Impact of positive surgical margins after radical prostatectomy. *Urology.* 2006;68:249–252.
12. Shikanov S, Al-Ahmadie H, Royce C, et al. Length of positive surgical margin after radical prostatectomy as a predictor of biochemical recurrence. *J Urol.* 2009;182:137–142.
13. Binder J, Kramer W. Robotically-assisted laparoscopic radical prostatectomy. *BJU Int.* 2001;87:408–410.
14. Rassweiler J, Frede T, Seemann O, et al. Telesurgical laparoscopic radical prostatectomy. *Eur Urol.* 2001;40:75–83.
15. Pasticier G, Rietbergen JB, Guillonneau B, et al. Robotically assisted laparoscopic radical prostatectomy: feasibility study in men. *Eur Urol.* 2001;40:70–74.
16. Patel VR, Tully AS, Holmes R, et al. Robotic radical prostatectomy in the community setting – the learning curve and beyond: initial 200 cases. *J Urol.* 2005;174:269–272.
17. Mikhail AA, Orvieto MA, Billatos ES, et al. Robotic-assisted laparoscopic prostatectomy: first 100 patients with 1 year of follow-up. *Urology.* 2006;68:1275–1279.
18. Bentas W, Wolfram M, Jones J, et al. Robotic technology and the translation of open radical prostatectomy to laparoscopy: the early Frankfurt experience with robotic radical prostatectomy and one year follow-up. *Eur Urol.* 2003;44:175–181.
19. Ahlering TE, Eichel L, Edwards RA, et al. Robotic radical prostatectomy: a technique to reduce pt2 positive margins. *Urology.* 2004;64:1224–1228.
20. Badani KK, Kaul S, Menon M. Evolution of robotic radical prostatectomy: assessment after 2,766 procedures. *Cancer.* 2007;110:1951–1958.

21. Patel VR, Palmer KJ, Coughlin G, et al. Robot-assisted laparoscopic radical prostatectomy: perioperative outcomes of 1,500 cases. *J Endourol*. 2008;22:2299–2305.

22. Wiltz AL, Shikanov S, Eggener SE, et al. Robotic radical prostatectomy in overweight and obese patients: oncological and validated-functional outcomes. *Urology*. 2009;73:316–322.

23. Murphy DG, Kerger M, Crowe H, et al. Operative details and oncological and functional outcome of robotic-assisted laparoscopic radical prostatectomy: 400 cases with a minimum of 12 months follow-up. *Eur Urol*. 2009;55:1358–1367.

24. Vickers AJ, Bianco FJ, Gonen M, et al. Effects of pathologic stage on the learning curve for radical prostatectomy: evidence that recurrence in organ-confined cancer is largely related to inadequate surgical technique. *Eur Urol*. 2008;53:960–966.

25. Vickers AJ, Bianco FJ, Serio AM, et al. The surgical learning curve for prostate cancer control after radical prostatectomy. *J Natl Cancer Inst*. 2007;99:1171–1177.

26. Liss M, Osann K, Ornstein D. Positive surgical margins during robotic radical prostatectomy: a contemporary analysis of risk factors. *BJU Int*. 2008;102:603–607.

27. Rocco B, Matei D, Melegari S, et al. Robotic versus open prostatectomy in a laparoscopically naïve centre: a matched-pair analysis. *BJU Int*. 2009;104:991–995.

28. Shikanov SA, Thong A, Gofrit ON, et al. Robotic laparoscopic radical prostatectomy for biopsy Gleason 8 to 10: prediction of favorable pathologic outcome with preoperative parameters. *J Endourol*. 2008;22:1477–1481.

29. Zorn KC, Gofrit ON, Orvieto MA, et al. Robotic-assisted laparoscopic prostatectomy: functional and pathologic outcomes with interfascial nerve preservation. *Eur Urol*. 2007;51:755–762.

30. Ahlering TE, Eichel L, Edwards R, et al. Impact of obesity on clinical outcomes in robotic prostatectomy. *Urology*. 2005;65:740–744.

31. Khaira HS, Bruyere F, O'Malley PJ, et al. Does obesity influence the operative course or complications of robot-assisted laparoscopic prostatectomy. *BJU Int*. 2006;98:1275–1278.

32. Castle EP, Atug F, Woods M, et al. Impact of body mass index on outcomes after robot assisted radical prostatectomy. *World J Urol*. 2008;26:91–95.

33. Herman MP, Raman JD, Dong S, et al. Increasing body mass index negatively impacts outcomes following robotic radical prostatectomy. *JSLS*. 2007;11:438–442.

34. Freedland SJ, Isaacs WB, Platz EA, et al. Prostate size and risk of high-grade, advanced prostate cancer and biochemical progression after radical prostatectomy: a search database study. *J Clin Oncol*. 2005;23:7546–7554.

35. D'Amico AV, Whittington R, Malkowicz SB, et al. A prostate gland volume of more than 75 cm3 predicts for a favorable outcome after radical prostatectomy for localized prostate cancer. *Urology*. 1998;52:631–636.

36. Levinson AW, Ward NT, Sulman A, et al. The impact of prostate size on perioperative outcomes in a large laparoscopic radical prostatectomy series. *J Endourol*. 2009;23:147–152.

37. Zorn KC, Orvieto MA, Mikhail AA, et al. Effect of prostate weight on operative and postoperative outcomes of robotic-assisted laparoscopic prostatectomy. *Urology*. 2007;69:300–305.

38. Gofrit ON, Zorn KC, Steinberg GD, et al. The Will ogers phenomenon in urological oncology. *J Urol*. 2008;179:28–33.

39. Tewari A, Srivastava A, Menon M. A prospective comparison of radical retropubic and robot-assisted prostatectomy: experience in one institution. *BJU Int*. 2003;92:205–210.

40. Laurila TA, Huang W, Jarrard DF. Robotic-assisted laparoscopic and radical retropubic prostatectomy generate similar positive margin rates in low and intermediate risk patients. *Urol Oncol*. 2008;27:529–533.

41. Smith JA Jr, Chan RC, Chang SS, et al. A comparison of the incidence and location of positive surgical margins in robotic assisted laparoscopic radical prostatectomy and open retropubic radical prostatectomy. *J Urol*. 2007;178:2385–2390.

42. White MA, De Haan AP, Stephens DD, et al. Comparative analysis of surgical margins between radical retropubic prostatectomy and RALP: are patients sacrificed during initiation of robotics program? *Urology*. 2009;73:567–571.

43. Ou YC, Yang CR, Wang J, et al. Comparison of robotic-assisted versus retropubic radical prostatectomy performed by a single surgeon. *Anticancer Res*. 2009;29:1637–1642.

44. Drouin SJ, Vaessen C, Hupertan V, et al. Comparison of mid-term carcinologic control obtained after open, laparoscopic, and robot-assisted radical prostatectomy for localized prostate cancer. *World J Urol*. 2009;27:599–605.

45. Rozet F, Jaffe J, Braud G, et al. A direct comparison of robotic assisted versus pure laparoscopic radical prostatectomy: a single institution experience. *J Urol*. 2007;178:478–482.

46. Parsons JK, Bennett JL. Outcomes of retropubic, laparoscopic, and robotic-assisted prostatectomy. *Urology*. 2008;72:412–416.

47. Watson RB, Civantos F, Soloway MS. Positive surgical margins with radical prostatectomy: detailed pathological analysis and prognosis. *Urology*. 1996;48:80–90.

48. Salomon L, Anastasiadis AG, Antiphon P, et al. Prognostic consequences of the location of positive surgical margins in organ-confined prostate cancer. *Urol Int*. 2003;70:291–296.

49. Eastham JA, Kuroiwa K, Ohori M, et al. Prognostic significance of location of positive margins in radical prostatectomy specimens. *Urology*. 2007;70:965–969.

50. Blute ML, Bostwick DG, Bergstralh EJ, et al. Anatomic site-specific positive margins in organ-confined prostate cancer and its impact on outcome after radical prostatectomy. *Urology*. 1997;50:733–739.

51. Aydin H, Tsuzuki T, Hernandez D, et al. Positive proximal (bladder neck) margin at radical prostatectomy confers greater risk of biochemical progression. *Urology*. 2004;64:551–555.

52. Obek C, Sadek S, Lai S, et al. Positive surgical margins with radical retropubic prostatectomy: anatomic site-specific pathologic analysis and impact on prognosis. *Urology*. 1999;54:682–688.

53. Ward JF, Zincke H, Bergstralh EJ, et al. The impact of surgical approach (nerve bundle preservation versus wide local excision) on surgical margins and biochemical recurrence following radical prostatectomy. *J Urol*. 2004;172:1328–1332.

54. Rosen MA, Goldstone L, Lapin S, et al. Frequency and location of extracapsular extension and positive surgical margins in radical prostatectomy specimens. *J Urol.* 1992;148:331–337.

55. Sofer M, Hamilton-Nelson KL, Civantos F, et al. Positive surgical margins after radical retropubic prostatectomy: the influence of site and number on progression. *J Urol.* 2002;167:2453–2456.

56. Kausik SJ, Blute ML, Sebo TJ, et al. Prognostic significance of positive surgical margins in patients with extraprostatic carcinoma after radical prostatectomy. *Cancer.* 2002;95:1215–1219.

57. Grossfeld GD, Chang JJ, Broering JM, et al. Impact of positive surgical margins on prostate cancer recurrence and the use of secondary cancer treatment: data from the CaPSURE database. *J Urol.* 2000;163:1171–1177.

58. Ochiai A, Sotelo T, Troncoso P, et al. Natural history of biochemical progression after radical prostatectomy based on length of a positive margin. *Urology.* 2008;71:308–312.

59. Weizer AZ, Ye Z, Hollingsworth JM, et al. Adoption of new technology and healthcare quality: surgical margins after robotic prostatectomy. *Urology.* 2007;70:96–100.

60. Roehl KA, Han M, Ramos CG, et al. Cancer progression and survival rates following anatomical radical retropubic prostatectomy in 3,478 consecutive patients: long-term results. *J Urol.* 2004;172:910–914.

61. Han M, Partin AW, Pound CR, et al. Long-term biochemical disease-free and cancer-specific survival following anatomic radical retropubic prostatectomy. The 15-year Johns Hopkins experience. *Urol Clin North Am.* 2001;28:555–565.

62. Touijer K, Secin FP, Cronin AM, et al. Oncologic outcomes after laparoscopic radical prostatectomy: 10 years of experience. *Eur Urol.* 2009;55:1014–1019.

63. Pavlovich CP, Trock BJ, Sulman A, et al. 3-Year actuarial biochemical recurrence-free survival following laparoscopic radical prostatectomy: experience from a tertiary referral center in the united states. *J Urol.* 2008;179: 917–922.

64. Krambeck AE, DiMarco DS, Rangel LJ, et al. Radical prostatectomy for prostatic adenocarcinoma: a matched comparison of open retropubic and robot-assisted techniques. *BJU Int.* 2009;103:448–453.

65. Bolla M, Poppel HV, Collette L, et al. Postoperative radiotherapy after radical prostatectomy: a randomised controlled trial (EORTC 22911). *Lancet.* 2005;366: 572–578.

66. Van der Kwast TH, Collette L, Bolla M. Adjuvant radiotherapy after surgery for pathologically advanced prostate cancer. *J Clin Oncol.* 2007;25:5671–5672.

67. Thompson IM Jr, Tangen CM, Paradelo J, et al. Adjuvant radiotherapy for pathologically advanced prostate cancer: a randomized clinical trial. *JAMA.* 2006;296:2329–2335.

68. Thompson IM, Tangen CM, Paradelo J, et al. Adjuvant radiotherapy for pathological T3N0M0 prostate cancer significantly reduces risk of metastases and improves survival: long-term followup of a randomized clinical trial. *J Urol.* 2009;181:956–962.

69. Wiegel T, Bottke D, Steiner U, et al. Phase III postoperative adjuvant radiotherapy after radical prostatectomy compared with radical prostatectomy alone in pt3 prostate cancer with postoperative undetectable prostate-specific antigen: ARO 96-02/AUO AP 09/95. *J Clin Oncol.* 2009;27: 2924–2930.

70. Stephenson AJ, Scardino PT, Kattan MW, et al. Predicting the outcome of salvage radiation therapy for recurrent prostate cancer after radical prostatectomy. *J Clin Oncol.* 2007;25:2035–2041.

71. Zorn KC, Gofrit ON, Steinberg GD, et al. Planned nerve preservation to reduce positive surgical margins during robot-assisted laparoscopic radical prostatectomy. *J Endourol.* 2008;22:1303–1309.

72. Guru KA, Perlmutter AE, Sheldon MJ, et al. Apical margins after robot-assisted radical prostatectomy: does technique matter? *J Endourol.* 2009;23:123–127.

73. Menon M, Shrivastava A, Kaul S, et al. Vattikuti institute prostatectomy: contemporary technique and analysis of results. *Eur Urol.* 2007;51:648–657.

Chapter 30

Techniques to Improve Urinary Continence Following Robot-Assisted Radical Prostatectomy

Pierre Mendoza, Saurabh Sharma, and David I. Lee

30.1 Introduction

Robot-assisted radical prostatectomy (RARP) is rapidly gaining popularity in the urologic community. Since its advent, this technique has benefited patients by achieving quicker convalescence. However, this improvement has also driven efforts to improve the functional outcomes after RARP with promising early results. This cutting edge approach provides advantages including enhanced visualization, dexterity, and instrumentation. However, specific techniques to minimize the anatomic and neuro-physiologic risks need to be further elucidated.

Postoperative incontinence after RARP is a bothersome complication, which carries the potential to have a tremendous impact on quality of life. Efforts to improve postoperative incontinence have led to many modifications in the surgical technique as well as preoperative and postoperative manipulations. This chapter highlights the various maneuvers described in the literature geared toward improving urinary incontinence post-RARP.

30.2 Definitions

The current International Continence Society (ICS) defines urinary incontinence as "the complaint of any involuntary leakage of urine".[1] However, patients experience different levels of continence as they recover from prostatectomy. As such, quantification of incontinence has been crudely defined by the number of incontinence pads per day (PPD). *Total continence* is often defined as the use of zero PPD and *social continence* as the use of a security pad or one PPD. When evaluating postoperative incontinence, one must consider the preoperative continence status of the individual patient.

30.3 Background

Historically, retropubic radical prostatectomy (RRP) has been considered the gold standard for the surgical treatment of prostate cancer. Both standard laparoscopic radical prostatectomy (LRP) and RARP involve the same basic anatomical relationships as RRP. However, refinements in minimally invasive techniques may translate into faster continence recovery.[2]

The data regarding postoperative incontinence from various series for RRP, LRP, and RARP is summarized in Table 30.1. Most series utilized validated questionnaires, including UCLA-PCI and EPIC, for the assessment of urinary incontinence. RARP studies included additional substratifications of "early continence" showing promising data as early as 1 week postoperatively.[3]

The studies of post-RRP demonstrate continence rates approximating 92–93% at 18-month follow-up.[4,5] Likewise, the best continence rates achieved by RARP are 93% with slightly shorter 12-month follow-up.[6] The LRP continence rates are 84% at 6-month follow-up.[7] Early continence data (3 months or less) following RRP data are not sufficiently available for comparison with RARP. Immediate postoperative

D.I. Lee (✉)
Division of Urology, Penn Presbyterian Medical Center,
University of Pennsylvania, Philadelphia, PA, USA
e-mail: david.i.lee@uphs.upenn.edu

A.K. Hemal, M. Menon (eds.), *Robotics in Genitourinary Surgery*,
DOI 10.1007/978-1-84882-114-9_30, © Springer-Verlag London Limited 2011

Table 30.1 Continence results following open, laparoscopic or robotic prostatectomy

Study	Year	Type	No. of cases	Method of assessment	Definitions used	Continence at 3 months	Continence at 6 months	Continence at 12 months	Continence at 18 months	Continence at 24 months
Benoit et al.[102]	2000	RRP, mixed pool data	25,651	Medicare claim	–	–	–	92	–	–
Catalona et al.[4]	1999	RRP	1,325	Questionnaire	0 PPD	–	–	–	92	–
Steiner et al.[103]	1991	RRP	593	–	0 PPD	47	75	89	–	92
Kundu et al.[5]	2004	RRP	2,737	Questionnaire	0 PPD	–	–	–	93	–
Kao et al.[104]	2000	RRP, multicentric	1,013	Questionnaire	Drops of urine	–	34	–	–	–
Rassweiler et al.[105]	2006	LRP, multicentric	5,824	Questionnaire	0 PPD	–	–	85		
Guillonneau et al.[106]	2002	LRP,	341	Questionnaire	0 PPD	–	73.3 ($n = 341$)	82.3 ($n = 255$)	–	–
Stolzenburg et al.[7]	2005	LRP	700		0 PPD	–	84($n = 500$)	92($n = 420$)	–	–
Badani et al.[6]	2007	RARP	1,110	Questionnaire	0 PPD	–	–	93		
Tewari et al.[3]	2008	RARP	214	Questionnaire	0 PPD	50	62	82	–	–

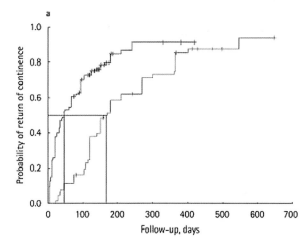

Fig. 30.1 Kaplan–Meier analysis of return of continence, in the RRP (*green*) and VIP (*red*) groups

continence (PoC) rates are promising for RARP. Tewari et al. showed a PoC of 35, 50, and 62% at the 1-, 3-, and 6-month time points, respectively ($n = 214$) [3]. Wang et al. have reported PoC rates of 82% at 3 months and 87% at 6 months ($n = 100$), respectively.[8] In comparison with LRP, results of RARP at 6 months are equal or inferior, but at 12-month follow-up the results are almost same.

In regard to comparative studies between RRP and RARP, Krambeck et al.[9] reported no significant difference in continence at 1 year between RARP and RRP patients (RARP 91.8%, RRP 93.7%, $P = 0.344$). Similarly, Ahlering et al.[10] reported that at 3-month follow-up there was no significant difference in continence (RARP 76%, RRP 75%, and $P \geq 0.05$). In contrast to the above studies, Tewari et al. with their VIP (Vattikuti Institute Prostatectomy) technique for RARP showed a significant difference between the RRP and RARP. Figure 30.1 shows the difference between the two groups (RARP/VIP vs. RRP). Patients achieved continence much quicker after VIP than after RRP. As shown in Fig 30.1, 50% of the follow-up population recovered continence in 44 days compared to 160 days, in VIP and RRP groups, respectively ($P < 0.05$).[11]

30.4 Mechanism of Urinary Incontinence After Radical Prostatectomy

Incontinence after radical prostatectomy can be due to intrinsic sphincter deficiency or dysfunction (ISD) or bladder dysfunction.[12] Sphincter dysfunction can be the result of direct trauma to sphincter, its nerve supply, or the supporting structures, or due to disuse atrophy. Increases in abdominal pressure or gravitational stress will result in stress urinary incontinence.

Bladder dysfunction can be due to pre-existing bladder outlet obstruction leading to detrusor instability in addition to age-related changes in detrusor function. Removal of the prostate and the obstruction can unmask the detrusor instability which may manifest as urge incontinence. Bladder dysfunction, caused by partial bladder denervation, may also result from surgical trauma.[13]

Many cases of post-prostatectomy incontinence will be a mixed picture with overlapping contributions from stress and urge components.[14] Ficazzola et al.[15] in their study using multichannel video urodynamics have shown ISD as the main culprit responsible for incontinence in post-prostatectomy patients. ISD was present in 90% of the patients. Bladder dysfunction was not always a significant contributor (45%). Overall incontinence due to ISD was 67%, combined ISD and bladder dysfunction was 23%, and pure bladder dysfunction was 3%. Another study by Chao et al.[16] showed that 57% had sphincter weakness alone, 39% had detrusor instability and/or decreased compliance combined with ISD, and only 4% had detrusor instability alone.

However, other studies such as those by Goluboff et al.[17] and Leach et al.[18] underscore bladder dysfunction as the predominant cause. According to Goluboff, the most common etiology for incontinence was detrusor instability alone, which was present in 40% after radical retropubic prostatectomy. Stress incontinence alone was present in only 8% after radical retropubic prostatectomy. Detrusor instability with stress incontinence was present in 52% after radical retropubic prostatectomy. Goluboff demonstrated that stress incontinence alone was a relatively rare cause of post-prostatectomy incontinence, with detrusor instability present in more than 90% of the patients. Leach et al. in a similar study reported stress incontinence to be present in 40%, stress plus bladder dysfunction in 42%, and bladder dysfunction alone in 14% of post-RRP patients.

Matsukawa et al.[19] in a retrospective urodynamics comparison demonstrated comparable degradations in both urethral sphincter function and bladder compliance between the RRP and LRP groups. Bladder function as measured by bladder compliance was significantly better in the laparoscopic group than the open group (45.7 vs. 25.8 ml/cm of water $P = 0.03$).

Obstruction after radical prostatectomy is usually the result of a narrowed vesicourethral anastomosis due to urethral stricture or bladder neck contracture. This obstruction can cause overflow incontinence and urge incontinence secondary to detrusor instability.[15] The incidence of bladder neck contracture after RARP is 1.1% at 1 year in a large series reported by Msezane et al.[20] In their study, there was no significant impact on urinary continence or QoL after appropriate management of the bladder neck contracture. This is remarkably low compared to other series of RRP that demonstrate bladder neck contracture rates of 2.5–32%.[21,22,23]

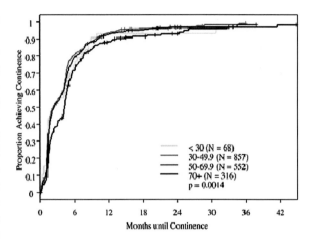

Fig. 30.2 Prostate size in grams and return to continence

30.5 Factors Influencing Continence After RARP

30.5.1 Age

Increasing age is an important predictor for post-prostatectomy incontinence. With advancing age there is atrophy of the rhabdosphincter and probable neural pathway degeneration. Several studies in patients with RRP have shown the negative impact of increasing age in recovering continence after surgery.[24,25,26]

Greco et al.[27] reported a comparative study between men older and younger than 70, and their continence outcome after RARP. Continence rates, as defined by requiring one precautionary pad or less per day, were equivalent between older and younger men at 1, 3, and 12 months after RARP. However, older men had a significant lower continence rate at 6 months (60 vs. 79%, $P = 0.04$). Older age is also associated with occasional urinary leaks after pad-free status has been achieved after RARP.[28] Mendiola et al.[29] reported in a follow-up of 300 patients that younger men have an earlier return of continence compared to older men after RARP. However, this difference disappeared after 1 year of follow-up.

30.5.2 Prostate Size

Although attractive as a factor, there is a general dearth on studies relating prostate size and its effect

on continence outcomes. Boczko et al.[30] in a series of 355 extra-peritoneal RARP patients reported the 6-month continence rate in patients with a prostate volume less than 75 g to be 97 vs. 84% in patients with prostate volumes greater than 75 g ($P<0.05$). In another study by Link et al.[31] increasing prostate size was associated with more postoperative urinary leaks but overall continence recovery was not affected as shown in Fig. 30.2.

30.5.3 Pathology

Most large RRP series have found no correlation between the stage of disease and incontinence rates.[4,24] In certain cases, the stage of disease may affect the surgical technique (i.e., nerve-sparing status), which may then have resultant effect on continence.[24]

30.5.4 Nerve Sparing

Eastham et al. have shown a positive impact of nerve sparing in regaining continence after RRP.[24] Similarly in a large series by Sacco et al.[32] recovery of continence was significantly worse in patients in whom both neurovascular bundles were resected during RRP ($P = 0.030$). In a study by Takenaka et al.[33] the continence rate in a group of patients without attempted nerve sparing was significantly lower at both 3 months ($P = 0.0046$) and 6 months postoperatively ($P = 0.0356$). However, Tseng conducted a multivariate analysis of an initial cohort of RARP patients and found in their series that nerve sparing was not significantly associated with the return of continence.[34]

30.5.5 Anastomotic Strictures

Several studies have reported that anastomotic stricture is an independent and significant risk factor for incontinence. The incidence of incontinence is directly proportional to the incidence of anastomotic strictures.[24,32] Chao et al.[16] reported anastomotic strictures in 26% of men with post-prostatectomy incontinence which they found to be associated with sphincteric dysfunction by video-urodynamic evaluation. Ahlering et al. noted a lower incidence of fossa navicularis stricture when using an 18 vs. 22 Fr catheter.[35] This simple maneuver decreased this risk of stricture from 6.9% in the 22 Fr catheter group to 0.9% in the 18 Fr catheter group in their experience ($P = 0.03$).

30.5.6 BMI (Body Mass Index)

BMI is associated with poor post-prostatectomy continence outcomes. Wiltz et al.[36] in a prospective study, using a validated questionnaire in 945 patients with RARP, found that men with normal weight had a significantly higher continence rate when compared with overweight and obese men, at both 12 months (70 vs. 68 vs. 57%, $P = 0.03$) and 24 months postoperatively (75 vs. 71 vs. 57%, $P = 0.04$). In a similar study

by Ahlering et al.,[37] using multivariate analysis, they demonstrated that only BMI predicted for pad-free continence at 6 months of follow-up ($P = 0.016$). Also, in this study, at 6-month follow-up, only 47% of obese patients vs. 91.4% of non-obese patients had achieved pad-free urinary continence ($P \leq 0.001$). Other studies, however, were unable to show similar predictive significance of BMI in recovery of postoperative continence.[38,39,40]

30.5.7 Effect of Previous Surgery

Menard et al.[41] in a comparative study of patients undergoing LRP with or without TURP reported 86 and 95.8% continence rates, respectively ($P = 0.77$). However, neurovascular bundle preservation was performed in only 56.5% in those with a prior history of TURP vs. 78.9% in those without a prior TURP ($P = 0.02$). There is considerable difference between two groups, though, not statistically significant. This may be accounted for the difference in nerve sparing in two groups to some extent. Colombo et al.[42] have shown superior continence results following RRP for those without any previous prostate surgery (Table 30.2).

30.6 Evaluation of Incontinence After RARP

30.6.1 History and Physical Examination

A thorough history is an important part in evaluation of men with postoperative incontinence. Symptoms such

Table 30.2 Difference in post prostatectomy continence recovery in patients with previous prostate surgery and those who had none

	Group 1 (43 pts)			Group 2 (120 pts)		
	Baseline	6 mos	12 mos	Baseline	6 mos	12 mos
No. complete continence (%)	100	32 (74)	37 (86)	0	110 (92)	114 (95)
No. incontinence (%)						
Mild (%)	0	16 (37)	4 (9)	0	5 (4)	5 (4)
Severe	0	10 (23)	3 (7)	0	3 (2.5)	0

Group 1 = previous prostate surgery (for BOO, TURP or open prostate surgery) and RRP.
Group 2 = only RRP.
Functional outcomes at baseline and 6- and 12-month follow-up.[42]

as leakage with maneuvers increasing intra-abdominal pressure, urgency, incomplete emptying, slow or split stream, frequency, dysuria may better characterize and elucidate specific causes for incontinence. The number of pads per day and relative degree of bother can also aid in the stratification of mild to severe incontinence. Stress incontinence defined as incontinence associated with a sudden increase in abdominal pressure (grade 1), incontinence with moderate activity (grade 2), and incontinence with minimal activity or gravitational incontinence (grade 3) may be suggestive of the presence of ISD.[15]

Preoperative voiding function should be used as a baseline measure. Significant voiding difficulties preoperatively may predispose to early postoperative continence issues. Past medical history should suggest any underlying neurological deficit and prior surgery and/or radiation therapy may contribute to treatment failure and frustration. Medication history is also important, particularly, tricyclic antidepressants (imipramine, amitriptiline), anticholinergics (atropine), cholinomimetics (bethanechol, neostigmine), and antihistaminics (diphenhydramine).

Physical examination will revolve around the standard urologic examination. Bladder palpation, rectal examination, Valsalva, and cough maneuvers as well as a neurologic exam will provide a comprehensive evaluation. A simple voiding diary may be an important objective measure of the degree and type of incontinence.

30.6.2 Further Investigation

Urinalysis and microscopy as an initial test should be performed in all cases. Concomitant infection should be excluded as a cause of irritative symptoms. In addition, a urodynamic investigation (UDS) may be warranted. Uroflowmetry and postvoid residual urine volumes are readily available in the office setting. UDS may help in objectively differentiating various causes of postoperative incontinence. In addition to detrusor pressure measurements, simultaneous fluoroscopy may prove to be a helpful adjunct in the evaluation of sphincteric dysfunction. Cystoscopic evaluation may be necessary in cases where stricture or bladder neck contractures are suspected as a cause of persistent incontinence.

30.7 Non-operative Strategies to Improve Continence Following RARP

30.7.1 Smoking Cessation

Cigarette smoke contains nicotine, which has well-studied pharmacological effects on the urinary bladder. Nicotine produces phasic contraction of isolated bladder muscles in vitro. These contractions may lead to increased detrusor activity that has been shown to be induced in vivo in the feline model. Another indirect mechanism may arise from the increases in intra-abdominal pressure caused by chronic coughing in smokers.[43]

Research has shown that smoking is strongly associated with lower urinary tract symptoms in men[44]; cessation may result in decreased symptoms.[44] Cigarette smoke has also been shown to have a strong relationship in the development of bladder neck contractures after RRP.[45] In a study by Borborogul et al.[45] smoking was the strongest predictor of bladder neck contracture when compared to coronary artery disease, hypertension, and DM.

In contrast, Wille et al.[39] could not find a statistically significant relation between smoking and postprostatectomy incontinence. Certainly, smoking cessation is also beneficial to general health and improved recovery in the perioperative period due to improved airway health and anesthesia tolerance.

30.7.2 Pelvic Floor Muscle Exercise/Therapy (PMFT)

The pelvic floor muscles such as levator ani are an important group of muscles that contribute to pelvic anatomy and physiology. Their proper function may be compromised in the post-prostatectomy patient due to the anatomic and physiologic distortion created by prostatectomy. PMFT therefore plays a very important role in augmenting the continence mechanism.

In a prospective study, using MRI as the imaging and measurement tool, Soong et al.[46] have shown that pelvic diaphragm thickness and the ratio of levator ani thickness to prostate volume are independent factors predictive of post-prostatectomy incontinence. They concluded that patients with better developed pelvic floor muscles, especially in relation to the size of the prostate, can be expected to achieve earlier recovery of continence after radical prostatectomy.

A randomized controlled trial by Manassero et al.[47] suggested that an early intensive and prolonged pelvic floor exercise can further increase the number of continent patients and this improvement persists in the first 12 months. Filocamo et al.[48] conducted a randomized controlled trial, with 300 consecutive patients who were to undergo standard RRP, and compared those with PMFT (group A) vs. no PMFT (group B). In their first treatment session, group A was taught how to perform a dominant pelvic muscle contraction while in the supine position without contracting the antagonist muscle group. At home, for 10 days, the patients performed three sets daily. In the second treatment session, patients were taught PMFT in all positions: sitting, standing, squatting, and going up and down stairs. After 1 month continence was achieved by 29 patients (19.3%) of group A as opposed to 12 (8%) patients of group B ($P = 0.006$). After 3 months 111 (74%) patients of group A and 45 (30%) of group B ($P<0.001$) were continent. At 6 months the rates were 144 (96%) and 97 (64.6%), respectively ($P<0.001$) (Fig. 30.3).

Several studies support the above fact that PMFT helps in early recovery of continence.[49,50,51] Pelvic floor exercise, with or without biofeedback enhancement, significantly improves continence rates in comparison to men not having undergone PMFT.[51]

30.7.2.1 Pharmacotherapy

There is no established pharmacotherapy for stress-related post-prostatectomy incontinence. Various available drugs such as impramine and tolterodine are being used with variable results in patients with evidence of bladder dysfunction as a cause of incontinence.

30.8 Intraoperative Techniques

30.8.1 Preservation of the Puboprostatic Ligaments

Some have advocated for a puboprostatic ligament-sparing technique to facilitate rapid return of urinary continence after RRP without compromising the oncologic efficacy of the procedure.[52,53] This can be combined with minimizing the endopelvic fascia incision during the apical dissection. In addition, preservation of the puboperinealis muscle and arcus tendineus may aid in return of early continence.[54,55] Stolzenburg after a comparative study proposed that the use of puboprostatic ligament sparing in endoscopic radical prostatectomy is beneficial in the recovery of early continence after nerve-sparing procedures, without any negative effect on margin status[56] (Fig. 30.4).

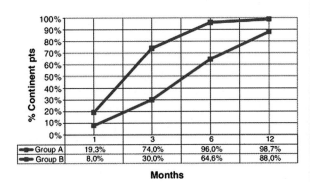

	1	3	6	12
Group A	19,3%	74,0%	96,0%	98,7%
Group B	8,0%	30,0%	64,6%	88,0%

Months

Fig. 30.3 Shows difference in return of continence between PMFT and non-PMFT groups. Group A = structured PFMT, Group B = no PFMT

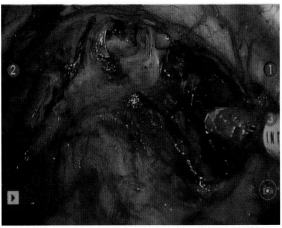

Fig. 30.4 Preservation of puboprostatic ligament

30.8.2 Suspension of the Dorsal Venous Complex

A periurethral suspension stitch has been used after DVC ligation. A 12 in. monofilament polyglytone suture on a CT-1 needle may be passed from the right to the left between the urethra and DVC, and then through the periosteum on the pubic bone. This can be done as a simple stitch or as a figure-of-eight fashion and then tied. Patel et al.[57] have shown that this approach yields statistically shorter continence recovery times and higher continence rates at 3 months.

30.8.3 Bladder Neck Preservation

Bladder neck preservation is an alternative maneuver. Careful dissection of the prostatovesical junction can maintain most of the circular muscle fibers of the bladder neck reducing the risk of anastomotic stricture and accelerating the return of urinary continence. Gaker et al.[58] have reported earlier return of continence without an adverse affect on oncologic outcomes when preserving the continence mechanism at the level of the bladder neck and prostatic urethra. Deliveliotis et al.[59] could not find a significant difference in the final continence outcome with bladder preservation but did report that the time to recovery of continence was reached earlier in the bladder preservation group. Surgical margins were unaffected. Selli et al.[60] reported similar continence outcomes. Sakai et al.[61] have also emphasized the importance of bladder neck preservation in promoting postoperative recovery of early continence.

30.8.4 Nerve Sparing

The rhabdosphincter is innervated by an intrapelvic branch of the pudendal nerve (somatic) and the mucosal and smooth muscle components by way of the urethral branch of the inferior hypogastric plexus (autonomic).[62] Preservation of an intrapelvic branch of the pudendal nerve (long pelvic nerve) has been shown to improve and maintain rhabdosphincter function after RRP.[63] Hollabaugh et al.[64] in a prospective comparative study reported the effect of

nerve preservation on recovery of continence after RRP. Although the overall continence rates were similar for the two groups (98.3% for nerve preservation vs. 92.1% without), nerve preservation decreased the time to achieve continence.

Montorsi described a nerve-sparing technique involving incision of the levator and prostatic fascia high anteriorly (1- and 11-o'clock positions) thereby developing the plane between the prostatic capsule and prostatic fascia thus sparing the neurovascular network. This allows for a minimal-touch dissection of the external urethral sphincter and a very efficient dissection of the neurovascular bundles at the level of membranous urethra and prostatic apex.[65]

Lunacek described modified 'curtain dissection' to improve preservation of the cavernosal nerves running in the neurovascular bundle based on fetal and adult studies. The cavernosal nerves running in the neurovascular bundle assume a concave curtain shape covering both lateral lobes of the prostate. Caudal to the prostate, the nerves are not only lateral but also dorsal to the membranous urethra. The lateral pelvic fascia must be incised and the dissection of the neurovascular bundle should be carried out more anteriorly.[66] Menon et al.[2] further described this technique as the "veil of Aphrodite" (Fig. 30.5). In their series they report encouraging continence recovery (95.2%) at 12 months. The potency rates were also very promising with 70 and 100% of the patients reported to have intercourse at 12 and 48 months, respectively. While the

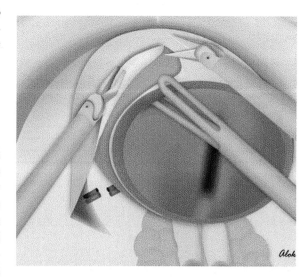

Fig. 30.5 Plane of dissection for veil of Aphrodite

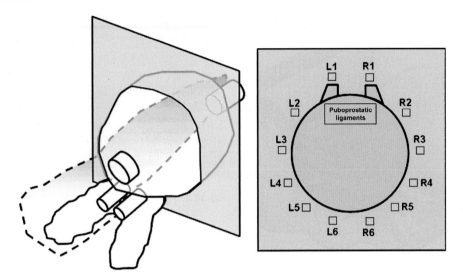

Fig. 30.6 Fascia preservation (FP) score scheme. The example shows preservation of L5 and L6 only, with a total FP score of 2

basic principle of the "veil" nerve-sparing technique is to improve potency rates, it appears to play a role in the recovery of continence as well. Kaul et al.[67] assessed 154 patients with the "veil" technique and reported excellent recovery of erectile function (both intercourse rates and return of normal erections) at 1 year after surgery, without compromising surgical margins and oncological outcomes.

In a prospective study of 151 patients, Van der Poel et al. found that the extent of fascial preservation at the lateral aspect of prostate is the best predictor of urinary continence at 6 and 12 months post-RARP.[68] They used a facial preservation scheme as depicted in Fig. 30.6. In their study the fascial preservation (FP) score is an important determinant of postoperative continence (FP score 6.4 vs. 4.4, $P = 0.001$).

In patients with low-risk disease, some have moved toward a seminal vesicle sparing approach. Limiting dissection toward the tips of the seminal vesicles minimizes injury to the visceral pelvic plexus coursing posterolateral to the prostate. John et al.[69] note a significant improvement in continence as well as potency recovery when employing this technique. Some investigators have suggested that the close approximation of the seminal vesicles to the neurovascular bundle, pelvic plexus, and vascular supply of the bladder neck blood may play a major role in postoperative urinary and erectile function and have developed algorithms to predict seminal vesicle involvement before surgery.[70]

30.8.5 Hypothermia of the Pelvic Floor

Hypothermic nerve sparing is novel concept described by Finley et al.[71] introducing the concept of limited iatrogenic injury to the neurovascular bundle by cooling the pelvic floor. Utilizing a 24 Fr three-way Foley catheter within an elliptical latex balloon the prototype endorectal cooling balloon system was created. Ice cold saline at 4°C was continuously infused at 40 cm of H_2O pressure. Additionally 4°C irrigation was used intracorporeally as an adjunct. In a prospective study patients were found to return to continence significantly earlier in the hypothermia group (median 39 days) compared with the control group (median 59 days, $P = 0.002$), representing a 33.9% improvement in the interval to continence. At 3 months, 86.8 ± 5.8% of the hypothermia group and 68.6 ± 2.0% of the control group were pad free. The use of traditional nerve sparing did not improve early continence rates (Fig. 30.7).

30.8.6 Apical Dissection

Myers[72] described the importance of prostatic apical anatomy, its variation, and implication of this variation in prostatectomy. He recognized two basic apical shapes: one with a "notch" and another without a "notch" (Fig. 30.8). Whether a notch exists depends on

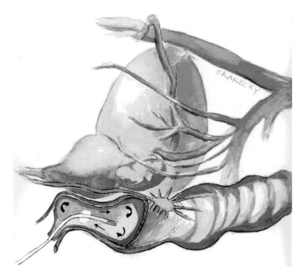

Fig. 30.7 Schematic depicting endorectal cooling balloon

the degree of lateral lobe development and the position of the anterior commissure. Excessive manipulation at the apex may lead to sphincter damage and is a risk factor for delayed recovery of continence. Thus meticulous dissection around the prostatic apex is of utmost importance.[24] Understanding the anatomy of

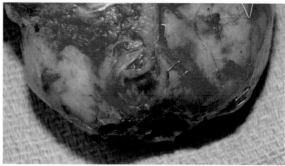

Fig. 30.8 Apical notch in a post-prostatectomy specimen

the apex and the surrounding structures is essential for fine apical dissection.[73] Lee et al.[74] studied the importance of prostatic apical anatomy and concluded that variations in the shape of the prostatic apex in relation to the membranous urethra may significantly affect the recovery of urinary continence after RRP. In their study, the group which was composed of patients with the prostatic apex not overlapping the membranous urethra at all on MRI (Fig. 30.9) had an early return to continence (83.3 vs. 66.7%, $P = 0.014$). In this context, Menon et al.[75] have described a technique

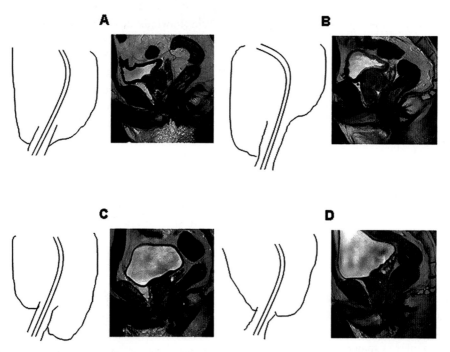

Fig. 30.9 Subjects were grouped according to the shape of prostatic apex observed on mid-sagittal MRI scan: (**a**) apex overlapping membranous urethra both anteriorly and posteriorly; (**b**) apex overlapping membranous urethra anteriorly; (**c**) apex overlapping membranous urethra posteriorly; and (**d**) no overlapping observed between apex and membranous urethra

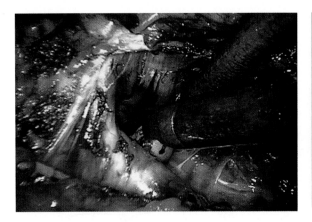

Fig. 30.10 A close view of the urethra at the prostatic apex, depicting the dorsal venous complex. The urethra is being freed posteriorly from the neurovascular bundles using blunt dissection

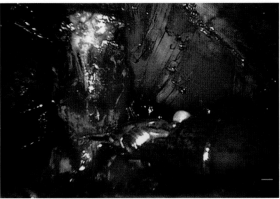

Fig. 30.11 Division of the urethra (*arrow*) distal to the prostatic apex (*arrow head*) with the help of articulated scissors

for apical dissection and have emphasized its significance in early recovery of continence. After exposure of the dorsal vein, urethra, and striated urethral sphincter, the puboperinealis muscle covering the urethra is dissected bluntly from the apex of the prostate. Next the urethra is freed at the apex with as little dissection as possible from underlying neurovascular bundle (Fig. 30.10). A #0 polyglactin suture on a CT-1 needle is used to ligate the deep dorsal vein while avoiding the puboprostatic ligaments. A second suture is placed through the anterior commissure of the prostate and the long tails of this suture are used as a traction handle. The distal complex is fixed by pulling the stay suture located over the proximal part of the prostate such that the exact plane on anterior surface of the prostate can be identified, which helps in avoiding inadvertent entry into the prostate and in ensuring appropriate excision of the striated sphincter musculature. This results in a good urethral stump (Fig. 30.11) without compromising positive apical margin rate (Fig. 30.12).

30.8.7 Preservation of Urethral Length

The membranous urethra is an important part of the continence mechanism. Several studies have emphasized that preservation of urethral length is an important determinant in the preservation of urinary continence.[76,77,78] Coakley et al.[79] employ the use of endorectal MRI in preoperative patients undergoing RRP, reporting that urethral length is directly related to

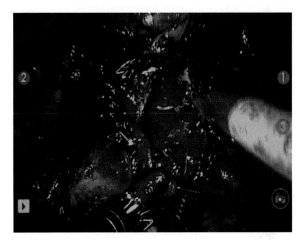

Fig. 30.12 Apical dissection. Note the staples in the edges of the dorsal vein in this case where the laparoscopic stapler was used

early recovery of continence postoperatively. Nguyen et al.[80] found that urethral length may be used as a predictive measure of time needed to achieve continence in patients undergoing RARP.

The challenge lies in precisely identifying the junction between the prostatic apex and the proximal urethra (Fig. 30.13); this will maintain maximal urethral length without compromising apical margin status. In their series, Ahlering et al.[81] describe a technique which combines precise transection of the apical–urethral junction with ligation of the puboprostatic ligaments during RARP. With this technical modification, positive margin rates decreased from 36 to 16.7%, and continence outcomes improved at 3 months (73 vs.

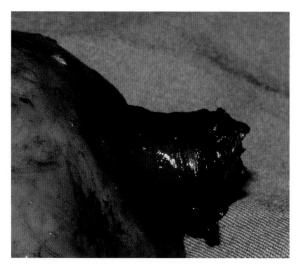

Fig. 30.13 Post-prostatectomy specimen showing well-defined urethro-prostatic junction

81%, $P = 0.24$). Of note, the authors utilized a laparoscopic stapler for control of the DVC which facilitated accurate apical–urethral transection. Van Randenborgh prospectively used a technique for preservation of the intraprostatic portion of urethral stump via craniodorsal retraction of prostate. They reported that this technique led to improve continence outcomes (89 vs. 76%, $P < 0.05$), without compromising surgical margins.

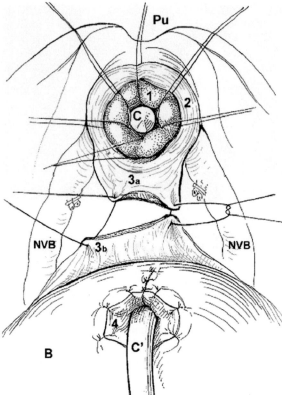

Fig. 30.14 Suturing the RS and median fibrous raphe to the remaining Denonvilliers' fascia. Pu = pubis; C = membranous urethral catheter; C' = bladder catheter; B = bladder; NVB = neurovascular bundle; 1 = membranous urethra; 2 = anterolateral wall of RS; 3a = sectioned posterior wall of RS and MFR; 3b = sectioned Denonvilliers' fascia; 4 = bladder-neck eversion

30.8.8 Posterior Repair

The rhabdosphincter is invested in a fascial framework which is supported below by a musculofascial plate that fuses with the midline raphe – a point of origin for the rectourethralis muscle.[82] Both the dorsal and ventral supports contribute to the competence of the sphincter.

Posterior rhabdosphincter repair is a novel technique first introduced by Rocco et al.[83] as a modification to ameliorate urinary incontinence after open radical prostatectomy. Reapproximation of the posterior semicircumference of the rhabdosphincter to the cut edge of Denonvilliers' fascia avoids caudal retraction of the urethrosphincteric complex prior to completion of the vesicourethral anastomosis. In addition, tension is taken off the anastomosis itself as an additional strength layer is added to the reconstruction

(Figs. 30.14, 30.15, and 30.16). In their study, patients with a posterior repair achieved significantly better continence at discharge (62.4 vs. 14.0%), at 1 month (74.0 vs. 30%), and at 3 months of follow-up (85.2 vs. 46%), though long-term recovery was similar in the two treatment groups (94 vs. 90%). Similar results in post-prostatectomy continence were demonstrated in LRP patients when the posterior reconstruction technique was added to the standard procedure.[84] Nguyen et al.,[85] in a prospective study, concluded that posterior repair contributes to improved urinary function outcomes in both LRP and RARP patients. Tewari et al.[3] also emphasized the importance of the posterior repair in continence recovery and reported improved outcomes.

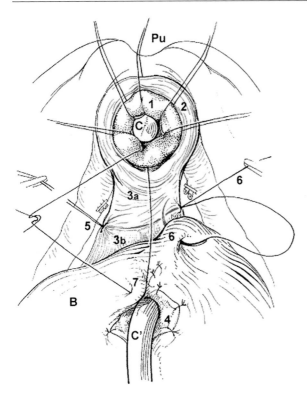

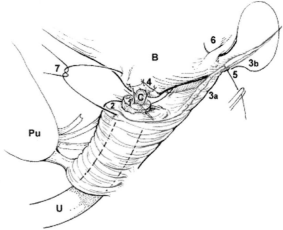

Fig. 30.16 Lateral view of action depicted in Fig 30.15. Fixation of the RS and DV (5) to the posterior wall of the bladder about 2 cm dorsocephalad to the new bladder neck (6). Pu = pubis; C = catheter; B = bladder; U = urethra; 1 = membranous urethra; 2 = anterolateral wall of RS; 3a = sectioned posterior wall of RS and MFR; 3b = sectioned Denonvilliers' fascia; 4 = bladder-neck eversion; 7 = posterior urethrovesical anastomosis

Fig. 30.15 Fixation of the RS and DV (5) to the posterior wall of the bladder about 2 cm dorsocephalad to the new bladder neck (6). Pu = pubis; C = membranous urethral catheter; C' = bladder catheter; B = bladder; 1 = membranous urethra; 2 = anterolateral wall of RS; 3a = sectioned posterior wall of RS and MFR; 3b = sectioned Denonvilliers' fascia; 4 = bladder-neck eversion; 7 = posterior urethrovesical anastomosis

we feel that there are fewer anastomotic leaks due to better support and improved ease of the urethrovesical anastomosis.

By comparison, Menon et al.,[86] in a randomized controlled trial, described a circumferential reconstruction of the periprostatic tissue, with an additional anterior layer, in comparison to the Rocco technique alone [[83]]. The continence rates at 1, 2, 7, and 30 days were 26 vs. 34%, 49 vs. 46%, 51 vs. 54%, and 74 vs. 80% for patients undergoing simple anastomosis and anastomosis with peri-anastomotic tissue reconstruction (double layer anastomosis), respectively (statistically not significant).

In a retrospective study at our institution, we found that the posterior rhabdosphincter repair is associated with a slight but statistically significant slower continence recovery. Patients were likely to achieve continence more slowly (HR = 0.65 [0.47, 0.91], $P = 0.01$) such that median time to continence was 36 weeks for the PRR group and 13 weeks for the control ($P = 0.007$). However, we continue to perform PRR as

30.8.9 Walsh Intussusception Stitch

Walsh in 2002 described buttressing sutures used to intussuscept the bladder neck to achieve early continence recovery after RRP. These sutures decrease the tension on the bladder neck as the bladder fills.[87] The described technique is as follows: a 2-0 Maxon suture is placed on the edges of the posterior bladder wall mainly in the adipose tissue, where the bladder was previously attached to the prostate, approximately 2 cm from the reconstructed bladder neck (Fig. 30.17). The suture is then tied in the midline. The next suture is a figure-of-eight 2-0 Maxon placed 2 cm lateral to the bladder neck on each side (Fig. 30.18). At this point, the bladder neck should protrude beneath the anterior hood of tissue created by the anterior stitch, similar to a turtle head outside its shell. After installation of saline, the bladder neck should be competent with very little leakage. Wille et al.[88] in a comparative study reported that intussusception of the bladder

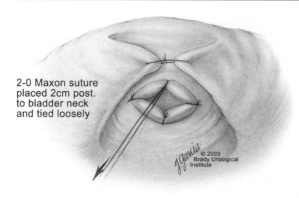

2-0 Maxon suture placed 2cm post. to bladder neck and tied loosely

Fig. 30.17 Intussusception of the bladder neck. A 2-0 Maxon suture is placed in the edges of the posterior bladder wall, where the bladder was previously attached to the prostate, about 2 cm from the reconstructed bladder neck and tied in the midline

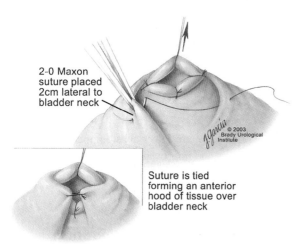

2-0 Maxon suture placed 2cm lateral to bladder neck

Suture is tied forming an anterior hood of tissue over bladder neck

Fig. 30.18 Intussusception of the bladder neck. A second figure-of-eight 2-0 Maxon suture is placed anteriorly about 2 cm lateral to the bladder neck on either side and tied

neck resulted in a significantly greater continence rate of 77 vs. 60% at 3 months postoperatively although the continence rates at 12 months were not significantly affected. In addition, overall urinary symptoms were significantly better in the intussusception group as compared to controls.

30.8.10 Creation of a Watertight Anastomosis

It has been proposed that excessive extravasation secondary to a poor vesicourethral anastomosis can lead to fibrosis and scarring at the vesicourethral junction.[89,90]

Van Velthoven has described a simple, running laparoscopic suture technique for accomplishing a watertight anastomosis during laparoscopic radical prostatectomy and is easily replicable in RARP[91] (see Fig. 30.19). The running suture is prepared by tying the ends of two 6 in. sutures of 3-0 polyglycolic acid: one suture is dyed and the other un-dyed to aid identification of either end. The running stitch is initiated by placing both needles outside-in through the bladder neck and inside-out on the urethra. The sutures are run from the 6:30 and 5:30 positions toward the 9- and 3-o'clock positions, respectively. After this, gentle traction is exerted on each thread simultaneously or alternately. This is an important step to ensure the water-tightness of the anastomosis by ensuring the integrity of the posterior layer. The suture line is continued up to the 12-o'clock position on either side and a single knot is tied at the top. Long-term continence and stricture outcomes are similar for the interrupted technique.[92,93] Poulakis has reported a decrease in dorsal leak rates with the running technique as compared to interrupted suturing.[93]

30.9 Postoperative Surgical Therapies for Post-prostatectomy Incontinence

30.9.1 Injection Therapy

Since its introduction in 1993, bovine glutaraldehyde crosslinked (GAX) collagen has been used extensively as a periurethral bulking agent in the treatment of ISD in men. Injection of a bulking agent beneath the urethral mucosa to improve competence of bladder outlet has been used successfully in women with sphincter deficiency. Transurethral collagen injections are a minimally invasive option in men with post-prostatectomy incontinence.

Westney et al.,[94] in a study of 307 patients with RRP, concluded that these patients (RRP) had a favorable response in terms of achieving continence after transurethral collagen injection. Quality of response correlated positively with duration of response with patients maintaining continence for a mean of 1 year after injection therapy. On an average three to four injections were required to achieve a plateau response.

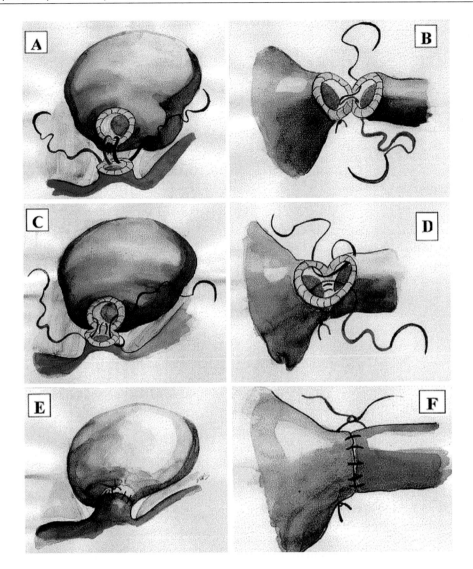

Fig. 30.19 Van Velthoven urethro-vesical anastomotic technique. **A.** A double armed stitch is started outside in on the bladder neck at the 6 o'clock position. **B.** These arms are then taken inside out on the urethra. **C.** After several throws, the slack is taken out to coapt the posterior wall. **D.** The separate arms are then run individually up to the 12 o'clock position. **E.** View of the completed anastomosis. **F.** Note that there is only a single pretied knot at the 6 o'clock position and one intracorporeal knot at the 12 o'clock position

30.9.2 The Male Sling

Slings are also a widely accepted treatment for ISD. The concept is based on the upward compression of the bulbous urethra. In contrast to the artificial urinary sphincter (AUS), the sling procedure allows physiological voiding. Commiter et al.,[95] in a prospective study in 48 men with stress incontinence, reported intermediate-term results of the bone-anchored male perineal sling with a median of 4 years and minimum of 2-year follow-up. They demonstrated the success rate comparable to that of the AUS (80% ≤1 pad daily) with very low morbidity. Similarly, Migliari et al.[96] reported 77, 67, and 63% of the patients to be socially continent at the 3-month, 1-year, and 3-year follow-up, respectively. Significant perineal pain was reported in the early postoperative period but this resolved in all patients. Infection was reported in three

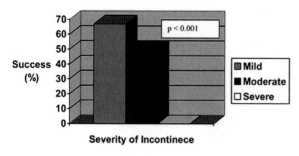

Fig. 30.20 Success after sling procedures was associated with the degree of preoperative incontinence

patients. The possibilities of progressive failure over time and significant perineal pain were the major issues of concern.

Castle et al. [97] in another study with post-prostatectomy patients found that success after sling procedures is associated with the degree of preoperative incontinence. Success with sling is more likely in patients with mild to moderate incontinence. Severely incontinent patients may benefit more from an AUS as compared to sling. Patients with a history of previous radiation or an artificial urinary sphincter were at high risk for failure (Fig. 30.20).

30.9.3 Artificial Urinary Sphincter

The artificial urinary sphincter is perhaps the most effective long-term treatment option for sphincter insufficiency. The AUS has the longest track record with the widest experience with respect to the number of patients treated over any other treatment. Leibovich et al.[98] in their experience with 458 AUS patients (417 men) reported an overall continence rate of 88.2%, a reoperation rate of 23.1%, and a mechanical reliability of 88%. Patient satisfaction rate was greater than 90%.

Trigo et al.[99] in a prospective study investigated the long-term efficacy of the AUS for post-prostatectomy incontinence. Forty consecutive patients were treated with follow-up ranging from 27 to 132 months (mean $= 53.4 \pm 21.4$ months). They found a significant reduction in pad count from 4.0 ± 0.9 to 0.62 ± 1.07 diapers per day ($P < 0.001$) leading to continence in 90%. Surgical revision rate was 20%.

Lai et al.[100] in a 13-year retrospective experience with 218 patients with a mean follow-up of 36.5 months (60 = prostatectomy and pelvic radiation,

116 = prostatectomy without radiotherapy) concluded that AUS is a safe and durable treatment for male intrinsic sphincter deficiency even in patients with a history of AUS complications, neurogenic bladder, pelvic radiation, bladder neck contracture, failed injectables, or male slings.

30.10 Conclusion

Postoperative incontinence after RARP is a major concern and is one of the direct predictors of postoperative satisfaction.[101] Important aspects in achieving improved continence rates include the following:

(1) Sound knowledge of the pelvic anatomy, especially of the prostatic apex, the surrounding musculature, and rhabdosphincter
(2) Meticulous dissection with emphasis on sphincter identification and preservation, hemostasis, and minimal distortion of the sphincter anatomy
(3) Specific technical modifications that show promise for improved results

While a comprehensive evaluation and targeted therapy should be instituted if incontinence occurs, the emphasis should be concentrated on improving surgical technique to minimize any unwanted morbidity and decreased quality of life. Further research is absolutely required to establish 'gold standard' techniques for optimizing post-RARP continence.

References

1. Abrams P, Cardozo L, Fall M, et al. The standardisation of terminology of lower urinary tract function: report from the standardisation sub-committee of the international continence society. *Neurourol Urodyn*. 2002;21(2): 167–178.
2. Menon M, Shrivastava A, Kaul S, et al. Vattikuti institute prostatectomy: contemporary technique and analysis of results. *Eur Urol*. March, 2007;51(3):648–657. discussion 657–648.
3. Tewari A, Jhaveri J, Rao S, et al. Total reconstruction of the vesico-urethral junction. *BJU Int*. April, 2008;101(7):871–877.
4. Catalona WJ, Carvalhal GF, Mager DE, Smith DS. Potency, continence and complication rates in 1,870

consecutive radical retropubic prostatectomies. *J Urol.* August, 1999;162(2):433–438.

5. Kundu SD, Roehl KA, Eggener SE, Antenor JA, Han M, Catalona WJ. Potency, continence and complications in 3,477 consecutive radical retropubic prostatectomies. *J Urol.* December, 2004;172(6 Pt 1):2227–2231.

6. Badani KK, Kaul S, Menon M. Evolution of robotic radical prostatectomy: assessment after 2,766 procedures. *Cancer.* November 1, 2007;110(9):1951–1958.

7. Stolzenburg JU, Rabenalt R, Do M, et al. Endoscopic extraperitoneal radical prostatectomy: oncological and functional results after 700 procedures. *J Urol.* October, 2005;174(4 Pt 1):1271–1275. discussion 1275.

8. Wang L, Chung SF, Yip SK, Lau WK, Cheng CW, Sim HG. The natural history of voiding function after robot-assisted laparoscopic radical prostatectomy. *Urol Oncol.* April 10, 2009.

9. Krambeck AE, DiMarco DS, Rangel LJ, et al. Radical prostatectomy for prostatic adenocarcinoma: a matched comparison of open retropubic and robot-assisted techniques. *BJU Int.* February, 2009;103(4):448–453.

10. Ahlering TE, Woo D, Eichel L, Lee DI, Edwards R, Skarecky DW. Robot-assisted versus open radical prostatectomy: a comparison of one surgeon's outcomes. *Urology.* May, 2004;63(5):819–822.

11. Tewari A, Srivasatava A, Menon M. A prospective comparison of radical retropubic and robot-assisted prostatectomy: experience in one institution. *BJU Int.* August, 2003;92(3):205–210.

12. Levy JB, Seay TM, Wein AJ. Post prostatectomy incontinence. *AUA update series.* 1996;XV: Lesson 8.

13. Hellstrom P, Lukkarinen O, Kontturi M. Urodynamics in radical retropubic prostatectomy. *Scand J Urol Nephrol.* 1989;23(1):21–24.

14. Carlson KV, Nitti VW. Prevention and management of incontinence following radical prostatectomy. *Urol Clin North Am.* August, 2001;28(3):595–612.

15. Ficazzola MA, Nitti VW. The etiology of post-radical prostatectomy incontinence and correlation of symptoms with urodynamic findings. *J Urol.* October, 1998;160(4):1317–1320.

16. Chao R, Mayo ME. Incontinence after radical prostatectomy: detrusor or sphincter causes. *J Urol.* July, 1995;154(1):16–18.

17. Goluboff ET, Chang DT, Olsson CA, Kaplan SA. Urodynamics and the etiology of post-prostatectomy urinary incontinence: the initial Columbia experience. *J Urol.* March, 1995;153(3 Pt 2):1034–1037.

18. Leach GE, Trockman B, Wong A, Hamilton J, Haab F, Zimmern PE. Post-prostatectomy incontinence: urodynamic findings and treatment outcomes. *J Urol.* April, 1996;155(4):1256–1259.

19. Matsukawa Y, Hattori R, Yoshikawa Y, Ono Y, Gotoh M. Laparoscopic versus open radical prostatectomy: urodynamic evaluation of vesicourethral function. *Int J Urol.* April, 2009;16(4):393–396.

20. Msezane LP, Reynolds WS, Gofrit ON, Shalhav AL, Zagaja GP, Zorn KC. Bladder neck contracture after robot-assisted laparoscopic radical prostatectomy: evaluation of incidence and risk factors and impact on urinary function. *J Endourol.* February, 2008;22(2):377–383.

21. Erickson BA, Meeks JJ, Roehl KA, Gonzalez CM, Catalona WJ. Bladder neck contracture after retropubic radical prostatectomy: incidence and risk factors from a large single-surgeon experience. *BJU Int.* December, 2009;104(11):1615–1619.

22. Davidson PJ, van den Ouden D, Schroeder FH. Radical prostatectomy: prospective assessment of mortality and morbidity. *Eur Urol.* 1996;29(2):168–173.

23. Park R, Martin S, Goldberg JD, Lepor H. Anastomotic strictures following radical prostatectomy: insights into incidence, effectiveness of intervention, effect on continence, and factors predisposing to occurrence. *Urology.* April, 2001;57(4):742–746.

24. Eastham JA, Kattan MW, Rogers E, et al. Risk factors for urinary incontinence after radical prostatectomy. *J Urol.* November, 1996;156(5):1707–1713.

25. Stanford JL, Feng Z, Hamilton AS, et al. Urinary and sexual function after radical prostatectomy for clinically localized prostate cancer: the prostate cancer outcomes study. *JAMA.* January 19, 2000;283(3):354–360.

26. Van Kampen M, De Weerdt W, Van Poppel H, et al. Prediction of urinary continence following radical prostatectomy. *Urol Int.* 1998;60(2):80–84.

27. Greco KA, Meeks JJ, Wu S, Nadler RB. Robot-Assisted Radical Prostatectomy In Men Aged >/=70 Years. *BJU Int.* March, 2010;105(6):886–887.

28. Rodriguez E Jr, Skarecky DW, Ahlering TE. Post-robotic prostatectomy urinary continence: characterization of perfect continence versus occasional dribbling in pad-free men. *Urology.* April, 2006;67(4):785–788.

29. Mendiola FP, Zorn KC, Mikhail AA, et al. Urinary and sexual function outcomes among different age groups after robot-assisted laparoscopic prostatectomy. *J Endourol.* March, 2008;22(3):519–524.

30. Boczko J, Erturk E, Golijanin D, Madeb R, Patel H, Joseph JV. Impact of prostate size in robot-assisted radical prostatectomy. *J Endourol.* February, 2007;21(2): 184–188.

31. Link BA, Nelson R, Josephson DY, et al. The impact of prostate gland weight in robot assisted laparoscopic radical prostatectomy. *J Urol.* September, 2008;180(3): 928–932.

32. Sacco E, Prayer-Galetti T, Pinto F, et al. Urinary incontinence after radical prostatectomy: incidence by definition, risk factors and temporal trend in a large series with a long-term follow-up. *BJU Int.* June, 2006;97(6): 1234–1241.

33. Takenaka A, Soga H, Sakai I, et al. Influence of nerve-sparing procedure on early recovery of urinary continence after laparoscopic radical prostatectomy. *J Endourol.* July, 2009;23(7):1115–1119.

34. Tseng TY, Kuebler HR, Cancel QV, et al. Prospective health-related quality-of-life assessment in an initial cohort of patients undergoing robotic radical prostatectomy. *Urology.* November, 2006;68(5):1061–1066.

35. Yee DS, Ahlering TE, Gelman J, Skarecky DW. Fossa navicularis strictures due to 22f catheters used in robotic radical prostatectomy. *JSLS.* July–September, 2007;11(3):321–325.

36. Wiltz AL, Shikanov S, Eggener SE, et al. Robotic radical prostatectomy in overweight and obese patients:

oncological and validated-functional outcomes. *Urology.* February, 2009;73(2):316–322.

37. Ahlering TE, Eichel L, Edwards R, Skarecky DW. Impact of obesity on clinical outcomes in robotic prostatectomy. *Urology.* April, 2005;65(4):740–744.

38. Boorjian SA, Crispen PL, Carlson RE, et al. Impact of obesity on clinicopathologic outcomes after robot-assisted laparoscopic prostatectomy. *J Endourol.* July, 2008;22(7):1471–1476.

39. Wille S, Heidenreich A, von Knobloch R, Hofmann R, Engelmann U. Impact of comorbidities on post-prostatectomy incontinence. *Urol Int.* 2006;76(3): 223–226.

40. Boczko J, Madeb R, Golijanin D, et al. Robot-assisted radical prostatectomy in obese patients. *Can J Urol.* August, 2006;13(4):3169–3173.

41. Menard J, de la Taille A, Hoznek A, et al. Laparoscopic radical prostatectomy after transurethral resection of the prostate: surgical and functional outcomes. *Urology.* September, 2008;72(3):593–597.

42. Colombo R, Naspro R, Salonia A, et al. Radical prostatectomy after previous prostate surgery: clinical and functional outcomes. *J Urol.* December, 2006;176(6 Pt 1):2459–2463. discussion 2463.

43. Koley B, Koley J, Saha JK. The effects of nicotine on spontaneous contractions of cat urinary bladder in situ. *Br J Pharmacol.* October, 1984;83(2):347–355.

44. Koskimaki J, Hakama M, Huhtala H, Tammela TL. Association of smoking with lower urinary tract symptoms. *J Urol.* May, 1998;159(5):1580–1582.

45. Borboroglu PG, Sands JP, Roberts JL, Amling CL. Risk factors for vesicourethral anastomotic stricture after radical prostatectomy. *Urology.* July, 2000;56(1):96–100.

46. Song C, Doo CK, Hong JH, Choo MS, Kim CS, Ahn H. Relationship between the integrity of the pelvic floor muscles and early recovery of continence after radical prostatectomy. *J Urol.* July, 2007;178(1):208–211.

47. Manassero F, Traversi C, Ales V, et al. Contribution of early intensive prolonged pelvic floor exercises on urinary continence recovery after bladder neck-sparing radical prostatectomy: results of a prospective controlled randomized trial. *Neurourol Urodyn.* 2007;26(7): 985–989.

48. Filocamo MT, Li Marzi V, Del Popolo G, et al. Effectiveness of early pelvic floor rehabilitation treatment for post-prostatectomy incontinence. *Eur Urol.* November, 2005;48(5):734–738.

49. Van Kampen M, De Weerdt W, Van Poppel H, De Ridder D, Feys H, Baert L. Effect of pelvic-floor re-education on duration and degree of incontinence after radical prostatectomy: a randomised controlled trial. *Lancet.* January 8, 2000;355(9198):98–102.

50. Burgio KL, Goode PS, Urban DA, et al. Preoperative biofeedback assisted behavioral training to decrease post-prostatectomy incontinence: a randomized, controlled trial. *J Urol.* January, 2006;175(1):196–201. discussion 201.

51. MacDonald R, Fink HA, Huckabay C, Monga M, Wilt TJ. Pelvic floor muscle training to improve urinary incontinence after radical prostatectomy: a systematic review of effectiveness. *BJU Int.* July, 2007;100(1):76–81.

52. Avant OL, Jones JA, Beck H, Hunt C, Straub M. New method to improve treatment outcomes for radical prostatectomy. *Urology.* October 1, 2000;56(4):658–662.

53. Poore RE, McCullough DL, Jarow JP. Puboprostatic ligament sparing improves urinary continence after radical retropubic prostatectomy. *Urology.* January, 1998;51(1):67–72.

54. Tewari AK, Bigelow K, Rao S, et al. Anatomic restoration technique of continence mechanism and preservation of puboprostatic collar: a novel modification to achieve early urinary continence in men undergoing robotic prostatectomy. *Urology.* April, 2007;69(4):726–731.

55. Takenaka A, Tewari AK, Leung RA, et al. Preservation of the puboprostatic collar and puboperineoplasty for early recovery of urinary continence after robotic prostatectomy: anatomic basis and preliminary outcomes. *Eur Urol.* February, 2007;51(2):433–440. discussion 440.

56. Stolzenburg JU, Liatsikos EN, Rabenalt R, et al. Nerve sparing endoscopic extraperitoneal radical prostatectomy–effect of puboprostatic ligament preservation on early continence and positive margins. *Eur Urol.* January, 2006;49(1):103–111. discussion 111–102.

57. Patel VR, Coelho RF, Palmer KJ, Rocco B. Periurethral suspension stitch during robot-assisted laparoscopic radical prostatectomy: description of the technique and continence outcomes. *Eur Urol.* September, 2009;56(3):472–478.

58. Gaker DL, Steel BL. Radical prostatectomy with preservation of urinary continence: pathology and long-term results. *J Urol.* December, 2004;172(6 Pt 2):2549–2552.

59. Deliveliotis C, Protogerou V, Alargof E, Varkarakis J. Radical prostatectomy: bladder neck preservation and puboprostatic ligament sparing–effects on continence and positive margins. *Urology.* November, 2002;60(5): 855–858.

60. Selli C, De Antoni P, Moro U, Macchiarella A, Giannarini G, Crisci A. Role of bladder neck preservation in urinary continence following radical retropubic prostatectomy. *Scand J Urol Nephrol.* 2004;38(1):32–37.

61. Sakai I, Harada K, Hara I, Eto H, Miyake H. Intussusception of the bladder neck does not promote early restoration to urinary continence after non-nerve-sparing radical retropubic prostatectomy. *Int J Urol.* March, 2005;12(3):275–279.

62. Steiner MS. Anatomic basis for the continence-preserving radical retropubic prostatectomy. *Semin Urol Oncol.* February, 2000;18(1):9–18.

63. van der Horst C, Hamann MF, Kuhtz Buschbeck JP, Kaufmann S, Junemann KP, Naumann CM. Functional impact of the rhabdosphincter branch of the pelvic nerve on the membranous urethra in comparison to that of the pudendal nerve in male rabbits. *Urol Int.* 2009;83(1): 80–85.

64. Hollabaugh RS Jr., Dmochowski RR, Kneib TG, Steiner MS. Preservation of putative continence nerves during radical retropubic prostatectomy leads to more rapid return of urinary continence. *Urology.* June, 1998;51(6):960–967.

65. Montorsi F, Salonia A, Suardi N, et al. Improving the preservation of the urethral sphincter and neurovascular

bundles during open radical retropubic prostatectomy. *Eur Urol.* December, 2005;48(6):938–945.

66. Lunacek A, Schwentner C, Fritsch H, Bartsch G, Strasser H. Anatomical radical retropubic prostatectomy: 'curtain dissection' of the neurovascular bundle. *BJU Int.* June, 2005;95(9):1226–1231.

67. Kaul S, Savera A, Badani K, Fumo M, Bhandari A, Menon M. Functional outcomes and oncological efficacy of Vattikuti Institute prostatectomy with veil of aphrodite nerve-sparing: an analysis of 154 consecutive patients. *BJU Int.* March, 2006;97(3):467–472.

68. van der Poel HG, de Blok W, Joshi N, van Muilekom E. Preservation of lateral prostatic fascia is associated with urine continence after robotic-assisted prostatectomy. *Eur Urol.* April, 2009;55(4):892–900.

69. John H, Hauri D. Seminal vesicle-sparing radical prostatectomy: a novel concept to restore early urinary continence. *Urology.* June, 2000;55(6):820–824.

70. Zlotta AR, Roumeguere T, Ravery V, et al. Is seminal vesicle ablation mandatory for all patients undergoing radical prostatectomy? a multivariate analysis on 1,283 patients. *Eur Urol.* July, 2004;46(1):42–49.

71. Finley DS, Osann K, Skarecky D, Ahlering TE. Hypothermic nerve-sparing radical prostatectomy: rationale, feasibility, and effect on early continence. *Urology.* April, 2009;73(4):691–696.

72. Myers RP, Goellner JR, Cahill DR. Prostate shape, external striated urethral sphincter and radical prostatectomy: the apical dissection. *J Urol.* September, 1987;138(3):543–550.

73. Soga H, Takenaka A, Murakami G, Fujisawa M. Topographical relationship between urethral rhabdosphincter and rectourethralis muscle: a better understanding of the apical dissection and the posterior stitches in radical prostatectomy. *Int J Urol.* August, 2008;15(8):729–732.

74. Lee SE, Byun SS, Lee HJ, et al. Impact of variations in prostatic apex shape on early recovery of urinary continence after radical retropubic prostatectomy. *Urology.* July, 2006;68(1):137–141.

75. Menon M, Hemal AK, Tewari A, Shrivastava A, Bhandari A. The technique of apical dissection of the prostate and urethrovesical anastomosis in robotic radical prostatectomy. *BJU Int.* April, 2004;93(6):715–719.

76. Paparel P, Akin O, Sandhu JS, et al. Recovery of urinary continence after radical prostatectomy: association with urethral length and urethral fibrosis measured by preoperative and postoperative endorectal magnetic resonance imaging. *Eur Urol.* March, 2009;55(3):629–637.

77. Majoros A, Bach D, Keszthelyi A, et al. Analysis of risk factors for urinary incontinence after radical prostatectomy. *Urol Int.* 2007;78(3):202–207.

78. Minervini R, Felipetto R, Morelli G, Fontana N, Fiorentini L. Urodynamic evaluation of urinary incontinence following radical prostatectomy: our experience. *Acta Urol Belg.* December, 1996;64(4):5–8.

79. Coakley FV, Eberhardt S, Kattan MW, Wei DC, Scardino PT, Hricak H. Urinary continence after radical retropubic prostatectomy: relationship with membranous urethral length on preoperative endorectal magnetic resonance imaging. *J Urol.* September, 2002;168(3):1032–1035.

80. Nguyen L, Jhaveri J, Tewari A. Surgical technique to overcome anatomical shortcoming: balancing post-prostatectomy continence outcomes of urethral sphincter lengths on preoperative magnetic resonance imaging. *J Urol.* May, 2008;179(5):1907–1911.

81. Ahlering TE, Eichel L, Edwards RA, Lee DI, Skarecky DW. Robotic radical prostatectomy: a technique to reduce pt2 positive margins. *Urology.* December, 2004;64(6):1224–1228.

82. Burnett AL, Mostwin JL. In situ anatomical study of the male urethral sphincteric complex: relevance to continence preservation following major pelvic surgery. *J Urol.* October, 1998;160(4):1301–1306.

83. Rocco F, Carmignani L, Acquati P, et al. Early continence recovery after open radical prostatectomy with restoration of the posterior aspect of the rhabdosphincter. *Eur Urol.* August, 2007;52(2):376–383.

84. Rocco B, Gregori A, Stener S, et al. Posterior reconstruction of the rhabdosphincter allows a rapid recovery of continence after transperitoneal videolaparoscopic radical prostatectomy. *Eur Urol.* April, 2007;51(4):996–1003.

85. Nguyen MM, Kamoi K, Stein RJ, et al. Early continence outcomes of posterior musculofascial plate reconstruction during robotic and laparoscopic prostatectomy. *BJU Int.* May, 2008;101(9):1135–1139.

86. Menon M, Muhletaler F, Campos M, Peabody JO. Assessment of early continence after reconstruction of the periprostatic tissues in patients undergoing computer assisted (robotic) prostatectomy: results of a 2 group parallel randomized controlled trial. *J Urol.* September, 2008;180(3):1018–1023.

87. Walsh PC, Marschke PL. Intussusception of the reconstructed bladder neck leads to earlier continence after radical prostatectomy. *Urology.* June, 2002;59(6):934–938.

88. Wille S, Varga Z, von Knobloch R, Hofmann R. Intussusception of bladder neck improves early continence after radical prostatectomy: results of a prospective trial. *Urology.* March, 2005;65(3):524–527.

89. Surya BV, Provet J, Johanson KE, Brown J. Anastomotic strictures following radical prostatectomy: risk factors and management. *J Urol.* April, 1990;143(4):755–758.

90. Popken G, Sommerkamp H, Schultze-Seemann W, Wetterauer U, Katzenwadel A. Anastomotic stricture after radical prostatectomy. Incidence, findings and treatment. *Eur Urol.* 1998;33(4):382–386.

91. Van Velthoven RF, Ahlering TE, Peltier A, Skarecky DW, Clayman RV. Technique for laparoscopic running urethrovesical anastomosis: the single knot method. *Urology.* April, 2003;61(4):699–702.

92. Teber D, Erdogru T, Cresswell J, Gozen AS, Frede T, Rassweiler JJ. Analysis of three different vesicourethral anastomotic techniques in laparoscopic radical prostatectomy. *World J Urol.* December, 2008;26(6):617–622.

93. Poulakis V, Skriapas K, de Vries R, Dillenburg W, Witzsch U, Becht E. Vesicourethral anastomosis during endoscopic extraperitoneal radical prostatectomy: a prospective comparison between the single-knot running and interrupted technique. *Urology.* December, 2006;68(6):1284–1289.

94. Westney OL, Bevan-Thomas R, Palmer JL, Cespedes RD, McGuire EJ. Transurethral collagen injections for male intrinsic sphincter deficiency: the University of Texas-Houston experience. *J Urol.* September, 2005;174(3):994–997.

95. Comiter CV. The male perineal sling: intermediate-term results. *Neurourol Urodyn.* 2005;24(7):648–653.

96. Migliari R, Pistolesi D, Leone P, Viola D, Trovarelli S. Male bulbourethral sling after radical prostatectomy: intermediate outcomes at 2 to 4-year followup. *J Urol.* November, 2006;176(5):2114–2118. discussion 2118.

97. Castle EP, Andrews PE, Itano N, Novicki DE, Swanson SK, Ferrigni RG. The male sling for post-prostatectomy incontinence: mean followup of 18 months. *J Urol.* May, 2005;173(5):1657–1660.

98. Leibovich BC, Barrett DM. Use of the artificial urinary sphincter in men and women. *World J Urol.* 1997;15(5):316–319.

99. Trigo Rocha F, Gomes CM, Mitre AI, Arap S, Srougi M. A prospective study evaluating the efficacy of the artificial sphincter AMS 800 for the treatment of postradical prostatectomy urinary incontinence and the correlation between preoperative urodynamic and surgical outcomes. *Urology.* January, 2008;71(1): 85–89.

100. Lai HH, Hsu EI, Teh BS, Butler EB, Boone TB. 13 Years of experience with artificial urinary sphincter implantation at Baylor College of Medicine. *J Urol.* March, 2007;177(3):1021–1025.

101. Schroeck FR, Krupski TL, Sun L, et al. Satisfaction and regret after open retropubic or robot-assisted laparoscopic radical prostatectomy. *Eur Urol.* October, 2008;54(4):785–793.

102. Benoit RM, Naslund MJ, Cohen JK. Complications after radical retropubic prostatectomy in the medicare population. *Urology.* July, 2000;56(1):116–120.

103. Steiner MS, Morton RA, Walsh PC. Impact of anatomical radical prostatectomy on urinary continence. *J Urol.* March, 1991;145(3):512–514. discussion 514–515.

104. Kao TC, Cruess DF, Garner D, et al. Multicenter patient self-reporting questionnaire on impotence, incontinence and stricture after radical prostatectomy. *J Urol.* March, 2000;163(3):858–864.

105. Rassweiler J, Stolzenburg J, Sulser T, et al. Laparoscopic radical prostatectomy–the experience of the German laparoscopic working group. *Eur Urol.* January, 2006;49(1):113–119.

106. Guillonneau B, Cathelineau X, Doublet JD, Baumert H, Vallancien G. Laparoscopic radical prostatectomy: assessment after 550 procedures. *Crit Rev Oncol Hematol.* August, 2002;43(2):123–133.

Chapter 31

Penile Rehabilitation After Robotic Radical Prostatectomy: The Best Strategy

Andrea Gallina, Alberto Briganti, Nazareno Suardi, Andrea Salonia, Umberto Capitanio, and Francesco Montorsi

31.1 Introduction

Radical prostatectomy (RP) is the most widely performed procedure for patients with clinically localized prostate cancer (PCa) and a life expectancy of at least 10 years.[1-6] In the past, this procedure was associated with a high rate of treatment-specific side effects affecting health-related quality of life.[7,8] Since the diagnosis of PCa is becoming ever more frequent in younger patients,[9,10] urologists are motivated to identify the best strategies in order to reduce the surgery-related sequelae concerning quality of life. Contemporary patients, due to their young age, are motivated to preserve their sexual function and the couple's sexual health. To date, the ideal outcome cannot be limited to oncologic freedom from recurrence but should achieve optimal continence and potency after surgery. Since the introduction of anatomical dissection of the prostate pioneered by Walsh in 1982,[11] surgeons have developed several techniques for erectile function (EF) preservation. The bilateral nerve-sparing radical prostatectomy for clinically localized PCa is currently the gold standard.

Erectile dysfunction (ED) represents the most significant side effect negatively impacting the overall sexual health in patients treated with RP.[12] Research in post-RP recovery indicates a prevalence of 25–75% of men complaining of ED after surgery.[13-19] This wide range of postoperative ED can be explained by several factors: different study design, including differences in baseline tumor and sexual health characteristics of the population, surgical approach or technique, length of follow-up from surgery, surgeons' surgical volumes, and the quality of study methodologies in assessing both prevalence and severity of male ED.[17,19-23]

The most important factor associated with erectile function recovery after surgery is preoperative potency. Patients who are candidates for a BNSRP should ideally be fully potent prior to the procedure.[22,24] The preoperative EF is the key factor as patients who report any degree of ED or patients who already use pharmacological aids prior to the procedure are more likely to develop severe ED postoperatively, independent from the surgical technique used.[22,24]

Another important factor for EF recovery after surgery is represented by comorbitidy. Comorbid conditions, such as ischemic heart disease, diabetes mellitus, hypertension, hypercholesterolemia, or history of cigarette smoking, identified at the time of the patient history evaluation, seem also to negatively affect the impact on baseline penile hemodynamics and, in turn, may limit the recovery of spontaneous erections postoperatively.[22,24]

When analyzing post-RP ED, several intraoperative pathophysiological aspects deserve attention. Indeed, radical excision of the prostate should be performed with the objective of achieving total cancer control, i.e., removing all cancer present in the prostatic tissue while, in suitable candidates, maintaining the integrity of the anatomical structures on which urinary continence and erectile function are based. A recently published article sets as an ideal outcome, the so-called trifecta, which consist of three factors: freedom from cancer recurrence, complete continence, and complete EF recovery.[25] In this context, in order to preserve

F. Montorsi (✉)
Department of Urology, Vita-Salute San Raffaele, Milano 20132, Italy
e-mail: montorsi.francesco@hsr.it

erectile function a rigorous NS technique is mandatory.[4,24,26–29]

From an anatomical point of view, the cavernous nerves join the small vessels forming the so-called neurovascular bundle (NVB), which course along the posterolateral margin of the prostate, bilaterally, and are located between the visceral layer of the endopelvic fascia and the prostatic fascia. Several recent studies demonstrated that the course of NVB might be more complex than what previously thought. New anatomical reports described an extensive distribution of the nerve fibers belonging to the NVBs, which are more spread all around the prostatic capsule.[30–35] These studies have clearly demonstrated a wide course of the fibres included in the NVB, which altogether contribute to create a neurovascular layer, more than neurovascular bundle.[36] Based on the latter findings, some authors advocate a modification of the standard nerve-sparing approach, considering an intrafascial RP, with the aim of maximizing the preservation of nerve fibres.[24,27–29,37] Any manipulation of the nervous tissue may lead to neural damages, which might be transitory (namely neuropraxia caused by the damage to the cavernous nerves inevitably occurring during the excision of the prostate leading to temporary ED) or permanent (where one or both neurovascular bundles are transected during surgery). At a histological level, this damage leads to several cavernosal biochemical, morphological, and functional changes at the level of both smooth muscle and endothelial cells. The first consequence of the transitory or prolonged neural injury is the corporeal hypoxia.[38] When the smooth muscle cell is exposed to prolonged hypoxic conditions, there is a significant increase in the expression of hypoxia-related profibrotic substances, like transforming growth factor-β1 (TGF-β1) and endothelin-1 (ET-1). Those molecules promote the deposition of collagen I and III within the corpus cavernosum.[38–40] The trabecular smooth muscle is then replaced with collagen, which alter the mechanical properties as well as the integrity of the corpora cavernosa.[38,41,42] Moreover, chronic hypoxia and denervation have been shown to stimulate apoptosis.[41,43] Klein et al.[44] developed the first animal model of cavernous nerve damage aimed at addressing the extent of apoptosis in rat models undergoing penectomy at specific time intervals after nerve damage. DNA fragmentation and condensed cell nuclei are characteristic of apoptotic cells seen in the glans penis and the corporal bodies of denervated rats. Conversely, this was not seen in the sham-operated controls. It is possible that cellular apoptosis leads to increased deposition of connective tissue that may in turn cause a decrease in penile distensibility which results in veno-occlusive dysfunction.[44]

The role of hemodynamics impairment as a responsible key factor in determining postoperative ED has been deeply investigated. While it is absolutely clear that preservation of the cavernous nerves is mandatory to obtain an EF recovery after surgery, the potential role of vascular insufficiency increasingly became of interest as a contributor to postoperative ED in the last years.[45] Combination of nerve damage with decreased arterial inflow may intensify hypoxia and ultimately lead to penile apoptosis. Lim et al.[46] demonstrated that the rat with cavernous nerve crush and bilateral internal iliac artery ligation had significant decrease of intracorporeal pressure, loss of cavernous smooth muscle, and neural staining. Several trials have shown that in order to preserve erectile tissue, oxygenation needs to be warranted.[47,48] The blood supply to the erectile tissue can be significantly affected if the arteries irrigating the cavernous bodies are damaged intraoperatively. Therefore, not only the nervous tissue needs to be preserved but also the impairment of penile vascularization has to be as limited as possible. In this context, a rigorous preservation of the accessory pudendal arteries has been advocated, although their role in functional outcomes still needs to be prospectively established.[47,48]

In conclusion, both a postoperative denervation and/or an ischemic process consequent to the ligation of artery branches may cause a progressive fibrosis in the corpora cavernosa.[38,41,49] Fibrosis and the subsequent loss in elasticity and function of erectile tissue probably together cause ED.[38,41,49] The decrease of smooth muscle in the corpora cavernosa due to the fibrosis is associated with an impairment in the veno-occlusive mechanism which lead to venous leakage and, in turn, to ED of venous etiology.

The progression of technology led to the introduction of robotic-assisted radical prostatectomy (RARP). This procedure has been recently developed, and the results are really promising. The main advantage of the RARP relies on high magnification: the enhanced visibility provided to the surgeon by magnification allows for a better definition of anatomical landmarks. This translates in a more accurate dissection of the prostatic gland and, in turn, to a more precise preservation of neurovascular bundles, where an intrafascial technique is applicable.[37,50]

The functional outcomes of RARP are intriguing. The most recent published series of a high-volume center reports an erectile function recovery higher than 90%.[37] However, despite the advantages of this new surgical approach, a significant proportion of patients might still experience ED, with different degrees of severity.

31.2 Rationale for PDE5-I Prophylaxis in the Prevention of Post-RP Erectile Dysfunction

The introduction of phosphodiesterase type 5 inhibitor (PDE5-I) in the clinical setting has clearly revolutionized the management of post-prostatectomy ED. This class of agents acts within the smooth muscle cell by inhibiting the enzyme PDE5 which naturally degrades cyclic guanosine monophosphate (cGMP). cGMP is an intracellular nucleotide which works as second messenger in the process of smooth muscle cell relaxation. Increased levels of cGMP cause the activation of cGMP-specific protein kinases which trigger further intracellular events leading to the final reduction of intracellular calcium and, in turn, to smooth muscle cell relaxation.

A potential role of PDE5-I in the prevention of endothelial damage related to ischemia–reperfusion and/or denervation has been suggested by several base science studies. Behr-Roussel and colleagues recently published their experimental data regarding the potential mechanisms involved in chronic administration of PDE5-I.[51] They tested the effect of an 8-week-long treatment with sildenafil (60 mg/kg/day sc) in male rats and evaluated the electrically induced erectile response in vivo before and after an acute injection of sildenafil (0.3 mg/kg iv). The authors demonstrated that endothelial relaxation induced by acetylcholine was significantly enhanced in rats treated chronically with sildenafil as compared to those who did not receive the drug. These results might imply that either the muscarinic receptors or the transduction mechanisms that are involved in the activation of endothelial nitric oxide synthase (eNOS) are upregulated by

chronic sildenafil administration. Moreover, functional in vivo evaluations showed that chronic administration of sildenafil significantly enhanced frequency-dependent erectile response and was associated with an increased response to an acute injection of sildenafil in treated rats compared to untreated controls. Kovanecz et al. demonstrated that a long-term single daily dose of tadalafil prevented corporal veno-occlusive dysfunction and the underlying corporal fibrosis in the rat caused by cavernous nerve injury.[52] The authors hypothesized that PDE5-I may prevent ED through a cGMP-related mechanism. This potential effect appears to be independent of inducible nitric oxide synthase (iNOS) induction. A recent paper by Vignozzi et al. corroborates those findings.[53] The authors demonstrated in vitro that bilateral cavernous nerve injury induced penile hypoxia shown by a significant increase in hypoxyprobe labeling (a generally accepted probe of hypo-oxygenation) after a 3-month interval from surgical neurotomy. Vignozzi and colleagues showed that chronic tadalafil administration was able to completely restore penile oxygenation and smooth muscle/fibrous tissue ratio at histology.[53] The same group demonstrated the reproducibility of their findings publishing similar results using sildenafil and vardenafil.[43,54] In a very recent report, Lysiak and colleagues demonstrate a protective role of chronic tadalafil administration on the cavernous tissue in mice subjected to cavernous nerve resection or sham surgery.[55] Their report demonstrated that the chronic treatment with tadalafil significantly reduced the number of apoptotic cells and increased the phosphorylation of the two survival-associated kinases Akt and extracellular signal-regulated kinase $\frac{1}{2}$.[55] Lysiak and colleagues conclude that their findings may provide a rationale for the early administration of PDE-5 inhibition following radical prostatectomy or extensive pelvic surgery, during which there may be injury to the cavernous nerves, in order to facilitate the return to a normal erectile function.

Taken together, base science reports suggest a role of chronic PDE5-I administration in the prevention and, potentially, the cure of post-prostatectomy ED by avoiding the development of fibrosis and the decrease in smooth muscle in the corpora cavernosa.

Although base science evidence provides solid basis for a potential protective role of PDE5-I on cavernous tissue, the rationale for the use of these drugs as ED prophylaxis is not completely understood in human beings. Recent studies have clarified some mechanisms potentially involved in the post-RP ED etiology. Iacono et al. demonstrated the histological alterations in cavernous tissue after radical prostatectomy.[49] They collected 19 potent patients treated with RRP and subjected to a biopsy of the corpora cavernosa before surgical procedure and at 2 and 12 months postoperatively. In all cases the authors were able to find a decrease in trabecular elastic fibers and smooth muscle fibers, while the collagen content was significantly increased when compared with preoperative biopsies. Twelve months after surgery, the fibrosis advanced with a further decrease in elastic fibers ($p < 0.0003$) and smooth muscle fibers, substituted by collagen content, as compared with the first postoperative biopsy. Moreover, organized collagen and trabecular protocollagen deposits were increased.

Schwartz and colleagues recently published an elegant study on a total of 40 volunteers diagnosed with prostate cancer. All patients were fully potent before surgery and were treated with RRP. Patients were divided into two treatment groups, namely group 1 (50 mg sildenafil) and group 2 (100 mg sildenafil), and instructed to assume the study drug every other night for 6 months, beginning the day of catheter removal. Percutaneous biopsy of the corpora cavernosa was performed prior to incision for RRP and 6 months later.[56] In their paper the authors demonstrated that the early chronic use of high dose of sildenafil after radical prostatectomy seems to be associated with preservation of smooth muscle content within human corpora cavernosa.

Recently, a prophylactic regimen with methylprednisolone has been used in an interesting trial involving 70 preoperatively young patients (40–60 years) undergoing BNSRRP who were randomized to receive either 6 days of placebo or escalating doses of methylprednisolone starting from postoperative day 1.[57] The rationale of steroids use early after surgery was based on the potential use of this treatment in reducing the surgical neural inflammation and local edema that might contribute to dysfunction of neurovascular bundles after surgery. Nevertheless, no clinical benefit has been reported in patients receiving steroids compared to the placebo group in terms of erectile function recovery based on IIEF evaluation at the 3-, 6-, and 12-month evaluation ($P = 0.08$, $P = 0.50$, $P = 0.71$, respectively).

31.3 Management of Post-RP Erectile Dysfunction

The management of post-RP erectile dysfunction is mainly represented by administration of pro-erectile drugs. Historically, patients affected by postoperative ED may choose between several therapeutic options in order to obtain erections sufficient for a satisfactory sexual intercourse, including intracavernous injections,[20,58–60] urethral microsuppository,[20,61] vacuum device therapy, and eventually penile implants.[20,62] The advent of PDE5-I, namely sildenafil, tadalafil, and vardenafil, has significantly influenced the clinical practice and the treatment of patients after radical surgery. The oral administration represented a revolution of the management of post-RP erectile dysfunction. Today, PDE5-I represents the first-line therapy in patients who underwent either a unilateral nerve-sparing (UNS) or a BNS surgical approach.[20] Surgical technique represents a crucial point, since PDE5-I has the greatest effectiveness in patients who have undergone a rigorous NS procedure. In this context, although still controversial, a key role for the preservation of postoperative erectile function is played by surgical volume surgeon's experience in open RP. Several authors demonstrated that surgical volume is as an independent predictor of erectile function recovery after surgery, even after adjusting for patient age and nerve-sparing technique.[63–66] Regarding RARP, no studies have yet to highlight a potential role of surgical volume in the rate of EF recovery after surgery.

With the advances in the knowledge of post-prostatectomy ED pathophysiology, including the concept of tissue damage induced by poor corporeal oxygenation and denervation, open the way to the application of therapeutic regimens with the specific aim of increasing the early postoperative blood supply at the corpora cavernosa. The concept of "penile rehabilitation" after radical prostatectomy was pioneered by Montorsi and colleagues in 1997.[66] Their study included 30 patients treated with BNSRP and randomized to receive intracorporeal injections of alprostadil early after surgery or no therapy. With their results, the authors demonstrate that the rate of recovery of spontaneous erections in the groups receiving intracavernous injections (ICI) was significantly higher than observation alone. Similarly, Brock et al.[67] showed that the chronic administration of intracavernous alprostadil was able to significantly improve penile hemodynamics and, in turn, to increase the return of spontaneous erections (either partial or total) in patients with long-term arteriogenic ED. These data were confirmed also in the PDE5-I era by Mulhall et al.[68] The authors showed that the prophylactic use of alprostadil ICI resulted in higher rates of spontaneous functional erections and erectogenic drug response 18 months after NSRP also in patients who did not respond to oral compounds. Another potential strategy to reduce penile hypoxia immediately after RP may be represented by the application of vacuum constriction device (VCD). In this context, Raina et al. collected 104 patients subjected to open RP, either nerve sparing or non nerve sparing. The patients were randomized to prophylactic application of vacuum device or observation. The authors reported a significantly higher proportion of patient recovering spontaneous erection in the VCD group as compared to observation. They conclude that an early penile rehabilitation program with VCD is able to promote an adequate cavernosal oxygenation and therefore to prevent penile fibrosis after surgery.[69]

31.4 Phosphodiesterase Type 5 Inhibitors in the Management of Post-prostatectomy ED

Phosphodiesterase type 5 inhibitors have acquired an established role in the treatment of post-prostatectomy ED. Since the mechanism of action of this class of drugs implies the presence of nitric oxide within the corporeal smooth muscle cells, only patients undergoing an NS procedure should be expected to respond to these. To date, three molecules, namely sildenafil, tadalafil, and vardenafil, are approved for clinical use in the USA and the European Union, and those compounds have been utilized also to treat post-prostatectomy ED.

Since their introduction in 1998, a huge number of studies have demonstrated that PDE5-Is are significantly effective in ED patients after BNSRP and several predictors of response have been clearly outlined.[20,70,71] The most important factors include patient's age, patient's erectile function before surgery, and rigorous preservation of the neurovascular bundles.

Sildenafil is the drug which has been studied most extensively in the RP population since its introduction in 1998. In general terms, sildenafil has been acknowledged to achieve the best results in patients younger than 60, in patients treated with a bilateral NS procedure, and in patients who show some degree of spontaneous erection in the postoperative follow-up.[20] Several trials have highlighted a time-dependent erectile response to sildenafil. The efficacy of sildenafil increases as time passes by after the procedure: the best results are seen from 12 to 24 months after surgery. Sildenafil has been tested in different trials, with a response rate to treatment for ED after RP ranging from 35 to 75% among patients who underwent NS surgery and from 0 to 15% among those who were treated with non-NS surgery.[71-73] Padma-Nathan and colleagues recently published the first randomized placebo-controlled multicenter trial assessing the efficacy of sildenafil in the treatment of post-RP erectile dysfunction.[74] Seventy-six men were randomized into three arms 4 weeks after NSRP: 23 patients in the sildenafil 50 mg/day group, 28 patients in the sildenafil 100 mg/day arm, and 25 patients in the placebo arm. After an 8-week washout period 27% of patients taking sildenafil (50 or 100 mg/day) were able to achieve a natural erection vs. 4% in the placebo group. Even in presence of a sevenfold improvement, this study has been strongly criticized for the high prevalence of baseline erectile dysfunction in both groups, for the low rate of EF recovery at 11 months from RP, and for the limited population of the study. Bannowsky et al. evaluate the effect of low-dose sildenafil for rehabilitating erectile function after NSRP.[75] Forty-three sexually active patients were randomized to receive either placebo or sildenafil 25 mg/day at night. In the group taking sildenafil, 47% achieved and maintained a penile erection sufficient for vaginal intercourse at 1 year after NSRP, compared with 28% in the control group with no low-dose sildenafil. Clinically, those men who report some degree of spontaneous penile tumescence after surgery were the most likely to respond to PDE5-I.[75]

Furthermore, effectiveness of both tadalafil and vardenafil as an on-demand treatment has been also evaluated in such a challenging population of patients. Tadalafil was evaluated in a large multicenter trial conducted in Europe and in USA. Montorsi and colleagues evaluated 303 potent men treated with BNSRP and randomized to receive either tadalafil 20 mg on demand or placebo.[76] Seventy-one percent of patients treated with tadalafil 20 mg reported an improvement of their erectile function as compared to 24% of those treated with placebo ($P < 0.001$). The erectile function domain score of the IIEF questionnaire was significantly higher after treatment with tadalafil 20 mg compared to placebo (21.0 vs. 15.2; $P < 0.001$), and this difference was clinically significant. Tadalafil 20 mg allowed to achieve a 52% rate of successful intercourse attempts which was significantly higher than the 26% obtained with a placebo ($P < 0.001$).

Moreover, vardenafil has been tested in patients treated with ED following a uni- or bilateral NS prostatectomy in a prospective, placebo-controlled, multicenter, randomized study including North American patients only.[77] This was a 12-week parallel arm study comparing placebo to vardenafil 10 and 20 mg. Respectively, 71 and 60% of patients treated with a bilateral NS procedure reported an improvement in the erectile function following the administration of vardenafil 20 and 10 mg. A positive answer to sexual encounter profile (SEP) 2 question (were you able to insert your penis into your partner's vagina?) was seen in 47 and 48% of patients using vardenafil 10 and 20 mg, respectively. A positive answer to the more challenging SEP 3 question (did your erections last enough to have successful intercourse?) was seen in 37 and 34% of patients using vardenafil 10 and 20 mg, respectively.[77] More recently, an elegant analysis focusing on the other domains of the IIEF of the same population of patients undergoing NSRP has underlined vardenafil's benefit over placebo regarding intercourse satisfaction, hardness of erection, orgasmic function, and overall satisfaction with sexual experience ($P < 0.0009$ for each of the variable studied both at 10- and 20-mg doses).[78] Very recently, Gallo and colleagues[79] evaluated the role of vardenafil in the recovery of erectile function following pelvic urologic surgeries (RRP and cystectomy). After 6 months of daily therapy, vardenafil therapy was able to significantly increase the mean IIEF-5 score to 12.9 points in the bilateral nerve-sparing group, to 8.0 points in the unilateral nerve-sparing group, and to 11.3 points in the bilateral nerve-sparing radical cystectomy group.

The adverse event profile of the three PDE5-I has been very similar, and the discontinuation from treatment with one of the PDE5-I is usually caused by lack of efficacy, while tolerability is overall more than satisfactory.

Surprisingly, the potential benefit induced by a continuous PDE5-I has rarely been compared to an on-demand PDE5-I administration schedule in methodologically rigorous studies. However, it is widely recognized that there are logistic difficulties in preparing such large placebo-controlled studies. The only report investigating the role of on-demand vs. daily administration of PDE5-I after BNSRP has been recently published by Montorsi and colleagues.[72,80] In this randomized, double-blind, double-dummy, multicentre, parallel-group study, 628 men were randomized to receive vardenafil nightly and vardenafil on-demand or placebo for 9 months. Surprisingly, in contrast to the prophylactic use of PDE5 inhibitors for penile rehabilitation and treatment of ED in men following NSRP surgery, this study suggests a paradigm shift toward on-demand dosing with PDE5 inhibitors for the treatment of ED in patient treated with BNSRP.

31.5 Other Treatments in the Management of Post-prostatectomy ED

Intracavernous injection (ICI) of pro-erectile compound represents a valid alternative for patients not responding to PDE5-Is. The main advantage of ICI is that alprostadil induces erections by directly stimulating the production of cyclic adenosine monophosphate (cAMP) within the smooth muscle cells and thus does not require a functioning nerve to induce smooth muscle relaxation.[81] The main disadvantage of ICI relies in the limited compliance to the treatment. Penile pain remains a major obstacle to its widespread adoption by patients which often discontinue the therapy.[82] However, the results in patients not responding to oral compounds demonstrated a high rate of effectiveness.[66–68]

A potential second-line treatment in post-RP patients is represented by intraurethral prostaglandin. The drug is delivered as a suppository of alprostadil with MUSE. Similarly to ICI, intraurethral alprostadil directly induces smooth muscle relaxation and increases the penile blood supply, even in the presence of local nerve trauma or nerve damage. However, intraurethral prostaglandin is associated with urethral pain and discomfort, low response rate, and inconsistent efficacy.[83] The discomfort experienced during administration may be explained by a prostaglandin's direct effect on pain receptors at the urethral level.[84,85] The results in patients complaining post-RP erectile dysfunction are encouraging. In a retrospective analysis of the MUSE clinical trial, Costabile and colleagues analyzed 384 men with ED after RP.[87] The study showed a high rate of efficacy independently from nerve preservation. The "in office" response rate was 70%, with a 57% "home success" rate. Similar results were obtained by Raina and colleagues in a prospective, non-randomized trial including 91 patients.[61] At a median follow-up of 6 months, 74% of the patients treated with MUSE were able to obtain erections sufficient for vaginal intercourse vs. 37% in the control group. However, 32% of patients receiving intraurethral alprostadil discontinued treatment, due to local pain.

Vacuum constriction devices (VCDs) are able to promote penile tumescence through negative pressure effects on the corporeal chambers. In order to obtain a valid erection, VCD need to be associated with a venous constriction ring to maintain tumescence. Lack of spontaneity, difficult mechanics, and complications have led to high discontinuation rates.[86]

31.6 Conclusions

Radical prostatectomy is the current gold standard in patients diagnosed with clinically localized prostate cancer. Since the mean age at prostate cancer diagnosis is progressively declining due to the advent of prostate-specific antigen testing and prostate cancer screening programs, the demand for optimal postoperative quality of life is becoming more important. Progression in surgical technique and in medical technology may further improve the quality of life after radical prostatectomy. To date, the use of on-demand or chronic oral treatments in patients subjected to RP has been shown to be effective and safe, with better results seen in select young patients treated with a bilateral NS approach. Pharmacological prophylaxis, with either oral or local therapies, may potentially have a significantly expanding role in the future strategies aimed at preserving postoperative erectile function. Large, multicentric, placebo-controlled trials are needed in order to identify the best regimen able to provide the

best strategy for the recovery of erectile function after radical prostatectomy.

References

1. Heidenreich A, Aus G, Bolla M, Joniau S, Matveev VB, Schmid HP, et al. European association of urology. EAU guidelines on prostate cancer. *Eur Urol.* 2008;53:68–80.
2. Oliver SE, Donovan JL, Peters TJ, Frankel S, Hamdy FC, Neal DE. Recent trends in the use of radical prostatectomy in England: the epidemiology of diffusion. *BJU Int.* 2003;91:331–336.
3. Cooperberg MR, Broering JM, Litwin MS, Lubeck DP, Mehta SS, Henning JM, et al. The contemporary management of prostate cancer in the United States: lessons from the cancer of the prostate strategic urologic research endeavor (capsure), a national disease registry. *J Urol.* 2004;171:1393–1401.
4. Eggener SE, Guillonneau B. Laparoscopic radical prostatectomy: ten years later, time for evidence-based foundation. *Eur Urol.* 2008;54:4–7.
5. Ficarra V, Cavalleri S, Novara G, Aragona M, Artibani W. Evidence from robot-assisted laparoscopic radical prostatectomy: a systematic review. *Eur Urol.* 2007;51:45–55.
6. Heidenreich A. Radical prostatectomy in 2007: oncologic control and preservation of functional integrity. *Eur Urol.* 2008;53:877–879.
7. Madalinska JB, Essink-Bot ML, de Koning HJ, Kirkels WJ, van der Maas PJ, Schroder FH. Health-related quality of life effects of radical prostatectomy and primary radiotherapy for screen-detected or clinically diagnosed localized prostate cancer. *J Clin Oncol.* 1628;2001(19):1619–.
8. Lubeck DP, Litwin MS, Henning JM, Stoddard ML, Flanders SC, Carroll PR. Changes in health-related quality of life in the first year after treatment for prostate cancer: results from capsure. *Urology.* 1999;53:180–186.
9. Gallina A, Chun FK, Suardi N, et al. Comparison of stage migration patterns between Europe and the USA: an analysis of 11 350 men treated with radical prostatectomy for prostate cancer. *BJU Int.* 2008 Jun;101(12):1513–1518.
10. Scales CD Jr, Moul JW, Curtis LH, et al. Investigators. Prostate cancer in the baby boomer generation: results from capsure. *Urology.* 2007;70:1162–1167.
11. Walsh PC, Donker PJ. Impotence following radical prostatectomy: insight into etiology and prevention. *J Urol.* 1982;128:492–497.
12. Glina S. How much are patients interested in erectile dysfunction treatment after radical prostatectomy? *Eur Urol.* 2008;53:461–462.
13. Eastham JA, Scardino PT, Kattan MW. Predicting an optimal outcome after radical prostatectomy: the trifecta nomogram. *J Urol.* 2008;179:2207–2210.
14. Stanford JL, Feng Z, Hamilton AS, Gilliland FD, Stephenson RA, Eley JW, et al. Urinary and sexual function after radical prostatectomy for clinically localized prostate cancer: the prostate cancer outcomes study. *JAMA.* 2000;283:354–360.

15. Schover LR, Fouladi RT, Warneke CL, Neese L, Klein EA, Zippe C, et al. Defining sexual outcomes after treatment for localized prostate carcinoma. *Cancer.* 1785;2002(95):1773–1785.

16. Matthew AG, Goldman A, Trachtenberg J, Robinson J, Horsburgh S, Currie K, et al. Sexual dysfunction after radical prostatectomy: prevalence, treatments, restricted use of treatments and distress. *J Urol.* 2005;174:2105–2110.

17. Dubbelman YD, Dohle GR, Schröder FH. Sexual function before and after radical retropubic prostatectomy: a systematic review of prognostic indicators for a successful outcome. *Eur Urol.* 2006;50:711–718.

18. Sanda MG, Dunn RL, Michalski J, Sandler HM, Northouse L, Hembroff L, et al. Quality of life and satisfaction with outcome among prostate-cancer survivors. *N Engl J Med.* 2008;358:1250–1261.

19. Giuliano F, Amar E, Chevallier D, Montaigne O, Joubert JM, Chartier-Kastler E. How urologists manage erectile dysfunction after radical prostatectomy: a national survey (REPAIR) by the French urological association. *J Sex Med.* 2008;5:448–457.

20. Briganti A, Salonia A, Gallina A, Chun FK, Karakiewicz PI, Graefen M, et al. Management of erectile dysfunction after radical prostatectomy in 2007. *World J Urol.* 2007;25:143–148.

21. Salonia A, Zanni G, Gallina A, Saccà A, Sangalli M, Naspro R, et al. Baseline potency in patients candidates to bilateral nerve sparing radical retropubic prostatectomy. *Eur Urol.* 2006;50:360–365.

22. Michl UH, Friedrich MG, Graefen M, Haese A, Heinzer H, Huland H. Prediction of postoperative sexual function after nerve sparing radical retropubic prostatectomy. *J Urol.* 2006;176:227–231.

23. Salonia A, Gallina A, Briganti A, Zanni G, Saccà A, Dehò F, et al. Remembered international index of erectile function domain scores are not accurate in assessing preoperative potency in candidates for bilateral nerve-sparing radical retropubic prostatectomy. *J Sex Med.* 2008;5: 677–683.

24. Montorsi F, Salonia A, Suardi N, Gallina A, Zanni G, Briganti A, et al. Improving the preservation of the urethral sphincter and neurovascular bundles during open radical retropubic prostatectomy. *Eur Urol.* 2005;48:938–945.

25. Bianco FJ Jr, Scardino PT, Eastham JA. Radical prostatectomy: long-term cancer control and recovery of sexual and urinary function ("trifecta"). *Urology.* 2005;66(5 Suppl):83–94.

26. Graefen M, Walz J, Huland H. Open retropubic nerve-sparing radical prostatectomy. *Eur Urol.* 2006;49:38–48.

27. Zorn KC, Gofrit ON, Orvieto MA, Mikhail AA, Zagaja GP, Shalhav AL. Robotic-assisted laparoscopic prostatectomy: functional and pathologic outcomes with interfascial nerve preservation. *Eur Urol.* 2007;51:755–762.

28. Menon M, Shrivastava A, Kaul S, Badani KK, Fumo M, Bhandari M, et al. Vattikuti Institute prostatectomy: contemporary technique and analysis of results. *Eur Urol.* 2007;51:648–657.

29. Stolzenburg JU, Rabenalt R, Do M, Schwalenberg T, Winkler M, Dietel A, et al. Intrafascial nerve-sparing endoscopic extraperitoneal radical prostatectomy. *Eur Urol.* 2008;53:931–940.

30. Costello AJ, Brooks M, Cole OJ. Anatomical studies of the neurovascular bundle and cavernosal nerves. *BJU Int.* 2004;94:1071–1076.

31. Lunacek A, Schwentner C, Fritsch H, Bartsch G, Strasser H. Anatomical radical retropubic prostatectomy: 'curtain dissection' of the neurovascular bundle. *BJU Int.* 2005 Jun;95(9):1226–1231.

32. Tewari A, Takenaka A, Mtui E, Horninger W, Peschel R, Bartsch G, et al. The proximal neurovascular plate and the tri-zonal neural architecture around the prostate gland: importance in the athermal robotic technique of nerve-sparing prostatectomy. *BJU Int.* 2006;98: 314–323.

33. Eichelberg C, Erbersdobler A, Michl U, Schlomm T, Salomon G, Graefen M, et al. Nerve distribution along the prostatic capsule. *Eur Urol.* 2007;51:105–110.

34. Ganzer R, Blana A, Gaumann A, Stolzenburg JU, Rabenalt R, Bach T, et al. Topographical anatomy of periprostatic and capsular nerves: quantification and computerised planimetry. *Eur Urol.* 2008;54:353–361.

35. Gianduzzo TR, Colombo JR, El-Gabry E, Haber GP, Gill IS. Anatomical and electrophysiological assessment of the canine periprostatic neurovascular anatomy: perspectives as a nerve sparing radical prostatectomy model. *J Urol.* 2008;179:2025–2029.

36. Sievert KD, Hennenlotter J, Laible I, et al. The periprostatic autonomic nerves–bundle or layer? *Eur Urol.* 2008;54:1109–1116.

37. Menon M, Shrivastava A, Bhandari M, Satyanarayana R, Siva S, Agarwal PK. Vattikuti Institute prostatectomy: technical modifications in 2009. *Eur Urol.* 2009 Jul;56(1): 89–96.

38. Leungwattanakij S, Bivalacqua TJ, Usta MF, Yang DY, Hyun JS, Champion HC, et al. Cavernous neurotomy causes hypoxia and fibrosis in rat corpus cavernosum. *J Androl.* 2003;24:239–245.

39. Granchi S, Vannelli GB, Vignozzi L, Crescioli C, Ferruzzi P, Mancina R, et al. Expression and regulation of endothelin-1 and its receptors in human penile smooth muscle cells. *Mol Hum Reprod.* 2002;8:1053–1064

40. Filippi S, Marini M, Vannelli GB, Crescioli C, Granchi S, Vignozzi L, et al. Effects of hypoxia on endothelin-1 sensitivity in the corpus cavernosum. *Mol Hum Reprod.* 2003;9:765–774.

41. User HM, Hairston JH, Zelner DJ, McKenna KE, McVary KT. Penile weight and cell subtype specific changes in a post-radical prostatectomy model of erectile dysfunction. *J Urol.* 2003;169:1175–1179.

42. Ciancio SJ, Kim ED. Penile fibrotic changes after radical retropubic prostatectomy. *BJU Int.* 2000;85:101–106.

43. Ferrini MG, Kovanecz I, Sanchez S, Umeh C, Rajfer J, Gonzalez-Cadavid NF. Fibrosis and loss of smooth muscle in the corpora cavernosa precede corporal veno-occlusive dysfunction (cvod) induced by experimental cavernosal nerve damage in the rat. *J Sex Med.* 2009;6: 415–428.

44. Klein LT, Miller MI, Buttyan R, Raffo AJ, Burchard M, Devris G, et al. Apoptosis in the rat penis after penile denervation. *J Urol.* 1997;158:626–630.

45. Mulhall JP, Slovick R, Hotaling J, Aviv N, Valenzuela R, Waters WB, et al. Erectile dysfunction after radical

prostatectomy: hemodynamic profiles and their correlation with the recovery of erectile function. *J Urol*. 2002;167: 1371–1375.

46. Lim KB, DeYoung L, Brock G. Chronic PDE5 inhibitor altered cavernosal protein expression-use in identifying protein biomarker for erectile recovery post trauma? *J Sex Med*. 2006;3(suppl 5):383.

47. Mulhall JP, Secin FP, Guillonneau B. Artery sparing radical prostatectomy-myth or reality? *J Urol*. 2008;179:827–831.

48. Secin FP, Touijer K, Mulhall J, Guillonneau B. Anatomy and preservation of accessory pudendal arteries in laparoscopic radical prostatectomy. *Eur Urol*. 2007; 51: 1229–1235.

49. Iacono F, Giannella R, Somma P, Manno G, Fusco F, Mirone V. Histological alterations in cavernous tissue after radical prostatectomy. *J Urol*. 1676;2005:173:1673.

50. McCullough TC, Barret E, Cathelineau X, Rozet F, Galiano M, Vallancien G. Role of robotics for prostate cancer. *Curr Opin Urol*. 2009 Jan;19(1):65–68.

51. Behr-Roussel D, Gorny D, Mevel K, Caisey S, Bernabè J, Burgess G, et al. Chronic sildenafil improves erectile function and endothelium-dependent cavernosal relaxations in rats: lack of tachyphylaxis. *Eur Urol*. 2005;47: 87–91.

52. Kovanecz I, Rambhatla A, Ferrini MG, Vernet D, Sanchez S, Rajfer J, et al. Chronic daily tadalafil prevents the corporal fibrosis and veno-occlusive dysfunction that occurs after cavernosal nerve resection. *BJU Int*. 2008;101: 203–210.

53. Vignozzi L, Filippi S, Morelli A, et al. Effect of chronic tadalafil administration on penile hypoxia induced by cavernous neurotomy in the rat. *J Sex Med*. 2006;3: 419–431.

54. Vignozzi L, Morelli A, Filippi S, et al. Effect of sildenafil administration on penile hypoxia induced by cavernous neurotomy in the rat. *IJIR*. 2008;20:60–67.

55. Lysiak JJ, Yang SK, Klausner AP, Son H, Tuttle JB, Steers WD. Tadalafil increases akt and extracellular signal-regulated kinase 1/2 activation, and prevents apoptotic cell death in the penis following denervation. *J Urol*. 2008;179(2):779–785.

56. Schwartz EJ, Wong P, Graydon J. Sildenafil preserves intracorporeal smooth muscle after radical retropubic prostatectomy. *J Urol*. 2004;171:771–774.

57. Parsons JK, Marschke P, Maples P, Walsh PC. Effect of methylprednisolone on return of sexual function after nervesparing radical retropubic prostatectomy. *Urology*. 2004;64:987–990.

58. Stephenson RA, Mori M, Hsieh YC, Beer TM, Stanford JL, Gilliland FD, et al. Treatment of erectile dysfunction following therapy for clinically localized prostate cancer: patient reported use and outcomes from the surveillance, epidemiology, and end results prostate cancer outcomes study. *J Urol*. 2005;174:646–650.

59. Matthew AG, Goldman A, Trachtenberg J, Robinson J, Horsburgh S, Currie K, et al. Sexual dysfunction after radical prostatectomy: prevalence, treatments, restricted use of treatments and distress. *J Urol*. 2005;174:2105–2110.

60. Giuliano F, Amar E, Chevallier D, Montaigne O, Joubert JM, Chartier-Kastler E. How urologists manage erectile dysfunction after radical prostatectomy: a national survey (REPAIR) by the French urological association. *J Sex Med*. 2008;5:448–457.

61. Raina R, Pahlajani G, Agarwal A, Zippe CD. The early use of transurethral alprostadil after radical prostatectomy potentially facilitates an earlier return of erectile function and successful sexual activity. *BJU Int*. 2007;100: 1317–1321.

62. Lane BR, Abouassaly R, Angermeier KW, Montague DK. Three-piece inflatable penile prostheses can be safely implanted after radical prostatectomy through a transverse scrotal incision. *Urology*. 2007;70:539–542.

63. Bianco F, Kattan M, Eastham J. Surgeon and surgical volume as predictors of erectile function outcomes following radical prostatectomy. *J Sex Med*. 2004;1(suppl 1):33.

64. Ayyathurai R, Manoharan M, Nieder AM, Kava B, Soloway MS. Factors affecting erectile function after radical retropubic prostatectomy: results from 1,620 consecutive patients. *BJU Int*. 2008;101:833–836.

65. Hollenbeck BK, Dunn RL, Wei JT, Montie JE, Sanda MG. Determinants of long-term sexual health outcome after radical prostatectomy measured by a validated instrument. *J Urol*. 2003;169:1453–1457.

66. Montorsi F, Guazzoni G, Strambi LF, et al. Recovery of spontaneous erectile function after nerve-sparing radical retropubic prostatectomy with and without early intracavernous injections of alprostadil: results of a prospective, randomised trial. *J Urol*. 1997;158:1408–1410.

67. Brock G, Tu LM, Linet OI. Return of spontaneous erection during long-term intracavernosal alprostadil (caverject) treatment. *Urology*. 2001;57:536–541.

68. Mulhall J, Land S, Parker M, Waters WB, Flanigan RC. The use of an erectogenic pharmacotherapy regimen following radical prostatectomy improves recovery of spontaneous erectile function. *J Sex Med*. 2005;2:532–545.

69. Raina R, Agarwal A, Ausmundson S, Lakin M, Nandipati KC, Montague DK, et al. Early use of vacuum constriction device following radical prostatectomy facilitates early sexual activity and potentially earlier return of erectile function. *Int J Impot Res*. 2006;18:77–81.

70. Montorsi F, Briganti A, Salonia A, Rigatti P, Burnett AL. Current and future strategies for preventing and managing erectile dysfunction following radical prostatectomy. *Eur Urol*. 2004;45:123–133.

71. Raina R, Lakin MM, Agarwal A, Mascha E, Montagne DK, Klein E, et al. Efficacy and factors associated with successful outcome of sildenafil citrate use for erectile dysfunction after radical prostatectomy. *Urology*. 2004;63: 960–966.

72. Zippe CD, Jhaveri FM, Klein EA, et al. Role of viagra after radical prostatectomy. *Urology*. 2000;55:241–245.

73. Raina R, Lakin MM, Agarwal A, Sharma R, Goyal KK, Montague DK. Long-term effect of sildenafil citrate on erectile dysfunction after radical prostatectomy: 3-year follow-up. *Urology*. 2003;62:110–115.

74. Padma-Nathan E, McCullough AR, Giuliano F, et al. Postoperative nightly administration of sildenafil citrate significantly improves the return of normal spontaneous erectile function after bilateral nerve-sparing radical prostatectomy. *J Urol*. 2003;4(Suppl):375.

75. Bannowsky A, Schulze H, van der Horst C, Hautmann S, Jünemann KP. Recovery of erectile function after

nerve-sparing radical prostatectomy: improvement with nightly low-dose sildenafil. *BJU Int.* 2008;101:1279–1283.

76. Montorsi F, Nathan HP, McCullough A, et al. Tadalafil in the treatment of erectile dysfunction following bilateral nerve sparing radical retropubic prostatectomy: a randomized, double-blind, placebo controlled trial. *J Urol.* 2004;172:1036–1041.

77. Brock G, Nehra A, Lipshultz LI, et al. Safety and efficacy of vardenafil for the treatment of men with erectile dysfunction after radical retropubic prostatectomy. *J Urol.* 2003;170:1278–1283.

78. Nehera A, Grantmyre J, Nadel A, Thibonnier M, Brock G. Vardenafil improved patient satisfaction with erectile hardness, orgasmic function and sexual experience in men with erectile dysfunction following nerve sparing radical prostatectomy. *J Urol.* 2005;173:2067–2071.

79. Gallo L, Perdona S, Autorino R, et al. Recovery of erection after pelvic urologic surgery: our experience. *Int J Impot Res.* 2005;17:484.

80. Montorsi F, Brock G, Lee J, Shapiro J, Van Poppel H, Graefen M, et al. Effect of nightly versus on-demand vardenafil on recovery of erectile function in men following bilateral nerve-sparing radical prostatectomy. *Eur Urol.* 2008;54:924–931.

81. Ruiz Rubio JL, Hernandez M, Rivera de los Arcos L, et al. Mechanisms of prostaglandin E1-induced relaxation in penile resistance arteries. *J Urol.* 2004;171:968–973.

82. Lakin MM, Montague DK, VanderBrug Medendorp S, et al. Intracavernous injection therapy: analysis of results and complications. *J Urol.* 1990;143:1138–1141.

83. Porst H. Transurethral alprostadil with MUSE (medicated urethral system for erection) vs. intracavernous alprostadil—a comparative study in 103 patients with erectile dysfunction. *Int J Impot Res.* 1997;9:187–192.

84. Lepor H, McCullough A. Penile rehabilitation post-prostatectomy: is there a role for MUSE? *Rev Urol.* 2008;10:1–5.

85. Costabile RA, Spevak M, Fishman IJ, et al. Efficacy and safety of transurethral alprostadil in patients with erectile dysfunction following radical prostatectomy. *J Urol.* 1998;160:1325–1328.

86. Sidi AA, Becher EF, Zhang G, et al. Patient acceptance of and satisfaction with an external negative pressure device for impotence. *J Urol.* 1990;144:1154–1156.

87. Zagaja GP, Mhoon DA, Aikens JE, Brendler CB. Sildenafil in the treatment of erectile dysfunction after radical prostatectomy. *Urology.* 2000;56:631.

Chapter 32

Laparoscopy or Robotic Radical Prostatectomy: Pros and Cons

Claude Abbou and Leticia Ruiz

32.1 Advantages of the Laparoscopic Approach

The cost of laparoscopic radical prostatectomy is lower than that of the robotic-assisted procedure, since there is no need for purchase or maintenance of the robot, and the instruments used are less expensive.[1] These advantages persist even if the operative time tends to be longer for the laparoscopic approach.

32.2 Disadvantages of the Laparoscopic Approach

The learning curve for laparoscopic radical prostatectomy is steep. It has been considered to be around 40–60 cases for the experienced laparoscopic surgeon.[2] Most of the initial series published considered the procedure technically demanding.[3–5] Some authors consider that around 200 cases are needed before reaching the learning curve, with the most technically challenging step being the urethro-vesical anastomosis.[6,7] It is also possible that second- and third-generation surgeons will acquire adequate skills with a smaller series of surgery, specially if mentorship is applied[8] compared to surgeons who started when the technique was just developing.

There is a limited range of movements, since surgery is performed with rigid instruments. This leads to difficulties in dissection and in performing the urethro-vesical anastomosis. Intracorporeal suturing is difficult to master. Investment in training by surgeon is time consuming and costly. The see one, do one, teach one concept does not apply to this technique.

Another disadvantage of the laparoscopic radical prostatectomy is its two-dimensional vision, and the lack of control of the laparoscope by the surgeon who relays on an assistant that must be familiar with the procedure to help the surgeon adequately. In lengthy procedures lack of assistance can lead to even higher increases on operative times. Some centers bypass this difficulty by using the AESOP voice-activated robotic arm to control the laparoscope.

32.3 Advantages of the Robotic-Assisted Procedure

The use of the da Vinci Surgical System (Intuitive Surgical, Sunnyvale, California) permits several advantages.

Ergonomy for the surgeon, who comfortably seats at a console: The console can be located in the operating room or in an adjacent room. Eventually, the console could be situated remotely from the patient. This opens the possibility of telesurgery at a distant site. The feasibility of telesurgery and telementoring using the da Vinci Surgical System was demonstrated, by performing four right nephrectomies in porcine models with surgeons operating a console at distances of 1,300 and 2,400 miles from the operating room.[9]

C. Abbou (✉)
Department of Urology, Henri Mondor Hospital, Creteil, France
e-mail: claude.abbou@hmn.ap-hop-paris.fr

A.K. Hemal, M. Menon (eds.), *Robotics in Genitourinary Surgery*,
DOI 10.1007/978-1-84882-114-9_32, © Springer-Verlag London Limited 2011

The console is integrated with three-dimensional display stereo viewer and provides 10- to 15-fold magnification. Improved image quality has the potential of improving functional results by permitting more accurate dissection of the neurovascular bundles.

Instruments are wristed, providing 7° of motion, resembling more closely the movements of the human hand and wrist. In addition, movements of the hand are scaled and tremor is corrected. These characteristics enable the laparoscopy-naïve surgeon to acquire the skills to migrate into minimally invasive surgery, since movements are intuitive.

The robot-assisted radical prostatectomy has a shorter learning curve, compared to the laparoscopic procedure, with surgeons without previous experience in laparoscopy acquiring proficiency with as few as 12 cases.[10] Since the definition of learning curve varies widely, so do the cases necessary to attain it, depending on the parameters considered and the studies that are evaluated. Some studies suggest that 20–25 cases are needed for proficiency.[11] Operative time to perform robotic radical prostatectomy is significantly reduced as the surgeon's experience increases. This was demonstrated in a series by Menon and colleagues[12] in which, after 18 procedures, operative times for the robotic procedure became shorter than those of laparoscopic procedures by experienced surgeons. An interesting study showed that intensive 5-day training enabled most participants to incorporate and maintain robotic-assisted prostatectomy into their practices.[13]

The presence of a computer between patient and surgeon opens the possibility of developing new applications, such as image-guided surgery (IGS). The potential benefit of adding image guidance to the da Vinci robotic surgical system, by improving dissection and surgical margins, has been demonstrated in a laboratory model.[14]

procedure. Also, the rest of the team does not benefit from the three-dimensional image.

Probably the most important disadvantage is the very high cost of the robot, its maintenance, and consumable equipment. Several studies have addressed this aspect. It has been estimated that 45% of the average direct cost, and a third of the average total cost, corresponds to medical and surgical supplies, while operating room services corresponded to 30 and 35%, respectively, to average direct and total costs.[16] A study of 643 consecutive patients who underwent radical prostatectomy by either open, robotic-assisted, or laparoscopic approach compared the cost of each modality and found that robotic-assisted radical prostatectomy direct cost (OR time, disposables) exceeded laparoscopic radical prostatectomy by more than $1,000, without including the cost of purchase and maintenance of the robot, which depends on case volume at each particular center. Depending on the model and year of purchase of the robot, this cost could approach $2,700 if 126 cases per year are performed.[1] If the robot is shared with other specialties, its cost per case could be around $900, considering a case load of 300 per year for 7 years.[17] Models have been developed to evaluate cost depending on operative time, length of stay, and local cost for room and board and demonstrated decreasing cost as operating room time and length of stay decrease, and higher advantages at high-cost hospitals.[18]

A study at Duke University Medical Center showed more regret and dissatisfaction among patients who underwent the robotic procedure, compared to the open approach (19.9 vs 12.9% of dissatisfaction, correspondingly) even if functional results were not statistically different in the laparoscopic and robotic-assisted groups.[19] Authors attributed this finding to higher expectations and different demographics in patients choosing the robotic approach.

32.4 Disadvantages of the Robotic-Assisted Procedure

When the procedure is performed by robotic assistance, there is a lack of tactile feedback.[15]

Communication among surgeon, assistant, and rest of the staff can be impaired during the robotic-assisted

32.5 Results

32.5.1 Perioperative Results

Regarding perioperative outcomes, cumulative analysis showed no significant difference in complication rates after RALP and LRP,[20] even if some studies reported contradictory results. Analysis of two studies[21,22] proved that operative time was shorter for RALP and complication rate was lower for RALP, so they hypothesized that increasing surgeon experience might have influenced these results. In contrast, a series from France[23] showed higher rate of complications and transfusion rate in the RALP group compared to the LRP. In centers with extensive laparoscopic experience, when the learning curve is excluded, operative time is similar in both approaches.[23]

In general, catheterization time and hospital stay are similar between RALP and LRP, although a study reported that 95% of patients operated by the robot-assisted procedure were discharged within 23 h.[24]

Median blood loss was comparable in both techniques in two studies[22,23] and lower for RALP in other two studies.[12,25]

Both techniques can be performed by either the transperitoneal or extraperitoneal approach.[15,26–28]

32.5.2 Oncologic Outcomes

According to studies reporting oncologic results of laparoscopic and robotic-assisted radical prostatectomy, no difference is noted regarding positive surgical margins.[20] Positive surgical margins ranged from 11 to 30% after laparoscopic radical prostatectomy and from 9.6 to 26% for robotic-assisted radical prostatectomy.[20] Some authors have looked at additional procedures or treatments (salvage radiotherapy, chemotherapy, or hormonal therapy) after radical prostatectomy to assess cancer control and concluded that unfavorable outcomes decrease with increasing surgical volume.[29,30]

A study at Tulane evaluated 100 patients who underwent robotic-assisted radical prostatectomy, according to the time of surgery. Patients were divided into three groups (I, first 33 cases; II, second 33 cases; and III, last 34 cases), and a statistically significant decrease in positive surgical margins was noted from 45.4 to 21.2 to 11.7%, respectively, as the series progressed.[31] Similar results regarding surgical margins have been observed in other series.

A comprehensive review of robotic and laparoscopic series found an overall weighted mean for positive margin rate of 12.5% for robotic radical prostatectomies and 19.6% for laparoscopic radical

prostatectomy. It must be considered that the robotic series had 77.4% pT2 tumors and 21.5% pT3 tumors; the laparoscopic series had 70.4% of T2 tumors.[32]

Biochemical recurrence-free survival at 5 years is similar, ranging from 82 to 100% for robotic-assisted prostatectomy[33,34] and 85% in a series of 1,115 extraperitoneal laparoscopic procedures,[35] and 90.5% at 3 years for a series of 1,000 transperitoneal prostatectomies.[36]

32.5.3 Functional Results

32.5.3.1 Urinary Continence

Continence outcomes have also been evaluated in reviews. At 3 months, urinary continence ranged from 73 to 91% for robotic-assisted prostatectomy and 51–94% for the laparoscopic group, while at 6 months it ranged from 82 to 97% and 73 to 96%, respectively.[32,37] A study comparing laparoscopic and robotic radical prostatectomy showed no difference in continence rates at 6 months.[25]

32.5.3.2 Erectile Function

Rates for erectile function vary among series, as do definitions for potency, rendering it difficult to compare results.[20] Potency rates for robotic series at referral centers vary from 70 to 80% and from 42 to 76% for laparoscopic series. A non-statistically significant trend favoring the robotic technique was observed in a comparative study.[25] A study of 1,151 of a mature series of robotic-assisted radical prostatectomy, using the superveil nerve-sparing technique, reported 94% potency at 6–18 months after surgery.[38] This result has not been reproduced in other series.

32.6 Conclusions

At this moment, there are no prospective multicenter trials comparing laparoscopic and robotic radical prostatectomy. Results from surgical series have not demonstrated significant differences in operative outcomes, cancer control, or functional results between laparoscopic and robotic-assisted radical prostatectomy. However, results improve as surgeons complete their learning curves. Taking this into account, it is expected that surgeons at high volume centers, regardless of the technique, will attain the best results.

References

1. Bolenz C, Gupta A, Hotze T, et al. Cost comparison of robotic, laparoscopic, and open radical prostatectomy for prostate cancer. *Eur Urol.* 2010 Mar;57(3):453–458.

2. Guillonneau B, Vallancien G. Laparoscopic radical prostatectomy: the Montsouris experience. *J Urol.* 2000;163: 418–422.

3. Schuessler WW, Schulam PG, Clayman RV, Kavoussi LR. Laparoscopic radical prostatectomy: initial short-term experience. *Urology.* 1997;50(6):854–857.

4. Abbou CC, Salomon L. Hoznek, et al. Laparoscopic radical prostatectomy: preliminary results. *Urology.* 2000;55: 630–633.

5. Stolzenburg JU, Do M, Pfeiffer H, Konig F, Aedtner B, Dorschner W. The endoscopic extraperitoneal radical prostatectomy (EERPE): technique and initial experience. *World J Urol.* 2002;20:48–55.

6. Rassweiler J, Sentker L, Seeman O, Hatzinger M, Rumpelt HJ. Laparoscopic radical prostatectomy with the Heilbronn technique: an analysis of the first 180 cases. *J Urol.* 2001;166:2101–2108.

7. Eden CG, Neill MG, Louie-Johnsun MW . The first 1000 cases of laparoscopic radical prostatectomy in the UK: evidence of multiple 'learning curves'. *BJU Int.* 2009;103(9):1224–1230.

8. Fabrizio MD, Tüerk I, Shellhammer PF. Decreasing the learning curve using mentor initiated approach. *J Urol.* 2003;169:2063–2065.

9. Sterbis JR, Hanly EJ, Barry C, Herman BC, et al. Transcontinental telesurgical nephrectomy using the da Vinci robot in a porcine model. *Urology.* 2008;71(5): 971–973.

10. Ahlering TE, Skarecky D, Lee D, Clayman R. Successful transfer of open surgical skills to a laparoscopic environment using a robotic interface: initial experience with laparoscopic radical prostatectomy. *J Urol.* 2003;170:1738–1741.

11. Patel VR, Tully AS, Holmes R, Lindsay J. Robotic radical prostatectomy in the community setting-the learning curve and beyond: initial 200 cases. *J Urol.* 2005;174:269–272.

12. Menon M, Shrivastava A, Tewari A, et al. Laparoscopic and robot assisted radical prostatectomy: establishment of a structured program and preliminary analysis of outcomes. *J Urol.* 2002;168:945–949.

13. Gamboa AJ, Santos RT, Sargent ER, et al. Long-term impact of a robot assisted laparoscopic prostatectomy mini fellowship training program on postgraduate urological practice patterns. *J Urol.* 2009;181:778–782.

14. Herrell SD, Kwartowitz DM, Milhoua PM, Galloway RL. Toward image guided robotic surgery: system validation. *J Urol.* 2008;181:783–790.

15. Abbou CC, Hoznek A, Salomon L, et al. Laparoscopic radical prostatectomy with a remote controlled robot. *J Urol.* 2001;165:1964–1966.

16. Palmer KJ, Lowe GJ, Coughlin GD, Patil N, Patel VR. Launching a successful robotic surgery program. *J Endourol.* 2008;22(4):819–824.

17. Lotan Y, Cadeddu JA, Gettman MT. The new economics of radical prostatectomy: cost comparison of open, laparoscopic and robot assisted techniques. *J Urol.* 2004;172:1431–1435.

18. Scales CD, Jones PJ, Eisenstein EL, Preminger GM, Albala D. Local cost structures and the economics of robot assisted radical prostatectomy. *J Urol.* 2005;174:2323–2329.

19. Schroeck FR, Krupski TL, Sun L, et al. Satisfaction and regret after open retropubic or robotic-assisted laparoscopic radical prostatectomy. *Eur Urol.* 2008;54:785–793.

20. Ficarra V, Novara G, Artibani W, et al. Retropubic, laparoscopic, and robot-assisted radical prostatectomy: a systematic review and cumulative analysis of comparative studies. *Eur Urol.* 2009;55:1037–1063.

21. Menon M, Shrivastava A, Tewari A. Laparoscopic radical prostatectomy: conventional and robotic. *Urology.* 2005;66(suppl 5A):101–104.

22. Hu JC, Nelson RA, Wilson TG, et al. Perioperative complications of laparoscopic and robotic assisted laparoscopic radical prostatectomy. *J Urol.* 2006;175:541–546.

23. Rozet F, Jaffe J, Braud G, et al. A direct comparison of robotic assisted versus pure laparoscopic radical prostatectomy: a single institution experience. *J Urol.* 2007;178:478–482.

24. Menon M, Tewari A, Peabody J, et al. Vattikuti institute prostatectomy: technique. *J Urol.* 2003;169:2289–2292.

25. Joseph JV, Vicente I, Madeb R, Erturk E, Patel HRH. Robot-assisted versus pure laparoscopic radical prostatectomy: are there any differences? *BJU Int.* 2005;96(1): 39–42.

26. Guillonneau B, Vallencien G. Laparoscopic radical prostatectomy: the Montsouris technique. *J Urol.* 2000;163:1643–1649.

27. Bollens R, Vanden Bossche M, Roumeguere T, et al. Extraperitoneal laparoscopic radical prostatectomy: results after 50 cases. *Eur Urol.* 2001;40:65–69.

28. Gettman MT, Hoznek A, Salomon L, et al. Laparoscopic radical prostatectomy: description of the extraperitoneal approach using the da Vinci robotic system. *J Urol.* 2003;170:416–419.

29. Hu JC, Wang Q, Pashos CL, Lipsitz SR, Keating NL. Utilization and outcomes of minimally invasive radical prostatectomy. *J Clin Oncol.* 2008;26(14):2278–2284.

30. Ploussard G, Xylinas E, Salomon L, et al. Robot-assisted extraperitoneal laparoscopic radical prostatectomy: experience in a high-volume laparoscopy reference centre. *BJU Int.* 2009;105(8):1155–1160.

31. Atug F, Castle EP, Srivastav S, Burgess SV, Thomas R, Davis R. Positive surgical margins in robotic-assisted radical prostatectomy: impact of learning curve on oncologic outcomes. *Eur Urol.* 2006;49:866–872.

32. Berryhill R, Jhaveri J, Yadav R, et al. Robotic prostatectomy: a review of outcomes compared with laparoscopic and open approaches. *Urology.* 2008;72:15–23.

33. Ficarra V, Cavalleri S, Novara G, Aragona M, Artibani W. Evidence from robot-assisted laparoscopic radical

prostatectomy: a systematic review. *Eur Urol*. 2007;51: 45–56.

34. Murphy D, Kerger M, Crowe H, Peters JS, Costello AJ. Operative details and oncological and functional outcome of robotic assisted laparoscopic radical prostatectomy: 400 cases with a minimum of 12 months follow-up. *Eur Urol*. 2009;55:1358–1367.

35. Paul A, Ploussard G, Nicolaiew N, et al. Oncologic outcome after extraperitoneal laparoscopic radical prostatectomy: midterm follow-up of 1,115 procedures. *Eur Urol*. 2010 Feb;57(2):267–272.

36. Guillonneau B, El-Fettouh H, Baumert H, et al. Laparoscopic radical prostatectomy: oncological evaluation after 1,000 cases at Montsouris institute. *J Urol*. 2003;169:1261–1266.

37. Mottrie A, Van Migen P, De Naeyer G, Schatteman P, Carpentier P. Fonteyne. Robot-Assisted laparoscopic radical prostatectomy: oncologic and functional results of 184 cases. *Eur Urol*. 2007;52:746–751.

38. Menon M, Shrivastava A, Bhandari M, Satyanarayana R, Siva S, Agarwal PK. Vattikuti institute prostatectomy: technical modifications in 2009. *Eur Urol*. 2009;56:89–96.

Chapter 33

Complications of Robotic Prostatectomy

Sameer Siddiqui, Akshay Bhandari, and Mani Menon

33.1 Introduction

Prostate cancer is the most common solid organ malignancy in men in the United States. Over the past 80 years, the radical prostatectomy has been the most common form of surgical treatment for prostate cancer. The technique has evolved over time including the establishment of the retropubic approach, routine ligation of the dorsal venous complex, and the sparing of the neurovascular bundles. In the last 8 years, the single greatest paradigm shift in surgically treated prostate cancer occurred with the adaptation of the robotic-assisted radical prostatectomy. In 2008, over 70,000 robotic prostatectomies were performed worldwide (intuitive surgical). To date, no randomized trials have compared the robotic and open approach. However, there is growing body of data suggesting that robotic prostatectomies may be associated with lower complication rates. The complication rates of radical retropubic prostatectomy reported from centers of excellence are low and range from 6 to 10%.[1,2] However, data from the analysis of population-based registries suggest a complication rate of around 30% of which 20% are medical and 10% surgical.[3,4] A recent population-based analysis comparing minimally invasive and retropubic radical prostatectomy during 2003–2005 concluded that men undergoing minimally invasive prostatectomy when compared to retropubic radical prostatectomy experienced significantly fewer 30-day complications, blood transfusions, anastomotic strictures, and shorter length of stay.[5] Comparative studies have shown decreased postoperative pain scores with minimally invasive prostatectomy compared to open surgery.[6,7] Multiple studies have also consistently shown decreased blood loss compared to the open technique and shorter days of hospitalization.[7,8]

The goal of this chapter is to provide a broad overview of the etiology and management of surgical and medical complications after robotic prostatectomy. The Vattikuti Urology Institute (VUI) has performed over 4,200 robotic prostatectomies as of this writing. Given this large body of experience, a significant portion of this chapter is based on our accumulated knowledge in managing complications from robotic prostatectomies.[7,9,10]

We started our robotic prostatectomy program in 2001 and have performed over 4,200 robotic prostatectomies as of this writing. Over this time period, our technique has undergone several modifications.[11–15] In the past we have published our complication rates for over 1,200 patients.[7,9,10] Although there have been some recent reports of complications from robotic prostatectomy, the overall literature addressing the complications of robotic prostatectomy is sparse. We currently hold the largest series of robotic prostatectomy and have therefore drawn heavily upon our own experience in preparing this chapter.

33.2 Technique of Vattikuti Institute Prostatectomy (VIP)

The VIP technique has undergone several modifications over the years.[11–13,15,16] In contrast to the

S. Siddiqui (✉)
Vattikuti Urology Institute, Henry Ford Health System, Detroit, MI, USA
e-mail: sameersiddiqui10@gmail.com

A.K. Hemal, M. Menon (eds.), *Robotics in Genitourinary Surgery*,
DOI 10.1007/978-1-84882-114-9_33, © Springer-Verlag London Limited 2011

Montsouris technique,[17] we approach the bladder neck via the antegrade approach. Earlier in our experience, we switched to a running urethrovesical anastomosis using a double-armed suture. In addition, we have abandoned bulk ligation of dorsal venous complex in favor of precise suturing of individual veins after urethral transection. We have also described the lateral prostatic fascia nerve-sparing technique (veil of Aphrodite).[12] Other modifications include endopelvic fascia sparing, extended pelvic lymph node dissection to include hypogastric nodes, two-layer anastomosis,[18] and, most recently, catheterless urethrovesical anastomosis.[13]

33.2.1 Patient Selection

We do not have specific exclusion criteria. Any patient who is a candidate for radical retropubic prostatectomy is considered a candidate for VIP. Relative contraindications for this procedure are the same as those for laparoscopy. These include advanced obstructive lung disease, abnormalities of cardiac output, and significant prior abdominal surgeries. That having said, 30% of the patients who presented to us for robotic prostatectomy had a history of prior abdominal or inguinal surgery.

33.2.2 Patient Positioning and Port Placement

Patient is placed in lithotomy position with the help of stirrups. Pressure points are carefully padded with foam pads. Patient is secured to the table with heavy tape and the table is then moved to a steep Trendelenburg position. Pneumoperitoneum is then established using a Veress needle. Ports are placed under direct vision. The abdomen is transilluminated in a dark room to outline abdominal vessels during port placement. We use a standard six-port technique.

33.2.3 Developing of the Extraperitoneal Space

Using a 30° angled up lens, a transverse peritoneal incision is made extending from one medial umbilical ligament to the other. The incision is extended in an inverted U to the level of the vasa on either side. The space of Retzius is entered through the areolar tissue anterior to the bladder.

33.2.4 Lymph Node Dissection

The extent of the lymph node dissection earlier on in our experience included the external iliac and obturator lymph nodes. However, we now routinely include the internal iliac nodes, overlying the hypogastric vein. This dissection is typically carried out caudal to the origin of the obliterated umbilical artery so as to avoid injury to the ureter.

33.2.5 Bladder Neck Transection and Posterior Dissection

We approach the bladder neck directly without opening the endopelvic fascia or ligating the dorsal vein complex. The Foley balloon is deflated while keeping it in the bladder. The anterior bladder wall is grasped in the midline by the assistant and lifted directly toward the ceiling. This simple maneuver aids in clearly identifying the bladder neck. A 1 cm incision is made in the anterior bladder neck in the midline to expose the Foley catheter. The left-sided assistant then grasps the tip of the Foley catheter with firm anterior traction, thus exposing the posterior bladder neck, which is then incised.

The posterior bladder neck is then dissected away from the prostate and the fascial layer anterior to the vasa and seminal vesicles is incised, thus exposing the vasa and seminal vesicles. The vasa are then dissected and transected and the distal end is held by the left assistant whereas the proximal end is held by the right assistant to provide the necessary exposure and counter-traction. The artery to the seminal vesicles is then controlled using clips or fine coagulation and the seminal vesicles are dissected away. This exposes the Denonvilliers' fascia, which is carefully incised, and a plane is developed between the prostate and the perirectal fat. This dissection is carried down to the apex of the prostate and laterally to the pedicles of the prostate.

Next, the seminal vesicle is retracted superome-dially by the contralateral assistant and the pedicle is placed on traction. The pedicles are controlled by either clipping or coagulating the vessels individually by bipolar coagulation.

33.2.6 Nerve Sparing

For standard nerve sparing, the major neurovascu-lar bundles that run posterolaterally are preserved in the usual fashion. Minimal bipolar coagulation or no cautery is used for this step. If a more extensive nerve sparing is planned, the prostatic fascia is incised ante-riorly to create the "veil of Aphrodite" that has also been described as "high anterior release"[19] or "curtain dissection"[20] by others. For this, the avascular plane between the prostatic fascia and the prostate is entered deep to the venous sinuses of the Santorini plexus.

33.2.7 Apical Dissection and Urethral Transection

Prior to performing apical dissection, we ensure that the Foley catheter is within the prostatic urethra. With the assistant firmly retracting the prostate toward the patients head, the dorsal venous complex is transected without bulk ligation. It is important not to skeletonize the urethra as minimal manipulation hastens return of continence. The urethra is transected using a cold

scissors about 5 mm distal to the prostatic notch and the free specimen is placed in a bag.

The dorsal venous complex is then controlled with a running 2-0 braided polyglactin suture on a 17 mm tapered needle. Pneumoperitoneum is lowered and per-ineal pressure is applied by the assistant to ensure good control of the dorsal venous complex as increased abdominal pressure may falsely mask any open venous sinuses.

33.2.8 Urethrovesical Anastomosis

We routinely perform a two-layer anastomosis. For this two, 3-zero double-armed monofilament sutures are used. The first suture of the outer layer is passed through the Denonvilliers' fascia and then through the posterior rhabdosphincter. After four passes from right to left which creates a posterior plate (Fig. 33.1a) the suture is then locked and its one end is held gently by an assistant.

Using the other double-armed suture the ure-throvesical anastomosis (inner layer) is then per-formed. The first suture is passed outside-in on the posterior bladder wall at the 4 o'clock position, contin-uing into the urethra at the corresponding site inside-out. After three passes in the bladder neck and two in the urethra the bladder is then cinched down to the urethra gently. After a few more throws, the direction of the stitch is then changed such that the passage is now inside-out on the bladder neck and outside-in on the urethra. The suture is then run clockwise to the 11 o'clock position. Next, the other end of the suture is

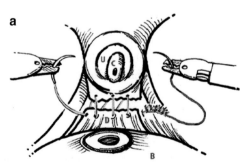
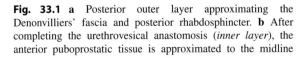
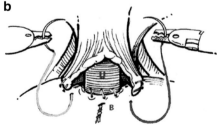

Fig. 33.1 a Posterior outer layer approximating the Denonvilliers' fascia and posterior rhabdosphincter. **b** After completing the urethrovesical anastomosis (*inner layer*), the anterior puboprostatic tissue is approximated to the midline bladder tissue to complete the anterior pubovesical collar recon-struction. B, bladder. C, Foley catheter. D, Denonvilliers' fascia. U, urethra

run in a counterclockwise fashion from the 4 o'clock position to the 11 o'clock position starting inside-out on the bladder and outside-in on the urethra. Both ends of the suture are then tied to each other to complete the inner layer of the anastomosis. A fresh 20 Fr Foley catheter is placed by the assistant and the integrity of the anastomosis tested by instilling 250 cc of saline.

Finally the outer layer is completed by suturing the puboprostatic ligament to the anterior pubovesical collar (Fig. 33.1b).

33.2.9 Suprapubic Catheter Placement

Under robotic visualization of the anterior abdominal wall, a 14 Fr Rutner (Bard Medical, Covington, GA) suprapubic catheter is percutaneously placed in the midline approximately one-third of the distance from the umbilicus to the pubic symphysis by the bedside assistant. Before placement in the bladder, the bedside assistant inserts a 2-0 nonabsorbable polypropylene suture on a straight needle through the skin and abdominal wall adjacent to the suprapubic catheter. The console surgeon grasps the needle and places a full-thickness horizontal mattress suture through the anterior bladder wall. The needle is then passed back through the anterior abdominal wall approximately 1 cm lateral to the initial needle puncture where it is grasped by the bedside assistant once it is through the skin. With the robotic surgeon maintaining tension on the suture, the anterior bladder wall is lifted and the bedside assistant places the suprapubic catheter (Fig. 33.2). Prompt drainage of irrigation fluid confirms proper placement of the catheter. The catheter balloon is then instilled with 4 cc sterile water. Once

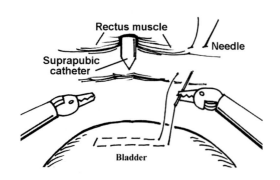

Fig. 33.2 Suprapubic catheter placement

the specimen is extracted and pneumoperitoneum is no longer present, the external suture is tied onto the skin with the help of a button, thereby anchoring the anterior bladder wall to the anterior abdominal wall. The Foley catheter is plugged and the suprapubic catheter is connected to gravity drainage.

33.2.10 Specimen Retrieval

A Jackson-Pratt drain is only placed if there is a persistent anastomotic leak. This is passed through the left assistant port in the iliac fossa and secured on the outside with a #3-0 nylon suture. The specimen that is already placed in an endobag is removed by enlarging the umbilical port incision as required. The fascia is closed with interrupted #1 polyester suture and the skin is closed with subcuticular sutures.

33.2.11 Postoperative Care

Patients receive a liter bolus in the recovery room. Intravenous ketorolac and oral acetaminophen with codeine are used for pain control. Antibiotics are only used perioperatively for 24 h. In the past, we had routinely used 5,000 units of unfractionated subcutaneous heparin every 8 h along with sequential compression devices for thromboembolic prophylaxis in the immediate postoperative period. However, in compliance with the recent DVT guidelines (reference) we now use heparin only in patients that are high risk for developing postoperative DVT/PE. Early ambulation is the key to minimizing thromboembolic episodes and is a major component of our postoperative pathway. Patients are encouraged to ambulate within 6 h of surgery.

Clear liquid diet is started on the day of surgery and advanced to a surgical diet on postoperative day 1 if patients tolerate clear liquids. In patients with suprapubic catheters, the urethral Foley is removed on postoperative day 1 as long as the urine is clear and draining well. Routine postoperative hematocrit is not drawn. Patients are discharged home with a catheter and follow-up in 7 days for a catheter removal under cystographic control. Patients with a suprapubic catheter are asked to clamp the catheter starting on postoperative day 5 and are asked to record postvoid residual volumes.

33.3 Data Collection

We used hospital claims data to analyze complications in all 4,000 patients undergoing VIP at our institute from 2001 to 2008. Data were cross-validated with a prospectively collected database as well as our monthly mortality and morbidity data. Preoperative and intraoperative patient data were also obtained from our database. Complications are graded into four groups using the original Clavien classification system[21] (Table 33.1). We also sub-categorized complications broadly into medical and surgical complications. In the following section, we discuss these complications in detail. The numbers in parentheses after each

Table 33.1 Complications of robotic prostatectomy using the original Clavien classification system

Complications	N (%)
Clavien grade I	151 (3.8)
Surgical	
Retention	59 (1.5)
CT-guided drainage	34 (0.9)
Ileus	29 (0.7)
Rectal injury	14 (0.4)
Other surgical	2 (<0.1)
Medical	
Neutropenia, arrhythmia, pneumonia	13 (0.3)
Clavien grade II	30 (0.8)
Surgical	
Re-exploration	22 (0.6)
Robotic	10 (0.3)
Open	*12 (0.3)*
Other surgical	5 (0.1)
Medical	
Respiratory distress	3 (<0.1)
Clavien grade III	17 (0.4)
Surgical	
Bowel injury	6 (0.1)
Recto-urethral fistula	1 (<0.1)
Medical	
Thromboembolic, cardiac	10 (0.3)
Clavien grade IV	1 (<0.1)
Total complications	199 (5)

complication represent the complications that we have had in our series of 4,000 patients.

33.4 Complications

33.4.1 Anesthesia-Related Complications (<0.1%)

While some anesthetic complications are common for both minimally invasive surgery and open surgery, others are unique to minimally invasive surgery. Most of these complications are related to insufflation of abdomen with carbon dioxide and the subsequent rise in intra-abdominal pressure.

Sinus bradycardia is frequently observed and is attributed multiple factors including insufflation with carbon dioxide, increased vagal response from stretching of the peritoneal structures, steep Trendelenburg position, and hypercapnia. This is usually managed successfully by promptly administering atropine, desufflating the abdomen, and reversing the Trendelenburg position. If not managed appropriately and in a timely manner asystolic cardiac arrest may develop. We report one such case where we had to abort a procedure due to asystole. Patient was appropriately resuscitated and underwent an uneventful procedure at a later date after undergoing a thorough cardiac evaluation.

Increased intra-abdominal pressure causes an increase in intra-thoracic pressure and increase in both pulmonary and systemic vascular resistance. This causes increased blood pressure and decreased cardiac output, which may be significant in patients with borderline cardiac output at baseline.

Fluid management can be very challenging in these patients due to inability to accurately measure urine output. Overhydration causes increased urine output that can obscure the operative field and make the anastomosis very challenging. Fluid overload in a steep Trendelenburg position can also cause significant facial edema, specifically early in the learning curve when operative times are in excess of 3 h. We typically prefer to limit intravenous fluids to less than 1,000 cc for the entire case till the point of anastomosis. We report one case of severe bronchial edema requiring emergent re-intubation.

We have experienced once the case of severe ana-phylaxis presumably from latex in a patient with no known allergies. We also report a case of infiltration of intravenous fluids into subcutaneous tissue lead-ing to significant swelling of the forearm. To prevent this complication, the bedside surgeon should ensure proper functioning of the intravenous line after the arms are tucked to the patient's side and secured, as it can be a challenge to troubleshoot once the patient is draped and the robot is docked.

Corneal abrasions are not an uncommon complica-tion and although not associated with any long-term sequelae in our experience can be a cause of signif-icant pain and discomfort in the immediate postop-erative period. Most cases are due to lagophthalmos (failure of eyelids to close) that leads to drying of the cornea. We have virtually eliminated this com-plication by carefully covering the eyes with an eye patch.

33.4.2 Non-vascular Access-Related Complications (0.1%)

Most of the access-related complications are the same for any laparoscopic procedure. These could range from minor bleeding to major vascular or visceral catastrophe. In a large study, Chandler et al.[22] reported that most of the access-related complications occur at the time of initial access and that 75% of these involved puncture to the bowel or retroperitoneal vessels. It cannot be adequately stressed that basic laparoscopic skills are an essential requirement prior to establish-ing a successful robotic prostatectomy program. At our institution we use the closed technique of establishing access, wherein a Veress needle is used to puncture the peritoneal cavity blindly followed by insufflation of carbon dioxide. Thereafter, the first trocar is intro-duced blindly into the peritoneal cavity. The camera is introduced through this trocar and subsequent tro-cars are placed under vision. Proponents of the open technique described by Hasson[23] consider it to be safer than the closed technique; however, there to our knowl-edge there are no studies that have confirmed this claim. Another alternative is to use an optical trocar to enter the abdomen under direct view.[24] In patients with significant abdominal surgeries we sometimes use a hybrid technique, wherein the Veress needle is used to establish pneumoperitoneum following which

a 5 mm optical trocar with a 0° lens is used to enter the abdomen under direct vision. In the end the surgeon should use the technique he/she is comfortable with.

33.4.2.1 Subcutaneous Emphysema and Air Embolism (0%)

Subcutaneous emphysema could be caused by improper placement of Veress needle or due to leakage of carbon dioxide around ports when the incisions are too large. Murdock et al.[25] reported that longer operative times and greater number of ports predispose to subcutaneous emphysema. While subcutaneous emphysema mostly involves a limited area and is largely inconsequential, rarely it can track all the way up to the neck and severely compromise oxygenation. Its incidence can be minimized by limiting the incision to the size of the port and also by avoiding multiple passes through the peritoneum while placing ports. Once discovered, it can be managed by placing a purse-string suture around the leaking port and by decreasing the intra-abdominal pressure. In our experience subcutaneous emphysema is an uncommon problem and has not yet been associated with any adverse event.

Carbon dioxide embolism is another rare but lethal complication of laparoscopy. When encountered, it is invariably caused by insufflation through a Veress nee-dle that has punctured a blood vessel or organ.[26,27] It is best avoided by simply confirming proper place-ment of the Veress needle prior to insufflation. This can be done using a syringe half filled with saline. The syringe is first aspirated and then saline injected and the water column is observed. If blood is aspirated or if the column does not drop freely, the needle should be repositioned. Carbon dioxide embolism results in sud-den onset bradycardia and hypotension. It manifests as an abrupt decline in oxygen saturation and a sud-den increase in end-tidal carbon dioxide followed by a rapid decrease. Management is immediate desuffla-tion of peritoneum, turning the patient to a left lateral decubitus while still in Trendelenburg position and hyperventilation with 100% oxygen.

33.4.2.2 Visceral Injury (0.1%)

Both solid and hollow visceral organs can be poten-tially injured during insertion of Veress needle or placement of trocars. Bowel injuries can be associated with a significant morbidity as well as mortality. In a large review carried out by van der Voort et al.[28] the incidence of laparoscopy bowel perforation was about 0.4%. Small bowel injuries were most frequent. A trocar or Veress needle caused most of the bowel injuries (42%). Approximately 70% of laparoscopy-induced bowel injuries were seen in patients with adhesions or previous laparotomy. While 67% of the bowel injuries were recognized within 24 h of surgery, the mortality rate associated with laparoscopy-induced bowel injury was almost 4%.

Of the six bowel injuries recorded in our cohort, four patients had a history of prior abdominal surgery requiring extensive lysis of adhesions. The other two were probably the result of instrument passage. However, approximately 30% of our patients had previous abdominal or inguinal surgery and the overall incidence of iatrogenic bowel injury in this cohort was about 0.2%. Proper patient selection is the key to establishing a successful minimally invasive program and it may be advisable to restrict robotic prostatectomy to patients who have not had prior abdominal surgery, during the learning phase. An extraperitoneal or perineal approach may be indicated in these patients. We have rarely performed adhesiolysis through a minilaparotomy in some of these patients. The robot is then docked after open port placement and the prostatectomy completed.

Injury to solid organs is uncommon. We report one case of renal hematoma from puncture of a pelvic kidney with a Veress needle. A small renal hematoma was noted, which was observed for sometime intraoperatively. It was stable and we therefore proceeded with the prostatectomy. Barring gross hematuria, there were no adverse sequelae.

Other potential organs that can be injured are the urinary bladder and stomach. Placing a Foley catheter and oro-gastric tube in all patients, prior to insertion of the Veress needle, may reduce the risk of occurrence of these injuries.

33.4.3 Vascular Complications (<0.1%)

33.4.3.1 Access Related (<0.1%)

The incidence of access-related vascular injuries reported in the laparoscopic literature is low, ranging from 0.03 to 0.2%.[29–31] Like visceral injuries, majority of access-related vascular injuries are caused either by the first trocar or by the Veress needle.[32,33] In fact Champault et al. reported that 83% of the serious vascular injuries occur during the placement of the first trocar.[34] The aorta and common iliac vessels are most frequently injured. It is generally recommended that the access phase of laparoscopy be performed with the patient lying level, without any Trendelenburg tilt. Trendelenburg rotates the sacral promontory and brings the aortic bifurcation close to the umbilicus, thus increasing the chances of vascular injury.[35] Also, intra-abdominal pressure rather than volume of carbon dioxide insufflated should be used as a guide to determine when to place the primary trocar. We insufflate the abdomen to 20 mmHg for port placement and then decrease the intra-abdominal pressure to 15 mmHg. We have thus far encountered one major vascular injury during access resulting in a contained, non-expanding retroperitoneal hematoma. The procedure was aborted, patient was managed conservatively, and the robotic prostatectomy was completed on a later date.

Injury to accessory abdominal vessels, such as inferior epigastric artery and vein, can occur during secondary port placement. Chandler et al. reported that injury during secondary port placement was to abdominal wall vessels in 35% of the cases and to the aorta or iliac artery in 30% of cases.[22] We recommend port placement under proper transillumination in a dark room to prevent injury to these accessory abdominal vessels. It is also recommended that all ports be removed under direct vision at the conclusion of the procedure and the port sites observed for arterial bleeders. If discovered, cauterizing these bleeders alone is usually insufficient. A figure-of-eight suture should be placed for adequate control.

33.4.3.2 Access Unrelated (<0.1%)

Majority of vascular injuries in radical prostatectomy occur during pelvic lymphadenectomy.[36,37] Commonly injured vessels are the external iliac and the obturator. As described in our technique, we routinely perform an extended node dissection to include the internal iliac group of lymph nodes and this puts the hypogastric vein at risk of injury. While we have never experienced any vascular injury as a direct cause of surgical dissection, we have had to explore one patient for bleeding from an accessory obturator artery presumably from an injury caused by a suture needle. The stereotactic vision and precision of the robotic instruments along with motion scaling help in preventing inadvertent movements. There is obviously no substitute for a thorough knowledge of vascular anatomy of the pelvis.

33.4.4 Rectal Injury (0.3%)

The reported rate for rectal injury in laparoscopic prostatectomy is 1–3.3%.[38–43] We report an incidence of about 0.3%, Patel et al.[44] reported an incidence of 0.1% in 1,800 patients, and Fischer et al.[45] reported an incidence of 1% in 210 patients undergoing robotic prostatectomy.

In our experience most of the rectal injuries occurred posterolaterally, close to the apex. Majority of these patients had aggressive apical cancer and were undergoing a planned wide excision. All rectal injuries were identified intraoperatively and repaired primarily in two layers, an inner mucosal and outer seromuscular with a running #3-0 polyglactin suture. Anal dilation is performed in all patients. Patients were kept on a clear liquid diet for 72 h and received broad-spectrum antibiotic coverage postoperatively.

Ten of the 11 patients were discharged home within 72 h with no complications. However, one patient developed a recto-vesical fistula that needed a diverting colostomy followed by delayed repair of fistula. This patient had locally extensive carcinoma and gross fecal spillage was noted at the time of injury. In patients with aggressive local disease we now routinely order a complete bowel preparation preoperatively.

33.4.5 Ureteral Injury (<0.1)

This is a rare complication but often missed intraoperatively. It can happen during extended lymphadenectomy and during posterior dissection. We have encountered two ureteral injuries thus far. One of these was presumably during extended pelvic lymphadenectomy during a salvage prostatectomy. The other occurred in a patient with prior inguinal hernia repair with mesh which resulted in a distorted anatomy. Both these injuries were missed intraoperatively and required delayed exploration and repair. The first patient underwent a transureteroureterostomy and the other was managed with a psoas hitch combined with a Boari flap. Hu et al. reported 1 ureteral injury in 322 patients undergoing robotic prostatectomy.[46] Several large open prostatectomy series have also reported a very low incidence of ureteral injury.[1,47]

We also report one case of obstruction of the ureteral orifice during urethrovesical anastomosis. Patient was explored the next day with robotic assistance. The anastomosis was taken down and it was discovered that he had a complete duplication on one side and the ectopic ureteral orifice was incorporated within the anastomosis. While we do not routinely use indigo carmine or methylene blue, some authors have found it helpful to locate the ureteral orifices. The ureteral orifices can be very close to the bladder neck in patients with large median lobes and the urethrovesical anastomosis should be performed using utmost care in these patients. We recommend the use of a small needle such as a 17 mm, $\frac{1}{2}$ circle tapered needle for anastomosis.

33.4.6 Postoperative Anemia and Blood Transfusion (1.9%)

Blood loss in minimally invasive prostatectomy is significantly lower than with open prostatectomy. Available robotic series report a mean blood loss in the range of 100–300 cc and a transfusion rate in the range of 0.3–2%.[45,48–50] Our mean blood loss is about 140 cc and transfusion rate is 1.9%. Only one patient had required intraoperative blood transfusion in our series.

The lower blood loss associated with robotic prostatectomy could be attributed to pneumoperitoneum and the superior vision and high magnification of the endoscopes. The dorsal vein complex can often be a source of troublesome bleeding. As our technique has evolved, we have abandoned bulk ligation of the dorsal venous complex in favor of precise suturing of individual veins after urethral transection. It is helpful to lower the intra-abdominal pressure and apply perineal pressure to identify all bleeding sinuses.

Meticulous hemostasis is also required during dissection of the pedicle and neurovascular bundles. In our experience patients undergoing a more aggressive nerve sparing such as the "veil of Aphrodite" experience a higher blood loss as thermal coagulation is used very sparingly. For this, the plane of dissection is between the prostatic capsule and the prostatic fascia which contains several venous sinuses. If these vessels are not carefully controlled then often result is troublesome pelvic hematomas that can jeopardize the urethrovesical anastomosis.

Patients on anticoagulation with warfarin often pose a unique set of challenges. We analyzed our data on patients with chronic anticoagulation undergoing robotic prostatectomy and found that patients on perioperative bridging therapy with subcutaneous low molecular weight heparin had a significantly higher transfusion rate (23 vs 2%) than patients not on perioperative bridging therapy.[51] However, this did not translate into increased complications or readmissions.

In general, patients on anticoagulation or antiplatelet agents, those with bleeding diatheses, large prostate volumes (>100 cc), and those who undergo a very aggressive nerve sparing or wide excision are at a higher risk of developing complications from bleeding postoperatively. A cystogram should be routinely performed in such patients. A sausage-shaped bladder is usually seen in patients who develop a large pelvic hematoma. These patients can sometimes develop a delayed leak. Therefore, our practice is to keep a Foley catheter in place for a minimum of 2 weeks in these patients. An organized pelvic hematoma can cause partial or complete disruption of the urethrovesical anastomosis. We have seen this in three patients, who were explored robotically. The anastomosis was completely taken down, clots were evacuated, and anastomosis was re-done.

33.4.6.1 Management of Acute Postoperative Hemorrhage After Robotic Prostatectomy

Acute post-surgical hemorrhage is a rare but life-threatening complication of radical prostatectomy and in many cases may require re-operation. Acute postoperative hemorrhage is defined as bleeding in the postoperative period requiring blood transfusions to maintain hemodynamic stability or severe bleeding necessitating immediate surgical exploration. We have explored 10 patients thus far for acute postoperative hemorrhage. Of these, seven patients were explored minimally invasively with robotic assistance and the other three underwent open exploration. We were able to identify a clear source of bleeding in six of the seven patients who underwent robotic exploration. Of these, three were in the pelvis and three were rectus sheath hematomas. Overall, the median hospitalization for patients that underwent robotic exploration was 3 days and these patients did better than those that underwent open exploration. Based on our experience, we have developed an algorithm for the management of postoperative hypotension following robotic prostatectomy (Fig. 33.3).

33.4.7 Urinary Ascites (0.7%)

This is perhaps one of the most disturbing complications in our series. Urinary ascites leads to chemical peritonitis and resulting ileus. These patients usually present with severe abdominal pain and distension, closely mimicking acute abdomen from bowel injury. The differentiation between a urinary leak and bowel injury is critical, as the management is vastly different. Patients with urinary ascites usually have an elevated serum creatinine secondary to urinary absorption and cystographic evidence of a urinary leak. While cystographic leaks are common with open approach, they seldom cause symptoms as they are extraperitoneal. A CT cystogram should be obtained emergently in these patients and any fluid collection should be drained percutaneously under CT or ultrasound guidance. Patients with urinary peritonitis appear desperately ill, but recover dramatically with drainage. If the patient does not improve immediately, he should be re-imaged and if needed, re-drained. On the contrary patients with unrecognized bowel injury are desperately ill and will not recover unless the injury is repaired. Figure 33.4 shows our algorithm of managing patients with unexplained postoperative pain that lasts >48 h.

Nine of the 26 patients (35%), who presented with urinary ascites, also required blood transfusions and had large pelvic hematomas on imaging. Pelvic hematomas tend to organize and distract the

Fig. 33.3 Algorithm of
management of postoperative
hypotension following robotic
prostatectomy

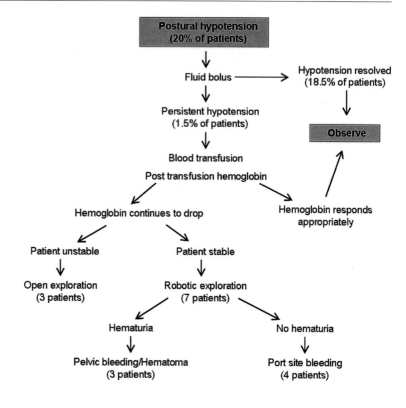

Fig. 33.4 Algorithm of
managing patients with
unexplained postoperative
pain lasting >48 h following
robotic prostatectomy

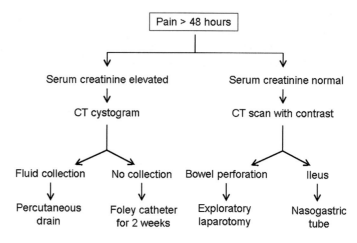

anastomosis. Thus some of these patients may have a normal initial cystogram and then present later with a delayed leak on repeat cystogram.

We adopted the two-layer anastomosis in an attempt to improve early continence but found no improvement in our hands.[18] However, we continue to perform a two-layer anastomosis as we have observed a lower incidence of cystographic leaks in these patients. We attribute this difference to better hemostasis and therefore fewer pelvic hematomas. Whether this will ultimately decrease the incidence of urinary ascites requiring CT-guided drainage is yet to be seen.

33.4.8 Postoperative Ileus (0.7%)

Certain patients present with typical postoperative ileus that is unrelated to urinary ascites. Etiologies include bleeding or peritoneal irritation from carbon dioxide. The patients are best managed with bowel rest and sometimes may require placement of a nasogastric tube until bowel function returns.

33.4.9 Bowel Complications (0.2%)

These include bowel injuries unrelated to access, incisional, and port site hernias and incarcerated hernias. Bowel can be injured during instrument passage by the bedside assistants. We report two such cases in our series. We also report three cases of incisional hernia. At the end of the procedure we extract the specimen through a vertical midline or paramedian incision. The fascia is then closed with interrupted #1 polyester suture. Using meticulous technique and taking adequate fascial bites, wound dehiscence can be minimized; however, one patient was on chronic steroids and had very weak fascia. His closure broke down twice and he ultimately required definitive closure with a dermal graft. The other two were not associated with any identifiable risk factors and were probably purely technical.

Port site hernias are a rare occurrence after laparoscopy. It is felt that port site hernia in adults is usually confined to port sizes >10 mm. We use dilating trocars as these are associated with a lower incidence of bleeding as well as port site hernias.[52] Two 12 mm ports are used. One port is placed periumbilically and the second one is placed in the right anterior to midaxillary line, slightly above the iliac crest. While the periumbilical port site is extended to for specimen extraction and its fascia then closed, we do not routinely close fascia on the other 12 mm port site given its location. We have encountered two port site hernias thus far and both of these were at the 8 mm robotic trocar sites.

Up to 5% of our patients have an incidental inguinal hernia that is discovered during robotic prostatectomy. Early in our experience we were not very compulsive in repairing these hernias. However, we have had two patients who presented with incarcerated inguinal hernia within a week from their robotic prostatectomy. Because of this, we have now changed our practice and are more aggressive in repairing these inguinal hernias with a simple plug and a mesh. This can be done relatively easily with the robot and it only adds 5 min to the operating time. Other robotic series have reported a 0.6–1% incidence of incisional/incarcerated hernias.[45,48]

Early recognition of bowel complications is particularly important as patients with laparoscopic bowel injuries or hernias will present with atypical signs and symptoms. Bishoff et al.[53] reported their experience with laparoscopic bowel injuries and found that majority of injuries (69%) were unrecognized intraoperatively. They also observed that interestingly majority of these patients initially presented with leukopenia rather than leukocytosis. A high index of suspicion is needed to diagnose this entity as patients may rapidly deteriorate due to overwhelming sepsis.

33.4.10 Lymphocele (0.2%)

This is a rare complication in our series. While only eight patients presented with symptomatic lymphocele requiring percutaneous drainage, the incidence of asymptomatic lymphoceles is probably greater. We attribute this low incidence to the transperitoneal nature of our procedure. In general, extended lymph node dissection and an extraperitoneal approach are associated with a higher incidence of lymphocele formation. Incidence of lymphocele causing deep venous thrombosis is also higher with extraperitoneal approach. Feicke et al. reported a 5% incidence of symptomatic lymphocele in 99 patients undergoing extended pelvic lymphadenectomy during robotic prostatectomy.[54] We occasionally observe lower extremity lymphedema in patients undergoing pelvic lymphadenectomy; however, it is a transient occurrence and usually resolves within 4–6 weeks.

33.4.11 Urinary Retention (1.5%)

Early in our experience, we were removing Foley catheters at 1–4 days postoperatively and experienced a high incidence of urinary retention (4.7%). While the anastomosis is watertight, there is significant edema at the urethrovesical anastomosis for the first few days. We have since modified our pathway and now leave catheters in for an average of 7 days. With this, we have noticed a significant decrease in urinary retention to 0.9%. Patel et al. report a retention rate of 0.4% in 1,800 patients.[44]

When patients present with urinary retention, a well-lubricated Coudé tip catheter is passed gently into the bladder. In certain cases an assistant could place a gloved finger in the rectum to support the urethrovesical anastomosis. If there is any suspicion about proper placement of the catheter, we recommend obtaining a limited cystogram to confirm location of the catheter. A flexible cystoscopy followed by passage of a guidewire may be used only as a second resort.

33.4.12 Medical Complications (0.5%)

In a population-based analysis comparing minimally invasive radical prostatectomy with radical retropubic prostatectomy, Hu et al.[5] reported that incidence of cardiac (1 vs 1.7%), respiratory (2.5 vs 4.6%), and other medical complications (4.8 vs 5.6%) was significantly lower for minimally invasive prostatectomy. Our results confirm these findings. Fourteen patients in our series had a major medical complication such as deep venous thrombosis or pulmonary embolism (seven patients), stroke (one patient), myocardial infarction (three patients), and respiratory (three patients). There were six minor medical complications. Other robotic prostatectomy series also report a similar low incidence of medical complications.[44]

We attribute this low incidence of medical complications to several factors:

1. The average time to ambulation in patients undergoing minimally invasive prostatectomy is significantly less than open prostatectomy. In fact majority of our patients are ambulating within 6 h of their surgery.
2. As previously described, due to the transperitoneal nature of our technique the incidence is significant lymphoceles and thus deep venous thrombosis and pulmonary embolism are very low.
3. The minimal blood loss associated with minimally invasive prostatectomy leads to less fluid electrolyte imbalance and therefore a low incidence of other medical complications such as cardiac arrhythmias.
4. Short operative times.
5. Decreased tissue trauma. A recent study from Fracalanza et al. demonstrated that markers for an acute phase reaction including IL-6, C-reactive protein, and serum lactate were higher in patients undergoing open prostatectomy vs the robotic

approach, supporting the notion that open surgery was associated with significantly more tissue trauma.[55]

We have experienced one death, presumably from a massive myocardial infarction on postoperative day 21.

33.5 Delayed Complications

The incidence of bladder neck contracture after robotic prostatectomy is low and is in the range of 0.1–1%.[44,45,50] The two most common delayed complications of radical prostatectomy are urinary incontinence and impotence. We have published outcomes of over 2,500 patients undergoing Vattikuti Institute Prostatectomy.[11,15]

33.5.1 Continence

At 12-month follow-up, 84% of the patients had total urinary control and 8% used a liner for security reasons or for occasional stress incontinence. About 95.2% of the patients were socially dry (≤1 pad/day) at 12 months and 23.7% of the patients reported having complete continence (0 pads) immediately after catheter removal; 50% of the patients reported continence within 4 weeks and 90% of the patients were continent at 3 months. In our analysis <1% of the patients were completely incontinent. Other robotic series have confirmed similar results.[49,50,56] While the overall continence rates at 12 months are comparable to those of open radical prostatectomy,[57,58] the median time to continence appears to be shorter for robotic prostatectomy. While there have been some recent reports of improvement in early continence by restoring Denonvilliers' fascia,[59–61] we found no such improvement in early continence rates in a randomized trial.[18] In our experience, early continence rates were high in both groups.

33.5.2 Potency

Potency rates were best in patients undergoing bilateral extended nerve sparing ("veil of Aphrodite"). We use the sexual health inventory for men (SHIM) questionnaire to measure sexual function. In patients with no preoperative erectile dysfunction (defined as

SHIM score >21) undergoing bilateral veil nerve sparing, intercourse was reported in 93% of the patients; however, only 73% of the patients reported return to baseline. In comparison, in patients with no preoperative erectile dysfunction undergoing bilateral standard nerve sparing, intercourse was reported in only 68% of the patients and only 39% of the patients reported return to baseline.[15] Other robotic series have reported overall potency at 12 months in the range of 70–80%.[50,56,62]

33.6 Conclusion

Robotic radical prostatectomy is a safe procedure with less blood loss and is associated with a low medical as well as surgical complication rate. Yet, it is still a major procedure with potentially major complications that require prompt diagnosis and management. Persistent pain after 48 h is the harbinger of a potential problem and warrants aggressive investigation. Patients who develop urinary peritonitis after a transperitoneal prostatectomy may present with acute abdomen and should be treated with percutaneous drainage: others should be explored to rule out a bowel injury. Patients with acute postoperative hemorrhage after robotic prostatectomy do well with prompt exploration using robotic or minimally invasive techniques where possible. Like any major procedure, certain complications of robotic prostatectomy can be minimized by proper patient selection and meticulous surgical technique.

References

1. Catalona WJ, et al. Potency, continence and complication rates in 1,870 consecutive radical retropubic prostatectomies. *J Urol.* 1999;162(2):433–438.
2. Lepor H, Nieder AM, Ferrandino MN. *Intraoperative and postoperative complications of radical retropubic prostatectomy in a consecutive series of 1,000 cases. J Urol.* 2001;166(5):1729–1733.
3. Alibhai SM, et al. 30-Day mortality and major complications after radical prostatectomy: influence of age and comorbidity. *J Natl Cancer Inst.* 2005;97(20):1525–1532.
4. Bianco FJ Jr, et al. Variations among high volume surgeons in the rate of complications after radical prostatectomy: further evidence that technique matters. *J Urol.* 2005;173(6):2099–2103.
5. Hu JC, et al. Patterns of care for radical prostatectomy in the united states from 2003 to 2005. *J Urol.* 2008;180(5):1969–1974.
6. Bhayani SB, et al. Laparoscopic radical prostatectomy: a multi-institutional study of conversion to open surgery. *Urology.* 2004;63(1):99–102.
7. Tewari A, Srivasatava A, Menon M. A prospective comparison of radical retropubic and robot-assisted prostatectomy: experience in one institution. *BJU Int.* 2003;92(3):205–210.
8. Farnham SB, et al. Intraoperative blood loss and transfusion requirements for robotic-assisted radical prostatectomy versus radical retropubic prostatectomy. *Urology.* 2006;67(2):360–363.
9. Bhandari A, et al. Perioperative complications of robotic radical prostatectomy after the learning curve. *J Urol.* 2005;174(3):915–918.
10. Menon M, Bhandari A Complications of robotic prostatectomy. In: Loughlin KR, ed. Complications of Urologic Surgery And Practice: Diagnosis, Prevention, And Management, Informa healthcare; New York, NY; 2007: 369–379.
11. Badani KK, Kaul S, Menon M. Evolution of robotic radical prostatectomy: assessment after 2,766 procedures. *Cancer.* 2007;110(9):1951–1958.
12. Kaul S, et al. Robotic radical prostatectomy with preservation of the prostatic fascia: a feasibility study. *Urology.* 2005;66(6):1261–1265.
13. Krane LS, Bhandari M, Peabody JO, Menon M. Impact of percutaneous suprapubic tube drainage on patient discomfort after radical prostatectomy. *Eur Urol.* 2009;56(2):325–330.
14. Menon M, Hemal AK. Vattikuti institute prostatectomy: a technique of robotic radical prostatectomy: experience in more than 1,000 cases. *J Endourol.* 2004;18(7):611–619. discussion 619.
15. Menon M, et al. Vattikuti institute prostatectomy: contemporary technique and analysis of results. *Eur Urol.* 2007;51(3):648–657. discussion 657–8.
16. Menon M, et al. Vattikuti institute prostatectomy, a technique of robotic radical prostatectomy for management of localized carcinoma of the prostate: experience of over 1100 cases. *Urol Clin North Am.* 2004;31(4):701–717.
17. Guillonneau B, Vallancien G. Laparoscopic radical prostatectomy: the montsouris technique. *J Urol.* 2000;163(6):1643–1649.
18. Menon M, et al. Assessment of early continence after reconstruction of the periprostatic tissues in patients undergoing computer assisted (robotic) prostatectomy: results of a 2 group parallel randomized controlled trial. *J Urol.* 2008;180(3):1018–1023.
19. Nielsen ME, et al. High anterior release of the levator fascia improves sexual function following open radical retropubic prostatectomy. *J Urol.* 2008;180(6):2557–2564. discussion 2564.
20. Lunacek A, et al. Anatomical radical retropubic prostatectomy: 'curtain dissection' of the neurovascular bundle. *BJU Int.* 2005;95(9):1226–1231.
21. Clavien PA, Sanabria JR, Strasberg SM. Proposed classification of complications of surgery with examples of utility in cholecystectomy. *Surgery.* 1992;111(5):518–526.
22. Chandler JG, Corson SL, Way LW. Three spectra of laparoscopic entry access injuries. *J Am Coll Surg.* 2001;192(4):478–490. discussion 490–1.

23. Hasson HM. Open laparoscopy: a report of 150 cases. *J Reprod Med*. 1974;12(6):234–238.

24. String A, et al. Use of the optical access trocar for safe and rapid entry in various laparoscopic procedures. *Surg Endosc*. 2001;15(6):570–573.

25. Murdock CM, Wolff AJ, Van Geem T. Risk factors for hypercarbia, subcutaneous emphysema, pneumothorax, and pneumomediastinum during laparoscopy. *Obstet Gynecol*. 2000;95(5):704–709.

26. Cobb WS, et al. Gas embolism during laparoscopic cholecystectomy. *J Laparoendosc Adv Surg Tech A*. 2005;15(4):387–390.

27. Scoletta P, et al. Carbon dioxide embolization: is it a complication of laparoscopic cholecystectomy? *Minerva Chir*. 2003;58(3):313–320.

28. van der Voort M, Heijnsdijk EA, Gouma DJ. Bowel injury as a complication of laparoscopy. *Br J Surg*. 2004;91(10):1253–1258.

29. Bonjer HJ, et al. Open versus closed establishment of pneumoperitoneum in laparoscopic surgery. *Br J Surg*. 1997;84(5):599–602.

30. Hashizume M, Sugimachi K. Needle and trocar injury during laparoscopic surgery in Japan. *Surg Endosc*. 1997;11(12):1198–1201.

31. Mac Cordick C, et al. Morbidity in laparoscopic gynecological surgery: results of a prospective single-center study. *Surg Endosc*. 1999;13(1):57–61.

32. Catarci M, et al. Major and minor injuries during the creation of pneumoperitoneum. A multicenter study on 12,919 cases. *Surg Endosc*. 2001;15(6):566–569.

33. Schafer M, Lauper M, Krahenbuhl L. Trocar and Veress needle injuries during laparoscopy. *Surg Endosc*. 2001;15(3):275–280.

34. Champault G, Cazacu F, Taffinder N. Serious trocar accidents in laparoscopic surgery: a French survey of 103,852 operations. *Surg Laparosc Endosc*. 1996;6(5):367–370.

35. Ahmad G, Duffy JM, Watson AJ. Laparoscopic entry techniques and complications. *Int J Gynaecol Obstet*. 2007;99(1):52–55.

36. Lazzeri M, et al. Iatrogenic external iliac artery disruption during open pelvic lymph node dissection: successful repair with hypogastric artery transposition. *Scand J Urol Nephrol*. 1997;31(2):205–207.

37. Safi KC, et al. Laparoscopic repair of external iliac-artery transection during laparoscopic radical prostatectomy. *J Endourol*. 2006;20(4):237–239. discussion 239.

38. Bollens R, et al. Extraperitoneal laparoscopic radical prostatectomy. Results after 50 cases. *Eur Urol*. 2001;40(1):65–69.

39. Gill IS, Zippe CD. Laparoscopic radical prostatectomy: technique. *Urol Clin North Am*. 2001;28(2):423–436.

40. Guillonneau B, Vallancien G. Laparoscopic radical prostatectomy: the montsouris experience. *J Urol*. 2000;163(2):418–422.

41. Hoznek A, et al. Laparoscopic radical prostatectomy. The Creteil experience. *Eur Urol*. 2001;40(1):38–45.

42. Rassweiler J, et al. Laparoscopic radical prostatectomy with the Heilbronn technique: an analysis of the first 180 cases. *J Urol*. 2001;166(6):2101–2108.

43. Turk I, et al. Laparoscopic radical prostatectomy. Technical aspects and experience with 125 cases. *Eur Urol*. 2001;40(1):46–52. discussion 53.

44. Dangle P, PalmerPatil N, Samavedi J, Coughlin S, PatelV. R G. Operative complications of robotic-assisted radical prostatectomy. *Eur Urol Suppl*. 2008;7:3.

45. Fischer B, et al. Complications of robotic assisted radical prostatectomy. *World J Urol*. 2008;26(6):595–602.

46. Hu JC, et al. Perioperative complications of laparoscopic and robotic assisted laparoscopic radical prostatectomy. *J Urol*. 2006;175(2):541–546. discussion 546.

47. Lepor H, Kaci L. Contemporary evaluation of operative parameters and complications related to open radical retropubic prostatectomy. *Urology*. 2003;62(4):702–706.

48. Ahlering TE, et al. Successful transfer of open surgical skills to a laparoscopic environment using a robotic interface: initial experience with laparoscopic radical prostatectomy. *J Urol*. 2003;170(5):1738–1741.

49. Patel VR, Thaly R, Shah K. Robotic radical prostatectomy: outcomes of 500 cases. *BJU Int*. 2007;99(5):1109–1112.

50. Zorn KC, et al. Robotic-assisted laparoscopic prostatectomy: functional and pathologic outcomes with interfascial nerve preservation. *Eur Urol*. 2007;51(3):755–762. discussion 763.

51. Krane LS, et al. Robotic-assisted radical prostatectomy in patients receiving chronic anticoagulation therapy: role of perioperative bridging. *Urology*. 2008;72(6):1351–1355.

52. Bhoyrul S, et al. A randomized prospective study of radially expanding trocars in laparoscopic surgery. *J Gastrointest Surg*. 2000;4(4):392–397.

53. Bishoff JT, et al. Laparoscopic bowel injury: incidence and clinical presentation. *J Urol*. 1999;161(3):887–890.

54. Feicke A, et al. Robotic-assisted laparoscopic extended pelvic lymph node dissection for prostate cancer: surgical technique and experience with the first 99 cases. *Eur Urol*. 2009;55(4):876–883.

55. Simonetta F, Vincenzo F, Stefano C, et al. Is robotically assisted laparoscopic radical prostatectomy less invasive than retropubic radical prostatectomy? Results from a prospective, unrandomized, comparative study. *BJU Int*. 2008;101(9):1145–1149.

56. Joseph JV, et al. Robotic extraperitoneal radical prostatectomy: an alternative approach. *J Urol*. 2006;175(3 Pt 1):945–950. discussion 951.

57. Graefen M, Walz J, Huland H. Open retropubic nerve-sparing radical prostatectomy. *Eur Urol*. 2006;49(1):38–48.

58. Walsh PC, et al. Patient-reported urinary continence and sexual function after anatomic radical prostatectomy. *Urology*. 2000;55(1):58–61.

59. Nguyen MM, et al. Early continence outcomes of posterior musculofascial plate reconstruction during robotic and laparoscopic prostatectomy. *BJU Int*. 2008;101(9):1135–1139.

60. Rocco B, et al. Posterior reconstruction of the rhabdosphincter allows a rapid recovery of continence after transperitoneal videolaparoscopic radical prostatectomy. *Eur Urol*. 2007;51(4):996–1003.

61. Tewari AK, et al. Anatomic restoration technique of continence mechanism and preservation of puboprostatic collar: a novel modification to achieve early urinary continence in men undergoing robotic prostatectomy. *Urology*. 2007;69(4):726–731.

62. Patel VR, et al. *Robotic radical prostatectomy in the community setting–the learning curve and beyond: initial 200 cases. J Urol*. 2005;174(1):269–272.

Part IV
Adrenal, Kidney, and Ureter

Chapter 34

Robotic Urologic Surgery: Robotic-Assisted Adrenalectomy

Vinod Narra, Craig G. Rogers, and Mani Menon

34.1 Introduction

Since the first description of a minimally invasive technique for removal of the adrenal gland by Gagner in 1992[1] numerous refinements and alternatives to this technique have evolved including a retroperitoneoscopic approach and robotic-assisted adrenalectomy. Minimally invasive adrenalectomy has now become the standard of care for benign lesions,[2–8] as well as instances of malignant lesions and has demonstrated a reduced morbidity, shorter hospital stays, and improved pain control over the conventional open techniques.[9–12]

The traditional approach to a laparoscopic adrenalectomy where the ports are placed in a subcostal position creates an unnatural stance for the operating surgeon and leads to tremendous stress on the surgeon's shoulders, back, and arms. Because an adrenalectomy is performed within a narrow operative field and requires precise dissection it has became an ideal indication for robotic surgery. The first robotic adrenalectomy was reported in 2001 by Horgan and Vanuno[13] and since that time numerous case-controlled studies have reported excellent outcomes.[13–23] The use of the robot provides a more comfortable operating environment with improved 3D optics in addition to reducing trauma and manipulation to the adrenal gland. And, as vascular injuries are the most often reported injury during laparoscopic surgery, robotic-assisted surgery allows for fine dissection necessary to avoid injury to the vena cava and renal vessels.

The purpose of this chapter is to detail the technique of both right and left transperitoneal robotic-assisted adrenalectomy. Although partial adrenalectomies have been performed robotically,[24–27] this chapter will focus on whole gland excision and steps can be taken to modify the approach should a partial excision be desirable.

34.2 Planning

Careful patient selection based on diagnosis and operative risk in addition to a thorough pre-operative radiographic evaluation allowing for a detailed understanding of the adjacent anatomy can significantly reduce morbidity associated with a robotic-assisted adrenalectomy. For hormone-secreting tumors, it is wise to enlist the endocrinology service not only for pre-operative control but also for a smooth post-operative course. Anti-platelet and anti-coagulants are held appropriately. Bowel cleansing is not necessary and in fact if performed should be brought to the attention of the anesthesiologist in order to ensure adequate volume resuscitation.

34.3 Operative Team and Positioning

The minimum operative team consists of a console surgeon, bedside assistant, surgeon, scrub nurse, circulating nurse, and anesthesiologist. The anesthesiologist

M. Menon (✉)
Professor of Urology, Columbia University, New York Director, Menon-Vattikuti Center, New York Presbyterian Hospital, USA
e-mail: mmenon1@hfhs.org

A.K. Hemal, M. Menon (eds.), *Robotics in Genitourinary Surgery*,
DOI 10.1007/978-1-84882-114-9_34, © Springer-Verlag London Limited 2011

Fig. 34.1 Patient placed in lateral decubitus position with pressure points padded

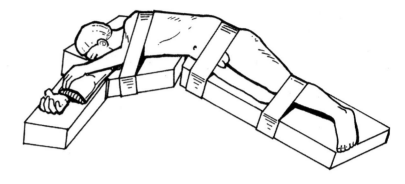

takes their place at the head of the bed, and the scrub nurse and assisting surgeon occupy a position opposite the robot.

The patient is initially placed in the supine position upon a beanbag on the operating table. After induction of general anesthesia, monitoring lines, a nasogastric tube, and a Foley catheter are inserted. Our practice is to place the patient in a lateral decubitus position with inner leg flexed and the outer leg extended (Fig. 34.1). The patient's abdomen is brought to the edge of the bed and the arms and pressure points are padded after placement of an axillary role. The bed is then flexed to increase the space between the ribs and the iliac crest after which the beanbag is hardened and the safety straps are applied. The bed is then placed in reverse trendelenburg.

34.4 Trocar Configuration

With respect to the left, the head would be on the left and for the right the head would be on the right:

AAL – Anterior axillary line
MCL – Midclavicular line
C   – Camera port
R_1 R_2 – 8 mm robotic arms
A_1 A_2 – 12 mm assistant ports

Insufflation is initiated by lifting the anterior abdominal wall with piercing towel clamps and inserting a Veress needle. The camera port is then placed lateral to the umbilicus after insufflation is completed. A 30° up scope is then inserted and the robotic ports are positioned as in Fig. 34.2. The robotic system is brought in from the back over the shoulder in a plane created by

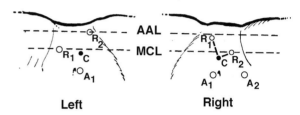

Fig. 34.2 Port placement for *left* and *right* robotic-assisted adrenalectomy

the camera port and target adrenal gland. The system is docked and inspected for appropriate range of motion without interference. If there is any resistance or interference the system should be de-docked and adjusted prior to commencing the operation. An additional port is used on the right side for liver retraction. If a fourth robotic arm is available this can be used as a substitute for this second assistant port. An alternative approach is placement of trocars to resemble a kidney resection with the robotic arms between the midclavicular line and the anterior axillary line, equidistant from the camera port which is placed lateral to the umbilicus.

34.5 Left Robotic-Assisted Adrenalectomy

34.5.1 Exposure of the Adrenal Gland

With a monopolar hook in the right hand and Maryland bipolar in the left the operation commences with mobilization of the splenic flexure along the white line of Toldt drawing the colon inferiorly and medially thereby exposing the left kidney (Fig. 34.3). The lienophrenic and lienorenal ligaments are then taken down releasing the spleen and taking it along with the

Fig. 34.3 Mobilization of splenic flexure along *dotted line*. Inset with colon reflected inferiorly exposing pancreatic tail and spleen

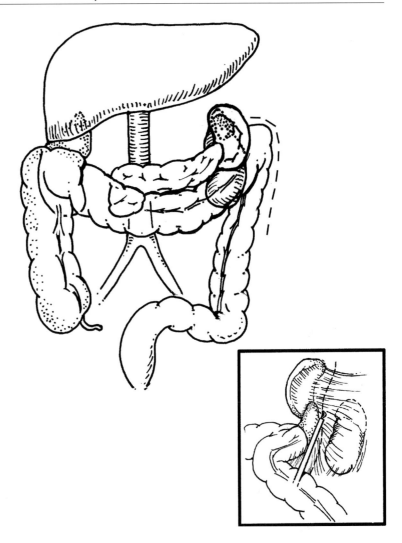

tail of the pancreas to a medial orientation. By releasing the spleen, a natural plane develops similar to an opening of a book and defines the inferior border of the pancreas and the superior border of the adrenal gland, which will be useful during final dissection and avoid injury to the pancreas (Fig. 34.4). Through the assistant port, a suction irrigator is placed to keep the operative field clean and to provide gentle traction.

34.5.2 Identification of the Adrenal Vein

Gerota's fascia is incised and with minimal use of electrocautery the renal vessels are identified and exposed. After identification of the renal vein, the adrenal vein is traced superiorly to the inferior border of the adrenal gland. The adrenal vein is then circumferentially dissected. It is the easy maneuverability of the robotic arms and the degrees of freedom that allow for ease in dissection around the vein. A clip applicator is then brought through the assistant's port and the vein is doubly clipped on the stay side and singly clipped on the go side. If the assistant has a difficult angle for placing these clips (or if your assistant is less experienced and you are not comfortable having them place the clip), one can use the robotic hem-o-lok clip applier. This gives the console surgeon full control of clip placement with the added precision and articulation that the robot provides. When using this, place a single clip (these are 10 mm) on the stay and a single go. The vein is then transected (Fig. 34.5).

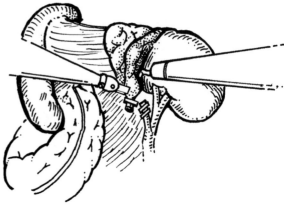

Fig. 34.6 Circumferential dissection of the *left* adrenal gland

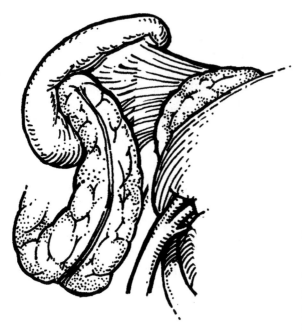

Fig. 34.4 Reflection of spleen and pancreas exposing the *left* adrenal gland

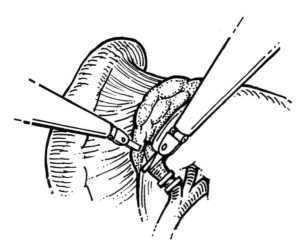

Fig. 34.5 The *left* adrenal vein is clipped and transected

34.6 Removal of the Gland

The final step is the circumferential dissection of the adrenal gland starting along the superior pole of the kidney and then defining the lateral and superior borders of the gland (Fig. 34.6). To prevent the gland from obscuring the dissection plane it is best to dissect medial to lateral terminating at the superior pole. The

vessels should easily be controlled with the hook electrocautery without the need for further clips or ties. If possible perinephric fat is preserved along the borders of the adrenal gland, which can be grasped with the forceps without rupturing the capsule of the gland. If there is minimal fat on the gland either the right or the left hand can be placed posterior to the adrenal gland and the gland displaced anteriorly allowing for a no touch dissection. The gland is then placed in a retrieval bag brought in from the assistant's port and bag is left within the abdomen until hemostasis is assured. No drains are necessary. The robot is de-docked, the specimen is removed, and the fascial defects are closed under direct vision.

In cases where the adrenal vein is difficult to identify because of the size of the adrenal gland then proceed with exposure of the lateral border of the adrenal gland and the superior pole of the kidney and following the inferior border of the adrenal gland medially the vein should be encountered.

34.7 Right Robotic-Assisted Adrenalectomy

34.7.1 Exposure of the Adrenal Gland

As in the left, the pneumoperitoneum on the right is first established with a Veress needle and an understanding of the fascial layers is critical to avoid injury to or CO_2 insufflation within the liver. After placement of the trocars and docking of the robot, the

Fig. 34.7 *Dotted line* indicates dissection *line* for retraction of liver and colon

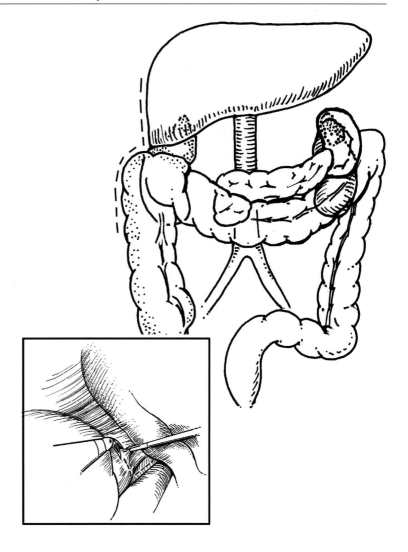

hepatic flexure is freed inferio-medially exposing the right kidney and duodenum (Fig. 34.7). The duodenum is kocherized to expose the infra-hepatic vena cava. In order to visualize the right adrenal gland the right lobe of the liver must be mobilized along the right triangular ligament allowing progressive displacement of the liver superiorly. We utilize a grasper through the second assistant's port to grasp a position superior along the lateral abdominal wall to provide this liver retraction. Caution should be exercised to avoid aggressive retraction superiorly or excessive dissection of the triangular ligament either of which can lead to a parenchymal injury or a tear of an accessory vein which is a direct branch off of the inferior vena cava.

After the exposure is completed, the focus of attention is then redirected inferiorly and orientation is established by identifying the superior pole of the kidney and the inferior vena cava (Fig. 34.8). The right hand utilizes the hook electrocautery or scissors while the left hand with bipolar forceps grasps the perinephric fat displacing it laterally. Dissection is initiated along the lateral border of the vena no lower than the right renal artery progressing superiorly until the adrenal vein is encountered. On occasion a smaller vein is first identified which can be controlled with ligaclips but unless it has a broad base a thorough search for the true adrenal vein should proceed until the apex of the gland is reached. Similar to controlling the left adrenal vein, the right adrenal is

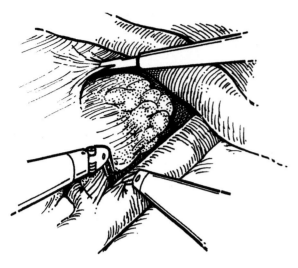

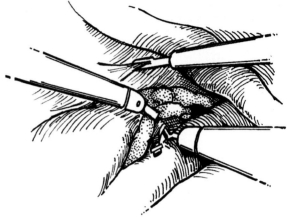

Fig. 34.10 Circumferential dissection of the adrenal gland

Fig. 34.8 With a grasper retracting the liver superiorly the lateral border of the inferior vena cava is defined

is removed, and the fascial defects are closed under direct vision.

circumferentially dissected without the need to change instruments. Ligating the vessel can be a challenge given the shortened length of the vein; however, any attempt at securing additional length should not be performed until the stay side has been secured with two ligaclips (Fig. 34.9). The adrenal gland is then reflected laterally and surrounding attachments taken down with electrocautery (Fig. 34.10).

The gland is then placed in a retrieval bag brought in from the assistant's port and bag is left within the abdomen until hemostasis is assured. No drains are necessary. The robot is de-docked, the specimen

34.8 Post-operative Management

Other than appropriate endocrine or blood pressure control, patients do not require post-operative nasal-gastric decompression and can in fact be advanced on their diet as tolerated. The foley catheter is removed the morning after surgery and activity is increased so the appropriate level of pain medication can be prescribed at discharge. In the absence of any pre-operative electrolyte abnormality post-operative labs can be restricted to a hematocrit.

34.9 Complications

Complications can occur at any step during this process but the sequelae can be minimized with immediate identification and management. The most common complication involves a direct vascular injury but bleeding can on rare occasions be associated with hepatic or splenic capsular disruption.[28] With the exception of the camera port all trocars and instruments should be inserted and removed under direct vision to ensure inadvertent injury. Unless extensive adhesions are present the use of electrocautery should be used judiciously to avoid thermal injury to the bowel.

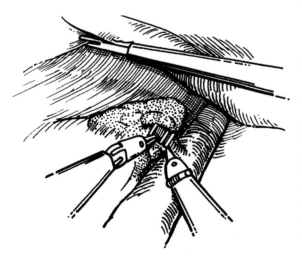

Fig. 34.9 The *right* adrenal vein is controlled with ligaclips

Table 34.1 Instrumentation used during robot-assisted adrenalectomy

Surgeon instrumentation			
Right arm	Left arm	Fourth arm (optional)	Assistant instrumentation
Monopolar hook or cold scissors	Maryland bipolar	Blunt tip grasper	Suction irrigator or blunt tip grasper

34.10 Conclusion

The advantages of a robotic-assisted adrenalectomy include improved depth perception with the 3D optics and increased degrees of freedom creating a wrist joint for improved precision around delicate vascular structures. These improvements provide the tools for meticulous surgical technique which in combination with thorough pre- and post-operative management enables a safe and effective adrenalectomy for a variety of clinical indications.

References

1. Gagner M, Lacroix A, Bolte E. Laparoscopic adrenalectomy in Cushing's syndrome and pheochromocytoma. *N Engl J Med.* 1992;327:1033.
2. Cyriac J, Weizman D, Urbach DR. Laparoscopic adrenalectomy for the management of benign and malignant adrenal tumors. *Expert Rev Med Devices.* 2006;3:777–786.
3. Guazzoni G, Cestari A, Montorsi F, et al. Laparoscopic treatment of adrenal diseases: 10 years on. *BJU Int.* 2004;93:221–227.
4. Hazzan D, Shiloni E, Golijanin D, et al. Laparoscopic vs open adrenalectomy for benign adrenal neoplasm. *Surg Endosc.* 2001;15:1356–1358.
5. Liao CH, Chueh SC, Lai MK, et al. Laparoscopic adrenalectomy for potentially malignant adrenal tumors greater than 5 centimeters. *J Clin Endocrinol Metab.* 2006;91:3080–3083.
6. Tsuru N, Ushiyama T, Suzuki K. Laparoscopic adrenalectomy for primary and secondary malignant adrenal tumors. *J Endourol.* 2005;19:702–708. discussion 708–9.
7. Valeri A, Borrelli A, Presenti L, et al. Adrenal masses in neoplastic patients: the role of laparoscopic procedure. *Surg Endosc.* 2001;15:90–93.
8. Zeh HJ 3rd, Udelsman R. One hundred laparoscopic adrenalectomies: a single surgeon's experience. *Ann Surg Oncol.* 2003;10:1012–1017.
9. Fazeli-Matin S, Gill IS, Hsu TH, et al. Laparoscopic renal and adrenal surgery in obese patients: comparison to open surgery. *J Urol.* 1999;162:665–669.
10. Hallfeldt KK, Mussack T, Trupka A, et al. Laparoscopic lateral adrenalectomy versus open posterior adrenalectomy for the treatment of benign adrenal tumors. *Surg Endosc.* 2003;17:264–267.
11. Jacobsen NE, Campbell JB, Hobart MG. Laparoscopic versus open adrenalectomy for surgical adrenal disease. *Can J Urol.* 2003;10:1995–1999.
12. Kirshtein B, Yelle JD, Moloo H, et al. Laparoscopic adrenalectomy for adrenal malignancy: a preliminary report comparing the short-term outcomes with open adrenalectomy. *J Laparoendosc Adv Surg Tech A.* 2008;18:42–46.
13. Horgan S, Vanuno D. Robots in laparoscopic surgery. *J Laparoendosc Adv Surg Tech A.* 2001;11:415–419.
14. Brunaud L, Bresler L, Ayav A, et al. Robotic-assisted adrenalectomy: what advantages compared to lateral transperitoneal laparoscopic adrenalectomy? *Am J Surg.* 2008;195:433–438.
15. Brunaud L, Bresler L, Zarnegar R, et al. Does robotic adrenalectomy improve patient quality of life when compared to laparoscopic adrenalectomy? *World J Surg.* 2004;28:1180–1185.
16. Desai MM, Gill IS, Kaouk JH, et al. Robotic-assisted laparoscopic adrenalectomy. *Urology.* 2002;60:1104–1107.
17. Gill IS, Sung GT, Hsu TH, et al. Robotic remote laparoscopic nephrectomy and adrenalectomy: the initial experience. *J Urol.* 2000;164:2082–2085.
18. Krane LS, Shrivastava A, Eun D, et al. A four-step technique of robotic right adrenalectomy: initial experience. *BJU Int.* 2008;101:1289–1292.
19. Moinzadeh A, Gill IS. Robotic adrenalectomy. *Urol Clin North Am.* 2004;31:753–756.
20. Rogers CG, Blatt AM, Miles GE, et al. Concurrent robotic partial adrenalectomy and extra-adrenal pheochromocytoma resection in a pediatric patient with von Hippel-Lindau disease. *J Endourol.* 2008;22:1501–1503.
21. Sung GT, Gill IS. Robotic renal and adrenal surgery. *Surg Clin North Am.* 2003;83:1469–1482.
22. Wu JC, Wu HS, Lin MS, et al. Robotic-assisted laparoscopic adrenalectomy. *J Formos Med Assoc.* 2005;104:748–751.
23. Young JA, Chapman WH 3rd, Kim VB, et al. Robotic-assisted adrenalectomy for adrenal incidentaloma: case and review of the technique. *Surg Laparosc Endosc Percutan Tech.* 2002;12:126–130.
24. Diner EK, Franks ME, Behari A, et al. Partial adrenalectomy: the national cancer institute experience. *Urology.* 2005;66:19–23.

25. Walther MM, Herring J, Choyke PL, et al. Laparoscopic partial adrenalectomy in patients with hereditary forms of pheochromocytoma. *J Urol.* 2000;164:14–17.
26. Janetschek G, Finkenstedt G, Gasser R, et al. Laparoscopic surgery for peochromocytoma: adrenalectomy, partial resection, excision of paragangliomas. *J Urol.* 1998;160: 330–334.
27. Julien JS, Ball D, Schulick R. Robot-assisted cortical-sparing adrenalectomy in a patient with von Hippel-Lindau disease and bilateral pheochromocytomas separated by 9 years. *J Laparoendosc Adv Surg Tech A.* 2006;16:473–477.
28. Strebel RT, Muntener M, Sulser T. Intraoperative complications of laparoscopic adrenalectomy. *World J Urol.* 2008;6:555–560.

Chapter 35

Robot-Assisted Laparoscopic Radical Nephrectomy and Nephroureterectomy

Ben R. McHone, Ronald S. Boris, and Peter A. Pinto

Significant advances have been made in the field of minimally invasive urologic surgery since the use of laparoscopy was initially described. Minimally invasive surgery was originally considered the realm of laparoscopic surgeons, often with additional subspecialty training. The development of robotic surgery broadened the field of urologic surgeons capable of using minimally invasive techniques for radical prostatectomy. With time, the applications of robot-assisted surgery expanded to include radical nephrectomy and nephroureterectomy. Though initial results are still too premature to come to a definitive conclusion with regard to oncologic outcomes, the benefits to patients with respect to morbidity and convalescence are readily apparent. This chapter will describe the surgical techniques involved in performing robot-assisted laparoscopic radical nephrectomy and nephroureterectomy.

35.1 Robot-Assisted Laparoscopic Radical Nephrectomy

35.1.1 Indications/Contraindications

The indications for robot-assisted laparoscopic nephrectomy (RALN) are the same as for open or traditional laparoscopic nephrectomy and include primarily renal masses not amenable to nephron-sparing

surgery. Additionally, RALN can be utilized in the setting of metastatic disease with or without lymph node dissection.[1] Contraindications to performing RALN include comorbid conditions precluding the administration of general anesthesia. T4 disease would be a relative contraindication depending on the site or extent of adjacent organ involvement.[2] However, previous abdominal surgery is not a contraindication to minimally invasive surgery and has been demonstrated to be safe.[3]

35.1.2 Patient Preparation

Patients eligible for surgery should provide a detailed history and receive a complete physical exam. Blood panel including a complete blood count, serum chemistry, coagulation studies, and alkaline phosphatase is obtained. A chest x-ray is recommended for preoperative screening as well as evaluation for pulmonary metastases; however, if the suspicion of distant metastasis is high then a chest CT may be obtained. A bone scan is recommended for an elevated alkaline phosphatase, for symptomatic bone pain, or to complete a metastatic evaluation. If possible a three-phase CT scan or MRI should be obtained to properly evaluate the renal mass. Attention should be paid to the number and position of renal vessels, retroperitoneal lymph nodes, or possible adjacent organ involvement. If there is any question regarding a caval or renal vein thrombus, an MR venogram is required.

Each patient undergoes a mechanical bowel preparation the evening before surgery. A single dose of intravenous antibiotics should be administered in the preoperative holding area. Before the induction of

P.A. Pinto (✉)
Urologic Oncology Branch, National Cancer Institute,
National Institutes of Health, Bethesda, MD, USA
e-mail: pintop@mail.nih.gov

general anesthesia, sequential compression devices are applied and activated.

35.2 Transperitoneal RALN

Step 1: The patient is turned onto the table in a modified lateral decubitus. We place a thin long gel pad on the operating room table prior to positioning and do not use bean bags or other stabilizing devices. The patient is shifted to the center of the table with his/her flank over the break. Two large jelly rolls are used for support of the neck, back, and hips as the body lays comfortably at about 30°–45° tilt. The lower leg is placed in a bent knee position and the upper leg remains naturally straight. Pillows are placed between the legs longitudinally and all pressure points are sufficiently padded and supported.

A small axillary roll is properly placed. Anesthesia assists in obtaining a comfortable height and position for the patient's head and neck. A traditional arm rest is used to secure the down (contralateral) arm roughly perpendicular from the patient's body. The abdomen, hips, and legs are padded and taped safely and securely to the operating room table. The table is flexed to the minimum angle that adequately opens up the flank to maximize operating space. A vascular arm rest is secured to the table and the ipsilateral shoulder and arm (upside) are rested without tension onto the arm rest. This arm is secured using a Kerlex wrap and tape (Fig. 35.1). Positioning safety is tested by rotating the table in either direction and ensuring that the patient is well secured and protected.

Step 2: A Pfannenstiel incision is marked on the patient prior to positioning, as skin distortion after the patient is positioned can lead to a curved incision. This site will be used to extract the specimen. Pneumoperitoneum is achieved with a Veress needle to a pressure of 15–20 mmHg. We recommend needle placement away from any previous incisions as bowel may be adherent in those locations. However, prior abdominal surgery is not a contraindication to entry with a Veress.[3] For those less comfortable with this approach, a Hasson technique can be used. A 12 mm umbilical port is placed and the abdominal

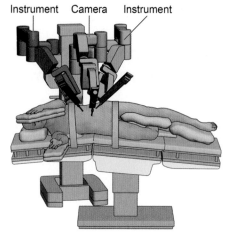

Instrument   Camera   Instrument

Transperitoneal approach

Fig. 35.1 Patient positioning and robot docking for transperitoneal radical nephrectomy

contents are inspected for signs of injury or adhesions. Two additional 8 mm robotic ports are placed, each at least 8 cm from the umbilical port and from each other. A 12 mm assistant port is placed approximately 8 cm inferior to the umbilical port. This port is often placed in the area of the premarked Pfannenstiel incision. An additional 5 mm assistant port is placed superior to the umbilical port if needed for organ retraction (Fig. 35.2). Port placement for renal surgery, unlike that for prostate surgery, may vary from patient to patient. This is especially true for obese patients where ports need to be displaced cephalad and laterally (Fig. 35.3). It is important to remember that the kidney is fixed and the ports

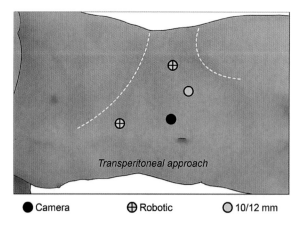

Transperitoneal approach

● Camera   ⊕ Robotic   ○ 10/12 mm

Fig. 35.2 Port placement for transperitoneal approach

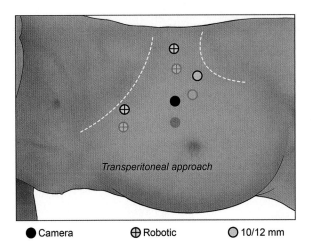

Fig. 35.3 Lateral shifting of transperitoneal port placement in obese patient

● Camera   ⊕ Robotic   ○ 10/12 mm

placed to optimize access to the renal hilum, which for obese patients may be far away from the umbilicus. When using the standard system, the ports need to be spaced out further to avoid robotic arm collisions. The fourth arm cannot be utilized for flank surgery with the standard system. When using the da Vinci S or Si systems (Intuitive Surgical Inc., Sunnyvale, CA), the slimmer profile of the robot allows the ports to be placed in closer proximity to each other. Additionally, the fourth arm can be brought in over the hip and placed a few fingers above the iliac crest. Once the ports are placed, the robot can be docked over the patient's back and ipsilateral shoulder at a 20° angle to the patient's head (Fig. 35.1). Hot-shears are used in the right hand while Maryland forceps or bipolar grasping forceps are used in the left (Table 35.1). The assistant

Table 35.1 Surgeon and assistant instrumentation

Surgeon instrumentation			
Right arm	Left arm	Fourth arm (optional)	Assistant instrumentation
• Curved monopolar scissors • 10 mm hem-o-lok clip applier	• Maryland bipolar grasper • 10 mm hem-o-lok clip applier	Prograsp dissector	• Suction-irrigator • Atraumatic grasper • 5 mm titanium clip applier • 10 mm hem-o-lok clip applier • Laparoscopic ultrasound • Laparoscopic DeBakey • Laparoscopic scissors

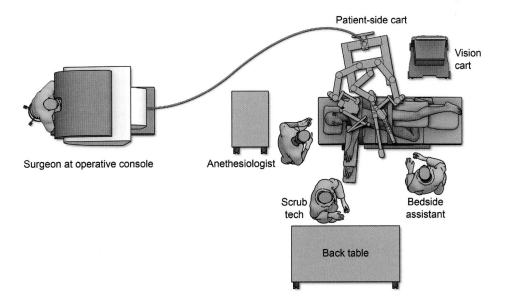

Fig. 35.4 Overhead view of operating room layout

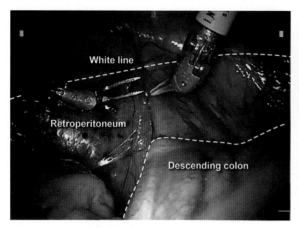

Fig. 35.5 Incising white line of Toldt

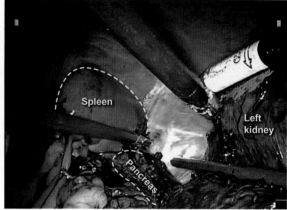

Fig. 35.6 Full mobilization of spleen with reflected tail of pancreas

stands/sits opposite the robot with an unimpeded view of a vision cart (Fig. 35.4).

Step 3: As with traditional laparoscopic nephrectomy, RALN commences by identifying and incising the white line of Toldt using the hot-shears and electrocautery away from the bowel to minimize thermal spread. The bowel is then mobilized from the iliac vessels to the respective hepatic or splenic flexure. During this time, the assistant can help provide medial traction using atraumatic graspers (Fig. 35.5). For a left nephrectomy, the line of dissection is carried cephalad by sharply dividing the splenophrenic ligaments. Blunt dissection around the spleen is avoided as it can lead to a tear or injury in the capsule of the spleen. Division of these ligaments is best performed with sequential left-handed bipolar and right-handed hot scissor maneuvers. This should be carried out until the diaphragm is visualized and the spleen is completely freed from the upper pole of the kidney. Full mobilization of the spleen, en bloc with the splenic flexure, is critical in rotating the tail of the pancreas medially in order to gain clear access to the left renal hilum (Fig. 35.6). For large renal tumors or cases that require a lymphadenectomy, this step becomes even more imperative.

During RALN for right-sided masses, the colon is mobilized from the iliac vessels to the hepatic flexure. This exposes the anterior surface of the duodenum. The duodenum, through a Kocher maneuver, is sharply mobilized in order to expose the anterior surface of the inferior vena cava. Although a useful dissection tool in laparoscopic surgery, use of

the irrigator-aspirator around the duodenum should be limited to minimize the risk for serosal tears. Such injuries, if unrecognized, can be devastating. Additionally, a 5 mm port can be placed in the subxiphoid position to allow for additional retraction of the liver and better exposure of the upper pole of the kidney and the right adrenal gland.

Step 4: The gonadal vessel and ureter to the diseased kidney are identified and traced cephalad. This is often best performed with identification of the psoas muscle which allows safe access to the posterior surface of the kidney. When tracing the right ureter to the right kidney, the gonadal vessels can be swept medially, separating them from the ureter and preventing avulsion of the gonadal vein from its insertion into the inferior vena cava. This maneuver can be performed by placing gentle lateral traction on the ureter with the Maryland bipolar and carefully sweeping the gonadal vein medially with the right robotic hand. Once the ureter has been traced to the inferior pole of the kidney it can be followed to the level of the renal hilum (Fig. 35.7). The assistant with the irrigator-aspirator or closed grasper can retract the kidney anteriorly, placing the hilum on stretch and allowing the robotic surgeon better access to the renal pedicle.

Step 5: Once the renal vein is identified the surgeon typically starts inferiorly to identify the renal artery. Exposure of the artery can be aided with division of hilar fat and fibrous tissue often covering the vessels. As mentioned previously hilar stretch can be provided with the assistant or alternatively the fourth

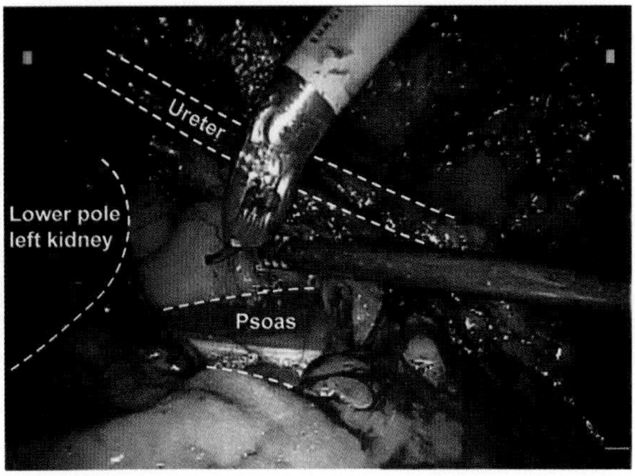

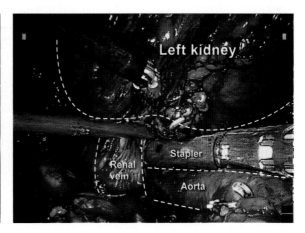

Fig. 35.7 Anterior retraction on ureter exposing psoas muscle

Fig. 35.9 Endoscopic stapling of renal artery

arm can be utilized by the console surgeon when the da Vinci S system is employed. In cases of a left nephrectomy, a lumbar vein and the gonadal vein are clipped and divided to allow better access to the renal artery. Once both vessels are adequately exposed, either an endovascular stapler or locking clips are applied to secure and divide the renal artery and vein, respectively (Figs. 35.8 and 35.9). If assistant access to the hilum is poor or the assistant lacks the skill set to ligate the hilum, the console surgeon can apply the locking clips himself/herself using a weck-application robotic instrument. One should observe prompt decompression of the renal vein after arterial ligation, as delayed decompression can indicate additional arteries or a potential renal vein thrombus. If there is any concern the laparoscopic ultrasound can be used to delineate any degree of

renal perfusion or to document the presence/absence of a renal vein thrombus.

Step 6: Generally, we do not recommend routine adrenal resection en bloc with the kidney. However, for T2 masses in the upper pole or clear radiologic documentation of mass extension into the adrenal, a concomitant adrenalectomy should be performed.[4] The left adrenal gland, after the adrenal vein is clipped and divided, can be easily taken with the left kidney. On the right, however, care needs to be used when approaching the adrenal vein. With the assistant placing lateral retraction on the kidney, the adrenal vein is exposed by tracing the inferior vena cava cephalad. The adrenal vein is then clipped and divided. Once the respective adrenal vein is secured and the renal hilum divided, the kidney and adrenal gland can be mobilized en bloc from the surrounding fossa. This is best performed with constant renal traction provided by the assistant. Both the surgeon and assistant should work in tandem to free the specimen from any remaining attachments. Liberal use of electrocautery can be used to cauterize any parasitic vessels. After clipping and dividing the ureter, the specimen is placed in an organ entrapment device (typically a 15 mm endocatch sack) and brought through the premarked Pfannenstiel incision.

Step 7: Robotic retroperitoneal lymph node dissection may be performed when indicated. In our experience, minimally invasive techniques have not precluded adequate lymphadenectomy. Current evidence does not support routine lymphadenectomies for T1 or T2 disease in the absence of clinically

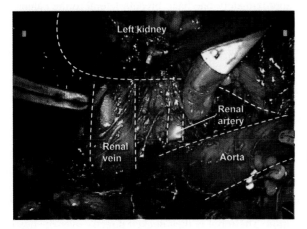

Fig. 35.8 Skeletonized aorta with exposed renal vein and artery

positive nodes.[5] However, retrospective data do suggest some benefit to improved staging in those with clinically detected nodal disease.[6] Pantuck et al. demonstrated improved survival in those patients with metastatic disease who underwent cytoreductive nephrectomy and lymphadenectomy prior to immunotherapy compared to those who did not receive an extended lymphadenectomy.[7] Intraoperative nomograms have been published to aid in the selection of patients who would most benefit from concomitant node dissection at the time of nephrectomy.[8]

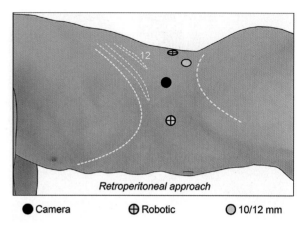

Camera   ⊕ **Robotic**   ○ **10/12 mm**

Fig. 35.10 Port placement for retroperitoneal approach

35.3 Retroperitoneal RALN

Advantages to the retroperitoneal robotic radical nephrectomy are similar to both open and laparoscopic nephrectomy, including the avoidance of entry into the peritoneum, easier access to the renal artery, and decreased ileus. It should be noted that retroperitoneoscopic surgery has been reported to have a steep learning curve and proper anatomic orientation can be challenging.[9,10] This can lead to inadvertent complications and even caval transection.[11] Furthermore, any history of previous retroperitoneal renal surgery can lead to significant scarring, and re-accessing that space may be particularly hazardous. Finally, particularly large renal masses adherent or adjacent to intra-abdominal organs are a contraindication to using this operative approach.

35.4 Patient Positioning, Retroperitoneal Access, and Port Placement

Immediately following endotracheal intubation and foley catheter placement, the patient is placed in the full flank position with the table flexed to increase the distance between the 12th rib and the iliac crest. After all pressure points are padded and the appropriate rolls and bolsters placed, the patient is secured to the bed using wide cloth tape. The flank and abdomen are prepped and draped sterilely. An incision is made off the tip of the 12th rib, large enough to accommodate one's index finger. Dissection is carried

down to the lumbodorsal fascia, which is incised and the retroperitoneum is entered. One's index finger is placed into the retroperitoneal space and the psoas muscle and lower pole of the kidney are palpated. Through this incision a balloon dilator is placed under direct vision. The balloon is expanded with sterile carbon dioxide to a volume of 800 cc to create the working space. After the working space is created, the balloon is removed and a port with a soft collar and low profile is placed into the incision. The soft collar prevents leakage of gas from the working space and the low profile limits any visual interference. Three additional ports are placed. An 8 mm robotic port is placed on similar horizontal axis (1–2 fingerbreadths inferiorly) with the camera port to the most medial extent possible without violating the peritoneum. This will function as the left robotic arm port. A second 8 mm port (right robotic arm) is placed on the same axis as the other 8 mm port approximately one hand breadth lateral to the camera port. A 12 mm assistant port should be triangulated inferiorly between the camera port and the right robotic arm (Fig. 35.10).

35.5 Docking of Robot

When performing retroperitoneal robotic renal surgery we typically rotate the foot of the table away from the robot approximately 45°. This allows anesthesia easier access to the head of the patient during the operation. The robot is then docked directly over the head and ipsilateral shoulder of the patient (Fig. 35.11).

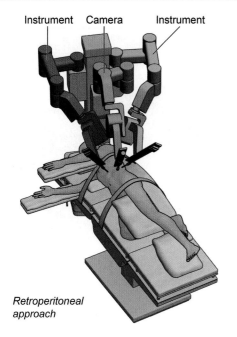

Instrument   Camera   Instrument

*Retroperitoneal
approach*

Fig. 35.11 Patient positioning and robot docking for retroperitoneal radical nephrectomy

Surgeons should pay special attention to insure a safe distance between the robotic arms and the body of the patient, particularly the left robotic arm which is typically directly over the neck of the patient. Once the robot is properly docked and final positioning is assessed, the surgeon can commence the operation.

The majority of steps for retroperitoneal nephrectomy are identical to the transperitoneal approach detailed above. Initial orientation can be achieved by identifying and following the psoas muscle to locate the ureter. The ureter is then traced to the renal hilum and the vessels are identified and ligated. If the specimen is small, the camera port can be extended for specimen retrieval. Extraction for retroperitoneal surgery can be more challenging with larger masses. In cases where the mass is prohibitively large, a modified Pfannenstiel incision is created as described by Matin and Gill.[12] After the incision is made in the lower abdomen, dissection is carried down to the anterior rectus fascia and a vertical incision is created along the lateral rectus border. With the fascia and rectus muscle retracted, the transversalis fascia is divided near the pubis and the extraperitoneal space is entered. Careful blunt dissection into the retroperitoneum then allows for delivery of the larger specimens through this lower abdominal incision.[12]

35.6 Robot-Assisted Nephroureterectomy

35.6.1 Indication

The indication for a robot-assisted nephroureterectomy is the same as for the open or laparoscopic approaches.

35.6.2 Patient Preparation

Patient preoperative workup and preparation for a nephroureterectomy includes the workup done for a radical nephrectomy. In addition to imaging, a pathological diagnosis establishing the presence of a high-grade, invasive urothelial carcinoma is required. Finally, a cystoscopy is performed before extirpation to rule out a concomitant bladder mass.

35.6.3 Procedure

The nephrectomy and proximal ureteral dissection is carried out as described for the transperitoneal nephrectomy. Initial series reporting on minimally invasive nephroureterectomy describe a hybrid technique utilizing traditional laparoscopy to perform the nephrectomy and docking the robot only for the distal ureterectomy and bladder cuff.[13,14] Other series have documented the feasibility of performing concurrent upper and lower urinary tract surgery successfully in limited numbers.[15,16] Recently, Rha and colleagues described a hybrid port technique where 12 mm ports are intubated with 8 mm robotic ports at various steps of the procedure, allowing greater port versatility for the robot. The entire procedure is done with the patient in modified flank position and without redocking the robot.[17] A similar method of hybrid port hopping has been described for robot-assisted retroperitoneoscopic nephroureterectomy.[18]

Step 1: Patients undergoing robot-assisted nephroureterectomy at our institution are initially prepared and positioned exactly as they would be for transperitoneal robot-assisted nephrectomy (Fig. 35.1).

Step 2: Port placement remains similar to the aforementioned procedure with the exception that the camera port and right robotic port may be shifted

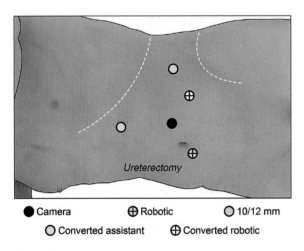

Fig. 35.12 Port placement for nephroureterectomy

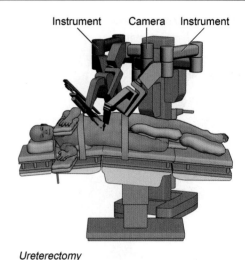

Ureterectomy

Fig. 35.13 Patient positioning and robot docking for nephroureterectomy

inferiorly, closer to the umbilicus (Fig. 35.12). This will allow better robotic access to the pelvis for the ureterectomy portion of the surgery.

Step 3: The robotic nephrectomy is performed in identical fashion as described in the steps above detailing the transperitoneal procedure. Once the kidney portion of the operation is complete, the specimen is mobilized into the pelvis for easier access prior to nephroureterectomy extraction (which is delayed until after ureterectomy and bladder cuff).

Step 4: The robot is de-docked and the table is rotated so that the patient is lying in a more supine fashion with slight Trendelenburg. An additional robotic port is placed just inferior and lateral to the umbilicus which will serve as the right robotic arm. A robot port can be "piggy-backed" through the 12 mm assistant port which serves as the left robotic arm. The remaining two ports (used as the left and right robot ports for the nephrectomy) can serve as converted assistant ports (Fig. 35.11).

Step 5: The robot is then redocked from below over the ipsilateral hip so that the "sweet spot" is now directed toward the ureterovesical junction (UVJ) (Fig. 35.13).

Step 6: The ureter is then identified and dissected inferiorly down to the level of the UVJ. Individual feeding vessels to the ureter are divided with bipolar electrocautery.

Step 7: Once the UVJ is approached the bladder is partially expanded with saline. This allows better identification of the UVJ as well as elevates the bladder out of the pelvis to facilitate cuff extraction. Vicryl

stay sutures are placed into the detrusor muscle on both sides of the junction for better exposure.

Step 8: The detrusor is incised longitudinally and the ureter circumferentially dissected until the mucosa of the bladder is visualized. With gentle cephalad retraction of the ureter the UVJ is dissected with cold scissors (Fig. 35.14) and then clipped prior to freeing the ureter and bladder cuff from the remnant bladder (Fig. 35.15). Alternatively, a vicryl suture can be placed at 6 o'clock into the mucosa prior to complete division of the ureter to insure that the first layer closure adequately incorporates the mucosa into the stitch (Fig. 35.16). The suture is then run from 6 to 12 o'clock including both the mucosa and the internal muscle into the running stitch (Fig. 35.17). Next, a second vicryl layer of superficial muscle is run to complete the bladder closure. Integrity of the closure is tested with bladder irrigation through the foley catheter (intraoperative bladder cuff images provided by Daniel Eun, MD, Assistant Professor, Division of Urology, University of Pennsylvania).

Step 9: A 15 mm endocatch bag is placed into the abdomen under direct vision and the specimen is placed inside. A port site is then extended to complete specimen extraction.

Preliminary data for lymphadenectomy in advanced upper tract urothelial carcinoma appear promising, though they are not as well established as the data for

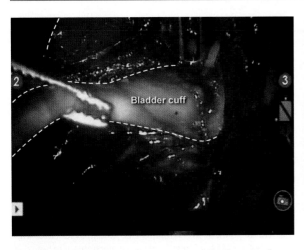

Fig. 35.14 Cephalad retraction on ureter while dissecting intramural ureter and bladder cuff

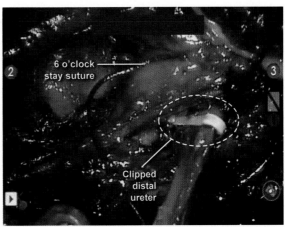

Fig. 35.16 Bladder cuff dissection with placement of stay suture at 6 o'clock position of ureteral orifice

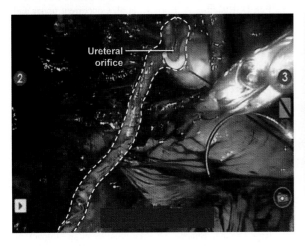

Fig. 35.15 Completed bladder cuff excision

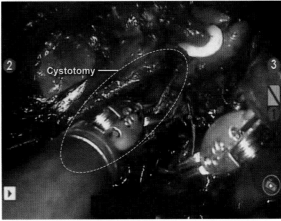

Fig. 35.17 Closure of cystotomy

lymphadenectomy in bladder cancer. Kondo et al. performed lymphadenectomies in their cohort of patients undergoing nephroureterectomies. Patients were categorized as having either complete or incomplete regional lymphadenectomies. Regional lymph nodes were defined based on tumor location within the upper urinary tract. For those with tumors in the right renal pelvis, upper, or mid-ureter, the hilar, paracaval, and retrocaval nodes were dissected. Tumors in either the left renal pelvis, upper or proximal ureter required renal hilar and para-aortic node dissections. Distal ureteral tumors required pelvic lymphadenectomies. Complete and incomplete lymph node dissections demonstrated a nonsignificant increase in cancer-specific survival within the entire group. However, in patients with pT3–4 disease, both complete and incomplete lymph node dissections demonstrated a statistically significant improvement in cancer-specific survival. Finally, on multivariate analysis, complete lymph node dissection was a significant prognostic factor in those with pT3–4 disease, whereas incomplete lymph node dissection was not, lending support that the extent of nodal dissection is important.[19] These data are supported by a more recent multi-institutional study also comparing pNx to pNo patients who underwent radical nephroureterectomy. Although no cancer-specific survival benefit was conferred in those with a pT1 primary tumor, those patients with pT2–4 primary tumors who underwent a lymphadenectomy were found to have significant improvement in cancer-specific survival.[20] Finally, minimally invasive techniques do not preclude the ability of urologic surgeons to perform adequate lymphadenectomies for upper tract urothelial carcinoma. Data comparing open lymphadenectomies to those performed laparoscopically demonstrated no difference in nodal yield or node density.[21]

Acknowledgments The authors would like to thank Dr. Daniel Eun with his assistance in completing this chapter.

References

1. Flanigan RC, Mickisch G, Sylvester R, et al. Cytoreductive nephrectomy in patients with metastatic renal cancer: a combined analysis. *J Urol.* 2004;171:1071–1076.
2. Karellas ME, Jang TL, Kagiwada MA, et al. Advanced-stage renal cell carcinoma treated by radical nephrectomy and adjacent organ or structure resection. *Br J Urol.* 2008;103:160–164.
3. Thomas MA, Rha KH, Ong AM, et al. Optical access trocar injuries in urological laparoscopic surgery. *J Urol.* 2003;170:61–63.
4. O'Malley RL, Godoy G, Kanofsky JA, et al. The necessity of adrenalectomy at the time of radical nephrectomy: a systematic review. *J Urol.* 2009;181:2009–2017.
5. Blom JHM, van Poppel H, Marechal JM, et al. Radical nephrectomy with and without lymph-node dissection: final results of European organization for research and treatment of cancer (EORTC) randomized phase 3 trial 30881. *Eur Urol.* 2009;55:28–34.
6. Canfield SE, Kamat AM, Sanchez-Ortiz RF, et al. Renal cell carcinoma with nodal metastases in the absence of distant metastatic disease (clinical stage txn1-2M0): the impact of aggressive surgical resection on patient outcome. *J Urol.* 2006;175:864–869.
7. Pantuck AJ, Zisman A, Dorey F, et al. Renal cell carcinoma with retroperitoneal lymph nodes: role of lymph node dissection. *J Urol.* 2003;169:2076–2083.
8. Blute ML, Leibovich BC, Cheville JC, et al. A protocol for performing extended lymph node dissection using primary tumor pathological features for patients treated withradical nephrectomy for clear cell renal cell carcinoma. *J Urol.* 2004;172:465–469.
9. Bachmann A, Ruszat R, Forster T, et al. Retroperitoneoscopic pyeloplasty for ureteropelvic junction obstruction (UPJO): solving the technical difficulties. *J Urol.* 2006;49:264–272.
10. Rassweiler JJ, Seemann O, Frede T, et al. Retroperitoneoscopy: experience with 200 cases. *J Urol.* 1998;160:1265–1269.
11. McAllister M, Bhayani SB, Ong A, et al. Vena cava transection during retroperitoneoscopic nephrectomy: report of the complication and review of the literature. *J Urol.* 2004;172:183–185.
12. Matin SF, Gill IS. Modified Pfannenstiel incision for intact specimen extraction after retroperitoneoscopic renal surgery. *Urology.* 2003;61:830–832.
13. Hu JC, Silletti JP, Williams SB. Initial experience with robot-assisted minimally invasive nephroureterectomy. *J Endourol.* 2008;22:699–704.
14. Nanigian DK, Smith W, Ellison LM. Robot-assisted laparoscopic nephroureterectomy. *J Endourol.* 2006;20:463–466.
15. Eun D, Bhandari A, Boris R, et al. Concurrent upper and lower urinary tract robotic surgery: strategies for success. *Br J Urol.* 2007;100:1121–1125.
16. Murphy D, Challacombe B, Olsburgh J, et al. Ablative and reconstructive robotic-assisted laparoscopic renal surgery. *Int J Clin Pract.* 2008;62:1703–1708.
17. Park SY, Jeong W, Ham WS, et al. Initial experience of robotic nephroureterectomy: a hybrid-port technique. *Br J Urol.* 2009;104:1718–1721.
18. Rose K, Khan S, Godbole H, et al. Robotic assisted retroperitoneoscopic nephroureterectomy – first experience and the hybrid port technique. *Int J Clin Pract.* 2006;60:12–14.
19. Kondo T, Nakazawa H, Ito F, et al. Impact of the extent of regional lymphadenectomy on the survival of patients with urothelial carcinoma of the upper urinary tract. *J Urol.* 2007;178:1212–1217.
20. Roscigno M, Shariat SF, Margulis V, et al. Impact of lymph node dissection on cancer specific survival in patients with upper tract urothelial carcinoma treated with radical nephroureterectomy. *J Urol.* 2009;181:2482–2489.
21. Busby JE, Brown GA, Matin SF. Comparing lymphadenectomy during radical nephroureterectomy: open versus laparoscopic. *Urology.* 2008;71:413–416.

Chapter 36

Robot-Assisted Partial Nephrectomy

Brian M. Benway, Robert S. Figenshau, and Sam B. Bhayani

36.1 Introduction

Since its introduction in 2004 by Gettman and colleagues,[1] robot-assisted partial nephrectomy (RAPN) has been steadily gaining acceptance as part of a new standard of care for the treatment of localized renal malignancy. However, this rise to prominence has not been without its share of difficulties.

Soon after the introduction of robot-assisted partial nephrectomy, initial studies evaluating operative parameters and immediate outcomes failed to find a significant advantage over other available techniques, namely open and laparoscopic partial nephrectomy,[2,3] leading some to suggest that RAPN had a limited role in the treatment of renal malignancy.

However, as the experience has matured, newer, more robust series have begun to demonstrate remarkable improvements in critical operative parameters, suggesting that robot-assisted partial nephrectomy does indeed have a place in the urologist's armamentarium.

In this chapter, we will discuss the evolution of renal surgery in general, and more specifically, the rising interest in robot-assisted partial nephrectomy, a technique which built upon the foundations forged by the pioneers of the late 20th century. We will then present a detailed atlas of technique for robot-assisted partial nephrectomy, detailing the methods employed by today's top robotic renal surgeons. Finally, we will explore the available literature pertaining to robot-assisted partial nephrectomy, detailing the outcomes associated with this burgeoning technique.

36.2 The Evolution of Renal Surgery

For many decades, open radical nephrectomy served as the gold standard for surgical treatment for renal cell carcinoma of any size. However, with the advent of high-resolution cross-sectional imaging, there has been a shift in the diagnosis of renal malignancy, away from large, generally symptomatic masses, to small, often serendipitously detected masses.[4–8]

Along with this shift in the diagnosis of renal cancer came increased interest in nephron-sparing techniques, which would allow for complete resection of the tumor while preserving the unaffected portions of the kidney. Partial nephrectomy gained acceptance as a new standard of care for clinical stage T1 lesions, demonstrating equivalent cancer control to radical extirpation, as well as equivalent perioperative morbidity.[9–14]

Moreover, long-term outcomes have demonstrated that preservation of the healthy, unaffected renal parenchyma is associated with a sharp decrease in the risk for long-term renal dysfunction and improved overall survival. Indeed, maximal preservation of renal functional reserve appears to be associated with a decreased risk of development of numerous diseases, including hypertension, diabetes mellitus, and cardiopulmonary diseases.[11,14,15]

In the early 1990s, Clayman and colleagues introduced laparoscopic techniques for radical nephrectomy, ushering in the era of minimally-invasive

S.B. Bhayani (✉)
Division of Urologic Surgery, Department of Surgery,
Washington University School of Medicine, St. Louis,
MO, USA
e-mail: bhayanisa@wudosis.wustl.edu

A.K. Hemal, M. Menon (eds.), *Robotics in Genitourinary Surgery*,
DOI 10.1007/978-1-84882-114-9_36, © Springer-Verlag London Limited 2011

renal surgery.[16] Soon after, Winfield et al. and McDougall et al. described the technique for laparoscopic partial nephrectomy, which rapidly gained acceptance at high-volume centers of excellence.[17,18] Laparoscopic partial nephrectomy represented a significant leap forward in the treatment of localized kidney cancer. Reports soon demonstrated operative parameters on par with its open counterpart, and reproducible reports of oncologic equivalence were followed.[9,11,19,20]

However, despite the clear advantages of laparoscopic partial nephrectomy, the technique has failed to make inroads outside of high-volume academic centers, owing in large part to the formidable technical challenge associated with the approach, namely with regard to tumor excision and renal reconstruction, aspects of the procedure which are performed under the duress of warm ischemia. In fact, two troubling studies published in 2006 found that laparoscopic partial nephrectomy was sorely underutilized by the urologic community at large, with only 12% of all renal masses and less than 50% of renal masses less than 2 cm in size being addressed with nephron-sparing techniques.[5,21]

The introduction of robotic technology into urologic surgery has prompted a renaissance in the minimally-invasive treatment of urologic disease. Offering a magnified stereoscopic view, along with fully articulating wristed instruments, motion scaling, and elimination of tremor, robot assistance allows for precise handling of tissues and instruments, allowing even laparoscopically naïve surgeons to replicate the success of open surgery through a minimally-invasive approach.[7,22]

Robotic surgery's initial applications for minimally-invasive prostatectomy have propelled robotic technology to the fore and have led to a rapid increase in the number of robotic systems available throughout the United States and the rest of the world. Much as robotic technology has refined the minimally-invasive treatment of prostate cancer, robot assistance stands to provide substantial improvements in minimally-invasive nephron-sparing surgery, eliminating much of the technical challenge associated with the laparoscopic approach, and thereby reducing the barrier of entry for the urologic community. These important steps forward may indeed equalize access to the standard of care for all patients who are diagnosed with renal cancer.

36.3 Atlas of Technique

Despite the relative ease and short learning curve of robot-assisted partial nephrectomy,[23] the technique remains quite challenging, especially to the novice renal surgeon. While the available robotic systems offer an enhanced three-dimensional view and an unprecedented range of instrument motion, there are significant limitations associated with the technique, chief among them the lack of haptic feedback. This loss of sensory perception requires the robotic surgeon to be intimately familiar with the strength of the robotic arms and to be able to rely largely upon visual cues to gauge the amount of tension being applied to delicate structures, as the robotic arms are capable of exerting an incredible amount of force, even when meeting resistance. Nowhere is this particular facet of robot-assisted renal surgery more critical than when dissecting near the hilar structures.

Therefore, it is recommended that any urologist considering robot-assisted renal surgery should first gain adequate experience with their robotic system. This would include sanctioned hands-on courses which provide the surgeon with thorough instruction in the handling of the robotic system, ideally in an environment which provides a live-animal model. Furthermore, it is recommended that the surgeon become facile with robot-assisted laparoscopic prostatectomy before attempting to employ robotic technology for the purposes of renal surgery.

It is also recommended that the initial transition to robot-assisted renal surgery be focused on radical nephrectomy. Beginning with radical nephrectomy will allow the surgeon to become familiar with the landmarks associated with robot-assisted renal surgery, while also affording the opportunity to become comfortable with hilar dissection using the robotic system.

36.3.1 Patient Selection and Other Considerations

Proper patient selection is critical to the success of robot-assisted renal surgery. While complex central and hilar tumors are capable of being addressed robotically, challenging cases such as these should not be attempted during the initial experience. As such, the ideal initial patients for the novice surgeon would be thin females with exophytic masses and uncomplicated renal vasculature. This particular patient will offer minimal interference from peri-renal fat, which will drastically reduce the difficulty of retraction and hilar dissection. Moreover, an exophytic renal mass is relatively simple to excise and reconstruct, which will minimize the risk of prolonged ischemic times during the initial experience.

It is critical to obtain a thorough patient history, paying special attention to prior abdominal and retroperitoneal surgery, as well as to medical renal disease and other comorbidities such as diabetes mellitus and hypertension. Patients who are on anticoagulation will generally require clearance to have their anticoagulants temporarily suspended in the perioperative period.

Proper informed consent is crucial. Patients must be counseled to the attendant risks of robot-assisted partial nephrectomy, including the risk for hemorrhage requiring transfusion, postoperative urine leak, and inability to completely resect the tumor. In addition, the patient must be counseled regarding the possibility of conversion to radical nephrectomy or to an open procedure.

As dissection of the hilar anatomy can be very difficult, it is recommended that a contrast-enhanced CT scan be performed whenever possible to identify the hilar anatomy. This will allow the surgeon to be prepared for multiple arteries and veins, as well as for anatomic aberrancy.

36.3.2 Patient Positioning and Trocar Placement

The patient should be placed in a flank position, in a manner nearly identical to that of a laparoscopic or open procedure. However, excessive flexion of the table is often not necessary when undertaking a robotic approach. In addition, the arms should be positioned as far cephalad as safely possible, to minimize collisions with the robotic arms. An axillary roll should be placed, and the patient should be secured to the table in a manner that will allow the table to be rolled if necessary.

Sequential compression devices should be placed to provide prophylaxis against deep venous thrombosis.

In addition, a preoperative dose of fractionated heparin can be administered for further prophylaxis and should not lead to increased risk of bleeding complications.

With regard to trocar placement, there are two generally accepted approaches. The first and most widely utilized is a medial trocar arrangement, which places the camera port near the umbilicus. This approach replicates a standard transperitoneal laparoscopic approach and should therefore be familiar to most renal surgeons. The alternative approach locates the camera laterally, providing a closer view that is more akin to a retroperitoneal approach, even though the camera and instruments remain in the peritoneal space. Both approaches have been extensively described and are capable of providing adequate visualization and instrument mobility.[1,23–30]

However, in our center's experience, we find the medial approach to be more favorable for a number of reasons, chief among them the wide viewing angle provided by the relatively greater distance between the camera and the target structures. Not only does this approach allow for easier visualization of the surrounding structures, but it also allows the camera to be panned for tracking of instruments passed by the assistant, thus lowering the potential for iatrogenic injury. Furthermore, the digital zoom of later model robotic systems allows for closer inspection of the surgical field, though this zoom feature is often not necessary. In addition, the medial approach often requires only one assistant port, whereas the lateral approach is generally described as using two assistant ports. In the latter, the assistant is placed at somewhat of a disadvantage, as he or she must work on both sides of the camera arm.[26] A detailed illustration of the medial and lateral approaches can be found in Figs. 36.1 and 36.2.

In patients with excessive peri-renal fat or in instances when a surgeon must work with an inexperienced assistant, the fourth arm can be utilized to allow the surgeon greater control over the retraction.[24,31] However, the novice surgeon must be cautioned that unlike robot-assisted laparoscopic prostatectomy, including the fourth arm in a robot-assisted partial nephrectomy is actually *more* technically demanding, due to crowding of the instruments and robotic arms into a comparatively smaller working space. As such, a four-arm approach should be considered an advanced procedure. An illustration of the four-arm approach can be found in Fig. 36.3.

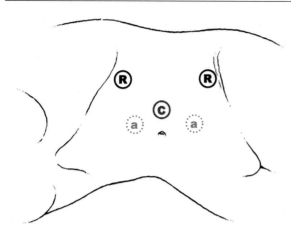

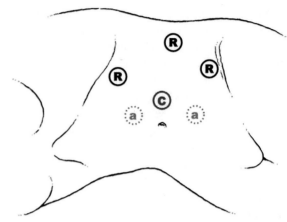

Fig. 36.1 Trocar configuration for the medial camera three-arm approach. A 30° downward-angled lens is used. R, robotic arm; C, camera; a, assistant port (12 mm). The *dotted line* indicates that the assistant port may be placed at either location; only one assistant port is generally necessary. For right-sided procedures, a 5 mm subxiphoid port may be used for placement of a liver retractor (not pictured)

Fig. 36.3 Trocar configuration for the medial camera four-arm approach. A 30° downward-angled lens is used. R, Robotic arm; C, Camera; a = assistant port (12 mm). The *dotted line* indicates that the assistant port may be placed at either location; only one assistant port is generally necessary. For right-sided procedures, a 5 mm subxiphoid port may be used for placement of a liver retractor (not pictured)

36.3.3 Robot Docking and Instrument Selection

The robot should be docked at an angle, on a line connecting the expected location of the renal hilum and the umbilicus. The elbows of the working arms should be pushed out as far laterally as the device will allow, in order to maximize the excursion of the arms and to minimize external collisions.

The right hand should be outfitted with the robotic scissors, which should be connected to monopolar electrocautery. The left hand should be outfitted with the ProGrasp forceps. The assistant should retract with a laparoscopic suction device. Other instruments to have available on the field for the assistant include a Weck (Teleflex, Research Triangle Park, NC, USA) Hem-o-lok clip applier, a LapraTy (Ethicon, Cincinnati, OH, USA) clip applier, a laparoscopic ultrasound probe, and a laparoscopic bulldog applier or Satinsky clamp. In addition, a vascular stapler device with multiple reloads should be readily available, in the event of misadventure requiring emergent nephrectomy.

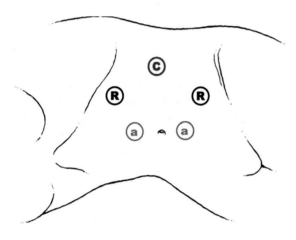

Fig. 36.2 Trocar configuration for the lateral camera approach. A 30° upward-angled lens is used. R, robotic arm; C, camera; a, assistant port (12 mm). Traditionally, two assistant ports are used. For right-sided procedures, a 5-mm subxiphoid port may be used for placement of a liver retractor (not pictured)

When placing the caudad port, the trocar should be introduced approximately 2 cm cephalad to the iliac crest in order to minimize external arm collisions with the hip. For right-sided tumors, an accessory subxiphoid port for a liver retractor is often necessary. This port should be placed as close to the midline as possible, so as not to interfere with the right robotic arm.

On the back table, the surgical assistant should prepare the renorrhaphy sutures, as well as sutures for collecting system repair. As we will discuss later, we strongly recommend the use of a sliding-clip technique

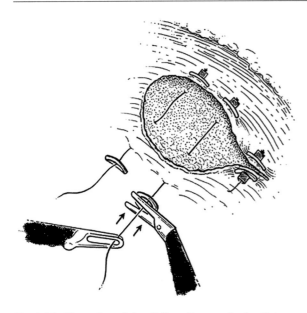

Fig. 36.4 Illustration of the sliding-clip renorrhaphy. Sutures are prepared on the back table by cutting an 0 polyglactin suture to a length of 12–15 cm. A knot is tied at the end, followed by a LapraTy clip and a Hem-o-lok clip. Once the suture has been placed through-and-through, the assistant places a second Hem-o-lok clip on the loose end of the suture, which is then slid into place by the surgeon. The repair is locked in place with a LapraTy clip

for renal reconstruction. As the required sutures can be time consuming to prepare, it is crucial that these sutures are fashioned beforehand.

The collecting system sutures should consist of one or two 2-0 polyglactin sutures, cut to a length of 12 cm. At the end, a knot should be tied, followed by a LapraTy clip. Hem-o-lok clips should not be used on these sutures, as they are non-degradable and could erode into the collecting system. The renorrhaphy sutures are 0 polyglactin sutures cut to a length of 12–15 cm. At the end, a knot is tied, followed by a LapraTy clip, then a Hem-o-lok clip (Fig. 36.4).

In addition, bolster material and tissue sealants should be immediately available, should either be necessary to achieve satisfactory closure and hemostasis.

36.3.4 Initial Dissection

The bowel is reflected along the white line of Toldt, thus exposing the retroperitoneum. For right-sided tumors, the duodenum must also be carefully reflected

in order to gain access to the hilum. Great care must be taken during this maneuver, as the vena cava lies directly inferior to the duodenum, and is therefore prone to iatrogenic injury.

The lower pole of the kidney should then be identified, and just off the lower pole, the ureter and gonadal vasculature should be identified. It is preferable to leave the gonadal vein intact if at all possible, and therefore, the vein should be dropped medially whenever possible. Great care must be taken to avoid excessive skeletonizing of the ureter, so as not to compromise the blood supply.

The pocket created by elevating the ureter should allow the kidney to be placed on gentle lateral stretch. Dissection should be carried carefully cephalad to reveal the hilar vessels. Astute surgeons may be able to detect the venous impulse which is the hallmark of the renal vein.[24] The artery should lie directly posterior to the vein.

The extent of hilar dissection should be largely dictated by the needs of the preferred method of vascular control. If a laparoscopic Satinsky clamp is to be used to clamp the hilum en bloc, then further dissection between the artery and the vein is not generally necessary. However, if laparoscopic bulldog clamps are to be used, separation of the artery and vein will be necessary. The ProGrasp forceps are best suited for this task, as they are able to bluntly dissect the plane between the vein and the artery. Great care should be taken to eliminate the posterior hilar fat from the field, to ensure that the bulldog clamps are able to fully close.

In some instances, it may be possible to isolate a segmental arterial branch which provides the entire blood supply to the tumor. Selective clamping of this artery may lead to less ischemic insult, as the unaffected portions of the kidney remain perfused. However, while effective for polar tumors, such dissection increases the risk of vascular injury and should be considered an advanced technique.[32,33]

36.3.5 Preparing for Excision

The fat surrounding the tumor should be reflected to expose a 1 cm margin of normal capsular tissue around the mass. This maneuver will greatly aid in reconstruction. The fat overlying the kidney should be left intact, but may be inadvertently released from the surface of the tumor. If this occurs, the fat should be immediately collected and placed with the specimen.

Intraoperative ultrasound should then be performed to assess the extent of the tumor and to delineate the margins of dissection, which should be marked by scoring the capsule. If selective clamping of a segmental renal artery is to be employed, color Doppler flow should be used to assess for complete cessation of flow after temporary occlusion of the segmental artery.

Once the stage is set for excision, the renal vasculature should be carefully occluded with either a Satinsky clamp or bulldog clamps. If a Satinsky clamp is to be used, it is imperative that the assistant closely monitors the clamp and takes steps to avoid external collisions which could lead to avulsion of the vasculature. Due to the inherent risks of the Satinsky clamp method, we prefer the use of bulldog clamps, which are used to occlude the vessels individually. As the bulldog clamps may weaken during reprocessing, it is recommended to clamp the artery doubly whenever possible to ensure complete occlusion. Clamping of the vein is left to surgeon preference, though it is highly recommended, especially for central, anterior, or hilar tumors.

36.3.6 Tumor Excision

The tumor is then sharply excised using the robotic scissors. The ProGrasp may be used to gently spread the tissues and present the underlying parenchyma for dissection. Great care should be taken to follow the expected curvature of the tumor. If the tumor is entered, the last steps should be retraced, and the tumor should be recaptured. Should this occur, it is recommended to repair this defect on the back table after extraction, to avoid an iatrogenic false-positive margin.

Dissection should be carried out from near to far, using the attachment of the far side as a hinge that will allow for relatively simple retraction as excision is carried out. Any entry into large venous channels or into the collecting system should be noted. Once excision is complete, the tumor should be placed out of the field nearby for later extraction. At this juncture, the assistant may collect a biopsy of the resection bed, if deemed necessary.

36.3.7 Renal Reconstruction

Reconstruction should be undertaken with all deliberate speed. The cortex should be cauterized for hemostasis; however, cautery should not be applied to the medulla. At this juncture, the robotic scissors should be replaced with a needle driver; the ProGrasp should remain on the left hand, as this instrument has the capacity to serve as a needle driver, if necessary. If there has been entry into the collecting system or into a large venous sinus, these areas should be oversewn using the 2-0 polyglactin suture in a running fashion. The repair should be secured with a LapraTy clip to obviate the need for knot tying. Should a bolster or tissue sealants be deemed necessary, they may be applied now or shortly after commencing the renorrhaphy.

Sliding-clip renorrhaphy should then be performed.[23–25,34–36] The prepared sutures should be placed at 1 cm intervals along the length of the defect. After completing the second throw, the assistant places a Hem-o-lok clip on the loose end. This clip need not be placed in direct apposition to the capsule, as it will be slid into position under tension by the surgeon. However, the assistant should take care to ensure that the suture is placed as close to the middle of the clip as possible, as this will allow the clip to be slid along the suture with greater ease.

The Hem-o-lok clip is then slid into position by straddling the suture with the jaws of the needle driver. Appropriate tension has been placed when the capsule dimples slightly. As this maneuver is being performed, the ProGrasp should hold tension on the loose end of the suture in a direction perpendicular to the capsule, so as to minimize the risk of tearing through the capsule. Once the Hem-o-lok clip has been slid into place, the repair is locked in place by a LapraTy clip. This clip, too, may be slid over the suture, though it does not slide as readily as the Hem-o-lok clip. Once all renorrhaphy sutures have been placed, they may be re-tightened by the surgeon to precisely calibrate the tension upon the repair.

The clamps should then be carefully removed from the hilum, and the repair should be inspected for hemostasis. Should slight bleeding be encountered, a period of observation is warranted, as reperfusion of the kidney will lead to an increase in mass which may further apply tension to the repair and can thus tamponade the bleeding. Should bleeding persist, the clips can be further re-tightened or additional sutures may be placed.

36.3.8 Extraction and Closure

Once hemostasis has been verified, the specimen should be placed in a retrieval bag and the robot should be undocked. The specimen should then be extracted through a widened incision in order to prevent undue compression of the often delicate tumor. A drain may be left in place if deemed necessary.

The fascia of the extraction site should be repaired, though repair of the remaining sites is generally not necessary, as the risk of herniation is low.[37] The skin incisions should be closed after irrigation.

36.3.9 Postoperative Care and Management of Perioperative Complications

Appropriate analgesia should be provided. Serum chemistries and hematocrit should be monitored in the immediate postoperative period and on a daily basis. Mild ileus should be expected, though most patients will tolerate a diet by postoperative day 1. Ambulation may safely be commenced on postoperative day 0.

Immediate postoperative complications may include cardiac events, deep venous thrombosis, acute renal insufficiency or failure, unrecognized bowel injury, and renal hemorrhage. The latter may be self-limited and may respond to observation and possible transfusion of blood products. On rare occasions, significant bleeding may prompt further intervention, such as selective embolization or return to the operating theatre for completion nephrectomy. Patients who develop renal insufficiency may require nephrology evaluation and may very rarely require dialysis. Provided that ischemic time did not exceed 30 min, it is very likely that renal insufficiency will be self-limited.[38]

Unrecognized bowel injuries often have an atypical presentation in the minimally-invasive setting. Unlike open procedures, patients may not develop the classic signs of leukocytosis, peritonitis, and ileus. Rather, they will often develop leukopenia, tenderness limited to the port site closest to the injury, and diarrhea.[39] If bowel injury is suspected, immediate evaluation with abdominal imaging and general surgery consultation is warranted.

Intermediate complications may include urine leak and development of an arteriovenous malformation. Urine leaks may have a delayed presentation and may be heralded by flank pain, excessive drainage from a port site, and fever. Abdominal imaging will confirm the diagnosis. Treatment requires the placement of a ureteral stent and percutaneous drainage of the urinoma; repair is rarely required.[40] Arteriovenous malformation or pseudoaneurysm is a rare complication which can occur at any time and often presents as painless gross hematuria. Arteriography confirms the diagnosis, and treatment often consists of selective embolization or, in rare instances, completion nephrectomy.[41-43]

36.3.10 Long-Term Follow-Up

Long-term follow-up consists of periodic imaging and laboratory evaluation, including abdominal CT, chest X-ray, complete blood count, basic metabolic panel, and hepatic function panel. It is of note that if a bolster was used in reconstruction, the material may persist with a defect that appears to contain air. This may often be confused with an abscess unless the radiologist is provided a proper history.

36.4 Outcomes of Robot-Assisted Partial Nephrectomy

Initial published reports on robot-assisted partial nephrectomy demonstrated respectable operative parameters and excellent short-term outcomes. Operative times in these series ranged from 142 to 279 min, while warm ischemic times ranged from 20 to 32 min. In addition, rates of positive margins were quite low, with only seven positive margins reported in a total of 256 patients across all series, representing only 2.7% of all patients evaluated. At a period of up to 16 months, no patient in any of the initial series developed disease recurrence.[1-3,22,29,30,44-46] It is of note that these series represented the initial experience of the early adopters of the technique and were therefore likely confounded by the learning curve of the procedure. Furthermore, each study except for one was hindered by the relatively small number of patients in each experience, with typical study sizes ranging from 8 to 13 patients. Nevertheless, these results provided evidence of feasibility for the procedure.

However, initial comparative analyses pitting robot-assisted partial nephrectomy against laparoscopic partial nephrectomy raised some understandable concern that the additional expense of robot assistance did not justify its inclusion in the renal surgeon's armamentarium. For instance, in the first published comparative analysis between robot-assisted partial nephrectomy and laparoscopic partial nephrectomy, Caruso et al. found that the robot assistance did not confer any specific advantage over a laparoscopic approach, including critical parameters such as overall operative time and warm ischemic time.[3] However, it is of note that the authors focused solely on patients with exophytic tumors, which are arguably relatively simple to address, regardless of approach. A larger and more recent comparative analysis, however, has found that the benefits of a robot-assisted approach become more apparent as tumor complexity increases.[34] Indeed, robot-assisted partial nephrectomy has been finding increased application in addressing complex central and hilar tumors that might otherwise recommend an open approach.[45,46]

More recent reports, however, have begun to demonstrate substantial improvements in operative parameters, with overall operative times ranging from 83 to 174 min. Perhaps more critical is the profound reduction in warm ischemic times, which range from 18 to 22 min in the most recent analyses.[23,28,34,47]

Likewise, contemporary comparative studies have begun to demonstrate a clear advantage of robot-assisted partial nephrectomy over a standard laparoscopic approach. In the largest single-surgeon series to date, Wang and Bhayani found that robot-assisted partial nephrectomy provides significantly shorter overall operative times as well as warm ischemic times, when compared with laparoscopic partial nephrectomy.[47] These results are further corroborated in a large multi-institutional series from Benway and colleagues,[34] who found that warm ischemic times were nearly 9 min shorter in the robot-assisted arm (19.7 vs 28.4 min for the laparoscopic approach, $p<0.0001$). A summary of the outcomes of contemporary comparative series is outlined in Table 36.1.

36.5 Learning Curve and Technical Refinements

The above-mentioned improvements in operative parameters for robot-assisted partial nephrectomy appear to be multifactorial, likely owing to refinements in technique, coupled with larger study sizes with a greater number of cases performed after the learning curve for the procedure has been surpassed.

As with any procedure, robot-assisted partial nephrectomy presents unique technical challenges during a surgeon's initial experience. As such, the procedure does carry with it a learning curve. A recent analysis evaluating 50 patients who underwent robot-assisted partial nephrectomy by a single surgeon, however, found that the learning curve for the procedure is quite modest. Evaluating by overall operative time, the learning curve could be surpassed in only 19 procedures. However, examining those portions which are performed under warm ischemia, including tumor excision and renal reconstruction, the learning curve is somewhat more substantial, requiring 26 cases to develop proficiency.[23]

These figures compare favorably, however, to laparoscopic partial nephrectomy, using the same parameters for evaluation. In a 2005 report from Link and colleagues, the authors found that while overall operative time did appear to decrease with surgeon experience, the learning curve for those portions of the procedure performed under the conditions of warm ischemia could not be identified, even after 200 procedures.[48] As will be discussed later, this striking contrast suggests that most surgeons will be able to develop proficiency with a robot-assisted approach within a relatively short period.

Another important factor in evaluating contemporary literature is an important refinement in technique, which greatly improves the efficiency of renal reconstruction. Sliding-clip renorrhaphy obviates the need for intracorporeal knot tying, which, though comparatively simple to perform using robot assistance, is nevertheless challenging and time consuming. The use of sliding clips allows the surgeon to quickly and efficiently close the renal defect, while exercising unprecedented control over the tension of the repair. A recent analysis evaluating the impact of this refinement found that adoption of a sliding-clip technique can provide reductions in warm ischemic times of up to 8 min.[23]

Table 36.1 Overview of contemporary series comparing RAPN to LPN

	Caruso et al. (2006)[3]		Aron et al. (2008)[2]		Deane et al. (2008)[22]		Wang and Bhayanl (2009)[47]		Benway et al. (2009)[23]		Jeong et al. (2009)[49]		Kural et al. (2009)[50]	
	LPN	RAPN	LPN	RAPN	LPN	RAPN	LPN	RAPN	LPN	RAPN	LPN	RAPN	LPN	RAPN
N	10	10	12	12	11	11	62	40	118	129	26	31	20	11
Tumor size	2.2	2	2.9	2.4	2.3	3.1	2.4	2.5	2.6	2.9	2.4	3.4	3.1	3.2
OR time	253	279	256	242	290	229	156	140 ($p = 0.04$)	174	189	139	169 ($p = 0.03$)	226	185
WIT	29	26	22	23	35	32	25	19 ($p = 0.03$)	28	19 ($p < 0.0001$)	17.2	20.9	35.8	27.3 ($p = 0.02$)
EBL	200	240	300	329	198	115	173	136	196	155 ($p = 0.03$)	208	198	388	286
Complications	1	1	1	1	1	1	9	8	8.60%	10.20%	1	1	1	1
Conversions	1	2	0	2	1	0	3	1	4.50%	1.60%	0	1	3	0
PSM	1	0	0	0	0	0	1	1	3.90%	1%	NR	NR	5%	0%
Recurrence	NR	NR	NR	NR	NR	NR	0	0	0	0	2	2	0	0

WIT, warm ischemic time; EBL, estimated blood loss; PSM, positive surgical margin; NR, not reported.

36.6 The Case for Robot-Assisted Partial Nephrectomy

As discussed earlier, there has been a striking shift in the diagnosis of renal malignancy toward smaller masses amenable to nephron-sparing surgery. Yet, despite its emergence as a standard of care, partial nephrectomy has struggled to make inroads in the urologic community at large in the laparoscopic era. Certainly, a major barrier to entry for most surgeons has been the formidable and likely forbidding learning curve of laparoscopic partial nephrectomy.

Robot-assisted partial nephrectomy stands to reduce and perhaps eliminate this barrier of entry, providing enhanced visualization and improved dexterity of the surgical instrumentation, compared to a traditional laparoscopic approach. Indeed, Deane and colleagues conclusively demonstrated that after just ten robot-assisted procedures, a laparoscopically naïve surgeon was able to perform robot-assisted partial nephrectomy with a level of competency equivalent to laparoscopic partial nephrectomy performed by experienced laparoscopic renal surgeons.[22] Certainly, these data, coupled with that of Benway et al., suggest that robot-assisted partial nephrectomy is a procedure which is rapidly learned, allowing for a relatively short learning curve to achieve technical competence.[23] This, in turn, indicates that the introduction of robotic technology may stand to level the playing field, allowing most urologists to offer their patients the current standard of surgical care.

Furthermore, the drastic reductions in overall operative times, and perhaps more critically, reductions in warm ischemic times with a robot-assisted approach could theoretically lead to improved long-term functional outcomes, though this particular facet of outcomes has yet to be explored in the robotic literature.

However, there are a few criticisms of the robot-assisted approach which warrant discussion. First, the adoption of robotic technology requires a substantial capital expense, which may render its adoption less attractive to lower volume centers. While comparative cost analysis is presently lacking in the literature, one must consider the potential for cost reductions, in terms of shorter overall operative times and shorter hospital stay,[23,47] as well as the potential for improved functional outcomes, which may reduce the overall cost burden upon the healthcare system.

Also, many authors have raised concerns over the reliance upon the bedside assistant for critical maneuvers, including those employed to establish and protect the means of hilar control.[3,31] Some authors have described techniques which may reduce the dependence upon the bedside assistant, including the use of the fourth arm for retraction, and even for hilar clamping.[31,32] However, it should be noted that in our institutional experience, we have not noted any untoward outcomes which could be attributed to the inexperience of the bedside assistant, and therefore, the veracity of these concerns has yet to be rigorously validated.[34]

36.7 Conclusions

Robot-assisted partial nephrectomy is a safe and efficacious procedure for patients diagnosed with localized renal masses. The relatively slight learning curve, coupled with the potential for drastic improvements in critical operative parameters, indicates that robot-assisted partial nephrectomy may represent the future standard of care for the surgical management of small renal masses.

References

1. Gettman MT, Blute ML, Chow GK, et al. Robotic-assisted laparoscopic partial nephrectomy: technique and initial clinical experience with da vinci robotic system. *Urology.* 2004;64:914.
2. Aron M, Koenig P, Kaouk JH, et al. Robotic and laparoscopic partial nephrectomy: a matched-pair comparison from a high-volume centre. *BJU Int.* 2008;102:86.
3. Caruso RP, Phillips CK, Kau E, et al. Robot assisted laparoscopic partial nephrectomy: initial experience. *J Urol.* 2006;176:36.
4. Chow WH, Devesa SS, Warren JL, et al. Rising incidence of renal cell cancer in the united states. *JAMA.* 1999;281:1628.
5. Hollingsworth JM, Miller DC, Daignault S, et al. Rising incidence of small renal masses: a need to reassess treatment effect. *J Natl Cancer Inst.* 2006;98:1331.
6. Jayson M, Sanders H. Increased incidence of serendipitously discovered renal cell carcinoma. *Urology.* 1998;51:203.
7. Shapiro E, Benway BM, Wang AJ, et al. The role of nephron-sparing robotic surgery in the management of renal malignancy. *Curr Opin Urol.* 2009;19:76.
8. Smith SJ, Bosniak MA, Megibow AJ, et al. Renal cell carcinoma: earlier discovery and increased detection. *Radiology.* 1989;170:699.

9. Lerner SE, Hawkins CA, Blute ML, et al. Disease outcome in patients with low stage renal cell carcinoma treated with nephron sparing or radical surgery. *J Urol*. 1996;155:1868.

10. Lerner SE, Hawkins CA, Blute ML, et al. Disease outcome in patients with low stage renal cell carcinoma treated with nephron sparing or radical surgery. *J Urol*. 1996;167:884. 2002.

11. Lau WK, Blute ML, Weaver AL, et al. Matched comparison of radical nephrectomy vs nephron-sparing surgery in patients with unilateral renal cell carcinoma and a normal contralateral kidney. *Mayo Clin Proc*. 2000;75:1236.

12. Mitchell RE, Gilbert SM, Murphy AM, et al. Partial nephrectomy and radical nephrectomy offer similar cancer outcomes in renal cortical tumors 4 cm or larger. *Urology*. 2006;67:260.

13. Senga Y, Ozono S, Nakazawa H, et al. Surgical outcomes of partial nephrectomy for renal cell carcinoma: a joint study by the Japanese society of renal cancer. *Int J Urol*. 2007;14:284.

14. Uzzo RG, Novick AC. Nephron sparing surgery for renal tumors: indications, techniques and outcomes. *J Urol*. 2001;166:6.

15. Thompson RH, Boorjian SA, Lohse CM, et al. Radical nephrectomy for pt1a renal masses may be associated with decreased overall survival compared with partial nephrectomy. *J Urol*. 2008;179:468.

16. Clayman RV, Kavoussi LR, Soper NJ, et al. Laparoscopic nephrectomy: initial case report. *J Urol*. 1991;146:278.

17. Winfield HN, Donovan JF, Godet AS, et al. Laparoscopic partial nephrectomy: initial case report for benign disease. *J Endourol*. 1993;7:521.

18. McDougall EM, Clayman RV, Chandhoke PS, et al. Laparoscopic partial nephrectomy in the pig model. *J Urol*. 1993;149:1633.

19. Gong EM, Orvieto MA, Zorn KC, et al. Comparison of laparoscopic and open partial nephrectomy in clinical T1a renal tumors. *J Endourol*. 2008;22:953.

20. Marszalek M, Meixl H, Polajnar M, et al. Laparoscopic and open partial nephrectomy: a matched-pair comparison of 200 patients. *Eur Urol*. 2009;55:1171.

21. Hollenbeck BK, Taub DA, Miller DC, et al. National utilization trends of partial nephrectomy for renal cell carcinoma: a case of underutilization? *Urology*. 2006; 67:254.

22. Deane LA, Lee HJ, Box GN, et al. Robotic versus standard laparoscopic partial/wedge nephrectomy: a comparison of intraoperative and perioperative results from a single institution. *J Endourol*. 2008;22:947.

23. Benway BM, Wang AJ, Cabello JM, et al. Robotic partial nephrectomy with sliding-clip renorrhaphy: technique and outcomes. *Eur Urol*. 2009;55:592.

24. Bhayani SB. Da vinci robotic partial nephrectomy for renal cell carcinoma: an atlas of the four-arm technique. *J Robotic Surg*. 2008;1:7.

25. Cabello JM, Benway BM, Bhayani SB. Robotic-assisted partial nephrectomy: surgical technique using a 3-arm approach and sliding-clip renorrhaphy. *Int Braz J Urol*. 2009;35:199.

26. Cabello JM, Bhayani SB, Figenshau RS, et al. Camera and trocar placement for robot-assisted radical and partial nephrectomy: which configuration provides optimal visualization and instrument mobility. *J Robot Surg*. 2009;DOI: 10.1007/s11701-009-0152-8.

27. Badani KK, Muhletaler F, Fumo M, et al. Optimizing robotic renal surgery: the lateral camera port placement technique and current results. *J Endourol*. 2008; 22:507.

28. Ho H, Schwentner C, Neururer R, et al. Robotic-assisted laparoscopic partial nephrectomy: surgical technique and clinical outcomes at 1 year. *BJU Int*. 2009;103:663.

29. Kaul S, Laungani R, Sarle R, et al. Da vinci-assisted robotic partial nephrectomy: technique and results at a mean of 15 months of follow-up. *Eur Urol*. 2007;51:186.

30. Phillips CK, Taneja SS, Stifelman MD. Robot-assisted laparoscopic partial nephrectomy: the NYU technique. *J Endourol*. 2005;19:441.

31. Rogers CG, Laungani R, Bhandari A, et al. Maximizing console surgeon independence during robot-assisted renal surgery by using the fourth arm and tilepro. *J Endourol*. 2009;23:115.

32. Figenshau R, Bhayani S, Venkatesh R, et al. Robotic renal hilar control and robotic clip placement for partial nephrectomy. *J Endourol*. 2008;22:2657.

33. Benway BM, Baca G, Bhayani SB, et al. Selective versus nonselective arterial clamping during laparoscopic partial nephrectomy: impact upon renal function in the setting of a solitary kidney in a porcine model. *J Endourol*. 2009;23:1127.

34. Benway BM, Bhayani SB, Rogers CG, et al. Robot assisted partial nephrectomy versus laparoscopic partial nephrectomy for renal tumors: a multi-institutional analysis of perioperative outcomes. *J Urol*. 2009;182:866.

35. Bhayani SB, Figenshau RS. The Washington university renorrhaphy for robotic partial nephrectomy: a detailed description of the technique displayed at the 2008 world robotic urologic symposium. *J Robot Surg*. 2008;2:2.

36. Agarwal, D,, O'Malley, P,, Clarke, D, et al. Modified technique of renal defect closure following laparoscopic partial nephrectomy. *BJU Int*. 2007;100:967.

37. Tonouchi H, Ohmori Y, Kobayashi M, et al. Trocar site hernia. *Arch Surg*. 2004;139:1248.

38. Simmons MN, Schreiber MJ, Gill IS. Surgical renal ischemia: a contemporary overview. *J Urol*. 2008;180:19.

39. Bishoff JT, Allaf ME, Kirkels W, et al. Laparoscopic bowel injury: incidence and clinical presentation. *J Urol*. 1999;161:887.

40. Meeks JJ, Zhao LC, Navai N, et al. Risk factors and management of urine leaks after partial nephrectomy. *J Urol*. 2008;180:2375.

41. Dzsinich C, Szabo Z, Dlustus B, et al. Arteriovenous fistula after partial nephrectomy–successful surgical repair. Report of a case. *Thorac Cardiovasc Surg*. 1984;32:325.

42. Negoro H, Kawakita M, Koda Y. Renal artery pseudoaneurysm after laparoscopic partial nephrectomy for renal cell carcinoma in a solitary kidney. *Int J Urol*. 2005; 12:683.

43. Albani JM, Novick AC. Renal artery pseudoaneurysm after partial nephrectomy: three case reports and a literature review. *Urology*. 2003;62:227.

44. Bhayani SB, Das N. Robotic assisted laparoscopic partial nephrectomy for suspected renal cell carcinoma:

retrospective review of surgical outcomes of 35 cases. *BMC Surg*. 2008;8:16.

45. Rogers CG, Metwalli A, Blatt AM, et al. Robotic partial nephrectomy for renal hilar tumors: a multi-institutional analysis. *J Urol*. 2008;180:2353.

46. Rogers CG, Singh A, Blatt AM, et al. Robotic partial nephrectomy for complex renal tumors: surgical technique. *Eur Urol*. 2008;53:514.

47. Wang, AJ,, Bhayani, SB. Robotic partial nephrectomy versus laparoscopic partial nephrectomy for renal cell carcinoma: single-surgeon analysis of >100 consecutive procedures. *Urology*. 2009;73:306.

48. Link RE, Bhayani SB, Allaf ME, et al. Exploring the learning curve, pathological outcomes and perioperative morbidity of laparoscopic partial nephrectomy performed for renal mass. *J Urol*. 2005;173:1690.

49. Jeong W, Park SY, Lorenzo EI, Oh CK, Han WK, Rha KH. Laparoscopic partial nephrectomy versus robot-assisted laparoscopic partial nephrectomy. *J Endourol* 2009;23:1457–1460.

50. Kural, AR, Atug, F, Tufek, I, Akpinar, H. Robot-assisted partial nephrectomy versus laparoscopic partial nephrectomy: comparison of outcomes. *J Endourol* 2009;23: 1491–1497.

Chapter 37

Robotic Urologic Surgery: Robot-Assisted Partial Nephrectomy

Manish N. Patel, Mani Menon, and Craig G. Rogers

37.1 Introduction

For renal masses smaller than 4 cm, open partial nephrectomy (OPN) has been the preferred surgical procedure to preserve renal function and minimize the long-term complications associated with renal insufficiency.[1] Laparoscopic partial nephrectomy (LPN) has emerged as a viable alternative to OPN with comparable long-term oncologic and functional outcomes, but with the convalescence benefits of a minimally invasive approach.[2] However, LPN is a technically challenging procedure, particularly in regard to intracorporeal sutured renal reconstruction under the time constraints of warm ischemia. Robotic assistance for partial nephrectomy with the da Vinci Surgical System (Intuitive Surgical, Sunnyvale, CA) may facilitate some of the technical challenges of LPN by giving the surgeon three-dimensional stereoscopic vision, a tremor-free platform, and wristed instruments which help recapitulate the open technique.

In this chapter, we present our technique for transperitoneal robotic partial nephrectomy (RPN).

37.2 Operative Setup

Operative setup is depicted in Fig. 37.1. The operating table is located in the center of the room with the anesthesiology team at the patient's head. The surgical

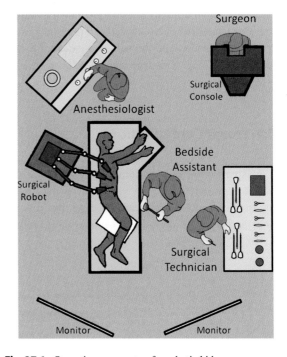

Fig. 37.1 Operating room setup for robotic kidney surgery

console and console surgeon are to the side of the room. Monitors are setup at the foot of the bed and the bedside assistant is positioned on the abdominal side of the patient next to the surgical technician. The robot is setup facing the patient's back.

37.3 Patient Positioning

General endotracheal anesthesia is administered and a Foley catheter is inserted. The patient is placed in flank position with the kidney over the table break as

C.G. Rogers (✉)
Vattikuti Urology Institute, Henry Ford Hospital, Detroit, MI, USA
e-mail: crogers2@hfhs.org

A.K. Hemal, M. Menon (eds.), *Robotics in Genitourinary Surgery*,
DOI 10.1007/978-1-84882-114-9_37, © Springer-Verlag London Limited 2011

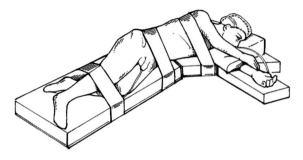

Fig. 37.2 Patient positioning for robotic kidney surgery

demonstrated in Fig. 37.2. We do not routinely flex the table, but a slight amount of table flexion may aid in increasing space for ports if needed. All pressure points are carefully padded and the patient is secured to the operating table with wide tape and velcro straps.

37.4 Trocar Configuration

As in laparoscopy, port placement is critical for the successful completion of RPN. Three primary configurations for port setup can be used for robotic kidney surgery, with the robotic camera placed either medially[3] (Fig. 37.3a), laterally[4,5] (Fig. 37.3b), or in between (Fig. 37.3c). Two robotic ports are placed under vision following placement of the camera port. With a medial camera position the robotic ports are triangulated toward the renal hilum in a wide V configuration. The medial camera placement offers a global view that simulates conventional laparoscopy. For the lateral camera position, the robotic ports and the assistant port are placed in a diamond-type configuration. This template may reduce arm collisions and provide more space for the assistant and the fourth arm. However, the camera is closer to the kidney resulting in a less global view. To obtain a global view, the camera can temporarily be moved to the medial assistant port. Placing the camera in an intermediate position combines the advantages of both the medial and the lateral camera positions. Ports are placed in nearly a straight line that is perpendicular to a line drawn between the camera port and the hilum. A 12 mm assistant port is placed periumbilically. A port for the fourth robotic arm may be placed approximately 4–5 fingerbreadths medially and caudally to the most caudal robotic instrument port. An optional 5 mm assistant port may be placed if necessary. For right-sided cases, a 5 mm subxiphoid port may also be placed for liver retraction (Table 37.1).

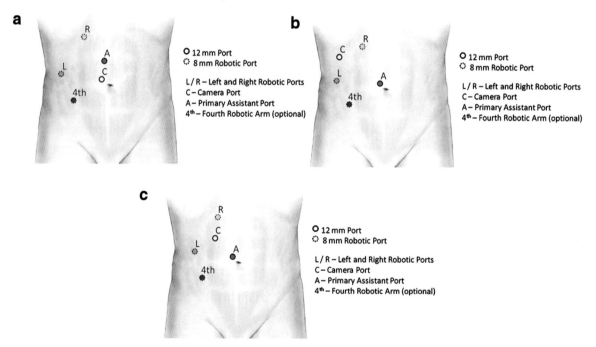

Fig. 37.3 Trocar placement for robotic kidney surgery. **a** Medial camera placement. **b** Lateral camera placement. **c** Intermediate camera placement

Table 37.1 Instrumentation used during robot-assisted partial nephrectomy

Surgeon instrumentation			Assistant instrumentation (blue)
Right arm (yellow)	Left arm (green)	Fourth arm (red)	• 5 mm laparoscopic grasper
• Monopolar curved scissors or monopolar hook	• Maryland bipolar forceps, fenestrated bipolar forceps, or Prograsp forceps	• Dual blade retractor or double fenestrated retractor	• 5 mm laparoscopic needle driver
• Large needle driver	• Large needle driver (optional)		• 5 mm laparoscopic scissors
			• Laparoscopic bulldog clamp applier
			• 5 and 10 mm Hem-o-lok clip applier
			• Suction tip and irrigator
			• 10 mm specimen extraction bag

37.5 Sutures

37.5.1 Inner Layer Reconstruction

3-0 or 4-0 Vicryl or monocryl suture on a RB-1 or SH needle is anchored with a Lapra-Ty (Ethicon, J & J, Piscataway, NJ) clip and knot (Fig. 37.4a).

37.5.2 Capsular Reconstruction

0-Vicryl suture on a CT-1 about 5–6 inches in length is anchored with a 10 mm Hem-o-lok (Teleflex Inc., Limerick, PA) clip and knot (Fig. 37.4b).

37.6 Step-by-Step Technique

37.6.1 Step 1: Trocar Placement

After the patient has been positioned and the abdomen has been prepped and draped, peritoneal access is achieved at the umbilicus using a Veress needle or the Hassan technique. Once access is achieved, the abdomen is insufflated to a pneumoperitoneum pressure of 20 mmHg. We place the 12 mm assistant port

first. The 12 mm assistant port is placed periumbilically or may be moved lateral to the rectus in obese patients. If using the lateral camera template, a 0 or 30° upward-angled scope is initially used, while a 0 or 30° downward-angled scope is used for the medial camera template. The robotic camera is placed though the 12 mm assistant port and the abdomen is inspected for the presence of adhesions and to assess the ability to place additional ports. If necessary, laparoscopic adhesiolysis can be performed to allow for safe port placement.

Camera and robotic working ports are placed under vision as depicted in Fig. 37.3a, b. Additional ports may be placed based on surgeon preference. The robot is docked posteriorly over the shoulder of the patient at approximately a 20° angle toward the head of the patient.

37.6.2 Step 2: Bowel Mobilization and Identification of Anatomic Landmarks

With either the permanent cautery hook or monopolar curved scissors in the right hand and forceps in the left hand, the colon is mobilized medially to expose the kidney (Fig. 37.5). The peritoneum is incised lateral to the colon along the white line of Toldt.

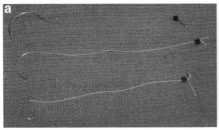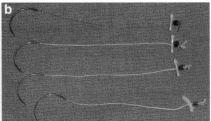

Fig. 37.4 Sutures for renal reconstruction. **a** Suture for inner layer renal reconstruction. **b** Suture for capsular reconstruction

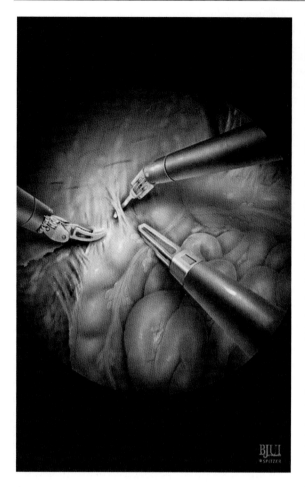

Fig. 37.5 Bowel mobilization to expose the kidney

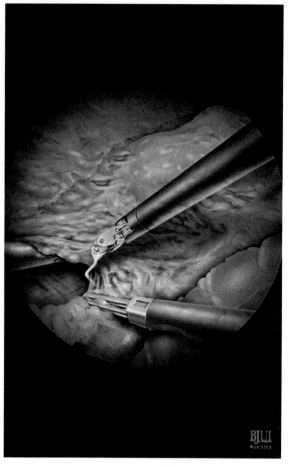

Fig. 37.6 Identification and retraction of the ureter and gonadal vein for posterior dissection

Using low cautery with sharp and blunt dissection, the colon is reflected medially. The bedside assistant helps retract the colon medially to develop an avascular plane between the posterior mesocolon and the anterior Gerota's fascia.

Bowel mobilization can be performed with complete robotic assistance without problems of sufficient reach with the da Vinci S system. During bowel mobilization, if the left-hand instrument is attached to cautery, care must be taken to avoid thermal injury to the bowel by inadvertently hitting the wrong pedal on the console.

Continued medial reflection and upward retraction of the bowel will expose the ureter and gonadal vein (Fig. 37.6). These structures are retracted anteriorly to expose the underlying psoas muscle. A plane along the psoas muscle is created and followed cranially toward the renal hilum.

37.6.3 Step 3: Hilar Dissection

The renal hilum is identified by tracing the gonadal vein cranially. For right-sided procedures, the gonadal vein is traced to its insertion into the vena cava and then followed cranially to the renal vein. For left-sided procedures, the gonadal vein is traced directly to its insertion in the renal vein. The renal vein is dissected. For left-sided procedures, it may be necessary to ligate and transect the gonadal vein to allow for exposure and dissection of the renal artery which is generally located posterior to the renal vein. The renal artery is then dissected.

To assist in hilar dissection, the fourth robotic arm instrument may be used to lift the kidney anteriorly by placing it under the ureter (Fig. 37.7). This places the renal hilum on stretch, allowing two-handed dissection of the renal hilar vessels.

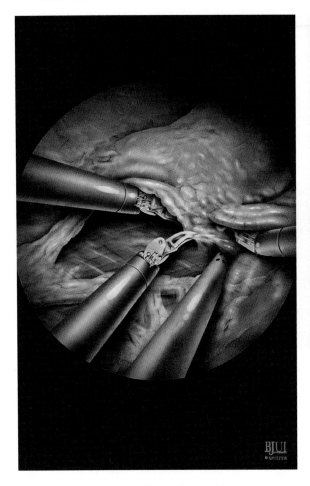

Fig. 37.7 Hilar dissection with fourth arm assistance

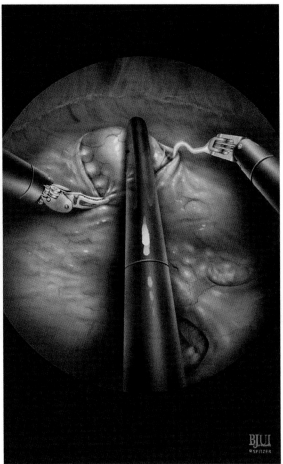

Fig. 37.8 Tumor identification with intraoperative ultrasound

A variety of robotic instruments may be used to dissect the renal hilum. In the right hand, the robotic hook is useful for blunt dissection of hilar vessels. The curved monopolar scissors may also be used for sharp dissection of the renal hilum and may be more cost-effective as they are utilized later in the case for tumor excision. In the left hand, the Maryland bipolar forceps allow for precise cauterization of small vessels, while the fenestrated bipolar and Prograsp forceps allow for spreading and isolation of tissues and can be used later in the case as a needle driver.

37.6.4 Step 4: Tumor Identification

Intraoperative ultrasound is useful to locate the tumor and delineate margins of resection. The assistant introduces a flexible laparoscopic ultrasound probe through the 12 mm assistant port (Fig. 37.8). The TilePro feature of the da Vinci S system (Fig. 37.9) allows the surgeon to view live intraoperative ultrasound footage and preoperative radiographic images as a picture-on-picture display on the console screen, guiding tumor localization without the need to leave the console to view external images.[6] Image sources are connected to the console and TilePro is activated by tapping the camera pedal to turn the images on or off. To more accurately delineate margins of resection, the console surgeon may guide the tip of the ultrasound probe to desired locations.

Gerota's fascia is opened to expose the tumor. Adjacent normal parenchyma is exposed to allow for placement of sutures during later capsular reconstruction. Intraoperative ultrasound is again used to demarcate margins of resection which are scored onto the

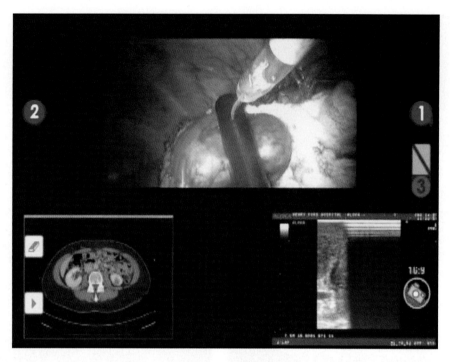

Fig. 37.9 TilePro image demonstrating ability to simultaneously view live intraoperative ultrasound image and preoperative radiographic images on the console screen during robotic partial nephrectomy

renal capsule using cautery (Fig. 37.10). The kidney maybe mobilized and positioned for optimal access to the tumor during excision and renal reconstruction. This may be accomplished by using a laparoscopic sponge placed behind the kidney or by using the fourth robotic arm to grasp perirenal fat.

37.6.5 Step 5: Hilar Clamping

To minimize warm ischemia time, ensure that all sutures, instruments, and materials necessary for renal reconstruction are available prior to clamping, and the monopolar scissors are available in the right hand for tumor excision. Intravenous mannitol (12.5 g) is routinely given prior to clamping for osmotic diuresis. Hilar occlusion is performed by the assistant using either laparoscopic bulldog clamps (Fig. 37.11) for occluding renal vessels individually or a Satinksy clamp for en bloc clamping of the entire renal hilum.

When using bulldog clamps the renal artery is occluded prior to the renal vein. For small or exophytic tumors, the renal artery alone may be clamped. For endophytic, hilar, or multiple tumors, we recommend

clamping both the renal artery and the renal vein to improve visualization. If a Satinsky clamp is used, care must be taken to avoid external collision of the robotic arms with the clamp to prevent injury to renal vessels. Excision and reconstruction may be attempted without hilar clamping for small or exophytic tumors; however, predissection of the renal hilum is recommended to allow for vascular control if needed.

During application of hilar clamps, the console surgeon may lift up the kidney to help expose the renal vessels and place them on stretch. The console surgeon may use the robotic instruments to help guide clamp placement.

37.6.6 Step 6: Tumor Excision

The tumor is excised sharply using curved robotic scissors along the previously scored margin (Fig. 37.12). The scissors are initially curved away from the tumor to initiate capsular incision and then curved toward the tumor for deeper resection. Robotic forceps are used to provide upward traction on the tumor during resection. Use of the blunt-tipped Prograsp or fenestrated bipolar

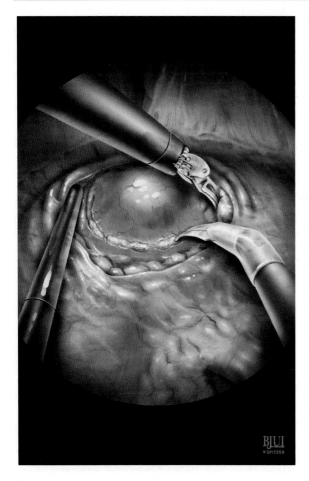

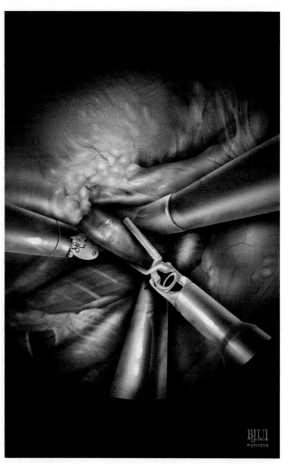

Fig. 37.10 Demarcation of tumor boundaries for subsequent tumor excision

Fig. 37.11 Renal hilar clamping with laparoscopic bulldog clamps

instruments during this step may help minimize trauma to the tumor during retraction. The assistant provides countertraction on the renal parenchyma and removes any blood from the field with the suction irrigator to help delineate the plane of resection. Once the tumor is excised, it is placed out of the way next to the kidney for later retrieval.

37.6.7 Step 7: Inner Layer Renal Reconstruction

For renal reconstruction, the curved scissors in the right hand are replaced with a robotic needle driver. The Prograsp or fenestrated bipolar forceps may be switched to a needle driver or kept in the left hand and used as a needle driver per surgeon preference.

To identify any entry into the collecting system, a ureteral catheter may be placed prior to surgery, allowing visualization of a retrograde injection of indigo carmine. This, however, is not routinely performed as the vision provided by the robotic camera generally allows visualization of any collecting system entry.

A 3-0 or 4-0 vicryl or monocryl suture on a RB-1 or SH needle is used to achieve hemostasis and repair any entry into the collecting system (Fig. 37.13). The suture may be anchored with a preplaced Lapra-Ty clip to avoid knot tying under warm ischemia. However, the suture may also be tied robotically per surgeon preference. When using a preplaced Lapra-Ty clip, a second Lapra-Ty clip is placed by the assistant to secure the stitch. The assistant passes the needles into the surgical field through the 12 mm assistant port. The assistant also helps provide visualization of small bleeding vessels by suctioning any blood in the

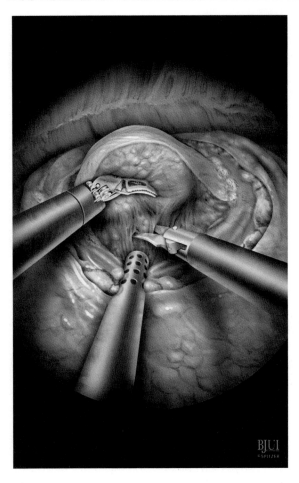

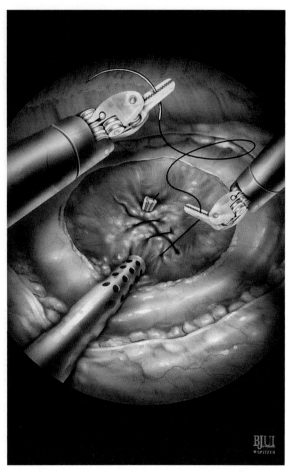

Fig. 37.12 Tumor excision

Fig. 37.13 Sutured reconstruction of the inner layer

surgical field. Additional sutures are placed as needed to obtain hemostasis and close any collecting system entry.

37.6.8 Step 8: Capsular Reconstruction and Clamp Removal

The renal capsular edges are reapproximated using interrupted stitches. 0-Vicryl suture on a CT-1 needle, cut to approximately 5–6 inches in length, is prepared prior to hilar clamping with a hemolock clip secured on the outer end with a knot. Large bites of capsule are taken to ensure that the suture does not rip through the renal parenchyma (Fig. 37.14).

On the opposite side of the capsule, the stitches are secured using large hemolock clips applied by the

assistant. The clips are slid down the suture by console surgeon to reapproximate capsular edges under tension (Fig 37.15).[7] The assistant must be careful to place the suture in the center of the clip before closing or it may be difficult for the console surgeon to cinch down. When cinching the clips down, the suture is held perpendicular to the renal capsule to ensure that the stitch does not rip through the renal parenchyma. Large hemolock clips are used to help spread the force of the suture over a larger surface area, allowing the console surgeon to cinch the clip down tighter resulting in closer capsular reapproximation and better hemostasis. The clips are tightened down until renal parenchymal dimpling is seen.

For wedge resections done on smaller tumors, the capsule often closes completely and bolsters and hemostatic agents may not be needed. For larger tumors leaving a broad defect, complete closure of the

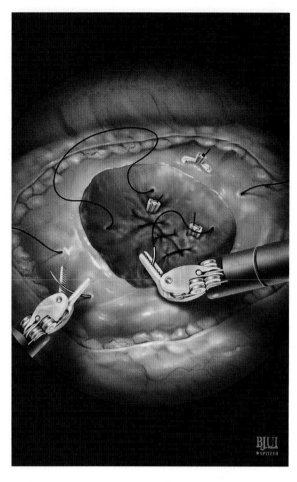

Fig. 37.14 Sutured capsular reconstruction

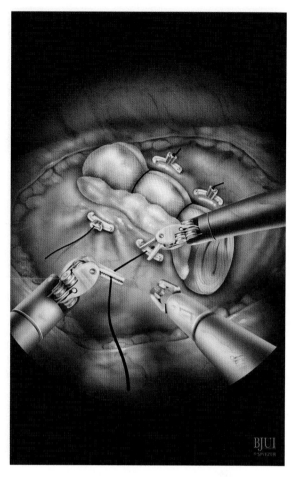

Fig. 37.15 Sliding hemolock clip technique over bolsters

capsular edges may not be possible. Surgicel (Ethicon, J & J, Piscataway, NJ) bolsters may be placed under the capsular stitches along with hemostatic agents, such as Floseal (Baxter, Deerfield, IL), for added hemostasis.

Once the hemolock clips are placed, the renal hilar clamps are removed. If bulldog clamps were used, the venous clamp is removed first, followed by the arterial clamp. To help the bedside assistant visualize the clamps, the console surgeon may lift up the kidney. The assistant may need to suction any blood or clot near the hilum that has accumulated during the procedure.

Lapra-Ty clips may be placed by the assistant next to the Hem-o-lok clips to help prevent them from eventually sliding back, although we have not yet seen this occur. The needles are cut and removed. A second dose of mannitol may be given after unclamping the renal hilum.

37.6.9 Step 9: Specimen Retrieval and Closure

The specimen is retrieved and placed into an extraction bag inserted through the periumbilical 12 mm port (Fig. 37.16). The periumbilical port incision is extended to remove the specimen. The fascia is closed with interrupted 0-braided polyester sutures. The skin is closed with subcuticular sutures and sterile strips.

37.7 Special Considerations

Complex tumors (hilar, endophytic, or multiple) and large tumors pose a particular challenge to a minimally invasive approach for partial nephrectomy. Complex

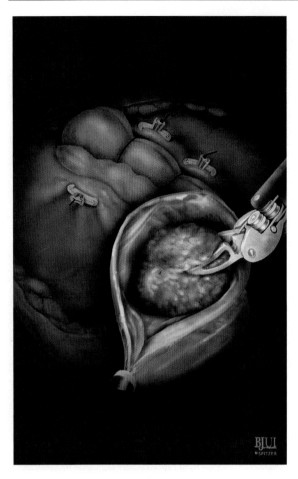

Fig. 37.16 Specimen retrieval

angles and proximity to critical structures make these tumors difficult for both minimally invasive and open approaches. To remove these difficult tumors robotically, specialized techniques are required for their dissection and excision. For hilar tumors, careful dissection along the renal vessels is necessary. Using a spreading technique with blunt-tipped forceps, a plane can often be created between the tumor and the critical hilar structures. If segmental vascular branches supplying the tumor are identified, these branches may be carefully dissected and clipped prior to excising the tumor. Enucleation of the base of endophytic tumors may also be necessary to avoid critical structures.

In the setting of multiple renal tumors, warm ischemia time may be reduced by excising smaller tumors without clamping. A laparoscopic sponge may be used to tamponade the defect prior to performing renal reconstruction.[3] PN for large tumors may also be performed with robotic assistance. For these tumors, positioning the kidney for optimal resection and reconstruction is key, as meticulous renorrhaphy technique is important to minimize the risk of bleeding or urine leak.

It is recommended that surgeons at the beginning of their learning curve with robotic partial nephrectomy start with small exophytic tumors and slowly progress to more complex tumors. Careful patient selection and surgeon experience are important when performing RPN for complex tumors.

37.8 Steps to Avoid Complications

Bleeding is the most serious and one of the most common complications during minimally invasive partial nephrectomy. During laparoscopic partial nephrectomy, the rate of intraoperative hemorrhage has been reported to be about 2–3.5%.[8,9] Bleeding during different steps in the procedure can be controlled using various techniques. Cautery can be used to stop isolated bleeding during dissection, but care must be taken to avoid thermal injury when near bowel or large vascular structures. If a specific bleeding vessel is identified, the assistant may use a locking grasper to occlude the vessel until cautery or clips to control the bleeding. Bleeding during dissection of the hilum can usually be controlled using a laparoscopic sponge or cottonoid to tamponade the bleeding. Leaving the sponge in place for a few minutes while working in another location will often result in hemostasis.

Bleeding while on clamp can occur due to a number of reasons. A main renal artery branch may have been missed during clamping. If this is suspected, a long straight bulldog clamp can be placed across the renal hilum to encompass all branches of the artery. An accessory artery, usually from the adrenal gland, may also perfuse the kidney. In this case, a bulldog clamp can be placed in the fat between the kidney and the adrenal gland to occlude perfusing vessels. Also, old bulldog clamps may lose their closing force over time, allowing flow to enter the kidney. In this case a second bulldog clamp may be placed across the renal artery. If there is still significant bleeding due to a suspected unoccluded arterial vessel, the renal vein can be unclamped which may help alleviate renal congestion and improve vision. Pneumoperitoneum can also be temporally increased to reduce bleeding as needed.

When coming off clamp, bleeding may occur from small vessels missed during renal reconstruction. When removing the clamps, the arterial clamp may be flashed to confirm that hemostasis has been obtained prior to its removal from the surgical field. If bleeding is noted, additional sutures may be placed, or the hemolock clips can be cinched down tighter, tamponading any bleeding vessels. Postoperatively, blood pressure is monitored closely and controlled to avoid hypertension which may potentially lead to bleeding.

37.9 Conclusions

Minimally invasive partial nephrectomy has demonstrated good functional and oncologic outcomes, as well as benefits in regard to convalescence. Laparoscopic partial nephrectomy, however, is a challenging procedure usually requiring advanced surgical training and skills. RPN is a new adaptation of this technique that addresses the technical challenges of LPN, potentially offering select patients the benefit of minimally invasive surgery that might otherwise receive total nephrectomy or open surgery.

References

1. Go AS, Chertow GM, Fan D, et al. Chronic kidney disease and the risks of death, cardiovascular events, and hospitalization. *N Engl J Med*. 2004;351:1296.
2. Porpiglia F, Volpe A, Billia M, et al. Laparoscopic versus open partial nephrectomy: analysis of the current literature. *Eur Urol*. 2008;53:732.
3. Rogers CG, Singh A, Blatt AM, et al. Robotic partial nephrectomy for complex renal tumors: surgical technique. *Eur Urol*. 2008;53:514.
4. Badani KK, Muhletaler F, Fumo M, et al. Optimizing robotic renal surgery: the lateral camera port placement technique and current results. *J Endourol*. 2008;22:507.
5. Kaul S, Laungani R, Sarle R, et al. Da vinci-assisted robotic partial nephrectomy: technique and results at a mean of 15 months of follow-up. *Eur Urol*. 2007;51:186.
6. Rogers CG, Laungani R, Bhandari A, et al. Maximizing console surgeon independence during robot-assisted renal surgery by using the fourth arm and tileprotrade mark. *J Endourol*. 2009;23:115.
7. Bhayani SB, Figenshau RS. The washington university renorrhaphy for robotic partial nephrectomy: a detailed description of the technique displayed at the 2008 world robotic urologic symposium. *J Robot Surg*. 2008;2:139.
8. Gill IS, Kavoussi LR, Lane BR, et al. Comparison of 1,800 laparoscopic and open partial nephrectomies for single renal tumors. *J Urol*. 2007;178:41.
9. Ramani AP, Desai MM, Steinberg AP, et al. Complications of laparoscopic partial nephrectomy in 200 cases. *J Urol*. 2005;173:42.

Chapter 38

Robotic Donor Nephrectomy: Technique and Outcomes – An European Perspective

J. Hubert and M. Ladrière

38.1 Introduction

Worldwide increase of renal insufficiency leads to try to develop kidney transplantation. Living donors are an increasing source of grafts, the incidence of them varying considerably from one country to the other (from 7% of renal transplants in France to 35–40% in northern Europe).[1] Legal extension of the potential kidney donors to non-genetically related persons or even in some countries possibility of altruistic, cross, or domino transplantation leads to consider how to increase the willingness to donate and therefore to reduce the physical postoperative consequences to the donor.

Although launched at the end of the 1990s, the development of robotics has rarely been applied to nephrectomies and furthermore to living donor nephrectomies,[2,3] as most urologic centers use the robotic technology exclusively for prostatectomies.

Multiple advantages of robotics which are now well-known and the mini-invasive approach may also be offered to living donors while allowing to get grafts of the same high quality than in open surgery.[4]

38.2 Preoperative Kidney Evaluation

Arteriography which was the former standard vascular investigation is no longer performed. Uro-angio-CT multislice scan allows now reliable evaluation of arteries (number, situation, potential calcifications, etc.), veins (number, possible aberrant situation, collateral veins such as lumbar, adrenal, and genital), and excretory system. This allows the surgeon to anticipate the preoperative difficulties. Kidneys with up to three arteries, two veins, or two ureters are not contraindicated for donation.

The preoperative biological investigations comprise serum creatinine and EDTA clearance (patients under 80 ml/mn/1.73 m^2 are excluded for kidney donation).

Mag 3 (or DMSA) scan is systematically performed to evaluate the respective renal functions. If these appear to be slightly asymmetric the best kidney is kept for the donor.

The left kidney is harvested unless it is contraindicated (mainly due to complex vascularization or asymmetric renal function), the length of the left renal vein facilitating the following transplantation.

38.3 Patient Positioning and Port Placement

The patient is installed in a supine position, the operative table not being flexed but laterally tilted, this allowing the patient to be placed in a 60° lateral position. Careful padding of leg, hip, thorax, and head is performed.

Pneumoperitoneum is created with the help of a Veress needle introduced subcostally when operating on the left side. An open approach at the umbilicus is performed when operating on the right side.

A first, 12 mm trocar is inserted at the umbilicus. Three other trocars are inserted under laparoscopic control after insufflation of carbon dioxide: a 10 mm

J. Hubert (✉)
Department of Urology, University Hospital of Nancy, CHU Nancy – Brabois Vandoeuvre les Nancy, France
e-mail: j.hubert@chu-nancy.fr

A.K. Hemal, M. Menon (eds.), *Robotics in Genitourinary Surgery*,
DOI 10.1007/978-1-84882-114-9_38, © Springer-Verlag London Limited 2011

trocar in the left iliac fossa, a second 10 mm trocar subcostally (on the midclavicular line), and a third 12 mm trocar at midway between the two working ports, slightly laterally for the 0° optic. A 5 mm trocar may be inserted on the midline under the xyphoid for introducing a grasper and help to recline the liver upward when operating on the right side.

The patient side assistant works through the 12 mm trocar placed at the umbilicus. His role consists in changing the instruments, sucking, introducing the necessary material (threads, gauzes, etc.).

A second trained surgeon is required during the short specific part of the procedure consisting in applying the Hem-o-lok (Weck Inc) clips, dividing the vessels, introducing the endobag, extracting the kidney, and cooling it.

After having placed the ports, the surgeon goes to the console. He uses a bipolar forceps in the left hand and the electrocautery hook in the right hand.

A backtable with Satinsky clamps is ready for an urgent conversion to open surgery if may be necessary.

38.4 Surgical Steps

Most of living donor nephrectomies are performed on the left side. The operation begins with mobilization of the colon, which allows identifying the genital vein, the ureter, and the psoas muscle. Cephalad dissection along this vein facilitates reaching the left renal vein. The renal artery is dissected behind the lower or upper margin of the renal vein depending on preoperative CT-scan data. On the left side, lumbar and adrenal veins are clipped and divided.

The kidney is then dissected in the extracapsular plane in order to remove all perirenal fats. Flipping the kidney forward may help to complete the pedicle dissection and its "skeletonization."

The genital vein is kept adherent to the ureter, this allowing to limit traction and it is devascularization. Dissection of the ureter goes down to the inferior aspect of the iliac vessels.

Once the kidney has been skeletonized, a Pfannenstiel incision is performed. A 3/0 Vicryl running suture creates a purse on the peritoneum, allowing pneumostasis around the 15 mm endobag which is introduced through that incision (Fig. 38.1).

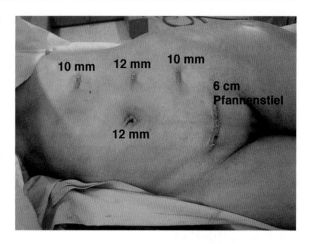

Fig. 38.1 Trocar placement on the midclavicular line

Gonadal vessels are clipped and divided; an Hem-o-lok clip is applied on the distal ureter before dividing it.

The opened endocatch helps to recline the colon toward the right side of the abdomen; two Hem-o-lok clips are applied on the renal artery next to the aorta and two on the renal vein, on the right side of the aorta, this leaving maximal length of vessels at the site of the kidney. The vessels are then divided and the kidney is entrapped in the endobag. It is extracted through the Pfannenstiel incision and immediately perfused and refrigerated.

Pneumostasis is reestablished by closing the purse on the peritoneum.

A complementary 6/0 non-absorbable running suture is then performed on the arterial stump for additional safety of the procedure (Fig. 38.2).

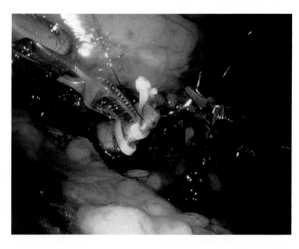

Fig. 38.2 Complementary suture on the arterial stump

Lowering of the insufflating pressure and checking for hemostasis are performed. No drainage is required.

Living donor nephrectomy is only rarely performed on the right side.

Its principles are similar to that of left nephrectomy, but with some specificities related to the shortness of the renal vein and retrocaval situation of the artery. Flipping of the kidney is required to allow the retrocaval dissection of the artery in order to get a maximum length. A sample of the gonadal vein may be taken with the intent of lengthening the renal vein during bench surgery.

Aponeuroses at the 12 mm trocar sites and at the suprapubic incision are closed with No. 2 Vicryl stiches. Ropivacaine aponevrotic infiltration at all incisions helps to limit the postoperative pain and the use of morphinic drugs.

38.5 Postoperative Care

Liquid intake is authorized at the evening of the operation.

Prevention of venous thrombosis begins within the 8 postoperative hours (Enoxaparin, etc.) and is carried on during 15 days. The antithrombotic socks are worn until return to normal physical activities.

A postoperative ultrasound control of the renal fossa is performed on po day 3 or 4 before the patient is discharged from the hospital.

38.6 Results

In a 79 patients series (32 males and 47 females, mean BMI 25.2), who underwent robotic-assisted laparoscopic live donor nephrectomy, left kidneys were mainly harvested (72 left/7 right). Renal vessels comprised two arteries 14 times and three in four cases.

Mean operative time, warm, and cold ischemia were 175, 4.98, and 204 min, respectively. No patient was converted nor required reintervention; the estimated blood loss was minimal (mean post-op Hb decrease: 0.78 g/dl; no transfusion was required). Postoperative complications included two phlebitides

and two peripheral pulmonary embolisms, one acute pyelonephritis, and 1 chylous ascites. Preoperative, day 5, and day 30 creatinine levels were 90 ± 17, 119 ± 22, and 110 ± 20.7 µmol/l, respectively. The mean hospital stay was 6 ± 1.7 days.

All of the donor kidneys functioned immediately in the recipients. Decrease of serum creatinine was superior to 10% at day 1 in 76 cases, at day 2 in 2 cases, and at day 9 in 1 case (requiring one postoperative session of hemodialysis). Mean creatinine levels were 72.3, 45.1, and 16.2 mg/l at day 0, D1, and D5, respectively.

38.7 Conclusion

Robotics is basically a natural evolution and expansion of laparoscopic surgery, enhancing the surgeon's dexterity. It offers to the patient the advantages of the laparoscopic parietal mini-invasive approach but also endocorporeal mini invasiveness which are the indirect consequences of meticulous pedicle, ureteral, and renal dissection, step-by-step excellent hemostasis, minimal hurting of any tissues. These advantages are related to the robotic technology: 3D vision, instrument's 7 degrees of freedom, motion scaling, tremor filtering, and ergonomic position reducing the surgeon's fatigue.

Robotics allows to offer the best of the technology, minimum invasiveness, and maximum quality of work to these specific patients who are healthy and generously offer one of their kidneys.

References

1. Kok NF, Weimar W, Alwayn IPJ, et al. The current practice of live donor nephrectomy in Europe. *Transplantation*. 2006;82:892–897.
2. Horgan S, Vanuno D, Sileri P, Cicalese L, Benedetti E. Robotic-assisted laparoscopic donor nephrectomy for kidney transplantation. *Transplantation*. 2002;73(9):1474–1479.
3. Hoznek A, Hubert J, Antiphon P, Gettman MT, Hemal AK, Abbou CC. Robotic renal surgery. *Urol Clin North Am*. 2004 Nov;31(4):731–736.
4. Reimer J, Rensing A, Haasen C, et al. The impact of living related kidney transplantation on the donor's life. *Transplantation*. 2006;81:1268–1273.

Chapter 39

Robotic Donor Nephrectomy

Kari J. Thompson and Santiago Horgan

39.1 Introduction

Renal transplantation remains the standard of care for end-stage renal disease (ESRD). Unfortunately, as the demand for donor kidneys has increased this has not been followed by an increase in organ availability. Thus, patients must wait for a long time for an organ with the appropriate blood type and tissue type. Live donor renal transplant allows a superior outcome and typically a shorter waiting time for transplant in comparison to cadaveric renal transplant.[1] According to the Organ Procurement and Transplantation Network, approximately 6,000 living donor renal transplants have been performed annually in the United States since 2000. Murray[2] performed the first successful living donor transplant between identical twins in 1954. Since then, with the advancement of surgical techniques and anti-rejection medications, thousands have had successful transplantation.

Although living renal donation has proven superior in graft survival compared to cadaveric transplantation, open donor nephrectomy offered the donor few benefits. The operation has a large amount of postoperative pain and a long recovery period. Thus, the donors are often hesitant to undergo this operation. The introduction of laparoscopic techniques by Ratner et al. in 1995[3] was an attempt at an alternative to the open technique to alleviate the shortage of kidneys available for transplantation. By offering an operation with a shorter recovery time, less postoperative pain, a superior cosmetic result, and shorter hospitalization, more patients would be willing to become donors. Shortly after Ratner began laparoscopic-assisted donor nephrectomy, other studies[4–7] confirmed that a minimally invasive approach doubled the number of living renal donor transplantation rate. Consequently, laparoscopic donor nephrectomy is considered the standard of care.

There remains a steep learning curve for this operation and the standard limitations of laparoscopy apply: limited degrees of freedom, two-dimensional imaging, difficulty with triangulation, and an unstable visual platform. Since the da Vinci Surgical System (Intuitive Surgical, Mountain View, CA) was approved by the Food and Drug Administration in July 2000, traditional laparoscopic surgery has been transformed. The advantages of the robot include camera stability, increased number of degrees of freedom, three-dimensional view, and improved surgeon's ergonomics. The robotic system allows for a precise dissection of the renal hilum, particularly in complex vascular anatomy, and the ureter. In 2002, we reported our first series of 12 patients who underwent a robotic donor nephrectomy.[8] The presumed advantages of the robot were confirmed at this time. The learning curve on the robot is shorter than laparoscopic procedures, even with an inexperienced surgeon. The robotic system provides all of the benefits of a minimally invasive approach without giving up the dexterity, precision, and intuitive movements of open surgery. We present our experience using the da Vinci Surgical system to perform robotic hand-assisted living related donor nephrectomy.

S. Horgan (✉)
Minimally Invasive Surgery, University of California San Diego, San Diego, CA, USA
e-mail: shorgan@ucsd.edu

A.K. Hemal, M. Menon (eds.), *Robotics in Genitourinary Surgery*,
DOI 10.1007/978-1-84882-114-9_39, © Springer-Verlag London Limited 2011

39.2 Surgical Anatomy

The kidneys are retroperitoneal organs measuring approximately 11 cm in length, 6 cm in width, and 3 cm in thickness. The right kidney is slightly lower than the left due to the liver. A dense fibrous capsule encases each kidney. Gerota's fascia is located between the kidneys and the psoas muscle and the lumbar spine.

Classically, each kidney is supplied by a single renal artery, arising from the abdominal aorta, and a single renal vein, entering the inferior vena cava. The left renal vein receives the left gonadal vein, left adrenal vein, and the left lumbar vein before crossing anterior to the aorta to join the inferior vena cava. The renal arteries typically originate from the aorta at the level of L2 below the superior mesenteric artery. Aberrant renal arteries may be seen in up to 25% of patients.

The ureter is a fibromuscular thick-walled tube, approximately 25 cm in length. The abdominal section lies behind the peritoneum on the medial aspect of the psoas major, and it is crossed obliquely by the internal spermatic vessels. It enters the pelvic cavity when it crosses the termination of the common iliac vessels.

In the presence of normal anatomy bilaterally, the left kidney is always preferred for donor nephrectomy because of the superior length and better quality of the wall of the left renal vein. Traditionally, the presence of multiple renal arteries was considered a contraindication to kidney transplant due to the increased risk of technical complications.[9] Currently, a variety of techniques have been described for management of multiple vessels.[10] Therefore, multiple arteries are not a contraindication for transplant. The initial experience with laparoscopic procurement of the right kidney was unfavorable due to venous complications.[11] Thus the left is always preferable.

In our practice, we routinely harvest the left kidney regardless of vascular abnormalities due to the longer left renal vein. In our experience, the use of grafts with multiple arteries did not increase arterial or urologic complications in the recipients nor did it affect graft survival or kidney function.

39.3 The Robotic System

The operations are performed using the da Vinci Surgical system (Intuitive Surgical, Mountain View, CA). This system includes three components:

1. Surgeon console: the surgeon operates while seated at a console, using four pedals, a set of console switches, and two master controls. The movements of the surgeon's fingers are transmitted by the master controls to the instrument located inside the patient. A three-dimensional image of the surgical field is obtained using a 12 mm scope, which contains two cameras that integrate images.
2. Control tower: monitor, light source, and cord attachments for the cameras.
3. Surgical arm cart: provides four robotic arms, three instrument arms, and one laparoscope arm, which executes the surgeon's commands.

39.4 Preoperative Evaluation

The initial evaluation is performed by the transplant nurse coordinator. The patients attend an information session where the risks of the operation and typical postoperative course are explained to them. A potential donor may be considered if he or she is at least 18 years of age and has a compatible blood type with the recipient. After this is confirmed, further testing is done including human lymphocyte antigen (HLA) tissue typing and a cross-match for reactive HLA. After eligibility is determined, the transplant surgeon evaluates the patient. A conscious preoperative evaluation ensures that the donor is left with normal renal function after nephrectomy. CT angiography is highly accurate for determining the renal vasculature and in detecting abnormalities. The left kidney is routinely selected, and surgical strategy is planned in advance.

39.5 Surgical Technique

39.5.1 Patient Positioning

The patient is placed onto the operating room on top of a beanbag. Pneumatic compression stockings are placed on both lower extremities. After induction of general anesthesia, a Foley catheter and oral gastric tube are placed. Preoperative antibiotics are administered prior to skin incision. The patient is then placed into right lateral decubitus position with an axillary role placed under the right axilla. The air from the beanbag is then removed allowing the patient secure positioning when the operating room table is fully flexed to open up the angle between the left costal margin and the superior iliac crest. Both the left arm and the left leg are cushioned to protect all joints and pressure points. Once this is established, the abdomen is prepped and draped in standard sterile fashion.

39.5.2 Port Placement

A 7 cm infraumbilical midline incision is performed. A Lap Disk hand port (Ethicon) is introduced, and pneumoperitoneum achieved with 14 mmHg CO_2 insufflation. This hand port is used by the transplant surgeon to place their own hand into the abdomen to facilitate retraction and dissection and, lastly, for removal of the kidney. Under direct visualization, a 12 mm trocar (Ethicon) is placed in the supraumbilical position close to the midline. The 12 mm trocar is used for the 30° robotic laparoscope. Two 8 mm robotic trocars are placed, one trocar to the left of the camera trocar in the junction between the mid-clavicular line and the subcostal margin and the other trocar is placed in the mid-clavicular line to the right of the camera trocar. These two trocars are for the surgeon's right and left hand. An additional 12 mm trocar (Ethicon) is placed in the left lower quadrant, to assist with suction, clipping, stapling, and cutting. The da Vinci Surgical system is then brought into position and the arms are connected to specific trocars (Fig. 39.1).

39.5.3 Mobilization of the Descending Colon and Identification of the Ureter

The assistant surgeon's hand is introduced into the abdomen via the hand port. This is done to expose the left colic gutter by providing countertraction on the descending colon. The operation is started by mobilizing the descending colon by incising the lateral peritoneal reflection along Toldt's fascia by using hook electrocautery. The splenic flexure is taken down systematically and the colon is rotated medially. This allows access to the kidney and the psoas muscle. At this point, we are able to easily identify the ureter. It is dissected free circumferentially in a cephalad direction, beginning at the level of the left common iliac artery (Fig. 39.2). Once isolated, a 6 cm Penrose drain is introduced through the assistant's trocar, looped around the ureter, and clipped to itself. The assistant uses a grasper to grab the Penrose drain and to retract the ureter lateral and anteriorly. Care must be taken not to alter the vascular supply of the ureter; this is accomplished by preserving generous amounts of fat around it.

39.5.4 Posterior Dissection of the Kidney

The posterior attachments of the kidney are taken down with the assistance of the hand of the transplant surgeon and the articulated robotic instruments. The robot is particularly helpful during this part of the operation

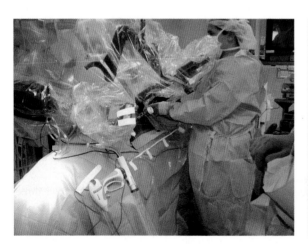

Fig. 39.1 Placement of the da Vinci

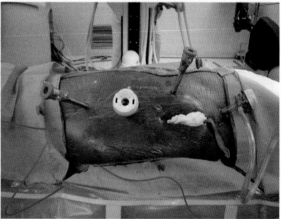

Fig. 39.2 Mobilization and dissection of the ureter

in dissection of the upper pole of the kidney from the spleen. The articulated arm reproduces the action of the human wrist.

39.5.5 Anterior Dissection of the Kidney

The gonadal vein is identified medial to the ureter and followed superiorly to its junction with the left renal vein. Gerota's fascia is incised superiorly, and the anterior kidney surface is identified. Then, following in a cephalad direction, a plane between the superior medial aspect of the kidney and adrenal gland is developed. This plane of dissection is then carried superiorly and laterally with hook cautery until the kidney is free from its superior pole attachments.

39.5.6 Dissection of the Renal Hilum

Next we turn our attention to the hilum of the kidney. The renal vein is circumferentially dissected using hook cautery (Fig. 39.3). Its tributaries (gonadal, lumbar, and left adrenal veins) are transected by the assistant using an ultrasonic dissector. The kidney is then retracted medially and the renal artery is identified and dissected free to the aorta. The entire kidney is now free from all of its attachments other than the vascular pedicles and the ureter. The robotic system is now detached from the patient and the remainder of the operation is continued laparoscopically.

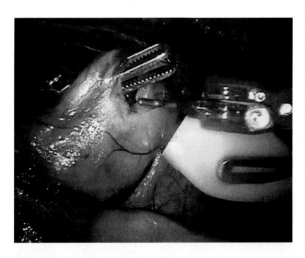

Fig. 39.3 Dissection of the renal hilum

39.5.7 Division of the Renal Hilum and Kidney Removal

The ureter is clipped twice distally at the level of the common iliac artery and sharply transected. At this point, i.v. heparin at 80 units/kg is administered. Immediately after that a locking clip (Hem-o-lok Ligation System) is placed on the renal artery at the level of the aorta take-off. The renal artery is then transected using a linear cutting vascular stapler (LCS, Ethicon). The renal vein is then transected with the stapling device. At this point, the kidney is removed through the midline incision and taken to the back table where it is flushed with cold infusion of University of Wisconsin solution (ViaSpan, Barr Laboratories, Pomona, NY). Laparoscopic inspection of the renal bed is performed to ensure hemostasis and i.v. protamine is administered. After evacuation of pneumoperitoneum and removal of the trocars, the lower midline incision is closed with a running #1 Maxon. The skin incisions are closed with subcuticular 4–0 absorbable monofilament and infiltrated with local anesthetic.

39.6 Postoperative Care

Patients are transferred to the floor after anesthetic recovery. They are encouraged to ambulate early and use an incentive spirometer ten times an hour. Clear liquid diet is typically started the evening of the operation. Toradol and morphine are used for pain control until the patient is tolerating a diet, at this time they are transitioned to oral medications. On postoperative day 1 a complete blood count and chemistry are performed. The Foley catheter is then removed based on urine output and the laboratory results. Patients are typically discharged within 2 days of their operation.

39.7 Management of Complications

At the beginning of our series we experienced three major intraoperative bleeds. All were due to failure of the stapling device, resulting in conversion to open procedure. We then modified our technique to first placing a locking clip on the renal artery prior to transection with the stapling device. The locking clip decreases the intraluminal pressure of the bloodstream, minimizing chances of failure of the stapling device.

We believe that using the hand-assisted technique is critical not only for retraction throughout the case but also for emergent situations. The bleeding can easily be managed with manual compression until the surgeon achieves hemostasis. In a case requiring immediate conversion to an open procedure, the abdominal cavity can be quickly accessed through the already existing midline incision.

Other vascular injuries may occur during dissection of the renal vein tributaries. Tears can be typically be repaired using a locking clip. If there is no stump remaining, a 5-0 prolene suture should control the bleeding.

39.8 Conclusion

The favorable outcome in the donors and recipients shows that robotic hand-assisted donor nephrectomy (RHADN) is safe and feasible. For this reason, the robotic-assisted donor nephrectomy has become our preferred approach. Further experience is needed to compare cost and outcomes of RHADN versus standard laparoscopic donor nephrectomy in order to determine which procedure is safer and more cost-effective.

References

1. Schulam PG, et al. Laparoscopic live donor nephrectomy: the initial 3 cases. *J Urol*. 1996;155:1857–1859.
2. Murray JE, Merrill JP, Harrison JH. Renal homotransplantations in identical twins. *J Am Soc Nephrol*. 1955;12: 201–204.
3. Ratner LE, et al. Comparison of laparoscopic and open donor nephrectomy: a randomized controlled trial. *BJU Int*. 2005;95:851–855.
4. Bettschart V, et al. Laparoscopic procurement of kidney grafts from living donors does not impair initial renal function. *Transplant Proc*. 2002;34:787–790.
5. Novotny MJ. Laparoscopic live donor nephrectomy. *Urol Clin North Am*. 2001;28:127–135.
6. Meng MV, et al. Laparoscopic live donor nephrectomy at the university of California San Francisco. *Clin Transpl*. 2001;113–121.
7. Flowers JL, et al. Comparison of open and laparoscopic live donor nephrectomy. *Anns Surg*. 1997;226: 483–489.
8. Horgan S, et al. Robotic-assisted laparoscopic donor nephrectomy for kidney transplantation. *Transplantation*. 2002;73:1474–1479.
9. Roza AM, et al. Living-related donors with bilateral multiple renal arteries: a twenty year experience. *Transplantation*. 1989;47:397–399.
10. Emiroglu R, et al. Multiple-artery anastomosis in kidney transplantation. *Transplant Proc*. 2000;32: 617–619.
11. Mandal AK, et al. Should the indications for laparoscopic live donor nephrectomy of the right kidney be the same as for the open procedure? anomalous left renal vasculature is not a contraindication to left donor nephrectomy. *Transplantation*. 2001;71:660–664.

Chapter 40

Robot-Assisted Laparoscopic Pyeloplasty

Iqbal Singh and Ashok Kumar Hemal

40.1 History and Introduction

In 1886, Trendelenburg described the first open surgical repair of a ureteropelvic junction obstruction (UPJO), and the first successful pyeloplasty was performed 5 years later by Kuster in 1891.[1] Over the next 100 years drastic changes occurred in the pyeloplasty techniques like Heineke-Mickulicz by Fenger, plication of the renal pelvis by Kelly, Finney pyloroplasty, Y-V pyeloplasty. Culp and de-Weerd introduced the spiral flap in 1951, followed by vertical flap by Scardino and Prince in 1953. Until 25 years ago, the gold standard for UPJO repair was an Anderson–Hynes dismembered pyeloplasty through a flank incision with reported success rates of 95–99%.[2] With the development of minimal access techniques, the treatment options available to the urologist have now broadened significantly. In 1983, Wickham[3] described the percutaneous technique of antegrade pyelolysis. Later in 1986 Smith et al.[4] described their initial series of "Endopyelotomy" in USA. Later in the same year Inglis and Tolley[5] also described the use of retrograde rigid uretero-renoscopy to relieve strictures causing secondary UPJO and in 1993 McClinton et al.[6] described their series of 49 retrograde balloon dilatation (Endoburst) in 42 patients of UPJO. Later in the same year Chandoke and Clayman[7] described the "Acuise ureteral cutting balloon device" for performing retrograde endopyelotomy. The drawbacks of open surgical pyeloplasty include significant postoperative pain and morbidity mainly on account of the flank incision and delayed convalescence. In an effort to overcome these disadvantages of traditional open pyeloplasty other minimally invasive options such as endopyelotomy and laparoscopic pyeloplasty came into existence.

Open surgical pyeloplasty through retroperitoneal access has traditionally been the reference standard for managing ureteropelvic junction obstruction (UPJO) with reported success rates exceeding 90%.[8] With recent advances and global trends toward a near universal adoption of minimally invasive access surgery for managing UPJO, endopyelotomy and laparoscopic pyeloplasty (LP) came into vogue.

Anderson and Hynes dismembered laparoscopic pyeloplasty using four ports in the pediatric patients was first described by Peters and Retik.[9] Later Sung and Gill in 1999 described the feasibility and efficacy of RALPP in a porcine study using the Zeus[TM] robotic system.[10] The same authors again compared the efficacy of Zeus[TM] versus daVinci[TM] robotic system for robot-assisted laparoscopic pyeloplasty (RALPP) in another porcine model demonstrating a shorter total operating room time (61.4 versus 83.4 min; $P = 0.10$) and anastomotic time (44.7 versus 66.4 min; $P = 0.110$) with the daVinci[TM] system. During RALPP anastomosis, the total number of suture bites/ureter was 13.0 for the daVinci[TM] system ($n = 6$) and 10.8 for the Zeus system ($n = 6$); they concluded that the intraoperative technical movements appeared inherently more intuitive with the daVinci system than with the Zeus[TM] robotic system.[11] Subsequently Lorincz and Mc Lorie described the technical feasibility of RALPP in a porcine study using the Zeus[TM] robot with acceptable morbidity.[12]

I. Singh (✉)
Clinical Instructor, Urology, Department of Urology,
Wake Forest Baptist Medical Centre, Wake Forest University
Medical School, Winston-Salem, NC, USA
e-mail: iqbalsinghp@yahoo.co.uk

A.K. Hemal, M. Menon (eds.), *Robotics in Genitourinary Surgery*,
DOI 10.1007/978-1-84882-114-9_40, © Springer Verlag London Limited 2011

Dismembered laparoscopic pyeloplasty (DLP) was first described and reported in the English literature way back in 1993 by Schuessler and coworkers.[13] In the same year Kavoussi et al.[14] and later Janetschek in 1994[15] also confirmed the safety and efficacy of laparoscopic pyeloplasty. Subsequently the results of laparoscopic pyeloplasty (LP) were found to be comparable to open surgery by other workers.[16–18] This prompted certain workers to rename LP as the new reference standard for managing UPJO.[19] The advantages of LP include shorter convalescence, reduced pain, briefer hospital stays, superior cosmesis, with success rates exceeding 90%. LP has traditionally been confined to the domain of high-volume centers of excellence with skilled laparoscopic surgeons.[20] While LP may also be performed safely, effectively, and efficiently in a cost-efficient manner,[21] the main current drawback of LP is the relative difficulty of performing intracorporeal suturing that demands significant training and expertise. However, with the emergence of robot assistance in laparoscopic urology, the daVinci[TM] robotic system and its three-dimensional vision, tremor filtering, Endowrist[TM] system with 6 degrees of freedom, reconstructive surgery and intracorporeal suturing have become technically easier.[22–24] Initial cases of robot-assisted laparoscopic pyeloplasty were reported by Graham,[25] Guilloneau,[26] and Gettman and colleagues.[23] Subsequently several workers have successfully described and reported larger series of robot-assisted laparoscopic pyeloplasty (see Table 40.1).

40.2 Surgical Technique of Robot-Assisted Laparoscopic Pyeloplasty (RALPP)

40.2.1 Pre-operative Assessment

The diagnosis of ureteropelvic junction obstruction (UPJO) is based on symptomatology and is subsequently confirmed by imaging studies such as computed tomographic (CT) urography or an ultrasound/intravenous urography, which also helps in diagnosing co-existing and secondary pathologies such as renal stones, crossing vessels, and megaureter. A pre-operative assessment of the UPJO with MAG3

renal dynamic scan (nuclear renography) is an essential step as it provides a more objective and definitive assessment of UPJO. It provides a baseline quantification of the pre-operative renal function in terms of both the split and the absolute glomerular filtration rate (GFR) that is essential for follow-up. The renogram also confirms the diagnosis of significant renal outflow tract function.

40.2.2 Indications

Symptomatic patients with evidence of significant outflow tract obstruction as evidenced by serial renal scans and/or worsening obstructive hydronephrosis are the candidates that are most likely in need of some form of pyeloplasty. Patients with large baggy pelvis may in addition need a reduction pyeloplasty in order to ensure a dependent drainage. Patients with equivocal UPJO are best observed and kept on regular follow-up with serial renograms.

40.2.3 Contraindications

Patients with prior major intraabdominal surgery/laparotomy should be excluded from undergoing a transperitoneal laparoscopic/robotic procedure. Patients of UPJO with extensive co-morbidity on account of general medical problems and/or cardio-pulmonary insufficiency are those in whom a laparoscopic procedure may serve to be a relative contraindication.

40.2.4 Pre-operative Preparation

The type of repair to be performed is dependent on the size of the pelvis, length of the UPJ stricture, the presence of a crossing vessel, and the degree of renal function. Sterile urine cultures must be obtained prior to surgery. Cystoscopy with retrograde pyelography (RGP) may be performed in select cases of renal outflow obstruction with equivocal findings where the diagnosis of UPJO is in doubt or in case concomitant pathological abnormalities co-exist.

Table 40.1 The salient features of cases of robot-assisted laparoscopic pyeloplasties that have been reported in the published English literature

Salient features of selected worldwide reported series of "robotic pyeloplasty"

Author (Year)	N	Approach	Mean ORT (CT) ST[a]	EBL	CV (%)	HS (D)	Complic	Follow-up (MTH)
Gupta et al. (2009)[27]	24	T/P-TM-ADP	125±24, 44±15[a]	38.7	–	2.5	1(PD)	12
Kaouk et al. (2008)[37]	10	RP-ADP (1°-4, 2°-6)	175	50	3(30)	2	Nil	30(24–36)
Yanke et al. (2008)[38]	29	T/P-RA-ADP	–	–	20(69)	–	Nil	19(13–25)
Murphy et al. (2008)[39]	15	T/P-RA-ADP	187	30	9(44)	2.2	Nil	–
Mufarrij et al. (2008)[40]	117	1° UPJ, T/PRA-ADP	217(80–510)	58(10–600)	62(53)	2.1(0.8–7)	9(M);4 (m)–(11%)	30(3–63)
	23	**2° UPJ, TPRA-ADP**	**216(110–345)**	**68(10–300)**	**15(65.2)**	**2.1(1–3)**	**1(M)–(4.2%)**	**24(5–51)**
Hemal et al.(2008)[41]	**9**	**2° UPJ, TPRA-ADP**	**106(95–150)**	**72.4(40–200)**	**2(22)**	**3.4(2–5)**	**Nil**	**7.4(2–15)**
Schwenter et al.(2007)[42]	80	1° UPJ, TP RA-ADP	108.3(72–215)	<50	45(48.9)	4.6(3–11)	3(RS:1, H:1, U:1)–3.2%	39.1
	12	**2° UPJ, TP RA-ADP**						
Olsen et al. (2007)[43]	67	RP(Peds) 8-NDP, 59-RA-ADP	146(92–300)	–	15(22.4)	1.5(1–6)	11(UTI:2, H:2, N:2, DJJ stent:3) 16.4%	12(0.9–49)
Lee et al. (2006)[44]	33	RP(Peds)	219(133–401)	3(0–50)	11(33.3)	2.3(0.5–6)	1(3%)	10
Weise et al. (2006)[45]	31	TP RA-ADP	271(76)	<100	23(74)	2(1–3)	Nil	10(1–31)
Yee et al. (2006)[46]	8	TP RA-ADP(Peds)	363(255–522)	13.1	–	2.4	1(Failed), 1 Ileus	14.7
Kutikov et al. (2006)[47]	9	TP RA-ADP(Peds)	123	–	0	1.4	Nil	–

Table 40.1 (continued)

Salient features of selected worldwide reported series of "robotic pyeloplasty"

Author (Year)	N	Approach	Mean ORT (CT) STᵃ	EBL	CV (%)	HS (D)	Complic	Follow-up (MTH)
Patel et al. (2005)[48]	50	RP-ADP	122(60–330)	40	30	1.1	–	11.7
Palese et al. (2005a)[49]	35	TP RA-ADP	216.4 ± 52.9	73.9 ± 58.3	10(28.6)	2.89	1(failed-nephrectomy)	7.9
Palese et al. (2005b)[50]	38	TP RA-ADP	225.6 ± 59.3 64.2 ± 14.6*	77.3 ± 55.3	10(26.3)	2.9(1.1–13)	4(UTI:1, PN:2, GPS:1)	12.2
Atug et al. (2005a)[51]	7	TP RA-ADP(Peds)	184(165–204) 39.5(30–46)ᵃ	31.4(10–50)	–	–	Prolonged drain:2	10.9(2–18)
Atug et al. (2005b)[52]	8	TP RA-ADP(Adult)	275.8(180–345)	48.6(10–100)	2(25)	1.1(1–2)	Nil	12.3(4–22)
Atug et al. (2006)[53]	37 **7**	1° UPJ, TP RA-ADP **2° UPJ, TP RA-ADP**	219.4(130–345) **279.8(230–414)**	49.5(10–200) **52.5(20–100)**	16(43%) **2(28%)**	1.1(1–2) **1.2(1–3)**	Nil **Nil**	13.5(3–29) **10.7(3–20)**
Mendez-Torres et al. (2005)[54]	32	RA-ADP(31) Fengerplasty(1)	300(120–510)	52	14(44)	1.1(1–3)	2(UTI:1, Stent migration:1)	8.6(1.5–16)
Bernie et al. (2005)[55]	7	T/P RA-ADP	324	60(50–100)	4(57)	2.5(2–6)	2(UTI:1, hematuria:1)	10(5–15)
Gettman et al. (2002a)[23]	6	TP RA-ADP(4)ᵃ RA Fengerplasty(2)~	140(80–215) 70(40–115)ᵃ 77.5(75–80)~	<50	–	4	(0)Nil	–
Gettman et al. (2002b)[24]	7 **2**	1° TP RA-ADP **2° TP RA-ADP**	138.8(80–215) **62.4(40–115)***	<50	–	4.7(4–11)	1(11%) open reop	4.1(1–8)
MEAN	703		202	50	45	3.4	6.0	14.9

Most figures are rounded of to the nearest decimal. 1/2°–denotes primary or secondary UPJ obstruction. *Bold font* denotes **2° UPJO** cases.

RP, retroperitoneoscopic; TP, transperitoneal; TM, transmesocolic; RA-AHDP, robotic-assisted Anderson–Hynes dismembered pyeloplasty; NDP, non-dismembered pyeloplasty; RAF, robotic-assisted fengerplasty; ᵃST, suture time; H, hematuria; U, urinoma; RS, restented; N, nephrostomy; DJJ, displaced JJ stent; PD, prolonged drainage; UTI, urinary tract infection; PN, pyelonephritis; GPS, gluteal compartment syndrome; M, major; m, minor.

In our experience pre-operative placement of a JJ ureteral stent is no longer a necessary step. Pre-operatively patients are advised a clear liquid diet for 24 h and a rectal suppository on the night prior to surgery. The procedure is performed under general anesthesia and prophylactic antibiotics. In the opinion of these authors, in confirmed cases the pre-placement of a ureteral stent is no longer required; in case any difficulty is anticipated in locating the ureteropelvic junction, 20 mg of furosemide may be administered intravenously in order to distend the renal pelvis and facilitate its identification intraoperatively. The robot is sterile draped and the console camera is re-calibrated prior to initiating the procedure.

40.2.5 Position

A Foley catheter is placed and clamped so as to ensure and confirm easy passage of the JJ stent into the bladder by seeing reflux of urine, when antegrade ureteral stenting is done that is removed later. The patient is positioned with the ipsilateral kidney facing upward in the standard kidney/flank position at an angle of 60° with a supplemental kidney bridge and an axillary roll over a flexed operating table (lateral decubitus position) with adequate back supports. The patient is secured by strapping with a wide surgical tape over a foam pad both at the level of the ipsilateral chest/shoulder and at the level of the thigh along with the anti-embolic pneumatic leg bags. Adequate care is taken to pad all the pressure points. The ipsilateral arm is fixed to another arm board rest over a stack of blankets that is securely taped to the arm rest over a foam pad in a manner so as to facilitate free movement of the robotic arms.

40.2.6 Surgical Approach

Robot-assisted laparoscopic pyeloplasty can be performed by transperitoneal or retroperitoneal approach.

(i) Transperitoneal approach is generally the preferred approach for RALPP. This allows clear visualization of all the anatomical structures with adequate space for optimal access and positioning of the robotic and assistant ports. It is also the preferred approach to repair of UPJO associated with the pelvic ectopic kidney and/or the horse shoe kidney. Transperitoneal access may be used for a robot-assisted laparoscopic pyeloplasty by using either the transmesocolic approach that has also been previously described by us elsewhere[27] or the classical colonic mobilization approach to the UPJ. The transmesocolic approach has the advantage of doing away with colonic mobilization, providing the most direct approach to the UPJ after incising the mesocolon through the relatively avascular transmesocolic window and precluding extensive renal mobilization. It is considered to be safe and feasible in patients with a large prominent hydronephrotic pelvis underlying a thin mesentery and is considered to be a highly effective technique.[26] The use of the transmesocolic approach is generally restricted to a left-sided UPJO, because anatomically the left colic flexure lies superior to the right colic flexure and the left UPJ lies beneath the left colonic mesentery. This approach should be avoided in patient with a high BMI and a thick mesentery. The traditional retrocolic access with mobilization of the colon to approach the UPJ is preferred by us in cases of UPJO associated in the right kidney, with morbid obesity, concomitant renal calculi, accessory renal vessels, retrocaval ureter, and/or prior renal surgery where renal mobilization would be needed.

Retroperitoneal laparoscopic approach on the contrary is the preferred surgical approach to the UPJ in patients with prior repetitive transabdominal intraperitoneal surgery where post-operative adhesions may preclude a safe laparoscopic/robotic intraperitoneal access. Retroperitoneoscopic surgery has the advantage of offering direct early surgical access to the ureteropelvic junction, and in case of any leak or infection the urinoma is contained within the retroperitoneum. The disadvantages of retroperitoneal access include lack of space and technical difficulty of intracorporeal suturing due to instrument/port collision/overcrowding. The retrocaval ureter can also be successfully repaired via this approach.

Port Placement: Figure 40.1 shows the port placement that is frequently used by us for a transmesocolic approach. Pneumoperitoneum is established by a Veress needle (Gyrus, ACMI, Inc) at a point just outside the lateral border of the rectus muscle above the umbilicus. Once adequate pneumoperitoneum has been achieved, Veress needle is removed, and the stab incision is extended for placement of a 12 mm

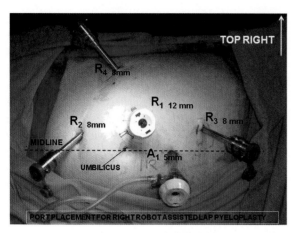

Fig. 40.1 Suggested port placement is depicted for a typical right robot-assisted pyeloplasty where R_1 is the primary 12 mm camera port placed just 2–3 cm lateral to the umbilicus. R_2 and R_3 are the secondary 8 mm robot ports placed about 7–8 cm on either side of the camera port in the same line. R_4 is the fourth robotic arm 8 mm port which is placed in the right iliac fossa. A1 is the assistant 5 mm port for suction which is placed supraumbilically in the midline equidistant from R_1 and R_3. In addition a distance of 7–8 cm should also be maintained in between the port sites to avoid arm collision

this incision, this serves as the primary 12 mm robotic camera port alternatively this may be placed just above the iliac crest. The left and right 8 mm robotic ports are inserted below and parallel to the 12th rib, at the anterior axillary line and at the costovertebral angle, the assistant 5 mm suction port is placed lateral to the camera port. In place of the latter alternatively a fourth port (12 mm) can also be placed anterior to the iliac crest into the ipsilateral retroperitoneal space for the assistant for retraction, suction, or introduction of sutures. The daVinci S^{TM} surgical robot system cart is docked from over the head of patient with a 0 or 30° up lens. The ureter is identified in the retroperitoneum, which is dissected proximally along with its periureteral tissue up to the pelvis and UPJ taking care to preserve any crossing vessels. The area of stenotic UPJ is excised and the ureter is spatulated with the robotic hot scissors. A watertight tension-free ureteropelvic anastomosis is performed over an antegrade JJ stent by using a pair of 4-0 Monocryl^{TM} or Vicryl^{TM} running sutures placed anteriorly and posteriorly in a manner similar to that used for transperitoneal robotic pyeloplasty that are finally tied together.

camera port. The endoscope is then introduced and the abdomen is inspected for any intraabdominal injury. Two working 8-mm robotic ports are also inserted under direct laparoscopic vision in the ipsilateral midclavicular line on either side of the camera port. In order to avoid any instrument collision between the robotic arms a working distance of about 7–8 cm is maintained with an obtuse docking angle and triangulation of the instruments. One or two additional 5 mm ports are also inserted infraumbilically either in the midline or on the contralateral side for retraction, suction, and suture handling. Alternatively with the four-arm robot (Prograsp^{TM}), the fourth robotic trocar may substitute for the additional trocar. After placing the trocars the robot is securely positioned and docked from the back of the patient.

Robot-assisted retroperitoneoscopic pyeloplasty:[28] An incision approximately 1.3 cm long is placed just below and lateral to the tip of the 12th rib. A spherical retroperitoneal balloon trocar PDB^{TM} system (OMSPDB^{TM} balloon 1000 – round shape or a OMSPDBS2^{TM} – kidney shape; Covidien, Autosuture) or (PDB^{TM}, US Surgical, Norwalk, CT) is used to dilate and develop the retroperitoneal space. Hasson's convertible trocar blunt tip trocar 12 mm is inserted via

40.3 Excision, Reduction Pyeloplasty, Stenting, and Ureteropyelostomy

RALPP: The robot is wheeled from the patient's back and it is then docked in a manner such that the laparoscope is aligned with the UPJ and robot (daVinci^{TM} robot comes in at an angle of 15° while the new daVinci-S^{TM} can come straight from the patients back). The colon is reflected at the level of the UPJ. One should avoid dissection of the ureter caudal into the pelvis so as to preserve the periureteral tissues (this is done using a monopolar curved scissors and a Maryland^{TM} fenestrated bipolar forceps or an endowrist^{TM} PK dissector). One should consider placing a stay suture on the pelvis both above and on the proximal ureter just below the UPJ. The renal pelvis is sharply incised and continued anterior and posterior to the UPJ. The ureter is then spatulated for 2–3 cm on its lateral (oriented anterior in flank position) border until it opens up after this dismemberment of the ureter from the pelvis is performed. While handling the UPJ, one should endeavor to make a pyelotomy first and then use the UPJ part of pelvis that will be discarded later as a handle to move the ureter. The anastomosis starts on the dependent wall beginning at the apex of spatulation using fine monofilament absorbable – usually 10–12 cm long 5-0 Monocryl™ sutures are used to perform a running or an interrupted (less efficient) watertight and tension-free anastomosis. The anastomosis stops at upper end of ureter and the portion of the UPJ stricture and pelvis is then resected and an interrupted suture is placed at the apex. Then second suture on either side of apex stitch is then run along the posterior and anterior rows as described.

The sequential intraoperative steps of robot-assisted laparoscopic pyeloplasty are illustrated in the series of endocamera images in Figs. 40.2, 40.3, 40.4, 40.5, 40.6, 40.7, 40.8, 40.9, 40.10, 40.11, 40.12, and 40.13. A brief 8 min operative video clip demonstrating the salient operative steps of robot-assisted technique of transperitoneal laparoscopic pyeloplasty performed by these authors is also appended to this chapter.

The robotic surgical system arms approach the patient from the back at an angle of 30° cephalad direction; however, with the availability of the new four-arm daVinci-S™ surgical robot it can be set up to directly approach from the back of the patient. The robot is docked in a manner such that the camera port is aligned with the UPJO. If the pelvis is grossly hydronephrotic, a transmesocolic approach is used to expose the pelvis. The basic surgical steps are mimicry of open surgery. The principles followed are (i) preservation of crossing vessels, (ii) dismembering the UPJO and excising the narrow portion, (iii) spatulating the ureter medially, (iv) subtracting the dilated pelvis, and (v) creating a watertight-dependent stented ureteropelvic anastomosis.

In the *transmesocolic approach*, the robotic monopolar scissors is used to make an incision, parallel to the mesenteric vessels, through a relatively avascular area in the mesentery overlying the UPJ in a manner so as to avoid injury to any major mesenteric vessel. With a combination of blunt and sharp dissection with the robotic monopolar hot scissors and the robotic bipolar forceps, the UPJ is dissected free from the surrounding soft tissue attachments through the mesenteric window. Excision of the UPJ, reduction pyeloplasty (if indicated), lateral spatulation of the ureter, and a stented anastomosis are performed with robotic assistance. The reduction pyeloplasty is performed by using the robotic hot monopolar robotic scissors and the bipolar forceps in a manner so as to subtract the redundant pelvis and achieve a proximal residual tapered renal pelvis. The ureteral spatulation is performed by holding the obliquely cut end of the ureter with the robotic bipolar forceps and inserting the robotic hot monopolar

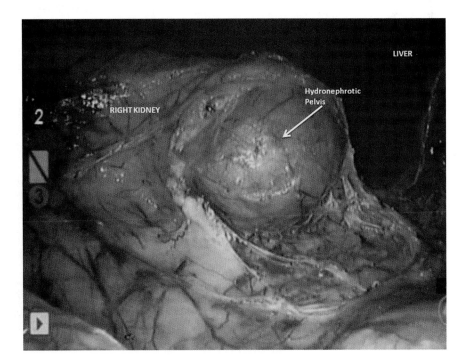

Fig. 40.2 An endocamera view of the hydronephrotic right kidney with a dilated renal pelvis

Fig. 40.3 An endocamera view of the dissected right renal hydronephrotic pelvis, the right ureteropelvic junction the right ureter with the crossing vessel at the right ureteropelvic junction

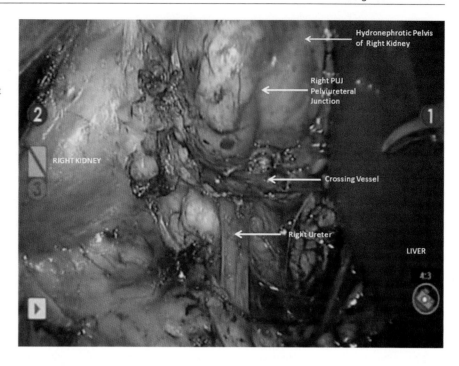

scissors and incising it on its lateral aspect for a length of about 1.5 cm. The technique of robot-assisted laparoscopic antegrade stenting has been described by us later in this chapter. After completion of the anastomosis (technique of anastomosis is detailed later in this chapter) the rent in the mesentery is finally closed with a continuous 3-0 vicryl™ sutures.

Under robotic control, by using a combination of blunt and sharp dissection with the right monopolar scissors and a left bipolar PK™ forceps the ipsilateral colon is reflected and retracted medially along the line of Toldt, in order to expose the kidney. In the robot-assisted technique of *Retroperitoneoscopic pyeloplasty*, the kidney is approached posteriorly; the

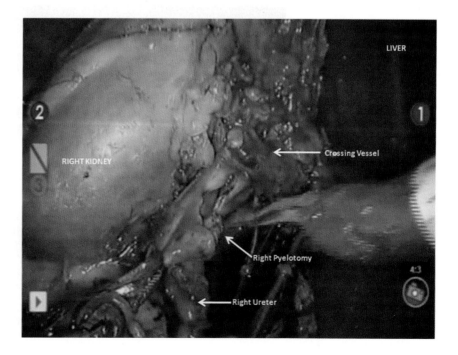

Fig. 40.4 An endocamera view of the redundant pelvis with pyelotomy in preparation for a dismembered Anderson–Hynes reduction pyeloplasty

Fig. 40.5 An endocamera view of the subtraction of the redundant pelvis in progress

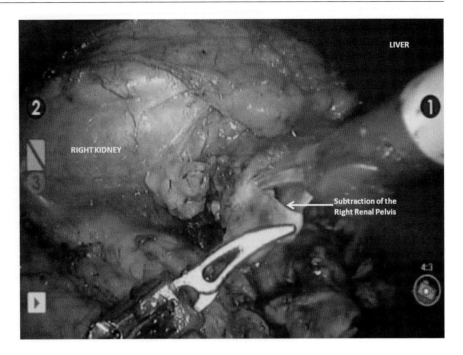

psoas muscle is identified with the ureter running anteriorly that is followed till the inferior pole of the kidney and the renal hilum. The renal hilum area is dissected identifying the renal vein, artery, and the renal pelvis. By using the landmark provided by the psoas muscle and the gonadal vein on the right (may be clipped if needed) the ureteropelvic junction is exposed down to the proximal ureter.

After placing stay sutures on the pelvis, the stenotic PUJ segment is transected, excised, and the divided ureteral end is spatulated on the lateral side for a length of 1 cm, and any redundant pelvis is also

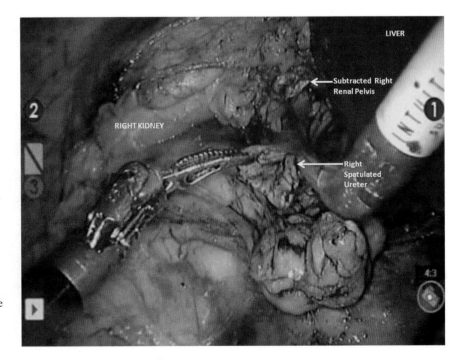

Fig. 40.6 An endocamera view of the subtracted right proximal renal pelvis with the right spatulated ureter fashioned for a dependent anastomosis

Fig. 40.7 The initiation of the apical stitch for the right ureteropyelostomy

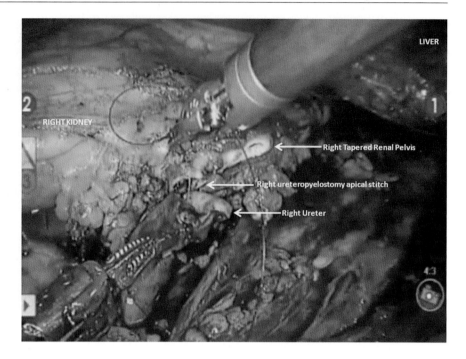

excised. A JJ ureteral stent pre-loaded on a guide wire is inserted with its floppy tip facing proximally in an antegrade fashion through one of the robotic/costovertebral area ports and is manipulated by the robotic graspers and guided under vision distally into the spatulated ureter first, and the guide wire is then disengaged taking care to grasp the stent with the robotic forceps while the guide wire is withdrawn out via the port by the assistant. The proximal coil of the JJ stent is then manipulated into the tapered

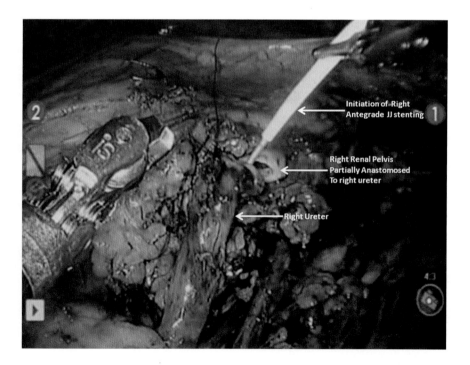

Fig. 40.8 An endocamera view of the partially re-anastomosed right renal pelvis with antegrade placement of the JJ stent in progress

Fig. 40.9 An endocamera view of the partially re-anastomosed right renal pelvis with antegrade placement of the JJ stent in progress

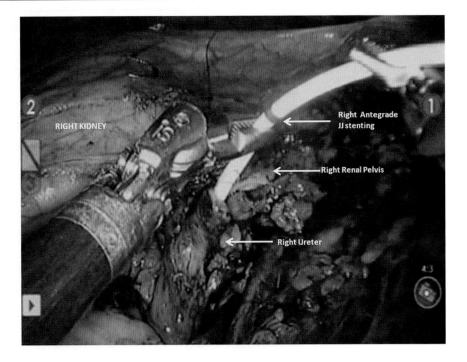

renal pelvis. In case any anterior crossing vessels are encountered all attempts are made to preserve them as far as possible and these are either repositioned posterior to the spatulated ureteropelvic anastomosis or the pelvis is simply translocated anterior to it.

For dilated baggy renal pelvis the excess of the endopelvic tissue is excised and by using 5-0 Monocryl® (Ethicon~poliglicaperone) sutures a *Dismembered Anderson–Hynes pyeloplasty* is performed in the usual manner. The initial throw of the same suture is used to secure the spatulated ureter

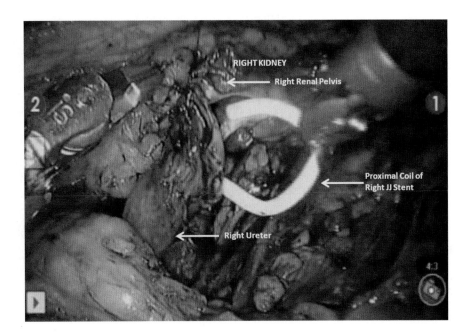

Fig. 40.10 An endocamera view of the partially re-anastomosed right renal pelvis with antegrade placement of the JJ stent in progress

Fig. 40.11 An endocamera view of the right anastomotic pyeloplasty in progress over a JJ stent

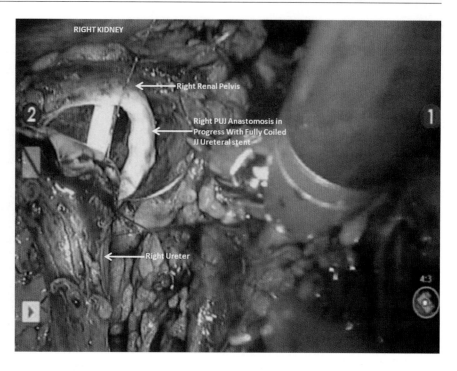

to the dependent part of the renal pelvis, and sub-sequently two additional running sutures are placed for completing the anterior and posterior wall of the anastomosis. After completing on one side of the anas-tomosis, a double-J ureteral stent is placed with a pre-loaded straight guide wire in an antegrade manner inserted through one of the assistant ports, manipulated

distally into the ureter and proximally into the pelvis and the rest of the anastomosis is then completed in a sequential manner. The renal pelvis is reposi-tioned behind the renal vessels, and Gerota's fascia is closed using 2-0 Vicryl® (Ethicon~polygalactin) sutures. Alternatively the suture may be prepared by tying two 5-0 monocryl™ (Ethicon~poliglicaperone)

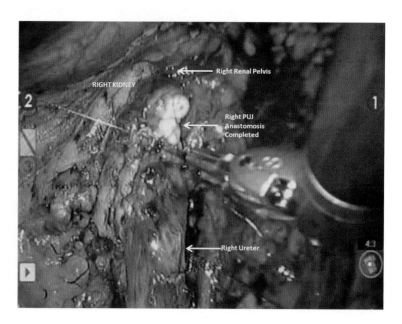

Fig. 40.12 An endocamera view of the completed right re-anastomotic pyeloplasty

Fig. 40.13 An endocamera view of the fully retroperitonealized right kidney at the termination of the procedure

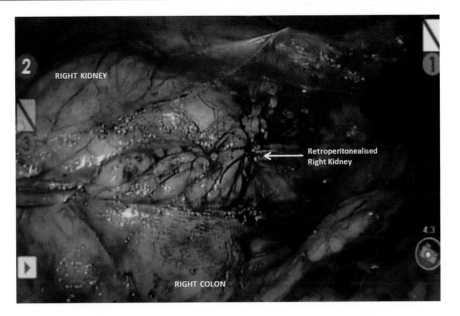

sutures (dyed and undyed) to make a single suture with two needles and the rest of the anastomosis is similarly completed in two hemi-circles. After completing the anastomosis the kidney is retroperitonealized by replacing the colon and suturing back the peritoneal fold with continuous 3-0 vicryl sutures and the robotic needle driver.

For patients with focal stenosis/without any crossing vessels, in whom a robot-assisted *Non-dismembered Fengerplasty* is intended, a 2 cm longitudinal incision is usually made through the stenotic area straddling the UPJO, extending to about a centimeter on either side of the stenotic area between two stay sutures placed medially and laterally, the incision is then closed transversely using 4-0 Vicryl™ interrupted sutures.

For UPJO associated with a high insertion of the ureter a *Foley Y-V plasty* is preferred where in a "V"-shaped flap is made on the pelvis with its base positioned on the medial aspect of the pelvis and its apex positioned at the UPJ. This is then extended laterally on to the proximal ureter across the UPJ stricture so that the apex of the flap lies alongside the ureterotomy. The anastomosis is then performed between the ureterotomy and the anterior wall of the pelvic flap.

In cases of UPJO associated with multiple and/or extensive proximal ureteric strictures, *Davis intubated ureterotomy* is the preferred surgical approach where in the stricture is incised and is allowed to heal by re-epithelialization over a JJ ureteral stent.

The robot is undocked and a JP® drain (optional) is placed in the perinephric space under laparoscopic vision brought out through a separate stab incision in the lower quadrant. In our opinion the placement of a perinephric drain in the presence of a JJ stent especially in the setting of transmesocolic approach to repair of the primary UPJO is not necessary in a majority of such cases, unless otherwise indicated in its own merit. However, we do advocate the placement of a drain in cases of repair of a secondary UPJO/salvage pyeloplasty due to higher risks of a possible urinary leak or breakdown of the anastomosis. In our opinion the placement of a drain may also be indicated in the setting of a retrocolic approach where colonic mobilization has been performed and also in the situation where extensive renal mobilization may have been performed. The bowel is repositioned and secured with a 2-0 Vicryl™ sutures. The ports are removed and closed at the fascia level using 0 Vicryl™ suture(s). The incisions are closed with 4-0 Monocryl® sutures and sealed with Dermabond™ (2-octyl cyanoacrylate-Ethicon, Inc., Somerville, NJ) adhesive.

Outcome & Follow-Up: In recent appraisal of a series of 24 cases of transmesocolic robot-assisted pyeloplasty reported from a single center, by Gupta and coworkers[27] these authors successfully reported on the safety and feasibility of the transmesocolic robot-assisted procedure with comparable operative times (mean ORT: 125.33± 23.48 and suturing time:43.58

±15.15 min), a mean hospital stay of 2.5 days and satisfactory long-term outcomes at a mean follow-up of 12 months. These authors had placed a drain in all their cases without any major complication being reported. One of their patients had fever with prolonged drainage due to a misplaced stent that later required an additional procedure for its cystoscopic repositioning.

40.4 Managing Concomitant Surgical Pathologies

(i) *Crossing Vessels*: In case(s) of UPJO associated with a crossing vessel(s) every attempt should be made to preserve them. This is done by either dismembering the pelvis and doing a posterior translocation of the crossing vessel and performing the pyeloplasty anterior to it or alternatively by a vascular relocation procedure that involves superior translocation and fixation of the crossing vessel proximal to the UPJO (*Hellstrom's procedure*). The robotic Hellstrom technique of vascular relocation involves mobilization of the crossing vessels and pexing the perivascular tissue to the Gerota's fascia with or without the perinephric fat.[29] Alternatively the crossing vein/artery is mobilized and then the dilated pelvis is folded over it using 5-0 sutures of Vicryl®.

(ii) *Concomitant renal/pelvic stones*: A concomitant robot-assisted laparoscopic pyelolithotomy can be easily accomplished at the time of the pyelotomy prior to the pyeloplasty. This has also been previously described by these authors[30,31] and others.
Robot-Assisted Laparoscopic Technique of Extended Pyelolithotomy: After exposing the renal pelvis a 'V' shaped incision (pyelotomy) is made away from the UPJ or for larger stones this incision can be extended into the intrarenal pelvis (extended pyelotomy). The stones are then extracted from the pelvis and/or the calyces by using the robotic Prograsp™ device. Alternatively a flexible cystoscope/ureterorenoscope device can also be introduced from one of the port sites to retrieve some of the otherwise inaccessible calyceal stone(s) by using a combination of one or more of the following; flushing,

helical nitinol stone extractor or holmium laser lithotripsy. The retrieved stones can be placed into an Endocatch™-10 mm (Covidien Autosuture) bag which can be removed later through the 12 mm assistant port. The pyeloplasty is then performed in the usual manner. The pyelotomy can then be closed after a reduction pyeloplasty intracorporeally over a JJ stent placed in an antegrade manner by a running suture as described above in the robot-assisted technique of laparoscopic pyeloplasty. According to these authors[29] transperitoneal stone surgery was safe as it was not associated with any adverse events like fever, peritonitis and prolonged ileus. Concomitant management of renal pelvic stones during a robotic-assisted laparoscopic pyeloplasty has also been described by Atug et al.[32] who had reported a 100% success rate without any delayed complications in eight of their patients with UPJO and nephrolithiasis

(iii) *Secondary ureteric stricture(s)/Periureteral granuloma*: Robotic-assisted laparoscopic surgery facilitates the dissection, excision and repair of secondary ureteral strictures. In our experience it is also well suited to the surgical management of periureteral granulomas that can be successfully managed by excision and a stented ureteropyelostomy. We have successfully performed a robot-assisted transperitoneal laparoscopic ureteropyelostomy in two such cases of UPJO due to post-SWL/post-URS periureteral granuloma.
Robotic-Assisted Laparoscopic Surgical Technique (Excision Ureteropyelostomy): Patient position and port placement are similar as for a right-sided pyeloplasty. Pure laparoscopy may be performed to take down some of the adhesions using the laparoscopic scissors and electrocautery. After docking the robot, the right colon is reflected medially and any more adhesions are taken down. Dissection is then continued down to the inferior vena cava (IVC) up to the point where the right gonadal vein was identified as it drained into the IVC. The right gonadal vein was mobilized and divided between Hem-o-Lock™ clips. After dissecting down to the psoas muscle the ureter can be more easily defined and followed more proximally until the periureteral calcified mass is seen to be intimately associated with

the proximal ureter. The dilated renal pelvis is identified and located. The calcified mass and the proximal ureter are then meticulously dissected free from surrounding structure and are subsequently excised en bloc. The distal ureter is mobilized along with the renal pelvis, spatulated and stented (antegrade manner) with a 8.2 × 26 double-J ureteral stent in order to ensure a tension-free and watertight ureteropyelostomy by placing 5-0 Monocryl™ sutures in a running fashion as described above earlier in this chapter. Periureteral and perirenal fat is then replaced over the anastomosis and secured with additional 5-0 Monocryl™ sutures. The specimen is then retrieved via an Endocatch™ bag and a closed-suction Jackson Pratt ™ drain is inserted to drain the right pericolic gutter at the termination of the procedure.

(iv) *Retrocaval ureter*: The Robot-assisted laparoscopic technique as well as the purely laparoscopic technique of excision and successful repair of the retrocaval ureter has been described below which has been previously reported and described by us before elsewhere.[33,34]

Robot-Assisted Laparoscopic Technique of Repair of Retrocaval ureter: The patient is positioned in a manner similar to that for a right transperitoneal pyeloplasty. Port position – A Veres needle is used to create a pneumoperitoneum, and 12 mm port is inserted for the camera at the level of the umbilicus at the lateral border of rectus abdominis muscle. After inspecting the peritoneum, two robotic 8 mm ports are inserted under vision beneath the costal margin in the mid-clavicular line and the other three fingers below the anterior superior iliac spine. Another assistant 5 mm port is inserted 5 cm below the camera port for retraction and suction. The robot is then docked. The right colon is mobilized medially to provide exposure to the right retroperitoneal structures. By a combination of blunt and sharp dissection the right renal pelvis, inferior vena cava, right gonadal vein, right ureter and duodenum are identified. The right renal pelvis is mobilized and right ureterolysis is performed till the level of its disappearance superiorly below the inferior vena cava. The renal pelvis is divided at the ureteropelvic junction and the retrocaval ureteric segment is transposed anterior to the inferior vena cava. A stented (stent with

the wire is introduced in an antegrade manner via the 5 mm port, which is grasped with a robotic needle driver, manipulated into the ureter, and passed down into the bladder) pyeloureterostomy is performed with 5-0 monocryl™ sutures in a manner similar to that described by us earlier in this chapter under the section of robot-assisted laparoscopic pyeloplasty. A JP™ drain is inserted via the 5-mm port and the robot is undocked. The ports are then closed at the facial level with 1-0 vicryl™ sutures.

(v) Giant Hydronephrosis and Nephroptosis: Concomitant laparoscopic nephroplication and nephropexy along with laparoscopic repair of the UPJO has also been previously described and reported in the literature by these authors.[35]

Robot-Assisted Laparoscopic Technique Nephrolysis and Nephropexy: For UPJO associated with significant nephroptosis robot-assisted laparoscopic nephropexy can also be performed that has been described by others.[36] The patient position and port placement are similar to as described by us previously in this chapter under the section for the robot-assisted transperitoneal technique of pyeloplasty. The colon is mobilized along the avascular line of "Toldt" and subsequently the proximal ureter, ureteropelvic junction, and the renal pelvis are also mobilized. The hepatorenal ligament is also divided in order to completely mobilize the kidney and be able to place the nephropexy fixation sutures as cranial as possible. In such cases after performing the dismemberment of the renal pelvis and transposing the pelviureteral junction anterior to the crossing vessels, complete nephrolysis is initially performed by using the right robotic monopolar scissors and a left robotic bipolar forceps for dissection in the perinephric space. A robot-assisted laparoscopic transperitoneal dismembered reduction pyeloplasty is performed in the usual manner as described above. The nephropexy is then performed using robotic assistance by using a 3-0 Vicryl sutures on a CT-1 needle, with three to four sutures placed through the renal capsule, that are tacked to the fascia of muscles in the bed of the kidney, over the quadratus lumborum muscle at the level of the hepatorenal ligament. Subsequently secondary suture(s) are also placed through the posterior aspect of the lower pole of the kidney which is transfixed and to the fascia of the psoas major muscle. The procedure is terminated by placing a JP™ drain in the perinephric space.

Follow-up: The Foleys catheter and the drain are generally removed at 48 h following surgery. When drainage is less than 30 ml/12 h the drain can be removed and the patient can generally be discharged with an indwelling bladder catheter that is removed 2–3 days later. Alternatively the bladder catheter can be removed first and in case the flank drainage is less than 30 ml/12 h the drain can be removed and the patient is discharged. Stent removal is generally done at 6–8 weeks. Subsequently they are followed up with a diuretic renogram initially at 3 and later at 6 months following surgery and annually thereafter provided the initial renogram(s) is/are satisfactory. A successful result is defined by a combination of patent ureteropelvic junction on the nuclear renogram and a subjective improvement in the patient analog pain scores.

40.5 Discussion

Table 40.1 shows the salient features of major published series of robot-assisted laparoscopic pyeloplasty reported and published in the English literature till date[11,37–55]. To date, Muffraiz et al. have reported the largest series of RALPL (140 cases) of RALPL demonstrating the overall safety and durability of robot-assisted repair of both the primary and the secondary UPJO.[40]

Approach to RALPL (Transperitoneal or Retroperitoneal): Most RALPLs have been commonly performed via transperitoneal access.[38–42,45–55] The advantages of the transperitoneal approach include availability of an adequate and considerably larger working space and a greater degree of familiarity with the traditional anatomical landmarks. The transmesocolic approach is anatomically and surgically well suited to lend itself to a robot-assisted laparoscopic repair of the left PUJO. Some workers have also described and reported on the safety and feasibility of robot-assisted retroperitoneoscopic pyeloplasty.[37,43,44] The advantages of the retroperitoneoscopic approach include direct access to the UPJO; confinement of any possible urinary leak (urinoma) to

the retroperitoneum; and the avoidance of peritoneal transgression, ileus, and minimal chance of bowel injury. Problems of the retroperitoneal approach include limited working space, difficult intracorporeal suturing due to lack of space, difficulty in identifying lower polar anterior crossing vessels, overcrowding of the ports, instrument collision, and the need to position the robot more cephalad than usual.[37]

In the opinion of these authors the retroperitoneal approach should be reserved for patients of UPJO with prior multiple transperitoneal surgeries. However, we feel that until more data emerge and long-term follow-up is available the retroperitoneoscopic (robot-assisted laparoscopic) approach should not be the preferred initial approach to repair the UPJO laparoscopically.

(A) Peri-operative Data/Outcomes:

(i) *ORT*: A review of some major selected published reports on robot-assisted laparoscopic pyeloplasty reveals that the mean ORT is about 207 (60–510) min and depending upon the level of expertise in experienced hands the robot/console time (CT) appears to be just above an hour (50–76) min. The ORT varied depending on whether it was a primary or a secondary (redo) pyeloplasty and whether a transperitoneal or retroperitoneal access was employed. Some workers have shown that the ORT may be longer in cases of secondary UPJ repair following prior failed pyeloplasty.[53] The initial surgeons learning curve may also impact the overall operating room times.[55] Moreover the ORT may vary depending on whether the duration of cystoscopy, retrograde uretero-pyelography, and/or stent placement was included or not. Most reported studies depicted in Table 40.1 have included these as a part of the overall operative duration. Additional procedures such as stone removal may prolong the ORT.[46] Nevertheless RALPL[17] has decreased the difficulty of intracorporeal suturing and considerably shortened the prolonged ORTs and the steep learning curve that were associated with laparoscopic pyeloplasty.[16,20,23,42,56,57] Schwenter et al. reported (in their single center 5-year experience with 92 cases of Robot-assisted AHD pyeloplasty) a mean anastomotic suturing time of 24.8 min.[42] Patel et al. also reported a mean anastomotic (suturing) time of 20 min (mean overall ORT of

91 min) in latter 10 of their 51 cases of RALPL.[48] This also signifies the fact that the operative duration of RALPL, including the suturing time tends to significantly decrease with increasing experience.

(ii) *Crossing Vessels*: The presence of crossing vessels is commonly known to be associated with the occurrence of UPJO and these may also influence the treatment of UPJO. A review of the selected published data on major cases of RALPL as shown in Table 40.1 reveals that crossing vessels were present in association with UPJO in almost half the cases, with a mean of 45(0–69)%. In our opinion as far as possible anterior crossing vessels should be preserved. In case these interfere with the anastomosis despite mobilization of the ureter and renal pelvis, it is better to transpose the ureter.[37]

(iii) *Estimated Blood Loss (EBL)*: A comparison of the published series depicted in Table 40.1 shows that the mean estimated blood loss in RALPL has been about 50 (0–600) mls.[23,24,37,39–42,44–46,48–55] Studies have shown that the EBLs are comparable to pyeloplasty performed conventionally/with robotic assistance, without any statistically significant difference.[23,45]

(iv) *Length of Hospital Stay (LOS)*: The average length of hospitalization according to major selected series of RALPL depicted in Table 40.1 is about 3.2 (1–11) days; however, in most of these series the duration of hospitalization was about 2 days.[37,39–50,52–55] Studies have shown that while the LOS appears to be similar following conventional pyeloplasty/RALPL, the general trend of LOS appeared to relatively shorter with the RALPL cases.[45,55]

(v) *Peri-operative Complications*: A review of the published literature on RALPL suggests that the average perioperative complication rate is about 6(0–16)%. Majority of these reported complications were minor related to stent displacement, hematuria, ileus, prolonged drainage, and urinary tract infections.[40,41,46,50,51,54,55] Others have also reported the occurrence of other complications like urinoma, pyelonephritis, compartment syndrome, and nephrectomy too.[24,40,49,50] In one of the largest series by Muffariz et al. comprising 140 cases of UPJO managed by

RALPL, the authors reported a 7.1% major and 2.9% minor complication rate.[40]

(B) *Functional Outcomes*: The mean follow-up of the selected series of RALPL as depicted in Table 40.1 is about 14.9 (1–51) months. Bernie et al. reported no difference in the outcomes following laparoscopic pyeloplasty performed with/without robotic assistance.[55] Weise et al. also reported a virtually similar short-term outcome of RALPL versus conventional laparoscopic pyeloplasty.[45] In a single center 5-year experience with 92 cases of RALPL that included 12 cases of secondary UPJO the authors reported a 100% patency rate (96.7 success rate) without any conversions, and appreciable cosmetic outcomes, during a mean follow-up of 39.1 months.[42] Patel et al. also reported a success rate of 100% in their 51 cases of RALPL during a mean follow-up of 11.7 months.[48] Open surgery continues to be the reference standard against which all current minimally invasive surgical technique(s) for the management of UPJO are likely to be compared against. The published global literature on robot-assisted laparoscopic pyeloplasty has been reviewed previously in detail by us elsewhere.[58]

(C) *Secondary Pyeloplasty*: Redo pyeloplasty is an overall technically difficult and challenging procedure.[59] RALPL[41,53] and/or laparoscopic pyeloplasty[60] may also be feasible for the repair of select patients of secondary UPJO due to prior failed open/endoscopic repair of primary UPJO. The challenges associated with secondary pyeloplasty are chiefly on account of adhesions and variable reactionary peripelvic fibrosis due to urinary leakage, bleeding, or excessive use of thermal energy (diathermy) in the region of the UPJ following its primary repair (endopyelotomy/open). These workers have shown that the ORT may be significantly greater by about an hour in such cases of secondary pyeloplasty. According to Hemal and colleagues[41] the actual benefits perceived to be associated with robot-assisted laparoscopic redo pyeloplasty were the relative ease of performing a thorough dissection, superior delineation of the prior scarred tissue, and better preservation of the periureteral sheath encompassing the blood supply to the ureter, with a clean and precise tailoring of ureteral and pelvic flaps for suturing a leakproof anastomosis. It is also prudent to be cautious of potential adhesions that may exist between the UPJO especially on the right side while attempting a redo right-sided UPJO repair, due to its anatomical proximity to the inferior vena cava. While secondary UPJO repair appears to be more prone to failure, RALPL appears to be a good modality even for these complicated cases in select situations, with the overall success rate being even higher (91.6%) in at least some series[42] than that has been reported in the past with pure laparoscopic pyeloplasty (80%).[59]

(D) *Robot-assisted Laparoscopic pyeloplasty in the children*: Robot-assisted laparoscopic pyeloplasty for UPJO has also been successfully performed both via the retroperitoneal and via the transperitoneal approach in the pediatric population, by several workers[43,44,46,47,51] attesting its feasibility and safety in the children. Though the laparoscopic technique to repair of the UPJO appeared to be technically a highly demanding procedure in the children, the availability of robotic assistance and equipment has considerably decreased the operating time due to the relative ease of intracorporeal suturing. In our opinion the transperitoneal approach should be the initial preferred approach for a robot-assisted laparoscopic pyeloplasty as it may be better suited in the infants and younger children. Due to intraoperative space constraints, we feel that the retroperitoneal approach to repair of the UPJO should be preferred only in the older children with prior history of transperitoneal surgery.

(E) *Advantages of Robot Assistance*: The advantages of robot-assisted laparoscopic pyeloplasty over pure laparoscopic pyeloplasty include motion scaling, tremor obliteration, three-dimensional stereoscopic vision, and greatly simplified precise suturing of the pelvis. Other workers[23] have also shown that RALPL is associated with overall shorter anastomotic and ORT. Depending on the center of excellence, the degree of expertise achieved and the economic viability of an institution affording a daVinci robot[TM] the laparoscopic pyeloplasty with or without robot assistance remains an effective and viable option for most cases of UPJO[61,62] that may even encompass to include patients with renal congenital anomaly,[63] presence

of a lower pole crossing vessel, failed previous endopyelotomy,[41,53,59] or even concomitant renal calculi.[40,52] One of the notable benefits of robot assistance is relative ease of spatulating the ureter, refashioning the pelvic flaps, and the suturing the ureteropelvic junction anastomosis. RALPL for UPJO complicated with concomitant stones, secondary UPJO, anomalous/horseshoe/ectopic kidney/duplex pelvis has also been shown to be feasible, safe, and effective, with durable success rates.[64] According to Leveillee et al. long-term data are now emerging for RALPP that appears to be a feasible and effective alternative to laparoscopy for reconstructive procedures of the ureter.[65] According to Peters et al.[66] the question whether RALPP is better than open surgery would be difficult to prove given overall success rate of above 95% in most series of open and laparoscopic pyeloplasty, as based on the current experience and ease of intracorporeal suturing with RALPP it may be not easy reverting to laparoscopic or open pyeloplasty especially in high-volume institutions where a robotic system may be currently available. In recent meta-analysis review by Bragga et al.[67] the authors suggested the take home message that RALPP appeared to be equivalent to traditional laparoscopic pyeloplasty with regard to operative time, complications, and success rates. However, Novara et al.[68] in an editorial comment to this meta-analysis also commented that strength of this meta-analysis was weak given the fact that the quality of their data, was quite poor, due to lack of any randomized trials and few published reports. Fornara et al.[69] also in an editorial comment to this meta-analysis suggested the actual advantage(s) lay probably for the surgeons who were laparoscopically naïve as RALPP, reduces the learning curve, and makes it simpler to learn the robotic surgical technique versus purely laparoscopic technique. RALPL is believed to be highly effective for managing PUJO, as it is associated with lower morbidity, faster recovery, and overall a durable success rate.[70]

(F) *Advances*: Recently Desai and colleagues have described and reported that their maiden case of a scar-less single-port transperitoneal laparoscopic pyeloplasty was performed by using a tri-port inserted through a single umbilical incision and a 2 mm sub-costal needlescopic port without any extra-umbilical incision(s). Their reported ORT, EBL, and LOS were 2.7 h, 50 cc, and 2 days, respectively.[71] Subsequently they also reported on two cases of bilateral simultaneous AHDP in bilateral primary UPJO that were performed after a pre-placed JJ ureteral stent, by using the same novel single-access multichannel tri-port (R-port[TM], Advanced Surgical Concepts, Dublin, Ireland) enabling a scar-less surgery through a single obscured infraumbilical incision.[72] Another multichannel port also available for similar single-port procedures includes the Uni-X[TM] port (Pnavel Systems, Morganville, NJ, USA). However, though the single-port transumbilical laparoscopy or embryonic natural orifice transumbilical endoscopic surgery (E-NOTES) appears to be encouraging, according to Canes and colleagues, these were plagued with the problems of triangulation, difficult retraction, instrument crowding, restricted vision, and patient limitations.[73] Robot-assisted laparoscopic pyeloplasty has also been successfully described with a transperitoneal approach without isthmusectomy, as a safe and feasible procedure in the management of UPJO in patients with anomalous or horseshoe kidneys.[74] Recently concurrent robot-assisted laparoscopic bilateral pyeloplasties in a group of five children have also been described in the literature.[75]

In a recent publication by Hemal and colleagues[76] while comparing the outcomes of RALPL (30 patients) versus pure laparoscopic pyeloplasty (30 patients) for UPJO concluded that RALPL was associated with more rapid dissection, reconstruction, and faster intracorporeal suturing with finer sutures with antegrade JJ stenting and shorter ORT though the long-term success rates were equivalent. Further, technical advances and improvements in the technique and instrumentation are likely to expand the entire spectrum of surgery including the way the future laparoscopic ablative and advanced reconstructive urological procedures such as these are likely to be performed. In future flexible (elephant trunk technology based) roof top, magnetic or miniaturized robotic systems may soon occupy the modern operating room.

40.6 Conclusion

A review of the recent selected series from the published English literature (Pubmed[TM]) reveals that currently more than 670 robot-assisted laparoscopic pyeloplasties have been successfully performed worldwide over the past 8 years. This testifies to the overall safety and efficacy of RALPL as a minimally invasive procedure. The short-term results appear to be similar as compared to those achieved with conventional laparoscopic pyeloplasty. The notable advantage of RALPL over laparoscopic pyeloplasty appears to be on account of the relative ease in acquiring skills needed for intracorporeal suturing, that is greatly simplified. The concomitant advantage of tremor-free meticulous dissection, precise suturing, and superior stereoscopic three-dimensional vision also contributes to the overall excellent results achieved following RALPL.

In keeping with the initial high current cost of the robot/equipment and consumables, RALPL apparently remains a costly procedure that outweighs the cost of standard laparoscopic pyeloplasty. The potential cost benefits of RALPL and long-term benefits remain to be ascertained, and this remains an area of ongoing concern.

References

1. Poulakis V, Witzsch U, Schultheiss D, Rathert P, Becht E. History of ureteropelvic junction obstruction repair (pyeloplasty). From Trendelenburg (1886) to the present Urologe A. 2004;43(12):1544–1559.
2. Anderson JC, Hynes W. Plastic operation for hydronephrosis. Proc R Soc Med. 1951;44(1):4–5.
3. Wickham JE, Kellet MJ. Percutaneous pyelolysis. Eur Urol. 1983;9(2):122–124.
4. Badlani G, Eshghi M, Smith AD. Percutaneous surgery for ureteropelvic junction obstruction (endopyelotomy): technique and early results. J Urol. 1986;135(1):26–28.
5. Inglis JA, Tolley DA. Ureteroscopic pyelolysis for pelviureteric junction obstruction. Br J Urol. 1986;58(3):250–252.
6. McClinton S, Steyn JH, Hussey JK. Retrograde balloon dilatation for pelviureteric junction obstruction. Br J Urol. 1993;71(2):152–155.
7. Chandhoke PS, Clayman RV, Stone AM, McDougall EM, Buelna T, Hilal N, Chang M, Stegwell MJ. Endopyelotomy and endoureterotomy with the acucise ureteral cutting balloon device: preliminary experience. J Endourol. 1993;7(1):45–51.

8. O'Reilly PH, Brooman PJ, Mak S. The long-term results of Anderson-Hynes pyeloplasty. BJU Int. 2001;87: 287–289.

9. Peters CA, Schlussel RN, Retik AB. Pediatric laparoscopic dismembered pyeloplasty. J Urol. 1995;153(6):1962–1965.

10. Sung GT, Gill IS, Hsu TH. Robotic-assisted laparoscopic pyeloplasty: a pilot study. Urology. 1999;53(6):1099–1103.

11. Sung GT, Gill IS. Robotic laparoscopic surgery: a comparison of the da Vinci and Zeus systems. Urology. 2001;58(6):893–898.

12. Lorincz A, Knight CG, Kant AJ, Langenburg SE, Rabah R, Gidell K, Dawe E, Klein MD, McLorie G. Totally minimally invasive robot-assisted unstented pyeloplasty using the Zeus Microwrist Surgical System: an animal study. J Pediatr Surg. 2005;40(2):418–422.

13. Schuessler WW, Grune MT, Tecuanhuey LV, Preminger GM. Laparoscopic dismembered pyeloplasty. J Urol. 1993;150: 1795–1799.

14. Kavoussi LR, Peters CA. Laparoscopic pyeloplasty. J Urol. 1993;150:1891–1894.

15. Janetschek G, Peschel R, Reissigl A. Laparoscopic dismembered pyeloplasty. J Endourol. 1994;8:S83.

16. Jarrett TW, Chan DY, Charambura TC, Fugita O, Kavoussi LR. Laparoscopic pyeloplasty: the first 100 cases. J Urol. 2002;167:1253–1256.

17. Inagaki T, Rha KH, Ono AM, Kavoussi LR, Jarrett TW. Laparoscopic pyeloplasty: current status. BJU Int. 2005;95:102–105.

18. Janetschek G, Peschel R, Frauscher F. Laparoscopic pyeloplasty. Urol Clin North Am. 2000;27:695–704.

19. Zhang X, Li HZ, Ma X. Retrospective comparison of retroperitoneal laparoscopic versus open dismembered pyeloplasty for ureteropelvic junction obstruction. J Urol. 2006;176:1077–1080.

20. Tan BJ, Rastinehad AR, Marcovich R, Smith AD, Lee BR. Trends in ureteropelvic junction obstruction management among urologists in the United States. J Urol. 2005;65:260–264.

21. Hemal AK, Goel R, Goel A. Cost-effective laparoscopic pyeloplasty: single center experience. Int J Urol. 2003;10(11):563–568.

22. Hemal AK, Menon M. Robotics in urology. Curr Opin Urol. 2004;14(2):89–93.

23. Gettman MT, Peschel R, Neururer R, Bartsch G. A comparison of laparoscopic pyeloplasty performed with the da Vinci robotic system versus standard laparoscopic techniques:Initial clinical results. Eur Urol. 2002a;42: 453–458.

24. Gettman MT, Neururer R, Bartsch G, Peschel R. Anderson-Hynes dismembered pyeloplasty performed using the *da vinci* robotic system. Urology. 2002b;60(3):509–513.

25. Graham RW, Graham SD, Bokinsky GB, Monahan MB. Urological upper tract surgery with the daVinci robotic system, pyeloplasty. J Urol. 2001;165:V74.

26. Guillonneau B, Jayet C, Cappele O, Navarre S, Martinez J, Vallancien G. Robotic-assisted laparoscopic pyeloplasty. J Urol. 2001;165:V75.

27. Gupta NP, Mukherjee S, Nayyar R, Hemal AK, Kumar R. Transmesocolic robot-assisted pyeloplasty: single center experience. J Endourol. 2009;23(6):945–948.

28. Kaouk JH, Hafron J, Parekattil S, Moinzadeh A, Stein R, Gill IS, Hegarty N. Is retroperitoneal approach feasible

for robotic dismembered pyeloplasty: initial experience and long-term results? J Endourol. 2008;22(9):2153–2159.

29. Meng MV, Stoller MI. Hellstrom technique revisited: laparoscopic management of UPJ obstruction. Urology. 2003;62(3):404–408.

30. Badani KK, Hemal AK, Fumo M, Kaul S, Shrivastava A, Rajendram AK, Yusoff NA, Sundram M, Susan Woo S, Peabody JO, Mohamed SR, Menon M. Robotic extended pyelolithotomy for treatment of renal calculi: a feasibility study. World J Urol. 2006;24:198–201.

31. Lee RS, Passerotti CC, Cendron M, Estrada CR, Borer JG, Peters CA. Early results of robot assisted laparoscopic lithotomy in adolescents. J Urol. 2007;177:2306–2310.

32. Atug F, Castle EP, Burgess SV, Thomas R. Concomitant management of renal calculi and pelvi-ureteral junction obstruction with robotic laparoscopic surgery. BJU Int. 2005;96:1365–1368.

33. Gupta NP, Hemal AK, Singh I, Khaitan A. Retroperitoneal ureterolysis and reconstruction of retrocaval ureter. J Endourol. 2001;15(3):291–293.

34. Hemal AK, Rao R, Sharma S, Clement RG. Pure robotic retrocaval ureter repair. Int Braz J Urol. 2008;34(6):734–738.

35. Jindal L, Gupta AK, Mumtaz F, Sunder R, Hemal AK. Laparoscopic nephroplication and nephropexy as an adjunct to pyeloplasty in UPJO with giant hydronephrosis. Int Urol Nephrol. 2006;38(3–4):443–446.

36. Boylu U, Lee BR, Thomas R. Robotic-assisted laparoscopic pyeloplasty and nephropexy for ureteropelvic junction obstruction and nephroptosis. J Laparoendosc Adv Surg Tech A. 2009;19(3):379–382.

37. Kaouk JH, Hafron J, Parekattil S, Moinzadeh A, Stein R, Gill IS, Hegarty N. Is retroperitoneal approach feasible for robotic dismembered pyeloplasty: initial experience and long-term results? J Endourol. 2008;22(9):2153–2159.

38. Yanke BV, Lallas CD, Pagnani C, McGinnis DE, Bagley DH. The minimally invasive treatment of ureteropelvic junction obstruction: a review of our experience during the last decade. J Urol. 2008;180:1397–1402.

39. Murphy D, Challacombe B, Olsburgh J, Calder F, Mamode M, Khan MS, Mushtaq I, Dasgupta P. Ablative and reconstructive robotic-assisted laparoscopic renal surgery. Int J Clin Pract. 2008;62:1703–1708.

40. Mufarrij PW, Woods M, Shah OD, Palese MA, Berger AD, Thomas R, Stifelman MD. Robotic dismembered pyeloplasty: a 6-year, multi-institutional experience. J Urol. 2008;180:1391–1396.

41. Hemal AK, Mishra S, Mukharjee S, Suryavanshi M. Robot assisted laparoscopic pyeloplasty in patients of ureteropelvic junction obstruction with previously failed open surgical repair. Int J Urol. 2008;15(8): 744–746.

42. Schwentner C, Pelzer A, Neururer R, Springer B, Horninger W, Bartsch G, Pesch R. Robotic Anderson-Hynes pyeloplasty: 5-year experience of one centre. BJUI. 2007;100:880–885.

43. Olsen LH, Rawashdeh YF, Jorgensen TM. Pediatric robot assisted retroperitoneoscopic pyeloplasty: a 5-year experience. J Urol. 2007;178(5):2137–2141.

44. Lee RS, Retik AB, Borer JG, Peters CA. Pediatric robot assisted laparoscopic dismembered pyeloplasty:

comparison with a cohort of open surgery. J Urol. 2006;175(2):683–687.

45. Weise ES, Winfield HN. Robotic computer-assisted pyeloplasty versus conventional laparoscopic pyeloplasty. J Endourol. 2006;20:813–819.

46. Yee DS, Shanberg AM, Duel BP, Rodriguez E, Eichel L, Rajpoot D. Initial comparison of robotic-assisted laparoscopic versus open pyeloplasty in children. Urology. 2006;4067(3):599–602.

47. Kutikov A, Nguyen M, Guzzo T, Canter D, Casale P. Robot assisted pyeloplasty in the infant-lessons learned. J Urol. 2006;176(5):2237–2239.

48. Patel V. Robotic-assisted laparoscopic dismembered pyeloplasty. Urology. 2005;66:45–49.

49. Palese MA, Stifelman MD, Munver R, Sosa RE, Philipps CK, Dinlenc C, Del Pizzo JJ. Robot-assisted laparoscopic dismembered pyeloplasty: a combined experience. J Endourol. 2005a;19:382–386.

50. Palese MA, Munver R, Phillips CK, Dinlenc C, Stifelman M, Delpizzo JJ. Robot-assisted laparoscopic dismembered pyeloplasty. JSLS. 2005b;9:252–257.

51. Atug F, Woods M, Burgess SV, Castle EP, Thomas R. Robotic assisted laparoscopic pyeloplasty in children. J Urol. 2005a;174(4 pt 1):1440–1442.

52. Atug F, Castle EP, Burgess SV, Thomas R. Concomitant management of renal calculi and pelvi-ureteric junction obstruction with robotic laparoscopic surgery. BJU Int. 2005b;96:1365–1368.

53. Atug F, Burgess SV, Castle EK, Thomas R. Role of robotics in the management of secondary ureteropelvic junction obstruction. Int J Clin Pract. 2006;60:9–11.

54. Mendez-torres F, Woods M, Thomas R. Technical modifications for robot-assisted laparoscopic pyeloplasty. J Endourol. 2005;19:393–396.

55. Bernie JE, Ramakrishna V, Brown J, Gardner TA, Sundaram CP. Comparison of laparoscopic pyeloplasty with and without robotic assistance. JSLS. 2005;9:258–261.

56. Soulie M, Thoulouzan M, Seguin P, Mouly P, Vazzoler N, Pontonnier F, Plante P. Retroperitoneoscopic laparoscopic versus open pyeloplasty with a minimal incision: comparison of two surgical approaches. Urology. 2001;57:443–447.

57. Chen RN, Moore RG, Kavoussi LR. Laparoscopic pyeloplasty indications, technique, and long term outcome. Urol Clin North Am. 1998;25:323–330.

58. Singh I, Hemal AK. Robot-assisted pyeloplasty: review of the current literature, technique and outcome. Can J Urol. 2010;17(2):5099–5108.

59. Rohrmann D, Snyder HM III, Duckett JW Jr, Canning DA, Zderic SA. The operative management of recurrent ureteropelvic junction obstruction. J Urol. 1997;158:1257–1259.

60. Sundaram CP, Grubb RL, Rehman J, Yan Y, Chen C, Landman J, McDougall EM, Clayman RV. Laparoscopic pyeloplasty for secondary ureteropelvic junction obstruction. J Urol. 2003;169:2037–2040.

61. Jarrett TW, Chan DY, Charambura TC, Fugita O, Kavoussi LR. Laparoscopic pyeloplasty: the first 100 cases. J Urol. 2002;167:1253–1256.

62. Turk IA, Davis JW, Winklemann B. Laparoscopic dismembered pyeloplasty-the method of choice in the presence of an enlarged renal pelvis and crossing vessels. Eur Urol. 2002;42:268–277.

63. Chammas M Jr, Feuillu B, Coissard A, Hubert J. Laparoscopic robotic-assisted management of pelvi-ureteric obstruction in patients with horseshoe kidneys:technique and 1-year follow-up. BJU Int. 2006;97:579–583.

64. Nayyar R, Gupta NP, Hemal AK. Robotic management of complicated ureteropelvic junction obstruction. World J Urol. 2010;28(5):599–602.

65. Leveillee RJ, Williams SK. Role of robotics for ureteral pelvic junction obstruction and ureteral pathology. Curr Opin Urol. 2009;19(1):81–88.

66. Peters CA. Robotic pyeloplasty-the new standard of care? J Urol. 2008;180(4):1223–1224.

67. Braga LH, Pace K, Demaria J, Lorenzo AJ. Systematic review and meta-analysis of robotic-assisted versus conventional laparoscopic pyeloplasty for patients with ureteropelvic junction obstruction: effect on operative time, length of hospital stay, postoperative complications, and success rate. Eur Urol. 2009;56(5):848–857.

68. Novara G. Editorial Comment on: systematic review and meta-analysis of robotic-assisted versus conventional laparoscopic pyeloplasty for patients with ureteropelvic junction obstruction: effect on operative time, length of hospital stay, postoperative complications, and success rate. Eur Urol. 2009;56(5):857–858.

69. Fornara P, Greco F. Editorial Comment on: systematic review and meta-analysis of robotic-assisted versus conventional laparoscopic pyeloplasty for patients with ureteropelvic junction obstruction: effect on operative time, length of hospital stay, postoperative complications, and success rate. Eur Urol. 2009;56(5):858.

70. Gupta NP, Nayyar R, Hemal AK, Mukherjee S, Kumar R, Dogra PN. Outcome analysis of robotic pyeloplasty: a large single-centre experience. BJU Int. 2010;105(7):980–983.

71. Desai MM, Rao PP, Pascal-Haber G, Desai MR, Mishra S, Kaouk JH, Gill IS. Scarless single port transumbilical nephrectomy and pyeloplasty: first clinical report. BJU Int. 2008;101:83–88.

72. Desai MM, Stein R, Rao P, Canes D, Aron M, Rao PP, Haber GP, Fergany A, Kaouk J, Gill IS. Embryonic natural orifice transumbilical endoscopic surgery (E-NOTES) for advanced reconstruction: initial experience. Urology. 2009;73(1):182–187.

73. Canes D, Desai MM, Aron M, Haber GP, Goel RK, Stein RJ, Kaouk JH, Gill IS. Transumbilical single port surgery: evolution and current status. Eur Urol. 2008;54:1020–1030.

74. Chammas M, Feuillu B, Coisard A, Hubert J. Laparoscopic robotic assisted management of pelvi-ureteral junction obstruction in patients with horseshoe kidneys:technique and 1 year follow up. BJU Int. 2006;97:579–583.

75. Freilich DA, Nguyen HT, Borer J, Nelson C, Passerotti CC. Concurrent management of bilateral ureteropelvic junction obstruction in children using robotic assisted laparoscopic surgery. Int Br J Urol. 2008;34(2):198–204.

76. Hemal AK, Mukherjee S, Singh K. Laparoscopic pyeloplasty versus robotic pyeloplasty for ureteropelvic junction obstruction: a series of 60 cases performed by a single surgeon. Can J Urol. 2010;17(1):5012–5016.

Chapter 41

Robotic Surgery for Urolithiasis

Rajeev Kumar and Ashok K. Hemal

The management of urolithiasis is one of the success stories of minimal invasive advancements in urology. This has been the result of improvements in technology and techniques that have included extra-corporeal lithotripters, miniaturized scopes, energy sources, and stone retrieval devices. These improvements have been reflected in the AUA guidelines for the management of urolithiasis which now recommend one or the other of these minimal invasive procedures as the first-line treatment for all varieties of stones.[1] However, open stone surgery remains one of the treatment modalities in most situations. This is due to the limitations of every minimal invasive technique and the less than perfect results possible even with combination therapies. Further, in certain situations, open stone surgery may even be the treatment modality of choice due to the poor outcomes expected with minimal invasive techniques.[1]

Robot-assisted laparoscopic surgery has become the minimal invasive modality of choice for a large number of reconstructive urology procedures where open surgery was the mainstay of management. This has been most evident in radical prostatectomy for prostate cancer and pyeloplasty for ureteropelvic junction obstruction.[2,3] In both these procedures, it has enabled precise reconstruction with all the benefits of minimal invasive surgery. The use of robotic assistance for urolithiasis is a natural extension of this combination of need for open surgery and reconstruction of the

pelvicalyceal system following stone extraction. In this chapter we review the current indications, technique, and published literature on the use of robotic surgery for the management of urolithiasis.

41.1 Indications

The common indications for robotic assistance in urolithiasis are given in Table 41.1.

41.1.1 Renal Calculi with Ureteropelvic Junction Obstruction

The most common indication for the use of robotic surgery in the management of urolithiasis is in patients with a concomitant ureteropelvic junction obstruction (UPJO). Ideal management of such patients requires a simultaneous stone removal and repair of the obstructed UPJ. Endoscopic treatments have less than optimal results in these cases. In a recent review, Eden concluded that the results of balloon dilatation and endopyelotomy techniques for the management of UPJO are about 15–20% inferior to open surgery while those of laparoscopic or robotic surgery match the open surgery outcomes.[4] The poor results of endopyelotomy have led to the search for alternative methods for management of renal stones in kidneys with a UPJO.

Agarwal et al.[5] recently described a combination of percutaneous nephrolithotomy (PCNL) and laparoscopic pyeloplasty for these cases. Two of their patients had failed a previous endopyelotomy.

R. Kumar (✉)
Department of Urology, All India Institute of Medical Sciences, New Delhi, India
e-mail: rajeev02@gmail.com

A.K. Hemal, M. Menon (eds.), *Robotics in Genitourinary Surgery*,
DOI 10.1007/978-1-84882-114-9_41, © Springer-Verlag London Limited 2011

Table 41.1 Indications for robotic assistance in urolithiasis surgery

Category	Procedure	Indication
Reconstructive procedures with stone removal	Pyeloplasty with pyelolithotomy	UPJ obstruction with secondary stone
	Ureteric reimplantation with stone extraction	Megaureter with stones
	Ureteropyelostomy with pyelolithotomy	Duplex PCS with UPJ obstruction in lower moiety with secondary stone
Stone-related features	Extended pyelolithotomy	Large stone/partial staghorn
	Ureterolithotomy	Impacted large ureteric stone
Kidney-related features	Pyelolithotomy	Ectopic kidney
	Nephrectomy/partial nephrectomy	Non-functioning kidney
	Nephrolithotomy	Stone in renal diverticulum
Patient-related features	Pyelolithotomy, extended pyelolithotomy	Pediatric patient

While they managed to execute both procedures simultaneously in 8 of their 10 patients, they needed to change positions between stone removal and pyeloplasty and had significant operative times. Shrivastava et al.[6] described their experience of combined laparoscopic pyelolithotomy and pyeloplasty in a cohort of 20 patients. They achieved complete stone clearance in 75% patients with the remaining achieving clearance with the aid of ancillary procedures. Nambirajan et al.[7] described a wide range of laparoscopic procedures in the management of renal calculi. Their series of 18 cases included patients who required a simultaneous pyeloplasty, partial nephrectomy, or extraction of stones in a diverticulum. Other authors have reported similarly good success rates using laparoscopy for the simultaneous management of renal calculi and ureteropelvic junction obstruction.[8,9]

Robotic assistance has proven to be of significant advantage in the management of UPJO.[3] It naturally follows that it may also be beneficial in the management of concurrent UPJO and stones. Atug et al.[10] reported the first series of eight cases undergoing simultaneous robotic pyeloplasty and pyelolithotomy. All cases had a retrograde catheter placed in the renal pelvis over a guide wire and this was used for the subsequent placement of a ureteric stent at the end of the procedure. Stone localization was achieved using a flexible nephroscope and all stones were retrieved intact without fragmentation. Stone extraction resulted in a mean prolongation of the surgery by 1 h. They achieved 100% stone clearance with no significant immediate or long-term complications at a mean follow-up of over 1 year.

41.1.2 Large/Staghorn Renal Calculi

Large renal calculi can be managed well using PCNL. A number of these stones are composed of calcium compounds, making them relatively hard. The bulk of the stones as well as their composition can often result in significantly long operative times with the possibility of residual calculi. Over a third of patients with large staghorn stones or with grossly dilated systems may have residual calculi following PCNL.[11] The large bulk may also preclude complete clearance in one session and require additional sessions of PCNL or ancillary procedures. A single open/laparoscopic/robotic procedure may allow the removal of an intact stone without fragmentation, thus minimizing the possibility of residual fragments and the need for extended or multiple procedures in these cases.[12] Badani et al.[13] described the use of robotic surgery in the management of patients with large partial or complete staghorn calculi. In 13 patients who underwent robotic extended pyelolithotomy, 12 had complete clearance while 1 patient with a complete staghorn had residual calculi. The authors concluded that robotic extended pyelolithotomy offered a useful one-time minimally invasive option for the management of patients with partial staghorn calculi.

41.1.3 Pediatric Renal Calculi

Renal calculi in children continue to pose a management dilemma. Despite the miniaturization of nephroscopes, it is often difficult to obtain satisfactory percutaneous renal access and complete clearance. Children require general anesthesia for most surgical procedures and also for extra-corporeal shock wave lithotripsy (ESWL). This makes it imperative that a procedure offering maximum possibility of a one-time clearance be chosen for the management of their calculi. In cases where open surgery would be considered a reasonable option to obtain these goals, laparoscopy or robotic assistance presents a feasible minimally invasive alternative.

Casale et al.[14] presented their experience of laparoscopic pyelolithotomy in eight children. The indication included failed percutaneous access, failed ESWL, and stone burden greater than 2.5 cm.[2] They were able to successfully remove the calculi in all eight children and all were rendered pain free.

The benefits seen on pure laparoscopy have been duplicated with robotic assistance. Lee et al.[15] reported their results in five children who underwent robotic-assisted pyelolithotomy and highlight the advantages of this procedure. Four of their five patients had a cystine staghorn calculus and all four had failed previous minimally invasive procedures (PCNL/ESWL). The fifth patient had a concomitant UPJ obstruction and was thus ideally suited for this procedure. The authors were successful in removing the stones in four of the five children and failed in one due to the inability of their electrohydraulic lithotripter to break the cystine stone. One patient had a residual calculus that required a subsequent ESWL.

41.1.4 Ectopic Kidneys

Stones in ectopic kidney are often difficult to access percutaneously. This is particularly true for kidneys located in the pelvis or close to the midline where a posterior access is not feasible. These kidneys per se are predisposed to stone formation and have poorer clearance rates following ESWL when compared with normally placed kidneys.[16] Such ectopic kidneys are generally malrotated with the pelvis pointing anteriorly. A transperitoneal laparoscopic/robotic approach affords direct access to these pelvises, making pyelolithotomy a relatively straightforward procedure.

41.1.5 Stones in Renal Diverticula

Stones located in renal diverticula are often small but respond poorly to ESWL. The narrow neck of the diverticulum makes clearance unlikely and PCNL with ablation of the lining of the diverticulum is often considered a more efficacious procedure.[17] In the upper pole, these diverticula are often located in the anterior renal cortex and this location makes a percutaneous access difficult and fraught with potential complications. Laparoscopy with the use of intraoperative ultrasound guidance allows a direct access to these diverticular stones with the possibility of thermal ablation of the diverticular cavity. Nambirajan et al.[4] described their successful use of laparoscopy in the management of such cases.

41.1.6 Calculi with Associated Anomalies

Apart from the ureteropelvic junction, another common site of obstruction in the urinary system which may be associated with calculi is the ureterovesical junction. Congenital megaureters with calculi require simultaneous stone removal and ureteric reimplant with or without tailoring of the redundant ureter. These patients form another indication for the use of robotic surgery.[18]

41.1.7 Non-functioning Segments/ Kidneys

Long-standing/impacted calculi may result in a nonfunctioning segment of the kidney or at times make the entire renal unit non-functional. If a decision is taken to perform a partial or complete nephrectomy, robotic assistance offers a minimal invasive option to open surgery. This is particularly true for partial nephrectomy where robotic assistance enhances the ability to perform closure of the opened pelvicalyceal system and renal parenchyma. The advantage of laparoscopy in such circumstances has been previously demonstrated.[4]

41.2 Operative Setup

41.2.1 Retrograde Catheter Placement

Pre-placement of an open-ended ureteric access catheter is an optional step practiced at a number of centers. In all cases except those where a nephrectomy is being planned, the patient is placed in a lithotomy position for the insertion of the ureteric catheter into the renal pelvis. A Foley's type catheter is placed in the bladder and the ureteric catheter is secured to this bladder catheter using a suture. Both catheters are kept within the sterile surgical field for intraoperative access. The bladder catheter is kept on continuous drainage.

The ureteric catheter aids in identification of the ureter and pelvis and may be useful during the placement of a ureteric stent. In case the ureteric access catheter is being placed, we do not recommend the placement of a ureteric stent at this stage of the procedure since this hinders stone extraction and the stent may get displaced during stone removal.

Our practice, however, is to proceed without this initial step. We place a Foley catheter into the bladder and clamp the outflow. This allows the bladder to distend with urine. When the JJ ureteric stent is placed intraoperatively, reflux of urine from the lower end of the stent as it enters the urine-filled bladder confirms correct positioning.

41.2.2 Patient Positioning

The patient position varies with the location of the kidney of interest. The following description will be for the more common normally located kidneys. The patient is placed in a 60° lateral decubitus position with the ipsilateral side up. The lower leg is flexed while the upper leg is kept extended. The kidney bridge is not raised. The upper shoulder is kept at 90° to the torso and the elbow flexed into a neutral position. All pressure points are padded with particular care being taken at the axilla and elbow.

The robot is docked over the back of the patient and is parked almost perpendicular to the table at the level of the umbilicus. Two monitors are used for the assistants, one cranial and one caudal to the surgical

cart on the same side as the cart. The assistant stands on the side opposite to the docked robot, in a position similar to that used during robotic pyeloplasty and is described in another chapter. The anesthesiology equipment remains at the head of the patient. In patients with a pelvic kidney, the patient position mimics that used during a radical prostatectomy with a Trendelenburg tilt of only about 30°. In all cases, an orogastric or nasogastric tube is placed at the beginning of the procedure to empty the stomach and to minimize chances of injury. This tube can be removed at the end of the procedure.

41.2.3 Trocar Configuration

Trocar placement is almost similar to that for a robotic pyeloplasty except for the assistant port which should be 12 mm for stone retrieval or insertion of an Endocatch® device. Pneumoperitoneum is created using a Veress® needle at the junction of the lateral and middle thirds of the line joining the anterior superior iliac spine and the umbilicus. This point is subsequently used for an 8 mm trocar for one of the robotic arms.

After the pneumoperitoneum has been created, the primary 12 mm camera port is placed lateral to the umbilicus. One robotic arm trocar is placed at the site of the Veress® needle insertion while another is placed lateral to the rectus cranial to the umbilicus. The assistant's port is 12 mm in size and is usually sited in the midline periumbilically or on the contralateral side. For right-sided surgeries, an additional liver retraction 5 mm port may be needed in the angle between the rib-cage and the xiphoid process.

While using a four-arm robot, certain tricks aid in avoiding robotic arm collision and optimizing port placements. The patient is maintained in a 60–75° decubitus position and the operating table is lowered to its minimum height. The inferior flexion of the table is maximized to open up the operating space and the fourth arm port is inserted laterally in the lower quadrant. Further, while using the four-arm setup, the camera arm setup joint must be maneuvered to the side opposite the fourth arm.

For pelvic kidneys, the trocar placement for the robotic arms and the camera are similar to those for a radical prostatectomy. The assistant's port is placed on the right side, 2 cm above, and medial to the anterior superior iliac spine.

41.2.4 Instrumentation List

The basic instruments required for this surgery are given in Table 41.2 below.

Additional instrumentation is required for the stone retrieval. This consists of

1. Flexible nephroscopes
2. Stone removal forceps and Nitinol N® baskets
3. Intracorporeal lithotripter
4. Nephroscopy vision cart
5. C-arm fluoroscope
6. Laparoscopic ultrasound probe

41.2.5 Step-by-Step Technique: Pyelolithotomy/Pyeloplasty

Step # 1: Kidney Exposure: Colon Mobilization

0 or 30° down lens
Right arm: Hook electrocautery/monopolar scissors
Left arm: Maryland grasper
4th arm (if used): Prograsp® forceps

The colon is mobilized by making an incision along the line of Toldt. The incision is carried from the cranial-most attachment down to the level of the pelvic brim to allow a generous mobilization and minimize the possibility of an inadvertent injury. This incision can be made using either the hook electrocautery or the monopolar scissors.

41.2.5.1 Trans-mesocolic Approach

For patients with left-sided surgery and a thin mesentery, a trans-mesocolic approach may also be attempted by creating a window through the mesocolon overlying the pelvis. However, this is recommended only if the stone retrieval is anticipated to be simple since the limited exposure does not allow extensive manipulation within the kidney.

Step #2: Pelvis Exposure, Retraction, and Pyelotomy

30° lens
Right arm: Monopolar scissors
Left arm: Maryland grasper

The pelvis can be identified by either following the ureter up to the point of its insertion or the gonadal vein cranially. If a ureteric catheter has been pre-placed, it may also be used to identify the ureter/pelvis. At times, in cases with previously scarred tissue, pelvis identification may be aided by distending it with saline or a colored dye through the ureteric catheter. Another alternative is to administer 20 mg of furosemide intravenously. This distends the pelvis with urine making it easier to identify. Once the pelvis is identified, it is carefully mobilized on all sides using a combination of blunt and sharp dissection. The lower pole of the kidney may also need to be mobilized. During mobilization of the upper anterior surface of the pelvis, care must be taken not to injure the renal vessels that lie in close proximity. Complete pelvis mobilization aids in subsequent lithotomy and also allows identification of any aberrant vasculature that may need to be treated, particularly in cases with a simultaneous UPJO. The posterior surface of the pelvis needs special mobilization right up to the sinus since an extension of the pyelotomy may be required in cases with large calculi.

The pyelotomy is made using the scissors – without electrocautery – on the posterior surface of the pelvis is a manner similar to that made in an open pyelotomy. The ends of the "smile" incision point toward the upper and lower calyx, respectively, with the curve of the smile facing the UPJ. This minimizes the risk of

Surgeon		Assistant
Right arm	**Left arm**	1. Suction irrigator
1. Hot shears (monopolar curved scissors)	1. Maryland bipolar forceps	2. Blunt tip grasper
2. Needle driver	2. Large needle driver	3. Needle driver
3. Permanent cautery hook		4. Laparoscopic scissors

Table 41.2 Instrumentation required

an uretropelvic avulsion and permits extension of the incision into the calyx for an extended pyelolithotomy if required.

Step #3: Stone Extraction

30° lens
Right arm: Maryland grasper
Left arm: Prograsp® forceps/Large needle driver
Assistant: Flexible/rigid nephroscope, stone graspers, stone basket

If the stone lies in the renal pelvis, the simplest method of removal is to grasp it directly with the robotic Maryland® bipolar forceps. In order to avoid using an extra instrument, the Maryland® bipolar forceps previously used in the left arm can be moved to the right arm and a needle driver can be used in the left arm to hold down the posterior lip of the opened pelvis and expose its interior. The anterior lip of the pelvis is held up by the previously placed hitch stitch. Once the stone is visible, it can be brought out by the right arm grasper. At times, the assistant may be able to use a sturdier laparoscopic stone grasper to remove the stone.

If the stones lie in the calyces and are not readily visible in the pelvis, a flexible nephroscope needs to be used. It is helpful if the assistant is facile in the use of these instruments. Otherwise the console surgeon will need to scrub and do the patient side manipulation. Another assistant will then be required to handle the console since both the robotic arms and the flexible nephroscope may require simultaneous manipulation. The most common technique of using the nephroscope is through the cranial robotic port after de-docking the robotic arm from this port. This port generally allows the most direct access into the pelvis. Inserting the nephroscope through the rubber seal of the port helps maintain the pneumoperitoneum and simultaneous robotic vision and assistance with the caudal robotic instrument can be achieved. The assistant may have to provide continuous suction of the nephroscope irrigation fluid through his port. The pyelotomy is kept open using the hitch stitch anteriorly and the instrument in the caudal robotic arm posteriorly. The nephroscope is gently advanced into the pelvis under direct visual guidance of the robotic camera. Once inside the pelvis, vision is obtained through the nephroscope camera itself and all the calyces can generally be inspected. Small stones may be retrieved intact using nephroscopic graspers or stone baskets. Larger stones may need intracorporeal fragmentation using any of the available energy sources. Pneumatic lithotripters, electrohydraulic generators, and the holmium laser have all been used without complications in these cases.

If a flexible nephroscope is not available, a rigid nephroscope may also be used in a similar fashion. However, this has limited intrarenal maneuverability and may be associated with a greater risk of bleeding from trauma during manipulation.

Small stones may be removed intact through the nephroscope or through the 12 mm assistant port. For larger stones, a specimen bag is used to keep the stones secure inside the abdomen till the end of the procedure. Intraoperative fluoroscopy is generally difficult due to the presence of the robotic cart. It is therefore advisable to have an exact count and localization of the stones before beginning surgery. If there are serious doubts about residual calculi, intraoperative laparoscopic ultrasound probes may be used to localize the stone without removing the robot. In desperate situations, the robot may need to be de-docked to allow fluoroscopy and then re-docked to complete the procedure.

Once the stones have been removed, the pelvicalyceal system is flushed with saline to wash out any gravel or debris. If the cranial robotic arm had been de-docked for nephroscopy, it is re-docked and the needle driver is moved to the right arm while the Maryland® grasper is returned to the left arm.

We prefer to place the JJ ureteric stent in an antegrade fashion by inserting a flexible guide wire through the cranial assistant port and threading the stent over it. An alternative technique is to place the guide wire through a 16Fr Venflon® directly pierced through the abdominal wall in line with the pelvis and the ureter.[19] Another option is to retain the ureteric access catheter instead of the stent and remove it in the postoperative period. However, this is fairly uncomfortable for the patient and is the least favored approach.

Step #4: Pyeloplasty/Pyelotomy Closure

30° lens
Right arm: Needle driver
Left arm: Maryland grasper/Needle driver

If a pyeloplasty is required, it is performed after the stone retrieval has been completed. The technique of pyeloplasty has been described elsewhere in this book and is similar for these cases. In case a pyeloplasty is not required, the pyelotomy is carefully closed using running or interrupted 5–0 Monocryl® or Vicryl® sutures. In children, 6–0 Poliglecaprone sutures on small needles may provide more precise approximation. The hitch stitch, if placed, is released and the pelvis may be wrapped in the peri-renal fat to minimize scarring/adhesions. A drain may be left by placing it through either the caudal robotic port or through a caudal assistant port. In case the stones are still within the abdomen, they are removed with the bag through the 12 mm assistant port. The robotic instruments are removed under vision and the abdomen desufflated completely. The port sites are closed.

Step #5: Postoperative Care

Postoperative care is similar to that for an open pyelolithotomy/pyeloplasty. The patient may be mobilized and allowed oral intake the same evening. In case the anastomosis/pyelotomy closure was deemed to be perfect and there is minimal drainage, the bladder catheter can be removed on day 1 following surgery and the drain may be removed the next day.

41.2.6 Step-by-Step Technique: Diverticular Stones

Step # 1: Kidney Exposure: Colon Mobilization

0° lens
Right arm: Hook electrocautery/Monopolar scissors
Left arm: Maryland grasper

The initial steps are similar to those previously described for a pyelolithotomy. However, the renal mobilization needs to be more extensive, particularly over the area of the diverticulum. Peri-renal fat and fat within the Gerota's fascia is completely removed in order to identify the diverticulum.

Step #2: Stone Localization and Removal

0° lens
Right arm: Hook electrocautery/Monopolar scissors
Left arm: Maryland grasper
Assistant: Laparoscopic ultrasound probe

Renal parenchyma is generally thinned out or scarred in the region overlying the diverticulum. It may also form a visible bulge on the renal surface. The laparoscopic ultrasound probe aids in its identification in difficult cases. Once the diverticulum is identified, a radial incision is made in the parenchyma overlying it using the hook electrocautery or the monopolar scissors. The incision is deepened to enter the diverticulum and visualize the stone. Once the stone is seen, it is held in the Maryland® grasper or by the assistant and removed. These stones are generally small and may be removed intact. The diverticular cavity can now be inspected and its lining fulgurated with the electrocautery hook. Peri-renal fat may also be placed within the marsupialized cavity.

41.2.7 Step-by-Step Technique: Partial/Simple Nephrectomy

The procedure for a partial or simple nephrectomy is similar to that described elsewhere in this book for other indications. For a partial nephrectomy, a laparoscopic ultrasound probe is useful in identifying the exact location of the stones to plan the incision.

41.3 Specific Situation: Pelvic Kidney

When a pyelolithotomy is being performed for stones in an ectopic/pelvic kidney, the operative steps have to be modified. These kidneys have aberrant vasculature and mobilization as for an orthotopic kidney cannot be performed. The kidney is often seen as a bulge behind the lower mesentery of the bowel. The bowel is mobilized off the anterior surface of the kidney. The pelvis is usually anteriorly located, right below the mesentery. Renal mobilization is difficult and unnecessary. The renal pelvis can be identified either by distending it with saline through the pre-placed ureteric catheter or

Table 41.3 Tips and tricks

Problem	Solution
Vascular or organ injury	Appropriate site selection for Veress® needle insertion
	Incision in skin/sheath wide enough to allow easy port insertion
	All secondary ports inserted under direct vision
	Confirm insulation of all cautery instruments
Emphysema	Ensure entry into peritoneum before insufflation
	Seal all port sites, avoid excessively large incisions
Difficulty identifying pelvis	Consider pre-placed ureteric catheter in initial cases
	Administer furosemide intravenously
Port crowding	Maintain 60° decubitus
	Inferior flex the operating table
	Place fourth port laterally and lower
Robotic arm clashing	Move the setup joint of camera port to the head end
Nephroscope unable to reach all calyces	Remove robotic instruments and desufflate the abdomen
Stone too large to grasp	Intracorporeal lithotripsy
Lost stones	Use of Endocatch® device to place stones
Incomplete stone retrieval	Laparoscopic ultrasound

by using a laparoscopic ultrasound probe. It is important to be aware of the aberrant renal vasculature that may course anterior to the pelvis. Once the pelvis is identified, a direct pyelotomy is made after placing the hitch stitch, usually caudal to the site of the incision. The remaining procedure is similar to that previously described.

41.4 Avoiding Complications

Four specific complications that should be avoided during robotic stone surgery are injury to the renal vessels, ureteropelvic junction avulsion, failure to localize the stones, and inability to extract the stones. Certain tips to optimize the outcome are given in Table 41.3.

Vessel injury: Robotic surgery for stones is performed transperitoneally due to the limited space available in the retroperitoneal approach. The transperitoneal approach means that the pelvis is the most posterior structure at the hilum and renal vessels are encountered during pelvis mobilization. The craniomedial and anterior dissection of the pelvis should be performed carefully to avoid vascular injury. It is usually not necessary to mobilize the vessels off the anterior pelvis wall since the major mobilization and pyelotomy are made on the posterior surface. Mobilization of the lower pole of the kidney improves visibility on the posterior surface of the pelvis, further minimizing the need for extensive dissection on the anterior surface.

Ureteropelvic junction avulsion: This usually occurs due to an incorrectly placed pyelotomy and an attempt to remove large stones through a limited pyelotomy. The principles of open surgery need to be rigorously followed. The ends of the pyelotomy should point toward the calyces and a generous lip of the pelvis must remain between the incision and the UPJ. Intracorporeal stone fragmentation should be performed for large stones to avoid tears during extraction.

Failure to localize the stones may occur particularly in patients with multiple calculi or after fragmentation. Intraoperative fluoroscopy is difficult in the presence of the surgical cart. Pre-operative careful assessment of the radiographic images and visual correlation of the extracted stones with the images will help minimize these problems. The availability of laparoscopic ultrasound probes would also help decrease the incidence of residual calculi.

Inability to extract the stones would result from their loss within the peritoneal cavity. This complication is easily avoided by placing all extracted stones within a specimen bag before retrieval.

41.5 Conclusions

Robotic surgery for urolithiasis is technically feasible and efficacious in specific situations. It allows the advantages on open surgery in conjunction with a minimally invasive approach.

References

1. Preminger GM, Assimos DG, Lingeman JE, Nakada SY, Pearle MS, Wolf JS Jr. AUA nephrolithiasis guideline panel. Chapter 1: AUA guideline on management of staghorn calculi: diagnosis and treatment recommendations. *J Urol.* 2005;173:1991–2000.

2. Tewari AK, Jhaveri JK, Surasi K, Patel N, Tan GY. Benefit of robotic assistance in comparing outcomes of minimally invasive versus open radical prostatectomy. *J Clin Oncol.* 2008;26:4999–5000.

3. Schwentner C, Pelzer A, Neururer R, et al. Robotic anderson-hynes pyeloplasty: 5-year experience of one centre. *Bju Int.* 2007;100:880–885.

4. Eden CG. Minimally invasive treatment of ureteropelvic junction obstruction: a critical analysis of results. *Eur Urol.* 2007;52:983–989.

5. Agarwal A, Varshney A, Bansal BS. Concomitant percutaneous nephrolithotomy and transperitoneal laparoscopic pyeloplasty for ureteropelvic junction obstruction complicated by stones. *J Endourol.* 2008;22: 2251–2255.

6. Srivastava A, Singh P, Gupta M, Ansari MS, Mandhani A, Kapoor R, et al. Laparoscopic pyeloplasty with concomitant pyelolithotomy – is it an effective mode of treatment? *Urol Int.* 2008;80:306–309.

7. Nambirajan T, Jeschke S, Albqami N, Abukora F, Leeb K, Janetschek G. Role of laparoscopy in management of renal stones: single-center experience and review of literature. *J Endourol.* 2005;19:353–359.

8. Ball AJ, Leveillee RJ, Patel VR, Wong C. Laparoscopic pyeloplasty and flexible nephroscopy: simultaneous treatment of ureteropelvic junction obstruction and nephrolithiasis. *JSLS.* 2004;8:223–228.

9. Ramakumar S, Lancini V, Chan DY, Parsons JK, Kavoussi LR, Jarrett TW. Laparoscopic pyeloplasty with concomitant pyelolithotomy. *J Urol.* 2002;167:1378–1380.

10. Atug F, Castle EP, Burgess SV, Thomas R. Concomitant management of renal calculi and pelvi-ureteric junction obstruction with robotic laparoscopic surgery. *Bju Int.* 2005;96:1365–1368.

11. Lam HS, Lingeman JE, Barron M, Newman DM, Mosbaugh PG, Steele RE, et al. Staghorn calculi: analysis of treatment results between initial percutaneous nephrostolithotomy and extracorporeal shock wave lithotripsy monotherapy with reference to surface area. *J Urol.* 1992;147:1219.

12. Nayyar R, Wadhwa P, Hemal AK. Pure robotic extended pyelolithotomy: cosmetic replica of open surgery. *J Robot Surg.* 2007;1:207.

13. Badani KK, Hemal AK, Fumo M, Kaul S, Shrivastava A, Rajendram AK, et al. Robotic extended pyelolithotomy for treatment of renal calculi: a feasibility study. *World J Urol.* 2006;24:198–201.

14. Casale P, Grady RW, Joyner BD, Zeltser IS, Kuo RL, Mitchell ME. Transperitoneal laparoscopic pyelolithotomy after failed percutaneous access in the pediatric patient. *J Urol.* 2004;172:680–683.

15. Lee RS, Passerotti CC, Cendron M, Estrada CR, Borer JG, Peters CA. Early results of robot assisted laparoscopic lithotomy in adolescents. *J Urol.* 2007;177:2306–2309.

16. Sheir KZ, Madbouly K, Elsobky E, Abdelkhalek M. Extracorporeal shock wave lithotripsy in anomalous kidneys: 11-year experience with two second-generation lithotripters. *Urology.* 2003;62:10–15.

17. Gross AJ, Herrmann TR. Management of stones in calyceal diverticulum. *Curr Opin Urol.* 2007;17:136–140.

18. Hemal AK, Nayyar R, Rao R. Robotic repair of primary symptomatic obstructive megaureter with intracorporeal or extracorporeal ureteric tapering and ureteroneocystostomy. *J Endourol.* 2009;23:2041–2046.

19. Kumar R, Yadav R, Kolla SB. Simultaneous bilateral robot-assisted dismembered pyeloplasties for bilateral ureteropelvic junction obstruction: technique and literature review. *J Endourol.* 2007;21:750–753.

Chapter 42

Ureteral Reconstruction Utilizing Robotic-Assisted Techniques

Patrick Mufarrij, Elias Hyams, and Michael Stifelman

42.1 Introduction

The role of robotics in urology has expanded dramatically over the last decade. This technology is especially useful for upper tract urinary reconstruction, which often necessitates intricate surgical manipulation. Advantages of robotic systems allow surgical maneuvers to be performed with extreme control and visualization, while still adhering to the basic tenets of open surgical technique, without the same morbidity.

This chapter reviews robotic surgical techniques for ureteral reconstruction. Herein, ureterolysis with omental wrapping, ureteroureterostomy, ureterocalicostomy, and ureteral reimplantation are described.

42.2 Preoperative Assessment

Crucial to the planning of ureteral reconstruction is appropriate imaging to elucidate the disease process. Three-phase computed tomography scans or magnetic resonance urograms are excellent in this regard. Diuretic nuclear renography is also utilized to document baseline renal function and confirm obstruction. Retrograde ureterography or ureteroscopy can also provide further anatomic information.

Patients receive a thorough informed consent regarding all possible options of ureteral reconstruction, as well as the need for long-term follow-up

and the possibility of disease recurrence, necessitating further interventions.

42.3 Operative Setup

For mid- to upper ureteral reconstructions, patients are positioned in a semi-lateral decubitus position with or without a modified low lithotomy in case access to the bladder is desired. We obtain peritoneal access for the camera trocars via a direct-vision, Hasson technique. Trocar configuration consists of the 12 mm origin trocar above the umbilicus and two 8 mm robotic trocars 2–4 cm lateral and 8–10 cm away from the origin in either direction. These three trocars create a "V"-shaped configuration. The fourth robotic 8 mm trocar is placed in the lower quadrant 2 cm above pubic bone in the mid-clavicular line. The 10 mm assistant trocar is placed just caudal to the umbilicus, midway between two of the robotic trocars. The robot surgical system is anchored at a 90° angle to the operating table, lining up the center beam of the robot with the camera trocar.

For lower ureteral reconstructions, such as reimplantation or distal ureteral reconstruction, patients are positioned in low lithotomy with steep Trendelenburg, similar to robotic prostatectomy positioning. Trocars are configured with a 12 mm origin trocar at the umbilicus and two robotic 8 mm trocars to the left, one just lateral to the umbilicus in the mid-clavicular line and the other one, 2 cm superior to umbilicus in the anterior axillary line. To the right of the umbilicus we place the fourth 8 mm trocar lateral to umbilicus in mid-clavicular line. The 10 mm assistant port is placed above and between the fourth robotic trocar and the

M. Stifelman (✉)
Langone Medical Center, New York University, New York, NY, USA
e-mail: michaelstifelman@nyumc.org

A.K. Hemal, M. Menon (eds.), *Robotics in Genitourinary Surgery*,
DOI 10.1007/978-1-84882-114-9_42, © Springer-Verlag London Limited 2011

12 mm origin port. The da Vinci robotic system is then anchored between the patient's legs.

For all procedures, once hemostasis is achieved and confirmed, all trocars are removed under laparoscopic or direct vision. The 8 and 5 mm trocars generally do not require fascial closure but are simply closed subcutaneously. The fascia of the 10 mm assistant trocar and the 12 mm origin trocar are closed with absorbable suture.

42.4 Robotic Ureterolysis

Exposing as much of the ureter as possible is paramount during these cases. This is accomplished by releasing the colon medially and, if operating on the right ureter, by also Kocherizing the duodenum. Rotating the table to maximize gravitational forces also helps with this exposure. The console surgeon typically uses the Gyrus PK bipolar graspers (ACMI/Olympus, Southborough, MA) in the left hand and the curved robotic scissors in the right. The assistant provides exposure with a suction/irrigator and helps to switch robotic instruments and place clips when necessary. After exposing the retroperitoneum, we locate structures such as the iliac vessels, gonadal vessels, and the lower pole of the kidney to help uncover the ureter. In areas of extreme disease, Doppler ultrasonography can help to distinguish the ureter from vascular structures.

Once identified, the healthy portions of the ureter are isolated with vessel loops and placed on traction to aid in the ureterolysis of the diseased ureteral segment. Frozen sections of the diseased tissue are routinely sent prior to proceeding with the ureterolysis to rule out malignancy. The diseased ureteral segment is dissected free by splitting the fibrous capsule anteriorly to reveal the ureteral adventitia. For this, the console surgeon may employ the robotic Potts scissors (Intuitive Surgical, Sunnyvale, CA). The remaining ureter is circumferentially released from disease using a combination of blunt and sharp dissection, avoiding the use of electrocautery to preserve the tenuous blood supply of the ureter.

After completing the ureterolysis, attention is directed to the omental wrapping. The console surgeon uses Gyrus PK bipolar graspers in the left hand and Prograsp graspers (Intuitive Surgical, Sunnyvale,

CA) in the right to isolate and harvest the omental flap. The distal portion of the pedicle is brought underneath the ureter and secured to the sidewall with clips or 2.0 absorbable suture. The lateral omental pedicle is then secured to the sidewall, allowing the entire omental flap to lay posterior to the ureter. The medial edge of the omentum is now wrapped anterior to the ureter and also secured to the sidewall. Finally, a surgical drain is placed near the omental wrap.

As the literature demonstrates, robotic techniques can be successfully applied to ureterolysis. Although laparoscopic ureterolysis can also be safely performed with comparable success rates to open surgery, a high rate of open conversion exist (17%).[1] Stifelman et al.[2] reported on five patients who underwent robotic ureterolysis (RU). Every patient demonstrated symptomatic and radiographic resolution of obstruction at a mean follow-up of 5.4 months. In the same report, five patients underwent laparoscopic ureterolysis (LU). Four of the five patients had symptomatic resolution, and two of nine renal units among these laparoscopic patients required stenting for recurrent obstruction. There were no intraoperative complications in either group, and no postoperative complications among RU patients. One patient undergoing LU, however, developed a perioperative ureteral urine leak, managed with prolonged Foley catheter drainage and stenting. Clearly, higher volume experiences and comparisons with open ureterolysis are necessary for definitive evaluation of RU.

42.5 Ureterocalicostomy

As was described for ureterolysis, exposure and isolation of the ureter are accomplished with a combination of sharp and blunt dissection. Dissection, avoiding cautery as much as possible, is continued up to the area of ureteral stricture, at which point the ureter is transected below the level of disease using Potts scissors. The healthy ureter is then spatulated laterally to prepare it for the anastomosis with the lower pole calyx.

Next, the renal hilum is isolated by identifying the psoas muscle, elevating the posterior surface of the kidney off this muscle, and then using a combination of dissection and the Doppler probe to examine the renal hilum, which is on stretch. The renal artery and vein are then dissected free and isolated. The most dependent lower pole calyx of the kidney is then identified using a laparoscopic Doppler ultrasound probe. In preparation for the resection of the renal lower pole to expose the calyx for anastomosis, Gerota's fascia is cleared off this segment of kidney circumferentially. Prior to clamping the renal artery, patients are appropriately volume resuscitated and given 12.5 g of mannitol.

The assistant surgeon then separately clamps the renal artery and vein using laparoscopic vascular bulldog clamps, while the console surgeon sharply transects the renal lower pole, using endoshears, to expose the calyx. Hemostasis is by suture ligating open vessels with 3-0 polyglactin sutures and by cauterizing the renal cortex with the Tissuelink device (Tissuelink, Dover, NH). After hemostasis is accomplished, bulldog clamps are removed, and another dose of 12.5 g of mannitol is administered. Areas of new bleeding are controlled. If necessary, a flexible nephroscope can be introduced through the assistant port to basket any stones in the collecting system using a 1.9 Fr tipless Nitinol basket (Boston Scientific, Natick, MA).

The anastomosis of the newly spatulated proximal healthy ureter to the isolated lower pole calyx is then performed using interrupted 4-0 polyglactin sutures. A tension-free anastomosis, with efficient apposition of ureteral and calyx urothelium, is essential to success of this reconstruction. To that end, a psoas hitch or nephropexy can be performed to reduce any possible anastomotic tension. Before completing the anastomosis, a stent is passed antegrade or retrograde, under laparoscopic vision, over a wire, such that the stent curls in the bladder and in the collecting system. The remaining proximal ureteral stump is ligated with 2-0 absorbable suture. The completed anastomosis is then covered with a vascularized pedicle of Gerota's fascia to promote healing, to add blood supply, and to protect from urine extravasation. Lastly, a self-suction drain is placed near the reconstruction.

Robotic-assisted laparoscopic ureterocalicostomy has been reported in the literature by Korets et al.[3] for a patient with a small intrarenal pelvis and 1.5 cm proximal ureteral stricture. The ureter was dissected free and spatulated for anastomosis as described above. Then, the lower pole was transected after clamping the renal artery. As this patient had renal stones, flexible nephroscopy was performed to basket them prior to completing the robotic anastomosis. There were no complications, and intravenous urography at 1 year postoperatively demonstrated no evidence of obstruction. The authors assessed that robotic assistance significantly facilitated intracorporeal suturing, which had been a reported limitation in previous feasibility studies of laparoscopic ureterocalicostomy.[4,5]

42.6 Ureteroureterostomy

With the patient positioned in semi-lateral decubitus with modified low lithotomy, retrograde pyelography can be performed to delineate the area of obstruction.

As described above, the ureter is isolated and exposed using a combination of sharp and blunt dissection, while avoiding thermal energy as much as possible. For cases of ureteral stricture, the diseased portion of the ureter is excised with Potts scissors. In obstruction from a retrocaval ureter, the ureter proximal and distal to the obstruction is transected, leaving the retrocaval segment in situ. Alternatively, if the retrocaval portion of the ureter can be easily removed from under the vena cava, the ureter distal to the retrocaval portion can be transected while the proximal ureter is gently retracted to liberate the retrocaval portion.

The anastomosis is prepared by spatulating the distal ureter medially and the proximal ureter laterally. A "handle" of diseased or redundant ureteral tissue can be used to manipulate the ureter without having to directly grasp the healthy ureteral tissue to be used for the anastomosis. This "handle" can be excised just prior to completing the anastomosis. Once again, a tension-free anastomosis is critical and various techniques, as described above, can be employed to prevent undue strain on the reconstruction. For the anastomosis, we use a dyed and an undyed 4-0 polyglactin suture. The dyed suture is secured laterally and the undyed suture is anchored medially. We perform the posterior wall anastomosis first by passing the medial undyed suture beneath the ureter to rotate the ureter 180° and display the posterior wall anteriorly. Next, the undyed suture is run along the posterior wall and tied to the dyed suture. The undyed suture is then passed back below the ureter, restoring the anatomical position and presenting the anterior wall. A stent is passed under laparoscopic visualization over a wire either antegrade or retrograde, and the anterior anastomosis is completed in a running fashion, lateral to medial, with the dyed suture. If desired, the anastomosis can be wrapped with a vascularized omentum flap as discussed above. Finally, a self-suction drain is placed near the reconstruction.

Investigators at NYU[6] have reported a case of robotic ureteroureterostomy for a ureteral stricture resulting from an impacted calculus. They excised the diseased ureteral segment with robotic Potts scissors and performed the tension-free anastomosis as described above. They also comment that omentum or a Gerota's fascia flap can be employed to protect and buttress the anastomosis. These authors also reported a case of robotic ureteroureterostomy for treatment of obstruction from a retrocaval ureter. Furthermore, robotic ureteroureterostomy has also been successfully executed in patients with complex, aberrant anatomy. Yee and associates describe this procedure for a patient with ureteral obstruction in the setting of crossed renal ectopia with fusion.[7]

42.7 Ureteral Reimplantation

As described above, the patient positioning is similar to that for robotic prostatectomy. Five trocars are placed as previously described, and the robotic system is brought between the patient's legs.

First, the posterior peritoneum is incised longitudinally at the level of the iliac vessels in order to locate the ureter, which, once identified, is isolated with a vessel loop. The ureter is then dissected bluntly and sharply, with minimal cautery until the diseased segment is identified. Next, the ureter is transected above the diseased area with curved endoshears and it is spatulated using robotic Potts scissors. For cases of segmental distal ureterectomy, the ureter must be dissected caudally to the posterior bladder wall. If transitional cell carcinoma has been confirmed or is suspected, bladder spillage is avoided after ureteral transection, and the bladder cuff oversewn with 3-0 absorbable suture.

Attention is now paid to the bladder, which is filled with approximately 300 mL of normal saline, via the indwelling urethral catheter. The bladder is mobilized from the anterior abdominal wall by incising the peritoneum lateral to the obliterated umbilical artery, thus entering the space of Retzius. This dissection is carried

caudal to the pubis, and the urachus is then transected allowing the space between the anterior abdominal wall and bladder to be further developed. In order to ensure a tension-free anastomosis between the distal ureter and bladder, the contralateral superior bladder pedicle may be ligated to improve bladder mobilization. In all cases, we recommend at least a psoas hitch, using 2-0 absorbable suture, to minimize anastomotic tension. Avoidance of the genitofemoral nerve is critical when performing the hitch.

At this point, an approximately 1.5 cm full-thickness incision is made in a portion of the lateral bladder dome, aided by having the bladder distended. The ureter is spatulated with robotic Potts scissors, and an extravesical anastomosis is performed using 4-0 monocryl sutures in an interrupted fashion, ensuring proper mucosal apposition. Prior to completing the mucosal apposition, a ureteral stent can be placed over a wire in a retrograde fashion with robotic assistance. Alternatively, the stent can be placed cystoscopically over a wire once the entire anastomosis is complete. The bladder is filled again with saline, and any leaks in the mucosal connection are closed with another interrupted anastomotic suture. If a non-refluxing anastomosis is desired, a longer submucosal tunnel can be created prior to reimplantation. A second anastomotic layer is performed between the serosa of the bladder and the adventitia of the ureter. We often will add a third layer of closure consisting of perivesical fat, which serves the same purpose as a Gerota's or omental flap as described above. Finally, a self-suction drain can be placed near the anastomosis.

Robotic ureteral reimplantation has been reported throughout the literature. The first reported case was from Yohannes and associates and was performed for distal ureteral stricture disease.[8] This group created a refluxing anastomosis, and postoperative excretory urography at 5 months showed no evidence of obstruction. Mufarrij et al.[6] described robotic reimplantation for three patients with iatrogenic distal ureteral injury and one patient with a congenital stricture. These authors performed a psoas hitch in each case, prior to a two-layer, extravesical refluxing anastomosis. In other reports, robotic ureteral reimplantation has been performed during robotic prostatectomy for unintended transection of the right ureter.[9] Tunneled ureteral reimplantation has also been accomplished in other reports.[10] These authors noted the enhanced ability to creating a submucosal tunnel using the robot's three-dimensional view, and postoperative imaging demonstrated no obstruction.

Distal ureterectomy using robotic techniques for ureteral transitional cell carcinoma has been reported, as well.[11] This group utilized a psoas hitch to provide a tension-free anastomosis between the ureter and bladder. In this case, cystoscopy was performed at the outset of the case to score the bladder mucosa surrounding the ureteral orifice, being careful not to carry the incision through the bladder wall to prevent spillage. Patients with low-stage, low-grade segmental ureteral TCC may be offered such robotic reconstructions; however, proper staging and counseling of such patients are necessary.

42.8 Conclusion

Although the experience with robotic-assisted reconstruction of the upper urinary tract is in its infancy, it has exhibited feasibility, safety, and excellent comparative outcomes for certain procedures. Recent studies continue to demonstrate the ability of this technology to be applied to almost any surgical situation, pushing the envelope even further with regards to the potential utility of robotics.[12–17] Nonetheless, larger, prospective studies comparing robotic techniques to the standard of care are warranted. The ultimate role of robotics for upper urinary tract reconstruction is yet to be defined and will likely depend on the evolution of other minimally invasive techniques, such as natural orifice and single port approaches, as well as improvements in the robot itself, such as introduction of haptic feedback. At this time, robotic reconstruction should be examined for its advantages over other minimally invasive techniques.

References

1. Srinivasan AK, RIchstone L, Permpongkosol S, Kavoussi LR. Comparison of laparoscopic with open approach for ureterolysis in patients with retroperitoneal fibrosis. *J Urol.* 2008;179(5):1875–1878.

2. Stifelman MD, Shah O, Mufarrij P, Lipkin M. Minimally invasive management of retroperitoneal fibrosis. *Urology.* 2008;71(2):201–204.

3. Korets R, Hyams ES, Shah OD, Stifelman MD. Robotic-assisted laparoscopic ureterocalicostomy. *Urology.* 2007;70:366–369.

4. Vanlangendonck R, Venkatesh R, Vulin C, et al. Laparoscopic ureterocalicostomy: development of a technique simplified by application of nitinol clips and a wet monopolar electrosurgery device. *J Endourol.* 2005;19(2):225–229.

5. Gill IS, Cherullo EE, Steinberg AP, et al. Laparoscopic ureterocalicostomy: initial experience. *J Urol.* 2007;171: 1227–1230.

6. Mufarrij PW, Shah OD, Berger AD, Stifelman MD. Robotic reconstruction of the upper urinary tract. *J Urol.* 2007;178:2002–2005.

7. Yee DS, Shanberg AM. Robotic-assisted laparoscopic ureteroureterostomy in an adolescent with an obstructed upper pole system and crossed renal ectopia with fusion. *Urology.* 2006;68(3):673.e5–7.

8. Yohannes P, Chiou RK, Pelinkovic D. Pure robot-assisted laparoscopic ureteral reimplantation for ureteral stricture disease: case report. *J Endourol.* 2003;17:891–893.

9. Dinlenc CZ, Gerber E, Wagner JR. Ureteral reimplantation during robot assisted laparoscopic radical prostatectomy. *J Urol.* 2004;172:205.

10. Naeyer GD, Van Migem P, Schatteman P, et al. Pure robot-assisted psoas hitch ureteral reimplantation for distal-ureteral stenosis. *J Endourol.* 2007;21(6):618–620.

11. Uberoi J, Harnisch B, Sethi AS, et al. Robot-assisted laparoscopic distal ureterectomy and ureteral reimplantation with psoas hitch. *J Endourol.* 2007;21(4): 372–373.

12. Hemal AK, Nayyar R, Gupta NP, Dorairajan LN. Experience with robotic assisted laparoscopic surgery in upper tract urolithiasis. *Can J Urol.* 2010;17(4):5299–5305.

13. Hemal AK, Nayyar R, Gupta NP, Dorairajan LN. Experience with robot assisted laparoscopic surgery for upper and lower benign and malignant ureteral pathologies. *Urology.* 2010;76(6):1387–1393.

14. Hemal AK, Nayyar R, Rao R. Robotic repair of primary symptomatic obstructive megaureter with intracorporeal or extracorporeal ureteric tapering and ureteroneocystostomy. *J Endourol.* 2009;23(12):2041–2046.

15. Singh I, Kader K, Hemal AK. Robotic distal ureterectomy with reimplantation in malignancy: technical nuances. *Can J Urol.* 2009;16(3):4671–4676.

16. Hemal AK, Rao R, Sharma S, Clement RG. Pure robotic retrocaval ureter repair. *Int Braz J Urol.* 2008; 34(6): 734–738.

17. Laungani R, Patil N, Krane LS, Hemal AK, Raja S, Bhandari M, Menon M. Robotic-assisted ureterovaginal fistula repair: report of efficacy and feasiblity. *J Laparoendosc Adv Surg Tech A.* 2008;18(5):731–734.

Chapter 43

Robotic or Laparoscopic Renal Surgery: Pros and Cons

Alexander Mottrie

43.1 Malignant Disease

43.1.1 Partial Nephrectomy (PN)

43.1.1.1 Introduction

The incidence of renal cell carcinoma (RCC) has increased in the last two decades[1] but up to 70% of these are small and localized tumors.[2] For most of these tumors, open or laparoscopic radical nephrectomy have proven to be an overtreatment also causing a significant risk factor for the development of chronic renal insufficiency with its specific morbidity including hip fractures and cardiovascular problems.[3–5] In the contemporary practice open partial nephrectomy (OPN) is the gold standard for a single small renal tumor but in the last decade many minimally invasive alternative treatments have been presented. In particular, laparoscopy has shown benefits over OPN like reduced postoperative pain or morbidity, improved cosmesis, shorter recovery and length of stay in the hospital, and earlier return to work, but with equivalent efficacy in terms of functional and oncological outcomes.[6,7] Moreover, in the past years, laparoscopy has gained popularity and laparoscopic partial nephrectomy (LPN) is nowadays considered as one of the standard treatments for renal cancer. The recent introduction of robotic surgery to urology and, later on, its application to renal surgery with robot-assisted partial nephrectomy (RAPN) has given us another option for minimally invasive nephron-sparing surgery.

43.1.1.2 Indications and Contraindications

In general, indications for partial nephrectomy in laparoscopy or robotics are the same originally described for open surgery: *absolute indications* for PN include localized lesion in solitary kidney, patients with bilateral renal lesions, or chronic renal insufficiency.[8–11] *Relative indications* include hereditary forms of RCC like Von Hippel–Lindau syndrome, hereditary papillary RCC, Birt–Hogg–Dubé syndrome, or tuberous sclerosis in which there is an high risk of future development of metachronous renal malignancies. *Relative indications* also exist for patients with unilateral lesion but with the risk of future renal insufficiency such as in hypertension, diabetes, nephrolithiasis, or chronic pyelonephritis.[12] An *elective indication* is considered PN for a localized, incidental, unilateral tumor with a normal contralateral kidney. There are also *contraindications* to PN like renal vein or inferior cava involvement, massive tumor size, or local invasion. As relative contraindications are considered lymphadenopathy or bleeding diathesis.[8] PN is well established and considered to be the standard management for all organ-confined tumors up to 4 cm in diameter, but recently several publications have shown the possibility to perform LPN in tumors larger than 4 cm with excellent operative efficacy and oncological outcomes. Simmons et al.[13] in a retrospective review of 425 LPN procedures, comparing three groups (control group 1: tumor <2 cm, control group 2: tumor 2–4 cm, and study group: tumor >4 cm), have proven

A. Mottrie (✉)
Urology Department, Onze Lieve Vrouw Hospital, Aalst, Belgium
e-mail: a.mottrie@telenet.be

A.K. Hemal, M. Menon (eds.), *Robotics in Genitourinary Surgery*,
DOI 10.1007/978-1-84882-114-9_43, © Springer-Verlag London Limited 2011

that the tumor size >4 cm as sole parameter does not increase significantly the risk for positive margins (0 vs 0.5 vs 6.5%, respectively, $p = 0.19$), intraoperative (9 vs 8 vs 7%, respectively, $p = 0.4$), or overall postoperative genitourinary complications (11 vs 24 vs 24%, respectively, $p = 0.03$); Simmons et al.[14] have also demonstrated equivalent outcomes in intermediate-term oncologic control for renal tumors >4 cm, comparing retrospectively laparoscopic partial and radical nephrectomy but all authors agree that a careful patient selection and adequate laparoscopic expertise are absolute prerequisites.

43.1.1.3 Oncological Outcomes

Oncological Outcomes in LP

The main aim of renal cancer surgery is removing the whole tumor. In many studies LPN and OPN have similar oncological outcomes, but morbidity is lower in LPN.

The long-term outcome for pT1a tumors treated with OPN in the study of Fergany et al.[15] was excellent with a cancer specific survival (CSS) at 5- and 10-years of 88 and 73%, respectively. In Permpongkosol's et al. paper,[16] comparing 85 LPNs with 58 OPNs, after a mean follow-up of 40.4 ± 18.0 and 49.68 ± 28.84 months for LPN and OPN, respectively, the disease-free survival (DFS) for pT1, was, respectively, 91.4 and 97.6% at 5 years.

Gill et al.,[17] reported a 3-year CSS for patients with a single cT1N0M0 renal cell carcinoma of 99.3 and 99.2% after LPN and OPN respectively. Moreover, based on multivariate analysis, hospital stay, operative blood loss and operative time were significantly shorter in the laparoscopic group. In the same series, the role of LPN for renal cancers over 4 cm has been proven, because 68 patients in the laparoscopic group and 66 in the open group had a pT1b tumor. Lane and Gill[18] reported the outcomes at 5 years for LPN with an overall survival (OS) and a CSS, respectively, equal to 86 and 100% and a DFS of 97% in 37 patients. Gill et al.[19] showed their LPN experience in solitary kidney: 22 patients had undergone LPN for renal tumor (median size 3.6 cm) in a solitary kidney: at a median follow-up of 2.5 years OS, CSS and DFS were 91, 100, and 100% respectively. A more recent study from the University of Chicago

reported 76 patients with T1a (<4 cm) tumors who underwent LPN over a 4-year period. This group was compared with a matched cohort who underwent OPN over an 8-year different time period. With approximately 20 months of follow-up there were no reported recurrences in either group and preservation of renal function as determined by serum creatinine was seen as equivalent.[20] Recently, a retrospective comparison between LPN and OPN for renal cancer is presented. The mean tumor size was 2.8 cm in LPN group and 2.9 cm in OPN group: the Kaplan-Meier estimate of 5-years OS for pT1 stage RCC was 96 and 85% ($p = 0.1$) in LPN and OPN group, respectively, and the Kaplan–Meier estimate of 5-year local recurrence-free survival (RFS) were 97 and 98% ($p = 0.9$) for LPN and OPN, respectively.[21]

Whether PN should be proposed and performed in all cases of renal tumor greater than 4 cm is still in debate. Until now, few studies report oncological outcomes after LPN for tumor larger than 4 cm. Simmons et al.[14] compared retrospectively the intermediate-term oncologic and renal functional outcomes of laparoscopic radical nephrectomy (LRN) and LPN for Stage T1b-T3N0M0 tumors >4 cm in size. First of all, they did not find any differences in total complication rates in both groups at 19–20% ($p = 0.85$). The median tumor size was 5.3 cm in the LRN group and 4.6 cm in the LPN group ($p = 0.03$) and there were no positive tumor margins in either group in the final pathological findings. If we look at the oncological outcomes after a median follow-up of 57 months in the LRN group and 44 months in the LPN group ($p = 0.14$), we find a RFS rate of 97 and 94% in LRN and LPN groups, respectively, ($p = 0.43$) and in both groups the same OS rate 89% ($p = 0.94$) and the CSS 97% ($p = 0.96$) (Table 43.1).

All these studies show that LPN has a similar oncological outcome in intermediate term for pT1 RCC as open surgery but furthermore they show that morbidity (blood loss, hospital stay, operative time, or postoperative complications) is less or at least comparable with open surgery.[16,17,20,21]

Oncological Outcomes in RAPN

Even if the data are new and the series sometimes small and longterm follow-up not presently available, the oncological outcomes from RAPN appear to be

Table 43.1 LPN oncological outcomes

Authors	No. of patients	Mean FU	TNM	OS	CSS	DSF
Permpongkosol et al.[16]	85	40.4 ± 18.0 months	pT1	93.75%[a]	NA	91.4%[a]
Gill[17]	771	1.2 years	pT1	NA	99.3%[b]	98.6%[b] (local recurrence)
Lane[18]	37	5.7 years	pT1	86%[a]	100%[a]	97.3%[a]
Gill et al.[19]	22	2.5 years	pT1	91%	100%	100%
Marszalek et al.[21]	100	3.6 years	pT1	96%[a]	NA	97%[a] (local recurrence)
Simmons[14]	35	44 months	pT1b	89%	97%	97%

[a]5 years Kaplan–Meier.
[b]3 years Kaplan–Meier.

similar to those reported in laparoscopic and open series. In five series with intermediate outcome data, no recurrences have been reported up to 28 months postoperatively. Deane et al.,[22] comparing retrospectively 11 patients undergone to conventional LPN with 10 patients to RAPN, did not find any statistical difference in terms of operating time, blood loss or positive margins at the frozen section, and after a mean follow-up of 16 months, there was no evidence of recurrences in both groups. Rogers et al.[23] with one of the largest multicenter series, showed that in 148 patients, undergone to RAPN between October 2002 and September 2007 at six different private and academic hospital centers, there was no evidence of tumor recurrence at a mean follow-up of 7.2 (range 2–54) months overall and no recurrence in six patients (4.0%) with positive margins after a mean follow-up of 18 months (range 12–23 months). Mottrie et al.[24] between September 2006 and October 2007 performed a total of 17 RAPNs for RCC (11 pT1a and 5 pT1b and 1 angiomyolipoma): after a mean follow-up of 19 months (range 14–24) no local or systemic recurrence has been reported (Table 43.2).

43.1.1.4 Positive Margins

Because the main aim of renal surgery is the removal of the whole tumor, incomplete excision of the neoplasm can leave tumor on the resection bed and this is considered a positive margin. During OPN, when a positive margin is found on frozen section, deeper resection is easier to be performed before closure of the parenchymal defect. In LPN or RALPN, by the time of the result of the frozen section, the parenchymal defect is already closed and the hilar vessels are already unclamped in order to reduce ischemia time.

Positive Margins in LPN

In literature the positive margin rate in LPN is comparable to OPN: Breda et al.[25] in retrospective multi-institutional survey of 17 centers performing LPN, have found a positive margin rate of 2.4% that is comparable to that reported in contemporary studies on LPN (2–3.5%)[26–28] and OPN (0.8–6.8%).[25,29–31] Permpongkosol et al.,[32] reported 511 LPNs performed by two surgeons and found nine patients (1.8%) with

Table 43.2 RAPN oncological outcomes

Authors	Dean[22]	Rogers[23]	Kaul[106]	Aron[60]	Mottrie[24]
No. of RAPN (No. of tumors)	10 (11)	8 (14)	10 (10)	12 (12)	17 (17)
Mean OR time	228.7 min (95–375)	192 min (165–214)	155 min (120–185)	242 min (130–360)	133 min (105–220)
WIT	32.1 min (30–45)	31 min (24–45)	21 min (18–27)	23 min (13–36)	24 min (16–35)
TNM (cm size)	pT1a (2.5–4)	12 pT1a, 2 pT1b (2.6–6.4)	pT1a (1.0–3.5)	pT1a (1.4–3.8)	11 pT1a, 5 pT1b (2.2–5.3)
Positive margins	None	None	None	None	None
Mean FU	16 months	3 months	15 months	7.4 months	19 months
Local recurrence	None	None	None	None	None

a positive margin. This is one of the series with the longest follow-up for patients with positive margins; seven of the nine patients were undergone to surveillance: one patient with von Hippel–Lindau disease, died 10 months later surgery for a metastatic RCC to the pancreas, but the other six patients had no evidence of local or systemic recurrence after a median follow-up of 32 months. In fact the management of positive margins after RCC is not yet standardized but data from literature suggest that a positive margin does not lead necessarily to a local recurrence or metastatic disease and does not impair the CSS: if there is absolute certainty that the resection has been completed and only a microscopic when positive margin is present, a vigilant monitoring with CT every 6–12 months could be an option.[33] Recently, several laparoscopic series have shown that the tumor size or even the position do not correlate with a positive margin rate: Simmons et al.[14] performed LPN in 35 patients with pT1b-pT3 RCC (mean size 4.6 cm; range 4.1–7.5 cm), without any positive margins. Okimura et al.[34] presented their experience with LPN in 21 patients with an incidentally detected stage pT2, pT3a, or pT3b renal mass (mean size pT2 6.5 cm, pT3a 3.2 cm, pT3b 5.8 cm), showing a CSS rate of 95% after a mean follow-up of 29 months (range 1–58), but the renal parenchymal and perirenal fat surgical margins were negative for cancer in all 21 patients (100%). Rais-Bahrami et al.[35] in a retrospective review of LPN compared 274 patients with tumor burden <4 cm (mean size 2.3 cm) with 34 patients with tumor burden >4 cm (mean size 5.8 cm); they reported no statistical differences in surgical margins ($p = 0.206$). Complex cases like multiple or large and centrally or hilar tumors are nowadays treated laparoscopically without increased of morbidity: Gill et al.,[36] performed 25 LPNs for hilar tumor (mean tumor size was 3.7 cm.) and laparoscopic surgery was successful in all cases without any open conversions or operative re-interventions. Histopathology confirmed RCC in 17 patients (68%), and in all surgical margins were negative. Latouff et al.[37] described 18 LPNs for hilar lesions: mean surgical time was 238 min (range 150–420 min) and only one patient had a positive margin (7.1%) on the surface that was adjacent to the renal artery but after a median follow-up of 26 months, no local or systemic progressions is occurred.

Anyway all efforts to avoid and prevent surgical margins should be attempted and although the positive margin rate is comparable between LPN and OPN, it continues to further improve by applying new surgical techniques.

Positive Margins in RAPN

Lam et al.,[38] performed an extensive review of literature and found that the risk of positive margins during partial nephrectomy could be minimized with a precise visualization of the tumor and tumor margins. With this exact purpose, the development of the da Vinci surgical system (Intuitive Surgical Corp., Sunnyvale, California, USA) allows for simple and complex procedures to be performed more easily by a greater number of surgeons than the conventional laparoscopic approach; its advanced characteristics are three-dimensional visualization, magnification, 7 degrees of freedom at the distal instrument wrist, the absence of the fulcrum effect, and the elimination of tremor. Rogers et al.[39] reported about 11 successful RAPNs for hilar RCC defined as a tumor located in the region of the renal hilum in physical contact with the renal vessels. The mean tumor size was 3.8 cm (range 2.3–6.4 cm) and the mean operative time was 202 min (range 154–253): in all cases the surgical margins were negative. Rogers et al.,[40] also showed the feasibility of RAPN for hilar, endophytic, and multiple renal tumors: 14 tumors were resected in eight patients (mean 2.4 cm, range 0.8–6.4 cm), with a mean operating time of 192 min (range 165–214 min). In all patients RAPN was successfully without any intraoperative complications and without positive surgical margins. Mottrie et al.[24] performed 5 of 17 RCC as an advanced challenge: 1 patient had a renal tumor of 5.3 cm that was very close to the hilum, 2 others had two synchronous ipsilateral tumors, and 2 more patients had a tumor, which was endophytic and close to the renal vascular supply. All the patients had negative margins and although the warm ischemia time of these patients was among the longest of the group, their postoperative laboratory results showed no deterioration of their renal function. For the authors, robotic assistance facilitated the laparoscopic approach especially in the crucial steps of the tumor resection and reconstruction; the magnified three-dimensional visualization, the articulating robotic instruments, and the elimination of tremor ease the maintenance of an accurate plane of tumor resection and renal reconstruction. This makes the whole procedure easier and probably faster, so avoiding positive surgical margins and in the same time reducing the warm ischemia time of the kidney and resulting in better preservation of the patients renal function. A recent review about the RAPN stated that the positive margin rates in robotic partial nephrectomy are rare (7/211, 3.3%) and no recurrences have been reported up to 54 months of follow-up in any studies reviewed.[41]

43.1.1.5 Risk of Tumor Spillage or Port-Site Seeding

Seeding during OPN is rare but can be correlated to a vigorous tumor handling and spillage during the operation. In recent years, with the widespread use of laparoscopy, not only local recurrence but also port-site metastasis has become a concern. Nevertheless, Rassweiler et al.[42] in a big review of over 1,000 laparoscopic procedures for urological malignancies, found only two cases of port-site metastasis (0.18%). Lee et al.[43] and Rane et al.[44] have reported five and six cases of port-site metastasis respectively, after LRN. Recently, the first case of port-site metastasis after a LPN was reported,[45] but the mechanism of the abdominal wall recurrence is still unclear and the incidence of port-site metastases (that is higher in TCC cancer), might reflect a cancer-related poor prognostic factors rather than the laparoscopic technique. In literature the incidence of port-site metastasis is similar to that of the abdominal incision scar (0.4%) after OPN.[46]

43.1.1.6 Functional Outcomes

Physiology of Renal Ischemia and Ischemia Time

The aim of PN is to remove completely the tumor obtaining adequate hemostasis in the shortest possible hilar clamping time. Determining the safe limit of ischemia time is essential to minimize the complications of acute renal failure (ARF) and chronic renal failure (CRF). The mechanism of ischemia–reperfusion injury depends on the metabolic properties of the kidney: oxygenation in the kidney parenchyma is graded with the highest O_2 levels in the cortical zone, a decrease in O_2 tension at the level of the outer medulla, and the lowest O_2 levels in the papillae. The outer cortex has a high O_2 reserve and, thus, cells in this region are relatively protected. Outer medullary epithelial cells are most susceptible to hypoxia because they rely heavily on oxidative metabolism and reside in an area with minimal O_2 reserve. Papillary epithelial cells reside in a constitutively hypoxic environment and they can survive on anaerobic metabolism during short periods of ischemia. Because renal dysfunction results from both vascular and tubular injury processes, and certain regions of the kidney being more susceptible to ischemic injury, renoprotective agents like intravenous furosemide and mannitol before both clamping and unclamping the renal vessels and a good hydration can promote diuresis and decrease the risk of reperfusion injury and the release of free radicals.[47]

In laparoscopy it is difficult to perform cold ischemia of the kidney. Efforts to obtain cold ischemia have been attempted like intrarenal cooling via a special endo-vascular catheterization of the renal artery or by using a ureteral catheter to irrigate the kidney with cold solution.[48,49] Guillonneau et al.,[50] using a ureteral catheter and cold saline irrigation, to decrease renal temperature, found that the postoperative creatinine level was higher in the group with cold ischemia as compared with no ischemia but not statistically significant. In another retrospective study Abukora et al.[51] comparing 12 patients who had warm ischemia with 14 patients who had cold ischemia, found loss of function in the group with cold ischemia. For these reasons and for some concerns about complications, in laparoscopy, mainly warm ischemia is used today.

The upper limit of warm ischemia time (WIT) has been accepted to be 30 min based on animal and anecdotal clinical data. Nevertheless, ARF or CRF has multifactorial causes: renal function preservation is not only related to the duration of WIT, but Fergany et al.,[52] in a solitary kidney series, found that in the long term, only the percent of parenchyma resected, the patient age, and the congenital solitary kidney or the timing of contralateral nephrectomy, had a statistical effect on postoperative creatinine level.

Functional Outcomes in LPN Compared to OPN

There are several studies suggesting that 30 min of WIT is not an absolute limit for ischemia during PN.[53,54] Bhayani et al.[53] compared patients who had no hilar clamping versus two groups of patients who had hilar clamping of less than and more than 30 min. The median creatinine did not change significantly postoperatively, and none of the 118 patients required dialysis. Porpiglia et al.,[55] in a prospective study, performed LPN in 18 patients with WIT >30 min. The glomerular filtration rate (GFR) was not significantly different 3 months after LPN with WIT >30 min. They evaluated renal function by nuclear scan and they found that contribution of the affected kidney decreased from 48 to 36% after 5 days from surgery and statistical analysis demonstrated that the loss of function was influenced only by the WIT. Nevertheless, contribution of the operated kidney to overall renal function increased to 40% at 3 months and to 43% at 1-year postoperatively. They observed that the maximum loss of renal function was between 32 and 42 min of WIT. Although the overall GFR was maintained and no patients required dialysis in the presence of a normal contralateral kidney, the authors concluded that efforts should be made to maintain the WIT under 30 min. Desai et al.[54] demonstrated similar results, but they found out that when WIT was >30 min, the risk of renal dysfunction was higher in presence of advancing age (age >70 years) and pre-existing renal insufficiency (creatinine serum level >1.5 mg/dL).

Nowadays there is ongoing debate on "safe" WIT. It is clear that WIT is one of the factors that has an impact on residual renal function, but other risk factors can influence the renal function as age, preoperative renal function, solitary kidney, comorbidities, and amount of normal parenchyma excised. In a solitary kidney cohort for LPN, Gill et al.[19] stated that the postoperative decrease in renal function was impacted by various factors, including patient age 60 years or older (serum creatinine increased by 19% in patients younger than 60 years vs 40% in those 60 years or older), 30% or greater kidney parenchyma excised (when comparing less than 30 vs 30% or greater excision of the kidney parenchyma, serum creatinine increased by 34 vs 53%) and warm ischemia time more than 30 min (when comparing 30 min or less vs more than 30 min of warm ischemia, serum creatinine increased by 15 vs 43%).

Gill et al.[17] in a multi-institutional study showed 5-year functional outcomes for patients undergone to OPN and LPN: patients in OPN were high risk (older, had greater comorbidities, decreased performance status, higher percentage with elevated baseline serum creatinine level), whereas patients undergone to LPN had longer warm ischemia time (WIT); the mean WIT in LPN group was higher comparing with OPN (30.7 min, range 4.0–68.0 vs 20.1 min. range 4.0–52.0 respectively, $p < 0.0001$); the mean operative time for

LPN and OPN was 3.3 and 4.3 h, respectively, and on multivariate analysis operative time for LPN was 0.78 times that of OPN ($p < 0.0001$). Nonetheless, only 0.9% of patients in each group required dialysis for acute renal failure and early functional outcomes were similar in two groups because after 3 months, 97.9 and 99.6% of patients in LPN and OPN groups, respectively, had a functioning kidney. However, LPN offered less operative time, decreased operative blood loss, and a shorter hospital stay.

Gong et al.[20] from University of Chicago, comparing a cohort of 76 patients having undergone LPN with 77 patients having undergone OPN for solitary tumors, reached the same conclusions showing, a mean follow-up of 20 months, a mean creatinine level of 1.3 mg/dL vs 1.2 mg/dL ($p = 0.272$) in LPN and OPN groups respectively. In a recent review Marszalek et al.[21] analyzed 200 patients after OPN and LPN for renal cancer, with a median follow -up of 3.6 years. Surgical time and hospitalization were shorter in the LPN group ($p < 0.001$); also warm ischemia time in LPN was shorter than cold ischemia time in OPN ($p < 0.001$) but the decline of postoperative GFR (24 h after surgery) was higher after LPN (8.8%) than after OPN (0.8%; $p < 0.001$). After a mean of 3.6 year, however, the decline in GFR was identical in both groups ($p = 0.8$). On preoperative evaluation, 12% of patients in the LPN group and 11% of patients in the OPN group had chronic kidney disease ($p = 0.8$). The respective percentages after 3.6 year were 21% after LPN and 18% after OPN ($p = 0.7$). This significant shift toward higher stages of chronic kidney disease after LPN ($p < 0.001$) and OPN ($p < 0.001$) was similar in both groups ($p = 0.8$). On multivariate regression analysis, preoperative GFR, ischemia time, and surgical access independently predicted the immediate postoperative (24–48 h) GFR decline; surgical access was not a predictor of long-term GFR. GFR at the last follow-up was similar in the LPN and OPN groups when stratified after ischemia times below and exceeding 30 and 20 min, respectively.

Reducing WIT in Laparoscopy

There is general consensus that "less is better" and nowadays not only the WIT for LPN is shorter in high-volume centers than some years ago but also many efforts have been attempted to reduce the ischemia

Table 43.3 Reducing WIT or providing regional ischemia

Author	No. of patients	Mean WIT	Technique
Baumert[56]	20 control group 20 study group (10 group 1a and 1b)	13.7 ± 4 vs 27.2 ± 5 min ($p < 0.01$)	Modified running suture and early hilar unclamp
Bollens[57]	39	9 min (range 6–40)	Pedicle clamping "on demand"
Nguyen[58]	50 control group 50 study group	31.1 vs 13.9 min ($p < 0.0001$)	Very early hilar unclamp
Verhoest[59]	5	NA	Regional ischemia by Satinsky clamp on parenchima

time during LPN. Baumert et al.[56] reported a decrease of ischemic injury in early unclamping after one or two running sutures on the tumor bed. The vascularized renal parenchyma is then closed over a surgical bolster. With this technique, warm ischemia time was reduced from 27.2 ± 5 (control group) to 13.7 ± 4 min (group 1). Bollens et al.[57] tried to reduce WIT with "on-demand clamping" of the hilum: in this technique, the hilum is dissected early but clamped only in the case of excessive bleeding. Out of 39 patients, 31 required on-demand clamping, with a mean ischemia time of 9 min. Nguyen et al.,[58] recently described their technique of early unclamping of the hilum to reduce WIT during LPN. According to this technique, only the initial parenchymal suturing is performed under ischemia, with the remainder of the bolstered renorrhaphy being performed in the revascularized kidney. They found that early unclamping significantly decreased ischemia time by >50%. Verhoest et al.[59] described an initial experience of compression of renal parenchyma by an endoscopic Satinsky clamp inserted percutaneously, without dissection of renal vessels: according to the authors the main advantage would be the reduction of operative time, and, by a regional ischemia, the preservation of the rest of the normal renal parenchyma and reduce the risk of microscopic lesions and acute tubular necrosis, as observed immediately after laparoscopic partial nephrectomy when the renal artery has been clamped (Table 43.3).

Functional Outcomes of RAPN in the Present Main Series

Robotic surgery is an emerging technique that offers a number of prospective advantages as magnified stereoscopic vision, elimination of tremor, and absence of the fulcrum effect. Nevertheless, Aron et al.[60] presented the results of a retrospective comparison between 12 patients undergone to RAPN with 12 LPNs. They found no differences between the two groups in terms of blood loss, operative time, length of stay, and WIT (23.0 min vs 22.0 min for RAPN vs LPN $p = 0.89$). Renal functional outcomes, as measured by 3-month serum creatinine and estimated GFR were comparable between the matched groups. The authors concluded that while technically feasible, RAPN offers no discernible clinical advantage for either tumor excision or sutured renorrhaphy. Dean et al.[20] and Caruso et al.[61] reached the same conclusion. It is to mention that in all these papers, they all compared their initial experience of RAPN in a small group of 10–12 patients, with a similar number of patients having undergone LPN performed by surgeons with an already vast experience in this matter. Nevertheless, Dean et al.[20] have mentioned the advantages of a clearly less steep learning curve with RAPN.

Remarkable improvements in operative parameters have been noted as the experience has matured and as the technique has been refined. By now, many papers have shown that robotic surgery allows complex procedures to be performed successfully, minimizing the technical challenges of laparoscopic approach and considerably reducing WIT. Rogers et al.[39] performed RAPN in 11 patients with hilar tumor: the mean WIT was 28.9 min (range 20–39 min), the mean operating time was 202 min (range 154–253 min), and the hospital mean stay was 2.6 days. Surgical margins were negative for malignancy in all cases and no patients experienced a significant postoperative increase in serum creatinine or estimated GFR. The authors concluded that not only LPN requires advanced skills in laparoscopy to accomplish tumor resection and renal reconstruction in an acceptable WIT but also tumors located near renal hilar structures significantly add to the technical challenges of LPN.

RAPN may now facilitate the advanced maneuvers required to successfully perform partial nephrectomy for renal hilar tumors using a minimally invasive surgical approach. The magnified, three-dimensional visualization, and articulating robotic instruments can facilitate precise tumor resection and renal reconstruction even for tumors near hilar structures. Comparing a single-surgeon experience of LPN and RAPN in 102 consecutive patients, Wang and Bhayani[62] found that operative time (140 vs 156 min, $p < 0.04$), WIT (19 vs 25 min $p < 0.03$), and length of stay were significantly shorter in robotic group (2.5 vs 2.4 days $p < 0.03$). Mottrie et al.[63] presented their experience with 50 patients undergone to RAPN. The mean tumor size was 25.6 mm (10–64 mm), the mean console time was 96.5 min (50–180 min), the mean warm ischemia time (WIT) was 21.2 min (10–40 min), and the mean hospital stay was 5.3 days. No major intraoperative complications were encountered. Mean GFR and hemoglobin levels at postoperative day 1 were 67.65 ml/min/1.73m^2 (20–140) and 12.16 g/dL (8.6–15.3) respectively. At 3 months, no patient experienced a significant change in GFR level. A subset analysis of the first 20, compared to the last 20 patients, showed a mean WIT of 26.1 vs 15.9 min, respectively ($p < 0.05$). Most importantly, they observed that with sliding-clip renorrhaphy of the tumor defect by sliding Hem-o-lok clips without coagulation sponge bolster, they could reduce WIT significantly. The same technique has been described by Benway et al.,[64] in order to reduce the ischemia time, with significant decrease of operating time and ischemia time (145.3 min and 17.8 min, respectively). Ho et al.[65] reported their results after RAPN in 20 patients for renal cell carcinoma less than 7 cm: for a mean tumor size of 30.2 mm, mean operation time and WIT were 82.7 min and 21.7 min respectively. Only in patients who require closing of pelvicalyceal system, the ischemia time was slightly higher (24.3 min) but after 1-year follow-up, no elevated serum creatinine level, local recurrence, or distant relapse were reported. Moreover, they focused on an important point: although the technique varies from surgeon to surgeon, it is generally felt that the sutures placed during LPN are larger and thus might theoretically result in greater damage to the surrounding parenchyma. In robotic surgery, the three dimensional magnified vision for the console surgeon enhanced the ability to detect any pelvicalyceal system entry and they concluded that most pelvicalyceal system entries could be identified in a very precise and accurate manner that only the excellent three dimensional vision offered by the da Vinci

robotic system could give. The possibility of rotating and articulating of the arm by endowrist system, allows the surgeon to be much more accurate and precise about the amount of healthy parenchyma taken during the suture. They also used absorbable sutures instead of laparoscopic clips for PCS closure, which eliminated the risk of erosion of the collecting system. These are the likely benefits of facilitated intracorporeal suturing with the da Vinci robotic system (Benway et al., 2009, "unpublished") showed their results of one of the first international experiences in RAPN: across four institutions 183 patients were undergone to RAPN between September 2006 and December 2008. Five patients had multiple tumors which were treated simultaneously, for a total of 191 tumors addressed with RAPN during the course of the study. A total of 191 tumors were excised in 183 patients. Mean tumor size was 2.87 cm (range 1.0–7.9 cm, median 2.50 cm), mean total operative time was 210 min (range 86–370 min, median 206 min), with a mean console time of 141.5 min (range 45–253 min, median 149 min). Mean warm ischemic times across the entire series averaged 20.7 min (range 0–51 min, median 22 min). Accounting only for those cases where the vessels were clamped, mean warm ischemic time was 23.9 min (range 10–51 min, median 23 min). Mean preoperative serum creatinine was 1.03 mg/dL (range 0.6–2.0 mg/dL, median 0.97 mg/dL) and the mean creatinine 24 h postoperatively was 1.18 mg/dL (range 0.6–2.4 mg/dL), accounting for a mean change of + 0.16 mg/dL; this difference was statistically significant ($p < 0.001$) but on last follow-up, serum creatinine in most cases returned to baseline, with a mean value of 1.04 mg/dL and this value was not significantly different from preoperative values ($p = 0.84$). there were a total of 18 complications (9.8%). Pathologic data were available for 173 patients: overall, 69% of tumors excised exhibited malignant features; positive surgical margins on final pathology were encountered in seven patients (3.8%) and two of these patients were found to have benign pathology (angiomyolipoma) while the remaining five patients had malignant tumors, for an overall positive surgical margin rate of 2.7% for malignancy. The authors concluded that RAPN, offering a magnified, three-dimensional view, and fully-articulating wristed instruments, the da Vinci Surgical System (Intuitive, Sunnyvale, CA USA) affords the surgeon unprecedented access and control during renal surgery, especially during the critical steps of tumor

Table 43.4 Overview of published series on RAPN

Authors	No. of pts	Mean tumor size (cm)	Mean OP time (min)	Mean WIT (min)	Mean hospital stay (days)	Positive margins	Mean FU (months)
Deane[22]	10	3.1	229	32.1	2.0	None	16
Aron[60]	12	2.4	242	23.0	4.7	None	7.4
Kaul[106]	10	2.3	155	21.0	1.5	None	15
Rogers[40]	8	3.6	192	31.0	2.6	None	3
Rogers[23]	148	2.8	197	27.8	1.9	1	7.2 and 18
Mottrie[63]	17	2.5	133	21.2	5.3	1	21
Wang[62]	40	2.5	140	19	2.5	1	NA
Benway[64]	50	2.7	145.3	17.8	2.5	1	12
Ho[65]	20	3.5	82.8	21.7	4.8	None	12
Rogers[39]	11	3.8	202	28.9	2.6	None	NA
Bhayani[107]	35	2.5	142	21	2.5	None	NA
(Benway et al., 2009, "unpublished")	191	2.8	210	20.7	NA	7	

excision and renal reconstruction. Moreover, RAPN appears to be associated with a relatively short learning curve, with the potential for technical proficiency in less than 30 procedures for experienced renal surgeons, even in those without prior laparoscopic experience (Table 43.4).[20,64]

43.1.1.7 Complications in LPN and RAPN

LPN is challenging and therefore the reported complication rate is higher compared to OPN. Nevertheless, the incidence of complications in recent series from centers with expertise range from 9 to 33%, which is not significantly different compared to OPN. As for OPN, almost 50% of overall complications are medical. In the combined analysis of the largest series of LPN, hemorrhage is the most common urologic complication (5%), followed by urine leak (4.2%).[31] Simmons and Gill recently[66] using a five-tiered scale based on National Cancer Institute Common Toxicity Criteria to assess complication severity, demonstrated a decrease of overall, non-urological, hemorrhagic, and urinary leakage complications by 44, 23, 53, and 56%, respectively, despite an increased tumor and technical complexity, comparing an initial LPN series of 200 patients with the most recent group. The same authors compared data of the OPN series from Memorial Sloan-Kettering Cancer Center with his own recent LPN cohort and proved an overall complication rate of 26.8% (OPN) and 19% (LPN), respectively.

Zimmermann and Janetschek[67] reported overall rates of postoperative bleeding necessitating transfusion and urinary leakage as 2.7 and 1.9%. These rates are significantly lower than in previous studies because of the introduction of sealants or glues and in the same way of the improvement of techniques of suturing and resection.

Shapiro et al.[41] analyzing series of RAPN, found that 211 patients major complications were 14 (6.6%) and the most common were being ileus ($n = 4$) and urine leak ($n = 3$). Laparoscopic partial nephrectomy (LPN) duplicates the principles of open surgery and after several technical modifications, it has been standardized to a great extent. Nevertheless, LPN is a challenging procedure.

43.1.1.8 Conclusion

We have to consider robot-assisted laparoscopic nephron-sparing surgery as a new laparoscopic procedure with the advantage of a new sophisticated technology. The 3-D vision associated with the endowrist technology allows for excellent vision of the operative field and the possibility of dissecting the tissue optimally and varying the degree of incidence with the target structures. Robotic technology may be associated with decreased ischemia time, which is basically related to the length of the dissection of the tumor. In particular, the suturing phase is faster with robotic da Vinci System. The three-dimensional vision and the endowrist should also help to decrease the positive surgical margins because they typically provide optimal dissection angles during the procedure. Moreover, robotic surgery allows an average laparoscopic surgeon to perform more difficult cases, such as large, intraparenchymal, or even perihilar tumors. Indeed, the robot-assisted PN was revealed to be not only a feasible option but also resulted in adequate resection margins and warm ischemia time for larger lesions. The procedure also provides the surgeon with the possibility to work in a more natural "intuitive" way which is, although not proven yet, a clear advantage that eases precise extirpation of the tumor, as well as the reconstructive part of the operation. Personally, we feel it to be more comfortable operating on complex tumors in this minimally invasive process. Using the robot, we were able to perform minimally invasive procedures with safety for the patient, respecting the oncologic principles and preserving as much renal function as possible. The robot provides the surgeon with better, high-definition stereoscopic, and enlarged vision that proves very helpful in tumor dissection or recognition of the calyceal defects. The fact that the surgeon, the assistant, and the scrub nurse are all sitting during the operation also contributes to less fatigue and consequently better efficacy of the surgical team. These advantages of the robot-assisted partial nephrectomy give us the potential to operate not only on small exophytic tumors but also on more complex cases. The main disadvantages of the robotic-assisted partial nephrectomy are the augmented cost, the need for extra setup time, and the lack of the haptic feedback for the surgeon. One more disadvantage, the need of the console surgeon to view CT, ultrasound, or MRI images and thus disengage from the console is overcome with the use of special equipment as described in the literature.[68] We hope that with the advent of new robotic systems, perhaps from other companies, the cost will reduce with time. The setup time can be minimized if the same team of surgeons, assistants, scrub nurses, and room nurses is used all the time so that they become accustomed to the complexity of the robotic setup. The need to have two fully trained surgeons, one on the patient side and one on the console so that in case of an emergency the bedside surgeon can react while the console surgeon is scrubbing, is one more disadvantage. It remains to be proven whether the advantages outperform the disadvantages and lead to better overall results.

43.1.2 Laparoscopic Nephrectomy (LN)

43.1.2.1 Introduction

In 1990 Clayman et al.,[69] reported their first laparoscopic nephrectomy for benign disease. Over the last 20 years, this procedure has gained popularity and the indications for LN expanded: initially LN was performed for removal of non-functioning kidneys but now it can be considered the preferred approach for many diseases of the kidney. Indeed, laparoscopy is considered a primary and well-standardized modality for managing renal tumors. LN can be performed as a "pure" laparoscopy procedure through a retroperitoneal, transperitoneal approach, or, since 2001,[70] robot-assisted (RALN). We describe LN with attention to indications, oncological outcomes, and complications.

43.1.2.2 Indications and Contraindications

LN is generally indicated for treatment of benign diseases like removal of multicystic kidneys, diseased kidneys causing renovascular hypertension, end-stage ureteropelvic junction obstruction, or non-functioning or chronically infected kidneys. For malignant diseases indications for LN are usually RCC in stage T1 or T2 although removal of tumors up to 12–18 cm has been described by skilled laparoscopists. It is possible to perform LN in RCC stage T3a (tumor beyond the capsule) but only if size limitations permit. Patients with a previous history of abdominal surgery should be treated preferentially with a retroperitoneal approach because this factor can increase the complication rate. *Relative contraindications* for LN consist in tumors with renal vein or caval vein tumor thrombi. *Absolute contraindications* for LN are uncorrected coagulopathy, sepsis, or hypovolemic shock.

43.1.2.3 Oncological Outcomes

Laparoscopic techniques for managing RCC, nowadays, are considered to be safe, following well-established guidelines for surgical dissection.

There are many studies that show that LN is a safe procedure that provides shorter hospital stay, reduced estimated blood loss, decreased pain medication requirements, faster return of bowel activity, improved cosmesis, and an earlier return to full activities compared with open approach.[71–74]

The long-term oncologic outcome of transperitoneal laparoscopic radical nephrectomy (LRN) is comparable to open radical nephrectomy for many authors.[75–79] Permpongkosol et al.[78] compared 67 patients undergone to LRN with 54 undergone to open radical nephrectomy; they reported, for transperitoneal LRN, 10-year DFS, CSS, and actuarial survival rates of 94, 97, and 76%, respectively, that were not statistically different with open surgery (87, 86, and 58%, respectively). When stratified into T1 and T2 categories, patients undergoing transperitoneal LRN had 10-year disease-free, cancer-specific, and actuarial survival rates of 98, 98, and 75%, respectively, compared to 84, 95, and 81%.

Desai et al.[80] published a prospective randomized trial comparing retroperitoneal LRN to transperitoneal LRN. The retroperitoneal technique was associated with more rapid arterial and venous control and decreased total operative time (150 vs 207 min). Both modalities were similar in estimated blood loss, complication rates, analgesia requirements, and length of hospital stay. Berglund et al.[81] demonstrated that retroperitoneal LRN could be performed successfully in obese patients. Obese patients undergoing retroperitoneal LRN had more favorable estimated blood loss, operative times, conversion rates, and hospital stay, although the outcome did not reach significance compared with obese patients managed with transperitoneal LRN.

43.1.2.4 Complications

Complication rates associated with laparoscopic surgery decrease as the experience of the operating surgeon expands. Pareek et al.[82] recently reviewed the reported complications of laparoscopic renal surgery. Overall, 10.7% of patients undergoing a pure LRN experienced a major complication compared with 9.3% of patients who underwent a hand-assisted LRN (no statistical significance). The most frequent major complications in the LRN group included venous and arterial bleeding (1.8 and 1.0%). In the hand-assisted LRN group, the most common major complications

included wound infection (1.5%) and arterial hemorrhage (1.0%). Although the complication rate between LRN and hand-assisted group was not statistically significant the wound infection rates were significantly higher in patients managed with hand-assisted LRN compared with patients treated with pure laparoscopic techniques. Steinberg et al.[73] compared complication rates in patients undergoing open surgery and LRN. Intraoperative complications occurred in 7.2% of patients who were treated with LRN for pT1 tumors, 7.7% of patients who underwent LRN for pT2 tumors, and 17.6% of patients who underwent surgery with standard open techniques for pT2 tumors. Although there was an apparent higher complication rate for the open group, the difference was not statistically significant. The most common intraoperative complication in each of the groups was vascular injury and hemorrhage. The rates of postoperative complications were similar (19.9, 21.5, and 26.5%, respectively).

43.1.2.5 Robot-Assisted Radical Nephrectomy (RAPN)

The first robot-assisted laparoscopic nephrectomy was performed in 2001 by Guillonneau et al.[70] using the Zeus system (Computer Motion). Since that initial report, we do not find significant large series of radical nephrectomy.[83,84] These studies concluded that there are not many advantages or differences over traditional laparoscopy. Nevertheless we are convinced that the technical advantages of the robot system can play a role also in radical nephrectomy. Potential advantages of robotic assistance for radical nephrectomy include a magnified, three-dimensional view, and the articulating robotic instruments that can facilitate precise dissection and ligation of the renal hilar vessels. Rogers et al.[85] presented their experience of 42 patients that underwent RAPN and they concluded that, although it is not possible to claim the superiority of robotic nephrectomy over traditional laparoscopy, it can offer some potential benefits as the use of the fourth robotic arm to do the upward retraction on the kidney, in order to have precise dissection of the renal hilar vessels or the use of the robot in nephrectomy as a training platform for acquiring the robotic skill and experience required for more complex robotic renal surgery cases, such as a partial nephrectomy.

43.2 Benign Disease

43.2.1 Laparoscopic or Robot-Assisted Pyeloplasty

43.2.1.1 Introduction

Up to few years ago, the "gold standard" for the treatment of the ureteropelvic junction (UPJ) obstruction was the open surgery because in "skilled surgeon's hands" it has a success rate of up to 100%.[86–88] Nevertheless, this procedure has shown to have complications and morbidity correlated to the flank incision, especially in young patients. At present, besides open surgery, many minimally invasive endourological procedures are available for the treatment of UPJ obstruction, but they have a long-term success rate lower and not comparable to open surgery (20–25%).[4,5]

Since it was described in 1990s, the laparoscopic approach for UPJ has maintained the high efficacy of the open surgery without the morbidity of the open incision.[89,90] In many centers the laparoscopic approach has completely taken over the open surgery in the treatment of this disease, but its availability is mainly in high-volume laparoscopic centers while it is still limited in urologic community overall.[91] This phenomenon is likely due to the technical demands, which require specialized training and advanced laparoscopic skills. With the introduction of robotic technology the situation has rapidly changed because its advanced characteristics like three dimensional high-definition vision and the great degree of rotation movements allow to overtake the limitations of classical laparoscopy, especially in reconstructive procedures. Robotic-assisted laparoscopic pyeloplasty (RALP) has been shown to be equally effective in the treatment of UPJ obstruction, with a 90–95% success rate.[92–94]

43.2.1.2 Indications

The indications for laparoscopical repair of UPJ obstruction include patients who have a physiologically significant obstruction, intermittent flank pain, hematuria or recurrent urinary tract infections, renal stones, or secondary hypertension. Crossing vessels or duplicated collecting system can be treated laparoscopically and even failed endopyelotomy or failed open pyeloplasty can be managed laparoscopically with excellent outcomes.

43.2.1.3 Laparoscopic Pyeloplasty (LP) vs Robot-Assisted Laparoscopic Pyeloplasty (RALP)

Over the last 20 years, we assisted to an emergent and increasing interest toward LP. Since 1993 to nowadays the laparoscopic technique and skills have improved remarkably, with a consequent reduction of operating time, complications, and conversion rate to open but with a long-term outcome improvement. In literature, there are some reports that compare LP with open approach. Although they are retrospective studies, all of them reach the conclusion that, while the complication rate or intraoperative blood loss was not statistically different, the postoperative pain and the time to return to normal activities were statistically lower in all laparoscopy groups (Table 43.5).[89–99] Over the last 2 decades, with the increasing interest to minimally invasive techniques, robotic assistance is now playing a pivotal role in minimally invasive surgery. LP still has a long learning curve, with limitations that are intrinsic to conventional laparoscopic surgery: laparoscopic suturing is technically demanding and traditionally requires a significant amount of time to master and sometimes a good ability may never be achieved in a reasonable amount of time, because of the infrequency of cases. Once again the robot was initially looked to as a tool to enable more easily transition of surgeons from open to laparoscopic surgery but studies soon showed that the robot was not just a transition tool but in many ways was an improvement compared with standard laparoscopy. Gettman et al.[100] later compared six robot pyeloplasty with six standard laparoscopic pyeloplasty. Mean operative time and suturing time was less for the robot pyeloplasties, but blood loss, hospital stay, and complications were similar. Short-term subjective and imaging results at 3 months were indicative of 100% success. Patel[101] in one of the largest series of complete robot-assisted laparoscopic pyeloplasties with at least 11 months of follow-up described 50 patients undergone to RALP. Crossing vessels were present in 30% of the patients and were preserved in all cases. The operative time

Table 43.5 Main comparative series LP vs open approach

Authors	No. of pts	Success rate	Mean FU (range)	OP. time	Hospital stay	Complication rate
Bauer[89]	Lap 42	98	22 (12–38)	NA	NA	12
	Open 35	94	58 (12–138)	NA	NA	11
Soulié[95]	Lap 26	86	14.3 (6–32)	165 (120–260)	4.5 (3–7)	11.5
	Open 28	86	14.3 (6–32)	145 (80–250)	5.5 (4–9)	14
Klingler[96]	Lap 40	96 (NDP) 73.3	23.4 ± 9.1	NA	5.9 ± 2.1	17.5
	Open 15	93.4	21.9 ± 8.8	NA	13.4 ± 3.8	40.0
Zhang[97]	Lap 56	98	30.2 ± 12.5	80 (70–90) $p < 0.001$	7 (7–8) $p < 0.001$	3.5
	Open 40	98	23.4 ± 9.8	120 (105–125) $p < 0.001$	9 (8–10) $p < 0.001$	7.5
Calvert[98]	Lap 49	98	9	$159 \pm 33\ p < 0.001$	5.4 ± 2.2	20
	Open 51	96	12	$95 \pm 31\ p < 0.001$	5.6 ± 2.1	24
Bonnard[99]	Lap 20	96	24 (12–60)	219 (140–310) $p < 0.001$	2.4 (1–5) $p < 0.001$	NA
	Open 17	100	21 (12–51)	96 (50–150) $p < 0.001$	5 (3–7) $p < 0.001$	NA

(NDP): non-dismembering pyeolplasty

averaged 122 min (range 60–330) overall and the time for the anastomosis averaged 20 min (range 10–100). Most patients were discharged on postoperative day one. The follow-up for UPJ was performed by diuretic renal scan at 1 month, then every 3 months in the first year, then every 6 months for the second year, and then yearly. There were no complications, and blood loss was minimal in all cases. Forty-eight of fifty patients (96%) had both objective and subjective improvement.

There are other comparative studies between LP and RALP showing a shorter hospital stay and operative time. The complication rate is similar and success rate is 100% in both groups[102–104] (Table 43.6). Passerotti et al.,[105] in a recent paper, evaluated the quality of the suture anastomosis and the associated learning curve in RALP, LP, and open surgery on animal models. This interesting study clearly showed that suture anastomosis of the UPJ with robotic assistance was completed in a shorter time compared with freehand laparoscopy and required fewer cases to approach the times of open surgery. The quality of the anastomosis (as measured by patency and minimal leakage) was better in the RALP group compared with the LP group. Moreover the evaluation of quality of anastomosis, by histological assessment of collagen deposition with inflammatory infiltrates and edema, was better in RALP group where the amount of collagen III appeared to be less. The authors concluded that these findings demonstrate how for the inexperienced surgeon, robotic assistance had many distinct advantages over freehand laparoscopy when performing a pyeloplasty.

43.2.1.4 Conclusion

Both robotic and laparoscopic pyeloplasties attempt to emulate open surgery, but, with its three-dimensional, enhanced vision, and greater degree of rotational movement, the robot assistance shows clearly the advantages in dissection and tissue handling. Moreover, RALP offers the same results of a minimally invasive technique in terms of morbidity but with the same functional outcomes of LP. Finally even for the inexperienced surgeon, laparoscopic suturing

Table 43.6 Operative and outcomes main RALP

Authors	No. of pts	OP time (min)	Suturing time (min)	Hospital stay (days)	Success rate (%)	No. of complications (%)	FU (months)
Gettman[100]	6	167.5 ± 8.3	74	4	83	1/6	3
Patel[101]	50	122	20	1.1	96	None	11.7
Bhayani[102]	8	210	NA	2.3	88	1/8	NA
Atug[103]	20	230 ± 21.6	NA	2.5 ± 0.3	95	1/20	3
Weise[104]	31	199 ± 30.5	76	2.6 ± 0.23	100	2/14 (14%)	6 ± 3.3

is easier to learn at the onset with robotic assistance compared with freehand laparoscopy, without compromising the outcomes.

References

1. Jemal A, Siegel R, Ward E, et al. Cancer statistics. *Ca Cancer J Clin.* 2008;58:71–96.
2. Kane CJ, Mallin K, Ritchey J, et al. Renal cell cancer stage migration: analysis of the national cancer data base. *Cancer.* 2008;113(1):78–83.
3. Huang WC, Levey AS, Serio AM, et al. Chronic kidney disease after nephrectomy in patients with renal cortical tumours: a retrospective cohort study. *Lancet Oncol.* 2006;7(9):735–740.
4. Go AS, Chertow GM, Fan D, et al. Chronic kidney disease and the risks of death, cardiovascular events, and hospitalization. *N Engl J Med.* 2004;351(13):1296–1305.
5. Thompson RH, Boorjian SA, Lohse CM, et al. Radical nephrectomy for pT1a renal masses May be associated with decreased overall survival compared with partial nephrectomy. *J Urol.* 2008;179(2):468–471.
6. Schiff JD, Palese M, Vaughan ED Jr, et al. Laparoscopic vs open partial nephrectomy in consecutive patients: the cornell experience. *BJU Int.* 2005;96(6):811–814.
7. Klingler HC, Remzi M, Janetschek G, et al. Benefits of laparoscopic renal surgery are more pronounced in patients with a high body mass index. *Eur Urol.* 2003;43(5):522–527.
8. Uzzo R, Novick A. Nephron-sparing surgery for renal tumors: indications, techniques, and outcomes. *J Urol.* 2001;166(1):6–18.
9. Williams CS, Pinto PA. Laparoscopic partial nephrectomy. In: Bishoff JA, Kavoussi LR, eds. *Atlas of Laparoscopic Urologic Surgery*, Philadelphia, PA: WB Saunders; 2007:110–120.
10. Janetschek G. Laparoscopic partial nephrectomy: how far have we gone? *Curr Opin Urol.* 2007;17(5):316–321.
11. Novick AC. Renal-sparing surgery for renal cell carcinoma. *Urol Clin North Am.* 1993;20(2):277–282.
12. Oakley NE, Hegarty NJ, McNeill A, et al. Minimally invasive nephron-sparing surgery for renal cell cancer. *BJU Int.* 2006;98(2):278–284.
13. Simmons MN, Chung BI, Gill IS. Perioperative efficacy of laparoscopic partial nephrectomy for tumors larger than 4 cm. *Eur Urol.* 2008;55:199–208.
14. Simmons MN, Weight CJ, Gill IS. Laparoscopic Radical Versus Partial Nephrectomy For Tumors >4 Cm: Intermediate-Term Oncologic And Functional Outcomes. *Urology.* 2009;73(5):1077–1082.
15. Fergany AF, et al. Long-term results of nephron sparing surgery for localized renal cell carcinoma: 10-year followup. *J Urol.* 2000;163(2):442–445.
16. Permpongkosol S, Bagga HS, Romero FR, et al. Laparoscopic versus open partial nephrectomy for the treatment of pathological T1N0M0 renal cell carcinoma: a 5-year survival rate. *J Urol.* 2006;176:1984–1988.
17. Gill IS, Kavoussi LR, Lane BR, Blute ML, Babineau D, Colombo JR Jr, et al. Comparison of 1,800 laparoscopic and open partial nephrectomies for single renal tumors. *J Urol.* 2007 July;178(1):41–46.
18. Lane BR, Gill IS. 5-Year outcomes of laparoscopic partial nephrectomy. *J Urol.* 2007 Jan;177(1):70–74.
19. Gill IS, Colombo JR, et al. Laparoscopic partial nephrectomy in solitary kidney. *J Urol.* 2006;175:454–458.
20. Gong EM, Orvieto MA, Zorn KC, et al. Comparison of laparoscopic and open partial nephrectomy in clinical T(1a) renal tumors. *J Endourol.* 2008;22:953–958.
21. Marszalek M, Meixl H, Polajnar M, Rauchenwald M, Jeschke K, Madersbacher S. Laparoscopic and open partial nephrectomy: a matched-pair comparison of 200 patients. *Eur Urol.* 2009;55:1171–1178.
22. Deane LA, Lee HJ, Box GN, et al. Robotic versus standard laparoscopic partial/wedge nephrectomy: a comparison of intraoperative and perioperative results from a single institution. *J Endourol.* 2008;22:947–952.
23. Rogers CG, Menon M, Weise ES, et al. Robotic partial nephrectomy: a multi-institutional analysis. *J Robotic Surg.* 2008;2(3):141–143.
24. Mottrie A, Koliakos N, DeNaeyer G, et al. Tuomor evinucleoresection in robot-assisted partial nephrectomy. *J Robotic Surg.* 2009;3(2):65–69.
29. Porpiglia F, Fiori C, Terrone C, Bollito E, Fontana D, Scarpa RM. Assessment of surgical margins in renal cell carcinoma after nephron sparing: a comparative study: laparoscopy vs open surgery. *J Urol.* 2005;173:1098.
26. Moinzadeh A, Gill IS, Finelli A, Kaouk J, Desai M. Laparoscopic partial nephrectomy: 3-year followup. *J Urol.* 2006;175:459.
27. Moinzadeh A, Gill IS, Finelli A, Kaouk J, Desai M. Laparoscopic partial nephrectomy: 3-year followup. *J Urol.* 2006;175:459.
28. Venkatesh R, Weld K, Ames CD, Figenshau SR, Sundaram CP, Andriole GL, et al. Laparoscopic partial nephrectomy for renal masses: effect of tumor location. *Urology.* 2006;67:1169.
29. Thompson RH, Leibovich BC, Lohse CM, Zincke H, Blute ML. Complications of contemporary open nephron sparing surgery: a single institution experience. *J Urol.* 2005;174:855.
30. Sutherland SE, Resnick MI, Maclennan GT, Goldman HB. Does the size of the surgical margin in partial nephrectomy for renal cell cancer really matter? *J Urol.* 2002;167:61.
31. Porpiglia F, Volpe A, Billia M, Scarpa RM. Laparoscopic versus open partial nephrectomy: analysis of the current literature. *Eur Urol.* 2008;53(4):732–742.
32. Permpongkosol S, Colombo JR Jr, Gill IS, Kavoussi LR. Positive surgical parenchymal margin after laparoscopic partial nephrectomy for renal cell carcinoma: oncological outcomes. *J Urol.* 2006;176:2401–2404.
33. Yossepowitch O, Thompson RH, Leibovich BC, et al. Positive surgical margins at partial nephrectomy: predictors and oncological outcomes. *J Urol.* 2008;179(6):2158–2163.
34. Ukimura O, Haber GP, Remer EM, Gill IS. Laparoscopic partial nephrectomy for incidental stage pt2 or worse tumors. *Urology.* 2006;68(5):976–982.

35. Rais-Bahrami S, Romero FR, Lima GC, Kohanim S, Permpongkosol S, Trock BJ, et al. Elective laparoscopic partial nephrectomy in patients with tumors >4 cm. *Urology*. 2008;72(3):580–583.

36. Gill IS, Colombo JR Jr, Frank I, Moinzadeh A, Kaouk J, Desai M. Laparoscopic partial nephrectomy for hilar tumors. *J Urol*. 2005;174:850.

37. Lattouf JB, Beri A, D'Ambros OF, Grull M, Leeb K, Janetschek G. Laparoscopic partial nephrectomy for hilar tumors: technique and results. *Eur Urol*. 2008;54(2):409–416.

38. Lam JS, Bergman J, Breda A, Schulam PG. Importance of surgical margins in the management of renal cell carcinoma. *Nat Clin Pract Urol*. 2008;5:308–317.

39. Rogers CG, Metwalli A, Blatt AM, Bratslavsky G, Menon M, Linehan WM, et al. Robotic partial nephrectomy for renal hilar tumors: a multi-institutional analysis. *J Urol*. 2008;180(6):2353–2356.

40. Rogers CG, Singh A, Blatt AM, et al. Robotic partial nephrectomy for complex renal tumors: surgical technique. *Eur Urol*. 2008;53:514–523.

41. Shapiro E, Benway B, Wang AJ, Bhayani S. The role of nephron-sparing robotic surgery in the management of renal malignancy. *Curr Opin Urol*. 2009;19:76–80.

42. Rassweiler J, Tsivian A, Kumar AV, et al. Oncological safety of laparoscopic surgery for urological malignancy: experience with more than 1,000 operations. *J Urol*. 2003;169(6):2072–2075.

43. Lee BR, Tan BJ, Smith AD. Laparoscopic port site metastases: incidence, risk factors, and potential preventive measures. *Urology*. 2005;65(4):639–644.

44. Rane A, Eng MK, Keeley FX. Port site metastases. *Curr Opin Urol*. 2008;18:185–189.

45. Castillo OA, Vitagliano G, Diaz M, et al. Port-site metastasis after laparoscopic partial nephrectomy: case report and literature review. *J Endourol*. 2007;21(4):404–407.

46. Uson AC. Tumor recurrence in the renal fossa and/or the abdominal wall after radical nephrectomy for renal cell carcinoma. *Prog Clin Biol Res*. 1982;100:549–560.

47. Simmons MN, Schreiber MJ, Gill IS. Surgical renal ischemia: a contemporary overview. *J Urol*. 2008;180: 19–30.

48. Beri A, Lattouf JB, Deambros O, Grull M, Gschwendtner M, Ziegerhofer J, et al. Partial nephrectomy using renal artery perfusion for cold ischemia: functional and oncologic outcomes. *J Endourol*. 2008;22(6):1285–1290.

49. Landman J, Rehman J, Sundaram CP, Bhayani S, Monga M, Pattaras JG, et al. Renal hypothermia achieved by retrograde intracavitary saline perfusion. *J Endourol*. 2002;16(7):445–449.

50. Guillonneau B, Bermudez H, Gholami S, et al. Laparoscopic partial nephrectomy for renal tumor: single-center experience comparing clamping and no clamping techniques of the renal vasculature. *J Urol*. 2003;169(2):483–486.

51. Abukora F, Albqami N, Nambirajan T, et al. Long term functional outcome of renal units after laparoscopic nephron-sparing surgery under cold ischemia. *J Endourol*. 2006;20(10):790–793.

52. Fergany AF, Saad IR, Woo L, Novick AC. Open partial nephrectomy for tumor in a solitary kidney: experience with 400 cases. *J Urol*. 2006;175(5):1630–1633. discussion 1633.

53. Bhayani S, Rha KH, Pinto PA, et al. Laparoscopic partial nephrectomy: effect of warm ischemia on serum creatinine. *J Urol*. 2004;72:1264–1266.

54. Desai MM, Gill IS, Ramani AP, Spaliviero M, Rybicki L, Kaouk JH. The impact of warm ischaemia on renal function after laparoscopic partial nephrectomy. *BJU*. 2005;95:377–383.

55. Porpiglia F, Renard J, Billia M, et al. Is renal warm ischemia over 30 minutes during laparoscopic partial nephrectomy possible? One-year results of a prospective study. *Eur Urol*. 2007;52(4):1170–1178.

56. Baumert H, Ballaro A, Shah N, et al. Reducing warm ischaemia time during laparoscopic partial nephrectomy: a prospective comparison of two renal closure techniques. *Eur Urol*. 2007;52(4):1164–1169.

57. Bollens R, Rosenblatt A, Espinoza BP, et al. Laparoscopic partial nephrectomy with on-demand clamping reduces warm ischemia time. *Eur Urol*. 2007;52(3):804–809.

58. Nguyen MM, Gill IS. Halving ischemia time during laparoscopic partial nephrectomy. *J Urol*. 2008;179: 627–632.

59. Verhoest G, Manunta A, Bensalah K, Vincendeau S, Rioux-Leclercq N, Guillé F, et al. Laparoscopic partial nephrectomy with clamping of the renal parenchyma: initial experience. *Eur Urol*. 2007;52(5):1340–1346.

60. Aron M, Koenig P, Kaouk JH, et al. Robotic and laparoscopic partial nephrectomy: a matched-pair comparison from a high volume centre. *BJU Int*. 2008;102:86–92.

61. Caruso RP, Phillips CK, Kau E, Taneja SS, Stifelman MD. Robot assisted laparoscopic partial nephrectomy: initial experience. *J Urol*. 2006;176:36–39.

62. Wang AJ, Bhayani S. Robot partial nephrectomy versus laparoscopic partial nephrectomy for renal cell carcinoma: single-surgeon analysis of > 100 consecutive procedures. *Urology*. 2009;73 (2):306–310.

63. De Naeyer G, Sangalli M, Schatteman P, Carpentier P, Fonteyne E, Mottrie A. Robot-assisted laparoscopic partial nephrectomy: results of first 50 cases with analysis of learning curve. Abstract WCE092724 presented at 27th World Congress of Endourology, 2009 Munich.

64. Benway B, Wang A, Cabello JM, Bhayani SB. Robotic partial nephrectomy with sliding-clip renorrhaphy: technique and outcomes. *Eur Urol*. 2009;55(3): 592–599.

65. Ho H, Schwentner C, Neururer R, Steiner H, Bartsch G, Peschel R. Robotic-assisted laparoscopic partial nephrectomy: surgical technique and clinical outcomes at 1 year. *BJU Int*. 2009;103(5):663–668.

66. Simmons MN, Gill IS. Decreased complications of contemporary laparoscopic partial nephrectomy: use of a standardized reporting system. *J Urol*. 2007;177(6):2067–2073.

67. Zimmermann R, Janetschek G. Complications of laparoscopic partial nephrectomy. *World J Urol*. 2008;26(6): 531–537.

68. Bhayani SB, Snow DC. Novel dynamic information integration during da Vinci robotic partial nephrectomy and radical nephrectomy. *J Robot Surg*. 2008;2: 67–69.

69. Clayman RV, Kavoussi LR, Soper NJ, et al. Laparoscopic nephrectomy: initial case report. *J Urol.* 1991;146: 278–282.

70. Guillonneau B, Jayet C, Tewari A, Vallancien G. Robot assisted laparoscopic nephrectomy. *J Urol.* 2001;166:200–201.

71. McDougall E, Clayman RV, Elashry OM. Laparoscopic radical nephrectomy for renal tumor: the Washington university experience. *J Urol.* 1996;155:1180–1185.

72. Dunn MD, Portis AJ, Shalhav AL, et al. Laparoscopic versus open radical nephrectomy: a 9-year experience. *J Urol.* 2000;164:1153–1159.

73. Steinberg AP, Finelli A, Desai MM, et al. Laparoscopic radical nephrectomy for large (greater than 7 cm, T2) renal tumors. *J Urol.* 2004;172 (6 pt 1):2172–2176.

74. Allan JD, Tolley DA, Kaouk JH, et al. Laparoscopic radical nephrectomy. *Eur Urol.* 2001;40:17–23.

75. Chan DY, Cadeddu JA, Jarrett TW, et al. Laparoscopic radical nephrectomy: cancer control for renal cell carcinoma. *J Urol.* 2001;166:2095–2099. discussion 2099–2100.

76. Ono Y, Kinukawa T, Hattori R, et al. The long-term outcome of laparoscopic radical nephrectomy for small renal cell carcinoma. *J Urol.* 2001;165 (6 pt 1):1867–1870.

77. Portis AJ, Yan Y, Landman J, et al. Long-term followup after laparoscopic radical nephrectomy. *J Urol.* 2002;167:1257–1262.

78. Permpongkosol S, Chan DY, Link RE, et al. Long-term survival analysis after laparoscopic radical nephrectomy. *J Urol.* 2005;174(4 pt 1):1222–1225.

79. Saika T, Ono Y, Hattori R, et al. Long-term outcome of laparoscopic radical nephrectomy for pathologic T1 renal cell carcinoma. *Urology.* 2003;62:1018–1023.

80. Desai MM, Strzempkowski B, Matin SF, et al. Prospective randomized comparison of transperitoneal versus retroperitoneal laparoscopic radical nephrectomy. *J Urol.* 2005;173:38–41.

81. Berglund RK, Gill IS, Babineau D, et al. A prospective comparison of transperitoneal and retroperitoneal laparoscopic nephrectomy in the extremely obese patient. *BJU Int.* 2007;16:871–874.

82. Pareek G, Hedican SP, Gee JR, et al. Meta-analysis of the complications of laparoscopic renal surgery: comparison of procedures and techniques. *J Urol.* 2006;175:1208–1213.

83. Klingler DW, Hemstreet GP, Balaji KC. Feasibility of robotic radical nephrectomy–initial results of single-institution pilot study. *Urology.* 2005;65:1086–1089.

84. Nazemi T, Galich A, Sterrett S, Klingler D, Smith L, Balaji KC. Radical nephrectomy performed by open, laparoscopy with or without handassistance or robotic methods by the same surgeon produces comparable perioperative results. *Int Braz J Urol.* 2006;32:15–22.

85. Rogers C, Laungani R, Krane LS, Bhandari A, Bhandari M, Menon M. Robotic nephrectomy for the treatment of benign and malignant disease. *BJU Int.* 2008;102(11):1660–1665.

86. Cogus C, Karamursel T, Tokatli Z, Yaman O, Ozdiler E, Cogus O. Long-term results of Anderson-Hynes pyeloplasty in 180 adults in the era of endourologic procedures. *Urol Int.* 2004;73:11–14.

87. O'Reilly PH, Brooman PJ, Mak S, et al. The long-term results of Anderson-Hynes pyeloplasty. *BJU Int.* 2001;87:287–289.

88. Arun N, Kekre NS, Nath V, Gopalakrishnan G. Is open pyeloplasty still justified? *Br J Urol.* 1997;80:379–381.

89. Bauer JJ, Bishoff JT, Moore RG, Chen RN, Iverson AJ, Kavoussi LR. Laparoscopic versus open pyeloplasty: assessment of objective and subjective outcome. *J Urol.* 1999;162:692–695.

90. Klinger HC, Remzi M, Janetschek G, Kratzik C, Marberger MJ. Comparison of open versus laparoscopic pyeloplasty techniques in treatment of ureteropelvic junction obstruction. *Eur Urol.* 2003;44: 340–344.

91. Eden CG. Minimally invasive treatment of ureteropelvic junction obstruction: a critical analysis of results. *Eur Urol.* 2007;52:983.

92. Atug F, Woods M, Burgess SV, et al. Robotic assisted laparoscopic pyeloplasty in children. *J Urol.* 2005;174:1440–1442.

93. Lee RS, Retik AB, Borer JG, et al. Pediatric robot assisted laparoscopic dismembered pyeloplasty: comparison with a cohort of open surgery. *J Urol.* 2006;175: 683–687.

94. Olsen LH, Rawashdeh YF, Jorgensen TM. Pediatric robot assisted retroperitoneoscopic pyeloplasty: a 5-year experience. *J Urol.* 2007;178:2137–2141.

95. Soulie M, Thoulouzan M, Seguin P, et al. Retroperitoneal laparoscopic versus open pyeloplasty with a minimal incision: comparison of two surgical approaches. *Urology.* 2001;57:443–447.

96. Klingler HC, Remzi M, Janetschek G, Kratzik C, Marberger MJ. Comparison of open versus laparoscopic pyeloplasty techniques in treatment of uretero-pelvic junction obstruction. *Eur Urol.* 2003;44:340–344.

97. Zhang X, Li HZ, Ma X, et al. Retrospective comparison of retroperitoneal laparoscopic versus open dismembered pyeloplasty for ureteropelvic junction obstruction. *J Urol.* 2006;176:1077.

98. Calvert RC, Morsy MM, Zelhof B, Rhodes M, Burgess. NA. Comparison of laparoscopic and open pyeloplasty in 100 patients with pelvi-ureteric junction obstruction. *Surg Endosc.* 2008;22(2):411–414.

99. Bonnard A, Fouquet V, Carricaburu E, Aigrain Y, El-Ghoneimi A. Retroperitoneal laparoscopic versus open pyeloplasty in children. *J Urol.* 2005;173(5): 1710–1713.

100. Gettman M, Peschel R, Neururer R. A comparison of laparoscopic pyeloplasty performed with the da Vinci robotic system versus standard laparoscopic techniques: initial clinical results. *Eur Urol.* 2002;42: 453–458.

101. Patel V. Robot-assisted laparoscopic dismembered pyeloplasty. *Urology.* 2005;66:45–49.

102. Bhayani SB, Link RE, Varkarakis JM, Kavoussi LR. Complete da Vinci versus laparoscopic pyeloplasty: cost analysis. *J Endourol.* 2005;19:327–332.

103. Atug F, Burgess S, Mendez-Torres F, Castle E, Thomas R. Laparoscopic pyeloplasty for ureteropelvic junction obstruction: comparing da Vinci robotic to classic laparoscopic pyeloplasty. *Eur Urol.* 2005;4(Suppl 3):196.

104. Weise ES, Winfield HN. Robotic computer-assisted pyelo-plasty versus conventional laparoscopic pyeloplasty. *J Endourol*. 2006;20:813–819.

105. Passerotti CC, Passerotti AM, Dall'Oglio MF, et al. Comparing the quality of the suture anastomosis and the learning curves associated with performing open, free-hand, and robotic-assisted laparoscopic pyeloplasty in a swine animal model. *J Am Coll Surg*. 2009;208:576–586.

106. Kaul S, Laungani R, Sarle R, et al. Da Vinci-assisted robotic partial nephrectomy: technique and results at a mean of 15 months of follow-up. *Eur Urol*. 2007;51: 186–192.

107. Bhayani SB, Das N. Robotic assisted laparoscopic partial nephrectomy for suspected renal cell carcinoma: retro-spective review of surgical outcomes of 35 cases. *Bmc Surg*. 2008;24;8(16):1–4.

Part V
Bladder

Chapter 44

Robot-Assisted Radical Cystectomy in Male: Technique of Spaces

Matthew H. Hayn, Piyush K. Agarwal, and Khurshid A. Guru

Robot-assisted radical cystectomy (RARC) is an alternative approach for treatment of bladder cancer. The technique of RARC allows precise and rapid removal of the bladder with minimal blood loss, which is theoretically translated into minimal morbidity with equivalent success to open surgery for the patient. Herein, we describe the operative technique of RARC in the male and robot-assisted extended pelvic lymph node dissection along with a brief review of the published literature. The potential advantages of robot-assisted surgery can be transferred in complex and advanced uro-oncologic surgery such as bladder surgery. However, long-term oncological and functional outcomes are yet awaited.

44.1 Introduction

Radical cystectomy and urinary diversion remain the cornerstone for the surgical management of bladder cancer.[1,2] Despite its effectiveness, the procedure is associated with significant morbidity with mortality rates approaching 2%.[1,3,4] Within urology, surgeons have embraced minimally invasive surgery to decrease the impact of disease treatment in our patients, which has been clearly seen by the shift in approach to radical nephrectomy[5] and radical prostatectomy.[6]

The first laparoscopic simple cystectomy was reported in 1992 by Parra et al. describing the removal of a benign retained bladder.[7] The first series of robot-assisted radical cystectomy (RARC) was published in 2003 by Menon et al.[8] Since that time, numerous other RARC series have been published.[9–14] Potential benefits of laparoscopic and robotic approaches include less surgical blood loss, early return of bowel function, and more rapid postoperative convalescence. Recently, Ng et al. reported decreased blood loss, transfusion rate, hospital stay, and complication rate with RARC compared to open radical cystectomy.[10]

In the last decade significant advances have been made in minimally invasive approach to surgical procedures. The use of the da Vinci® surgical system (Intuitive Surgical, Sunnyvale, California) with its 10 × magnification and 3D view of the pelvis has provided the opportunity to appreciate the pelvic anatomy beyond what has been previously possible. The primary goal of a radical oncologic procedure is to not only extirpate the tumor with negative margins but also attempt to best preserve the relevant important anatomic structures. A detailed knowledge of the surgical anatomy and application of contemporary technology has redefined pelvic surgery and made it much easier to achieve a balance. This has allowed for a more precise definition of anatomic structures than has been described by open techniques for procedures like prostatectomy, hysterectomy, or cystectomy. Modifications in techniques have been possible because of better visualization and appreciation of anatomy. This approach of robot-assisted radical cystectomy has been developed based on personal experience of over 150 consecutive cases at Roswell Park Cancer Institute. The pelvic cavity is wide and enclosed with important structures such as vessels, nerves, and viscera. The use of the pelvic anatomic spaces helps one in avoiding dissection close

K.A. Guru (✉)
Roswell Park Cancer Institute, Buffalo, NY, USA
e-mail: khurshid.guru@roswellpark.org

A.K. Hemal, M. Menon (eds.), *Robotics in Genitourinary Surgery*,
DOI 10.1007/978-1-84882-114-9_44, © Springer-Verlag London Limited 2011

to the pelvic viscera and makes the procedure onco-logically sound. This report summarizes the anatomic basis and provides a detailed explanation of the steps used in our technique. The new era of robot-assisted surgery dictates standardization of anatomical land-marks which could help the novice robotic surgeon approach the pelvis in the correct fashion and avoid scattered personal trials and failed attempts.

44.2 Surgical Technique

44.2.1 Pelvic Anatomy Overview

Male surgical anatomy of the pelvis in view of robot-assisted radical cystectomy (RARC) is divided into three avascular spaces: the periureteral space, the lat-eral pelvic space, and the anterior rectal space.

44.2.2 Periureteral Space

The periureteral space is formed by the space con-tained within the edges of the incised posterior peri-toneum proximally to the bifurcation of the iliac vessels and distally up to the ureterovesical junc-tion (Fig. 44.1). The pelvic ureters are contained within the space with the vascular pedicle to the blad-der located laterally (superior vesical artery and the obliterated umbilical ligament) and proximally bor-dered by the angle formed by the bifurcation of the iliac vessels. The pelvic portion of the ureter con-stitutes the landmark to initiate the dissection for RARC.

44.2.2.1 Lateral Pelvic Space

The lateral pelvic space is bordered medially by the lateral wall of the bladder, laterally by the pelvic side wall, anteriorly by the iliac vessels, and posteriorly by the obturator vessels and nerves which pass into the obturator foramen (Fig. 44.2). The limit of the depth of the space can be identified by the perirectal fat seen lateral and posterior to the bladder and distally by the endopelvic fascia. This space may occasionally contain the accessory pudendal artery which ideally needs to be preserved.

44.2.2.2 Anterior Rectal Space

The space constitutes the rectum posterior and the bladder with the prostate and the seminal vesicles ante-rior. The lateral boundary is constituted by the vascular pedicles and the neurovascular bundles. This space is separated typically between the anterior and the posterior Denonvillier's fascia (Fig. 44.3).

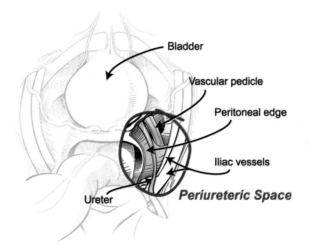

Fig. 44.1 Periureteric space

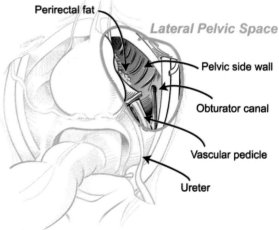

Fig. 44.2 Lateral pelvic space

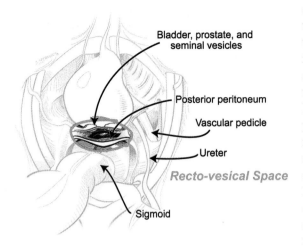

Bladder, prostate, and
seminal vesicles

Posterior peritoneum

Vascular pedicle

Ureter

Recto-vesical Space

Sigmoid

Fig. 44.3 Recto-vesical space

44.2.3 Positioning

RARC is performed under general endotracheal anesthesia. The patient is placed in supine position with adequate padding of pressure points. Gel pads are used across the chest in a crisscross manner. Foam crates are placed under the elbow and the hand which is kept in flexed position with a gauze roll inside the palm. The arms are tucked inside the side of the bed with help of a transversely placed sheet. The legs are placed in a modified lithotomy position in stirrups. At this point the patient is placed in steep Trendelenburg position. This position elevates the pelvis on a fulcrum at the level of the greater trochanter making the pelvic cavity less deep.

44.2.4 Port Placement

After draping the patient, a Foley catheter is inserted in a sterile fashion. We prefer to place all ports in the final steep Trendelenburg position. Pneumoperitoneum is achieved using a periumbilical incision with a Veress needle. Once a pressure of 12–14 mmHg is reached the 12 mm camera port is introduced preferably in the left supra-umblical area and the abdominal and pelvic cavities are inspected. A 30° up lens is used to place other five ports under direct vision. Two 8 mm ports are placed for the right and left robotic arms, respectively, 8–10 cm laterally on a line joining the umbilicus

and the anterior superior iliac spine. The right assistant port uses a 15 mm port which is placed two to three finger breadths above the anterior iliac spine and is used for retraction, suture exchange, application of staplers, and hemostatic clips. We prefer a 15 mm port to ease the introduction of a vascular stapler and a larger specimen bag to accommodate the radical cysto-prostatectomy specimen. The fifth port is the 5 mm right upper quadrant port which is placed between the camera port and the right robotic arm and is used for suction purposes. The sixth port is placed on the left lateral aspect as mirror image from the right lateral assistant port, two to three finger breadths above the anterior superior iliac spine (Fig. 44.4). The fourth robotic arm should not be placed in the same line as the left robotic arm as they tend to clash during the procedure. The robot is docked and camera is switched to a 0° lens for the remainder of the case. Occasionally we have utilized a 30° down lens for deeper pelvises.

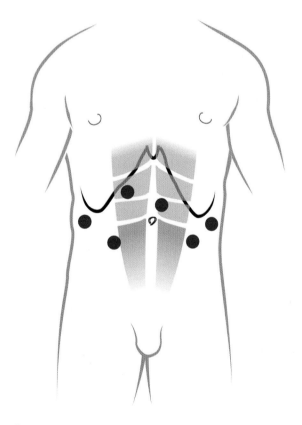

Fig. 44.4 Port placement

44.2.5 Surgical Steps

Once the ports are placed the key landmarks in the pelvis are examined. Examining and freeing the lateral paracolic space especially sigmoid adhesions is helpful. The goal is to define three avascular spaces (periureteral, lateral pelvic space, and anterior rectal spaces) and complete anatomic dissection of all critical portions of RARC.

44.2.5.1 Development of Periureteral Space

The peristalsis of the ureter with aid of magnification and 3D vision help in defining the landmarks for separating out the spaces. The incision of the posterior peritoneum is carried out with separation of the visceral fascia and identification of the ureter in the loose areolar tissue. The periureteral space is opened with mobilization and dissection of the ureter distally up to the ureterovesical junction. Preservation of the periureteral adventitial tissue is critical to ensure viability. Proximal mobilization of the ureter is carried out up to the aortic bifurcation which will later aid in completion of an extended lymph node dissection. One of the caveats in this technique is to avoid early clipping of the ureter during initial dissection. The intact distal ureters serve as a landmark in identifying the lateral pedicles and help optimize negative surgical margins.

44.2.5.2 Development of Lateral Pelvic Space

After completion of development of the periureteral space, an incision of the posterior peritoneum is carried parallel and lateral to the umbilical ligaments onto the anterior abdominal wall above the superior pubis ramus, which helps one in developing the second space, the lateral pelvic space. This avascular, areolar space is opened following the medial curve of the rami of the pubic bone. The vas deferens is seen traversing across underneath the posterior peritoneum and is divided to access the lateral pelvic space. The bladder is still left attached to the anterior abdominal wall as it provides natural anterior retraction. Once the avascular lateral pelvic space is developed one is able to identify the levator ani muscle on the lateral pelvic side wall and the lateral and posterior aspects of the bladder

can be identified medially. Blunt cold division of the tiny vessels traversing through the fat can cause annoying bleeding and these should be point cauterized. Occasionally, an accessory pudendal artery is encountered in the space and is preferably preserved. Once dissection of periureteral and lateral pelvic spaces is complete one should be able to identify the distal ureter up to the ureterovesical junction at the medial edge of the dissection and the vascular pedicle arising from the anterior division of the internal iliac (hypogastric) artery. The external iliac vessels as well as the obturator nerve and vessels are recognized on the lateral aspect of the pelvic space. Both the periureteral and lateral pelvic spaces are separated by the ureter and the posterolateral pedicle arising from the internal iliac vessels. The external iliac vessels, obturator nerve, and vessels constitute the lateral boundary of both the spaces.

44.2.5.3 Development of Anterior Rectal Space

Once the periureteral and lateral pelvic spaces are defined bilaterally the anterior rectal space is developed. The two lateral incisions of the posterior peritoneum are joined together at the peritoneal reflection of the pouch of Douglas. The dissection of this space is carried distally to the apex of the prostate. The plane between the anterior sheath of Denonvillier's fascia and the rectum is easily accessible. Blunt dissection following the anterior rectal wall is continued caudally. This plane is difficult to access if dissection is directed more proximally closer to the seminal vesicles and the prostate. This plane has been used in patients with tumors away from this area and who desire maximal preservation of sexual function. Using a 0° lens, the anterior rectal fibers which are adherent to the apex of the prostate can be clearly seen. Careful blunt and sharp dissection using a cold round tip scissors is preferred to separate the rectum from the prostatic apex. Use of the electrocautery hook or a hot scissors in this area may result in rectal injury.

44.2.5.4 Control of Vascular Pedicles and Mobilization of Neurovascular Bundles

The bladder is left suspended from the anterior abdominal wall while posterior dissection is completed.

Anterior and lateral traction on the bladder using the fourth arm with a cobra grasper would help expose the lateral vascular pedicles of the bladder. The distal UV junction is identified and the ureters are ligated with two Weck Hem-o-lok® clips (Teleflex Medical, Research Triangle Park, North Carolina). The distal ureteral margins are sent for frozen pathologic section. Other surgeons place pre-tagged Weck clips on the distal ureters that help with later identification. For those patients undergoing extracorporeal urinary diversion, both ureteral tags can then be clipped to the tag on the specimen bag to allow easy identification once the open incision is made. Based on the tumor stage and need for nerve preservation the dissection is either carried near the base of the bladder at the tip of the seminal vesicles or behind the planes of the Denonvillier's fascia. An endovascular stapling device or Hem-o-lok® clips can be used to secure the lateral pedicles in an expeditious fashion. In patients with locally advanced disease and the need for non-nerve-sparing radical excision we advocate wider excision of pedicle with the endovascular stapler. The landmark for identifying the inferior vesical pedicle is the appearance of the "fat pad." After controlling the inferior vesical vessels, the endopelvic fascia is opened bilaterally. Some surgeons advocate opening the endopelvic fascia earlier as they finish the lateral pelvic space dissection. This is done in order to help define the end of the vascular pedicle and provide a good landmark when doing the posterior dissection near the apex.

44.2.5.5 Anterior Exposure and Apical Dissection

Incision of the median and medial umbilical ligaments to release the bladder from the anterior abdominal wall is carried out once the posterior dissection is complete. The bladder will drop posteriorly. Dissection of the retropubic fat is performed and the superficial dorsal vein is cauterized. Suture ligation of the deep venous complex is performed; further release of the prostate is accomplished once the deep dorsal complex is incised. Once the proximal membranous urethra is skeletonized, the urethral catheter is removed. A Hem-o-lok® clip is applied just distal to the apex to prevent urine spillage. After incision of the urethra the specimen is placed in a retrieval bag and removed from the pelvic cavity. The pelvic cavity is irrigated and

the area is examined for any bleeding. Control of any bleeding and irrigation of the pelvis with sterile water is thoroughly performed with approximately 1 L of irrigation.

44.2.5.6 Crossing of the Ureter

Once the extended lymph node dissection is completed the ureters are evaluated for length and further mobilization. The ureters are mobilized as proximal as possible with the ureter held retracted with the fourth robotic arm or the right assistant. Occasionally one may need to sacrifice the branch of the common iliac vessels feeding the ureter for further mobilization. The lateral edge of the right side of the posterior peritoneum is lifted and dissection carried with the mobilization of the sigmoid. The sigmoid is left suspended by the fourth robotic arm while performing the posterior dissection. After the dissection the right assistant passes a MicroFrance grasper underneath the dissected space and the console surgeon is able to see the protruding tips of the grasper on the left side. The tag of the ureter is passed into the jaws of the MicroFrance grasper and transferred underneath the sigmoid colon across to the right side. The point of ureteral crossing is closely inspected to make sure that the ureter is not kinked or twisted.

44.2.6 Extended Lymph Node Dissection (Release and Roll Technique)

Once the cystectomy specimen is moved away from the pelvic cavity, adequate space is available for the node dissection. We prefer to perform this after completion of the cystectomy based on more available space to work freely, especially after resecting larger exophytic tumors. The ureter has already been mobilized proximally allowing one to view the vessels below the aortic bifurcation. Our initial approach starts with retraction of the posterior peritoneum by the right-sided assistant with a MicroFrance grasper. The gonadal vessels and the genitofemoral nerve are identified. The nodal tissue is mobilized off the psoas muscle by dividing the fibro-areolar attachments while paying attention and avoiding any injury to the genitofemoral nerve. The nodal tissue is lifted off the muscle and swept medially by point cauterizing the small fibrovascular attachments, which are controlled and incised by the round tip scissors.

Once this tissue package is dissected medially en bloc in what we describe as the "release and roll" technique. The edge of the common and external iliac artery can be identified. Distally the node of Cloquet is dissected with the lymphatic channels cauterized or clipped using small Weck clips, while paying attention to the confluence of circumflex iliac vessels, accessory obturator, and the inferior epigastric artery. Once the nodal package is dissected off the common and external iliac artery attention is paid to identify the iliac vein which typically appears flat due to pneumoperitoneum. In case of difficulty the right assistant can decrease the pneumoperitoneum to distend the iliac vein for better visualization. The whole package is mobilized and rolled medially as each vascular structure is identified and visualized.

Once this is completed attention is paid to the obturator package medial to the iliac vein. The nodal package is gently mobilized to identify the pubic bone and this helps define the plane of the dissection. Further medial mobilization is used to clear the nodal package off the pubic bone after which the obturator nerve is identified and skeletonized. Occasionally the obturator vessels may need to be sacrificed in order to completely clean out the obturator fossa. Once this package is mobilized, the obturator package is removed from underneath the proximal external iliac vein around the obturator nerve. The nodal package is skeletonized off the iliac vessels, nerve, and the pelvic side wall and rolled medially into the pelvis. We believe that the whole package has to be left en bloc without cutting into the package in order to optimize oncologic care. The vessels of the anterior division of the iliac vessels are then identified and skeletonized.

The cobra grasper is used to retract the sigmoid colon medially and clearly identify the common iliac vessels up to and around the bifurcation of the aorta. After identifying the vessels the nodal package is lifted and dissected away from the vessels and clipped proximally at the aortic bifurcation. After the dissection one should be able to identify the underlying common iliac vessels especially the vein. Once this is completed attention is paid to define the Triangle of Marcille.[15] The investing fascia is dissected off the psoas fascia in order to mobilize the iliac vessels medially. The fascia

is dissected distally for easy mobilization. Arterial branch of the common iliac artery needs to be controlled as it enters the psoas muscle. Once this vessel is controlled attention is paid to the collapsed hidden iliac vein from which the nodal package has been removed without injuring the obturator nerve. At completion of the definition of the "space of Marcille" one should clearly observe the obturator nerve exiting the psoas muscle. The nodal package from each side is placed in Endocatch® bags and removed when incision for the diversion is made. After completion of the node dissection aggressive sterile water irrigation is carried out again and thorough hemostasis is achieved before proceeding to the lymph node dissection on the other side.

44.3 Postoperative Care

A nasogastric tube is routinely left in place for 24 h. The patients are maintained on broad-spectrum antibiotics for at least 24 h and can be transitioned to oral regimens based on surgeon preference. Epidural catheters are not routinely used. Intravenous narcotics and/or ketorolac is usually adequate for pain management and can be promptly switched to oral narcotics once the patient is tolerating a diet.

It is important to increase patient activity as early as the day of surgery. Patients are encouraged to sit in a chair the same night of surgery. They are ambulated on the first postoperative day if not sooner. A liquid diet is started once bowel function returns which may be as early as the second or third postoperative day. Daily serum chemistry and hematocrits may be followed until discharge based on surgeon preference. Most patients do not seem to have significant third spacing and will rarely require additional fluid replacement other than standard maintenance fluids. Although postoperative hemorrhage and delayed bowel injury are rare, patients need to be monitored closely for these complications, as the incidence with RARC is unknown.

Ureteral stents and abdominal drains should be managed according to surgeon preference. Currently, the authors remove stents from a urostomy at 14 days when they return to clinic for their first postoperative visit when an ileal conduit is performed. Foley catheters are removed from orthotopic neobladders in

Table 44.1 RARC series reported in English literature

Author	N	Urinary diversion	Age	Mean OR time (min)	EBL (mL)	Hosp LOS (days)	Complications
Menon et al.[8]	17	Ileal conduit (3) Neobladder (14)	–	260 308	150	–	Re-exploration for postop bleed (1) Bilharziasis (13)
Hemal et al.[16]	24	Ileal conduit (4) W pouch (16) T pouch (2) double chimney (2)	–	290	200	–	Minimal blood loss and morbidity
Galich et al.[17]	13	Ileal conduit (6) Neobladder (5) Indiana pouch (2)	70	697	500	8	Enterovesical fistula + SBO (1) Abscess (1)
Abraham et al. (2007)	14	Ileal conduit (14)	76.5	419	212	5.8	42.8% Transfusion rate 28% Complication rate: Ileus (2) Urine leak (1) MI (1) Incomplete transection of L obturator nerve
Murphy et al.[18]	23	Ileal conduit (19) Studer pouch (4)	64.8	368	278	11.6	23% complication rate. Transfusion (1), rectal injury/colostomy (1), anastomotic stricture, ureter leak (1), b/l femoral neuropathy, postop bleed
Wang et al.[9]	33	Ileal conduit (17) Indiana pouch (3) Neobladder (12)	66	390	400	5	4 (12%) minor complications. Ileus (4) 3 (9%) major complications. Conversion to open (1); percutaneous drainage of abscess (1); EC fistula (1)
Guru et al.[15]	67	Ileal Conduit	67	–	520	–	Postop bleed/ transfusion/return to OR (1)
Ng et al.[10]	83	Ileal conduit (47) Indiana pouch (10) Neobladder (26)	70.9	375	460	5.5	Cellulitis, dehiscence, renal failure, ureteral obstruction, urinary fistula/ leak, FUO, PNA, UTI, abscess, pyelonephritis, ileus, fungal infn, SBO, *Clostridium difficile* colitis, GI bleed, hematemesis, EC fistula, arrhythmia, MI, transfusion (1), rash, dehydration, DVT, PE
Pruthi et al.[14]	100	Ileal conduit (61) Neobladder (38) None (1)	65.5	4.6 h	271	4.9	41 complications in 36 patients; 8% major complications; 30-day readmission rate 11%

EBL: estimated blood loss; Hosp LOS: length of hospital stay; FUO: fever of unknown origin; PNA: pneumonia; UTI: urinary tract infection; infn: infection; SBO: small bowel obstruction; EC fistula: enterocutaneous fistula; MI: myocardial infarction; DVT: deep vein thrombosis; PE: pulmonary embolism.

14–21 days. The decision to perform a cystogram at the time of foley catheter removal is based on individual surgeon preference.

44.4 Results

The results of larger RARC series currently in the literature are summarized in Table 44.1.

Our institutional RARC results were recently reviewed for 146 patients who underwent the procedure from October 2005 to July 2009. Of these, 32 (22%) were female and 114 (78%) were male. The average age was 68 years old. The mean overall operative time was 375 min, with a mean pelvic lymph node dissection time of 61 min. The mean lymph node yield was 22 nodes. The estimated blood loss was 577 mL, with an intraoperative transfusion rate of 20 (14%).

44.5 Conclusions

The results of current published reports of robotic-assisted radical cystectomy are encouraging and demonstrate the technical feasibility of RARC in the management of invasive bladder cancer. All forms of urinary diversions can be created and offered to patients. There are several steps in performing this procedure that can be mastered by any surgeon skilled in laparoscopic and robotic surgery. With advantages such as decreased morbidity, decreased blood loss, and improved convalescence robotic surgery is well suited for radical cystectomy. Once long-term oncologic efficacy is confirmed, urologists will be able to add robotic-assisted radical cystectomy to their armamentarium of treatment modalities for bladder cancer.

References

1. Huang GJ, Stein JP:. Open radical cystectomy with lymphadenectomy remains the treatment of choice for invasive bladder cancer. *Curr Opin Urol.* 2007;17:369.

2. Stein JP, Lieskovsky G, Cote R, et al. Radical cystectomy in the treatment of invasive bladder cancer: long-term results in 1,054 patients. *J Clin Oncol.* 2001;19:666.

3. Lowrance WT, Rumohr JA, Chang SS, et al. Contemporary open radical cystectomy: analysis of perioperative outcomes. *J Urol.* 2008;179:1313.

4. Ghoneim MA, el-Mekresh MM, el-Baz MA, et al. Radical cystectomy for carcinoma of the bladder: critical evaluation of the results in 1,026 cases. *J Urol.* 1997;158:393.

5. Portis AJ, Yan Y, Landman J, et al. Long-term followup after laparoscopic radical nephrectomy. *J Urol.* 2002;167:1257.

6. Badani KK, Kaul S, Menon M:. Evolution of robotic radical prostatectomy: assessment after 2766 procedures. *Cancer.* 2007;110:1951.

7. Parra RO, Andrus CH, Jones JP, et al. Laparoscopic cystectomy: initial report on a new treatment for the retained bladder. *J Urol.* 1992;148:1140.

8. Menon M, Hemal AK, Tewari A, et al. Nerve-sparing robot-assisted radical cystoprostatectomy and urinary diversion. *BJU Int.* 2003;92:232.

9. Wang GJ, Barocas DA, Raman JD, et al. Robotic vs open radical cystectomy: prospective comparison of perioperative outcomes and pathological measures of early oncological efficacy. *BJU Int.* 2008;101:89.

10. Ng CK, Kauffman EC, Lee MM, et al. A comparison of postoperative complications in open versus robotic cystectomy. *Eur Urol.* 2009;57:274–281.

11. Guru KA, Kim HL, Piacente PM, et al. Robot-assisted radical cystectomy and pelvic lymph node dissection: initial experience at Roswell park cancer institute. *Urology.* 2007;69:469.

12. Pruthi RS, Wallen EM:. Robotic assisted laparoscopic radical cystoprostatectomy: operative and pathological outcomes. *J Urol.* 2007;178:814.

13. Martin AD, Nunez RN, Pacelli A, et al. Robot-assisted radical cystectomy: intermediate survival results at a mean follow-up of 25 months. *BJU Int.* 2010;105:1706–1709.

14. Pruthi RS, Nielsen ME, Nix J, et al. Robotic radical cystectomy for bladder cancer: surgical and pathological outcomes in 100 consecutive cases. *J Urol.* 2010;183: 510–514.

15. Guru KA, Sternberg K, Wilding GE, et al. The lymph node yield during robot-assisted radical cystectomy. *BJU Int.* 2008;102:231.

16. Hemal AK, Abol-Enein H, Tewari A, et al. Robotic radical cystectomy and urinary diversion in the management of bladder cancer. *Urol Clin North Am.* 2004;31:719.

17. Galich A, Sterrett A, Nazemi T, et al. Comparative analysis of early perioperative outcomes following radical cystectomy by either the robotic or open method. *JSLS.* 2006;10:145.

18. Murphy DG, Challacombe BJ, Elhage O, et al. Robotic-assisted laparoscopic radical cystectomy with extracorporeal urinary diversion: initial experience. *Eur Urol.* 2008;54:570.

Chapter 45

Robotic-Assisted Laparoscopic Anterior Pelvic Exenteration for Bladder Cancer in the Female

Raj S. Pruthi, Matthew E. Nielsen, and Eric M. Wallen

45.1 Introduction

Radical cystectomy remains one of the most effective oncologic treatments for patients with muscle-invasive bladder cancer and for those with high-grade, recurrent, noninvasive tumors. Recently, there have been an increasing number of anecdotal reports and case series for minimally invasive approaches to cystectomy. Laparoscopic and robotic-assisted techniques have been shown to be viable approaches to cystectomy, and recent reports have demonstrated acceptable surgical and perioperative results.[1–5] Potential benefits of laparoscopic and robotic approaches that have been described include lower surgical blood loss, early return of bowel function, and more rapid postoperative convalescence.[3–5] The majority of these series have reported techniques and outcomes in a predominantly male patient population. The applications of such novel techniques to female cystectomy and anterior exenterative procedures have not been well documented and described. However, given the successful application of robotic techniques in male patients and given the recent experience of robotic approaches to hysterectomy, salpingo-oophorectomy, and other female pelvic procedures in the gynecologic literature, the stage has been set for the application of robotic approaches to anterior pelvic exenteration for female patients with bladder cancer.[6,7]

Cystectomy in male and female patents is different with regard to the surgical approach. Female patients have a broader pelvis with more ready access to the apical/urethral dissection than the male.[8] On the other hand, female pelvic anatomy may be less familiar to urologic surgeons due to the wealth of surgical experience in male patents, primarily owing to the treatment of prostatic diseases and malignancies. Even with bladder cancer, the preponderance of patients is male by a ratio of 3:1.[9] Furthermore, the female cystectomy procedure includes exenteration of the anterior pelvic organs including the uterus, fallopian tubes, ovaries, and occasionally part or all of the anterior vaginal wall. Such procedures can be associated with increased blood loss and added morbidity that has been observed in female patients vs. male patients in open radical cystectomy series by experienced surgeons.[10]

Herein we describe our technique and experience with robotic-assisted laparoscopic radical anterior pelvic exenteration in the female including preoperative preparation, surgical steps, postoperative care while also describing our perioperative and pathologic outcomes of this novel procedure. We describe the stepwise approach to the robotic-assisted laparoscopic radical anterior pelvic exenteration for urothelial carcinoma in the female allowing the urologic surgeon to more readily overcome the procedural learning curve.

45.2 Methods

45.2.1 Pre-operative Evaluation

All patients should undergo appropriate pre-operative lab work, imaging studies (chest x-ray, abdominal/pelvic cross-sectional imaging), and endoscopic

R.S. Pruthi (✉)
Division of Urologic Surgery, The University of North Carolina at Chapel Hill, Chapel Hill, NC 27599, USA
e-mail: rpruthi@med.unc.edu

A.K. Hemal, M. Menon (eds.), *Robotics in Genitourinary Surgery*,
DOI 10.1007/978-1-84882-114-9_15, © Springer-Verlag London Limited 2011

resection (i.e., transurethral resection of bladder tumor (TURBT)). Decisions for neoadjuvant chemotherapy should be made at the discretion of the treating medical team. At our institution, neoadjuvant chemotherapy is typically utilized in patients with clinical T3–T4 tumors or suspected node-positive disease. Overall, indications and pre-operative decisions should not be changed by the surgical tool or approach utilized. Bladder cancer is an unforgiving disease and despite the novelty of such minimally invasive procedures and the potential short-term surgical and perioperative benefits, it remains imperative that any such procedure abide to the indications, standards, and principles of the open operation. It is paramount to observe and maintain the oncologic principles of radical cystectomy irrespective of surgical modifications.

45.2.2 Patient Selection

Appropriate patients include those who generally are in good health and performance status. We tend to avoid the robotic approach in patients with severe cardiopulmonary compromise – which is not an uncommon comorbidity due to the risk factor of tobacco abuse that contributes to development of both urothelial carcinoma and cardiopulmonary disease. Limitations for patients in poor cardiopulmonary health status are primarily due to the positioning that includes extreme Trendelenburg that may exacerbate ventilatory difficulties and cardiac function. In one's early experience, prolonged OR times may not be suitable for such patients. We recommend careful patient selection in one's initial experience with robotic anterior pelvic exenteration including patient characteristics as follows:

- Good performance status
- Non-obese patients (BMI <30)
- Healthy: age <70, few comorbidities
- No previous intra-abdominal or pelvic surgery
- No prior chemotherapy or pelvic radiotherapy
- Low-volume disease (non-bulky tumors)

45.2.3 Bowel Preparation

If a bowel preparation is desired, we recommend an outpatient, mechanical-only, bowel preparation with the use of a single 8 oz bottle of magnesium citrate solution along with a clear liquid diet the day prior to surgery and a Fleets® enema the morning of the procedure. However, the overall benefits of the mechanical bowel preparation have come into question in the colorectal surgical literature (i.e., vs. no bowel preparation at all).[11,12] To this end, in all patients undergoing radical cystectomy including those undergoing a robotic approach, we currently no longer perform a mechanical or antibiotic bowel preparation and patients are allowed a regular diet until midnight before surgery. We still use a Fleets® enema the morning of the procedure in order to evacuate the rectum and thereby reduce bowel distension in the deep pelvis.

45.2.4 Intraoperative Considerations

Intraoperative preparation includes shaving the patient from the costal margin to the pubis. The abdomen, perineum, vagina, upper thighs, and peri-anal area are prepped and draped in the usual sterile fashion. A 20 Fr urethral catheter is inserted. Intraoperative fluids are restricted to 500 ml/h as tolerated by the patient. This minimizes the risk of edema of the face and neck that can occur due to fluids and the steep Trendelenburg position. A nasogastric or orogastric tube is inserted at the start of the procedure and removed at the end of the case. Occasionally the use of a uterine manipulator is employed and this is placed at the beginning of the case with the patient in the lithotomy position.

45.2.5 Steps of the Procedure

45.2.5.1 Positioning and Port Placement

1. *Patient positioning*
   After positioning, padding, securing, and preparing the patient in the supine position, the table is then placed in a steep Trendelenburg (>20°) position – identical to that of the robotic prostatectomy. For females, we use stirrups and the low lithotomy position with slight hip extension. Great care is taken to adequately pad and support the patient to avoid neuromuscular injury. Sequential compression devices are applied to the legs for DVT prophylaxis. We utilize a beanbag and cross-body taping to secure the

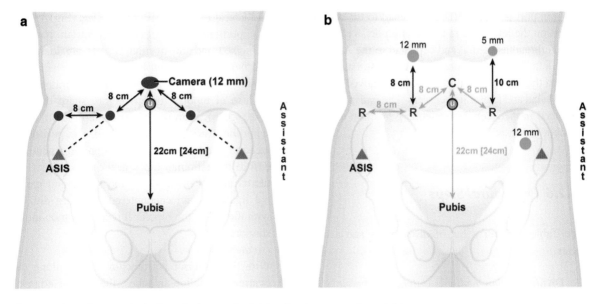

Fig. 45.1 Port placement including robotic ports (*red*) (**a**) and assistant ports (*green*) (**b**)

patient adequately and test the positioning by tilting the table prior to the skin prep.

2. *Port placement*

Port placement is similar to robotic prostatectomy with the addition of a 12 mm port on the side opposite of the assistant. Figures 45.1a, b and 45.2 demonstrate port placement based on a left-sided assistant. Veress insufflation is achieved through a vertical skin incision above the umbilicus, 22 cm above the symphysis pubis on the deflated abdomen. (In cases in which a more extended lymphadenectomy is anticipated (e.g., para-aortic dissection) or where an intracorporeal diversion is planned, this camera port is placed slightly higher at 24 cm above the symphysis.) The 12 mm camera port is placed here, and the remaining ports are placed under direct vision. Two 8 mm robotic ports are placed 8 cm away from the camera port, along the line from the camera port to the anterior spine of the iliac crest (ASIS) bilaterally. An additional 8 mm robotic port for the 4th arm is placed 8 cm directly lateral to the right-sided robotic port. A 12 mm port for retraction and stapling is placed 8 cm cephalad to the robotic port on the right. A

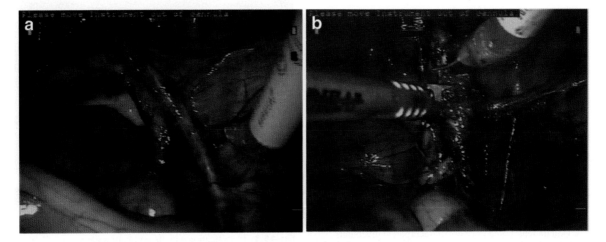

Fig. 45.2 Dissection (**a**) and bipolar fulguration and division (**b**) of ovarian pedicles (IP ligament)

5 mm port is placed 10 cm cephalad to the robotic port on the left. A 12 mm assistant port is placed 2 fingerbreadths medial and cephalad to the ASIS on the left. The port must be placed at least 8 cm away from the left robotic port and can be moved farther cephalad and lateral if necessary. The patient is then placed in the steep Trendelenburg position and the robot is docked.

45.2.6 Procedural Steps

(See Table 45.1 for a list of instruments and accessories.)

1. *Divide ovarian pedicles (infundibulopelvic [IP] ligament)*

   After any sigmoid adhesions of the left side bladder and pelvis are released sharply, all of the small bowel is vacated from pelvis. The ovarian pedicles (IP ligaments) are identified on each side superior

Table 45.1 Instruments and accessories

A. Recommended laparoscopic instruments
- 5 mm endoscopic long suction irrigator (45 mm)
- 5 mm endoscopic scissors
- 5 mm endoscopic locking grasper
- 5 mm endoscopic needle driver (for passing suture)
- 10 mm specimen retrieval bag

B. Recommended sutures/clips
- Dorsal vein stitch
  o 0 Vicryl on CT-2 (6 in.)
- Ureteral and terminal ileum tags
  o 3-0 Vicryl on SH (full length)
- Anastomosis stitch (for orthotopic diversion)
  o 3-0 Vicryl (or Monocryl) suture on RB-1
- Neobladder creation (intracorporeal diversion)
  o 2-0 Vicryl suture on SH
  o Stapler with vascular load
- Ureteroenteric anastomosis (intracorporeal diversion)
  o 4-0 Vicryl suture on RB-1 suture
- Hem-o-lok® (Weck Closure Systems, RTP, NC) large and extralarge clips with endoscopic applier
- Endovascular stapler/cutter with 60 mm vascular loads (e.g., Endo-GIA, Covidien, Mansfield, MA)

C. Recommended robotic instruments
- Two large needle drivers
- Hot shears (monopolar curved scissors)
- Maryland bipolar forceps
- Cadiere bipolar graspers
- Double fenestrated graspers (intracorporeal diversion)

and lateral to the ovaries themselves (Fig. 45.2a). The peritoneum overlying the ovarian pedicles is incised and the ovarian vessels are identified and isolated. They can be ligated with the use of Hem-o-lok clips or alternatively fulgurated with the use of bipolar forceps before sharp division (Fig. 45.2b). With the posterior peritoneum overlying the ovarian pedicles incised, this peritoneal incision is extended along the broad ligament lateral to the fallopian tubes in the direction of the uterus and bladder. When the round and cardinal ligaments are encountered, they are divided with the aid of the bipolar forceps and monopolar scissors.

2. *Isolate ureters*

   With the posterior peritoneum incised along the ovaries and fallopian tubes, the medial edge of that incised peritoneum is grasped and lifted. The ureter can be found underlying and somewhat adhered to the posterior peritoneum along this medial leaflet. The ureter is encircled and the ureter is bluntly and sharply dissected distally down toward the level of the bladder (Fig. 45.3). One should avoid grasping the ureter with the robotic instruments to avoid crush injury and resultant devascularization to the ureter itself. As one approaches the bladder they will encounter the uterine vasculature crossing a lateral to medial toward the level of the cervix. Overly aggressive distal dissection in this area can result in some bleeding. Hem-o-lok clips are used to ligate the ureters and they are divided at this level on each

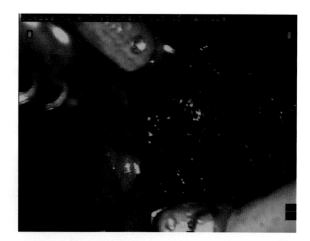

Fig. 45.3 Identification and dissection of ureters

side. The transected ureters are tucked into the upper quadrants away from the pelvic dissection.

3. *Posterior bladder dissection*

   The peritoneum is incised between the level of the uterus and vagina (posteriorly) and the bladder (anteriorly): this incision can be made right at the level of the peritoneal reflection. With this lateral ("east to west") incision made, the plane between the bladder and the vagina can be developed bluntly. With the uterine manipulator or a vaginal sponge stick in place, the dissection is carried along the vaginal wall to create an adequate wide margin on the level of the posterior bladder wall. In cases where a vaginal-sparing procedure is anticipated, this dissection can be taken down to the level of the bladder neck and urethra. If any aspect of the anterior vaginal wall is to be removed the vagina can be entered and the anterior vaginal wall taken en bloc with the bladder, thus creating the plane of dissection within the vagina itself.

4. *Lateral dissection*

   The peritoneum is incised just lateral to the medial umbilical ligaments on each side. This incision is carried laterally alongside the bladder and extending posteriorly to the previously made peritoneal incisions overlying the ureter and between the bladder and uterus/vagina. (Of note, the urachal and medial umbilical attachments are left intact to help suspend the bladder and facilitate the posterior and lateral dissection and the stapling of the bladder pedicles.) Blunt dissection can be used to develop the lateral perivesical space without much difficulty down to the level of the endopelvic fascia. In a non-orthotopic diversion, the endopelvic fascia can be incised at this point. The lateral vascular pedicles of the bladder including the superior vesical artery can now be readily visualized.

5. *Securing bladder pedicles*

   A laparoscopic endovascular stapler is used to ligate and transect the vascular pedicles to the bladder (Fig. 45.4a and 45.4b). Usually a single fire of a 60 mm stapler/cutter is sufficient to secure the bladder pedicles on each side. Alternatively these pedicles can be secured using the bipolar cautery or with the use of Hem-o-lok clips and then sharply divided. In cases where the anterior vaginal wall is to be taken en bloc with the bladder, the posterior plane of this dissection can be within the vagina itself – as opposed to between the bladder and vagina in a vaginal-sparing procedure. Vaginal entry can result in loss of pneumoperitoneum. To maintain insufflation pressure a moist laparotomy pad or large occlusive dressing (e.g., Tegaderm dressing, 3 M Corp., St. Paul, MN) is used to occlude the vaginal outlet and prevent loss of pneumoperitoneum.

6. *Anterior dissection*

   With the posterior and lateral dissections complete, attention is then turned anteriorly. The peritoneum is incised anteriorly through the medial umbilical ligament and the urachus thereby "dropping" the bladder. The anterior prevesical space is bluntly developed down to the level of the pubis and exposing the endopelvic fascia on each side. In an orthotopic diversion the endopelvic fascia is

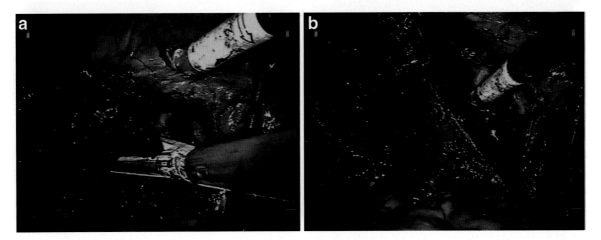

Fig. 45.4 Placement of endovascular stapler to divide pedicles (**a**) and image of divided bladder pedicle (**b**)

left intact to avoid any perturbance of the underlying continence mechanism in the female. In a non-orthotopic diversion the endopelvic fascia is incised, as noted previously, to allow for complete distal dissection of the bladder neck and urethra.

7. *Bladder neck/urethral dissection*

The bladder neck is then approached anteriorly. In an orthotopic diversion, great care is made to create this transection precisely at the level of the bladder neck (Fig. 45.5a). Careful and continued evaluation at the location of the bladder neck is performed with the Foley catheter balloon in place to help visualize and identify the bladder neck. This will help maximize intrapelvic urethral length and hopefully decrease risk of urinary incontinence (Fig. 45.5b).

In the non-orthotopic diversion, the urethra can be dissected quite distally. When a complete urethrectomy is desired, we circumferentially incise the urethra at the beginning of the case before docking the robot. Bovie electrocautery on cutting current can help release the urethra from the vaginal mucosa and allow for a more complete urethrectomy when approached transperitoneally with the robotic dissection. Before transecting or delivering the urethra, we will typically place an extralarge Hem-o-lok clip on the bladder (specimen) side to avoid any urine spillage.

After urethral transection, some remaining posterior lateral attachments will remain and these can often be divided with blunt and sharp dissection and with the use of monopolar and bipolar cautery. If the anterior vaginal wall has been incised en bloc, the entire bladder and anterior vaginal wall specimen can be removed through the vagina or placed in an impermeable bag.

8. *Specimen retrieval*

In cases of an orthotopic diversion after the bladder neck has been transected at the appropriate level, the Foley catheter is left in place and the remainder of the bladder specimen is completely freed dividing any remaining posterior lateral attachments. The catheter is clipped with an extralarge Hem-o-lok clip (to avoid any urinary spillage and contamination), the Foley is transected, and the cut end brought into the pelvis (Fig. 45.6a). The specimen is then placed in an impermeable retrievable bag that is moved out of the pelvis (Fig. 45.6b). The pelvis is irrigated, vaginal surface inspected, and hemostasis ensured. A urethral margin is sent for frozen section evaluation.

9. *Vaginal reconstruction/hysterectomy/oophorectomy*

This portion of the procedure can either be performed before or after the cystectomy. Blunt and sharp dissection allows for complete freeing up of fallopian tubes and ovaries down to the level of the cervix. The uterus is lifted and the peritoneum is incised circumferentially at the level of the cervix. The lateral tissue at the level of the cervix is fulgurated with the liberal use of the bipolar forceps as this is the site of much of the uterine blood supply. The uterus can then be transected at the level

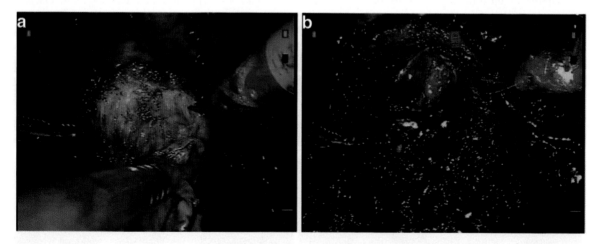

Fig. 45.5 Transection of urethra at the level of the bladder neck (**a**) in an orthotopic diversion. The bladder neck–urethral junction can be visualized and confirmed with catheter movement. Adequate urethral length remains after transection (**b**)

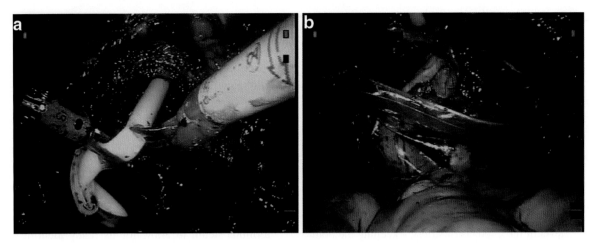

Fig. 45.6 Division of catheter (**a**) and placement of bladder in specimen bag (**b**)

of the cervix again with liberal use of monopolar and bipolar cautery. With the transection complete the uterus, fallopian tubes, and ovaries are freed and removed out of the pelvis. In a vaginal-sparing procedure, the small os at the level of the cervix remains the only opening into the vagina and this is closed with a figure-of-eight 0 Vicryl suture on a CT2 needle. If the anterior vaginal wall was excised en bloc with the bladder, this defect can be closed in continuity with the reapproximation of the vaginal walls. We typically use a 0 Vicryl suture on a CT2 needle to reconstruct the vagina typically in a caudad to cephalad (i.e., north to south) manner. Depending on the remaining vaginal anatomy this can also be done in a transverse manner if appropriate.

10. *Pelvic lymphadenectomy*

The initial surgical step is to identify and expose the external iliac artery and vein. On occasion, these vessels are readily visualized laparoscopically. In some cases, particularly in obese patients, the vessels need to be located and exposed from within the overlying retroperitoneal fat. In such cases, the external iliac artery can be located by noting its pulsations along its anticipated course. Blunt dissection (e.g., with the closed scissor tips by the surgeon or with the suction irrigator by the assistant) along the external iliac artery and vein exposes these structures. Blunt and sharp dissection is carried down to the anterior surface of the external iliac artery. The vein can then be found lying immediately adjacent (posterior and medial) to the artery. It is important

to dissect into the correct fibroalveolar plane just overlying the artery and the vein. This will allow for easier and more precise dissection of the lymph node packets for the remainder of the procedure. Margins of lymphadenectomy vary according to the discretion of the surgeon and generally include the obturator nodes, the external iliac nodes, and the common iliac nodes. Para-aortic lymphadenectomy is also possible, particularly with the use of the da Vinci S system which allows for more range of motion of the robotic arms.

The obturator and hypogastric lymph node dissection is begun by locating and developing the medial border of the external iliac vein, thereby exposing the obturator fossa posteriorly. Dissection along the external iliac vein must be done with great care to avoid a venous injury, because the vein is decompressed due to the steep Trendelenburg position. With the medial edge of the external iliac vein identified, the plane between the vein and the obturator packet can be extended to the pubic bone distally. Care must be made to identify the circumflex vein distally and any aberrant branches of the external iliac or obturator veins. Blunt and sharp dissection with the aid of monopolar scissors and fenestrated bipolar graspers – and with the appropriate counter traction placed by the assistant or the surgeon's nondominant hand – can be used to facilitate this dissection by retracting the vein laterally and the obturator node packet medially. Once the dissection off the external iliac vein is complete, the nodal packet can be dissected bluntly off the obturator nerve and vessels posteriorly. In a transperitoneal approach it is not necessary to ligate every lymphatic channel. Monopolar and bipolar cautery can aid in division of smaller lymphatic channels and the laparoscopic clips (e.g., Hem-o-lok™ clips) can be used to ligate larger lymphatic channels, pedicles, and vein branches as necessary. The pubic bone and anterior surface of obturator nerve and vessels mark the distal margin of the nodal packet. With the obturator packet freed and divided distally (down to and including the so-called node of Cloquet), it is peeled backed in the cephalad direction to the level of the hypogastric artery – keeping the obturator nerve, medial border of the external iliac vein, and the medial umbilical ligament in clear view. The medial umbilical ligament should be retracted medially to achieve proper exposure for the hypogastric dissection.

The base of the node packet near the internal iliac artery must be dissected with care as the internal iliac artery does not have the same fibroalveolar sheath as the external vessels. Consequently, the nodal tissue can be somewhat adherent with greater need for sharp dissection and coagulation of lymphatic and vascular attachments before division of the cephalad aspect of the packet near the level of the internal iliac artery.

Once the obturator/hypogastric dissection is complete, the extended dissection is undertaken, beginning distally, cephalad to and along the external iliac artery. Again, it is crucial to dissect down to the correct fibroalveolar plane over the artery. While avoiding the circumflex vein distally, all lymphatic tissue is taken between the external iliac vein and artery and laterally on the psoas muscle to the genitofemoral nerve. With this packet divided distally, this lymph tissue is teased and dissected in the cephalad direction with blunt and sharp dissection, occasionally using monopolar and bipolar cautery. Unlike the external iliac vein, it is quite rare to encounter aberrant branches off of the artery, and this dissection is readily performed proximally up to and along the common iliac vessels. One needs to remain cognizant that the ureter will be encountered crossing over the common iliac vessels. If desired, a para-aortic dissection can be accomplished robotically (particularly with the new-generation – da Vinci S –

robot). If a para-aortic dissection is anticipated and the classic da Vinci platform is used, it may be necessary to place the robotic ports approximately 2 cm superior or cephalad than the typical configuration.

11. *Tagging the Ureters*

Before undocking the robot, the ureters are returned to the pelvis. At the distal end of each ureter, a full length 3-0 Vicryl stitch on an SH needle is placed as a tag, and the ends are brought out through the assistant ports on each side. This allows for ready identification and localization of both ureters. A 3-0 Vicryl stitch is placed in the terminal ileum to allow for its ready identification during the urinary diversion. In the case of an orthotopic neobladder, 3-0 Vicryl sutures (on RB-1 needles) are placed at the 5 and 7 o'clock positions in the urethra and left in the pelvis. These posterior sutures are sometimes the most difficult to place in an open fashion and preplacement under robotic guidance is easier. The robot is then undocked. The robot is not re-docked later for the anastomosis, as this portion of the operation is easily accomplished through the small incision made next.

12 *Urinary Diversion*

After the robot is undocked, all ports are removed. The ureteral sutures are kept through their corresponding port sites and tagged. It is important to keep the patient in the Trendelenburg position initially in order to prevent the intestine from descending into the pelvis. A 6–8 cm incision is made midway from umbilicus to the pubis to perform the urinary diversion. Typically, an abdominal wall retractor is not required, and minimizing abdominal wall retraction may help reduce postoperative incisional musculoskeletal pain. Through this incision any further mobilization of the ureters can be carried out if needed. For an ileal conduit, the left ureter is tunneled under the sigmoid mesentery. In the case of an orthotopic neobladder where the afferent limb lies on the left side, the right ureter is tunneled underneath the sigmoid mesentery. The terminal ileum is identified with the assistance of the preplaced stitch, and the segment of bowel is harvested. The planned urinary diversion is then performed extracorporeally and the ureteroenteric anastomosis completed. For an orthotopic neobladder, the preplaced posterior urethral stitches are placed in their proper position in the neobladder neck. Anterior anastomotic sutures are placed thereafter. After the anastomotic sutures are placed and tagged, the patient is taken out of the Trendelenburg position.

More recently in certain cases we have performed the urinary diversion intracorporeally – including both ileal conduits and orthotopic ileal neobladders (Fig. 45.7). In such cases, the specimen is extracted through the vagina – either through the anterior vaginotomy in cases in which the anterior vaginal wall is removed or through a separate incision in the posterior vaginal wall in a vaginal-sparing procedure. A posterior incision is used in such cases to avoid the potential for overlapping suture lines in cases of orthotopic neobladder creation.

A pelvic drain (10 Fr Jackson-Pratt drain) is placed, and the incisions are closed. Of note, we do not typically re-approximate the fascia on laparoscopic or robotic ports ≤12 mm.

45.2.7 Postoperative Care

During closure of incisions, fluids are liberalized with the goal of a 1 l bolus of intravenous fluids before leaving the OR. Postoperative care is routine and at the discretion of the surgeon. In our practice we had found no added benefit of leaving the NG tube even overnight and now routinely employ an OG tube intraoperatively that is removed at the end of the case.

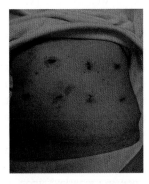

Fig. 45.7 Postoperative picture of female patient who has undergone robotic anterior pelvic exenteration, bilateral pelvic lymphadenectomy, and intracorporeal orthotopic ileal neobladder

After completing the procedure, all patients were taken to the urology inpatient ward and underwent routine postoperative care per our cystectomy care pathway which has previously been reported and which includes the use of prokinetic agents and non-narcotic analgesics. In addition we employ a "fast track" program of early diet advancement irrespective of status of flatus or bowel movement (see Table 45.2).[13]

The pelvic drain is typically removed prior to discharge. The patient returns at 10–14 days postoperatively for removal of the ureteral stents. In addition, in the case of an orthotopic neobladder, they will return 17–21 days after surgery for a cystogram and catheter removal. Clinical and oncologic follow-up is thereafter performed in stage-specific manner.

45.3 Results

We have performed robotic cystectomy in 110 cases and applied it to female patients in 30 procedures. Our experience and perioperative outcomes with robotic anterior pelvic exenteration in the first 30 consecutive female cases are shown in Table 45.3 with comparisons made to 80 male patients also undergoing a robotic

Table 45.2 Cystectomy fast track program

Preoperative
Counseling/expectations
No outpatient mechanical bowel prep or oral antibiotics (day before surgery)
Regular diet until midnight then NPO (day before surgery)
Surgical
– Perioperative antibiotics (second- or third-generation cephalosporin) × 24 h
– Removal of OG tube at end of procedure
Postoperative
Prokinetic agents (e.g., metoclopramide 10 mg i.v. q 8 h × 48 h)
Non-narcotic analgesics (e.g., ketorolac 30 mg i.v. q 6 h × 48 h. Convert to celecoxib 200 mg bid if no contraindications)
Early ambulation
Fast track diet (advanced irrespective of bowel function)
– POD#1 – chewing gum initiated (ad libitum) otherwise NPO
– POD#2 – clear liquids – 8 oz per 8 h
– POD#3 – unrestricted clear liquids
– POD#4 – regular diet

Table 45.3 Perioperative Outcomes

	Female ($n = 30$)	Male ($n = 80$)
Mean age	69.4 years*	63.4 years
Mean BMI	26.3 kg/m^2	27.8 kg/m^2
Mean ASA score	2.8	2.7
Diversion		
Conduit	22	44
Neobladder	8	35
None	0	1
Mean EBL (range)	234 ml	283 ml
Mean OR time (range)	4.4 h*	4.8 h
Postoperative		
Mean time to flatus	2.0 days	2.1 days
Mean time to BM	2.7 days	2.8 days
Mean time to discharge	5.1 days	4.7 days
Mean LN yield	18.8	19.1

*$p < 0.05$

cystectomy. Female patients were older (69.4 vs. 63.4 years; $p = 0.006$) and had shorter OR time (4.4 vs. 4.8 h; $p = 0.046$), but were not different with regard to other perioperative outcomes. It should be noted that our initial learning curve with robotic cystectomy of 20 cases were all male patients and these were included in this comparison.

Pathologic outcomes have also demonstrated an appropriate extirpative procedure in that no patient has a positive margin, and a mean number of lymph nodes removed is 19 (range 9–34) with our standard and extended dissection. Short-term (within 30 days of surgery) complication rate was 23%. Complications included ileus,[2] a fever of unknown origin,[1] anastamotic urine leak,[1] DVT,[1] acute renal failure,[1] and stent obstruction.[1]

45.4 Comment

Despite the novelty of such minimally invasive procedures, several principles and standards must be rigorously evaluated and maintained. First, it remains paramount to observe and maintain the oncologic principles of this operation irrespective of surgical modifications. That is, pathologic end points, and consequently oncologic outcomes, must never be compromised with such newer techniques. Second, such procedures should have appropriate perioperative outcomes with regard to operative time, surgical blood loss, and length of hospital stay. Such measures may reflect and impact on patient morbidity and recovery

and may also indicate operative difficulty (i.e., the learning curve) for the surgeon. For example, in robotic prostatectomy procedures, operative times have been used as an indirect measure of surgical difficulty and of progress in overcoming the learning curve.[14] Accordingly, novel procedures should not result in insurmountable difficulties or excess morbidities for surgeon or patient alike. Last, any such new procedures should not expose patients to any undue or excessive complications.

In our experience, the oncologic principles and pathologic outcomes appear to be maintained with a robotic approach. In no case has a positive margin been observed. In addition, the pelvic lymphadenectomy remains an important aspect of radical cystectomy, and, in our experience, an external iliac and even common iliac lymph node dissection can be readily performed robotically. Indeed, our mean lymph node count of 19 with the robotic approach compares favorably to the mean lymph node count of 16 observed in our open cystectomy experience.[5]

Indeed, with regard to perioperative outcomes, the robotic approach to anterior exenteration is associated with a relatively low surgical blood loss. Our low operative blood loss of 234 ml compares favorably to our own open experience and that of other reports in the literature.[10,15,16] Indeed, in the report by Lee et al. for open radical cystectomy, blood loss and transfusion requirements in females were significantly higher than that of males.[10] In addition, postoperative outcomes including time to flatus, time to bowel movement, and time to hospital discharge are also favorable in our experience.

In our experience, we only attempted the robotic cystectomy after a wealth of experience and sense of proficiency in both open cystectomy and robotic prostatectomy. And, it is only after an initial robotic cystectomy experience of 20 men did we initiate our robotic series in female patients. It is interesting to note that no differences were observed in the subsequent male series and the concurrent initial female experience.[17] It appears that a new learning curve for robotic anterior exenteration does not appear to have clinical difficulties or complications with regard to OR time, blood loss, and postoperative convalescence when the female experience is embarked upon after an initial approach in male patients. In other words, transition to proficiency in anterior pelvic exenteration occurred readily with near-identical outcomes as the concurrent male experience. It is unclear as to how these outcomes would have differed if female patients were part of that initial learning curve.

In conclusion, in our experience, the robotic anterior exenteration has been readily adapted to the surgical treatment of bladder cancer. The approach appears to achieve the clinical and oncologic goals of radical cystectomy in the female.

References

1. Cathelineau X, Arroyo C, Rozet F, Barret E, Vallancien G. Laparoscopic assisted radical cystectomy: the Montsouris experience after 84 cases. *Eur Urol.* June, 2005;47(6): 780–784.

2. Simonato A, Gregori A, Lissiani A, Bozzola A, Galli S, Gaboardi F. Laparoscopic radical cystoprostatectomy: our experience in a consecutive series of 10 patients with a 3 years follow-up. *Eur Urol.* 2005 Jun;47(6):785–790.

3. Rhee JJ, Lebeau S, Smolkin M, Theodorescu D. Radical cystectomy with ileal conduit diversion: early prospective evaluation of the impact of robotic assistance. *BJU Int.* November, 2006;98(5):1059–1063.

4. Guru KA, Kim HL, Piacente PM, Mohler JL. Robot-assisted radical cystectomy and pelvic lymph node dissection: initial experience at Roswell Park Cancer Institute. *Urology.* March, 2007;69(3):469–474.

5. Pruthi RS, Wallen EM. Robotic assisted laparoscopic radical cystoprostatectomy: operative and pathological outcomes. *J Urol.* September, 2007;178(3 Pt 1):814–818.

6. Advincula AP, Song A. The role of robotic surgery in gynecology. *Curr Opin Obstet Gynecol.* August, 2007;19(4):331–336.

7. Nezhat C, Saberi NS, Shahmohamady B, Nezhat F. Robotic-assisted laparoscopy in gynecological surgery. *JSLS.* July–September, 2006;10(3):317–320.

8. Stein JP, Skinner DG. Radical cystectomy – technique and outcomes. stein – textbook. In Lerner SP, Schoenberg MP, Sternberg CN, eds. *Textbook of Bladder Cancer.* Boca Raton, FL: Taylor and Francis; 2006:pp 445–469.

9. Hall MC, Chang SS, Dalbagni G, et al. Guideline for the management of nonmuscle invasive bladder cancer (stages Ta, T1, and Tis): 2007 update. *J Urol.* December, 2007;178(6):2314–2330.

10. Lee KL, Freiha F, Presti JC Jr, Gill HS. Gender differences in radical cystectomy: complications and blood loss. *Urology.* June, 2004;63(6):1095–1099.

11. Wille-Jorgensen P, Guenaga KF, Castro AA, Matos D. Clinical value of preoperative mechanical bowel cleansing in elective colorectal surgery: a systematic review. *Dis Colon Rectum.* August, 2003;46(8): 1013–1020.

12. Guenaga KK, Matos D, Wille-Jorgensen P. Mechanical bowel preparation for elective colorectal surgery. *Cochrane Database Syst Rev.* January, 2009;21(1):CD001544.

13. Pruthi RS, Chun J, Richman M. Reducing time to oral diet and hospital discharge in patients undergoing radical cystectomy using a perioperative care plan. *Urology.* October, 2003;62(4):661–665.

14. Herrell SD, Smith JA Jr.. Robotic-assisted laparoscopic prostatectomy: what is the learning curve? *Urology.* November, 2005;66(5 Suppl):105–107.

15. Chang SS, Smith JA Jr, Wells N, Peterson M, Kovach B, Cookson MS. Estimated blood loss and transfusion requirements of radical cystectomy. *J Urol.* December, 2001;166(6):2151–2154.

16. Novotny V, Hakenberg OW, Wiessner D, et al. Perioperative complications of radical cystectomy in a contemporary series. *Eur Urol.* February, 2007;51(2):397–402.

17. Pruthi RS, Stefaniak H, Hubbard JS, Wallen EM. Robotic anterior pelvic exenteration for bladder cancer in the female: outcomes and comparisons to their male counterparts. *J Laparoendosc Adv Surg Tech A.* February, 2009;19(1):23–27.

Chapter 46

Robotic-Assisted Laparoscopic Extended Pelvic Lymph Node Dissection for Bladder Cancer

A. Karim Kader and Ashok K. Hemal

46.1 Introduction

In the late 1800s Halstead first described the metastasis of primary tumors through lymphatics to regional lymph nodes.[1] In Urologic Oncology we know too well the dire consequences associated with the malignancies that we treat. We and particularly our patients are fortunate that a well-performed lymph node dissection can not only help stage patients but also provide benefits to local control and survival especially in testes and bladder cancer.

In this chapter we will describe the indications, techniques, and outcomes associated with extended pelvic lymph node dissection in the treatment of bladder cancer patients with a view of emphasizing the low morbidity and excellent cancer control of the robotic-assisted, laparoscopic approach.

Bladder cancer is the fourth most common cancer in men in the United States with nearly 53,000 new cases expected in 2009.[2] The vast majority of patients, approximately 70%, present with a non-muscle invasive form of the disease for which trans-urethral resection with possible intravesical therapy is usually sufficient. However, the remaining 30% of patients present with a muscle invasive form of the disease which risks metastases and death. In the absence of demonstrable metastases these patients warrant aggressive therapy as 50% of those undergoing definitive treatment die of the

disease at 5 years and over 85% of those not undergoing therapy for their disease will die within 2 years.[3] Due to the aggressive nature of muscle invasive bladder cancer, some have advocated "early cystectomy" for individuals with high-grade urothelial bladder cancers in the absence of muscle involvement if they do not respond to intravesical therapy.[4]

The current widely accepted standard of care for the treatment of this disease is radical cystectomy (cystoprostatectomy in the male patient and anterior exenteration in the female) with pelvic lymphadenectomy. Some argue for the use of neoadjuvant and/or adjuvant platinum-based chemotherapy in conjunction with surgery.[5–7] An alternative is the "bladder sparing" approach of platinum-based chemotherapy in conjunction with external beam radiation therapy which in North America has been typically reserved for individuals who are felt not to be surgical candidates.[6,7]

The 50% 5-year survival rates and the incidence of metastases which are undetectable by standard staging methods including laboratory investigations, chest X-ray, and CT scanning and bone scans, highlight the need for aggressive treatment of these patients.

Therefore, a carefully performed, pelvic lymph node dissection will provide the best possible staging of patients undergoing cystectomy and, as illustrated in this chapter, is likely to provide a therapeutic benefit in those with minimally positive lymph node disease and even in some with grossly positive lymph node disease.[8]

Surgery for urologic malignancy has a storied past plagued with the infliction of significant morbidity and mortality. The perioperative mortality rate for the cystectomy was 20% prior to the 1970s.[9] Thankfully, our understanding of anesthetic care, our appreciation of

A.K. Kader (✉)
Department of Urology, Comprehensive Cancer Center, Center for Cancer Genomics, Winston-Salem, NC, USA
e-mail: kkader@wfubmc.edu

A.K. Hemal, M. Menon (eds.), *Robotics in Genitourinary Surgery*,
DOI 10.1007/978-1-84882-114-9_46, © Springer Verlag London Limited 2011

the anatomy, and surgical technique together with a stage migration have helped to drop this rate down to approximately 2.5%.[10,11] Despite this, the contemporary complication rate for patients undergoing this surgery is approximately 50%, even at high volume centers.[12] In an ongoing attempt to decrease surgical mortality and morbidity associated with this procedure, a laparoscopic approach has been attempted and we have recently begun extending this to employ robotic assistance.[13]

Robotic-assisted laparoscopic surgery has revolutionized the world of urologic oncology. However, the concepts are not new and its beginnings are in laparoscopic surgery. Thanks to comfort levels with endoscopy and an understanding of anatomy, many urologists have embraced laparoscopy. Laparoscopic pelvic lymph node dissections for prostate cancer were at one point, in the early 1990s, the most commonly performed laparoscopic procedure performed in adults.[14] As the laparoscopic prostatectomy began development, the lymph node dissection continued. Now laparoscopic surgery is commonly employed for the treatment of renal cell carcinoma, testes cancer, and upper tract urothelial cancers. For all of these diseases the lymph node dissection has played an important role.

For some, especially for those not trained in laparoscopic surgery, it is inconceivable that a surgeon could provide comparable oncologic outcomes to their patients as an open surgeon. However, there are several examples where this has been demonstrated in urology namely with the laparoscopic nephrectomy and prostatectomy. Due to the challenges of laparoscopic surgery, especially with respect to surgeon comfort and difficulties with suturing, robotic-assisted laparoscopic surgery has emerged. These challenges have clearly been overcome and now we are in an era whereby, after a comparable learning curve to open surgery, oncologically sound treatment can be provided by many surgeons who felt ill equipped to perform laparoscopy. This is an exciting development for our patients and the surgeons providing their care.

In this chapter, attention will focus on the lymph node dissection performed at the time of radical cystectomy. Specifics regarding the indications, benefits, boundaries, and complications will be provided which will be applicable to open, laparoscopic, and robot-assisted laparoscopic approaches. We will then go further to discuss the evolution of the minimally

invasive technologies for performing this dissection and will provide data to support the use of the robotic-assisted approach for this procedure. Finally, technical points will be provided so that maximal lymph node yields can be achieved while avoiding complications.

46.2 Anatomy of Lymphatic Drainage of the Bladder

The seminal paper by Leadbetter and Cooper in the early 1950s summarized our understanding of the lymphatic drainage of the bladder.[15] Smith and Whitmore extended these initial descriptions and found in their series that the common iliac, external iliac, and obturator node packages were positive in 19, 65, and 74% of the time, respectively.[16]

Leissner and colleagues, who performed a large multicenter analysis of 290 patients undergoing an extended pelvic lymph node dissection at the time of radical cystectomy, described 12 anatomical locations or zones involved in bladder cancer patients. They used the IMA, genitofemoral nerve, and the pelvic floor as the margins of their dissection.[17] The zones include (1) pre-caval, (2) inter-aorto-caval, (3) pre-aortic to the level of the IMA, (4 & 5) right common and external iliac, (6 & 7) left common and external iliac, (8) pre-sacral, (9) right internal iliac, (10) right perivesical, (11) left internal iliac, and (12) left perivesical. In this series, 30% of patients had lymph node metastases. In those with only one positive node, that node was never present above the level of the bifurcation of the aorta. Further analysis looking at three levels, level I below the bifurcation of the iliac vessels, level II below the bifurcation of the aorta to level I, and level III below the IMA (internal mesenteric artery) to level II. Only 6.6% of positive nodes can be seen in level III. Therefore, given the fact that only 30% of the overall patient population had positive nodes, less than 2% of overall patients undergoing cystectomy with extended pelvic lymph node dissections had positive lymph nodes above the aortic bifurcation, and none of those in the single lymph node category (i.e., those individuals who are likely to derive most of the clinical benefit from a node dissection). We therefore advocate stopping the node dissection at the level of the aortic bifurcation.

From these studies, some attempts at standardizing the language used to describe the extent of the lymph node dissection have emerged. All nodal dissections include a lateral margin of the genitofemoral nerve, the obturator lymph node package, and the distal margin of Cloquet's node. As far as proximal extent of dissection and inclusion of pre-sacral nodes, there are essentially three broad categories.[15,18-20]

1. Modified PLND – Bifurcation of common iliac
2. Standard PLND – 2 cm above the common iliac
3. Extended PLND – Aortic Bifurcation with inclusion of the pre-sacral nodes

By way of separate areas we will use the following definitions in this chapter:

1. IMA – Nodes surrounding the aorta from the aortic bifurcation to the IMA
2. Aortic bifurcation – Nodes surrounding the aortic bifurcation
3. Common Iliac – Nodes surrounding the common iliac artery and vein
4. External Iliac – Nodes surrounding the external iliac artery and vein
5. Internal Iliac – Nodes surrounding the internal iliac artery and vein
6. Obturator – Nodes surrounding the obturator nerve
7. Iliacus – Nodes surrounding the iliacus muscle
8. Pre-sacral – Nodes anterior to the sacrum

46.3 Incidence of Lymph Node Metastases Identified at Cystectomy

The incidence of positive lymph nodes at the time of cystectomy for those individuals who are felt to be free of nodal metastases preoperatively is approximately 25%.[11,21] This relatively high rate of positive lymph nodes at the time of cystectomy points to the rather crude preoperative staging studies that are available for this disease. There are, however, some encouraging new technologies such as ultrasmall iron particle MRI which may more accurately predict those patients with occult metastases who may benefit from neoadjuvant chemotherapy.[22]

Other efforts with PET scanning have been met with frustration as demonstrated by the well-designed analysis by Swinnen and colleagues. In their study they obtained preoperative CT and PET scans on 51 patients undergoing radical cystectomy with a standardized extended pelvic lymph node dissection with pathologic analysis of eight separate nodal packages. Results of the pathologic, PET, and CT scans were then compared. Unfortunately, PET scanning, with an accuracy of 84%, sensitivity of 46%, and specificity of 97%, was no better that CT scanning for the 13 patients with positive nodes.[23]

Despite the poor performance of CT scans at detecting low-volume metastases, it may be sensitive enough, as those with minimal lymph node burden only detectable at the time of cystectomy may enjoy a 5-year cancer-specific survival of approximately 35%.[11,24] It is possible, however, that these survival rates could be improved if neoadjuvant chemotherapy was utilized in those patients whose preoperative staging demonstrated suspicious lymph nodes.[25]

There is mounting evidence that even standard pathologic analysis misses some occult metastases as noted when careful dissection, RT-PCR, and staining are used[26,27] or with the improved survival with extended pelvic lymph node dissections in the absence of lymph node metastases read by traditional means.[28]

46.4 Implications of Bladder Cancer Lymph Node Metastases

Unfortunately, there is a dramatic fall in survival rates once bladder cancer has spread to the regional lymph nodes. In their classic paper examining outcomes on 1,054 patients following cystectomy with median 10-year follow-up, Stein and colleagues demonstrated that in the 23% of patients with lymph node positive disease, the 5- and 10-year recurrence-free survival rates were 35 and 34%, respectively. This compares to the node negative patients in whom those with extravesical disease had 5- and 10-year recurrence-free survival rates of 50–60% and those with organ confined disease having rates nearing 85%.[11] Comparable results have been seen by others with 5-year recurrence-free survival rates ranging from 21 to 33% in those bladder cancer patients with nodal metastases noted following radical cystectomy with pelvic lymph node dissection.[29-32]

Number of lymph nodes involved is felt by some to play a role in prognosis. In the Stein paper those with

<5 nodes involved had a 10-year recurrence-free survival nearing 40%. Those with greater than or equal to five positive nodes had a recurrence-free survival rate of only 25% at 10 years.[11] A similar phenomenon with a six node cutoff was seen by Lerner and colleagues[32] and an eight node cutoff with Stein and colleagues.[33]

When thinking about the number of positive nodes it is also important to consider lymph node density which is an assessment of the degree of node positivity. Lymph node density is calculated by dividing the number of positive lymph nodes by the total number of lymph nodes sampled. Stein and colleagues demonstrated in their series of 1,054 patients following cystectomy that those patients with a lymph node density of 20% or less had a 43% 10-year recurrence-free survival compared with only 17% survival at 10 years when lymph node density was greater than 20% ($p < 0.001$).[33] Kassouff and colleagues obtained comparable results in their cohort of 248 cystectomy patients treated by radical cystoprostatectomy at M.D. Anderson cancer center. In this series, there was a comparable 5-year disease-specific survival of 54.6 and 15.3% in patients with lymph node densities of less than 20% compared to those above 20%. Furthermore, in a multivariate analysis of this population only lymph node density greater than 20% held as a predictor of disease-specific survival in this population.[34]

Extracapsular extension is a very powerful predictor of outcome following cystectomy as demonstrated by Fleischmann and colleagues.[35] In this study 507 consecutive cystectomy patients were analyzed for lymph node parameters including number of nodes positive, node density, and the presence of extracapsular extension. Extracapsular extension of disease outside the confines of the lymph node was identified as the most powerful predictor of outcome in the multivariate model. Interestingly, number of positive nodes and percent positive nodes were not significant in this analysis.

46.5 Extent of Lymph Node Dissection at Time of Cystectomy

Despite an acknowledgement of the importance of the pelvic lymph node dissection at the time of cystectomy, there is a lack of consensus on the extent of dissection needed to provide the maximum benefit.

We only have to look back to Jewett's initial description of outcome with this disease to know that pelvic nodal metastases occur in this disease without distant spread.[36] In addition, for over a half century we have known that a pelvic lymph node dissection can decrease local recurrence rates as demonstrated by Kerr et al.[37]

In a retrospective analysis looking at 68 patients treated between 1990 and 1993, Poulsen and colleagues compared outcomes in 68 patients undergoing a standard lymph node dissection (the iliac bifurcation to Cloquet's node including the obturator fossa) to 194 patients undergoing an extended lymph node dissection (including common iliac nodes to the aortic bifurcation, pre-sacral nodes, and the obturator fossa). They demonstrated an increased number of nodes in the extended lymph node dissection group consistent with the concept of "seek and you shall find." Furthermore, they demonstrated that the extended node dissections resulted in markedly improved survival for those with organ confined disease (<T3b, 85 vs 64%) and even in those without nodal metastases (<T3b/N0, 90 vs 71%).[38]

In the USC population, a benefit was seen with node dissections exceeding a yield of 15 nodes.[33] There was only a 25% 10-year recurrence-free survival in those patients who had 15 or less lymph nodes removed compared with a 36% 10-year recurrence-free survival in those individuals who had greater than 15 lymph nodes removed. In a SEER-based analysis of over 1900 cystectomy patients Konety et al. found a lymph node yield of 10–14 nodes to have the greatest impact on survival.[39]

Therefore, there appears to be a benefit to a more extensive node dissection with those patients having nodal yields of more than 10–15 nodes deriving the most significant benefit. However, we feel strongly that the nodal yield, as determined by the absolute nodal count, is just a surrogate for a carefully performed nodal dissection as the number can fluctuate greatly from 0 to 45 nodes or above. Every attempt should be made to completely clear all of the soft tissue within the boundaries outlined above as lymph node numbers are based on a variety of factors including

1. Boundaries of dissection
2. Inherent anatomical diversity
3. Diligence of the pathology team

With respect to assisting the pathology team, there may be a benefit when separate nodal packages, corresponding to the nodal areas are sent individually. Bochner and colleagues demonstrated a greater than threefold increase in nodal counts following a conversion from sending en bloc to sending separate nodal packages for analyses.[40]

46.6 Robotic-Assisted Laparoscopic Radical Cystectomy

Robotic-assisted laparoscopic radical cystectomy is a new, emerging extension of the well-described laparoscopic approach to the management of patients with muscle invasive or superficial bladder cancer refractory to intravesical therapy. As mentioned previously, the dawn of pelvic laparoscopy was the pelvic lymph node dissection.

From there, it is only logical that this technique expanded to include patients with bladder cancer as demonstrated by Hemal and colleagues.[41] Currently there are now greater than 500 cases of laparoscopic cystectomy in the literature.[42]

A pioneering series of robot-assisted laparoscopic radical cystectomy by Menon et al. has rekindled interest in "robot-assisted radical cystectomy worldwide.[43–45]

As outlined above a critical component of the radical cystectomy is the lymph node dissection. In the next section we will outline our technique and results in performing the robotic-assisted laparoscopic lymph node dissection as well as results of our colleagues. We will then discuss briefly complications and their management.

46.7 Technique for the Robotic-Assisted Laparoscopic Extended Lymph Node Dissection at Wake Forest University

(I) Port placement

As with any laparoscopic procedure optimal port placement allows for the best possible surgical outcomes. As opposed to the prostatectomy the extended lymph node dissection of the radical cystectomy requires a wider surgical field thus requiring more proximal placement of the robotic

ports. Typically, the camera port is placed two finger breadths above the umbilicus, the two robotic ports 17 cm from the pubis, and 10 cm from the camera port. Two further 12 mm assistant ports are placed on the right and the fourth arm or 5 mm assistant port on the left if a third arm robot is being used. In general care must be taken to place the ports higher, which helps in obtaining more proximal nodal tissue.

In our experience with the standard daVinci and daVinci-S systems, we have found the later system more conducive to a better lymph node dissection.

A 0 or 30° lens is used with the bipolar Maryland or plasma kinetic Maryland in the left hand, curved monopolar scissors in the right hand, and the prograsp in the fourth arm. Note, the suction assistant port is placed between the right robotic port and the camera port at a location of the pre-marked ileal conduit site.

(II) Nodal dissection

The first part of the dissection depends on the operating surgeon and school of thought. At WFUBMC we will often start with the dissection with the lymph node for several reasons:

1. One is "freshest" at the start of the case.
2. The lymph node dissection "sets-up" the rest of the case through the identification of the boundaries of dissection and important structures namely the genitofemoral nerves, the ureters, and the iliac vessels.
3. Many of the nodes may be sent along with the bladder specimen reducing the number of cumbersome instrument passages or expensive endocatch bags used in the procedure.

There is, however, controversy as some feel that the lymph node dissection is facilitated by having the bladder "out of the way."

When starting with the lymph node dissection, the initial step involves incision of peritoneum on the left lateral aspect of the sigmoid colon and early identification of the left ureter. This early identification allows for protection of this important structure. A concomitant left ureteral dissection is performed at the time of the nodal dissection. A proximal mobilization of the peritoneum and ureter are taken to the level of the IMA so as to facilitate passage of the left ureter

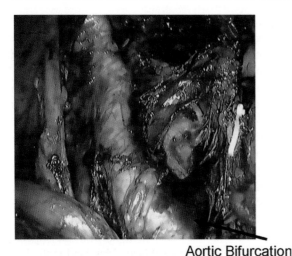

Fig. 46.1 Proximal extent of pelvic lymph node dissection demonstrating the aortic bifurcation. The left ureter can be seen in the *left* lower quadrant of the figure

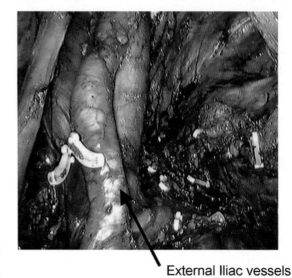

Fig. 46.3 Bifurcation of the left common iliac artery demonstrating the left external iliac artery and vein as well as the left internal iliac artery

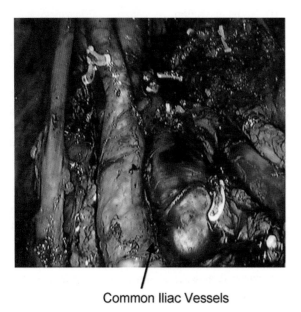

Fig. 46.2 More distal aspect of the dissection demonstrating the left common iliac artery

under the sigmoid mesentery. The iliac artery is identified at the level where the ureter crosses. A "split and roll" technique is used to incise the nodal tissue overlying the aorta from the IMA proximally (Fig. 46.1) down the left common (Fig. 46.2) and external iliac arteries (Fig. 46.3)

to Cloquet's node distally to the level of the circumflex iliac vein. The genitofemoral nerve is identified lateral to the common iliac artery and is preserved. All of the nodal tissue between the genitofemoral nerve and the artery are then harvested with careful attention to clip significant lymphatic vascular structures with Hem-O-Lok clips running longitudinally.

At this point it is critical to initiate a dissection lateral to the artery and medial to the pelvic musculature in the so-called space of Marseille. Very shortly upon entering this space the iliac vein will become apparent therefore caution and awareness are key to avoid injury to this structure. Further dissection lateral to the vein will further increase nodal yield. Perforating vessels from the pelvic side wall can be dealt with by judicious use of bipolar cautery. Upon deeper dissection, eventually one will come upon the obturator nerve which marks the end of the lateral dissection (Fig. 46.4) and underneath this level, we extend our dissection over the iliacus muscle.

A medial dissection on the artery is carried out and nodal tissue between the artery and vein is then harvested. This will initiate the "split and roll" on the vein which again is carried distally to Cloquet's node and Cooper's ligament.

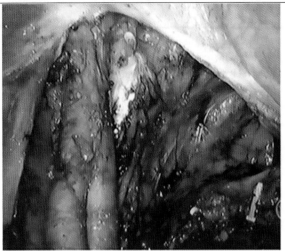

Obturator group of lymph nodes

Fig. 46.4 Left obturator nerve just deep to the left external iliac vein. Obturator lymph node packet has already been dissected out

The obturator nerve is again identified just deep to the pubic bone at which point the external iliac vein crosses it. The obturator package is harvested and dissected proximally to the bifurcation of the iliac arteries. The most proximal obturator tissue is then dissected free from the lateral aspect of the vessels in the "space of Marseille."

A "split and roll" technique is then used to dissect the nodal tissue overlying the left internal iliac artery. Identification and early clipping of the median umbilical and superior vesical arteries are possible during this dissection.

A comparable dissection is performed on the right; however, further dissection is carried out medial to the proximal aspect of the internal iliac artery in order to harvest the pre-sacral lymph nodes.

(III) Specimen retrieval

Separate packages vs right and left

Nodal packages are sent off as "right and left pelvic lymph nodes" in two separate packages. An Endocatch bag can work well to assist with LN removal, otherwise nodes can be removed from the abdomen using a microfrance grasper or a laparoscopic scoop under direct vision. Often the seat of the 12 mm port is removed to facilitate extrusion of some of the larger nodal packages.

46.8 Results at Our Institution and Others with the Robotic-Assisted Laparoscopic Lymph Node Dissection

Despite a motivated group of experienced pelvic surgeons whose pathologic specimens were being examined as part of a trial, only 73% of surgeons performed a complete dissection of all 12 pre-defined lymphadenectomy fields of the radical cystectomy.[17]

It takes experience, a knowledge of the anatomy, effort, and commitment in order to complete a thorough lymph node dissection. This can be said for both the open and robot-assisted laparoscopic approach.

We began our robotic program at Wake Forest University in January of 2008. In the intervening 18 months 65 RARCs were performed. As can be seen in Table 46.1, our median lymph node count was 16 which compares well with our most recent 45 open radical cystectomies with a median lymph node yield of 15.

There are several other centers using the robotic-assisted approach to radical cystectomy and as standard of care to perform pelvic lymph node dissections. A comparison of median lymph node yields between some of the largest RARC and ORC series can be seen in Table 46.1.

These series represent some of the largest series in the English language literature. As can be seen, there

Table 46.1 Lymph node counts in cystectomy series

Robot-assisted laparoscopic series

Group	Number of patients	Median LN	References
UNC	100	19	53
Cornell	83	17.9	54
RPMI	67	18	55
WFUBMC	45	16	56
Mayo Clinic	27	12.3	57

Open cystectomy series

Group	Number of patients	Median LN	References
USC	1,349	31	58
MSKCC	553	14	59
Mansoura	418	17.9	21
Vanderbilt	279	7	59
U Michigan	210	9	59

does not appear to be any significant difference in the number of median nodes collected at the time of cystectomy. This leaves little doubt that with typical lymph node dissections performed at leading institutions, there is no difference in absolute lymph node counts. Whether or not comparable recurrence-free survival rates are possible remains to be seen. There is, however, suggestion from a recent paper from the Mayo clinic in Arizona that in 59 patients with at least 6 months of follow-up (mean 25 months) the 12- and 36-month overall survival rates were comparable to open series at 82 and 69%, respectively.[46]

46.9 Complications of Robot-Assisted Lymph Node Dissection for Bladder Cancer

Complications associated with lymph node dissections are low with the open procedure and are limited to nerve-related injury to the genitofemoral or obturator nerves, lymphocele, or vascular injury. In a recent report of surgical complications associated with open and robotic cystectomies neither of these complications were described. In fact the robotic-assisted cystectomy patients had less overall (41 vs 59%) and less major complications (10 vs 30%).[46]

Nerve damage can come in the form of a neuropraxia or contusion which are self-limiting injuries that normally resolve within 6 weeks, axonotmesis where neural elements distal to the area of injury degenerate where symptoms take up to 6 months to resolve and complete transection.

The genitofemoral nerve (L1–L3) has both motor and sensory function. It has a genital branch which supplies the scrotal skin, cremasteric muscles, and lower abdominal muscles and a femoral branch which innervates the femoral triangle. Significant clinical sequelae of damage to the nerve are rare but can include paresthesia and pain.[47] Typically the nerve lies just lateral to the iliac artery and can be a fan of nerves rather than a single nerve. It typically represents the lateral dissection margin for the pelvic lymph node dissection for bladder cancer patients.

The obturator nerve (L2–L4) innervates the medial thigh adductor muscles (gracilis, pectineus, adductor longus, brevis, magnus, and obturator externus)

and provides sensation to the medial thigh. Disability can include problems with gait in some but not all patients who can compensate without too much difficulty. However, it can affect one's ability to drive with a decreased ability to shift from gas to break on the affected side. Therefore deficits can be motor or sensory and patients can even suffer from pain.

Injury to the obturator nerve is rare in robotic-assisted cystectomy with no reported cases in the literature. Although the reported rates are low, it is possible that rates are higher due to a lack of reporting or a lack of recognition especially in cases without transection.

For neuropraxic and axonotmetic injuries, time and physical therapy are best due to the self-limiting nature of these injuries. Following transection, complete recovery can reach 90% when primary repair is performed.[48] Primary repair can even be performed at the time of transection laparoscopically.[49]

Most of the literature on symptomatic lymphocele following laparoscopic pelvic lymph node dissection comes from the prostate cancer literature. The incidence is low, approximately 1% given the fact that these procedures are intraperitoneal and the lymphatic fluid can thus be absorbed by the peritoneal cavity.[50] The incidence of asymptomatic lymphoceles is likely higher but is difficult to ascertain as most of these patients are not imaged in the perioperative period. Symptoms relate to the mass effect of the lymphocele and can include pain from pelvic nerve compression, leg swelling from venous compression, hydronephrosis secondary to ureteral obstruction, and impact on bladder giving frequency or bowel giving constipation.

Management can come in the form of aspiration, drainage, sclerotherapy, or laparoscopic/open internal marsupialization. Risk factors associated with the development of lymphoceles include heparin, lack of lymphostasis (lack of clipping), metastatic lymph nodes, steroid, and diuretic use.[51]

As discussed earlier in this chapter, there is a growing body of evidence to support an increased node dissection. With an increase in the complexity of this part of the procedure it is fair to ask whether or not this increased dissection results in an increased complication rate. Brossner and colleagues compared 46 patients undergoing an open extended pelvic lymph node dissection at the time of radical cystectomy to a comparable group of 46 patients undergoing the standard dissection. Within a 30 day period there was no difference in complication rate between the two groups. The extended lymph node dissection did, however, increase the procedure time by 63 min.[52] There is no reason to believe that this data is not applicable to the robot-assisted laparoscopic series.

Therefore, complications stemming from pelvic lymph node dissections performed at the time of robotic-assisted laparoscopic cystectomy are rare. Careful attention to surgical technique, clipping of lymphatics and gentle dissection close to the genitofemoral and obturator nerves, and an understanding of the anatomy result in decreased complication rates. Thanks to the magnified image and dexterity provided by the robot, a further decrease in an already low complication rate should be achievable.

46.10 Conclusions

Robotic cystectomy is a new, minimally invasive technique which appears to result in less blood loss, shorter hospital stays, and potentially less complications. Furthermore, with careful attention to detail, comparable oncologic results are achievable with this procedure and the open procedure in terms of negative margins and total node counts. Definitive claims regarding oncologic outcomes await long-term follow-up.

References

1. Halstead WS. The treatment of wounds. *Johns Hopkins Hosp Rep.* 1891;2:279.
2. Jemal A, Siegel R, Ward E, et al. Cancer Statistics. *CA Cancer J Clin.* 2009;caac.20006:2009.
3. Prout GR, Marshall VF. The prognosis with untreated bladder tumors. *Cancer.* 1956;9:551.
4. Herr HW, Sogani PC. Does early cystectomy improve the survival of patients with high risk superficial bladder tumors? *J Urol.* 2001;166:1296.
5. DeVere White RW, Katz MH, Steinberg GD. Opposing Views. *J Urol.* 2009;181:1994.
6. Sengelv L, von der Maase H. Radiotherapy in bladder cancer. *Radiot oncol.* 1999;52:1.
7. Tonoli S, Bertoni F, De Stefani A, et al. Radical radiotherapy for bladder cancer: retrospective analysis of a series of 459 patients treated in an Italian institution. *Clin Oncol (R Coll Radiol).* 2006;18:52.
8. Herr HW, Donat SM. Outcome of patients with grossly node positive bladder cancer after pelvic lymph node dissection and radical cystectomy. *J Urol.* 2001;165:62.
9. Glantz GM. Cystectomy and urinary diversion. *J Urol.* 1966;96:714.
10. Ghoneim MA, Abdel-Latif M, El-Mekresh M, et al. Radical cystectomy for carcinoma of the bladder: 2,720 consecutive cases 5 years later. *J Urol.* 2008;180:121.
11. Stein JP, Lieskovsky G, Cote R, et al. Radical cystectomy in the treatment of invasive bladder cancer: long-term results in 1,054 patients. *J Clin Oncol.* 2001;19:666.
12. Shabsigh A, Korets R, Vora KC, et al. Defining early morbidity of radical cystectomy for patients with bladder cancer using a standardized reporting methodology. *Eur Urol.* 2009;55:164.
13. Hemal AK. Role of robot-assisted surgery for bladder cancer. *Curr Opin Urol.* 2009;19:69.
14. Wolf JS. Indications, technique, and results of laparoscopic pelvic lymphadenectomy. *J Endourol.* 2001;15:427.
15. Leadbetter WF, Cooper JF. Regional gland dissection for carcinoma of the bladder; a technique for one-stage cystectomy, gland dissection, and bilateral uretero-enterostomy. *J Urol.* 1950;63:242.
16. Smith JA Jr, Whitmore WF Jr. Regional lymph node metastasis from bladder cancer. *J Urol.* 1981;126:591.
17. Leissner J, Ghoneim MA, Abol-Enein H, et al. Extended radical lymphadenectomy in patients with urothelial bladder cancer: results of a prospective multicenter study. *J Urol.* 2004;171:139.
18. Herr H. Surgical factors in the treatment of superficial and invasive bladder cancer. *Urol Clin North Am.* 2005;32:157.
19. Skinner DG. Management of invasive bladder cancer: a meticulous pelvic node dissection can make a difference. *J Urol.* 1982;128:34.
20. Wishnow K, Johnson D, Ro J, et al. Incidence, extent and location of unsuspected pelvic lymph node metastasis in patients undergoing radical cystectomy for bladder cancer. *J Urol.* 1987;137:408.
21. Abdel-Latif M, Abol-Enein H, El-Baz M, et al. Nodal involvement in bladder cancer cases treated with radical cystectomy: incidence and prognosis. *J Urol.* 2004;172:85.
22. Thoeny HC, Triantafyllou M, Birkhaeuser FD, et al. Combined ultrasmall superparamagnetic particles of iron oxide-enhanced and diffusion-weighted magnetic resonance imaging reliably detect pelvic lymph node metastases in normal-sized nodes of bladder and prostate cancer patients. *Eur Urol.* 2009;55:761.
23. Swinnen G, Maes A, Pottel H, et al. FDG-PET/CT for the preoperative lymph node staging of invasive bladder cancer. *Eur Urol.* 2010;57:641.
24. Mills RD, Turner WH, Fleischmann A, et al. Pelvic lymph node metastases from bladder cancer: outcome in 83 patients after radical cystectomy and pelvic lymphadenectomy. *J Urol.* 2001;166:19.
25. Grossman HB, Natale RB, Tangen CM, et al. Neoadjuvant Chemotherapy plus cystectomy compared with cystectomy alone for locally advanced bladder cancer. *N Engl J Med.* 2003;349:859.
26. Retz M, Lehmann J, Szysnik C, et al. Detection of occult tumor cells in lymph nodes from bladder cancer patients by MUC7 nested RT-PCR. *Eur Urol.* 2004;45:314.
27. Theodorescu D, Frierson HF. When is a negative lymph node really negative? molecular tools for the detection of lymph node metastasis from urological cancer. *Urol Oncol: Seminars and Original Investigations.* 2004;22:256.

28. Herr HW. Extent of surgery and pathology evaluation has an impact on bladder cancer outcomes after radical cystectomy. *Urology*. 2003;61:105.

29. Gschwend JRE, Dahm P, Fair WR. Disease specific survival as endpoint of outcome for bladder cancer patients following radical cystectomy. *Eur Urol*. 2002; 41:440.

30. Hautmann RE, Gschwend JRE, de Petriconi RC, et al. Cystectomy for transitional cell carcinoma of the bladder: results of a surgery only series in the neobladder era. *J Urol*. 2006;176:486.

31. Madersbacher S, Hochreiter W, Burkhard F, et al. Radical cystectomy for bladder cancer today-a homogeneous series without neoadjuvant therapy. *J Clin Oncol*. 2003;21:690.

32. Lerner SP, Skinner DG, Lieskovsky G, et al. The rationale for en bloc pelvic lymph node dissection for bladder cancer patients with nodal metastases: long-term results. *J Urol*. 1993;149:758.

33. Stein JP, Cai JIE, Groshen S, et al. Risk factors for patients with pelvic lymph node metastases following radical cystectomy with en bloc pelvic lymphadenectomy: the concept of lymph node density. *J Urol*. 2003;170:35.

34. Kassouf W, Agarwal PK, Herr HW, et al. Lymph node density is superior to TNM nodal status in predicting disease-specific survival after radical cystectomy for bladder cancer: analysis of pooled data from MDACC and MSKCC. *J Clin Oncol*. 2008;26:121.

35. Fleischmann A, Thalmann GN, Markwalder R, et al. Extracapsular extension of pelvic lymph node metastases from urothelial carcinoma of the bladder is an independent prognostic factor. *J Clin Oncol*. 2005;23:2358.

36. Jewett HJ, Strong GH. Infiltrating carcinoma of the bladder: relation of depth of penetration of the bladder wall to incidence of local extension and metastases. *J Urol*. 1946;55:366.

37. Kerr WSJ, Colby FH. Pelvic lymphadenectomy and total cystectomy in the treatment of carcinoma of the bladder. *J Urol*. 1950;63:842.

38. Poulsen AL, Horn T, Steven K. Radical cystectomy: extending the limits of pelvic lymph node dissection improves survival for patients with bladder cancer confined to the bladder wall. *J Urol*. 1998;160:2015.

39. Konety BR, Joslyn SA, O'Donnell MA. Extent of pelvic lymphadenectomy and its impact on outcome in patients diagnosed with bladder cancer: analysis of data from the Surveillance, epidemiology and end results program data base. *J Urol*. 2003;169:946.

40. Bochner, et al. *J Urol*. 2004;172:1286.

41. Hemal AK, Kolla SB, Wadhwa P, et al. Laparoscopic radical cystectomy and extracorporeal urinary diversion: a single center experience of 48 cases with three years of follow-up. *Urology*. 2008;71:41.

42. Andrew J, Stephenson ISG. Laparoscopic radical cystectomy for muscle-invasive bladder cancer: pathological and oncological outcomes. *BJU Int*. 2008;102:1296.

43. Hemal AK, Abol-Enein H, Tewari A, et al. Robotic radical cystectomy and urinary diversion in the management of bladder cancer. *Urolo Clin North Am*. 2004; 31:719.

44. Menon M, Hemal AK, Tewari A, et al. Robot-assisted radical cystectomy and urinary diversion in female patients: technique with preservation of the uterus and vagina. *J Am Coll Surg*. 2004;198:386.

45. Menon M, Hemal AK, Tewari A, et al. Nerve-sparing robot-assisted radical cystoprostatectomy and urinary diversion. *BJU Int*. 2003;92:232.

46. Martin A, Nunez R, Pacelli A, et al. Robot-assisted radical cystectomy: intermediate survival results at a mean follow-up of 25 months. *BJU Int*. 2010;105:1706.

47. Murovic J, Kim D, Tiel R, et al. Surgical management of 10 genitofemoral neuralgias at the Louisiana state university health sciences center. *Neurosurgery*. 2005;56:298.

48. Vasilev S:. Obturator nerve injury: a review of management options. *Gynecol Oncol*. 1994;53:152.

49. Spaliviero M, Steinberg A, Kaouk J, et al. Laparoscopic injury and repair of obturator nerve during radical prostatectomy. *Urology*. 2004;64:1030.

50. Chow C, Daly B, Burney T, et al. Complications after laparoscopic pelvic lymphadenectomy: CT diagnosis. *AJR Am J Roentgenol*. 1994;163:353.

51. Karcaaltincaba M, Akhan O. Radiologic imaging and percutaneous treatment of pelvic lymphocele. *Eur J Radiol*. 2005;55:340.

52. Brössne RC, Pycha A, Toth A, et al. Does extended lymphadenectomy increase the morbidity of radical cystectomy? *BJU Int*. 2004;93:64.

53. Pruthi R, Nielsen M, Nix J, et al. Robotic radical cystectomy for bladder cancer: surgical and pathological outcomes in 100 consecutive cases. *J Urol*. 2010;183:510.

54. Ng C, Kauffman E, Lee M, et al. A comparison of postoperative complications in open versus robotic cystectomy. *Eur Urol*. 2010;57:274.

55. Guru K, Sternberg K, Wilding G, et al. The lymph node yield during robot-assisted radical cystectomy. *BJU Int*. 2008;102:231.

56. Richards K, Hemal AK, Kader A, et al. Robot assisted laparoscopic pelvic lymphadenectomy at the time of radical cystectomy rivals that of open surgery: single institution report. *Urology*. 2010;76:1400.

57. Woods M, Thomas R, Davis R, et al. Robot-assisted extended pelvic lymphadenectomy. *J Endourol*. 2008; 22:1297.

58. Stein JP, Penson DF, Cai J, et al. Radical cystectomy with extended lymphadenectomy: evaluating separate package versus en bloc submission for node positive bladder cancer. *J Urol*. 2007;177:876.

59. Herr H, Lee C, Chang SAM, et al. Standardization of radical cystectomy and pelvic lymph node dissection for bladder cancer: a collaborative group report. *J Urol*. 2004;171:1823.

Chapter 47

Robot-Assisted Intracorporeal Ileal Conduit

Alexander Mottrie, Jamil Rehman, Mattia N. Sangalli, Geert de Naeyer, Peter Schatteman, Paul Carpentier, Matthew H. Hayn, and Khurshid A. Guru

47.1 Introduction

Radical cystectomy with extended pelvic lymph node dissection is the most effective treatment for patients with organ-confined, muscle-invasive, or recurrent high-grade bladder cancer; data suggest that in the appropriately selected patient, early cystectomy is associated with superior oncologic outcomes.[1] Open radical cystectomy, however, is known to have significant morbidity.[2,3] With the broader approach of laparoscopic and robotic techniques for the treatment of renal and prostate cancer, the application of robotic approaches to the surgical treatment of bladder cancer is a logical progression. Since the first published report in 2003,[4] numerous surgical series have been published regarding the feasibility and outcomes of robot-assisted radical cystectomy (RARC).[5–9]

At many centers, urinary diversion after RARC is performed by an extracorporeal technique. Since a few years, in different institutes, this closed approach has been followed by the robot-assisted total intracorporeal ileal conduit reconstructions with promising results. This allows the patients to have full impact of the advantages of the minimal-invasive approach as the full procedure can now entirely be performed closed. Since 1992, various authors have reported their experience, using both robotic and laparoscopic approaches.[10–17]

47.2 Historical Background

In 1992, Kozminski and colleagues published a case report of laparoscopic-assisted ileal conduit, although a significant portion of the procedure was performed extra-corporeally.[10] Gill et al. in 2000 reported on two patients who underwent pure laparoscopic radical cystectomy with complete intra-corporeal ileal conduit creation.[11] In 2000, Potter et al. reported 5-year follow-up on a patient in whom a laparoscopic intracorporeal ileal conduit was performed.[12]

In 2003, Yohannes et al. used a dual approach utilizing both laparoscopic and robotic assistance.[13] In their series, robot-assisted cystectomy was performed followed by disengagement of the da Vinci robot and completion of the urinary diversion using standard laparoscopic approach with reintroduction of the robot to complete the ureteroileal anastomosis.[13] In 2004, Balaji et al. reported on using robotic assistance in the completion of intracorporeal laparoscopic ileal conduit urinary diversion, specifically in the completion of the ureteroileal anastamosis.[14] In 2006, Hubert et al. published the first report of successful robotic simple cystectomy with complete intracorporeal ileal conduit construction in two patients with neurogenic bladder.[16] Most recently, Pruthi et al. report on 12 patients who underwent robot-assisted laparoscopic intracorporeal urinary diversion, of whom 9 underwent creation of an ileal conduit.[17]

A. Mottrie (✉)
Department of Urology, Onze-Lieve-Vrouw (OLV) Clinic, Moorselbaan 164-9300 Aalst, Belgium
e-mail: a.mottrie@gmail.com

European Technique: Alexander Mottrie, Jamil Rehman, Mattia N. Sangalli, Geert de Naeyer, Peter Schatteman, and Paul Carpentier
Marionette Technique: Matthew H. Hayn and Khurshid A. Guru

A.K. Hemal, M. Menon (eds.), *Robotics in Genitourinary Surgery*,
DOI 10.1007/978-1-84882-114-9_47, © Springer-Verlag London Limited 2011

47.3 Surgical Technique

After obtaining experience with robotic radical prosta-tectomy, we embarked on robotic radical cystectomy with extracorporeal urinary diversion and then we pro-gressed to total intracorporeal technique. Our robotic cystectomy and urinary diversion technique is pre-viously described (18) and provides an anatomic approach, very familiar to most urologists. Our goal is to transfer the technical steps that we usually use in our open technique. Herein we describe our robotic urinary diversion (Ileal conduit).

Since February 2008, we routinely perform robotic-assisted cystectomy and ileal conduit (RACIC) for muscle-invasive urothelial carcinoma. The entire pro-cedure, including radical cystoprostatectomy, extended PLND, ileal conduit urinary diversion including isola-tion of the ileal loop (20 cm ileal segment) 15 cm from the ileocecal junction, restoration of bowel continuity with stapled side-to-side anastomosis, retroperitoneal transfer of the left ureter to the right side, and bilateral stented (8F feeding tube) ileoureteral anastomoses in a Wallace-type fashion, was performed intracorporeally with robotic assistance and the stoma was fashioned in an open fashion.

Preop preparation: Mechanical bowel preparation preoperatively comprises clear liquids for the 24 h prior to surgery and oral self-administration of 2–5 L of electrolyte lavage solution in the afternoon before the surgical procedure. Sequential compression stock-ings, subcutaneous low-molecular heparin, and broad-spectrum antibiotics are given before the surgical pro-cedure. The position for an external stoma is evaluated and marked on the skin of the patient. (*Alternatively, the patient may undergo outpatient, mechanical-only, bowel preparation with the use of magnesium citrate or fleets phosphosoda and a fleets enema the morning of surgery, along with a clear liquid diet a day prior to surgery.*)

The patient is positioned in a lithotomy position with both arms fixed along the body. There is about 10° of Trendelenburg. It is important to place the robotic laparoscopic ports appropriately. This is one of the most critical steps for successful use of the robotic tool with precision and accuracy facilitates, along with the cystectomy in the small pelvis, PLND, ureter mobilization, and transferring the left ureter to the right under the sigmoid mesentery without

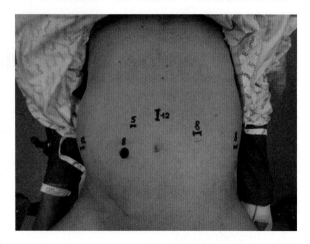

Fig. 47.1 Ports and stoma sites marked preop

collision of the arms. The patient's stature, body mass index (BMI), pelvis girdle configuration, and positioning also have an important bearing on the robotic arm ergonomics, length, and mobility that impact the movements inside the body. The 12 mm camera trocar is placed at the midline approximately 3–5 cm (dependent on size of the patient) cranial to the umbilicus. The three robotic 8 mm trocars are inserted in the abdominal wall as described in Fig. 47.1. One assistant 12 mm trocar is placed 5 cm cranial to the right iliac crest. Through this trocar, the Endo-GIAs will be inserted, thus necessitating sufficient distance to the pubis. Another 5 mm trocar is placed between camera trocar and right robotic arm.

It is also equally important that all elements of the patient setup are consistent and reproducible. After completing the extirpative portion of the pro-cedure (radical cystoprostatectomy, extended PLND), the specimen is trapped in a large endobag and the total intracorporeal ileal conduit urinary diversion is performed as described below.

47.3.1 Operative Steps

The radical cystectomy is performed in the same way as described for invasive bladder cancer previ-ously by our group,[18] except the ports are shifted 3–5 cm cranially, that helps in ileal conduit urinary diversion.

Step 1: Isolation, dissection, ligation, and tagging of both ureters

The left paracolic gutter is incised along the line of Toldt, and the left ureter is identified over the left common iliac artery. The ureter is freed distally with respect to its vascularization, clipped above the left vesicoureteral junction (VUJ) using Weck locking clips, and divided. The right ureter is mobilized and divided in a similar fashion. Both ureters can be tagged with sutures. Generous periureteral fat is maintained to keep adventitial blood supply of the ureter. The single clip on the proximal cut end of the ureter prevents urine leakage onto the surgical field and creates ureteral hydrodistension, thus facilitating the subsequent ureteroileal anastomosis.

(*Technical consideration*: If the available length of both ureters is considered too short by the surgeon, the former dissection is continued cranially and ureter mobilized proximally up the lower pole of the kidney and brought to the right side cranial to the inferior mesenteric artery.)

Step 2: Retroperitoneal transfer of the left ureter to the right side

Mobilization begins with dissection of the lateral attachments of the sigmoid colon. An atraumatic forceps is passed lifting the posterior peritoneum caudally toward the aortoiliac bifurcation. The posterior attachments (mesocolon) of the colon are then freed beginning at the sacral promontory in the presacral space providing an unobstructed passage or tunnel. This plane opens easily, as long as dissection remains in the avascular plane just adjacent to the vessels. The sigmoid colon is retracted superiorly and anteriorly, the blunt tip grasper is passed under the surface of the mobilized colon at the level of the sacral promontory, and the ureter is grasped (with its tagged suture) and is passed underneath the sigmoid loop and brought to the contralateral side. Care is taken not to twist the ureter nor to cause kinking.

Step 3: Bilateral ureteral spatulation and ureteral anastomosis in a Wallace fashion (Fig. 47.2)

A Prograsp forceps placed through the fourth arm grasps the end of both ureters in a fashion that they are nicely lined up one next to the other. After a 3 cm longitudinal incision is made along the anterior aspect of the distal ends (spatulation), a wide

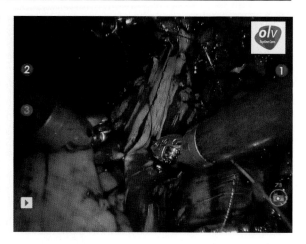

Fig. 47.2 Wallace-type spatulated ureteral anastomosis

anastomosis is formed in Wallace fashion. This is done using a monocryl 4-0 running suture.

(*Technical consideration*: The silk suture is used to stabilize the ureter with the fourth arm as it is partially transected and spatulated.)

Step 4: Identification, isolation, and suture marking of caecum 20 cm long ileal bowel segment for ileal conduit 15 cm from ileocecal segment

Bowel including cecum, ileocecal junction, and ileum is identified. A 20 cm ileal loop segment is isolated about 15 cm proximal to the ileocecal valve by placing marking sutures. The length of the bowel is determined by running the bowel an inch at a time, the tip of the instruments being used as a measuring stick.

(*Technical consideration*: The use of a string of known length can also facilitate this process.)

Step 5: Anchoring and tenting the selected ileal loop segment to the anterior abdominal wall (alternatively two-pulley sutures, aka Marionette technique) (Fig. 47.3)

Care is taken to maintain good vascularity of the isolated bowel segment by visual inspection of the mesentery, as well as transillumination in order to help to identify the mesenteric vessels. Three transparietal holding sutures are placed (on both extremities of the selected ileal loop and one on its midportion) to fix the bowel on the abdominal wall allowing improved presentation to the mesenterium. The sutures are fixed with Weck locking clips, making change of tension to the threads possible.

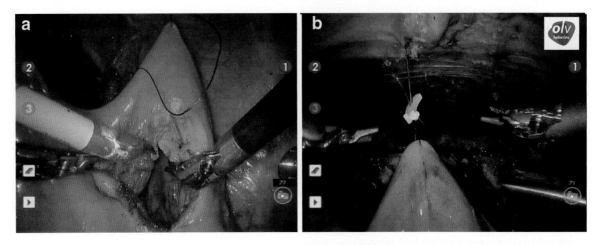

Fig. 47.3 a, b Anchoring stitches of ileal segment to abdominal wall and creation of window in mesentery

The transversal mesenteric vessels are gently coagulated with the Gyrus forceps as needed. Alternatively, sutures can be used before cutting them. (*Technical consideration*: (1) A cystoscope or laparoscope can be used from one of the assistant ports in order to help identify the mesenteric vessels with transillumination. (2) Instead of fixed holding sutures on both extremities of the selected ileal loop pulley sutures can be applied percutaneously with the help of Keith needle to pull, tent, and relax the either end of isolated bowel.)

Step 6: Bowel resection and isolation of the ileal conduit

A 20 cm segment of selected small bowel is now isolated using Endo-GIA visualizing vascularity and integrity. The ileal conduit is put caudal to the two bowel ends. The isolated bowel segment has oral and aboral ends, which can be marked to keep orientation.

Step 7: Restoration of bowel continuity with stapled side-to-side ileoileal anastomosis (Fig. 47.4)

The small bowel continuity is re-established by side-to-side anastomosis using laparoscopic Endo-GIA stapler (tissue load). The ends of the small bowel are secured together with an interrupted silk suture placed anti-mesenterically 5 cm from the stapled ends. The fourth arm grasps this suture to hold the bowel ends under tension caudally to ease the right positioning of the Endo-GIA jaws. The Endo-GIA stapler is fired along the adjacent anti-mesenteric sides of the small bowel. One transverse firing of

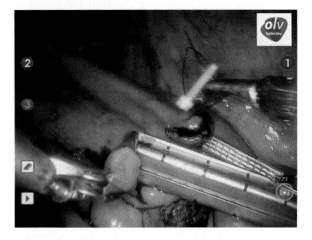

Fig. 47.4 Ileoileal bowel anastomosis

the Endo-GIA stapler is used to close the open ends of the ileal limbs. Interrupted sutures may be used to imbricate over the staple lines. The mesenteric trap (defect in the mesentery or mesenteric window) is closed using running 4-0 vicryl sutures. The distal ileum is relocated in the abdomen.

Step 8: Deanchoring the ileal segment (lateralized)

The ileal segment is released by cutting the anchoring or pulley sutures and this isolated bowel segment used for ileal conduit is outside the continuity of bowel. The oral and aboral sides are defined. The staplers are excised on both sides.

Step 9: Ureteroileal tension-free anastomosis (proximal or oral end and posterior layer anastomosed first) (Fig. 47.5)

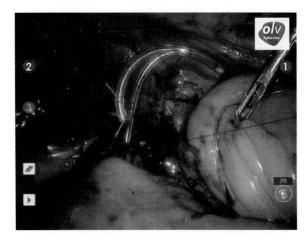

Fig. 47.5 Ureteroileal anastomosis

The ureteroileal anastomosis is fashioned in a refluxing manner. First the posterior anastomosis is performed starting proximal at the spatulation site of the right ureter. Running 4-0 monocryl sutures are used for the anastomosis. This step of the procedure is facilitated when the Prograsp brought through the fourth arm fixes the Wallace plate by stretching it.

Step 10: Passage of ureteral stents

Prior to completing the anterior layer of the ureteroileal anastomosis, ureteral stents (8F feeding tubes or 8F single-pigtail ureteral stents inserted over a 0.035 in. guide wire) are introduced through the aboral or distal end of the isolated ileal loop. They are introduced through the ipsilateral lateral assistant port and guided into the ileal conduit using a fenestrated grasping forceps, delivered near the oral or butt of the loop at the prospective ureteroileal anastomotic site, and then advanced into the ureters. The stents are secured with an absorbable stitch to the conduit (at the site of ileoureteral anastomosis) to prevent the stents from falling out during manipulation and in the postoperative period.

Step 11: Ureteroileal watertight anastomosis (anterior layer)

The ureteroileal anastomosis is performed using 4-0 monocryl running sutures is completed over 8F ureteric stents.

(*Technical consideration*: The parietal peritoneum should be sutured around the base of the conduit to cover the urinary anastomosis with peritoneum. This will also prevent the ureteroileal anastomosis from twisting.)

Step 12: Delivery of the aboral end through the marked stoma site and fashioning of conduit stoma (Fig. 47.6)

The distal or aboral end of the ileal conduit loop is delivered directly through the anterior abdominal wall through the 8 mm port preselected stoma site, corresponding to the inferior port placement site (in the right lower quadrant of the abdomen during cystectomy). The robotic arm is dislocated from the trocar, a grasping forceps is brought through that trocar, and the distal end is grasped. A lunar incision is made around the trocar and the fascia is incised in the form of a cross as far that the opening allows a two-finger dilation of the abdominal wall musculature. The conduit end is delivered. With four vicryl 2/0 stitches on the fascia, the muscularis of the conduit is fixed at about 3 cm proximal to its end. The ileal conduit is then secured to the skin and stoma matured using absorbable sutures in an everted fashion by grabbing also 2 cm proximal at its musculature in each stitch. The abdomen is irrigated and inspected for bleeding and inadvertent visceral injuries, the specimen is extracted in its organ bag through a supraumbilical incision, the trocars are removed under direct vision, and the port sites are closed with staples. A 10 mm drain is placed near the ileoureteral anastomosis to help detect urinary drainage.

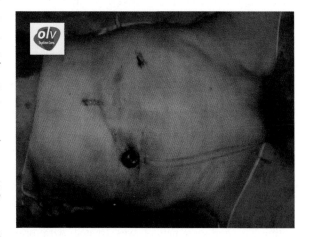

Fig. 47.6 Postop with stoma fashioned

47.3.2 Postoperative Care

After completing the procedure, all patients undergo routine care according to our radical cystectomy care pathway. The nasogastric tube is removed when flatus starts. Parenteral nutrition is commenced from the first day after RRC for 4–5 days. The patient can then begin solid nutrition. The drains are normally removed after 3 days, when the drainage is <100 mL. On the eighth day the ureteric stents are removed. Patient activity was encouraged as soon as possible, with most patients out of bed the night of surgery and ambulating on the first postoperative day. Patients are discharged once they are fully ambulant and tolerate oral nutrition. Serum creatinine and electrolytes are measured before hospital discharge.

47.4 Results

From February 2008 through September 2009 and from May 2009 until December 2009 in the O.L.V. Robotic Centre and in the Roswell Park Cancer Institute, respectively, a total of 35 patients underwent robot-assisted intracorporeal ileal conduit. Table 47.1 summarizes the results. The RACIC was technically successful in all patients without open conversion needed in any of the patients. The mean age was 72 (range 55–86), mean BMI was 28 (range 19–41), and median ASA score was 2.5 (range 2–3). Of the cohort, 16 (46%) had undergone previous surgery, and 5 (14%) were female. The mean operative time including PLND and urinary diversion was 346.2 min (range 210–480), mean operative time of diversion was 122 min (range 52–212), mean estimated blood loss (EBL) was 358 mL (range 200–3,900), and the median hospital stay was 14 days (range 10–27). In the five female patients, the specimen was extracted through the vagina. There were 8 complications among the 35 patients: one patient developed a small bowel obstruction that required exploratory laparotomy and lysis of adhesions, one patient developed a urine leak that resolved with nephrostomy tube drainage, and one patient had a non-specific colitis. Two patients developed urinary tract infections postoperatively; one patient required inpatient admission and intravenous antibiotics, and one patient was treated with oral antibiotics. One patient developed a deep venous

Table 47.1 Results

Demographics	
Number of patients	35
Male (*n*)	30
Female (*n*)	5
Mean age (years)	72 (55–87)
Operative parameters	
Mean overall OR time (min)	346.2 (210–480)
Mean diversion time (min)	122 (52–212)
Mean EBL (mL)	358 (200–3900)
Complications	
Intraoperative (*n*)	
Bladder injury	0
Rectal injury	0
Bowel injury	0
Blood transfusions	0
Conversion to laparoscopic	0
Conversion to open	0
Death	0
Postoperative (*n*)	
Urinary leakage	1 (nephrostomy tube)
Small bowel obstruction	2 (open adhesiolysis, conservative)
Non-specific colitis	1
Urinary tract infection	2
Deep venous thrombosis	1
Postoperative necrosis of ileal conduit (iatrogenic injury of conduit pedicle)	1

OR, operative; EBL, estimated blood loss; LOS, length of stay.

thrombosis, and one patient had a partial small bowel obstruction that resolved with bowel rest. There was one postoperative iatrogenic necrosis of the ileal conduit caused by uncareful retraction of the organ bag and thereby probably injuring the conduit pedicle, as the ileal conduit was well vascularized at the end of the operation, requiring an open revision.

A clear liquid diet was started on the third postoperative day. Postoperative renal function was normal (mean postoperative creatine 0.99 mg/dL) and excretory urography revealed unobstructed upper tracts.

47.5 Discussion

To date, there have been two series comparing intracorporeal versus extracorporeal urinary diversion after RARC. Pruthi et al. recently reported outcomes on

12 patients who underwent intracorporeal urinary diversion including ileal conduit ($n=9$) and orthotopic ileal neobladder ($n=3$). These patients were then compared to consecutive historical controls who underwent RARC and extracorporeal urinary diversion.[17] They report a longer mean OR time for the intracorporeal group (5.3 vs. 4.2 h, $p<0.001$), but no difference in mean EBL, time to flatus, bowel movement, or discharge. The intracorporeal group also had less mean inpatient narcotic usage. In addition, they reported similar complication rates between the two groups.[17]

47.6 Conclusions

Robot-assisted radical cystectomy is now being performed at many centers worldwide, especially those with significant prior robotic experience. Robotic cystectomy with intracorporeal urinary diversion has demonstrated to be a feasible, safe, reproducible technique without increased complications. As surgeons become more comfortable with robotic-assisted cystectomy, a natural progression is to attempt a completely intracorporeal procedure. Based on two small single-institution series, robot-assisted intracorporeal ileal conduit can be accomplished safely with acceptable operative times and postoperative outcomes. Larger series with longer follow-up and favorable results will be required to add this new paradigm to minimally invasive surgery for bladder cancer.

References

1. Sanchez-Ortiz RF, Huang WC, Mick R, Van Arsdalen KN, Wein AJ, Malkowicz SB. An interval longer than 12 weeks between the diagnosis of muscle invasion and cystectomy is associated with worse outcome in bladder carcinoma. *J Urol*. January, 2003;169(1):110–115; discussion 115.
2. Ghoneim MA, el-Mekresh MM, el-Baz MA, el-Attar IA, Ashamallah A. Radical cystectomy for carcinoma of the bladder: critical evaluation of the results in 1,026 cases. *J Urol*. August, 1997;158(2):393–399.
3. Huang GJ, Stein JP. Open radical cystectomy with lymphadenectomy remains the treatment of choice for invasive bladder cancer. *Curr Opin Urol*. September, 2007;17(5):369–375.
4. Menon M, Hemal AK, Tewari A, et al. Nerve-sparing robot-assisted radical cystoprostatectomy and urinary diversion. *BJU Int*. August, 2003;92(3):232–236.
5. Guru KA, Kim HL, Piacente PM, Mohler JL. Robot-assisted radical cystectomy and pelvic lymph node dissection: initial experience at Roswell Park Cancer Institute. *Urology*. March, 2007;69(3):469–474.
6. Ng CK, Kauffman EC, Lee MM, Otto BJ, Portnoff A, Ehrlich JR, Schwartz MJ, Wang GJ, Scherr DS. A comparison of postoperative complications in open versus robotic cystectomy. *Eur Urol*. 2010;57(2):274–281.
7. Nix J, Smith A, Kurpad R, Nielsen ME, Wallen EM, Pruthi RS. Prospective randomized controlled trial of robotic versus open radical cystectomy for bladder cancer: perioperative and pathologic results. *Eur Urol*. 2010;57(2):196–201.
8. Pruthi RS, Wallen EM. Robotic assisted laparoscopic radical cystoprostatectomy: operative and pathological outcomes. *J Urol*. September, 2007;178(3 Pt 1): 814–818.
9. Wang GJ, Barocas DA, Raman JD, Scherr DS. Robotic vs open radical cystectomy: prospective comparison of perioperative outcomes and pathological measures of early oncological efficacy. *BJU Int*. January, 2008;101(1): 89–93.
10. Kozminski M, Partamian KO. Case report of laparoscopic ileal loop conduit. *J Endourol*. 1992; 6:147–150.
11. Gill IS, Fergany A, Klein EA, et al. Laparoscopic radical cystoprostatectomy with ileal conduit performed completely intracorporeally: the initial 2 cases. *Urology*. July, 2000;56(1):26–29; discussion 29–30.
12. Potter SR, Charambura TC, Adams JB, 2nd, Kavoussi LR. Laparoscopic ileal conduit: five-year follow-up. *Urology*. July, 2000;56(1):22–25.
13. Yohannes P, Puri V, Yi B, Khan AK, Sudan R. Laparoscopy-assisted robotic radical cystoprostatectomy with ileal conduit urinary diversion for muscle-invasive bladder cancer: initial two cases. *J Endourol*. November, 2003;17(9):729–732.
14. Balaji KC, Yohannes P, McBride CL, Oleynikov D, Hemstreet GP, 3rd Feasibility of robot-assisted totally intracorporeal laparoscopic ileal conduit urinary diversion: initial results of a single institutional pilot study. *Urology*. January, 2004;63(1):51–55.
15. Haber GP, Campbell SC, Colombo JR, Jr., et al. Perioperative outcomes with laparoscopic radical cystectomy: "pure laparoscopic" and "open-assisted laparoscopic" approaches. *Urology*. November, 2007;70(5):910–915.
16. Hubert J, Chammas M, Larre S, et al. Initial experience with successful totally robotic laparoscopic cystoprostatectomy and ileal conduit construction in tetraplegic patients: report of two cases. *J Endourol*. February, 2006;20(2):139–143.
17. Pruthi RS, Nix J, McRackan D, Hickerson A, Nielsen ME, Raynor M, Wallen EM. Robotic-assisted laparoscopic intracorporeal urinary diversion. *Eur Urol*. 2010;57(6):1013–1021.
18. Buffi N, Mottrie A, Lughezzani G, et al. Surgery illustrated–Surgical Atlas. Robotic radical cystectomy in the male. *BJU Int*. September, 2009;104(5):726–745.

Chapter 48

Robotic Urinary Diversion: Technique, Current Status, and Outcomes

Abolfazl Hosseini, Martin C. Schumacher, Martin N. Jonsson, and N. Peter Wiklund

48.1 Introduction

The creation of the urinary diversion is a challenging surgical part after radical cystectomy and holds a special place in the development of urological practice. Following cystectomy, urine can be diverted either into an incontinent stoma, into a continent urinary reservoir catheterized by the patient or controlled by the anal sphincter, or into an orthotopic bladder substitute so that the patient voids per urethra.

The history of urinary diversion is almost more than one and half centuries old. Simon was the first to describe a urinary diversion, using intestinal segments in 1852.[1]

Ureterocutaneostomy or transuretero-ureterocutaneostomy, the simplest form of urinary diversion, was the first diversion which has been tried initially. Strictures and scarring of the ureters were common problems, which later led to the use of intestinal segments of ileum or colon to create conduits.

In the late nineteenth and early twentieth centuries, in the absence of prophylactic antibiotic treatment, urinary diversion using bowel segments carried a high risk for peritonitis. When Coffey in 1911[2] introduced a new method for ureteric implantation, ureterosigmoidostomy became the most frequently used technique. With increasing concern over secondary colonic malignancy, fewer ureterosigmoidostomies were performed, as it became unpopular because of the high incidence of tumor occurrence at the anastomosis between the ureters and the colon.[3]

The ileal conduit, first described by Zaayer in 1911, was established as a standard technique by Bricker in 1950.[4] At the same time, Ferris and Oedel demonstrated that hyperchloremic metabolic acidosis was common in 80% of the patients treated with ureterosigmoidostomy.[5] Thus the ileal conduit became the preferred form of urinary diversion. Longer follow-up has shown that ileal conduits do have significant physical and psychological morbidity, and this has stimulated the increasing use of continent urinary diversion and orthotopic bladder substitutes.

The first attempts to create a continent urinary diversion were undertaken by Tizzoni and Foggi in 1888.[6] They replaced the bladder in a female dog by an isoperistaltic ileal segment. Mauclaire, in 1895, used the isolated rectum as a urinary reservoir.[7] Sinaiko was the first to use the stomach for the creation of a urinary reservoir in 1956.[8] Two findings were essential for the development of modern continent urinary diversion: Kock established the principle of bowel detubularization to create a low-pressure reservoir, and Lapides popularized the use of clean intermittent catheterization.[9] In 1969, Kock published his first results obtained with an ileal continent fecal reservoir in patients after total proctocolectomy[10] and in 1975 he transferred the principle of this technique to urinary diversion.[11] In the 1980s as surgical outcomes of cystectomy continued to improve, emphasis was directed toward improving long-term quality of life. The pioneering work of Nils Kock and Maurice Camey[12] led to a variety of continent urinary reservoirs. The majority of these used either ileal segments, like the Hautmann and Studer neobladder,[13,14] or ileocecal segments, like 'Le Bag' MAINZ II pouch[15] and the modified rectal bladder of Ghoneim.[16] These are only a few examples of continence reservoirs which are still commonly used.

N.P. Wiklund (✉)
Department of Urologic Surgery, Karolinska University Hospital, Stokholm, Sweden
e-mail: Peter.Wiklund@karolinska.se

A.K. Hemal, M. Menon (eds.), *Robotics in Genitourinary Surgery*,
DOI 10.1007/978-1-84882-114-9_48, © Springer-Verlag London Limited 2011

In the 1990s with development of minimally invasive techniques and advances in instrumentation design the interest in laparoscopic urinary diversion following cystectomy increased dramatically. The first simple laparoscopic cystectomy for pyocystis was performed by Parra et al. in 1992.[17] In 1993 de Badajoz et al. published the first study on laparoscopic radical cystectomy (LRC) for muscle-invasive bladder cancer, wherein the ileal conduit urinary diversion was performed extracorporeally.[18]

In 1995 Puppo et al.[19] described five cases of a combined laparoscopic and transvaginal anterior pelvic exenteration for bladder cancer. In 2001 Turk et al. described a completely intracorporeal LRC with a continent urinary diversion (rectal sigmoid pouch).[20] A completely intracorporeal reconstruction of the entire LRC and urinary diversion procedure was reported by Gill et al., who also performed the first purely laparoscopic ileal conduit urinary diversion and laparoscopic orthotopic Studer neobladder in 2000 and 2002, respectively.[21,22]

During the last decade, urologists worldwide have witnessed a tremendous development of laparoscopic surgical treatment due to the development of robot-assisted surgery in many urological diseases. In parallel the interest in expanding the role of robot-assisted radical cystectomy (RARC) for the management of urinary bladder cancer has risen during last years and continues to grow. Robotic-assisted laparoscopic techniques have emerged allowing surgeons to more readily overcome the difficult learning curve and shorten operative times in minimally invasive abdominal and pelvic operations.[23]

The da Vinci Surgical System® (Intuitive Surgical, Inc., Sunnyvale, CA) was first introduced in 2000.[24] After the initial report of robot-assisted radical cystectomy,[25] several investigators have described the feasibility of RARC in the management of urinary bladder cancer.[26–28]

RARC has been grown steadily during last years and has replaced LRC in centers where the robot is available. The neobladder can be formed intracorporeally[25,29,30] but operative time may be reduced if this is done extracorporeally through the same incision used to deliver the cystectomy specimen. Dasgupta et al.[31] reported that RARC is a minimally invasive procedure with short- to medium-term follow-up which is oncologically and functionally equivalent to open radical cystectomy. Haber et al.[32] reported in a review article that minimally invasive techniques, LRC and RARC, were associated with significantly reduced blood loss, hospital stay, marginally higher operative time, similar postoperative complication rates, and adequate oncological outcome on early and intermediate follow-up analysis as compared with open surgery.

Herein we describe step by step the method used at Karolinska Institutet for robot-assisted urinary diversion with ileal conduit and orthotopic neobladder by intra- and extracorporeal technique.

48.2 Patient Selection

Care should be taken for patient selection. The selection process includes preoperative investigation to ensure fitness for surgery as well as specific counseling regarding robotic technology. Patients with decreased pulmonary compliance that would not tolerate Trendelenburg position are not candidates for the robot-assisted technique. Furthermore, patients with a history of previous extensive abdominal surgery may be a relative contraindication.

48.3 Preoperative Preparation

In patients scheduled for intracorporeal orthotopic neobladder, mechanical bowel preparation (osmotic laxative) should be used the day prior to surgery. Patients scheduled for an extracorporeal urinary diversion receive a clysma early in the morning. A stoma site is also marked the day prior to surgery. Broad spectrum intravenous antibiotics are administrated at the start of the procedure.

48.4 Operative Setup

48.4.1 Patient Position

After induction of general endotracheal anesthesia a naso-gastric tube and an 18 Ch Foley urinary catheter are inserted. The patient is placed in lithotomy position with arms adducted and padded. The legs are also abducted and slightly lowered on spreader bars. The table is placed in 25° Trendelenburg position during the cystectomy and lymph node dissection. For the urinary diversion the Trendelenburg position is decreased to 10–15°.

48.5 Equipment

The technique is challenging, requiring conventional laparoscopic infrastructure as well as an assistant with high skills in conventional laparoscopy. Standard laparoscopic surgical equipment with some extra instruments is required (Ligasure® Covidien, surgical endoscopy clip applicators, laparoscopic endo-catch bags, and laparoscopic stapler for intestinal stapling).

48.6 Surgical Steps

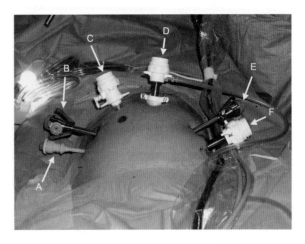

Fig. 48.1 Trocar placement for standard da Vinci system. *A.* 5 mm trocar. *B.* 8 mm trocar, *right* robot instrument. *C.* 12 mm trocar, suction, bowel grasping, LigaSure. *D.* camera trocar. *E.* 8 mm trocar, *left* robot instrument. *F.* 15 mm four robotic arm, specimen retrieval and stapling

Surgical step	Lens	Right robotic instrument	Left robotic instrument	Fourth robotic arm	Right assistant port
Anastomosis between urethra and ileum	0°	Needle driver	Cadiere	Cadiere	Bowel grasper
Isolation of 50 cm ileum	0°	Cadiere	Cadiere	Not in use	Endo-GIA 60 mm
Detubularization of ileal segment	0°	Scissors	Cadiere	Not in use	Suction device
Suturing of the posterior wall	0°	Needle driver	Cadiere	Cadiere	Grasper and hook
Folding of the neobladder and suturing the anterior wall	0°	Needle driver	Cadiere	Cadiere	Grasper and hook
Anastomosis between ureters and afferent limb	0°	Needle driver	Cadiere	Cadiere	Suction device
Placement of ureteric stents	0°	Cadiere	Cadiere	Not in use	Not in use
Closing of the neobladder	0°	Needle driver	Cadiere	Cadiere	Hook and suction device

48.6.1 Trocar Configuration

Port placement is critical for successful robotic surgery. After insufflation of the abdomen according to the Hasson technique,[33] a total of six ports are placed (Fig. 48.1). The 12-mm camera port placed supra-umbilical, although a higher pressure of 20 mmHg is helpful in providing additional abdominal wall tension while inserting the ports. Supra-umbilical position is

preferred in order to stay proximal to the urachus. This helps in performing an easier dissection of the proximal part of the ureters. The second (right) and third (left) robotic arm ports (8 mm) are placed a centimeter below the camera port, just lateral to the respective rectus muscles bilaterally and symmetrically. The fourth port (5 mm right assistance port) is placed approximately 5 cm above the right anterior superior iliac spine in the mid-axillary line. The fifth (15 mm) port is positioned approximately 5 cm above the left anterior superior iliac spine for the insertion of the fourth robotic arm instrument. During the intracorporeal construction of the urinary diversion the fourth arm port will be removed from the 15 mm port above the left anterior superior iliac spine allowing intestinal stapling through this port. The sixth (12 mm) assistant port is placed midway between the right robotic arm port and the camera port approximately 2.5 cm above the camera port.

48.6.2 Urinary Diversion

48.6.2.1 Orthotopic Neobladder, Intracorporeal Technique

Anastomosis Between the Urethra and Ileum

After the cystectomy and the lymph node dissection are finished the urinary diversion is performed. The first step is to perform an anastomosis between the

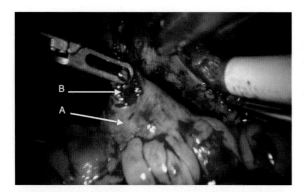

Fig. 48.2 An opening (*B*) in ileum (*A*) is performed to allow the passing of a 20 Ch catheter

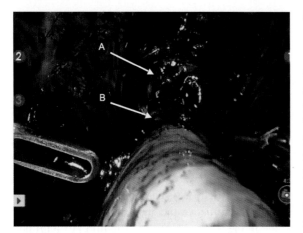

Fig. 48.3 Anastomosis between urethra (*A*) and ileum (*B*)

ileum and the urethra. The 0° lens is used for this initial step. The ileum is sufficiently mobilized in order to reach down to the urethra. This is important for two reasons, first the anastomosis between the neobladder and urethra can be performed without tension, and second the neobladder will be placed correctly in the small pelvis during the whole procedure. This will help during construction of the neobladder by running suture. A 20 Ch opening (Fig. 48.2) is made in the antimesentric site of ileum, using robotic scissor. The anastomosis is performed according to the Van Velthoven technique with a two times 18 cm 4-0 Biosyn® suture, allowing for 10–12 stitches (Fig. 48.3). A needle driver and a cadiere are used to establish the anastomosis.

Isolation of 50 cm Ileum

The orthotopic neobladder is fashioned from a 50 cm segment of terminal ileum. The intestine is isolated

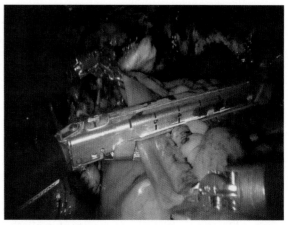

Fig. 48.4 Stapling of ileum using Endo-GIA 60 mm

using laparoscopic Endo-GIA with a 60 mm intestinal stapler (Fig. 48.4). The staple is inserted by the assisting surgeon, using the 15 mm port on the left side. The ileum is stapled 40 cm proximal to the urethral–ileal anastomosis. The continuity of the small bowel is restored by using Endo-GIA with a 60 mm intestinal stapler, positioning the distal and proximal end of the ileum side to side with the anti-mesentery part facing each other (Fig. 48.5). An additional transverse firing of the Endo-GIA staple is used to close the open ends of the ileal limbs (Fig. 48.6). Stay sutures may be used to attach the intestines before stapling them together.

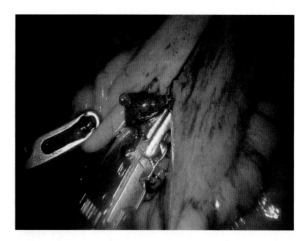

Fig. 48.5 Side-to-side anastomosis of ileum by Endo-GIA 60 mm

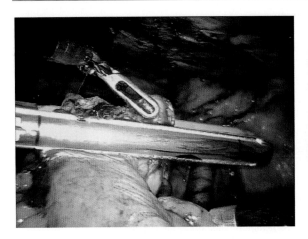

Fig. 48.6 Closing of the open end of ileal limbs using the Endo-GIA staple

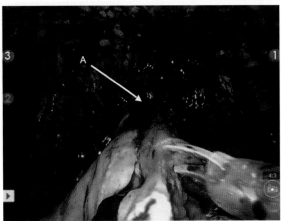

Fig. 48.8 Detubularization close to the ileourethral anastomosis (*A*), special care is taken not to interfere with the anastomotic suture

Detubularization

The distal 40 cm of the isolated ileal segment is detubularized along its antimesenteric border with cold scissors (Fig. 48.7), leaving a 10 cm intact proximal isoperistaltic afferent limb. Care is taken not to interfere with the sutures used for the anastomosis to the urethra (Fig. 48.8).

Formation of Studer Neobladder

After detubularization the posterior part of the Studer reservoir is closed using multiple running suture (25 cm 3-0 Biosyn®) in a seromuscular fashion,

avoiding suturing the mucosa. After the posterior part is sutured, the distal half of the anterior part of the reservoir is sutured, using the same suture. The 0° or 30° lens can be useful for this part of procedure. The proximal half of the anterior part of the reservoir is left open and is closed in the last part of the procedure.

Ureteric Entero-anastomosis

The anastomosis between the ureters and the afferent limb is performed using the Wallace technique[34] using a 0° lens. A 3-0 Biosyn® stitch is placed at the distal end of each ureter. The left ureter is tunneled under the sigmoid mesentery to the right side. The ureters are then incised and spatulated 2 cm (Fig. 48.9). The posterior walls of ureters are sutured

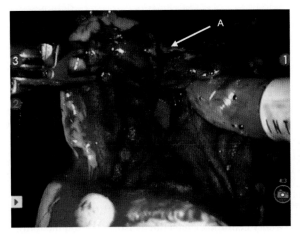

Fig. 48.7 Detubularization of ileum, antimesentricaly (*A*) in order to create the neobladder

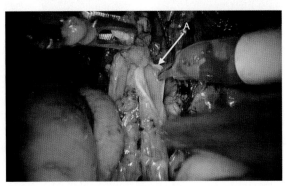

Fig. 48.9 Spatulation of the right ureter (*A*)

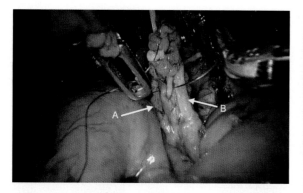

Fig. 48.10 Suture of left (*A*) and right (*B*) ureter side to side, according to the Wallace technique

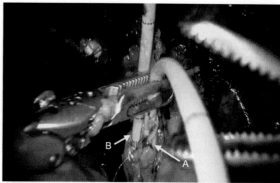

Fig. 48.12 Placement of stent up through the right ureter (*A*). The *left* uretric stent is already in place (*B*)

side to side, using 15 cm running 4-0 Biosyn® suture (Fig. 48.10). Before to anastomosis between the ureters and the intestinal loop is performed two Single-J 40 cm ureteric stents are introduced with Seldinger technique[35] through two separate 4 mm incision at the lower part of abdominal wall (Fig. 48.11). The stents are pulled through the afferent limb and pushed up in to the ureters on each side (Fig. 48.12). The ureters are then sutured to the afferent limb of the Studer pouch, using a two times 15 cm 4-0 Biosyn® suture (Fig. 48.13). After the ureteric entero-anastomosis is completed the stents are sutured and fixed to the skin.

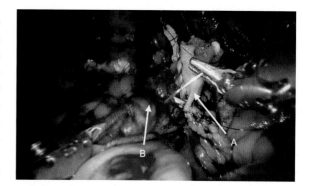

Fig. 48.13 Anastomosis between Wallace plate (*A*) and afferent limb (*B*) of the Studer reservoir, using seromucosal suturing technique

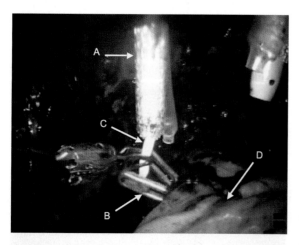

Fig. 48.11 Placement of uretric stent through a 3 mm port (*A*). *Right* robotic instrument (*B*) grasps the tip of the stent (*C*) and pulls in upward through the afferent limb of Studer reservoir (*D*)

Closure of the Studer Reservoir

The remaining part of the reservoir is then closed with a running 3-0 Biosyn® suture, using a 0° lens. The balloon of the indwelling catheter is filled with 10 cc. The neobladder is then filled with 50 cc of saline to check for leakage (Fig. 48.14). If leakage is observed extra sutures will have to be considered. A 21 Ch passive drainage is introduced and placed in the small pelvis.

48.6.2.2 Ileal Conduit, Intracorporeal Technique

Twenty centimeter intestine is isolated from the terminal ileum, using Endo-GIA with a 60 mm intestinal stapler. The continuity of the small bowel is restored as

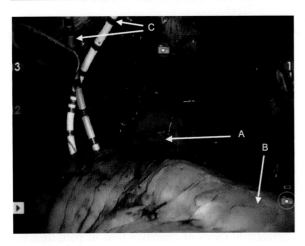

Fig. 48.14 After the neobladder (*A*) is completed it is filled with 50 cc saline to check for leakage. The anastomosis between ureters and afferent limb (*B*) is also checked for leakage. The uretric stents (*C*) are placed separately in the Studer reservoir

described above. The distal end of the conduit is fashioned as a stoma by surgical assistant at a previously marked site on the abdominal wall. The left ureter is tunneled under the sigmoid mesentery to the right side. The ureters are then incised and spatulated 2 cm. The Wallace technique is used here as described above. Single-J 40 cm ureteric stents are then introduced through the isolated ileal segment (ileal conduit), using a suction tube for a protective channel avoiding intestinal perforation. The stents are then pushed up into the ureters on each side and the ureteroenteric anastomosis is completed, using a two times 15 cm 4-0 Biosyn® suture.

48.6.2.3 Orthotopic Neobladder, Extracorporeal Technique

After completing of the radical cystectomy and lymphadenectomy the robot is undocked and all ports are removed. The orthotopic neobladder is fashioned through a 6–8 cm lower abdominal midline incision as described by Studer.[14] The posterior urethral sutures may be placed laparoscopically prior to undocking the da Vinci robot or via an open approach. Then the neobladder is created extracorporeally and placed into the pelvis. A Foley catheter is passed through the urethra into the neobladder. The abdominal incision is closed and da Vinci robot is docked again. The

urethral-neobladder anastomosis is performed robotically, using a two times 18 cm 4-0 Biosyn® suture, allowing for 10–12 stitches according to the Van Velthoven technique.

48.6.2.4 Ileal Conduit, Extracorporeal Technique

As described above the robot is undocked, all ports are removed. The urethral sutures are kept through their corresponding port sites and tagged. It is important to keep the patient in the Trendelenburg position initially to prevent the intestine from descending into the pelvis. A 5–7 cm muscle-splitting incision in the right iliac fossa incorporating a port site or a midway incision from umbilicus to the pubis is made. The midway incision facilitates any further mobilization of the ureters especially in obese patients. The left ureter is tunneled under the sigmoid mesentery. The ureters are then spatulated and sutured together according to the Wallace technique as described above. The terminal ileum is identified with the assistance of the preplaced stitch, and a 15–20 cm segment of bowel is isolated. Re-establishing intestinal continuity is performed, using multiple running 30 cm 3-0 Biosyn® suture in a seromuscular fashion, avoiding suturing the mucosa. The urinary diversion is then performed extracorporeally and the ureteroenteric anastomosis completed as described above.

48.6.2.5 Special Consideration

Patient Position

Care should be taken for using a pneumatic leg compression system due to risk of decreased vascular perfusion during the procedure. To avoid cardiovascular complications the patient is started on anticoagulant treatment with low molecular weight heparin according to his body weight the evening before surgery until the patient is fully mobilized. It is feasible to perform the urinary diversion with 10–15° Trendelenburg, since higher degree of Trendelenburg is to be avoided in order to minimize the risk for cardiopulmonary complications.

Port Position

It is always important to make sure that the fourth arm port and the left robotic arm port are not in a same alignment to avoid clashing of robotic arms.

Urethral-Neobladder Anastomosis

The anastomosis between the urethra and the ileum (Fig. 48.2) should be the first step in the formation of an intracorporeal orthotopic neobladder. This is a critical step because the anastomosis can be performed without tension, and the neobladder will be placed correctly in the small pelvis during the whole procedure.

48.7 Steps to Avoid Complication

Shoulder pads should be avoided due to high risk for plexus damages. Care should be taken during the tunneling of left ureter behind the colon sigmoid in order to avoid damaging any vascular structures. It is important to check for leakage after the neobladder has been created. Extra suturing to secure a watertight reservoir and anastomosis is fundamental to decrease postoperative complications.

48.8 Current Status and Outcomes

Construction of the urinary diversion after RARC is probably the most challenging part of the procedure, especially using a totally intracorporeal approach. Since the first robot-assisted radical cystectomy by Beecken et al. in 2003[25] results from more than 200 RARC worldwide have been published[36] and more than 700 patients are included in the database of IRCC (International Robotic Cystectomy Consortium; Khurshid Guru, personal communication). The feasibility of this technique has been reported by several investigators and the preferred method of elaborating the neobladder intracorporeally or extracorporeally is based on the respective surgeon's choice. The operative time used for the reconstruction is one of the important factors in the decision between

performing the diversion extra- or intracorporeally. Robot-assisted intracorporeal ileal conduit, orthotopic neobladder, and neobladder urethral anastomosis have been performed and well described in the literature.[26–29,31,37,38] Table 48.1 presents data from some small series of extracorporeally and intracorporeally performed urinary diversion. Some authors have successfully completed total intracorporeal reconstruction with operative time of 8.5 h for a Hautmann neobladder,[25] a mean of 11.5 h for a series of three ileal conduits,[30] and 12 h for an ileal neobladder.[29] Using a totally intracorporeal urinary diversion we obtained results which is comparable with the extracorporeal approach in terms of operative time as published by others.[39] However, most centers worldwide have preferred to perform the urinary diversion extracorporeally by extending the mini-incision used for removal of the specimen.[26,38,40–44] The completely intracorporeal approach would certainly be advantageous in the female patient where transvaginal specimen extraction is the most elegant way to extract the specimen. Those favoring the extracorporeal urinary diversion argue that a larger space allows a faster reconstruction and reduces operative time. Besides intracorporeal urinary diversion is very demanding from a technical point of view.

Evaluation of functional outcomes is impossible at present because of the lack of published data. So far the outcomes that are published are comparable to data from open series.[44] Murphy et al. reported that three of four patients who underwent nerve-sparing technique were potent with Tadalafil at 6 months follow-up. He reported also that all four patients with orthotopic neobladder were fully continent during daytime. Jonsson et al.[39] also reported that eight of nine patients who underwent attempted nerve-sparing cystectomy with total intracorporeal urinary diversion were potent with or without the use of tadalafil. They also reported that 11 of 12 patients were fully continent during daytime at 6 months [Table 48.1].

With time and increased experience, operative times, functional and oncological outcomes will continue to improve. Selection of appropriate urinary diversion following robot-assisted cystectomy in the form of intracorporeal or extracorporeal approach needs more studies. At this point in time intracorporeally performed urinary diversion may be recommended only in the hands of experienced surgeons at high-volume centers.

Table 48.1 Robotic-assisted radical cystectomy and urinary diversion

Authors (ref.)	Number of patients	Type of urinary diversion	Extracorporeal or intracorporeal	Mean operative time (min)	Mean perioperative blood loss (mL)	Mean postoperative hospital stay (days)	Erectile function and continence
Menon et al.[26]	17	Ileal conduit (3) Orthotopic neobladder (14)	Extracorporeal	140 260 308	150	n.a.	n.a.
Galich et al.[40]	13	Ileal conduit (6) Orthotopic neobladder (5) Indiana pouch (2)	Extracorporeal	697	500	8	n.a.
Guru et al.[41]	20	Ileal conduit (18) Orthotopic neobladder (2)	Extracorporeal	442	555	10	n.a.
Pruthi et al.[42]	50	Ileal conduit (29) Orthotopic neobladder (21)	Extracorporeal	306	271	n.a	n.a.
Wang et al.[43]	32	Ileal conduit (17) orthotopic neobladder (12) Indiana pouch (3)	Extracorporeal	390	400	5	n.a.
Murphy et al.[44]	23	Ileal conduit (19) Orthotopic neobladder (4)	Extracorporeal	397	278	12	Three patients potent with tadalafil Four patients continent daytime
Sala et al.[29]	1	Orthotopic neobladder	Intracorporeal	720	100	5	Continent daytime
Balaji et al.[30]	2	Ileal conduit	Intracorporeal	600 720	435 1,800	6	n.a.
Dasgupta et al.[31]	20	Ileal conduit (17) Orthotopic neobladder (3)	Extracorporeal	330	450	10	Three patients potent with tadalafil
Jonsson et al.[39]	18	Ileal conduit (5) Orthotopic neobladder (13)	Intracorporeal	501	525	12	11 of 12 patients were continent at daytime. 8 of 9 were potent with tadalafil

References

1. Simon J. Ectopia vesicae; operation for directing the orifices of the ureters into the rectum; temporary success; subsequent death; autopsy. *Lancet*. 1852;2:568.
2. Coffey RC. Physiologic implantation of the severed ureter or common bile duct into the intestine. *JAMA*. 1911;56:397.
3. Wear JB, Barquin OP. Ureterosigmoidostomy. Long-Term results. *Urology*. 1973;1:192–200.
4. Bricker EM. Bladder substitution after pelvic evisceration. *Surg Clin North Am*. 1950;30:1511.
5. Ferris DO, Odel HM. Electrolyte pattern of the blood after bilateral ureterosigmoidostomy. *JAMA*. 1950;142:634–641.
6. Tizzoni G, Foggi A. Die Wiederherstellung der Harnblase. *Zentralbl Chir*. 1888;15:921.
7. Mauclaire P. De quelques essais de chirurgie expérimentale applicables au traitement de l'exstrophie de la vessie et des anus de nature complexe. *Ann Mal Org Génitourin*. 1895;13:1080–1081.
8. Sinaiko E. Artificial bladder from segment of stomach and study of effect of urine on gastric secretion. *Surg Gynecol Obstet*. April, 1956;102(4):433–438.
9. Lapides J, Diokno AC, Silber SM, Lowe BS. Clean, intermittent self-catheterization in the treatment of urinary tract disease. *J Urol*. 1972;167(4):1584–1586, April, 2002.
10. Kock NG. Continent ileostomy. *Prog. Surg*. 1973;12:180.
11. Kock NG, Nilson AE, Nilsson LO, et al: . Urinary diversion via a continent ileal reservoir: clinical results in 12 patients. *J Urol*. 1982;128:469–475.
12. Camey M, Le Duc A. L'enterocystoplastie après cystoprostatectomie pour cancer de vessie. *Ann Urol*. 1979;13:114.
13. Hautmann RE, Miller K, Steiner U, Wenderoth U. The ileal neobladder: 6 years of experience with more than 200 patients. *J Urol*. 1993;150:40–45.
14. Studer UE, Ackermann D, Casanova GA, Zingg EJ. A newer form of bladder substitute based on historical perspectives. *Semin Urol*. 1988;6:57.
15. Fisch M, Wammack R, Muller SC, Hohenfellner R. The Mainz pouch II (sigma rectum pouch). *J Urol*. 1993;149:258–263.
16. Ghoneim MA, Ashamallah AK, Mahran MR, Kock NG. Further experience with the modified rectal bladder (the augmented and valved rectum) for urine diversion. *J Urol*. 1992;147:1252–1255.
17. Parra RO, Andrus CH, Jones JP, Boullier JA. Laparoscopic cystectomy: initial report on a new treatment for the retained bladder. *J Urol*. 1992;148:1140–1144.
18. Sanchez de Badajoz E, Gallego Perales JL, Reche Rosado A, Gutierrez de la Cruz JM, Jimenez Garrido A. Radical cystectomy and laparoscopic ileal conduit. *Arch Esp Urol*. 1993;46:621–624.
19. Puppo P, Perachino M, Ricciotti G, Bozzo W, Gallucci M, Carmignani G. Laparoscopically assisted transvaginal radical cystectomy. *Eur Urol*. 1995;27:80–84.
20. Turk I, Deger S, Winkelmann B, Schonberger B, Loening SA. Laparoscopic radical cystectomy with continent urinary diversion (rectal sigmoid pouch) performed completely intracorporeally: the initial 5 cases. *J Urol*. 2001;165:1863–1866.
21. Gill IS, Fergany A, Klein EA, et al. Laparoscopic radical cystoprostatectomy with ileal conduit performed completely intracorporeally: the initial 2 cases. *Urology*. 2000;56:26–30.
22. Gill IS, Kaouk JH, Meraney AM, et al. Laparoscopic radical cystectomy and continent orthotopic ileal neobladder performed completely intracorporeally: the initial experience. *J Urol*. 2002;168:13–18.
23. Schumacher MC, Jonsson MN, Wiklund NP. Robotic cystectomy. *Scand J Surg*. 2009;98:1–17.
24. Binder J, Kramer W. Robotically-assisted laparoscopic radical prostatectomy. *BJU Int*. 2001;87:408–410.
25. Beecken WD, Wolfram M, Engl T, et al. Robotic-assisted laparoscopic radical cystectomy and intra-abdominal formation of an orthotopic ileal neobladder. *Eur Urol*. 2003;44:337–339.
26. Menon M, Hemal AK, Tewari A, et al. Nerve-sparing robotassisted radical cystoprostatectomy and urinary diversion. *BJU Int*. 2003;92:232–236.
27. Hemal AK, Abol-Enein H, Tewari A, et al. Robotic radical cystectomy and urinary diversion in the management of bladder cancer. *Urol Clin North Am*. November, 2004;31(4):719–729.
28. Shah NL, Hemal AK, Menon M. Robot-assisted radical cystectomy and urinary diversion. *Curr Urol Rep*. March, 2005;6(2):122–125.
29. Sala LG, Matsunaga GS, Corica FA, Ornstein DK. Robotassisted laparoscopic radical cystoprostatectomy and totally intracorporeal ileal neobladder. *J Endourol*. 2006;20:233–236.
30. Balaji KC, Yohannes P, McBride CL, Oleynikov D, Hemstreet GPIII. Feasibility of robot-assisted totally intracorporeal laparoscopic ileal conduit urinary diversion: initial results of a single institutional pilot study. *Urology*. 2004;63:51–55.
31. Dasgupta P, Rimington P, Murphy D, et al. Robotic assisted radical cystectomy: short to medium-term oncologic and functional outcomes. *Int J Clin Pract*. November, 2008;62(11):1709–1714.
32. Haber GP, Crouzet S, Gill IS. Laparoscopic and robotic assisted radical cystectomy for bladder cancer: a critical analysis. *Eur Urol*. 2008;54:54–62.
33. Hasson HM. Open laparoscopy vs. closed laparoscopy: a comparison of complication rates. *Adv Plan Parent*. 1978;13:41–50.
34. Wallace DM. Ureteric diversion using a conduit: a simplified technique. *Br J Urol*. 1966;38:522.
35. Bigongiari LR. The Seldinger approach to percutaneous nephrostomy and ureteral stent placement. *Urol Radiol*. 1981;2(3):141–145.
36. Guru KA, Nyquist J, Perlmutter A, Peabody JO. A robotic future for bladder cancer? *Lancet Oncol*. February, 2008;9(2):184.
37. Menon M, Hemal AK, Tewari A, et al. Robot-assisted radical cystectomy and urinary diversion in female patients: technique with preservation of the uterus and vagina. *J Am Coll Surg*. 2004;198:386–393.
38. Hemal AK. Role of robot-assisted surgery for bladder cancer. *Curr Opin Urol*. January, 2009;19(1):69–75.
39. Jonsson NM, Schumacher CM, Hosseini A, et al. Robot-assisted radical cystectomy with totally intracorporeal

urinary diversion in patients with transitional cell carcinoma of the bladder. Abstract 796, AUA 2009. *J Urol.* April, 2009;181(4):284.

40. Galich A, Sterrett S, Nazemi T, Pohlman G, Smith L, Balaji KC. Comparative analysis of early perioperative outcomes following radical cystectomy by either the robotic or open method. *JSLS.* April–June, 2006;10(2):145–150.

41. Guru KA, Kim HL, Piacente PM, Mohler JL. Robot-assisted radical cystectomy and pelvic lymph node dissection: initial experience at Roswell Park Cancer Institute. *Urology.* March, 2007;69(3):469–474.

42. Pruthi RS, Wallen EM. Robotic assisted laparoscopic radical cystoprostatectomy: operative and pathological outcomes. *J Urol.* September, 2007;178(3 Pt 1):814–818.

43. Wang GJ, Barocas DA, Raman JD, Scherr DS. Robotic vs. Open radical cystectomy: prospective comparison of perioperative outcomes and pathological measures of early oncological efficacy. *BJU Int.* January, 2008;101(1):89–93.

44. Murphy DG, Challacombe BJ, Elhage O, et al. Robotic-assisted laparoscopic radical cystectomy with extracorporeal urinary diversion: initial experience. *Eur Urol.* September, 2008;54(3):570–580.

Chapter 49

Robotic Bladder Surgery Complications: Prevention and Management

Erik P. Castle, Rafael Nuñez-Nateras, Michael E. Woods, and Paul E. Andrews

Surgical complications are potentially encountered with all surgical procedures. Surgeons have the task of being aware of all potential complications, taking every effort to prevent them, identifying them when they do occur, and having the knowledge and skill to manage them. Complications can compromise patient outcomes and expectations, as well as present a significant source of anxiety for patient and surgeon alike. Robotic surgery of the bladder is not immune to the potential of surgical complications. In and of itself, bladder surgery can be a technically demanding procedure due to patient variability and the potential need for urinary diversion. Radical cystectomy, for example, is well recognized as a procedure associated with significant risks of complications. It has an associated morbidity that is reported in the literature to range from 28 to 64% and a mortality as high as 5.7%.[1-10]

With the increasing application of the robotic approach, bladder surgery has been added to the arsenal of the robotic surgeon. The robotic approach may have the potential to effect the outcomes of bladder procedures as far as perioperative complications are concerned. Procedures that traditionally employed large incisions or may have been associated with postoperative ileus and bleeding may benefit from the minimally invasive approach. This has been demonstrated in some early reports comparing open and robot-assisted radical cystectomy, showing a diminished complication rate of 30–50% in the robotic approach.[10-12] In our own experience,

perioperative complications for robot-assisted radical cystectomy have decreased from 68 to 28%.[13] Furthermore, robotic surgical systems may allow surgeons to perform complex procedures such as radical cystectomy on a regular basis which may not have been possible due to the steep learning curve for the purely laparoscopic approach.

Robotic technology in bladder surgery has been predominately limited to radical cystectomy for the management of bladder cancer. Due to the positive impact on morbidity, there is a trend to apply robotic techniques to a wider variety of bladder procedures, such as bladder augmentation, partial cystectomy, and bladder diverticulectomy.[14] There are some complications that are inherent to the use of laparoscopic/robotic techniques such as port placement, positioning, the pneuomoperitoneum, and instrumentation. On the other hand, there are complications that are attributable to the specific procedure and independent to the approach and are seen with open bladder surgery. Factors that play a role in these types of complications include the use of bowel segments for urinary diversion, bladder suture lines, drains and stents, and overall bowel function.

The purpose of this chapter is to asses the most common complications and to discuss their prevention, recognition, and management on patients undergoing robot-assisted bladder surgery. The complications will be divided into those inherent to the robotic approach and those attributable to the specific nature of the operation being performed. Reported incidence and outcomes will be discussed while prevention and management will be specifically outlined. For example, in some cases, management may include conversion to a laparoscopic or open approach while prevention may be a modification to patient preparation.

E.P. Castle (✉)
Mayo Clinic, Department of Urology, Phoenix, AZ, USA
e-mail: castle.erik@mayo.edu

A.K. Hemal, M. Menon (eds.), *Robotics in Genitourinary Surgery*,
DOI 10.1007/978-1-84882-114-9_49, © Springer-Verlag London Limited 2011

49.1 Current Literature on Robot-Assisted Bladder Surgery

Although there is a plethora of published reports on robot-assisted radical prostatectomy, the current available published literature on robot-assisted bladder surgery is scant. Most are limited to small- to moderate-sized case series as well as some scattered case reports. Robot-assisted radical cystectomy (RARC) outcomes have received the most attention and subsequently have been more frequently reported on in comparison to other bladder procedures. Fifteen reports were identified accounting for a total of 294 cases. Fifty-one complications were reported (Table 49.1). Ileus (10 patients) followed by urinary leak (3 patients), small bowel obstruction (3 patients), and port site bleeding (3 patients) were the most common complications identified. One death was reported.[15-29] To the authors knowledge, there are three reports of robot-assisted bladder augmentation, one of which is an animal series. In all reports no complications were identified during or after the procedure.[30-32] Four reports of robot-assisted bladder diverticulectomy were identified comprising a total of 10 patients. No complications were reported.[33-36] For robot-assisted partial cystectomy, four reports were identified including a total of eight patients between all four reports. The indication for partial cystectomy was a history of transitional cell carcinoma (2), bladder endometriosis (2), and urachal anomalies (4). Intraoperative bowel perforation accounts for the only complication reported in those series.[36-39]

Interpreting published series on complications can be difficult regardless of approach. Complication reporting is fraught with inherent bias primarily due to definitions of complications. Unless standardized categorization is utilized such as the Clavien classification system,[40] readers are left with rates that may vary dramatically from one series to another. For example, one surgeon may consider a urinary tract infection that occurs 3 months after surgery in a patient with an ileal conduit as a long-term complication while another may consider it an expected event in any patient with an incontinent urinary diversion. Despite the lack of uniformity within the published literature for open and robotic surgery, the current available literature provides us with the

Table 49.1 Current published robot-assisted radical cystectomy complications data

	Type of complication	Number	%[a]
1.	Gastrointestinal	17	33
	Ileus	10	
	Small bowel obstruction	3	
	Rectal injury	2	
	Enterocutaneous fistula	1	
	Intra-abdominal bleeding	1	
2.	Infection	11	22
	Percutaneous abscess	1	
	Abdominal abscess	1	
	Sepsis	1	
	Septic shock	1	
	Pyelonephritis	1	
	Wound infection	1	
	Fever of unknown origin	2	
	Urinary tract infection	3	
3.	Wound	7	14
	Dehiscence	1	
	Incisional hernia	1	
	Peristomal hernia	2	
	Port site bleeding	3	
4.	Genitourinary	7	14
	Misplaced ureteral stent	1	
	Enterovesical fistula	1	
	Anastomosis stricture	2	
	Urinary leak	3	
5.	Cardiovascular	3	6
	Deep vein thrombosis	1	
	Myocardial ischemia	1	
	Atrial fibrillation	1	
6.	Miscellaneous	3	6
	Dehydration	1	
	Conversion	1	
	Robot malfunction	1	
7.	Neurologic	2	4
	Bilateral femoral neuropraxia	1	
	Delirium tremens	1	
8.	Death	1	1

[a]Percentage based on total number of complications.

knowledge of the types of complications that may be encountered as well as the relative rates to expect to see them occur. This knowledge should allow for surgeons to modify technique and patient care if indicated to hopefully decrease the incidence of these complications, particularly the more severe ones.

49.2 Complications Inherent to the Robotic Approach

49.2.1 Equipment Malfunction

When utilizing and depending on mechanical devices or instruments, the surgeon is partially at the mercy of rates of equipment malfunction. This can be seen even with common instruments used in the operating room such as the electrical generator for the cautery or even the overhead lights. Having a "back-up" or contingency plan is crucial. This is evidence by the presence of auxiliary generators in all hospitals to handle interruptions in power. The same forethought needs to be employed when using robotic surgical instrumentation.

To ensure proper functioning, the robotic technology must be supported by a well-trained staff. They should be capable not only of quickly recognizing any equipment malfunction but also of providing an immediate and appropriate response to address problems. In the current literature, one bladder surgery complication was related to robot malfunction. It was related to camera/lens and required conversion to open surgery. Fortunately, non-recoverable robot failures occur in less than 0.5% of cases as reported by Lavery et al.[41]

Although the exact incidence is unknown, some of the older standard robotic systems had a relatively large number of "recoverable" faults. These are faults in the system that are hallmarked by an alarm sounding and disengagement of the masters in the console until the fault was addressed. The disengagement was presumably to prevent inappropriate continued movement of instruments and hopefully prevented injury to the patient. The surgical team then would follow specific steps such as contacting the support services as well as removing and reinserting instruments and replacing instruments in some cases. Some of these faults may be attributable to the age and version of the robotic systems but may also be a product of inappropriate use and positioning. In truth, many robotic techniques were being developed and perfect arm and robot positioning may not have been completely delineated. As evidenced by Lavery et al. non-recoverable faults can be kept to a minimum.

Prevention:

- Well-trained and seasoned surgical team;
- Inspection of instruments to ensure integrity of the cable system and servos;

- Ensure that start-up procedures of the system are normal to avoid underlying system errors;
- Ensure appropriate number of "uses" are left in each instrument.

Management:

- Stop activity that caused the malfunction;
- If the malfunction is specific to the instrument (e.g., scissors), replace with a fresh instrument;
- Robotic arm malfunction: If recoverable may be due to brief and unexpected movement. If continues, contact support services to review error codes associated with the event and identify if can be managed intraoperatively. One may consider disengaging arm and using addition "fourth arm" if available to complete the procedure;
- Write down and record error codes to have for support technician.
- Undocking the instrument/arm and re-docking in a different orientation. Evaluate the "boot" of the arm or camera and determine if orientation is appropriate for the arm;
- If equipment failure is not recoverable, conversion to a laparoscopic or open approach is the ultimate management.

49.2.2 Positioning

Attention to detail when positioning a patient for robot-assisted bladder surgery is extremely important to prevent complications. Early in the surgeon's experience, long surgical times may be encountered and may expose patients to neurologic injury, compartment syndrome, rhabdomyolysis, and ventilatory difficulties.[42–45] Neurologic injuries including ulnar, brachial, femoral, and peroneal neuropraxias as well as cerebral edema have also been described.[42,43] For most robot-assisted bladder procedures, a low-lithotomy position with the arms tucked at the side and extreme Trendelenburg will be used. This is the same position used during robot-assisted radical prostatectomy. In almost all reports of positioning complications, the common denominator is surgical operative time. Most often, such complications are encountered early in the learning curve when operative times are longer.[20] Simply put, one should limit the time a patient is in a non-ergonomic position.

Positioning problems may present immediately in the post-anesthesia recovery room. In the case of rhabdomyolysis, the patient will complain of severe pain in a large muscle group exposed to prolonged pressure. A compartment syndrome is often encountered as well. During open radical cystectomy the common area to be affected are the gluteal muscles. A clinical sign to note is the presence of brown urine and may signify urine myoglobin. The serum creatine phosphokinase (CPK) will invariably exceed 5,000 IU/dL. The treatment consists of hydration and alkalinization and needs to be instituted immediately to prevent subsequent renal failure. Prevention of renal failure is essential and may require a multidisciplinary approach. Adequate padding at all pressure points during surgery and aggressive fluid replacement play a crucial roll on its prevention. Early diagnosis may have a significant impact on the outcome by preventing or reducing the severity of complications from rhabdomyolysis. When suspected or risk factors are present (e.g., obese patients, prolonged operating time), measurement of the CPK level during the postoperative period is recommended. Preventive therapy is indicated if the CPK rises >5,000. Myoglobinuric acute renal failure complicates approximatively 30% of cases of rhabdomyolysis. Mortality from rhabdomyolysis can be as high as 5%.[46]

If a compartment syndrome is suspected, immediate orthopedic surgical consultation should be sought and compartment pressures measured. Measurement can be performed at the bedside with appropriate equipment. It is important to remember that peripheral pulses and capillary refill may be normal in acute compartment syndrome. Pain out of proportion is the hallmark and is likely due to neuropathy of the sensory nerve in that compartment. Therefore the surgeon should not take comfort in observing normal pulses if there is severe pain. Compartment syndrome can have severe consequences including loss of limb and death making immediate recognition key to its management. There have been anecdotal reports of compartment syndromes being identified in the upper extremities due to aggressive arm tucking and subsequent peripheral IV infiltration. It is important for the anesthesia team to ensure proper functioning of all IV infusions and periodically check the arms under the drapes if the operation is lasting more than 4–6 h.

Early in the robotic experience, some surgeons used shoulder sleds due to the concern for extreme Trendelenburg. The thought was that the shoulder sleds would prevent the patient from falling off the bed. In most cases, the patients will not fall off the bed due to the low lithotomy positioning of the legs. Furthermore, once the robot is docked to the patient, it is unlikely for the patient to move. The problems with the shoulder sleds are the anecdotal reports of shoulder impingement and pain along the superior aspect of the shoulder and acromium process. Use of foam and padding, arm tucking, and leg harnesses prevents slippage or significant movement of the patient. The areas to be sure are adequately padded include the popliteal fossa, peroneal surface, arms and wrists, back and buttocks, and the head and neck.

Prevention:

- Adequate padding of the legs, arms, hands, back, buttocks, head and neck;
- Ergonomic orientation of the wrists, arms, and legs;
- Keep operative times to a minimum and consider open conversion early in the learning curve at a specified time such as 4 h;
- Periodic examination of the arms and wrists for long cases (>4 h);
- Try to place peripheral IVs away from potential pressure points.

Management:

- Early identification is a key to minimizing poor outcomes;
- Early orthopedic surgical consultation if patient complains of pain out of proportion in a limb or location away from the surgical site;
- Measurement of compartment pressures if compartment syndrome is suspected;
- Measure serum creatine phosphokinase (CPK) and urine myoglobin if rhabdomyolysis is suspected;
- IV fluid hydration and alkalinization if myoglobinuria is identified.

49.2.3 Creation of Pneumoperitoneum, Port Placement, and Insertion of Trocars

Establishing the pneumoperitoneum and port placement are often the initial steps of any robotic procedure. There are potential complications of laparoscopic access into the abdominal cavity and are similar to what is found in the standard laparoscopy literature. The severity of these complications ranges from localized bruising from subcutaneous bleeding to perforation of major visceral and vascular structures. Reports from the laparoscopic literature have demonstrated that access-related injuries may have significant consequences, conferring a mortality of 13%. Bowel and retroperitoneal vascular injuries comprise 76% of all access-related injuries during the process of establishing a primary port.[47,48]

There are a variety of techniques of port placement including the use of a Veress needle, the Hasson open technique, and the use of dilating ports. When using a Veress needle, inadvertent injury to bowel or vascular structures may be encountered. Important points when using the Veress needle include the sense of easy passage with the classic "pop" felt through the peritoneum. Initial aspiration before insufflation to identify any bowel or visceral contents such as bile should be performed. If a blood vessel is entered, blood may be seen in the aspirate. Some surgeons advocate the "drop test" which involves the visualization of fluid through the needle with lift on the abdominal wall. This can be misleading in some cases due to appropriate dropping of the fluid whether or not the needle is in the peritoneal cavity. Probably one of the most important steps when using the Veress needle is achieving adequate lift with either towel clamps or direct lift on the fascia. Observation of a low pressure and high flow status during initial insufflation is critical. In most cases, a pressure less than 8 mm of Hg is observed if the needle is within the peritoneal cavity.

In most cases of vascular injury with a Veress needle, management involves removal of the needle and either applying pressure to the vessel or suture ligation. In cases of unidentified entry into a vessel, air embolus could be the end result. The injection of large volumes of carbon dioxide (CO_2) rapidly into the vascular system can result in a significant embolism. This can cause mechanical obstruction of the right ventricle outflow track with resultant pulmonary obstruction, right ventricular dilatation, and failure. Survival depends on immediate recognition, stopping the insufflation, and if necessary, placing the patient in left lateral decubitus with head down. Immediate intraoperative echocardiography and possible aspiration via a central venous catheter may be the next step.

Visceral injury from a Veress needle or other ports is a potential complication with any laparoscopic or robotic approach. The most common organs include the liver, spleen, small intestine, and large intestine. The liver is the most resilient of the structures, and a single puncture with a small needle or port can often be managed expectantly. In some cases argon beam coagulation may be used as well as the application of surgical hemostatic agents. The spleen is less forgiving, and management depends on the degree of injury and bleeding. Laparoscopic splenectomy or open conversion with splenectomy is dependent on the skills of the surgeon and the degree of bleeding encountered. Small bowel injuries that are small and do not appear to compromise the vascular integrity of the segment may be repaired using the robot with attention to appropriate closure of the mucosa and serosa as one would do in open fashion. If the duodenum is the segment injured, it is wise to obtain general surgical consultation and receive confirmation that simple two-layer closure is all that is needed due to the significant consequences of a postoperative duodenal leak. Colon injury can often be managed with simple two-layer closure even in the setting of unprepared bowel. However, general surgical consultation is advised due to the significant consequences of bowel leak from the large intestine.

One of the most common access injuries encountered is injury to the inferior epigastric vessels below the level of the umbilicus. Surprisingly, this occurs with secondary port placement most often. The injury is most common between the takeoff of the vessels from the external iliac and its passage through the rectus muscles. Although less common with robot-assisted radical cystectomy as most ports are above the level of the umbilicus to facilitate a complete lymphadenectomy, some assistant ports may be in the area in question with other bladder procedures. It is important to try to transilluminate the abdominal wall when placing the secondary ports, particularly if they are below the level of the umbilicus. It has been suggested that routine spreading of the subcutaneous tissues of the proposed port site with a blunt clamp is also helpful; this is likely more important if bladed trocars are being used. The use of only blunt and dilating trocars reduces the chance of vascular wall injury nearly fivefold.[49]

Management of an injury to the inferior epigastric vessels includes direct identification and clipping robotically or cutting down to the vessel and ligating it. In most cases, identification of the injury occurs when blood is seen dripping around a port. In these cases, the surgeon can put a large "figure-of-eight" suture through and through the abdomen to compress the vessels. The surgeon can then complete the operation and address the vessel at the end of the operation. The suture is unlikely to be adequate in the long run, and the authors suggest that one should cut down on the port site and formally ligate the vessels to avoid the delayed development of a rectus sheath hematoma or even intraperitoneal hemorrhage.

Port placement is one of the most critical steps in performing a successful robotic surgery. Appropriate placement prevents internal and external collision of the arms and allows for maximal movement needed for specific steps in bladder procedures such as ureteral mobilization and extended pelvic lymph node dissections. To avoid a poor port placement, surgeons can follow the port collocation to perform robot-assisted bladder surgery described by different authors.[50–52] Although much attention is given to port orientation and location, inappropriate port placement can also result in immediate need for conversion to open procedure due to emergent hemorrhage. Therefore the most important aspects in port placement include direct visualization whenever possible, use of blunt or dilating trocars when possible, and judicious use of conversion whenever necessary to handle vascular or visceral injuries.

Prevention:

- Adequately lift up the abdominal wall during Veress needle passage;
- Aspiration of the Veress needle before insufflation;
- Observe a low pressure–high flow status during initial insufflation;
- Direct visualization and transillumination during placement of secondary ports.

Management:

- Identification of all injuries as there may be more than one if not directly visualized passage of trocar;
- Robotic repair of small bowel enterotomies using appropriate open principles;
- Appropriate hemostatic agents and argon beam when necessary on liver and splenic injuries and open conversion of splenectomy may be needed for uncontrolled hemorrhage;

- Duodenal and large intestinal injuries should prompt intraoperative general surgical consultation during repair;
- Vascular injury management should be based on size of the vessel and degree of hemorrhage;
- Inferior epigastric vascular injury should be compressed initially with a transabdominal wall suture to complete the operation, ultimate cut down, and/or formal ligation recommended.

49.2.4 Cardiopulmonary Complications

Although cardiopulmonary complications are inherent to any major surgical procedure, it deserves mention here due to the cardiopulmonary effects of the pneumoperitoneum. The most common arrhythmia is sinus tachycardia; bradyarrhythmias (e.g., atrioventricular dissociation, nodal rhythm, sinus bradycardia) may also develop independently or in combination with tachycardia during the same procedure.[53] Conditions leading to development of arrhythmias are CO_2 insufflation, hypercapnia, increased vagal tone owing to traction on pelvic or peritoneal structures, Trendelenburg position, anesthetic drugs (especially halothane in combination with spontaneous ventilation), preoperative patient anxiety, endobronchial intubation, and gas embolism.[53] The role of the anesthesiologist throughout the robotic procedure is of paramount importance. Continuous monitoring of cardiovascular (electrocardiogram, arterial blood pressure, central venous pressure) and pulmonary (capnometry, in-line oxygen, airway pressures and tidal volume, frequent arterial blood gas analyses) parameters is essential. Invasive cardiac monitoring may be instituted in patients with heart disease (using a Swan–Ganz catheter) or in high-risk (i.e., ASA 3 or 4) patients when prolonged and complicated laparoscopic procedures are expected, especially since a central venous pressure line may not be as reliable in laparoscopic procedures as in open procedures.

Because hypercapnia is one of the most common underlying causes of cardiac arrhythmias, it is essential to monitor and control this problem. Overall, hypercapnia can be corrected rapidly by adjustment of ventilatory rate, tidal volume, use of positive end-expiratory pressure as needed, and reduction of intra-abdominal pressure to 10 mmHg. Exsufflation of the pneumoperitoneum for 5–10 min may allow the anesthesiologist to "catch up" and correct the hypercapnia; the pneumoperitoneum may then be reinitiated at a lower pressure (5–10 mmHg).[53,54]

In the event of any cardiac compromise, the surgeon should immediately exsufflate the abdomen. If cardiac arrest is encountered, one should provide cardiac massage (compressions) while the anesthesiologist administers 100% oxygen and appropriate drug therapy. If a CO_2 embolus is suspected, additional maneuvers, such as turning the patient to a left lateral decubitus position and attempting to aspirate the embolus, can be attempted.

Prevention:

- Limit intra-abdominal pressures to 15 mmHg and in some cases to 10 mmHg in patients with COPD;
- Avoidance of certain anesthetic agents and combinations (e.g., halothane and spontaneous ventilation) has been reported as well as premedication with atropine may prevent excessive vagal stimulation.[53]

Management:

- Immediate exsufflation of the pneumoperitoneum;
- Follow appropriate cardiac and resuscitation measures.

49.2.5 Unidentified Bowel Injury

Unidentified bowel injury is an inherent risk of minimally invasive surgery and presumably due to "blind" passage of instruments as well as thermal spread of energy. Specific mention of this potential complication is important due to the significant complications associated with delayed identification. Bowel injury is generally categorized into those resulting from thermal energy and those resulting from direct puncture.

49.2.6 Electrosurgical Etiology

Electrical and thermal burns to patient are usually predictable and preventable. Electrosurgically induced thermal injury may occur because of one of four mechanisms:

1. Active electrode trauma by unintended activation causing direct bowel or other organ injury. It may be seen when coagulation extends beyond the intended site to other adjacent structures (e.g., bowel, blood vessels, nerves, ureter).
2. Direct coupling may occur when the active electrosurgical instrument makes an unintended contact with another instrument that is in direct contact with unintended tissue (e.g., bowel). This may happen out of the field of view.
3. Capacitive coupling injury, in monopolar mode, occurs when the surrounding charge is not allowed to conduct back to and disperse via the abdominal wall.[55] This condition may develop when a metal cannula is anchored to the skin with a nonconductive plastic grip, which should never be done. As a result, the electrical field, which builds up around the activated electrosurgical instrument, cannot be conducted to the abdominal wall because the plastic retainer acts as an insulator. Capacitively coupled currents are eliminated in bipolar instruments since they travel in opposite directions and cancel the flow of current.[56]
4. Insulation breakdown may allow current to escape along the shaft of the instrument, thereby harming tissues that are otherwise outside the field of view of the laparoscope. Insulation breakdown along the shaft of the instrument may be a result of repeated use, resterilization, or mechanical damage to the instrument during repeated insertion through a trocar.[57]

Although thermal injuries to the bowel can occur via any of the aforementioned ways, the most common way is felt to be due to stray currents that are not apparent initially. Postoperatively, the patient with unrecognized bowel trauma may not develop fever, nausea, or signs of peritonitis for many days.[58] Accordingly, bowel injury must be ruled out for any patient who develops unexplained fever and has signs of peritonitis. Laparoscopic surgery affords patients decreased postoperative pain; therefore any patient with abdominal pain greater than expected should raise the suspicion for an acute abdomen. The most sensitive test is an abdominal CT scan with oral contrast accompanied by delayed films, usually 6 or more hours after the initial oral contrast load. Laboratory values may be remarkable for leukocytosis with an associated left shift (i.e., increased percentage of neutrophils). In some patients, a normal or even low leukocyte count is encountered, making the "left shift" a more reliable sign than the absolute white cell count.[56]

Minor postoperative thermal injuries of the bowel, discovered late in the postoperative period (i.e., >5–7 days postoperatively), may have to be managed conservatively, aided by administration of antibiotics and an elemental diet. Indeed, a closed fistula may develop that will heal with this approach. However, if the patient does not respond rapidly or develops worsening peritonitis, open surgical exploration is mandatory. Thermal injury caused by monopolar cautery often results in tissue damage that extends beyond the visible area of necrosis. With this in mind, the surgeon should perform a bowel resection with a safety margin of on either side before completing an end-to-end anastomosis. General surgical consultation should be sought in this setting.

Thermal injury caused by bipolar electrosurgery is more confined to the visible area of damage. These injuries only occur due to direct firing of the instrument on the bowel. If the injury is small, it can be managed by simple excision of the defect and closure of the bowel wall. Bipolar injuries that involve more than half of the circumference of the bowel should be treated by excision of the affected segment of the bowel followed by reanastomosis.[59]

49.2.7 Mechanical Etiology

Mechanical injury involving the bowel is usually caused by trocar insertion or operative trauma. This is one of the most important complications of robotic surgery because it is potentially life threatening, especially if the injury is not recognized at the time of the operation. Inadvertent mechanical damage can be caused by a wide variety of sharp and blunt instruments (e.g., graspers, scissors, retractors). This type of injury is usually visible to the surgeon and discovered intraoperatively. Direct visual identification during the procedure allows the surgeon to repair the injury robotically in standard fashion adhering to established principles for repair of enterotomy. Given its localized nature, bowel resection is rarely necessary. The abdomen may irrigated copiously at the end of the procedure with an antibiotic-containing solution; but in cases of small bowel enterotomy, infection is rare

due to the relatively sterile nature of small intestinal contents. If the situation is missed during the procedure, then postoperative symptoms develop much earlier than with an electrosurgical injury. Fever, nausea, ileus, and peritonitis develop in the very early postoperative period. Diagnosis is confirmed by an abdominal CT scan with oral contrast material. This type of injury should be managed with immediate return to the operating room to correct the problem by local excision or resection of bowel with subsequent reanastomosis and copious irrigation of the abdomen. Once again, general surgical consultation is recommended in this setting to ensure multidisciplinary management.

Prevention:

- Ensure appropriate insulation and integrity of instrumentation;
- Avoid blind passage of instrumentation whenever possible;
- Assistants should carefully pass sharp instruments such as laparoscopic scissors as such instruments are able to blindly puncture the bowel;

Management:

- CT of the abdomen and pelvis with oral contrast should be obtained in any patient with suspected bowel injury or signs of peritonitis;
- Immediate open repair and resection may be needed to avoid continued leakage of bowel contents;
- In rare cases, percutaneous drainage may be used to create a controlled leak resulting in a fistula. Usually in cases of very delayed presentation;
- General surgical consultation recommended in all cases.

49.3 Complications Inherent to Bladder Surgery

49.3.1 Vascular Injury

Fortunately, direct vascular injury during laparoscopic dissection is a rare event. The use of blunt trocars, small nature of the instrumentation, limitations on surgical speed, and magnification of the surgical field combine to decrease this potential problem. Vascular injury can include abdominal wall vessels such as the inferior epigastric, intraperitoneal, or retroperitoneal vasculature. The majority of these injuries can be avoided by direct visualization.

In almost all cases of radical cystectomy for bladder cancer, a standard or extended pelvic lymphadenectomy is performed. It is during this portion of the operation when a vascular injury may occur. This is particularly the case when gross, bulky lymphadenopathy is encountered. When vessel injury occurs, the surgeon can undertake several steps to resolve the bleeding and these steps are based on whether a vein or an artery is injured. In almost all cases of venous injury, control can be achieved via the robotic approach even with injury to larger vessels such as the iliac veins or even the vena cava. The fact that the pneumoperitoneum far exceeds central venous pressure allows robotic control. First, the pneumoperitoneum pressure can be raised to 20 mmHg, thereby slowing or stopping any venous bleeding. If the injury is small, it may respond to simple tamponade and formal repair may not be necessary. Injuries to larger vessels and even large venotomies should be repaired with a 4-0 or 5-0 vascular prolene suture. The first step is simply to apply pressure to the opening. With 5 min of continuous pressure, a suitable platelet plug will form and allow for suture repair of any venotomy, including the vena cava. In addition, a hemostatic patch, fibrin glue, or other laparoscopically applied hemostatic agents can be used.

In cases of small arteriotomies or small artery avulsion, clipping or suture ligation may be possible. In most cases of significant arterial injury, laparoscopic control is not possible and should not be undertaken due to the brisk bleeding that is encountered as well as decreased visualization due to the pressure of the bleeding encountered in the arterial system. In these cases, immediate conversion to an open approach with rapid vascular control is recommended. Open conversion should not be avoided or thought of as failure, but instead should be considered good judgment. Vascular surgical consultation may be required. Fortunately, this scenario is rare as the arterial vessels are very resilient and more forgiving than the venous structures.

Prevention:

- Be aware of the vascular anatomy of the pelvis;
- Sharp dissection along the pelvic vessels when bulky lymphadenopathy is encountered;

- Directly visualize all movements along the pelvic vessels.

Management:

- Have a laparoscopic vascular tray including laparoscopic bulldogs and clamps as well as vascular suture close by when encountering difficult anatomy;
- Intracorporeal repair and suturing may be attempted on venous injuries after 5 min of compression in cases of large injuries or large vessels. Repair as one would in an open approach using similar principles of suturing;
- Immediate open conversion and vascular control is recommended if significant hemorrhage is encountered.

49.3.2 Incisional Hernia

The occurrence of an incisional hernia is usually confined to port sites larger than 5 mm or any open wound for specimen extraction.[60,61] The patient presents with complaints of localized discomfort accompanied by nausea and signs of an ileus. A smaller number of patients will present with diffuse abdominal pain and/or signs of a complete bowel obstruction. On examination, there is tenderness and, at times, swelling overlying a port site. The diagnosis may be established with a plain film of the abdomen that may show an ileus pattern; however, the definitive study is an abdominal CT scan with oral contrast, which can actually reveal the bowel protruding above the fascial level.

Laparoscopic repair with dissection of the hernia and subsequent intra-abdominal closure can be attempted if the surgeon is familiar with this approach. In complicated cases in which a strangulated hernia is suspected or confirmed laparoscopically, open surgical repair is indicated. In most cases, general surgical consultation may be required.

This problem is most easily avoided by careful closure of the fascia whenever a $\geq$10 mm trocar is used. In children, it is advisable to perform fascial closure of any port site 5 mm or larger. Although dilating ports may be utilized, the authors recommend at least attempting closure of the 10-mm port sites using S-retractors and an Allis clamp to visualize the external oblique or rectus fascia. It can then be approximated with a single 0-vicryl suture. The fascial layer of larger wounds should be closed using standard wound closing principles. Although surgeons have their own preferences of suture material and technique (interrupted vs. running), the authors usually close with a number 1-vicryl suture on a CTX needle in running fashion. The most important factor for closure is visually identifying the fascial edge and recognizing that muscle and fat add little to the closure in the way of strength. Overall, employing standard wound closure principles for both trocar and open incisions is a key to success.

Prevention:

- Appropriate approximation of fascial edges;
- Closure of ≥ 10 mm ports, particularly if using bladed trocars.

Management:

- Observation and conservative management is an option if the bowel is not compromised;
- Laparoscopic or open surgical repair.

49.3.3 Postoperative Ileus

Postoperative ileus (POI) is the most common reported postoperative complication after open radical cystectomy. It is often defined as delay of return of bowel function greater than 4 days.[62,63] Although robotic surgery theoretically minimizes peritoneal irritation, surgical manipulation of the abdominal contents, activation of the spinal reflex arc and has a lower generalized sympathetic hyperactivity (depression of gastrointestinal motility), POI is still the most common complication. Delayed return of gastrointestinal motility may result in pain, abdominal distension, nausea, and vomiting. In addition, POI often results in an increased length of hospital stay.[62] Different factors have been postulated to contribute to the induction and maintenance of the ileus; however, the etiology is incompletely known. In cases where a urinary diversion is created, urine leak is often the cause of a POI.[63]

Recent literature has described novel measures and modifications to traditional preoperative management to prevent or diminished POI. Maffezzini et al.

analyzed the elimination of mechanical bowel preparation and fasting before surgery with an early artificial nutrition, combining parenteral nutrition, and enteral nutrition. Houba et al. studied the effect of chewing gum on postoperative return of bowel function. Donat et al. analyzed the use of intravenous metoclopramide combined with early nasogastric tube removal. All have shown to varying degrees a positive impact on diminishing the time to recover of bowel activity. However, they have not been widely adopted.

It has been the authors' experience that the robotic approach, such as robot-assisted radical cystectomy, has shortened the length of POI and in many cases eliminated it entirely. In our experience, elimination of mechanical and antibiotic bowel preparation is potentially helpful as well. Patients are likely to be less volume depleted the day of surgery and require less aggressive fluid resuscitation intraoperatively. In some cases, however, there is nothing that can be done to prevent the onset of POI and it is simply a function of a bowel anastomosis and creation of a urinary diversion. Some people have postulated that "urine in the wound" whether through microscopic leaks of the ureteral–ileal anastomosis or reabsorption via the intestinal segment may play roles in the development of POI.

Regardless of the cause, the management is most often conservative including increased ambulation, gum chewing, and waiting. In some cases, gastric decompression is needed with a nagogastric tube. In most cases it is important to rule out any electrolyte abnormalities such as hypokalemia, hypomagnesemia, hypercalcemia, and hypocalcemia. Most importantly, the surgeon must rule out a partial or complete small bowel obstruction in cases of severely prolonged ileus. A CT scan of the abdomen and pelvis with oral contrast should be ordered if either is suspected. In addition to the above potential causes, a urine leak should be ruled out. In cases of severe ileus or prolonged ileus, a urine leak may be the cause. Analysis of any drain fluid available for creatinine can provide quick determination of urine leakage. Finally, drainage of any intra-abdominal fluid collection may be necessary in prolonged ileus if infection, lymphocele, or urinoma is suspected.

Prevention:

- Possibly eliminate mechanical and antibiotic bowel preparation in cases of urinary diversion;

- Early ambulation in the postoperative setting, as early as the same day of surgery;
- Gum chewing has been shown to help in some reports;
- Maintain normal electrolyte levels.

Management:

- Correct any electrolyte abnormalities;
- Increase ambulation;
- Rule out any potential bowel obstruction with a CT scan of the abdomen and pelvis with oral contrast;
- Possibly insert a nasogastric tube for stomach decompression in cases of severe discomfort, airway compromise, or extremely prolonged ileus;
- Percutaneous drainage of any intra-abdominal fluid collection felt to be a potential source such as a lymphocele, ileus, or abscess.

49.3.4 Lymphocele and Lymph Leak

Lymphocele formation is commonly associated with pelvic procedures, such as pelvic lymph node dissection (2–9%).[64] The lymphocele may take weeks to develop and may even occur despite a transperitoneal approach. Presentation most often includes lower extremity edema secondary to local compression of the pelvic vasculature on the side of the lymphocele. In rare cases, the presenting findings may be venous thrombosis and pulmonary embolism. The lymphocele is readily diagnosed by CT.

There are numerous options for treatment and management. In the asymptomatic patient, observation may be elected in the absence of any evidence of infection or vascular compromise. In the presenting symptomatic patient, treatment is either immediate percutaneous drainage or intraperitonealization which can be performed via a laparoscopic approach in some cases. Sclerosing therapy can be used to treat the lymphocele in some cases, but it is not as successful as some of the other techniques.

During intraperitonealization, a tag of omentum can be placed into the opening made in the lymphocele to try and prevent recurrence. Prevention of lymphocele formation requires close attention to clipping suspected lymphatic structures. The impact of bipolar or harmonic devices on lymphatic patency is unreported to date.

Prolonged lymph leak has been observed by the authors in patients undergoing robot-assisted radical cystectomy with extended lymphadenectomy. Male patients may complain of fluid leaking from the native urethra and feel as if they are voiding. Female patients may complain of leakage from the vagina requiring pads in their undergarments. Although disconcerting in some cases, this is self-limiting. In all cases it will resolve but can take several weeks in patients requiring systemic anticoagulation or those with nutritional compromise. We feel that this may be due to the extensive nature of the lymphadenectomy as well as the use of cautery for much of the dissection.

Prevention:

- Use of meticulous clipping at proximal and distal borders of lymphadenectomy;
- Avoid subcutaneous heparin in the lower extremities and give in the upper extremities;
- Improve nutritional status of patient as soon as possible to promote healing.

Management:

- Percutaneous drainage with ultrasound or CT guidance often the initial step of a symptomatic lymphocele;
- Sclerosing therapy is an option but may result in an infected lymphocele, may be preferred in the nonsurgical candidate;
- Intraperitonealization of the lymphocele by creating a surgical window;
- Lymph leaks via the urethra or vagina are self-limiting and need no intervention other than improving nutritional status.

49.3.5 Wound Infection

Wound infection is actually quite rare in the setting of laparoscopic or robotic procedures. This is likely due to the percutaneous nature of the surgery and the lack of open wounds exposed in the operating room. Nevertheless, this may be encountered in some patients either at a port site or at an extraction site.

Prevention:

- Appropriate preoperative IV antibiotic infusion (within 30 min of incision);
- Use of appropriate sterile technique.

Management:

- IV antibiotics;
- Open and drainage of any localized purulence or infection;
- Typical wound care.

49.3.6 Deep Venous Thrombosis

Signs of deep venous thrombosis include localized calf tenderness with associated swelling. However, many patients with postoperative deep venous thrombosis have a subclinical course. The most common clinical scenario is detection of a deep venous thrombosis only after a patient has developed a pulmonary embolus. Subsequent evaluation of the pelvic and leg veins is undertaken most commonly with Doppler ultrasonography. Treatment is immediate anticoagulation, initially with heparin and then with warfarin. In patients with a pulmonary embolus who are not candidates for anticoagulation, a caval filter is placed under radiographic control. In many cases a retrievable filter can be placed if only temporary management is expected.

The problem can be avoided utilizing standard measures such as pneumatic sequential compression devices and/or mini-dose heparin and early postoperative ambulation. Currently the American College of Chest Physicians recommends either pneumatic compression stockings or heparin (i.e., mini-dose heparin or low molecular weight heparin) for all major pelvic urologic procedures.[65] Pneumatic compression stockings should be placed preoperatively and continued for 48–72 h postoperatively or until ambulatory. Some surgeons use low molecular weight heparin (Lovenox®) in addition to stockings in high-risk patients. Ultimately, early ambulation and risk stratification are recommended in all patients. The robotic approach lends itself to early ambulation in contrast to its open counterpart due to the minimally invasive nature of the surgery.

Prevention:

- Early ambulation;
- Use of lower extremity stockings or sequential compression devices initially in the preoperative holding area throughout the first 48–72 h;
- Use of unfractionated or low molecular weight heparin in prophylactic doses in addition to lower extremity measures in high-risk patients.

Management:

- Systemic anticoagualtion in almost all cases for at least 3–6 months;
- Placement of an inferior vena caval filter in cases when anticoagulation is contraindicated.

49.4 Complications of Urinary Diversion and Urine Leak from the Bladder

Whether an operation is performed open or robotically, there are complications that are inherent to the creation of the urinary diversion. These complications include problems at the bowel anastomosis such as a bowel leak or complications at the diversion site including urine leak and uretero-ileal strictures. In addition to mechanical problems, patients with urinary diversions may suffer electrolyte and acid–base problems with urine reabsorption. The most common disturbance is a hyperchloremic metabolic acidosis associated with the use of ileum. In most cases it is mild not requiring treatment, but in some cases it may require systemic alkalinization if bone resorption or fatigue are associated with the syndrome. Other bowel segments result in other disturbances depending on the type of mucosa in contact with urine, gastric, or jejunal. Furthermore, absorption problems such as B12 deficiency are known complications of the use of intestinal segments for urinary diversion. The full range of complications and management of these potential complications are beyond the scope of this chapter but are well established in the urologic literature.[66] As most of the urinary diversions reported in the literature employ extracorporeal creation of the diversion, the same open surgical principles such as tissue handling and bowel anastomotic and uretero-ileal anastomotic techniques should be used. The surgeon performing robot-assisted bladder surgery with urinary diversion should be aware of the potential complications, be able to manage them, and be able to fully inform the potential patient of these outcomes.

Robot-assisted procedures of the bladder that do not employ a urinary diversion can still produce a urine leak from the bladder itself. Although not specifically covered in the small case series' in the literature, such urine leaks are potential problems anytime the bladder is opened and closed such as with diverticulectomy, partial cystectomy, and ureteral reimplantation.

Prevention of such complications is via the application of standard urologic surgical principles such as appropriate closure of the bladder in multiple layers as well as adequate catheter drainage of the bladder. It is also important to place a surgical drain the field, especially since most of the robotic procedures will be performed via a transperitoneal approach. This of course introduces the potential for an intraperitoneal leak that may not have been a problem with standard extraperitoneal open approaches.

Prevention:

- Use of standard open surgical principles of tissue handling, suturing, and techniques of anastomosis;
- Appropriate drainage with ureteral and bladder catheters when appropriate;
- Appropriate use of surgical drains in the surgical field;
- Watertight closure of the bladder or any other anastomosis.

Management:

- Percutaneous drainage of any uncontrolled leak;
- Maximal bladder drainage with urethral or suprapubic catheters when appropriate;
- Percutaneous renal access and diversion when an uncontrolled leak persists.

49.5 Summary

Robot-assisted surgery continues to increase in application and acceptance throughout all surgical fields. Although the application of the robot to procedures such as radical cystectomy, bladder diverticulectomy, and partial cystectomy may introduce new potential complications inherent to the robotic nature of the procedure, the early literature supports a decrease in rates of overall complications. While the benefits of the minimally invasive nature of robot bladder surgery are apparent, it is important for any surgeon performing this operation to be well versed in complications associated with use of the robot.

Interestingly, most of the complications reported in the literature are similar to what is seen in the equivalent open procedure. This is largely due to the complex nature of procedures such as radical cystectomy. The very fact that a urinary diversion is being performed as well as the fact that it is done through a small open incision translates into similar complications to the open procedure. Therefore, it is also important for the surgeon to be aware of the standard complications associated with open pelvic surgery and urinary diversion. With knowledge in the prevention and management of all potential complications, robot-assisted bladder surgery will be successfully added to the armamentarium in the management of urologic diseases.

References

1. Chang SS, Cookson MS, Baumgartner RG, et al. Analysis of early complications after radical cystectomy: results of a collaborative care pathway. *J Urol*. 2002;167: 2012–2016.
2. Hollenbeck BK, Miller DC, Taub D, et al. Identifying risk factors for potentially avoidable complications following radical cystectomy. *J Urol*. 2005;174:1231–1237.
3. Konety BR, Allareddy V, Herr H. Complications after radical cystectomy: analysis of population-based data. *Urology*. 2006;68:58–64.
4. Quek ML, Stein JP, Daneshmand S, et al. A critical analysis of perioperative mortality from radical cystectomy. *J Urol*. 2006;175:886–889.
5. Studer UE, Burkhard FC, Schumacher M, et al. Twenty years experience with an ileal orthotopic low pressure bladder substitute–lessons to be learned. *J Urol*. 2006;176: 161–166.
6. Novotny V, Hakenberg OW, Wiessner D, et al. Perioperative complications of radical cystectomy in a contemporary series. *Eur Urol*. 2007;51:397–401.
7. Fairey A, Chetner M, Metcalfe J, et al. Associations among age, comorbidity and clinical outcomes after radical cystectomy: results from the Alberta Urology Institute radical cystectomy database. *J Urol*. 2008;180: 128–134.
8. Pycha A, Comploj E, Martini T, et al. Comparison of complications in three incontinent urinary diversions. *Eur Urol*. 2008;54:825–832.
9. Boström PJ, Kössi J, Laato M, et al. Risk factors for mortality and morbidity related to radical cystectomy. *BJU Int*. 2009;103:191–196.
10. Ng CK, Kauffman EC, Lee MM, et al. A comparison of postoperative complications in open versus robotic cystectomy. *Eur Urol*. 2010;57:274–281.
11. Novara G, Marco VD, Aragona M, et al. Complications and mortality after radical cystectomy for bladder transitional cell cancer. *J Urol*. 2009;182:914–921.
12. Hemal AK. Role of robot-assisted surgery for bladder cancer. *Curr Opin Urol*. 2009;19:69–75.
13. Nunez R, Andrews PE, Martin AD, et al. Comparison of open and robot assisted radical cystectomy. *J Urol*. 2009;181(Suppl 4):360–361.

14. Challacombe B, Dasgupta P. Reconstruction of the lower urinary tract by laparoscopic and robotic surgery. *Curr Opin Urol.* 2007;17:390–395.

15. Ak H, Kolla AB, Wadhwa P. First case series of robotic radical cystoprostatectomy, bilateral pelvic lymphadenectomy, and urinary diversion with the da Vinci S system. *J Robotic Surg.* 2008;2:35–40.

16. Sala LG, Matsunaga GS, Corica FA, et al. Robot-assisted laparoscopic radical cystoprostatectomy and totally intracorporeal ileal neobladder. *J Endourol.* 2006;20:233–235.

17. Rhee JJ, Lebeau S, Smolkin M, et al. Radical cystectomy with ileal conduit diversion: early prospective evaluation of the impact of robotic assistance. *BJU Int.* 2006;98:1059–1063.

18. Menon M, Hemal AK, Tewari A, et al. Robot-assisted radical cystectomy and urinary diversion in female patients: technique with preservation of the uterus and vagina. *J Am Coll Surg.* 2004;98:386–393.

19. Hemal AK, Abol-Enein H, Tewari A, et al. Robotic radical cystectomy and urinary diversion in the management of bladder cancer. *Urol Clin North Am.* 2004;31:719–729.

20. Pruthi RS, Smith A, Wallen EM. Evaluating the learning curve for robot-assisted laparoscopic radical cystectomy. *J Endourol.* 2008;22:2469–2474.

21. Wang GJ, Barocas DA, Raman JD, et al. Robotic vs open radical cystectomy: prospective comparison of perioperative outcomes and pathological measures of early oncological efficacy. *BJU Int.* 2008;101:89–93.

22. Abraham JB, Young JL, Box GN, et al. Comparative analysis of laparoscopic and robot-assisted radical cystectomy with ileal conduit urinary diversion. *J Endourol.* 2007;21:1473–1480.

23. Pruthi RS, Wallen EM. Robotic-assisted laparoscopic radical cystoprostatectomy. *Eur Urol.* 2008;53:310–322.

24. Guru KA, Kim HL, Piacente PM, et al. Robot-assisted radical cystectomy and pelvic lymph node dissection: initial experience at Roswell Park Cancer Institute. *Urology.* 2007;69:469–474.

25. Beecken WD, Wolfram M, Engl T, et al. Robotic-assisted laparoscopic radical cystectomy and intra-abdominal formation of an orthotopic ileal neobladder. *Eur Urol.* 2003;44:337–339.

26. Murphy DG, Challacombe BJ, Elhage O, et al. Robotic-assisted laparoscopic radical cystectomy with extracorporeal urinary diversion: initial experience. *Eur Urol.* 2008;54:570–580.

27. Galich A, Sterrett S, Nazemi T, et al. Comparative analysis of early perioperative outcomes following radical cystectomy by either the robotic or open method. *JSLS.* 2006;10:145–150.

28. Balaji KC, Yohannes P, McBride CL, et al. Feasibility of robot-assisted totally intracorporeal laparoscopic ileal conduit urinary diversion: initial results of a single institutional pilot study. *Urology.* 2004;63:51–55.

29. Menon M, Hemal AK, Tewari A, et al. Nerve-sparing robot-assisted radical cystoprostatectomy and urinary diversion. *BJU Int.* 2003;92:232–236.

30. Passerotti CC, Nguyen HT, Lais A, et al. Robot-assisted laparoscopic ileal bladder augmentation: defining techniques and potential pitfalls. *J Endourol.* 2008;22:355–360.

31. Gundeti MS, Eng MK, Reynolds WS, et al. Pediatric robotic-assisted laparoscopic augmentation ileocystoplasty and mitrofanoff appendicovesicostomy: complete intracorporeal–initial case report. *Urology.* 2008;72:1144–1147.

32. Al-Othman KE, Al-Hellow HA, Al-Zahrani HM, et al. Robotic augmentation enterocystoplasty. *J Endourol.* 2008;22:597–600.

33. Macejko AM, Viprakasit DP, Nadler RB. Cystoscope- and robot-assisted bladder diverticulectomy. *J Endourol.* 2008;22:2389–2391.

34. Myer EG, Wagner JR. Robotic assisted laparoscopic bladder diverticulectomy. *J Urol.* 2007;178:2406–2410.

35. Meeks JJ, Hagerty JA, Lindgren BW. Pediatric robotic-assisted laparoscopic diverticulectomy. *Urology.* 2009;73:299–301.

36. Tareen BU, Mufarrij PW, Godoy G, et al. Robot-assisted laparoscopic partial cystectomy and diverticulectomy: initial experience of four cases. *J Endourol.* 2008;22:1497–1500.

37. Sener A, Chew BH, Duvdevani M, et al. Combined transurethral and laparoscopic partial cystectomy and robot-assisted bladder repair for the treatment of bladder endometrioma. *J Minim Invasive Gynecol.* 2006;13:245–248.

38. Madeb R, Knopf JK, Nicholson C, et al. The use of robotically assisted surgery for treating urachal anomalies. *BJU Int.* 2006;98:838–842.

39. Chammas MF Jr, Kim FJ, Barbarino A, et al. Asymptomatic rectal and bladder endometriosis: a case for robotic-assisted surgery. *Can J Urol.* 2008;15:4097–4100.

40. Dindo D, Demartines N, Clavien PA. Classification of surgical complications: a new proposal with evaluation in a cohort of 6336 patients and results of a survey. *Ann Surg.* 2004;240:205–213.

41. Lavery HJ, Thaly R, Albala D, et al. Robotic equipment malfunction during robotic prostatectomy: a multi-institutional study. *J Endourol.* 2008;22:2165–2168.

42. Winfree CJ, Kline DG. Intraoperative positioning nerve injuries. *Surg Neurol.* 2005;63:5–18.

43. Kretschmer T, Heinen CW, Antoniadis G, et al. Iatrogenic nerve injuries. *Neurosurg Clin N Am.* 2009;20:73–90.

44. Bocca G, van Moorselaar JA, Feitz WF, et al. Compartment syndrome, rhabdomyolysis and risk of acute renal failure as complications of the lithotomy position. *J Nephrol.* 2002;15:183–185.

45. Choi SJ, Gwak MS, Ko JS, et al. The effects of the exaggerated lithotomy position for radical perineal prostatectomy on respiratory mechanics. *Anaesthesia.* 2006;61:439–443.

46. Bosch X, Poch E, Grau JM. Rhabdomyolysis and acute kidney injury. *N Engl J Med.* 2009;36:62–72.

47. Champault G, Cazacu F, Taffinder N. Serious trocar accidents in laparoscopic surgery: a French survey of 103,852 operations. *Surg Laparosc Endosc.* 1996;6:367–370.

48. Chandler JG, Corson SL, Way LW. Three spectra of laparoscopic entry access injuries. *J Am Coll Surg.* 2001;192:478–490.

49. Bhoyrul S, Payne J, Steffes B, et al. A randomized prospective study of radially expanding trocars in laparoscopic surgery. *J Gastrointest Surg.* 2000;4:392–397.

50. Pruthi RS, Stefaniak H, Hubbard JS, et al. Robot-assisted laparoscopic anterior pelvic exenteration for bladder cancer in the female patient. *J Endourol.* 2008;22: 2397–2402.

51. Hemal AK, Kumar R, Seth A, et al. Complications of laparoscopic radical cystectomy during the initial experience. *Int J Urol.* 2004;11:483–488.

52. Palmer KJ, Shah K, Samavedi S, et al. Robot-assisted radical cystectomy. *J Endourol.* 2008;22:2073–2077.

53. Gerges FJ, Kanazi GE, Jabbour-Khoury SI. Anesthesia for laparoscopy: a review. *J Clin Anesth.* 2006;18:67–78.

54. Rauh R, Hemmerling TM, Rist M, et al. Influence of pneumoperitoneum and patient positioning on respiratory system compliance. *J Clin Anesth.* 2001;13:361–365.

55. Li TC, Saravelos H, Richmond M, et al. Complications of laparoscopic pelvic surgery: recognition, management and prevention. *Hum Reprod Update.* 1997;3:505–515.

56. Nduka CC, Super PA, Monson JR, et al. Cause and prevention of electrosurgical injuries in laparoscopy. *J Am Coll Surg.* 1994;179:161–170.

57. Montero PN, Robinson TN, Weaver JS, et al. Insulation failure in laparoscopic instruments. *Surg Endosc.* 2009;doi:10.1007/s00464-009-0601-5.

58. Wu MP, Ou CS, Chen SL, et al. Complications and recommended practices for electrosurgery in laparoscopy. *Am J Surg.* 2000;179:67–73.

59. van der Voort M, Heijnsdijk EA, Gouma DJ. Bowel injury as a complication of laparoscopy. *Br J Surg.* 2004;91: 1253–1258.

60. Reardon PR, Preciado A, Scarborough T, et al. Hernia at 5-mm laparoscopic port site presenting as early postoperative small bowel obstruction. *J Laparoendosc Adv Surg Tech A.* 1999;9:523–525.

61. Tonouchi H, Ohmori Y, Kobayashi M, et al. Trocar site hernia. *Arch Surg.* 2004;139:1248–1256.

62. Chang SS, Baumgartner RG, Wells N, et al. Causes of increased hospital stay after radical cystectomy in a clinical pathway setting. *J Urol.* 2002;167:208–211.

63. Maffezzini M, Campodonico F, Canepa G, et al. Current perioperative management of radical cystectomy with intestinal urinary reconstruction for muscle-invasive bladder cancer and reduction of the incidence of postoperative ileus. *Surg Oncol.* 2008;17:41–48.

64. Naselli A, Andreatta R, Introini C, et al. Predictors of symptomatic lymphocele after lymph node excision and radical prostatectomy. *Urology.* 2009;doi:10.1016/j.urology.2009.03.011.

65. Goldhaber SZ. Prevention of recurrent idiopathic venous thromboembolism. *Circulation.* 2004;14:IV20–IV24.

66. Hautmann RE, Abol-Enein H, Hafez K, et al. Urinary diversion. World Health Organization (WHO) Consensus Conference on Bladder Cancer. *Urology.* 2007;69:17–49.

Part VI
Pediatric Urology

Chapter 50

Robotic Surgery for Ureteral Anomalies in Children

Rita Gobet and Craig A. Peters

50.1 Introduction

The advantages of robot-assisted minimal invasive surgery are particularly useful for ureteral surgery. Wristed instruments allow surgeons to perform extravesical and intravesical anti-reflux surgery as well as delicate high and low uretero-ureterostomies with precision and relative ease. The detailed descriptions of these procedures following in this chapter hopefully allow surgeons with or without laparoscopic experience to easily learn this new technique and to enable them to adapt these standard procedures for more complex cases.

50.1.1 Operating Room Setup

a. Drawing from overhead position
   – high ureteral surgery (Fig. 50.1)
   – low ureteral surgery (Fig. 50.2)
   – extravesical surgery (Fig. 50.2)
   – intravesical surgery (Fig. 50.2)

50.1.2 Patient Positioning

a. Intra-operative pictures
   – high ureteral surgery (Fig. 50.3)
   – low ureteral surgery (Fig. 50.4)

C.A. Peters (✉)
Division of Surgical Innovation, Technology and Translation, Sheikh Zayed Institute for Pediatric Surgical Innovation, Children's National Medical Center, Washington, DC, USA
e-mail: crpeters@cnmc.org

Robotic Ureteroureterostomy (proximal)

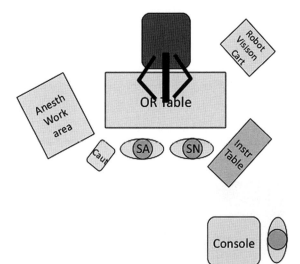

Fig. 50.1 OR setup for renal case

   – extravesical surgery: Trendelenburg
   – intravesical surgery

b. Highlights

For nearly all children, the robot can be brought to the foot of the bed and the patient's legs do not need to be split. The patient is placed in Trendelenburg position to provide exposure to the posterior aspect of the bladder without further retraction.

50.1.3 Trocar Configuration

a. Images
   – high ureteral surgery (Fig. 50.5)
   – low ureteral surgery (Fig. 50.6)

A.K. Hemal, M. Menon (eds.), *Robotics in Genitourinary Surgery*,
DOI 10.1007/978-1-84882-114-9_50, © Springer-Verlag London Limited 2011

Robotic Ureteral Reimplant

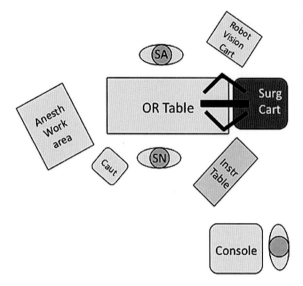

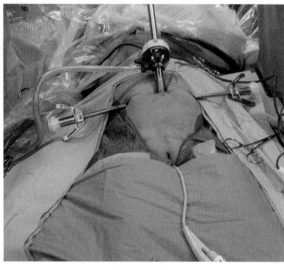

Fig. 50.4 Cannulae in position for bladder case in infant

Fig. 50.2 OR setup for bladder case

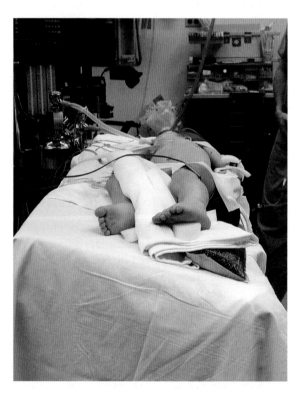

Fig. 50.3 Patient positioning and setup for renal case

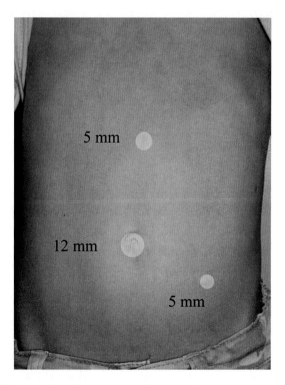

Fig. 50.5 Port sites for renal or high ureteral surgery

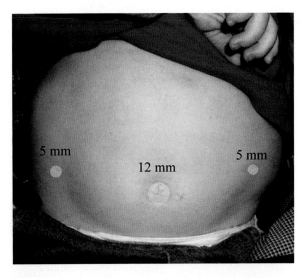

Fig. 50.6 Port sites after extravesical bladder procedure

– extravesical surgery: umbilicus, left and right
   working port at same umbilical level
– intravesical surgery (Fig. 50.7)

b. Highlights

Port placement for upper ureteral surgery is identical to that for robotic pyeloplasty in children. In small infants, ports for extravesical reimplant should

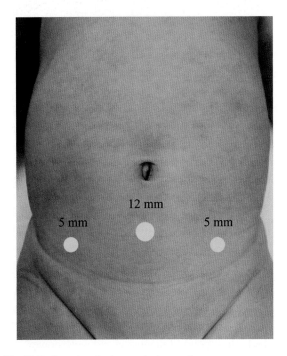

Fig. 50.7 Port sites for intravesical procedure

be moved slightly above the umbilicus to permit adequate intra-corporeal room. The mid-clavicular ports are placed symmetrically for one- or two-sided reimplants.

50.1.4 Instrumentation List

c. For all ureteral procedures (Table 50.1)
d. Sutures: Monocryl 5-0 for closure of any mucosal defects
   Vicryl 3-0 for the hitch stitch and 4-0 for the closure of the detrusor tunnel

50.2 Step-by-Step Technique

e. Ureteral reimplantation—extravesical (Lich-Gregoir)

Step 1. Placement of a transurethral bladder catheter to control bladder volume. For trocar placement the bladder should be empty and then filled to one-third to half the capacity for detrusor tunnel creation.

Step 2. We use a mini-laparotomy (modified Hassan technique) to insert the 12 mm camera port at the umbilicus, then the abdomen is insufflated (pressure 8–12 mmHg according to the age of the patient), and two robotic working ports (5 or 8 mm) are inserted at the umbilical level in the midclavicular line bilaterally under direct vision. An optional assistant working port (standard 5 or 8 mm port) can be inserted lateral to the robotic ports, although it is rarely used.

Step 3. In the vesicorectal or vesicouterine pouch the peritoneum is incised after identification of the ureter crossing the iliac vessels and the ductus deferens or the uterine vessels crossing the ureter (Fig. 50.8).

Step 4. The ureter is mobilized primarily toward the bladder to achieve about 4–5 cm of length. There is frequently a crossing vessel about 1 cm from the hiatus that will need to be ligated with cautery. Excessive dissection should be avoided to limit any injury to the perivesical nerves, particularly with a bilateral procedure. In boys the vas deferens should be left attached to and swept cranially with the peritoneum (Fig. 50.9).

Table 50.1 Instrumentation for all ureteral reconstructive procedures

Surgeon instrumentation			Assistant instrumentation
Left arm	Right arm	Fourth arm	• Suction-irrigator • Blunt tip grasper • Needle driver • Laparoscopic scissors
• De Bakey forceps or Maryland grasper • Curved monopolar scissors	• Curved monopolar scissors (8 mm) • Electrocautery hook • Needle driver • De Bakey forceps or Maryland grasper	Not used	• A separate instrument port is rarely used • Needles and suction are passed through one of the working ports

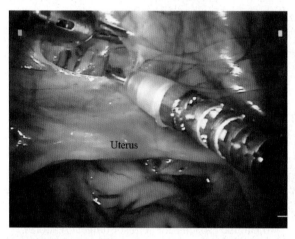

Fig. 50.8 Incising peritoneum over left ureter on the posterior aspect of the bladder

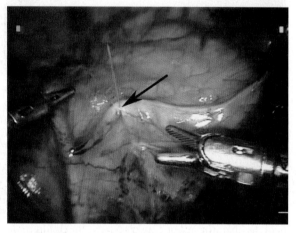

Fig. 50.10 Placement of a hitch stitch to lift the bladder superiorly and stabilize function

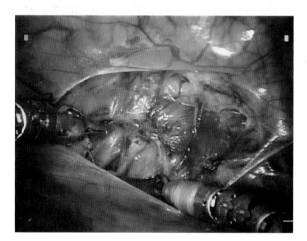

Fig. 50.9 Exposure of the ureter as it enters the detrusor

Step 5. A hitch stitch of 3-0 Vicryl is placed through the bladder wall above the planned tunnel in order to straighten the tissue and thereby facilitating tunnel creation. The stitch can be placed through the abdominal wall allowing easy adjustment of the tension applied (Fig. 50.10).

Step 6. Tunnel creation: The electrocautery hook is usually used for the incision of the detrusor muscle above the entrance of the ureter into the bladder wall. The direction of the tunnel should be slightly toward lateral to avoid kinking of the ureter. Using the hook or blunt graspers all fibers of the detrusor are divided until the bladder mucosa bulges through the incision showing the typical blue color. Care should be taken to completely divide the fibers (Waldeyer sheath) at the ureteral insertion. The edges of the detrusor layers should be undermined for 2–3 mm on both sides. If the mucosa is perforated, a 5-0 or 6-0 chromic, 8 cm in length, or monocryl suture is used to close the defect with a figure-of-eight stitch (Fig. 50.11).

Step 7. Closing tunnel: It is most efficient to start at the highest point of the tunnel and work downward; the first stitch will keep the ureter in place. A 4-0

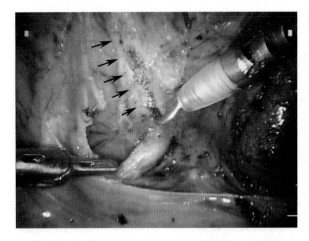

Fig. 50.11 Creation of detrusor tunnel with arrows marking the line of the detrusor tunnel

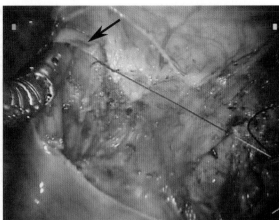

Fig. 50.13 Closing the detrusor tunnel over the mobilized ureter

Vicryl suture is used, cut to a 14 cm length. Grab a good bit of detrusor on one side, then lift the ureter up, pass the needle underneath, and then grab a bit of the other side of the detrusor, pass the needle back underneath the ureter, and tie. Subsequent sutures are placed without tension or having to pass the needle under the ureter. Four or five interrupted stitches are usually enough to get an adequate tunnel of about 3–4 cm (Figs. 50.12, closing tunnel start and 50.13, closing tunnel end).

Step 8. The hitch stitch is removed, closure of the peritoneum with 4-0 Vicryl is optional. In bilateral cases proceed with the same steps on the opposite side. Otherwise remove cannulae, evacuate the

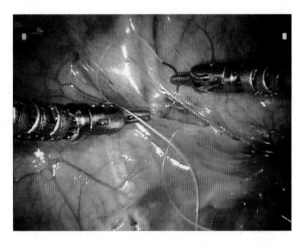

Fig. 50.14 Closing the peritoneum over the repair

pneumoperitoneum, and close the trocar sites. The bladder catheter is optional for unilateral cases, and for bilateral procedures is left in place for 24 h (Fig. 50.14).

50.3 Ureteral Reimplantation – Intravesical

Step 1. Port placement to gain access to the bladder for minimal invasive procedures remains a challenge since the bladder easily separates from the abdominal wall. The bladder will be filled with carbon

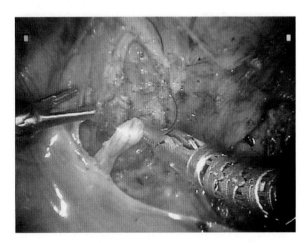

Fig. 50.12 Mobilizing the ureter into the intravesical tunnel that will be closed over to create an anti-reflux mechanism

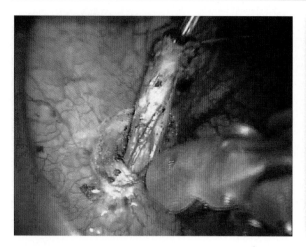

Fig. 50.15 Intravesical view of ureteral mobilization for cross-trigonal reimplantation

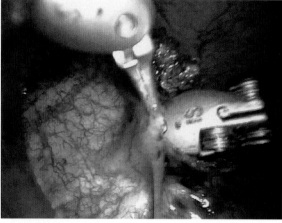

Fig. 50.16 Creating the submucosal tunnel

dioxide. In the event of a port site leak, the gas will fill the peritoneum and retroperitoneum thereby reducing the working field significantly. Moreover, closure of the bladder wall after the procedure is important but not trivial. The placement of the camera port at the umbilicus includes skin incision and then blunt dissection to mobilize the bladder dome while the bladder is distended with saline. Two sutures are then placed to facilitate opening of the bladder and placement of the port, they will be used later to close the bladder after the procedure. Under direct vision the working ports are placed just above the level of a Pfannenstiel incision in the midclavicular line. After all three ports are placed and the bladder is sealed, the saline is drained, and the bladder is filled with carbon dioxide. A feeding tube is placed in the urethra to suction blood and urine during the procedure.[1]

Step 2. Ureteral mobilization with stent: After identification of the ureteral orifices a 5 cm segment of a 5 Fr feeding tube is inserted into the ureter and sutured in place using needle holders on both arms. The electrocautery hook is then used to mobilize the ureter by incising the mucosa around the orifice and then dividing the muscular and fibrous bands between ureteral and bladder wall and retroperitoneum more proximally. To facilitate mobilization traction is provided by pulling the feeding tube with a needle holder. At this point hiatal repair is performed by re-approximating the detrusor with one or two stitches inferior to the ureter (Fig. 50.15).

Step 3. Tunnel dissection: Dissection and development of tunnels using scissors can be performed more proficiently than the open approach, given the articulation of the instruments. As in open surgery, care needs to be taken to stay strictly in the submucosal plane (Fig. 50.16).

Step 4. Anastomosis: The ureters are brought through the tunnels using the feeding tubes. The ureters are then sutured in the tunnel using 4-0 or 5-0 Monocryl suture. The path of the ureter is checked with a feeding tube to demonstrate patency (Fig. 50.17).

Step 5. The bladder is closed with the previously placed sutures, and fascia and skin are closed at the port sites. A bladder catheter is left in place for 1–2 days.

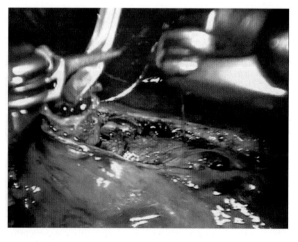

Fig. 50.17 Suturing the tunneled ureter to the opposite side of the trigone

50.4 Uretero-ureterostomy – High

Step 1. We recommend placement of a double J catheter into the recipient ureter which will be placed across the anastomosis. To achieve this we cystoscopically place a double J catheter of adequate length and size partially into the recipient ureter, and cross it to the donor ureter after completion of the back wall of the anastomosis. Radiological control of the correct position at the end of surgery is recommended.

Step 2. We use a minilaparotomy (Hassan technique) to insert the 12 mm camera port at the umbilicus, then the abdomen is insufflated (pressure 8–12 mmHg according to the age of the patient), and two robotic working ports (5 or 8 mm) are inserted, one in the midline half-way between the xyphoid and umbilicus, the second half-way between the anterior superior iliac spine and the umbilicus under direct vision. An optional assistant working port (standard 5 or 8 mm port) can be inserted contralateral to the midline robotic working port.

Step 3. Access to the ureter(s) is achieved by mobilizing the colon or by a transmesenteric approach on the left near the lower pole of the kidney. The ureter(s) are adequately mobilized (1–2 cm) avoiding trauma by direct handling of the ureteral tissue and minimizing devascularization. The recipient ureter is incised vertically; the donor ureter is transected obliquely or spatulated depending on its caliber (Figs. 50.18 and 50.19).

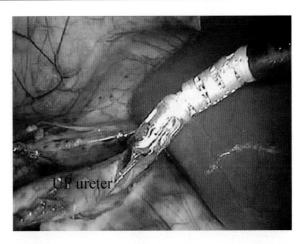

Fig. 50.19 Incising the upper pole ureter at the proposed site of the U–U

Step 4. The back wall of the anastomosis is performed using running or interrupted stitches. A monofilament absorbable suture, such as Monocryl is used. For children under 4 years, a 6-0 suture is employed; and for older children, a 5 0 suture is used (Figs. 50.20 and 50.21).

Step 5. The double J catheter is now placed across the anastomosis and into the upper pole.

Step 6. The anastomosis is completed. An intra-abdominal drain can be placed, but is not routinely used as the stent provides adequate drainage (Fig. 50.22).

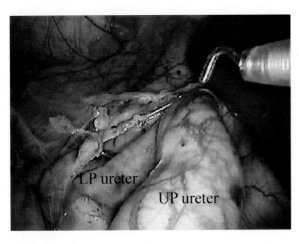

Fig. 50.18 Exposure of the dilated upper pole ureter and the normal lower pole ureter in preparation for a proximal uretero-ureterostomy for an ectopic ureter with upper pole function

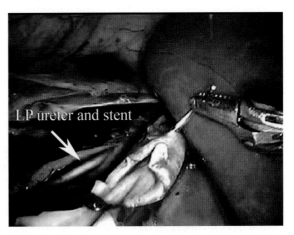

Fig. 50.20 The initial anastomotic stitch into the upper pole ureter after spatulation

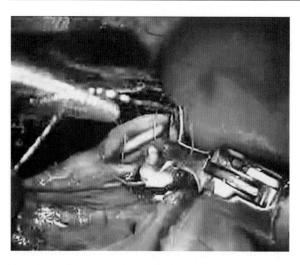

Fig. 50.21 Completing the back wall suture line of the U–U. The stent is visible in the lower pole ureter

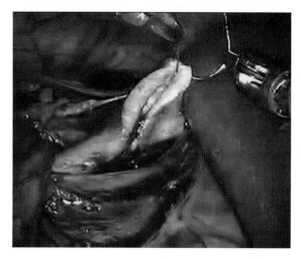

Fig. 50.22 Beginning the anterior wall suture line of the U–U

50.5 Uretero-ureterostomy – Low

Step 1. We recommend placement of a double J catheter via the recipient ureter into the donor renal pelvis, thereby stenting the anastomosis. To achieve this we cystoscopically place a double J catheter of adequate length and size partially into the (recipient) distal ureter, without removing the guide wire, and attach it to a transurethral bladder Foley catheter with tape. It should be kept sterile and within reach of the surgeon to manipulate and advance it during

completion of the anastomosis. Radiological control of the correct position at the end of surgery is recommended.

Step 2. We use a minilaparotomy (Hassan technique) to insert the 12 mm camera port at the umbilicus, then the abdomen is insufflated (pressure 8–12 mmHg according to the age of the patient), and two robotic working ports are inserted (5 or 8 mm), one in the midclavicular line half-way between the ribs and umbilicus, the second in the midline between symphysis and the umbilicus (avoiding bladder injury), under direct vision. An optional assistant working port (standard 5 or 8 mm port) can be inserted contralateral to the midline robotic working port.

Step 3. Access to the ureter(s) is achieved by opening of the peritoneum at the crossing of the ureter(s) over the iliac vessels. The ureter(s) are adequately mobilized (1–2 cm) avoiding trauma by direct handling of the ureteral tissue and minimizing devascularization. The recipient ureter is incised vertically, the donor ureter is transected obliquely or spatulated depending on its caliber (Figs. 50.23 and 50.24).

Step 4. The back wall of the anastomosis is performed using running or interrupted stitches. An absorbable monofilament suture such as Monocryl is our preference. For small children a 6-0 size would be employed while for school age and older, a 5-0 is used. We have not used a holding stitch, but this can facilitate suturing (Fig. 50.25).

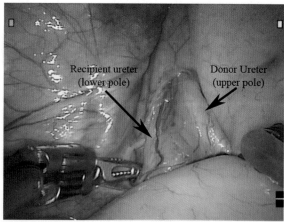

Fig. 50.23 Exposure of duplex ureters at the level of the iliac vessels in a child with incontinence from bilateral upper pole ectopic ureters in preparation for bilateral distal uretero-ureterostomies

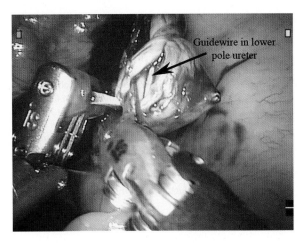

Fig. 50.24 Ureterotomy in the recipient, lower pole ureter showing the guidewire in place

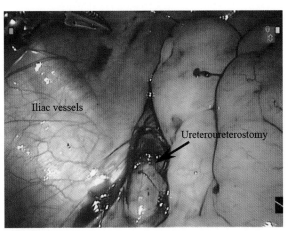

Fig. 50.26 Completion of the distal U–U

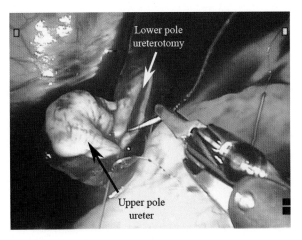

Fig. 50.25 Beginning of the anastomosis at the superior vertex of the recipient ureterostomy

Step 5. The double J catheter with side holes is advanced across the anastomosis. This can be facilitated by having the guide wire and pre-loaded stent accessible to the sterile field. The wire in the recipient ureter is backed out until the tip can be positioned into the donor ureter and advanced with the stent up to the pelvis.

Step 6. The anastomosis is completed. An intra-abdominal drain may be placed, but this is not routine as a ureteral stent is in place. A bladder catheter is left in place overnight and removed the next day at discharge (Fig. 50.26).

50.6 Special Considerations

We have performed unilateral extravesical ureteral reimplantations opposite to a nephrectomy using modified port placement and two positionings of the robot, one for kidney work to perform the nephrectomy and then in the bladder position for the reimplantation.[2] The change can be made efficiently if the team understands the strategy.

50.7 Steps to Avoid Complications

Complications associated with ureteral reimplantation surgery in specific are few.[3] Clearly an adequate tunnel length and ureteral mobility are important to ensure a successful result, although no clear parameters for length of the tunnel are defined. We have typically used the tip of the needle driver, which is about 1 cm in length as a marker and aim for 2.5–3 cm of length. This must factor in the degree of stretch the bladder wall is subject to. The ureter must be mobilized at least 5 cm. Avoiding excessive mobilization to prevent ischemia is important as well.

Urinary retention post-operatively after bilateral extravesical ureteral reimplantation is described and can occur in laparoscopic cases as well. This is likely, but not proven to be due to injury to posterolateral bladder nerves. These are microscopic and form a sheet-like plexus rather than being discrete nerves. Some will certainly be damaged in any peri-ureteral dissection, but this can be minimized by limiting the dissection too close to the ureter and the tunnel and avoiding excessive cautery during the dissection.[4]

Bladder leak after intravesical ureteral reimplantation has been experienced and is likely due to inadequate bladder port site closure. Secure, figure-of-eight sutures are needed to prevent leakage as the catheter will be removed in only 1 or 2 days. If leakage occurs, replacing the catheter is an effective treatment.

References

1. Peters CA, Woo R. Intravesical robotically assisted bilateral ureteral reimplantation. *J Endourol*. 2005;19:618–621.
2. Lee RS, Sethi AS, Passerotti CC, et al. Robot-assisted laparoscopic nephrectomy and contralateral ureteral reimplantation in children. *J Endourol*. 2010;24:123–128.
3. Passerotti CC, Nguyen HT, Retik AB, et al. Patterns and predictors of laparoscopic complications in pediatric urology: the role of ongoing surgical volume and access techniques. *J Urol*. 2008;180:681–685.
4. Casale P, Patel RP, Kolon TF. Nerve sparing robotic extravesical ureteral reimplantation. *J Urol*. 2008;179:1987–1989.

Chapter 51

Robotic Surgery of the Kidney in Children

Sanjeev A. Kaul and Jack S. Elder

51.1 Introduction

Minimally invasive surgery in pediatric urology has undergone a paradigm shift with the incorporation of the da Vinci surgical system. Following the popularity of robotic radical prostatectomy, several pediatric urological surgeries have been performed successfully with the da Vinci robot, including pyeloplasty, nephrectomy, partial nephrectomy, ureteral reimplantation, and appendicovesicostomy. Most are in various stages of refinement (partial nephrectomy, transureteroureterostomy, augmentation cystoplasty) but some are well established (nephrectomy, pyeloplasty, ureteral reimplantation). Robotics decreases the learning curve for pediatric reconstructive procedures. With a combination of three-dimensional vision, intuitive movements, visual immersion, and magnification robotic assistance can enable an experienced laparoscopist to expand his armamentarium to complex reconstructive procedures and a novice to explore the realm of minimally invasive pediatric urology.

This chapter explores the current status of robotic surgery of the kidney in children. A detailed step-by-step description of technique is provided, including operative setup and positioning, instrumentation and pearls, for preventing complications. The relevant contemporary literature is also reviewed. The transperitoneal approach will be described. These operative procedures can also be performed with a retroperitoneal approach, but the space is limited, particularly in small children. In contrast, the working space and visualization with the transperitoneal approach are much greater and easier to develop.

For purposes of organization, the procedures discussed are grouped into two categories: extirpative – nephrectomy, heminephrectomy, and nephroureterectomy and reconstructive – pyeloplasty, transposition of vessels for ureteropelvic junction obstruction, ureterocalicostomy, and pyelolithotomy.

Children pose an interesting dilemma regarding robotic instrumentation. An advantage of minimally invasive surgery is that small instruments are used. Although 5 and 8 mm instruments are available, the 5 mm instruments need a much wider range for movement. Consequently, in small infants, 8 mm instruments generally are necessary, whereas in older children 5 mm instruments usually are sufficient.

51.2 Extirpative Surgery

51.2.1 Nephrectomy, Heminephrectomy, and Nephroureterectomy

51.2.1.1 Indications

As congenital anomalies of the urinary tract are commonly diagnosed antenatally or in early childhood, the need for removal of the kidney or part of the kidney with/without the ureter is most common in infants and young children. Common indications for nephrectomy include renal non-function resulting

J.S. Elder (✉)
Vattikuti Urology Institute, Henry Ford Hospital, Children's
Hospital of Michigan, Detroit, MI, USA
e-mail: jelder1@hfhs.org

A.K. Hemal, M. Menon (eds.), *Robotics in Genitourinary Surgery*,
DOI 10.1007/978-1-84882-114-9_51, © Springer-Verlag London Limited 2011

from severe ureteropelvic junction (UPJ) obstruction, obstructive megaureter, vesicoureteral reflux, and multicystic dysplastic kidney (MCDK). Removal of the entire ureter is necessary for refluxing or obstructive/refluxing megaureter or posterior urethral valves (PUV) with the VURD ("valves, ureteral reflux, renal dysplasia") syndrome and a non-functioning kidney to prevent recurrent infections in the remnant ureteral stump. Less commonly nephrectomy may also be necessary for Wilms tumor, although robotic-assisted laparoscopic nephrectomy for Wilms tumor has not been reported. While laparoscopic nephrectomy generally is straightforward in children, robotic-assisted laparoscopic nephrectomy allows individuals developing a robotic pediatric program to develop their robotic skills and achieve a comfort level, as well as familiarize the robotic team with the unique aspects of robotic surgery in children. In our experience, however, in situations with previous renal surgery, robotics allows the identification and development of tissue planes around much more accurately than with conventional laparoscopic surgery.

Heminephrectomy is most commonly performed for a non-functioning hydronephrotic upper or lower pole moiety of a duplicated system or localized multicystic nephroma. Children with an abnormal duplicated upper urinary tract are ideal candidates for robotic-assisted laparoscopic surgery. The primary conditions include ectopic ureter, ectopic/orthotopic ureterocele, and vesicoureteral reflux. In girls, an ectopic ureter drains into the bladder neck, urethrovaginal septum, or vagina (approximately one-third each). If the ureter drains into the bladder neck, typically the affected ureter is obstructed at rest but refluxes during voiding. If the ureter drains into the distal urethra or vagina, it does not reflux. Most of these ectopic ureters are obstructive and associated with upper pole hydroureteronephrosis. In boys the ectopic ureter typically drains into the prostate, bladder neck, or seminal vesicle. If there is complete upper tract duplication, at times there is vesicoureteral reflux into the lower pole ureter and the upper ureter drains normally. Management generally is based on the function of the affected moiety; if there is non-function, then the moiety is removed, whereas if there is satisfactory function to that portion of the kidney, a ureteroureterostomy may be performed, anastomosing the upper pole ureter to the nonobstructed lower pole ureter, in the case of an ectopic ureter.

51.2.1.2 Operative Setup

The operative room setup is similar for the three procedures with minor modifications (Fig. 51.1). The surgical assistant helps the surgeon with organ retraction, changing instruments, and introducing and cutting sutures. Individual video monitors for the assistant and nurse facilitate smooth progress of the surgery, as everyone involved can monitor the procedure. The lowest electrocautery settings that provide adequate cutting/coagulation should be used. Higher settings may cause the current to dissipate and cause damage to adjacent tissues. The robot is docked from the patient's shoulder along a line from the kidney to the umbilicus.

a. Patient Positioning
   Small children present challenges to positioning and require individual customization and sometimes use novel techniques to provide optimum position. The patient is placed at 60–90° lateral tilt using a foam wedge or folded blanket to provide posterior support. A rolled-up blanket is placed below the flank to simulate the effect of the kidney bridge to "prop up" the kidney. A Foley catheter is left in place during the procedure. *It is important to bring the patient to the very edge of the table to facilitate movements of the robotic arms and the assistant's instruments.* The child's hips and shoulders need to be secured carefully to the table.

b. Trocar Configuration
   Trocar placement is critical and needs to be individualized to the size of the patient. Neonates and infants have limited surface area externally for port placement. Since it is mandatory to keep a fixed amount of the cannula within the abdomen, the limited space causes two bothersome situations:(1) the camera and instruments may be too close to the target organ to permit efficient movement and (2) the cannulae may fall out of the abdomen causing loss of pneumoperitoneum and interruption of the operation. On the other hand, little patients need relatively smaller excursion of the robotic arms to reach from the upper pole to the lower pole of the kidney and the distance to the bladder is shorter than in older children and these considerations provide some compensation for the challenging port placement. *A prudent principle is to keep the skin incisions for ports as far away from the operative site as possible to give the maximum permissible*

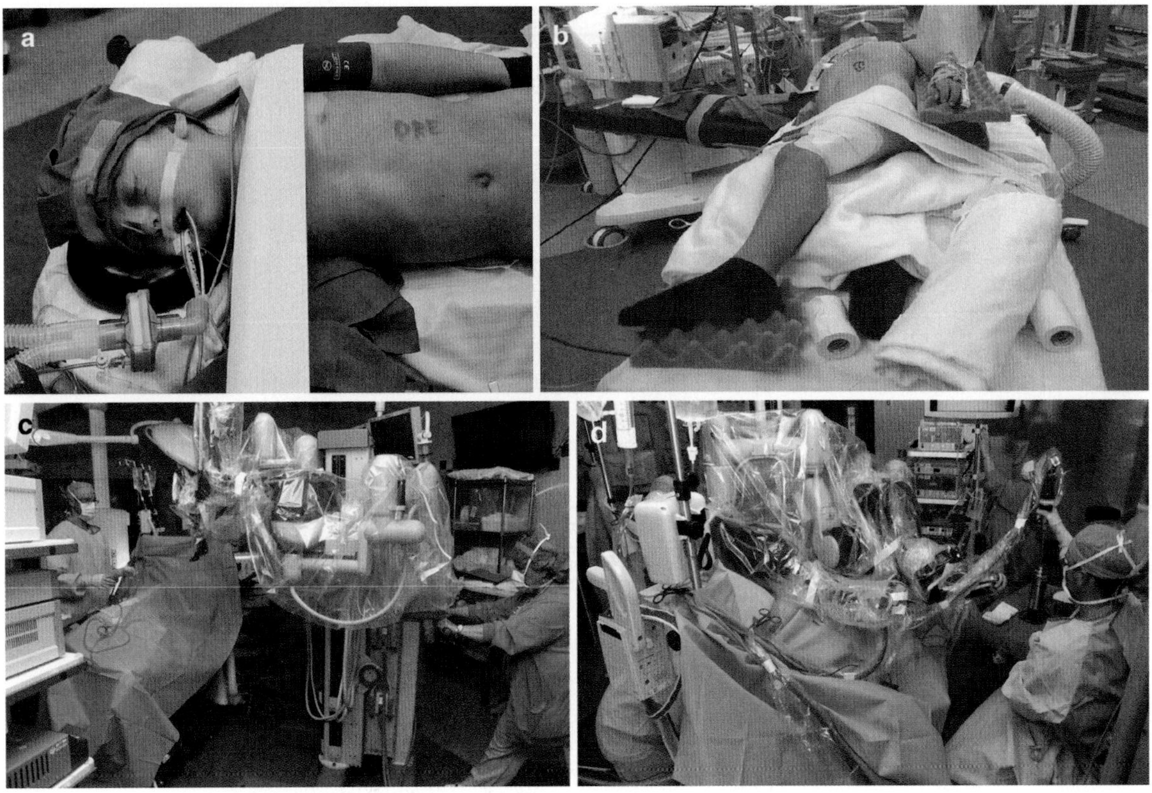

Fig. 51.1 Positioning for child undergoing robotic renal procedure. **a** Positioning for left renal procedure. Note left arm secured parallel to spine; **b** Different patient. Child should be in 15–45° lateral decubitus. Note left arm resting on gel pad. **c** da Vinci robot rolled in behind patient. **d** Assistant positioned in front of patient between anesthesia equipment (at *head of table*) and robotic equipment (at *foot of table*)

working space within the body. This issue is less critical in older children and adolescents.

Generally a four-port template is used (Fig. 51.2); one 12- or 8.5 mm camera port at the umbilicus, two 8 mm (or 5 mm in neonates and infants) robotic working ports, and one 5 mm assistant port (for clip application, suction/irrigation, introducing/removing and cutting sutures, and retraction). However, if limited bowel or liver retraction is necessary and there is limited bleeding, the assistant port can be avoided.

Pneumoperitoneum is created using either the Veress needle or the Hassan technique. The initial pressure is raised to 20 mmHg for port placement (the higher pressure provides rigidity to the abdominal wall and facilitates entry of the cannula with minimal indentation of the abdominal wall). Once the ports are placed, the pressure is decreased to 12 mmHg. The camera port is placed along the lateral aspect of the umbilical fold. In children, given the limited space within the abdomen, it is prudent to place the index finger along the port as a guard to prevent sudden entry and inadvertent damage to intra-abdominal organs. After surveying the abdomen the two robotic working ports are placed such that the three ports are triangulated to the working area. For a nephrectomy or heminephrectomy the ports are centered on the hilum and triangulated to the kidney. Therefore the upper port is placed in the ipsilateral upper quadrant close to the midline and midway between the umbilicus and xiphoid while the lower port is placed in the lower quadrant 2–3 in. medial and superior to the anterior superior iliac spine. For a nephroureterectomy ports are centered on the flank and the lower port is moved more medially and inferiorly to permit access to the pelvis. The assistant port is placed in the midline infraumbilically at a suitable distance

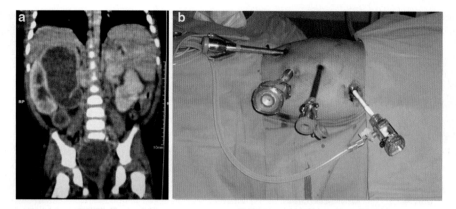

Fig. 51.2 A 16-month-old girl with duplicated right collecting system and hydroureteronephrosis of upper pole system secondary to ectopic ureter. **a** CT urogram. **b** Port positioning for right upper pole heminephroureterectomy

Table 51.1 Instrumentation for robotic extirpative renal surgery

Surgeon instrumentation		Assistant instrumentation
Right arm (yellow)	Left arm (green)	
• Monopolar hook • Needle driver • Scissors	• Maryland bipolar grasper • Needle driver	• Suction-irrigator • Atraumatic grasping forceps • Laparoscopic needle driver • Laparoscopic scissors

from the umbilicus to permit easy access for the assistant.

c. Instrumentation List (Table 51.1)

51.2.1.3 Step-by-Step Technique (Nephrectomy)

a. Exposure

The steps of nephrectomy are similar to those described for adults with some important differences. A zero degree lens is used for the procedure. The intra-abdominal and perinephric fat are minimal in children and the kidneys are readily visible through the colon. An incision is made along the line of Toldt using the hook and carried inferiorly to the pelvic brim, ensuring the colon is completely reflected medially. On the left it may be necessary to incise the lienorenal ligament and reflect the spleen superiorly, especially while dissecting the superior pole of the kidney. On the right, retraction of the liver may be required in children; a 5 mm port may be placed just below the xiphoid for this purpose. Attention should be directed to the duodenum on the right as it may overlap the renal artery and vein. The lateral aspect of the kidney should not be mobilized at this point, as the fascia holds the kidney against the posterior abdominal wall.

b. Identification of ureter

The ureter is readily visible on the iliopsoas after the colon is reflected. It may be identified by noting ureteral peristalsis. Rarely an extremely large megaureter may cause some confusion with bowel and the inferior vena cava on the right. If identification is difficult, it may be necessary to look for it at the pelvic brim overlying the iliac vessels and trace it back upward. The gonadal vessels are not as well developed in children as in adults, but may be a source of confusion with the ureter.

c. Hilar dissection and control

The renal vessels are apparent just below the spleen on the left and below the liver on the right. They may also be identified by tracing the ureter up to the hilum. The renal vein is usually apparent first and the artery is situated superiorly to the vein and may be hidden behind the vein. The renal artery is extremely delicate in children and vigorous manipulation (especially during partial nephrectomy) may cause vasospasm of the artery. In infants and small children, both the artery and the vein may be secured with 5 mm metallic clips or hem-o-lok clips. In older children it may be necessary to use the endoGIA stapler for the vein. Alternatively, the vessels may be tied off with sutures.

d. Mobilization of the kidney

Once the renal artery and vein are clipped, the kidney is avascular and can be dissected off the posterior abdominal wall and inferiorly using the hook. The last step is dissection of the superior pole. At this point, care should be taken to identify and protect the adrenal gland. Proceeding with the dissection on the capsule of the kidney is the safest option to protect the adrenal gland. Finally, the ureter is clipped doubly and cut to deliver the specimen. The operative site should be inspected to confirm adequate hemostasis.

e. Removal of specimen and closure of ports/skin

The specimen is removed through the 12 mm camera port. The 12 mm endocatch bag may be used in older children; however, it is usually too large for infants. Alternatively, a 5 mm laparoscope is introduced through the robotic port or assistant port and the ureter is held with a grasper introduced through the 8 mm cannula. The endocatch bag is inserted through the 12 mm cannula, placed around the specimen, and then removed. If required, the incision in the fascia is extended under vision. The 12 mm incision is closed with a 2-0 or 3-0 polyglycolic acid (PGA) suture. The 5 and 8 mm fascial incisions are closed with 4-0 PGA. Half inch steristrips are used to maintain skin closure.

f. Post-operative care

The patient is admitted for overnight observation with intravenous hydration. Intravenous ketoralac 0.5 mg/kg is administered as the operative procedure is finishing, and 0.25 mg/kg is given intravenously every 6 h, with a maximum of seven post-op doses. A regular diet is resumed as tolerated. Patients are usually discharged on post-operative day 1.

Other measures may reduce the need for post-operative analgesia. The port sites may be infiltrated with 0.25% bupivacaine before port insertion or during wound closure. In addition, a small retrospective study of children undergoing pyeloplasty suggested that intraperitoneal aerosolized bupivacaine reduces the need for post-operative narcotic analgesia.[1]

51.2.1.4 Step-by-Step Technique (Partial Nephrectomy)

During heminephrectomy with a duplicated kidney, there are five important clinical considerations:

(1) With an ectopic ureter or ureterocele, there is usually hydroureteronephrosis, and the ureter is generally easy to identify. However, it is extremely important to maintain the integrity of the normal lower pole ureter, which is adherent to the upper pole ureter. Cystoscopy is recommended at the beginning of the procedure to verify the lower urinary tract anatomy. In addition, a 3 or 4 Fr ureteral catheter may be inserted into the lower pole ureter to facilitate its identification.

(2) The hydronephrotic upper pole always has a distinct artery and vein, which may arise from the aorta or the renal artery. Although they may seem atretic, almost always they need to be ligated. When these vessels are clipped, the tissue demarcation between the upper and lower poles becomes obvious. On the other hand, if a refluxing lower pole is going to be removed, there is often not a distinct artery and vein.

(3) With an ectopic ureter or ureterocele and upper pole hydronephrosis, the upper pole ureter always passes posterior to the renal artery and vein, and these vessels will need to be mobilized to allow the dilated ureter to be passed behind them.

(4) With an ectopic ureter or ureterocele and upper pole hydronephrosis, the extent of involvement is quite variable. In some cases there is a large hydronephrotic moiety with overlying dysplastic parenchyma, whereas in other cases there is simply a dilated upper pole ureter with little overlying parenchyma. The pre-operative imaging studies should be reviewed at the beginning of the operative procedure to help plan the procedure.

(5) If the ureter is refluxing, then the vast majority, if not all, of the ureter should be removed during the partial nephrectomy, and it should be ligated, either with clips or with a suture ligature, or both. On the other hand, if it is non-refluxing, the ureter can be divided just below the pelvic brim and it does not need to be tied off. A caution, however, is the ectopic ureter draining into the bladder neck – these nearly always reflux during voiding – and, consequently, these ureters should be removed in their entirety and tied off.

Port placement and kidney exposure are as described for nephrectomy. The upper pole ureter is medially located at the hilum and passes posteriorly and laterally to the lower pole ureter at the lower pole of the kidney. The vascularity of the normal ureter should be protected. The dilated ureter is dissected proximally to the main renal pedicle. The pedicle is then gently separated from the underlying ureter; the hook is gentle and helps develop this plane. The kidney should be inspected periodically to be certain that it is remaining vascularized. The space superior to the pedicle then should be inspected. If there is sufficient room, then the dilated ureter should be transected at the level of the lower pole of the kidney and the ureter should be pushed behind the main renal vessels. The surgeon should then grasp the ureter above the renal pedicle. Traction on the ureter helps identify the upper pole artery and vein; until these vessels are transected, the upper pole of the kidney remains relatively fixed. The upper pole vessels are then mobilized and secured with 5 mm metallic clips or suture ligated and divided. The renal parenchyma is incised with electrocautery along the line of demarcation and any bleeding is controlled with electrocautery or suture ligature. The parenchyma generally is very thin and minimal bleeding is the norm. Once the affected pole is removed, the capsule generally is approximated over the raw area with mattress sutures of 3-0 PGA and an inlay of fatty tissue can be used. It is not necessary to drain the operative area.

Removal of the specimen and wound closure is as described for nephrectomy.

51.2.1.5 Step-by-Step Technique (Nephroureterectomy)

The operation proceeds as described in nephrectomy until the kidney is completely mobilized. The ureter is then dissected inferiorly to the pelvic brim. At the pelvic brim there are two structures that are encountered. First, the gonadal vessels cross the ureter from medial to lateral and should be protected. Second, care should be exercised as the iliac vessels are in close proximity to the ureter laterally. Within the pelvis the vas deferens is seen coursing across the ureter from a lateral to medial direction and should be carefully preserved. Dissection is continued until the junction of the ureter and bladder is identified. Superior traction is exerted on the ureter and a transfixation suture is placed at the ureterovesical junction. The ureter is then divided at the ureterovesical junction. At this point the entire kidney and ureter is delivered superiorly and the entire specimen is ready to be extracted.

Extraction of the specimen and closure of the abdomen are as described for nephrectomy.

51.2.1.6 Results of Heminephrectomy

Lee et al. described nine children who underwent robotic-assisted laparoscopic partial nephrectomy.[2] Mean patient age was 7.2 years. Mean operative time was 275 min. Mean hospitalization was 2.9 days. The authors did not compare their results to an open cohort.

51.2.1.7 Steps to Avoid Complications

In children there is less operative room and having expert assistance and pediatric anesthesia is critical, particularly in infants.

If the port placement seems suboptimal, then the port should be removed and placed in a different site.

Attention should be directed to the location of the bowel, because the tip of the camera is hot and the bowel can be injured easily.

On the right side, an enlarged ureter may be confused as small bowel or the inferior vena cava.

During occlusion of the renal artery or the polar vessels, 5 mm clips may be applied. Two clips should be placed through an assistant port proximally and distally and then the vessel may be transected. Alternatively, the main renal artery or vein may be tied off with a suture ligature or a circular tie. In general, pediatric vessels should not be transected with a stapled device.

During a heminephrectomy, the main renal artery may undergo vasospasm during ureteral dissection. Application of topical paparverine along the renal artery through a small spinal needle often causes the vasospasm to subside.

51.3 Reconstructive Surgery

51.3.1 Pyeloplasty

Pyeloplasty is an ideal procedure to perform with robotic assistance because the advantages of the robot are most apparent; the magnification helps in visualization of the ureteropelvic junction and upper ureter, the endowristed movements permit accurate suturing of the ureter to the pelvis, and the three-dimensional vision and intuitive movements significantly decrease the degree of difficulty and hence the learning curve for this procedure. As a result, robotic pyeloplasty has become the most commonly performed robotic urologic procedure in the pediatric population.

51.3.1.1 Indications

The indications for robotic-assisted pyeloplasty are similar to those for open pyeloplasty. These include grade 4 (severe) hydronephrosis with reduced function or poor drainage on diuretic renography, worsening hydronephrosis, deterioration of renal function, upper urinary tract infection, and recurrent flank or abdominal pain. Infants generally need to be at least 3 months old to accommodate the robotic instrumentation.

51.3.1.2 Operative Setup

The setup of the room is similar to that described for robotic nephrectomy.

a. Patient Positioning and Trocar Configuration
Principles of patient positioning remain the same as described for robotic nephrectomy. The patient is placed at 60° lateral tilt using a foam wedge or folded blanket to provide posterior support. A rolled up blanket is placed below the flank to simulate the effect of the kidney bridge to "prop up" the kidney. A Foley catheter is inserted at the beginning of the procedure, the bladder is drained, and then the tubing is clamped to distend the bladder for antegrade stent placement during the operative procedure. Cystoscopy and retrograde pyelography rarely are necessary. In addition, insertion of a double-J stent at the beginning of the case is not advised, as it may distort the anatomy of the ureteropelvic junction and make it difficult to identify the exact location and extent of the obstructed segment.

Since the operative steps for robotic pyeloplasty are mostly directed around the renal hilum, trocar placement should be centered to this location. A three-port template is ideal (Fig. 51.2); a 12 or 8.5 mm camera port at the umbilicus and two 5 mm (or 8 mm in neonates and infants) robotic working ports. Assistant ports usually are unnecessary. The handing and removal of sutures can be accomplished through the robotic working cannula. Pneumoperitoneum is achieved as described above. The ports are centered on the renal hilum and triangulated to the kidney. Therefore, the upper port is placed in the ipsilateral upper quadrant close to the midline and midway between the umbilicus and xiphoid, while the lower port is placed in the lower quadrant 2–3 in. medial and superior to the anterior superior iliac spine. An attempt is made to maintain at least 6 cm distance between the ports. However, this may not always be feasible, especially in infants. This arrangement provides an ideal working environment for both infants and older children. If the renal pelvis is extremely large, ports must be placed further away from the target area to permit smooth movement of the robotic arms.

b. Instrumentation List (Table 51.2)

51.3.1.3 Step-by-Step Technique

c. Exposure
Access to the kidney for pyeloplasty is achieved through a transperitoneal technique. Although a retroperitoneal access for laparoscopic pyeloplasty is described in children, the authors used 5 mm camera and 3 mm instruments. Given the bulkiness of the robot and the limitation of larger camera port (12 mm), this approach is not feasible in children with robotic assistance. The ureteropelvic junction may be approached in one of the two ways. *On the left side, the renal pelvis may be approached through the mesocolon.* Division of mesocolic vessels should be avoided. Advantages include obviating the need for colonic dissection and possibility of

Table 51.2 Instrumentation for robotic pyeloplasty

Surgeon instrumentation		
Right arm (yellow)	Left arm (green)	Assistant instrumentation
• Monopolar hook	• Maryland bipolar grasper	• Laparoscopic needle driver
• Needle driver	• Needle driver	• Laparoscopic scissors
• Scissors		

bowel injury; however, the disadvantage may be an inadequate exposure for sufficient ureteral dissection to provide a tension-free anastomosis. *On the right side and in older patients with more mesenteric fat it is usually necessary to mobilize the colon by incising along the line of Toldt.*

d. Identification of renal pelvis and ureter
The dilated renal pelvis is readily visible, although it may be decompressed if a ureteral stent has been placed pre-operatively. The renal pelvis is dissected and isolated and is carried down to identify the UPJ and the ureter. Attention is directed to the presence/absence of a crossing vessel and these should be carefully preserved. It is often helpful to place a "hitch stitch" percutaneously through the flank using 4-0 PGA on an RB-1 needle. The needle is straightened to simulate a Keith needle, passed through the flank, grasped by the surgeon, passed through the upper renal pelvis, and then back through the flank, where it is grasped by the assistant. The hitch stitch allows counter-traction for the surgical mobilization of the UPJ and the pyeloplasty. The ureter should be dissected for 2–3 cm to provide for a tension-free anastomosis. It is preferred to hold the periureteral tissues and not the ureter directly while this dissection proceeds to avoid devascularization of the ureter. After the renal pelvis and ureter are well mobilized one may proceed to the reconstruction.

e. Excision of redundant pelvis and pelviureteral anastomosis
Several techniques for pyeloplasty are described and the choice in an individual patient depends on the presence of crossing vessels, configuration, and size of the renal pelvis. Anderson–Hynes dismembered pyeloplasty is preferred because it permits excision of the redundant renal pelvis, excision of abnormal the UPJ segment, and transposition of crossing vessels. The lateral wall of the renal pelvis (which is oriented anteriorly) is divided first at the superior margin and carried downward to the lower border. This maneuver exposes the interior of the pelvis and the lateral wall (which is posteriorly oriented); this can then be divided, leaving the excess renal pelvis attached to the ureter. Leaving the pelvis attached to the ureter has two advantages: it helps to maintain the orientation of the ureter, preventing twisting and spiraling of the ureter and it provides a handle to hold the tissues while placing

the first anchoring stitch at the apex of the ureter. If there is significant redundancy to the renal pelvis, trimming is recommended, because leaving a large renal pelvis may cause the reconstructed UPJ to kink post-operatively. The ureter is then spatulated until normal ureteral mucosa is identified (usually 2–3 cm).

f. Pelviureteral anastomosis and stent placement
The anastomosis should be performed with a monofilament suture. The anchoring stitch is placed first; a 5-0 or 6-0 PDS on an RB-1 needle is used to approximate the apex of the spatulated ureter to the most dependent part of the dismembered pelvis. The needle travels from outside in on the pelvis and then from inside out on the ureter thereby placing the knot on the outside. *Care must be exercised at this step to ensure that the ureteral mucosa has been included in the stitch and that the back wall of the ureter has not been inadvertently included.* At this point the redundant renal pelvis and abnormal segment of ureteropelvic junction and ureter are excised. The medial wall of the renal pelvis is first approximated to the medial wall of the ureter and the suture tied to itself.

The ureteral stent is placed in an antegrade fashion prior to approximation of the lateral wall. An 18 Fr Angiocath is introduced through the abdominal wall in the region of the upper quadrant and a 0.028"/0.035" guide wire is threaded through the angiocath into the peritoneal cavity. The surgeon threads the guide wire through the anastomosis into the bladder and an appropriate stent is threaded over the guide wire. The appropriate stent length in centimeters generally is 10+ age in years (i.e., in a 4 years old, the stent should be 14 cm). The guide wire should be marked at this level, so that the surgeon can determine when the appropriate length of wire has been inserted. Next, the stent is passed over the guide wire, with the aid of the pusher. The Foley catheter in the bladder should have been clamped at the beginning of the case, and the surgeon should visualize urine coming back into the operative field. Injection of methylene blue into the bladder makes it obvious that urine is coming back, implying that the tip of the stent is in the bladder. Recently intraoperative sonography has been described to image the stent within the bladder.[3] Another 5-0 PDS suture is then used to approximate the lateral wall of the ipsilateral pelvis to the lateral wall of the ureter. Any remaining renal pelvis is then sutured together. Drains are not recommended routinely, because of the stent and the fact that the pyeloplasty is transperitoneal.

g. Closure of ports

The excised segment of renal pelvis and UPJ are removed and may be sent for histopathological examination and the cannulae removed. The fascia of the 12 mm port incision is closed with 3-0 PGA figure-of-eight stitch, the fascia for the operative ports is closed with 4-0 PGA, and the skin is approximated with Steristrips.

h. Post-operative care

This is similar to that described for nephrectomy. The ureteral stent is removed 4–6 weeks later.

51.3.1.4 Results

Robotic-assisted pyeloplasty has a favorable success rate compared with open pyeloplasty.[4] In a retrospective series of 33 children undergoing robotic-assisted pyeloplasty compared with open pyeloplasty, with a mean age of 7.8 years, operative time was 38 min less for open pyeloplasty, but analgesic requirements and length of stay were less in the robotic group, and success rate was similar in both groups. Kutikov et al. reported a series of nine infants, ages 3–9 months, who underwent a pyeloplasty.[5] Mean operative time was 123 min, with a mean console time of 73 min. Of the nine, seven demonstrated improvement in hydronephrosis. The long-term results of the remaining two infants were unclear at the time of the report. Franco et al. compared a robotic-assisted pyeloplasty to a laparoscopic anastomosis and found no significant differences in operative time or outcomes in 29 patients.[6]

51.3.2 Transposition of Lower Pole Crossing Vessel ("Vascular Hitch")

One of the most controversial procedures involving the upper urinary tract involves UPJ obstruction with a crossing vessel. There is evidence that in selected pediatric (as well as adult) patients with a UPJ obstruction and a crossing vessel, mobilizing the UPJ and separating it from the vessel, and then hitching the vessel

to the renal pelvis, is often curative. The pathology is that the UPJ is draped over the lower pole vessel; at rest, there is normal urine transport through the UPJ, but during diuresis, the renal pelvis may become overdistended and become kinked over the vessel, creating virtually complete upper urinary tract obstruction. Traditional teaching is that these patients have both the crossing vessel and the ureteropelvic narrowing. However, in a recent series of children who underwent the vascular hitch procedure and not a concurrent pyeloplasty, there was a 95% success rate.[7]

51.3.2.1 Indications

Typical patients include those with intermittent severe flank or abdominal pain. Typically these children have severe hydronephrosis during a symptomatic attack, but when asymptomatic have mild to moderate hydronephrosis with thick renal parenchyma. A diuretic renogram usually demonstrates good renal function in the involved kidney, but there may be satisfactory drainage following the administration of furosemide, although it is slower than the normal kidney. Infants or patients with antenatally diagnosed hydronephrosis rarely have this finding. Intraoperatively, if the UPJ appears widely patent and the pelvis is nondistended, then the vascular hitch procedure is appropriate. Consequently, operative setup, patient positioning, instrumentation, and operative approach to the UPJ are identical to that described for pyeloplasty. Pre-operatively it is impossible to determine whether a vascular hitch procedure will be appropriate.

51.3.2.2 Step-by-Step Technique

The UPJ is typically extrarenal and a crossing vessel is identified going to the lower pole of the kidney; the vessel crosses anterior to the UPJ. Using the hook, the renal pelvis is separated from the crossing vessel. The upper 2 cm of ureter is mobilized. A hitch stitch through the superior aspect of the renal pelvis as described for pyeloplasty may be helpful. If the renal pelvis is decompressed and appears widely patent with magnification, then a vascular hitch procedure may be considered.

The lower pole vessels are mobilized carefully; vasospasm may cause devascularization of the lower pole. The renal pelvis is mobilized and the UPJ is moved away from the vessels. The vessels are then fixed to the midportion of the renal pelvis. Two techniques are appropriate. Three or four 4-0 interrupted PGA sutures can be placed between the adventitia of the vascular complex and the seromuscular layer of the renal pelvis. Alternatively, the midportion of the renal pelvis may be wrapped around the vessels with three or four 4-0 PGA sutures. No ureteral stent is necessary.

a. Closure of ports
   Port closure is identical to that described for nephrectomy.
b. Post-operative care
   Post-operative care is identical to that described for nephrectomy.

51.3.2.3 Results

In a series of 20 patients, Gundeti et al.[7] described their results with robotic-assisted laparoscopic vascular hitch in 20 patients: 7- to 16-years old (mean 12.5 years), mean operative time was 90 min, and median hospital stay was 1 day. At a mean follow-up of 22 months, 19 of 20 patients were successfully treated. The single failure had recurrent flank pain and was cured by laparoscopic pyeloplasty.

51.3.3 *Ureterocalicostomy*

Ureterocalicostomy involves excision of the hydronephrotic lower renal pole parenchyma and anastomosis of the dismembered ureter directly to the lower pole calyx, providing urinary drainage. The procedure traditionally has been performed via open surgery through a flank incision or transabdominally, necessitating an extended hospital stay and convalescence. Today, with the availability of robotic assistance minimally invasive alternatives have gained popularity, with experienced centers offering these approaches preferentially as first-line therapy in appropriate patients.

51.3.3.1 Indications

Ureterocalicostomy is an attractive option for patients with UPJ obstruction *and* significant lower pole caliectasis. It is reserved for patients who have failed pyeloplasty, who have minimal pelvis, or those with a predominantly intrarenal pelvis. It is also an attractive option for patients with a long upper ureteral stricture that precludes tension-free anastomosis to the renal pelvis.

51.3.3.2 Operative Setup

The setup of the room is similar to that described for robotic pyeloplasty. Cystoscopy and placement of a ureteral stent may be helpful in patients with previous failed pyeloplasty.

a. Patient Positioning and Trocar Configuration
   Principles of patient positioning and trocar configuration remain the same as described for robotic pyeloplasty.
b. Instrumentation List (Table 51.3)

51.3.3.3 Step-by-Step Technique

a. Exposure
   A transperitoneal approach is used and the renal pelvis and ureter are approached by mobilizing the colon. In children with a failed pyeloplasty, there may be intraperitoneal adhesions and a Hassan technique may be preferred to avoid injury to bowel

Table 51.3 Instrumentation for robotic ureterocalicostomy

Surgeon instrumentation		Assistant instrumentation
Right arm (yellow)	Left arm (green)	
• Monopolar hook	• Maryland bipolar grasper	• Suction irrigator
• Needle driver	• Needle driver	• Atraumatic grasping forceps
• Monopolar scissors		• Laparoscopic needle driver
		• Laparoscopic scissors

during establishment of pneumoperitoneum. Also, in those undergoing re-operation the renal anatomy and orientation may be altered and this should be considered when the kidney, UPJ, and ureter are mobilized.

b. Identification of renal pelvis, ureter, and lower pole
The hydronephrotic kidney is readily visible on entry. The renal pelvis is isolated and dissected and the dissection is carried down to identify the fibrotic UPJ and the upper ureter. A long segment of normal ureter should be mobilized to facilitate a completely tension-free anastomosis. If there is significant fibrosis from prior surgery, it may be necessary to identify the virgin segment of ureter at a lower level and trace the same back to the UPJ and pelvis. The lower pole of the kidney is also mobilized circumferentially.

c. Transection of the ureter and lower pole segment
The ureter is tied and transected below the region of fibrosis and the normal ureter is widely spatulated. A segment of the lower pole of the kidney is then excised with monopolar scissors or the hook to expose the dilated lower pole calyx. As for the ureter, a wide opening should be made in the lower pole calyx to provide for a wide anastomosis and prevent stricture formation. In the presence of significant hydronephrosis, the lower pole parenchyma is thin, bleeding is minimal, and bovie coagulation suffices for hemostasis. As described for pyeloplasty, a holding stitch may be placed on the anterior surface of the lower pole to provide retraction and separation of the mucosa during anastomosis.

d. Ureterocalyceal anastomosis and stent placement
5-0 PDS on a RB needle is used to approximate the apex of the spatulated ureter to the most dependent part of the dismembered lower pole calyx and the knot is placed on the outside as described for robotic pyeloplasty. *Care must be exercised at this step to ensure that the ureteral mucosa has been included in the stitch and that the back wall of the ureter has not been inadvertently included.* The anastomosis is then continued using interrupted stitches approximating the calyx to the lateral wall of the ureter. Once the lateral half of the anastomosis is completed, the ureteral stent is placed in an antegrade fashion as described in the section on robotic pyeloplasty. The remaining portion of the anastomosis is then completed using interrupted stitches. On completion of the anastomosis, a segment of omentum

may be used to reinforce the anastomosis. Drains are unnecessary.

e. Closure of ports and post-operative care
This is similar to that described for robotic pyeloplasty. The ureteral stent is removed 6 weeks later.

51.3.3.4 Results

Past results with open ureterocalicostomy were fair, approximately 67% success, significantly lower than with pyeloplasty. These results were due in large part to challenging case selection. Casale et al. reported on nine children, 3 to 15 years old (mean 6.5 years) who underwent robotic-assisted ureterocalicostomy.[8] Of the patients, six had undergone a previous pyeloplasty, while three had an exaggerated intrarenal collecting system not amenable to standard dismembered pyeloplasty. Two of the patients underwent concurrent pyelolithotomy. Mean operative time was 168 min for the ureterocalicostomy portion. Mean post-operative stay was 21 h. Diuretic renography was performed at 6 and 12 months and was satisfactory in all patients.

51.3.4 Robotic Pyelolithotomy

51.3.4.1 Indications

Although extracorporeal shock wave lithotripsy and ureteroscopic or percutaneous extraction remain the gold standard for treatment of renal calculi in children, there are situations in which robotic-assisted laparoscopic pyelolithotomy may be particularly efficacious. Potential indications include obstructive or symptomatic cystine stones, concomitant calculi, and UPJ obstruction, and large renal pelvic calculi deemed not suitable for PCNL, such as the infant kidney. Calyceal calculi can be retrieved using flexible ureteroscopy introduced through the 8 mm cannula and guided using the robotic instruments.

51.3.4.2 Operative Setup

This setup is identical to that for robotic pyeloplasty.

a. Patient positioning and port placement
Patient positioning and three-port template used are similar to that described for robotic pyeloplasty.

Table 51.4 Instrumentation for robotic pyelolithotomy

Surgeon instrumentation		Assistant instrumentation
Right arm (yellow)	Left arm (green)	
• Monopolar hook	• Maryland bipolar grasper	• Laparoscopic needle driver
• Needle driver	• Needle driver	• Laparoscopic scissors
• Monopolar scissors	• Atraumatic grasper	• Flexible ureteroscope

An additional 5 mm assistant port may be helpful to provide traction/retraction and suction/irrigation, especially in cases with a history of recurrent pyelonephritis. In addition, an assistant port is ideal for extraction of the calculus after the surgeon has removed it from the renal pelvis.

b. Instrumentation List (Table 51.4)

51.3.4.3 Step-by-Step Technique

a. Exposure

A transperitoneal approach is used as described for pyeloplasty, and the renal pelvis and ureter are approached by mobilizing the colon. On the left side, a transmesenteric approach can be considered.

b. Identification of renal pelvis, ureter, and lower pole

The ureter is identified overlying the psoas muscle and followed superiorly to the renal pelvis. Gerota's fascia is incised to identify the renal pelvis, which is located lateral to the artery and vein and requires careful dissection to separate the overlying fat. The fat may be adherent to the pelvis if there has been prior episodes of pyelonephritis, and some bleeding may be encountered while mobilizing the pelvis.

c. Pyelotomy and extraction of calculi

A traction suture with 4-0 PGA on the superior aspect of the renal pelvis should be considered. A U-shaped incision is made on the renal pelvis extending from the inferior to the superior calyx. The calculus is visualized in the renal pelvis and if necessary gentle probing with the Maryland forceps within the pelvis may be necessary to sound the stone and retrieve it. In patients with multiple calculi a 7.5 Fr flexible ureteroscope is introduced through the assistant port and guided with the help of atraumatic robotic graspers into the renal pelvis. The pelvis and calyces are visualized to confirm that all calculi have been removed and if necessary a stone basket may be utilized to remove small calculi within the calyces. In selected cases an intraoperative x-ray may be considered to confirm that the kidney is stone free. Alternatively, intraoperative

sonography may be performed with the hand-held ultrasound probe.

d. Closure of pyelotomy

Once complete clearance of calculi is confirmed, the pyelotomy is closed with interrupted sutures of 4-0 or 5-0 PGA on an RB-1 needle. It is not necessary to place a ureteral stent. Gerota's fascia is approximated over the renal pelvis to complete the procedure.

e. Closure of ports and post-operative care

This step is identical to that described for robotic pyeloplasty.

51.3.4.4 Results

There are few reports of robotic-assisted pyelolithotomy in children. Lee et al. described five adolescents, mean age 16.6 years, who underwent robotic pyelolithotomy.[9] Of the patients, four had a staghorn cystine stone and one had calcium oxalate calculi and concurrent UPJ obstruction. Mean operative time was 315 min and mean hospital stay was 3.8 days. The calculi were removed by a robotic grasper or by a flexible cystoscope introduced through a robotic port. One patient with a staghorn calculus underwent open conversion. Of the remaining four patients, three were rendered stone free.

References

1. Freilich DA, Houch CS, Meier PM, et al. The effectiveness of aerosolized intraperitoneal bupivacaine in reducing postoperative pain in children undergoing robotic-assisted laparoscopic pyeloplasty. *J Pediatr Urol*. 2008;4:337–340.
2. Lee RS, Sethi AS, Passerotti CC, et al. Robotic assisted laparoscopic partial nephrectomy: a viable and safe option in children. *J Urol*. 2009;181:823–828.
3. Ginger VA, Lendvay TS. Intraoperative ultrasound: application in pediatric pyeloplasty. *Urology*. 2009;73:377–379.

4. Lee RS, Retik AB, Borer JG, Peters CA. Pediatric robotic assisted laparoscopic dismembered pyeloplasty: comparison with a cohort of open surgery. *J Urol*. 2006;175:683–687.

5. Kutikov A, Nguyen M, Guzzo T, et al. Robot assisted pyeloplasty in the infant – lessons learned. *J Urol*. 2006;176:2237–2239.

6. Franco I, Dyer LL, Zelkovic P. Laparoscopic pyeloplasty in the pediatric patient: hand sewn anastomosis versus robotic assisted anastomosis – is there a difference? *J Urol*. 2007;178:1483–1486.

7. Gundeti MS, Reynolds WS, Duffy PG, Mushtaq I. Further experience with the vascular hitch (laparoscopic transposition of lower pole crossing vessels): an alternative treatment for pediatric ureterovascular ureteropelvic junction obstruction. *J Urol*. 2008;180:1832–1836.

8. Casale P, Mucksavage P, Resnick M, Kim SS. Robotic ureterocalicostomy in the pediatric population. *J Urol*. 2008;180:2643–2648.

9. Lee RS, Passerotti CC, Cendron M, et al. Early results of robotic assisted laparoscopic lithotomy in adolescents. *J Urol*. 2007;177:2306–2309.

Chapter 52

Robotic Bladder Surgery in Children

Pasquale Casale and Yoshiyuki Kojima

Minimally invasive surgery has revolutionized many aspects of urological surgery, and the indications for laparoscopic and robotic surgeries have expanded to include not only adults but also children. The da Vinci surgical system (Intuitive Surgical, Sunnyvale, CA, USA) provides the advantages of simplification and precision of exposure and suturing because of allowing movements of the robotic arm in real time with increased degree of freedom and magnified three-dimensional view. Therefore, robotic surgery has the ability to perform pediatric reconstructive procedures with smaller learning curve and shorter operative time than conventional laparoscopic surgery.[1,2] Although the robotic approach most performed in pediatric urology is pyeloplasty for ureteropelvic junction obstruction, robotic bladder surgeries, such as ureteral reimplantation for vesicoureteral reflux (VUR), appendicovesicostomy and/or bladder augmentation for neurogenic bladder, and the management of urachal anomalies, recently have gained increasing acceptance. Although long-term outcome analysis has remained largely unexplored, robotic bladder surgery will be rapidly taking the place of open and conventional laparoscopic bladder surgery in children.

52.1 General Technique of Robotic Bladder Surgery in Children

The patient is usually supine on the table with the legs apart or in low lithotomy if they are adolescents. Trendelenburg is appropriate to allow the abdominal contents to fall in a cephalad manner away from the pelvis and get a fine view of the bladder. Typically, an open access technique is used for the 12- or 8-mm camera port or a Veress needle can be used if a 5-mm camera is preferred. The abdomen is insufflated with CO_2 at a pressure of 10–13 mmHg to observe the inside of the abdominal or 8–10 mmHg for the bladder cavity. Two additional working 5-mm trocars are usually inserted for the vesicoscopi approaches directly into the bladder where the 5- or 8-mm ports can be used for a transperitoneal approach. The robotic device is docked from the foot of the bed, and the robotic arms are engaged. We utilize bipolar forceps as a grasper and as either monopolar hook device or curved scissors during dissection.

52.2 Robotic Surgery for Vesicoureteral Reflux (Ureteral Reimplantation)

Vesicoureteral Reflux (VUR) is defined as the abnormal, retrograde flow of urine from the bladder into the upper urinary tract. It can be primary, caused by an anatomically insufficient vesicoureteric junction. Children with urinary tract infection may have VUR, which must be classified according to severity before it can be treated. The International Study Classification has established levels of severity from grade I–V.

P. Casale (✉)
Children's Hospital of Philadelphia, University of Pennsylvania School of Medicine, Philadelphia, PA, USA
e-mail: casale@email.chop.edu

Robotic Urologic Surgery

A.K. Hemal, M. Menon (eds.), *Robotics in Genitourinary Surgery*,
DOI 10.1007/978-1-84882-114-9_52, © Springer-Verlag London Limited 2011

Fig. 52.1 Robotic ureteral reimplantation (intravesical approach). Urethral catheter to be used as a suction device

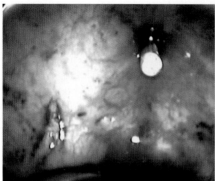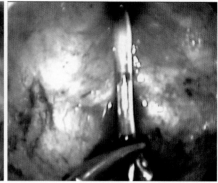

Generally, mild-grade cases are likely to resolve spontaneously. Antibiotic prophylaxis is a common practice in the management of children with VUR, as recommended in the guidelines of the American Urological Association. On the other hand, high-grade cases may require surgical management. The indications of ureteral reimplantation include breakthrough infections, worsening reflux, and higher grade reflux. Open ureteral reimplantation is still the gold standard with a success rate exceeding 95%. Subureteral injection of implant materials has shown much promise in recent years, with success rates of 72–99% after one or more injections.[3] Although successful conventional laparoscopic ureteral reimplantation has been described,[4] robotic ureteral reimplantation has a possibility to overcome many impediments of conventional laparoscopic ureteral reimplantation. Different techniques of ureteral reimplantation, i.e., extravesicle and vesicoscopic are considered to be options of robotic surgery.[3–7]

52.2.1 Vesicoscopic Approach (Transvesical Approach)

The vesicoscopic approach can be performed unilaterally or bilaterally, usually following the same steps as the open Cohen technique. This approach is not advocated in bladders with cystographic capacity less than 130 mL because of limitation of working space.

52.2.1.1 Technique

The bladder is filled with saline solution through the urethra. Using an open technique or visualization via a pediatric cystoscope, the 12-mm camera port is placed in the midline at the bladder dome. A 3-0 absorbable traction suture under cystoscopic vision secures the bladder wall and skin to the trocar. This helps to maintain pneumo-vesicum during the operation. A urethral catheter is inserted to drain the saline (Fig. 52.1), and the bladder is filled with CO_2 to the pressure of 8–10 mmHg. The working ports, either 8 or 5 mm, are positioned midway between the umbilicus and pubis at the midclavicular line. Ports are fixed to the abdominal wall using a stitch which is also used to close the bladder. The robotic device is then brought over the patient's feet. Similar to the open technique, ureteral dissection starts after placement of a 6-cm segment of a 5-Fr feeding tube or a 4-Fr open-ended ureteral catheter, secured to the ureter with a 4-0 absorbable suture. Mobilization of the ureters is done as in the laparoscopic pneumo-vesical procedure using the hook or scissor cautery. The submucosal tunnels are created by dissecting with scissors from the original hiatus to the other side of the trigone and incising the mucosa at the site of the new mucosal hiatus. Anastomosis of the ureters is performed after bringing them through the mucosal tunnel. Anchoring sutures of 4-0 absorbable suture are used to secure the ureter to the bladder musculature and the mucosal cuff is attached with 5-0 absorbable suture. The mucosa over the original hiatus is closed with running 5-0 absorbable. The working ports are removed and the bladder holding stitches are then tied. The flexible cystoscope is used to inspect the inside of the bladder. The port sites are also closed at the fascial level. The bladder catheter is kept overnight.

52.2.1.2 Clinical Results

The laparoscopic Cohen technique using CO_2 pneumo-vesicum was first described in a pig model in

2003.[8] After this animal trial, the clinical applications of this approach for children with VUR were reported. Yeung et al. reported the experiences of vesicoscopic Cohen's cross-trigonal ureteral reimplantation with pneumo-vesicum for children with primary VUR with a success rate of 96%.[4] We also reported our experiences with vesicoscopic Cohen's ureteral reimplantation for bilateral VUR with a success rate of 92.6%.[9] On the other hand, only one using robotic assistance is reported.[6] The technique may yield better results when refined using robot to assist in tissue manipulation and suturing. Peters et al. reported their five case experiences of robotic-assisted vesicoscopic Cohen's cross-trigonal ureteral reimplantation. Laparoscopic and robotic approaches make visualization and control excellent, and harbor, the potential for decreased postoperative bladder spasms, reduced incision pain, and shorter convalescence. Therefore, it might be developed as an alternative to open transvesical reimplantation such as Cohen, Glenn-Anderson, and Politano–Leadbetter techniques. This approach may be also an option for primary obstructing megaureter (ureterovesical junction obstruction; UVJO), although caution should be taken for children who require ureteral tapering. Additionally, the modification of this approach may permit development of more complex bladder surgeries including management of ureterocele, bladder neck repair, and local excision of unusual benign mesenchymal tumors, such as pheochromocytomas/paragangliomas or leiomyoma, in the posterior bladder wall; however, maintaining pneumo-vesicum is difficult and we need some trocar tricks. Small capacity bladders are difficult to navigate. This approach is still challenging, and we must continue to develop this approach.

52.2.2 Extravesical Approach

The extravesical approach can be also performed unilaterally or bilaterally, following the same steps as the open Lich–Gregoir technique.

52.2.2.1 Technique

Cystoscopy can be performed, and open-ended ureteral catheters are placed and secured to the urethral catheter to aid in the dissection. An open technique is used to place the first trocar, the 12-mm camera port, in the umbilicus. The working ports, 8 or 5 mm, are positioned in the midclavicular line bilaterally, about 1 cm below the umbilical line. If the child has a pubo-umbilical length less than 8 cm, then the midline camera port must be placed above the umbilicus between the xyphoid and umbilicus to prevent robotic arm collision. The robotic is docked over the patient's feet. The technique starts by dissecting the ureter after opening the peritoneum anterior to the uterus and just over the posterior bladder wall. A clear understanding of the anatomical differences in the pelvis between the boys and girls is required to expose the bladder and ureter. The ureter is freed from the surrounding tissue keeping its vessels intact. At this step, avoiding injury to the vas deferens in the boy or uterine artery in the girl, which transverses on the ureter, is required. The pelvic plexus is readily identified medial and caudal to the ureter. Care is taken to identify the pelvic plexus, avoiding injury to the area and allowing ureteral mobilization at the hiatus. The nerves can be seen entering and branching into the trigone distal to the ureteral hiatus (Fig. 52.2a). Approximately 4–5 cm is dissected to permit mobility and to prevent kinking as the bladder tunnel is created for the ureter (Fig. 52.2b). A detrusor trough is created by incising the muscularis of the bladder for about 3 cm and developing flaps with the cautery scissors. Fixation of the ureter with the bladder muscularis makes easier to perform subsequent muscularis closure using a 4-0 absorbable suture. The bladder muscularis is then closed over the ureter, using a 4-0 absorbable interrupted or running suture (Fig. 52.2c). Care must be taken to avoid any kinking or excessive compression of the ureter to prevent obstruction. Closure is performed proximal to distal or vice versa. In the latter, the ureter is well visualized but the needle needs to be passed under the ureter each time the suture is placed. We catch the adventitia of the ureter with each suture to ensure it does not slip back during the healing process. The urethral catheter is removed the next morning and the child is discharged after voiding.

52.2.2.2 Clinical Results

Open extravesical ureteral reimplantation was reported to be an effective method for repairing reflux without ureteral obstruction, but it can also result in a high rate of transient postoperative urinary retention even

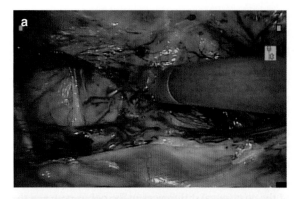

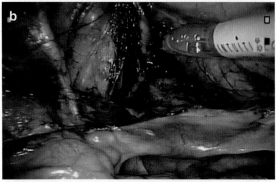

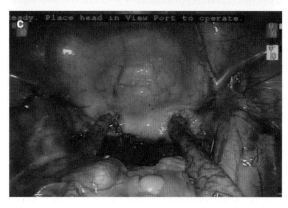

Fig. 52.2 a Robotic ureteral reimplantation (extravesical approach). The nerves entering and branching into the trigone distal to the ureteral hiatus. **b** Creation of detrusor tunnel for extravesical ureteral reimplant. **c** Closure of the bladder muscularis over the ureter

when detrusor dissection is minimized.[10] However, we reported that a total of 41 patients underwent robotic-assisted laparoscopic extravesical reimplantation for bilateral VUR with a success rate of 97.6% and without complication including urinary retention or exacerbation of dysfunctional voiding.[7] The improved visualization can avoid the injury of the pelvic plexus

and might decrease the incidence of postoperative urinary retention. This approach may also apply for the management of primary UVJO.

52.3 Robotic Surgery for Neuropathic Bladder

Neurologic conditions in children leading to neuropathic bladder dysfunction are predominantly congenital neural tube defects, including myelomeningocele, lipomeningocele, sacral agenesis, and occult lesions causing tethered cord. Patients with neuropathic bladder frequently exhibit mixed patterns of voiding dysfunction and/or urinary incontinence. Treatments can be proposed and combined according to not only the symptoms and urodynamic findings but also the patient's gender, age, and social environment. Although most of these children can be treated medically or with minimally invasive intervention, in some of them a continent catheterizable channel, usually appendicovesicostomy, and/or bladder augmentation are necessary. Robotic surgery can provide the ability to perform these complex and difficult reconstructive procedures in children. The children need mechanical preparation, intravenous hydration, and administration of broad-spectrum antibiotics before surgery.

52.3.1 Robotic Appendicovesicostomy

Appendicovesicostomy, which is performed by tunneling the appendix submucosally into the bladder, is an option in the treatment for patients with voiding dysfunction that needs clean intermittent catheterization (CIC) but without easily, catheterizable native urethra. Robotic appendicovesicostomy with or without other simultaneous reconstructive procedures can be one of the options for these children.

52.3.1.1 Technique

The patient is placed in the supine position in Trendelenburg. Three ports are utilized. The 12-mm camera port is placed in the umbilicus; and the other two 8-mm working ports on the right and left sides, in the midclavicular line at the level of the anterior superior iliac spines. The procedure commences with cecal mobilization. Care is taken to protect the appendiceal mesentery and mobilize with an adequate length. Once the cecum is mobilized, the appendix is separated from the cecum, leaving a small cuff of cecum with the appendix. The most challenging part of the procedure is creating the appendicovesical anastomosis. The robotic approach makes it easier than the conventional laparoscopic approach in this reconstruction. The bladder is filled with saline so one can measure the best position for the appendix due to its length, mobility of the bladder, and location of the stoma. A 4-cm detrusorrhaphy is made. The appendix is anastomosed to a small mucosal opening in the apex of the detrusor trough and the defect is closed using 4-0 absorbable interrupted suture (Fig. 52.3). The base of the appendix is brought up to reach the umbilicus or the right lower quadrant. We prefer the right lower quadrant trocar site to create a catheterizable stoma using a V-flap technique.

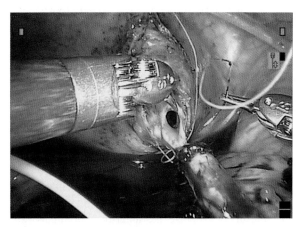

Fig. 52.3 Robotic appendicovesicostomy. Anastomosis of the appendix to a small mucosal opening in the apex of the detrusor trough

52.3.2 Robotic Bladder Augmentation (Ileocystoplasty)

Patients with both low bladder capacity and high pressure characteristics (low compliant bladder) are scheduled for bladder augmentation, because they have the risk of urinary tract infection and upper tract deterioration. Bladder augmentation is very reliable in expanding the capacity and lowering storage pressures of the poorly compliant bladder. Ileum is the most commonly used bowel segment for bladder augmentation. Although initial reports of conventional laparoscopic bladder augmentation generally involved laparoscopic bowel mobilization and harvesting, followed by extracorporeal bowel reconstruction, the current laparoscopic and robotic procedures have been successfully performed in a completely intracorporeal manner.[11,12] Conventional laparoscopic bladder augmentation is possible but not practical because of some difficulties with suturing for reconstruction and long operative time; however, robotic bladder augmentation has been expected to overcome these difficulties and allow shorter operative times.

52.3.2.1 Technique

Cystoscopy can be performed, and open-ended ureteral catheters should be placed for easy intraoperative identification of ureters. The patient's position and port placement are basically same as those in robotic appendicovesicostomy. Additional robotic and/or laparoscopic assistant ports are placed to introduce sutures easily into the abdomen and assist with retraction (Fig. 52.4). A 20-cm ileal segment chosen should be 15 cm proximal to the ileocecal valve and it is then isolated and detubularized. An endoscopic stapler devise, which is introduced through a laparoscopic assistant port, may be useful for isolation of ileum. Care is taken to protect the ileal mesentery and mobilize with an adequate length. Intracorporeal irrigation of the ileal segment with sterile saline can be done after detubularization of ileum. Bowel continuity is re-established in two layers with an end-to-end ileoileostomy using intracorporeal running 3-0 absorbable sutures followed by a Lembert suture and the mesenteric window is closed. After opening the native bladder, the anastomosis of the simple ileal on-lay patch[12] or U-shaped configuration[11] to the native bladder is performed from a posterior to anterior direction using complete intracorporeal 4-0 absorbable running sutures. Care must be taken to avoid twisting the ileal mesentery as the ileal segment is brought down to the bladder. If an appendicovesicostomy is needed, the appendix is anastomosed to the posterior

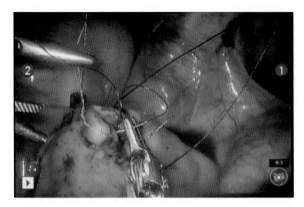

Fig. 52.4 Robotic augmentation. Bowel anastomosis with an end-to-end ileoileostomy using intracorporeal running sutures

wall of the native bladder in an extravesical fashion, as described above. A suprapubic catheter usually is placed. A water-tight anastomosis is confirmed by irrigation with sterile saline through the Foley catheter. Open-ended ureteral catheters can be removed after surgery.

52.3.2.2 Clinical Results

There are several case reports of robotic appendicovesicostomy and/or bladder augmentation for children with a neuropathic bladder,[12–16] as well as conventional laparoscopic procedures.[17,18] These preliminary reports suggest that the robotic approach provides satisfactory, safe, and successful clinical results. Additionally, the robotic bladder neck dissection and placement of bladder neck sling procedures for children with urinary incontinence caused by intrinsic sphincter deficiency have been reported.[19] All these reports show that robotic approach is technically feasible for complex bladder reconstructive surgeries and may be achieved with minimally invasive surgery in the pediatric population. Since conventional laparoscopic ileal conduit for children with neurogenic bladder was also reported previously,[20] robotic approach for this procedure may be also one of the options; however, whether robotic approach for children with neurogenic bladder can provide any significant advantages over open procedures remains controversial, a large case series studies will be needed.

52.4 Robotic Surgery for Urachal Anomalies

The urachus lies in the space of Retzius between the peritoneum and transversalis fascia and is encased between two layers of umbilicovesical fascia. There are several types of urachal anomalies including patent urachus, urachal cyst, alternating urachal sinus, and urachal diverticulum. The most common type of urachal anomalies is an urachal cyst, where there is an isolated section of patent urachus that communicates with neither the bladder nor the umbilicus. Most urachal anomalies are asymptomatic, but when they do become symptomatic, such as lower abdominal pain, fever, voiding symptoms, mass, umbilical discharge, and evidence of urinary tract infection, surgical treatment is usually needed. Treatment consisting of complete extraperitoneal excision of the urachus with an attached bladder cuff is recommended to avoid recurrence or development of carcinoma in unresected tissue.

52.4.1 Technique

Cystography and cystoscopy are usually performed to identify a possible diverticulum at the bladder dome and there is no communication between the bladder dome and urachus. The patient is placed in the supine position. The 12-mm camera port is placed in the midline between the umbilicus and the xyphoid process; and the other two 8- or 5-mm working ports on the right and left sides, in the midclavicular line above the level of the umbilicus. The 30° angle camera may be helpful to visualize the anterior abdominal wall. After pushing the umbilicus on the abdomen with the assistant's hand to confirm its position and to avoid the incomplete excision of the urachal remnant, the urachal duct is detached just caudal to the umbilicus, dissected from the anterior abdominal wall, and mobilized toward the bladder dome using monopolar hook device or curved scissors. The peritoneum is incised along the plane above the bladder dome to enter the space of Retzius. A segment of bladder cuff is resected circumferentially with the specimen using curved scissors and then the bladder defect is closed in a running fashion with two separate layers by 4-0 absorbable suture. The specimen can be removed through the port without wound enlargement. The bladder is distended via the Foley catheter to ensure a water-tight anastomosis.

52.4.2 Clinical Results

Successful management of urachal anomalies by conventional laparoscopic[21,22] and robotic approaches[23,24] have been reported in adults and children. Conventional laparoscopic and robotic approaches provide better visualization of urachal anomalies than open surgery, and a radical dissection can be achieved through the small incisions secondary to the wide visualization of the anterior abdominal wall. Since the closure of the bladder opening is needed after resection of a segment of bladder cuff, the advantage of the robotic approach over conventional laparoscopic management for the urachal anomalies is the ability to perform suturing with minimal difficulty.

52.5 Conclusion

Robotic pediatric bladder surgery is still in its infancy. The dexterity allowed with the robotic platform makes it an ideal approach to reconstruct the bladder with minimal manipulation and trauma to the bladder. If three ports are utilized, all the ports added together are a maximum equal to 2.8 cm (two 8-mm and one 12-mm ports). If an assistant port is utilized for procedures such as augmentation and appendicovesicostomy, the total added incision length is 4 cm (two 8-mm and two 12-mm ports). One must also take into consideration that the length of the individual incisions affects overall pain more than the number of incisions. Therefore, a single 4-cm incision will more likely generate more pain than four incisions all close to 1 cm. We must also take into consideration that most bladder procedures cannot be accomplished safely with a 4-cm incision.

References

1. Peters CA. Laparoscopy in pediatric urology: adoption of innovative technology. *BJU Int*. 2003;92(Suppl 1):52–57.
2. Peters CA. Robotic assisted surgery in pediatric urology. *Pediatr Endosurg Innov Tech*. 2003;7:403–413.
3. Hayn MH, Smaldone MC, Ost MC, Docimo SG. Minimally invasive treatment of vesicoureteral reflux. *Urol Clin North Am*. 2008;35:477–488.
4. Yeung CK, Sihoe JD, Borzi PA. Endoscopic cross-trigonal ureteral reimplantation under carbon dioxide bladder insufflation: a novel technique. *J Endourol*. 2005;19:295–299.
5. Lendvay T. Robotic-assisted laparoscopic management of vesicoureteral reflux. *Adv Urol*. 2008;2008:732942.
6. Peters CA, Woo R. Intravesical robotically assisted bilateral ureteral reimplantation. *J Endourol*. 2005;19:618–621.
7. Casale P, Patel RP, Kolon TF. Nerve sparing robotic extravesical ureteral reimplantation. *J Urol*. 2008;179:1987–1989.
8. Olsen LH, Deding D, Yeung CK, Jorgensen TM. *Computer assisted laparoscopic pneumovesical ureter reimplantation a.m. Cohen: initial experience in a pig model*. APMIS. 2003;109:23–25.
9. Kutikov A, Guzzo TJ, Canter DJ, Casale P. Initial experience with laparoscopic transvesical ureteral reimplantation at the children's hospital of Philadelphia. *J Urol*. 2006;176:2222–2225.
10. Lipski BA, Mitchell ME, Burns MW. Voiding dysfunction after bilateral extravesical ureteral reimplantation. *J Urol*. 1998;159:1019–1021.
11. Lorenzo AJ, Cerveira J, Farhat WA. Pediatric laparoscopic ileal cystoplasty: complete intracorporeal surgical technique. *Urology*. 2007;69:977–981.
12. Gundeti MS, Eng MK, Reynolds WS, Zagaja GP. Pediatric robotic-assisted laparoscopic augmentation ileocystoplasty and mitrofanoff appendicovesicostomy: complete intracorporeal–initial case report. *Urology*. 2008;72:1144–1147.
13. Pedraza R, Weiser A, Franco I. Laparoscopic appendicovesicostomy (mitrofanoff procedure) in a child using the da Vinci robotic system. *J Urol*. 2004;171:1652–1653.
14. Thakre AA, Yeung CK, Robot-assisted Mitrofanoff PC. Malone antegrade continence enema reconstruction using divided appendix. *J Endourol*. 2008;22:2393–2396.
15. Lendvay TS, Shnorhavorian M, Grady RW. Robotic-assisted laparoscopic mitrofanoff appendicovesicostomy and antegrade continent enema colon tube creation in a pediatric spina bifida patient. *J Laparoendosc Adv Surg Tech A*. 2008;18:310–312.
16. Storm DW, Fulmer BR, Sumfest JM. Laparoscopic robot-assisted appendicovesicostomy: an initial experience. *J Endourol*. 2007;21:1015–1017.
17. Casale P, Feng WC, Grady RW, Joyner BD, Lee RS, Mitchell ME. Intracorporeal laparoscopic appendicovesicostomy: a case report of a novel approach. *J Urol*. 2004;171:1899–1900.
18. Hsu TH, Shortliffe LD. Laparoscopic mitrofanoff appendicovesicostomy. *Urology*. 2004;64:802–804.
19. Storm DW, Fulmer BR, Sumfest JM. Robotic-assisted laparoscopic approach for posterior bladder neck dissection and placement of pediatric bladder neck sling: initial experience. *Urology*. 2008;72:1149–1152.

20. Ramalingam M, Senthil K, Ganapathy Pai M. Laparoscopy-assisted ileal conduit in sacral agenesis. *J Laparoendosc Adv Surg Tech A*. 2008;18:335–339.

21. Cutting CW, Hindley RG, Poulsen J. Laparoscopic management of complicated urachal remnants. *BJU Int*. 2005;96:1417–1421.

22. Turial S, Hueckstaedt T, Schier F, Fahlenkamp D. Laparoscopic treatment of urachal remnants in children. *J Urol*. 2007;177:1864–1866.

23. Madeb R, Knopf JK, Nicholson C, et al. The use of robotically assisted surgery for treating urachal anomalies. *BJU Int*. 2006;98:838–842.

24. Yamzon J, Kokorowski P, De Filippo RE, Chang AY, Hardy BE, Koh CJ. Pediatric robot-assisted laparoscopic excision of urachal cyst and bladder cuff. *J Endourol*. 2008;22:2385–2388.

Part VII
Female Urology and Infertility

Chapter 53

Robotic Surgery in Urogynecology

Mark S. Shimko and Daniel S. Elliott

53.1 Introduction

The da Vinci© robotic surgical system (Intuitive Surgical, Inc., Sunny Vale, CA) was approved for use in gynecologic procedures in the United States in 2005, although procedures had been performed prior to this time. There is a growing body of literature evaluating the feasibility of robotic assistance for laparoscopic urogynecologic and gynecologic procedures. Procedures performed robotically cover the whole spectrum of gynecology and urogynecology and include benign and radical hysterectomy, lymphadenectomy, myomectomy, and sacrocolpopexy. Although less well established, robot assistance has been used for vesicovaginal fistula repairs and treatment of endometriosis.[1-3]

As with other surgical fields, the need for and adoption of robotic assistance can best be understood in the context of standard laparoscopy, of which robotics is a technologic derivative. In general, laparoscopy was introduced as a minimally invasive method of performing established open procedures. The benefits include reduced hospital stay, decreased pain, and faster recovery. The costs include longer operative time, the need for specialized equipment, and skilled training with a significant learning curve. Robotic assistance represents a technical advancement that attempts to reproduce (and improve upon) the benefits of standard laparoscopy while decreasing the operative time and the learning curve associated with standard laparoscopy.

Two major obstacles to the wide-spread acceptance of laparoscopy in urogynecology have been the increased operative time associated with the procedures and technical skill required for complex procedures including intracorporeal suturing. With regard to the first obstacle, individual study results vary, but there appears to be a trend toward shorter operative time with robotic assistance over the standard laparoscopic procedures.[4-7] For the technical obstacle, robotic assistance is ergonomic with intuitive movements, tremor filtering, and three-dimensional imaging which may enable less-skilled laparoscopists to perform a procedure with robotic assistance, such as sacrocolpopexy or myomectomy, that has significant intracorporeal reconstruction and suturing.[8,9]

The past decade has seen a rapid increase in the literature on standard and robotic-assisted laparoscopy in urogynecology. Procedures such as transabdominal sacrocolpopexy and hysterectomy have well-established literature showing results comparable to the open procedure with a minimal hospital stay and low complication rates.[1,5-7,10-15] Following is a brief overview of the multiple urogynecologic and gynecologic procedures currently being performed with robotic assistance. A detailed view of robotic sacrocolpopexy is presented as a demonstration of the potential benefit of robotic assistance in urogynecology.

53.2 Hysterectomy

Hysterectomy is the most common major gynecologic procedure with about 600,000 procedures performed in the United States annually.[16] Although laparoscopic

D.S. Elliott (✉)
Department of Urology, Mayo Clinic, Rochester, MN, USA
e-mail: elliott.daniel@mayo.edu

A.K. Hemal, M. Menon (eds.), *Robotics in Genitourinary Surgery*,
DOI 10.1007/978-1-84882-114-9_53, © Springer-Verlag London Limited 2011

hysterectomy has been associated with a shorter hospital stay and faster recovery, it represents only about 10% of the hysterectomy population.[17]

Multiple studies have compared open hysterectomy to the laparoscopic and robot-assisted procedures for both benign and malignant disease, including cervical, ovarian, and endometrial cancer. Although it did not reach statistical significance, the robotic-assisted procedure was repeatedly associated with a shorter operative time compared to the laparoscopic procedure but still longer than the open procedure. For malignant disease, it yielded lymph node counts that equaled or surpassed those routinely obtained by open lymphadenectomies.[5,7]

53.3 Myomectomy

There are two principle stages to myomectomy: enucleation of the leiomyomas, which open surgeons rely heavily upon haptic feedback to accomplish, and repair of the uterine wall, which requires a strong, multilayer closure. Uterine rupture in future pregnancies and recurrence are particular concerns. Laparoscopic removal of leiomyomas is a technically challenging procedure which has not gained wide-spread acceptance in part due to a slightly higher recurrence rate.[18] Bedient et al. showed a trend toward a shorter operative time with the robot and otherwise the procedure was comparable to standard laparoscopy.[4] Despite these shortcomings, it is likely that more of these procedures will be performed robotically as the surgeons' robotic skill set expands.

53.4 Tubal Reanastomosis

Tubal reanastomosis has been performed with robotic assistance, with the gold standard being the open, microsurgical reconstruction. The robotic procedure has been reported in small series, with the initial feasibility studies published over a decade ago.[19] Robotic assistance has been shown to have comparable results in terms of pregnancy rates with a shorter hospital stay and longer operative time compared to open microsurgical reconstruction, although both procedures are associated with a brief hospital stay.[20]

53.5 Sacrocolpopexy

53.5.1 Introduction

Approximately one in nine women will undergo a hysterectomy for benign or malignant disease in their lifetime. Of these, approximately 10% will develop symptomatic vaginal vault prolapse.[21,22] Multiple corrective procedures are possible through transvaginal or transabdominal routes, as well as a combination of the two. The common goals for all surgical repairs of vaginal vault prolapse include restoration of proper anatomy; maintenance of sexual, bowel, and urinary function; and long-term durability.[12] The vaginal approach has historically been associated with decreased morbidity, including shorter hospitalization and convalescence.[23,24] Unfortunately, the vaginal approach is associated with lower long-term durability than the transabdominal procedure.[25]

Laparoscopic sacrocolpopexy was introduced in an attempt to combine the reduced morbidity and hospital stay of the transvaginal sacrocolpopexy with the long-term durability and success of the open transabdominal procedure. From this standpoint, the laparoscopic procedure is a huge success.[13–15] However, similar to hysterectomy, it has not gained wide-spread use due to the technical challenge required to perform a reconstructive procedure laparoscopically as well as the lengthened operative time.

Robotic-assisted sacrocolpopexy is perhaps one of the most effective uses of the da Vinci robotic system. Operative times from experienced surgeons are comparable to that reported in most open series. Complication rates are low and hospital stays are typically overnight. The advantages of a robotic system (ergonomic controls, intuitive motions, wrist movement, tremor filtering, and three-dimensional imaging) make intracorporeal reconstruction much easier.[1,6,11–15,26] As more robotic systems become available and more surgeons become technically skilled at their use, we expect a continued adoption of this procedure.

53.5.2 Preoperative Evaluation

The cohort of patients that are candidates for robotic-assisted laparoscopy has expanded in recent years. In past years, morbid obesity was seen as a relative contraindication but with the advent of longer instruments, the robotic approach is indicated in these patients due to few wound complications and easier access.

Contraindications to the robotic approach are the same as those for standard laparoscopy. Conditions that preclude steep Trendelenburg positioning and pneumoperitoneum such as right-sided heart failure and pulmonary hypertension exclude people from a procedure with robotic assistance.

53.5.3 Patient Preparation and Positioning

The patients are instructed to follow routine preoperative recommendations including no food or drink after midnight and discontinuation of anti-platelet and blood thinning medications whenever possible. The patients are given a mechanical bowel prep the evening prior to surgery to decompress the bowels and increase the working space within the abdomen.

The patient is placed under a general anesthetic, and a urethral catheter and nasogastric (or orogastric) tube are placed to decompress the bladder and stomach, respectively. The patient is placed in a dorsal lithotomy position with the legs in Allen stirrups for the entire procedure. Pressure points are appropriately padded. Special attention should be paid to the lateral part of the head of the fibula as the common peroneal nerve courses lateral to this bony structure and

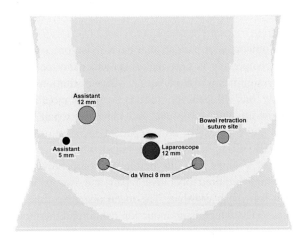

Fig. 53.1 Port placement for robotic sacrocolpopexy

is prone to pressure injury. The arms are tucked beside the torso. The patient is then prepped from the nipples to proximal thigh, including the vagina.

The patient's head is lowered so that they are in steep Trendelenburg position (30–45°) so that the abdominal contents fall out of the pelvis, if possible. Abdominal insufflation is accomplished using a Veress needle periumbilically. After adequate insufflation, a 12 mm periumbilical camera port is placed under direct visualization to avoid vascular or bowel injury. The remainder of the ports are then placed using the camera port for direct vision. Two additional 8 mm robot ports are then placed lateral to the rectus belly approximately 3 cm superior to the iliac crest. If using the da Vinci S system, the third robotic arm is tucked away from the patient and not used for this procedure. A 10 mm standard laparoscopic port for the assistance is then placed several centimeters subcostally just lateral to the right rectus belly. Another 5 mm assistant's port is placed approximately one hand's breadth inferiolaterally to the first assistant's port (see Fig. 53.1).

The robot is brought between the patients' legs and docked. A retracting suture is then placed through the skin in the left lateral abdomen to retract the sigmoid colon. The bladder is dissected from the anterior vaginal wall using forceps and cautery scissors. Posteriorly, the peritoneal reflection is then incised to mobilize the vagina. These planes should be relatively bloodless. A customized hand-held vaginal retractor manufactured at the Mayo Clinic (see Fig. 53.2) provides countertraction to facilitate the dissection. Both of these dissections should be carried out as distal (toward the introitus) as possible.

After the vagina is mobilized, sacral periosteum should be dissected free of overlying presacral tissue. The sigmoid colon was previously retracted, but this may be adjusted if necessary to obtain the proper exposure. Care should be taken to avoid the sacral venous complexes.

Based on visual inspection, the polypropylene Y-graft (IntePro® American Medical Systems, Minnetonka, MN) can have one and/or both of its armed shortened to approximate the patient's anatomy. It is then brought into the field through the 10 mm port. In our experience, the aforementioned steps are usually able to be accomplished within 30 min.

The robot is then used for intracorporeal suturing of the Y-graft to the vagina and sacrum. This is one of the steps that the robotic assistance can save

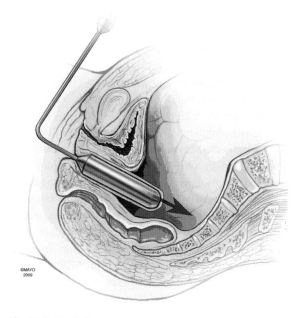

Fig. 53.2 Vaginal retractor

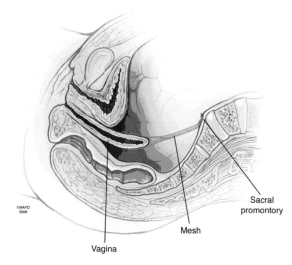

Fig. 53.3 Completed reconstruction with restoration of native vaginal position and axis

significant amounts of time over the standard laparoscopic approach. The posterior arm of the Y-graft is the more difficult anatomic position to suture, so this is usually sutured first with three to four interrupted Gore-Tex sutures (W. L. Gore and Associates, Inc., Newark, Delaware). The tension on the suture should be tight enough to overcome the small amount of elasticity of the material. Next, the anterior portion of the Y-graft is sutured in a similar fashion. The hand-held vaginal retractor is used to re-align the axis and position of the vagina to near-native configuration. The tail of the graft is then sutured to the sacral promontory (see Fig. 53.3). Care should be taken not to place tension on the vagina, which can cause erosion and failure of the repair. The posterior peritoneum is then closed to retroperitonealize the graft. The ports are then removed and the fascia of the ports, 8 mm and larger ports, are closed using a interrupted 2-0 polyglactin (Vicryl).

For the patients that require an anti-incontinence procedure at the same time, the change in vaginal access with the sacrocolpopexy can affect sling tension. To this end, dissection and sling placement may be carried out at any point but the tension on the sling should not be set until the sacrocolpopexy is complete.

53.5.4 Postoperative Course

The routine postoperative course is similar with only minor variations, regardless of the procedure.

Postoperatively, pain is managed with scheduled ketorolac intravenously with 15–30 mg every 6 h. The majority of these procedures are Type II wounds (clean-contaminated) and antibiotics are continued for 1–2 days postoperatively. The diet can be advanced immediately and the patients should be encouraged to ambulate the evening of the procedure. Patients with mesh or vaginal surgery are discharged home on 3 months of vaginal estrogen to prevent wound breakdown and mesh erosion.

53.5.5 Results

The outcomes of patients that have undergone robotic sacrocolpopexy is now maturing with many patients with significant follow up.[6,11] Our institution currently has 40 patients with at least 36 months of follow-up with subjective and objective repair success rates of 100% and a patient satisfaction rate of 95%. Complications were minor with the exception of a single port site hernia at postoperative day 5 which required operative repair and two patients that had mesh erosions. The mean operative time in this series, which is an induction cohort and therefore incorporates the learning curve, was 186 minutes, which compares favorably with open series.[27] Many of the most recent procedures were accomplished in about 2 h.

53.6 Potential Pitfalls

As with any robotic or laparoscopic procedure, there are certain situations that may lead to complications. Almost all of these patients have a history of hysterectomy, and therefore many patients have had previous abdominal operations. Dense adhesions may make port placement and access to the pelvis difficult or impossible. The bladder may be draped over the vaginal cuff and lead to the wrong plane of dissection. Inadvertent cystotomies may be created and can be closed primarily.

53.7 Conclusion

Robotic-assisted laparoscopy is emerging as a powerful tool for urogynecologists. It allows completion of complex procedures with a faster operative time than standard laparoscopy and results are comparable to the gold-standard open procedures. This has all been accomplished within the first decade of robotic assistance. As technologic advances and improved designs continue to be developed at a rapid pace, we expect these trends to continue and the robotic-assisted procedures to begin to show superiority over other methods with a decreased learning curve and improved outcomes. Also, robotic training is becoming standard in many residencies and the number of surgeons with this experience is growing.

53.8 Future Directions

There are still clearly limitations to the use of robotic technology. The introduction of teaching consoles and improved simulators will continue to decrease the learning curve and training burden of robotic procedures. Incorporating three-dimensional radiographic images into the console view and error-preventing algorithms are just two of the many advances on the horizon.

References

1. Elliott DS, Chow GK, Gettman M. Current status of robotics in female urology and gynecology. *World J Urol.* June 2006;24(2):188–192.
2. Nezhat C, Saberi NS, Shahmohamady B, Nezhat F. Robotic-assisted laparoscopy in gynecological surgery. *JSLS.* July–September 2006;10(3):317–320.
3. Liu C, Perisic D, Samadi D, Nezhat F. Robotic-assisted laparoscopic partial bladder resection for the treatment of infiltrating endometriosis. *J Minim Invasive Gynecol.* November-December 2008;15(6):745–748.
4. Bedient CE, Magrina JF, Noble BN, Kho RM. Comparison of robotic and laparoscopic myomectomy. *Am J Obstet Gynecol.* December 2009;201(6):566, e561–565.
5. Boggess JF, Gehrig PA, Cantrell L, et al. A comparative study of 3 surgical methods for hysterectomy with staging for endometrial cancer: robotic assistance, laparoscopy, laparotomy. *Am J Obstet Gynecol.* October 2008;199(4):360, e361–369.
6. Elliott DS, Krambeck AE, Chow GK. Long-term results of robotic assisted laparoscopic sacrocolpopexy for the treatment of high grade vaginal vault prolapse. *J Urol.* August 2006;176(2):655–659.
7. Magrina JF, Kho RM, Weaver AL, Montero RP, Magtibay PM. Robotic radical hysterectomy: comparison with laparoscopy and laparotomy. *Gyneco Oncol.* 2008;109(1):86–91.
8. Jayaraman S, Quan D, Al-Ghamdi I, El-Deen F, Schlachta CM. Does robotic assistance improve efficiency in performing complex minimally invasive surgical procedures? *Surg Endosc.* March 2010;24(3):584–588.
9. Stefanidis D, Wang F, Korndorffer JR Jr., Dunne JB, Scott DJ. Robotic assistance improves intracorporeal suturing performance and safety in the operating room while decreasing operator workload. *Surg Endosc.* February 2010;24(2):377–382.
10. Boggess JF, Gehrig PA, Cantrell L, et al. A case-control study of robot-assisted type III radical hysterectomy with pelvic lymph node dissection compared with open radical hysterectomy. *Am J Obstet Gynecol.* October 2008;199(4):357, e351–357.
11. Di Marco DS, Chow GK, Gettman MT, Elliott DS. Robotic-assisted laparoscopic sacrocolpopexy for treatment of vaginal vault prolapse. *Urology.* February 2004;63(2):373–376.
12. Elliott DS, Frank I, DiMarco DS, Chow GK. Gynecologic use of robotically assisted laparoscopy: sacrocolpopexy for the treatment of high-grade vaginal vault prolapse. *Am J Surg.* 2004;188(Suppl 1):52–56.
13. Ganatra AM, Rozet F, Sanchez-Salas R, et al. The current status of laparoscopic sacrocolpopexy: a review. *Eur Urol.* May 2009;55(5):1089–1103.
14. Paraiso MF, Walters MD, Rackley RR, Melek S, Hugney C. Laparoscopic and abdominal sacral colpopexies: a comparative cohort study. *Am J Obstet Gynecol.* May 2005;192(5):1752–1758.
15. Rozet F, Mandron E, Arroyo C, et al. Laparoscopic sacral colpopexy approach for Genitourinary prolapse: experience with 363 cases. *Eur Urol.* February 2005;47(2):230–236.
16. Keshavarz H, Hillis SD, Kieke BA, Marchbanks PA. Hysterectomy surveillance–united states, 1994–1999. *MMWR CDC Surveill Summ.* 2002;51:1–8.
17. Wu JM, Wechter ME, Geller EJ, Nguyen TV, Visco AG. Hysterectomy rates in the United States, 2003. *Obstet Gynecol.* November 2007;110(5):1091–1095.
18. Nezhat C, Lavie O, Hsu S, Watson J, Barnett O, Lemyre M. Robotic-assisted laparoscopic myomectomy compared with standard laparoscopic myomectomy – a

retrospective matched control study. *Fertil Steril.* February 2009;91(2):556–559.

19. Degueldre M, Vandromme J, Huong PT, Cadiere GB. Robotically assisted laparoscopic microsurgical tubal reanastomosis: a feasibility study. *Fertil Steril.* November 2000;74(5):1020–1023.

20. Dharia Patel SP, Steinkampf MP, Whitten SJ, Malizia BA. Robotic tubal anastomosis: surgical technique and cost effectiveness. *Fertil Steril.* October 2008;90(4): 1175–1179.

21. Marchionni M, Bracco GL, Checcucci V, et al. True incidence of vaginal vault prolapse. Thirteen years of experience. *J Reprod Med.* August 1999;44(8):679–684.

22. Olsen AL, Smith VJ, Bergstrom JO, Colling JC, Clark AL. Epidemiology of surgically managed pelvic organ prolapse and urinary incontinence. *Obstet Gynecol.* April 1997;89(4):501–506.

23. Karram M, Goldwasser S, Kleeman S, Steele A, Vassallo B, Walsh P. High uterosacral vaginal vault suspension with fascial reconstruction for vaginal repair of enterocele and vaginal vault prolapse. *Am J Obstet Gynecol.* December 2001;185(6):1339–1342.

24. Podratz KC, Ferguson LK, Lee RA, Symmonds RE. Abdominal sacral colpopexy for posthysterectomy vaginal vault descensus. *Obstet Gynecol.* 1995;50(10):719–720.

25. Benson JT, Lucente V, McClellan E. Vaginal versus abdominal reconstructive surgery for the treatment of pelvic support defects: a prospective randomized study with long-term outcome evaluation. *Am J Obstet Gynecol.* December 1996;175(6):1418–1421.

26. Hsiao KC, Latchamsetty K, Govier FE, Kozlowski P, Kobashi KC. Comparison of laparoscopic and abdominal sacrocolpopexy for the treatment of vaginal vault prolapse. *J Endourol.* August 2007;21(8):926–930.

27. Kramer BA, Whelan CM, Powell TM, Schwartz BF. Robot-assisted laparoscopic sacrocolpopexy as management for pelvic organ prolapse. *J Endourol.* April 2009;23(4): 655–658.

Chapter 54

Robotic Repair of Vesico-vaginal Fistula

Pankaj Wadhwa and Ashok K. Hemal

54.1 Introduction

Iatrogenic gynecological procedures account for majority of the genitourinary fistulae in developed countries[1] while inadequate obstetric care, usually obstructed labor, remains the predominant cause of vesico-vaginal fistulae (VVF) in developing countries.[2] Most urinary fistulae present 1–6 weeks after gynecologic or obstetric surgery.[2] Majority of VVF can be repaired transvaginally; an abdominal approach is usually preferred in patients with a large (>3 cm) fistula, supratrigonal fistula, fistula in close proximity to or involving ureteric orifices, and in patients with recurrent fistula following a transvaginal repair.

During the last decade laparoscopic approach for repair of VVF has been increasingly employed to off-set the morbidity of the 'open' abdominal repair, with similar success rates.[3–7] Despite the lesser morbidity allowing quicker convalescence, laparoscopic VVF repair has not gained widespread popularity, possibly due to the technical challenge associated with laparoscopic dissection of the fistula and intracorporeal suturing. The advent of robotic assistance, allowing fatigue-free ergonomic maneuverability of the instruments, accuracy, and magnified three-dimensional vision has helped overcome these technical difficulties.[8] The robotic approach has helped achieve excellent results, allowing smaller cystotomy, limiting the need for extensive dissection and placement of suprapubic cystostomy, even in cases of recurrent fistula surgery.[9]

54.2 Operative Setup

Outlay of the operating room is as follows. The anesthetist occupies the cranial end of the table; the laparoscopic assistant is by the right-hand side of the table with the video cart comprising the video monitor (2D), CO_2 insufflator, and cold light source at the caudal end on the right-hand side. The nurse assistant with instrument trolley is positioned caudal and further to the right of the laparoscopic assistant. The robot is placed at the caudal end of the table and is positioned between the legs of the patient after lithotomy with steep Trendelenburg tilt is done. The robotic console is on the left-hand side of the table.

54.3 Patient Positioning

After induction of general anesthesia and insertion of a naso-gastric tube, extended length intravenous lines are connected to allow the anesthetist 'remote access' and permit placing of the patients' hands by the side. The patient is placed supine in a low lithotomy position using stirrups. Adequate padding is applied around the knees and the shoulders. Additionally a cross-shoulder restraint is tied to prevent the patient from sliding cranially once the steep Trendelenburg position is employed.

A.K. Hemal (✉)
Department of Urology, Comprehensive Cancer Center, Institute for Regenerative Medicine, Robotics and Minimally Invasive Surgery, Baptist Medical Center, Wake Forest University School of Medicine, Wake Forest University Health Sciences, Winston-Salem, NC, USA
e-mail: ashokkhemal@gmail.com

A.K. Hemal, M. Menon (eds.), *Robotics in Genitourinary Surgery*,
DOI 10.1007/978-1-84882-114-9_54, © Springer-Verlag London Limited 2011

Vaginoscopy, cystoscopy, and stent placement are performed at this time; the patient is catheterized with a 14-Fr Foley's catheter. The catheter is placed transvaginally in cases with large VVF as it helps prevent leakage of pneumoperitoneal gas when vesicotomy is performed. The abdomen is then prepared and pneumoperitoneum is established using a Veress needle in the left hypochondrium, to avoid adhesions due to previous surgeries. Alternatively, an 'open technique' is employed supraumbilically and the trocars are placed. Thereafter, the table is tilted to a steep (50–60°) Trendelenburg position and the robot is docked; this facilitates the small bowel loops to gravitate away from the pelvis to the upper abdomen.

54.4 Trocar Configuration

A five-port transperitoneal approach is used; the camera port (12 mm) is placed in the midline supraumbilically and two 8-mm robotic ports are placed on either side at the pararectus muscle over the spinoumbilical line. A 5-mm port is placed on the right side 1 in. above and medial to anterior superior iliac spine for assistance and another 5-mm port on the right side between the camera and the robotic port for suction. Suture transfer is performed either through the robotic or the camera port after taking out the respective instrument, thus avoiding the need for another 12-mm port.

54.5 Instrumentation List

Table 54.1 lists the robotic and laparoscopic instruments required for the procedure. Sutures required include a 2-0 vicryl or monocryl, two 3-0 vicryl or monocryl, and 4-0 monocryl for port closure suture. Additionally, a 15-G Jakson Pratt or multi-pore abdominal drain is used at the end of the procedure.

54.6 Step-by-Step Technique

54.6.1 Vaginoscopy, Urethro-cystoscopy, and Bilateral Ureteric Double J Stenting or Catheterization

Vaginoscopy and urethro-cystoscopy are performed in the initial lithotomy position to study the location, size, and proximity of the fistula to the ureteric orifices and place double J stents or 6-F ureteric catheters bilaterally; this aids locating the orifices intra-operatively. In large VVF, a Foley's catheter is placed transvaginally through the fistula into the bladder and the balloon is inflated to plug the leak and allow bladder distension during cystoscopy.

54.6.2 Adhesiolysis

Trocar placements are performed as described above; laparoscopic adhesiolysis of omentum/bowel is often required to aid robotic trocar placement due to prior surgery. Subsequent robotic adhesiolysis is performed with robotic instruments.

54.6.3 Robotic Dissection of VVF

The Trendelenburg position is assumed and the robot is docked to the patient. The initial part of the dissection includes further adhesiolysis using a combination of sharp and blunt dissection with a Maryland-fenestrated bipolar forceps and a monopolar-curved scissors, to expose the anterior surface of the uterus and posterior superior aspect of the bladder. In the posthysterectomy cases, the small bowel loops or the sigmoid colon are required to be carefully dissected from the underlying bladder. Gentle tug on the Foley's catheter passed through the fistula further helps locate the approximate site of the fistula as seen from within the abdominal cavity allowing the placement of a

Table 54.1 Robotic and laparoscopic instruments utilized for robotic VVF repair

Surgeon instrumentation			Assistant instrumentation
Right arm (yellow)	Left arm (green)	Fourth arm (red)	
• Curved monopolar scissors	• Maryland bipolar grasper	Not required	• Suction irrigator
• Needle driver	• Needle driver		• Blunt tip grasper
			• Laparoscopic scissors

'minimal' vertical cystotomy near the area of interest, close to the midline, above the 'stuck area.' Once, cystotomy is made, the vaginally placed Foley's or ureteric catheter can be seen, which can be deflated and pulled out, thus facilitating visualization of the fistula and the stented ureteric orifices (Fig. 54.1a, b). If there is substantial leakage of pneumoperitoneum, the vagina is packed with a wet sponge to prevent the loss. The bladder is then mobilized from the anterior aspect of the lower uterine segment/vagina. The pre-placed stents or ureteric catheters provide an anatomic bearing of the ureteric orifices and help prevent or identify inadvertent injury to the ureters. The fistula is then circumscribed, disconnecting the bladder from the anterior vaginal wall (Fig. 54.2a, b). The key to a successful outcome is slow and careful sharp dissection of the fistulous edges as the trigone and ureteric orifices are invariably lying in close proximity, and also to avoid wide excision,which may hamper subsequent closure. Fistulous edges are freshened and bleeding is controlled with bipolar cautery. However, it is not essential to excise the rim of fistulous edge, as it becomes raw in any case.

54.6.4 Repair of the Fistula

The vagina is then sutured with 3-0 polyglactin as a running watertight stitch in either a transverse or

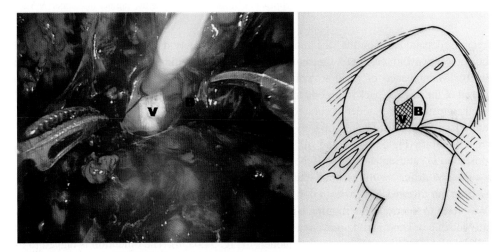

Fig. 54.1 Intraoperative photograph and diagrammatic representation showing minimal vertical midline cystotomy with a large VVF (packed with white sponge pad). The Foley's catheter is splinting open the cystotomy. B-Bladder; V-Vagina

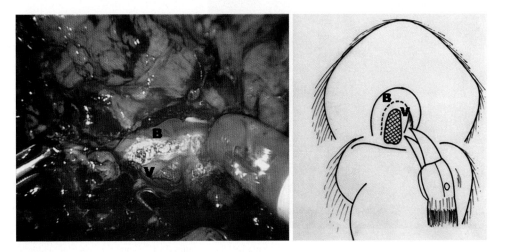

Fig. 54.2 Intraoperative photograph and diagrammatic representation shows dissection of the fistula. B-Bladder; V-Vagina

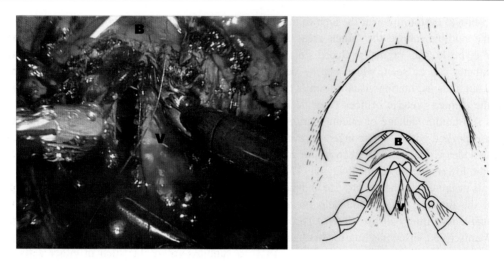

Fig. 54.3 Intraoperative photograph and diagrammatic representation shows suturing of the vagina. B-Bladder; V-Vagina

vertical direction (depending upon the size and orientation of the defect) to avoid tension on the suture line (Fig. 54.3a, b). Maintenance of pneumoperitoneum despite removal of the vaginal pack indirectly tests the adequacy of the closure. The bladder is sutured vertically or transverse in two layers using 3-0 polyglactin or poliglecaprone suture (Figs. 54.4a, b and 54.5). A Z-plasty modification in suturing is required if the fistula is close to a ureteric orifice, with the final suture line appearing zigzag, an inverted Y, or with a dog-ear on one side. We prefer to interrupt this running stitch by intermittently locking or knotting it to prevent laxity of the suture. To check for integrity of closure, the bladder

is moderately distended with sterile water through an 18-Fr indwelling trans-urethral catheter. In the event of any minor leakage, additional interrupted sutures are applied.

54.6.5 Interposition of the Tissue Between Two Suture Lines

A well-vascularized, pedicled omentum is interposed between the bladder and the vaginal suture lines (Fig. 54.6a, b). The omentum is tagged to the resilient

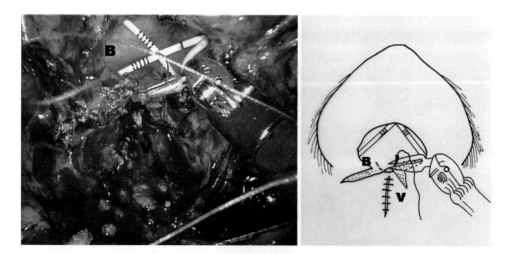

Fig. 54.4 Intraoperative photograph and diagrammatic representation shows sutured vagina and first layer of bladder closure. Both the ureteral stents are visible. B-Bladder; V-Vagina

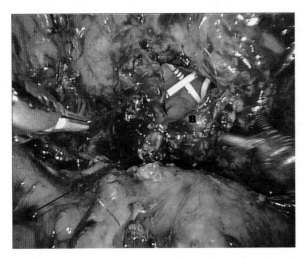

Fig. 54.5 Intraoperative photograph showing continuous suturing of the bladder. Both the distal ends of the ureteral stents can be seen through the remaining cystotomy. B-Bladder; V-Vagina

vaginal wall, which provides stability. In case the omentum is unavailable or cannot be adequately mobilized, the appendices epiploicae of the sigmoid colon or a local peritoneal flap is used for interposition between the suture lines. A drain is then placed in the rectovaginal pouch.

54.7 Special Considerations

One of the important steps to be considered is the transvaginal catheterization of the VVF. This is achieved by placement of a ureteric catheter placed from the bladder, cystoscopically, cannulating the fistula and retrieving it from the vagina. Tugging the catheter aids locate the approximate site of the fistula as seen from within the abdominal cavity allowing the placement of a 'minimal' cystotomy near the area of interest, close to the midline.

In larger fistulae, a Foley's catheter is placed transvaginally to achieve the same. Additionally, the catheter plugs the fistulae allowing bladder distension during cystoscopy.

During the fistula dissection phase of the procedure the catheter is pulled intra-abdominally (if required), which retracts open the vesicotomy, improving visualization of the fistula.

The ease of suturing and dexterity provided by the robot assistance allows concomitant ureteric reimplantation to be performed in cases wherein the fistula is too close to the ureteric orifice.

54.8 Step to Avoid Complications

a. Ureteric catheterization is an important step to prevent inadvertent ureteral injury during dissection as well as during reconstruction. It allows visualization of the ureteric orifices within the bladder, preventing taking a stitch too close to them during bladder reconstruction.

b. Adequate adhesiolysis is mandatory prior to performing a vesicotomy. The primary causative procedure will invariably lead to intraperitoneal

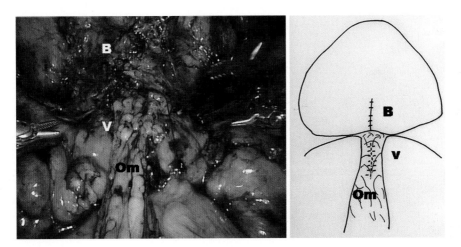

Fig. 54.6 Intraoperative photograph and diagrammatic representation shows omentum interposition between the two suture lines. B- Bladder; V-Vagina; Om-Omentum

adhesion. These could be parietal in nature, where adhesiolysis may be necessary to allow appropriate port placement or could be visceral wherein bowel loops may obscure the area of interest in the pelvis. Gentle and sharp dissection to aid the bowel to fall away is imperative to prevent a bowel injury during fistula dissection and allow tension-free closure of the vagina and bladder.

c. 'Stay midline' is probably the safest dictum to follow to prevent ureteric injury during dissection.

d. It is important to make available interposing tissue (omentum, sigmoid epiploacae, or peritoneal flap) which can be applied in between the suture lines.

References

1. Miller E, Webster GD. Current management of vesicovaginal fistulae. *Curr Opin Urol*. 2001;11:417–421.

2. Hilton P, Ward A. Epidemiological and surgical aspects of urogenital fistulae: A review of 25 years experience in southeast Nigeria. *Int Urogynaecol J*. 1998;9: 189–194.

3. Sotelo R, Mariano MB, Garcia-Segui A, et al. Laparoscopic repair of vesicovaginal fistula. *J Urol*. 2005;173: 1615–1618.

4. Chibber PJ, Shah HN, Jain P. Laparoscopic O'Conor's repair for vesico-vaginal and vesico-uterine fistula. *Br J Urol*. 2005;96:183–186.

5. Wong C, Lam PN, Lucente VR. Laparoscopic transabdominal transvaginal vesicovaginal fistula repair. *J Endourol*. 2006;20:24–43.

6. Nabi G, Hemal AK. Laparoscopic repair of vesicovaginal fistula and right nephrectomy for nonfunctioning kidney in a single session. *J Endourol*. 2001;15(8):801–803.

7. Hemal AK, Kumar R, Nabi G. Post-cesarean cervicovesical fistula: technique of laparoscopic repair. *J Urol*. 2001;165(4): 1167–1168.

8. Sundaram BM, Kalidasan G, Hemal AK. Robotic repair of vesicovaginal fistula: Case series of five patients. *Urology*. 2006;67:970–973.

9. Hemal AK, Kolla SB, Wadhwa P. Robotic reconstruction for recurrent supratrigonal vesicovaginal fistulas. *J Urol*. 2008;180(3):981–985.

Chapter 55

Robotic Surgery in Male Infertility (Robotic-Assisted Microsurgery)

Georges A. de Boccard and Alexander Mottrie

55.1 Introduction

Robot-assisted laparoscopic surgery allows very fine suturing in parts of the body that are usually inaccessible. Its advantages in terms of instrument manipulation, absence of vibrations, and console ergonomics have been demonstrated,[1] bringing up the question of applying robotics to open access.[2]

The feasibility of micro-sutures appeared to be limited by a lack of suture resistance and the da Vinci system's lack of tactile feedback.

In fact, the sensation of force feedback is visually obtained in the same way as in manual microsurgery. The instruments are manipulated with light pressure to avoid mashing the thread or bending the needle. The pressure of the forceps jaws is the lowest at the tips, which is the only part of the instrument used. It is possible to perform vaso–vaso and epididymo–vaso anastomosis with sutures as thin as 11/0, using two Black Diamond microforceps, one Potts scissors, and a Goldstein's microspike approximator. The duration of the procedure, including the robot installation, is not increased. This has been demonstrated in animal models first[3] and then in man[4, 5]

Use of the fourth arm shortens the procedure, since the operator can maintain focus during an instrument change. HD camera gives a very fine and precise vision.

G.A. de Boccard (✉)
Robot-Assisted Laparoscopic Surgery Center, Clinic Generale Beaulieu, Geneva, Switzerland
e-mail: boccard@iprolink.ch

Vasovasostomy and Vasoepididymostomy: Use of the da Vinci Robot in a Complete Extracorporeal Way to Perform Micro-Sutures

55.2 Installation in the Operating Room

(a) Important points

i. The robot is prepared on the left side of the table. Arm 3 is placed on the right side. The scrub nurse stays on the right of the patient with the instrument table (Fig. 55.1).

ii. Only one screen is necessary. It allows the scrub nurse to follow the intervention. An assistant is not necessary.

iii. The anesthesiologist stays at the patient's head and his movements are not restricted.

iv. The console location is not important.

55.3 Patient's Position

The patient is in dorsal decubitus, with legs together. The robot is placed perpendicularly on his left side with the camera centered on the scrotal incision. Proper placement of the camera arm is mandatory to obtain adequate mobility of the camera, which must permit access to both sides without repositioning of the robot or the patient (Fig. 55.2).

55.4 Trocars Placement

Important points:

v. Three #8 metal trocars are used to maintain the instruments and a plastic #12 trocar is used for the camera (Fig. 55.3).

A.K. Hemal, M. Menon (eds.), *Robotics in Genitourinary Surgery*,
DOI 10.1007/978-1-84882-114-9_55, © Springer-Verlag London Limited 2011

Fig. 55.1 Position of the surgeon and the robot

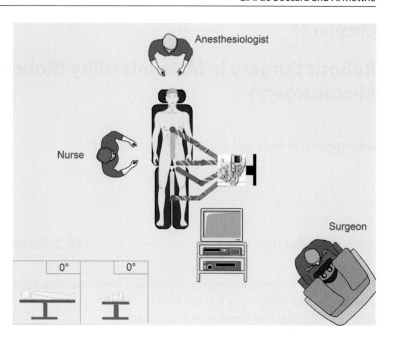

vi. The trocars are used only to maintain the instruments, but do not have any proper function such as ensuring tightness as in case of laparoscopy. Arms 1 and 2 are mounted with two Black Diamond microforceps and placed at 45° on both sides of the optic. Arm 3 holds a Potts scissors and is placed on the right with an angle of 30° with respect to the patient, facing the camera.

vii. The trocar tips are placed 10 cm from the operative field in order to allow very precise instrument movements without the risk of collision among the arms. The camera will be at 3 cm from the field. (There is no heat effect at this distance)

55.5 Instrumentation List

(b) Table of instruments used: (An assistant is not necessary.) (Table 55.1).

(c) The sutures used for anastomosis are Ethilon 9/0 and 10/0 with a BV4 round needle. A white multitubular drain is placed in the back of the operative field.

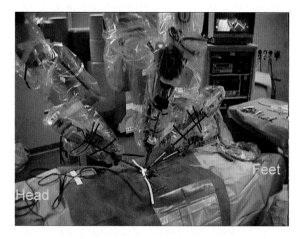

Fig. 55.2 Patients position

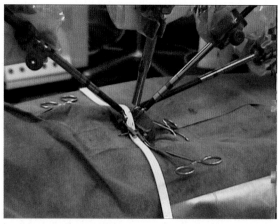

Fig. 55.3 Trocars configuration

Table 55.1 Instrument used

Surgeon instruments			Special instruments
Right arm (yellow)	Left arm (green)	Fourth arm (red)	
• Black diamond microforceps	• Black diamond microforceps	• Potts scissors	• Goldstein's microspike approximator

A white multitubular drain is placed in the back of the operative field.

55.6 Technique

(d) Technique for vasovasostomy

   i. Preparation of the operative field

The patient is preferably under general anesthesia, in order to avoid involuntary movements, which would disturb the proper course of the intervention and prolong it needlessly. Antibiotic prophylaxis (cephalosporin) is given. The scrotum is shaved and the skin is disinfected with aqueous betadine solution. The drapes are installed as a square, allowing only the scrotum to emerge. The verge is attached by the upper field to the abdominal skin.

   ii. Skin incision and preparation of spermatic structures.

This part is the same as for the classical microsurgery. The surgeon stays to the right of the patient and is assisted by a scrub nurse. A median scrotal incision starting from the penoscrotal angle is made over the length of 5 cm. The subcutaneous tissue is incised with an electric scalpel and then the left spermatic cord is dissected by spreading with scissors. The vas is located and its distal part is pulled out on a lacet. The proximal part is prepared in the same way and the fibrous portion separating the extremities is freed and then excised. It is not necessary to exteriorize the testicle. All bleeding must be controlled by bipolar coagulation, avoiding damaging the epididymal artery. The permeability of the distal segment is tested by injecting 2 mL of saline solution using a G 22 Venflon.

The fluid coming from the proximal segment is examined on the spot to look for spermatozoids. However, the absence of spermatozoids does not mean that the passage is blocked, but that recovery will probably take longer.

The two prepared segments are marked with a thread and placed back in the scrotum. The same procedure is performed on the other side. Then, the two straight vas ends are placed in the Goldstein's microspike approximator with a white multi-tubular drain at the bottom.

   iii. Robot installation

The robot must be prepared in advance on the left side of the patient. It is moved forward perpendicularly to the operating field, centered on the right vas presented in the Goldstein's microspike approximator (Fig. 55.4). The 0° optic is placed in a #12 trocar at an angle of 80°. The arm position should allow movement of a few centimeters to the left of the patient without changing the angle for the second anastomosis. Arms 1 and 2 have #8 trocars as in a laparoscopic intervention, but these are used only to support the instruments. They should not be too close to the field, as if they were in the abdominal cavity, and keep a distance of 10 cm between the black band at their

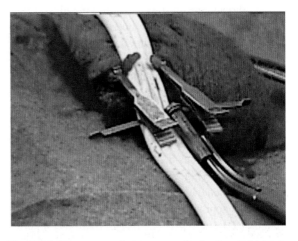

Fig. 55.4 Placement of the vas ends in the Goldstein's microspike approximator

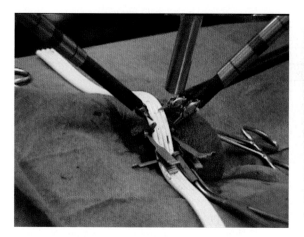

Fig. 55.5 Position of the instruments and the optic

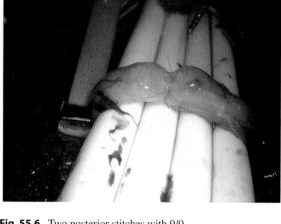

Fig. 55.6 Two posterior stitches with 9/0

tip and the vas. Trocars 1 and 2 hold Black Diamond microforceps (Fig. 55.5). They are placed at an angle of 45° with respect to the optic. Arm 3 is placed on the right. It also carries a #8 trocar holding Potts scissors and is placed in front of the camera at an angle of 30° with respect to the patient.

Then the surgeon can reach the console.

iv. Anastomosis

The console is set to perform ultrafine surgery. The light is adjusted if necessary using the "gain" buttons on the camera module. The vas ends can be re-cut and prepared in a fine way. The anastomosis is performed in the same way as in microsurgery:

The scrub nurse gives the microsurgical thread. She must wear magnifying glasses. She should not touch the operating field and shall continuously rinse the anastomosis with saline, using a syringe. While placing the stitches the operator maintains and stabilizes the vas deferens with help of one of the microforceps without pinching it. However, he can handle the fine peripheral aponeurosis without damage. Two separate posterior stitches are placed on the serous membrane with a 9/0 suture, cut at 4 cm (Fig. 55.6).

Then the mucous membrane is anastomosed by approximately six separate stitches using 10/0 sutures (Fig. 55.7). Then the anterior serous membrane is further strengthened using six separate 9/0 stitches. In some cases, it is

necessary to turn over the microapproximator in order to place a few extra posterior supporting stitches.

The two vas ends, which are now anastomosed, are delicately lifted by the robot forceps and the nurse cuts and then removes the drain away from the operating area (Fig. 55.8). She removes the microapproximator and the surgeon replaces the reconstituted right vas deferens in the scrotum.

The robot arms are discarded from the field and the left vas is pulled out of the scrotum with help of the marking suture left in place. It is placed in the microapproximator by the scrub nurse under control of the surgeon who leaves temporarily the console, but has not

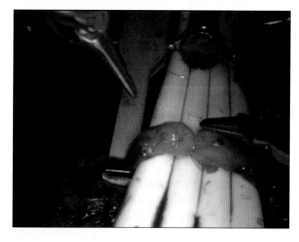

Fig. 55.7 Inner layer with 10/0

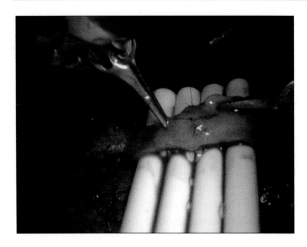

Fig. 55.8 Goldstein's microspike approximator is removed

rescrubbed. A white tubular drain is placed again at the bottom, facilitating the view of the threads.

The optics and the arms are moved a few centimeter to the left of the patient without changing their angle and the surgeon returns to the console for the second anastomosis.

After putting the second reconstituted vas deferens back in place, the robot is removed. The surgeon scrubs, after checking the hemostasis he closes the scrotal opening with one deep and one cutaneous running sutures with absorbable sutures.

(e) Technique for end-to-end vasoepididymostomy

  i. Preparation of the operating field
  The preparation is the same as for vasovasostomy

  ii. Incision and preparation of spermatic structures
  Following a medial incision of the scrotal skin, the testicle is taken out with its membranes. An incision is made in the vaginal membrane and the epididymis is exposed. If there is an obstruction, the epididymis tubules may appear dilated, but this is not always the case. The epididymis body is separated from the testicle and mobilized, making sure to preserve its vascularization. The vas is approached at the level of the epididymis head. It is dissected upward from the end of its circumvoluted part and cut. Its patency is tested by injecting 2

mL of saline, which should flow freely without any resistance. The cut end is passed through the top of the vaginal membrane and brought close to the epididymis, the circumvoluted part is ligated.

The second testicle is prepared in the same way and then replaced in the scrotum, making sure to locate the vas deferens end with the help of a 3/0 thread.

The first testicle is grasped and the distal part of epididymis is ligated and the body is sectioned. The spermatic liquid that leaks out is analyzed on the spot for the presence of spermatozoids. Presence of spermatozoids in this area is essential to continue the intervention. The Goldstein's microapproximator specially designed for end-to-end vasoepididymostomy is set up and the vas and epididymis are placed one end to the other.

  iii. Robot installation
  The position and installation of the arms are the same as for vasovasostomy.

  iv. Anastomosis

The first phase consists in observation of the cut epididymal tubules in order to identify the one from which the seminal liquid leaks periodically (Fig. 55.9). If necessary, it can be recut with the Potts scissors. After a few minutes of observation, the tubule is located and marked with a 10/0 suture.

Two separate stitches are placed on the posterior side with 9/0 sutures between the serous layer of the vas and epididymis without touching the marked

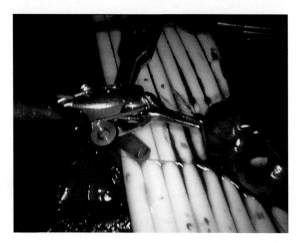

Fig. 55.9 Observation of the efferent tubule

tubule. The sutures are cut after each knot using the Potts scissors.

The mucous anastomosis is then performed with three 10/0 sutures placed in a triangle (Figs. 55.10 and 55.11). The anastomosis is completed by six 9/0

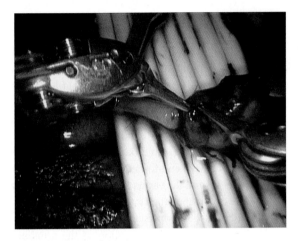

Fig. 55.10 Inner layer with three 10/0 sutures placed in a triangle

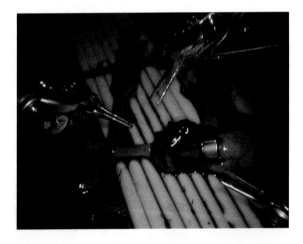

Fig. 55.11 Completion of the inner layer

stitches, closing the aponeurosis of the epididymis on the vas deferens serous membrane. Two PDS 7/0 stitches are finally placed to avoid traction of the anastomosis.

The surgeon scrubs again and returns to the operating field to place the operated side back in the scrotum. He pulls out the second testis and prepares the second anastomosis. It is not advisable to prepare both sides at once since, if the epididymis is cut too early, this may result in emptying of the tubules what makes it difficult to locate the efferent one.

The robot arms and camera are repositioned and the second anastomosis is performed in the same way.

After completing it, the surgeon scrubs again and returns a last time to the operating field. The robot is disconnected and various layers are closed with 4/0 absorbable sutures.

55.7 Important Points

(f) The sutures

The way the knots are placed is essential. The sutures must be knotted alternatively with the right hand and with the left hand.

The suture ends must be grasped by crossing the forceps and the knot shall be placed flat, without tension. The left hand must grasp the right end of the suture. The right hand must roll around the suture twice then grasp the other end of the suture on the left side. The knot is placed flat by pulling apart the two forceps horizontally (Fig. 55.12).A second knot is placed in the same way. A third knot is not always necessary.

The needle or the suture must be grasped by the forceps along the axis of the instrument, without making an angle with respect to the suture or twisting the needle in order to avoid rupture of the thread.

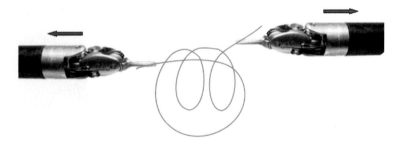

Fig. 55.12 Placing a flat knot

The thread or the needle must be held by the forceps tip in order to avoid applying too much force on the thread.

Before pressing the clutch pedal, the needle must be held in the right hand, at a slight distance from the field. Arm 3 with the Potts scissors is then activated and the thread is cut. Then, arm 3 is put back in its waiting position with the scissors pointing toward the field and arm 2 is activated again with the needle ready for the next suture.

The vas must never be grasped with the forceps, it should only be supported. Only the external membrane can be grasped.

In absence of mechanical tactile feedback, the suture's tension is appreciated by the apparent stretching (elasticity) of the suture and by the deformation of the tissue caused by the pressure exercised on it.

(g) Assistance and environment

The operating assistant or scrub nurse should never touch the field with an instrument. No pads or compresses are used. Constant rinsing with saline solution with a syringe and a Venflon is required.

Nobody should touch the patient, the operating table, or the robot during the procedure, since each movement or vibration will be felt by the surgeon, due to the very small size of the operating field.

55.8 How to Avoid Complications

(h) Prophylactic antibiotic therapy (Cephalosporin)
(i) Very thorough hemostasis
(j) Sufficient incision length
(k) Sufficient length of vas segments

References

1. Schiff J, Li PS, Goldstein M. Robotic microsurgical vaso-vasostomy and vasoepididymostomy: a prospective randomized study in a rat model. *J Urol*. 2004;171(4): 1720–1725.
2. Hemal AK, Menon M. Robotics in urology. *Curr Opin Urol*. 2004;14:89–93.
3. Kuang W, Shin PR, Oder M, Thomas AJ Jr. Robotic-assisted vasovasostomy: a two-layer technique in an animal model. *Urology*. 2005;65(4):811–814.
4. De Boccard G.Robotic vasectomy reversal. Geneva Foundation for Medical Research. 2006. http://www.gfmer. ch/Presentations_Fr/Vaso-vasostomie_robot_2006.htm. Accessed July 30, 2009
5. De Nayer G, Van Migen P, Schatteman P, Carpentier P, Fonteyne E, Mottrie A. Robotic assistance in urological microsurgery: initial report of a successful in-vivo robot-assisted vasovasostomy. *J Robotic Surg*. 2007;1: 161–162.

Part VIII
Patient's Perspective

Chapter 56

Treater to Target: Experiences of a Prostate Cancer Participant

Paul F. Schellhammer

Words matter. Therefore I have substituted "cancer participant" for the much more common term, "cancer survivor." Webster's dictionary defines survivor as: *One who lives through affliction, One who outlives another.* Survivor is the most common identifier for any individual who carries the diagnosis of a particular disease and is still alive. It is specifically applied in the cancer community to imply a victory over the declared enemy – the cancer cell. It also implies a certain degree of rigor and determination that a particular individual demonstrates in the cancer battle, and, consciously or subconsciously, implies that the nonsurvivors, the patients who have succumbed to their disease process, perhaps did not fight hard or long enough. Is the survivor a more positive thinker, a more active seeker of care, or imbued with whatever number of attributes that resulted in apparent victory? I use the word apparent because for the physician community, survivorship is time limited and measured in increments, whether 2, 3, 5, 10 years or beyond. For the patient community, it frequently is optimistically equated with cure. It is interesting here to recall the derivations of the word cure from the Latin word *curare* which is translated "to care." Caring for the patient with disease over the centuries, because of the increasing success of medical interventions, has translated to curing the patient with the disease. It has been inappropriately translated as a fix for the problem so that the problem is solved and relegated to an unpleasant and better forgotten memory of past history. However, since disease is a process and

caring for the patient with the disease is also a process and the first priority of a physician, we ought not condense all that this involves into the single endpoint – "the cure" – and thereby run the risk of minimizing "the caring."

The term survivor also conjures up the picture of an ongoing battle, long term or short term. Meriting and preserving that survivor state or designation, like in any battle, requires a state of hypervigilance and attention to the enemy. This constant state of hypervigilance can be exhausting and energy depleting. It tends to consume all of one's attention. It can be very non-productive and debilitating and adversely impact quality of life. This scenario is magnified in the case of prostate cancer, where very long life expectancy measured in years and even decades after diagnosis can be expected. Therefore, I have again chosen the descriptive "participant." The initial and specifically the subsequent treatments for cancer involve a process and I believe being a participant in the process provides a more productive outcome than that described by a combatant and survivorship mode. Participation encourages an attitude of living well with cancer which, in my opinion, is a primary objective. To paraphrase a statement to make this point – the patients who do best are those who don't battle disease but dance with it.

The mantra of today's medicine is to follow evidence-based principles which are based on well-conducted randomized controlled trials. In the case of prostate cancer few such trials exist to guide evidence-based decision making. Therefore we rely on retrospective reviews, observational series, and case reports which have a much lower pedigree of evidence. But a great deal can be learned from case series and case reports. Furthermore, a case report can imprint in our

P.F. Schellhammer (✉)
Sentara Medical Group, Eastern Virginia Medical School,
Urology of Virginia, Norfolk, VA, USA
e-mail: PFSCHELL@sentara.com

A.K. Hemal, M. Menon (eds.), *Robotics in Genitourinary Surgery*,
DOI 10.1007/978-1-84882-114-9_56, © Springer-Verlag London Limited 2011

memories a story which is more easily recalled than a series of summaries or reviews. In telling my story, in discussing my case report, I am articulating and repetitively clarifying the discussions I have had multiple times with patients in a similar situation. In fact, every clinic is an exercise in my thinking about the subject – from my personal perspective and from the prospective of the patient that I am counseling.

For the rest of this chapter I will discuss the treatment decisions and steps in which I have participated, my approach to these decision points, and, where available, provide references to studies that supported the decision. I trust the story, although officially only a level 4 case report is informative.

As a brief aside, I would like to quote a statement made by Malcolm Moore, one of the founders of Intel, when describing our age of technology. He said the power of information technology would double every 18 months into the foreseeable future. We have witnessed these leaps in our own lifetime. As an example, the current I-phone has many more times the computing power of the entire North American strategic air command in the 1960s. In the field of medicine, the characterization of the human genome which was begun in 1980 was predicted to consume extraordinary resources and have an unachievable timeline. However, it was completed earlier and at less cost because of high-throughput technology – and indeed it may not be too far in the future where individual genomic characterizations can be done for $100 or less. But technology is not biology and while technology will drive the accumulation of scientific knowledge as illustrated by the genome project – meaningful correlations and applications to cancer therapy in humans will proceed at a slower, sometimes frustratingly slower, pace.

56.1 Diagnosis

PSA was approved in 1986 as a marker to monitor for disease returns after radical prostatectomy and subsequently in 1996 as a diagnostic or screening marker. Intrigued by the possibility of PSA as a test for early detection, I became an early adopter and in 1990, at age 50, I began personal annual PSA testing. My first PSA was 2.4 ng/mL. I was quite content as this represented a result well below the accepted norm at

that time of 4.0 ng/mL. Annual PSA's through 1996 remained between 2.5 and 3.0 ng/mL. In 1995, Gann was the first to point out that absolute cutpoints were perhaps inappropriate and that PSA levels should be assessed as a continuous variable with increasing levels between 0 and 4 ng/mL, predicting for an increased risk of prostate cancer.[1] His data showed that a PSA level of 2–3 ng/mL represented a threefold risk for cancer when compared to a PSA of less than 1.0 ng/mL. This first foray into questioning the established level of 4 did not garner my attention and, furthermore, I had begun Proscar to combat bothersome LUTS. As anticipated, my PSA fell by greater than 50% and in 1998 was 1.0 ng/mL. My next PSA, 2 years later, was in 2000 and was recorded at 2.7 ng/mL. The alarm bell rang. I discontinued Proscar. My PSA rose to 6.5 ng/mL and TRUS-guided biopsies revealed Gleason 4+3 adenocarcinoma. The hiatus between 1998 and 2000 for PSA determination is explained by the fact that I suffered a myocardial infarction in 1998. Although there existed a strong family history for heart disease, my lipid profile was in the low-risk category. Furthermore, I had never had any symptoms and I had passed all the stress testing without incident. With this event, PSA concerns were put very much to the side as I engaged in cardiac rehabilitation. However, I think it is worth noting that the visceral reaction to my cardiac event versus that experienced with the cancer diagnosis was remarkably different. After the cardiac event, I vowed to partner with my heart in an exercise and dietary regimen and move forward toward better health. The diagnosis of cancer filled me with a sense of dread and betrayal. Destruction of the alien by whatever means was my immediate goal. All this in spite of the fact that I well knew that the greatest threat to my quality of life and longevity was heart disease and not prostate cancer. Even among the most well informed, and I consider myself well informed, emotions constitute a powerful driving force which override reason and measured deliberations. Urologists, all physicians, are asked by patients when they are confronted with a diagnosis: "Doc, what would you do?" "What would you advise your father or brother to do?" It is important to remember that, however, long and diligently we have weighed the question in our hypothetical situation, these hypothetical decisions do not include the emotional overlay of reality testing. The practice field differs from the playing field and we cannot assume that our measured assessments of pros and cons, risks and benefits would necessarily play out in similar fashion when personally faced with the facts.

The year was 2000 – available treatments for localized prostate cancer were surgery, external beam radiation, or brachytherapy. The laparoscopic and robotic-assisted approaches had not yet been introduced in the USA. I favored surgery not only because I was a practitioner of radical prostatectomy, but also because of its ability to remove billions of cancer cells in a 2–3 h procedure and to provide the additional information of pathologic staging that might direct further therapy. A ECOG trial[2] had been published demonstrating a survival benefit for adjuvant androgen deprivation when nodal metastases were present. The role of adjuvant radiation was being tested in a randomized controlled trial but results were not yet available. Analysis of this trial, recently published, demonstrating that adjuvant radiation therapy confers a survival benefit for patients with PT3 disease.[3] When patients ask me, "What is the best treatment currently available for localized prostate cancer?", I discuss with them the recommendations of the recent AUA prostate cancer guideline[4] which suggests that for low-, intermediate-, and high-risk disease, surgery, radiation, or active surveillance are appropriate choices with the caveat that with high-risk disease, active intervention is favored. A recent agency for health care and research assessment of treatment modalities for localized prostate cancer catalogues the risks and benefits of all therapies and emphasizes the importance of a well-informed patient.[5] After they consider all options, I tell them my rationale for choosing surgery but that I can well understand and support another choice.

The firm advice I can give with confidence is that time is on the side of the patient to review information, seek other opinions, and evaluate the risk benefit ratio of treatments. Often the most dissatisfied patients are those that propel themselves to urgent therapy without having given the time to evaluate the playing field. Before leaving the discussion of diagnosis, I will comment about the subject of screening and chemoprevention.

The urology community has digested the somewhat conflicting results of the PSA screening studies from the USA and Europe. The AUA has published a best practice statement encouraging patient education and consideration of baseline and subsequent interval PSAs for early detection. Urologists have disputed the US task force for prevention statement that PSA testing for patients over 75 years of age is inadvisable. If we are to pursue the diagnosis of prostate cancer with screening, we ought, with equal vigor, to employ a strategy that has been demonstrated through the RCT process to reduce the incidence/prevalence of the disease. The PCPT together with the recently reported results of the Reduce trial provides Level I evidence that opens the door for urologists to pre-empt early detection with disease prevention.*

56.2 Life After Radical Prostatectomy

My immediate postoperative course was uneventful. I say immediate because 6 weeks postoperative I developed fatigue, leg and abdominal pain, followed by fever and chills. A CT scan revealed a psoas abscess which was promptly drained percutaneously with eventual recovery. An example, however, that no procedure is complication free and that 30-day morbidity and mortality figures don't include operation-related problems arising day 31 and beyond.

Pathology was favorable reporting pT2, margin negative, N0, but Gleason 4+4 with a tertiary pattern of 5 (more about pathology reports later). Postoperative PSA's were undetectable at less than 0.01 ng/mL at 6 weeks and 6 months. Recovery of urinary continence and sexual function was satisfactory. However, I make it a point to advise patients that it is highly unlikely that sexual function will recover to match preoperative baseline, and that even urinary function; in the best of circumstances may have occasional lapses. At 1 year, my PSA returned to 0.09 ng/mL. Several months later it had climbed to 0.2 and 0.35 ng/mL. I could see nothing but a continued upward trend and that I would take action sooner or later. The question was, should it be sooner? At the time there were data from salvage radiation series that men whose PSA's were less than 1 ng/mL[6] had better outcomes than those whose PSA's were greater than 1 ng/mL. The larger multi-institutional cohort reported by Stephenson showing a clear correlation

---

* On 12/2/10 a ODAC panel overwhelmingly (17-0 & 14-4) voted against the approval of 5 alpha-reductase inhibitors for prostate cancer chemoprevention.

of postsalvage radiation PSA recurrence-free survival to pre-salvage PSA level had not yet been reported.[7] Some series advocated androgen deprivation together with salvage radiation for patients with high-risk features.[8] A Phase III trial comparing salvage radiation with or without Casodex 150 ng for 2 years (RTOG 9601) was ongoing but had not been unblinded for analysis (and remains unblinded to this date). I conferred with several "experts" most of whom advised against immediate therapy and specifically against radiation. This is in keeping with the general urologic practice as reported by an AUA survey in 1996 whereby only 13% of urologists stated that they employed salvage radiation therapy. Almost 10 years later in 2004, the CAPSure database assessment noted an increase to 20%.[9] However, the significant majority of urologists were not enamored with salvage radiation on the assumption that failure after radical prostatectomy is distant. But is PSA recurrence after radical prostatectomy due to local failure or distant failure, or both? Scans were normal and, as is usually the case, were not helpful in making this determination. I made the decision to receive 6 months of androgen deprivation along with prostate bed radiation.[8] The bone mineral density preserving effects of zoledronic acid had just been reported and I opted to receive zoledronic acid pre-androgen deprivation and at its completion in 6 months.

How can "early" salvage radiation plus androgen deprivation be supported? The evidence for local failure after radical prostatectomy has been documented with biopsy studies showing cancer in up to 40% of PSA failure cases.[10,11] The 10-year clinical local failure rate in the SPG4 trial and the control arm of SWOG 8794 approached 20%, higher than the distant failure rate.[12,13] Studies using MRI have shown a much higher incidence of bone metastatic disease than would be found by the traditional bone scan,[14] and disseminated tumor cells are present in the bone marrow in men with PSA failure with alarming frequency.[15] These findings also support the distant failure component of PSA recurrence. Observational studies from Stanford demonstrated a benefit using androgen deprivation and whole pelvic radiation versus prostate bed radiation alone.[8] Fortunately a number of trials are in process that will resolve uncertainties concerning mono versus combination therapy and the benefit of extended field radiation. The RTOG trial 0534 is a three-arm trial which will test prostate

bed radiation only versus prostate bed radiation plus androgen deprivation versus whole pelvic radiation plus prostate bed radiation plus androgen deprivation. The UKNCI Canadian Radicals trial will test adjuvant versus salvage radiation each with no, short-, or long-term androgen deprivation. The Stampede trial is a multi-armed sequential trial that will test at androgen deprivation ± docetaxel, zoledronic acid, or Celebrex.[16] It is encouraging that level 1 evidence will be available in the future upon which to base decisions. But currently Level 4 evidence from a large cohort gathered from a number of cancer centers supports salvage radiation initiated when the PSA level is < 0.5 ng/mL for a 48% PSA progression-free response at 6-year follow-up.[7]

As already noted, SWOG 8794 provides Level I evidence that postradical prostatectomy adjuvant radiation offers a statistically significant benefit in cancer-specific and overall survival for patients with pT3 disease.[3] Currently the question is: "Can salvage radiation at PSA rise provide benefits equal to that of adjuvant radiation while avoiding unnecessary therapy in the pT3 cohort who will never experience clinical or biochemical failure?" But a bright line distinguishing adjuvant from salvage radiation does not exist and what might be identified as adjuvant in some cases is more appropriately classified as salvage. Radiation is classified as salvage when given for a PSA rising above an identified undetectable cutpoint. This undetectable cutpoint is a moving target. On their review of the literature, the prostate cancer guidelines committee identified 54 cutpoints used to identify PSA failure after radical prostatectomy.[7] For uniformity of reporting, they established ≤0.2 ng/mL as an undetectable PSA. Others have supported a higher level of ≤ 0.4 ng/mL.[17] Patients receiving radiation identified as "adjuvant" within the first 4–6 months after radical prostatectomy when their PSA is undetectable by these definitions would be receiving radiation identified as salvage when lower PSA failure cutpoints are utilized. In the SWOG 8794 adjuvant trials 30% of patients had detectable PSAs and, therefore, by definition, were in reality receiving salvage radiation.

For accuracy of reporting and analysis, postradical prostatectomy radiation might be better calibrated to a PSA trigger and time boundary after surgery, than to the terms "adjuvant" or "salvage." And I believe that urologists who would prefer to apply radiation only for evidence of a rising PSA should consider using reliable ultra-sensitive PSA levels. The success of salvage radiation is PSA sensitive and is most successful when delivered at lower absolute PSA levels.[18] The initiation of postradical prostatectomy radiation at the earliest indication of a PSA rise might narrow any gap of benefit that might separate "adjuvant" from "salvage" therapy.

56.3 Postradiation

Radiation was delivered in a traditional four-field box technique to a dose of 64 Gy and was not carried beyond to the currently recommended 70 Gy because of urinary and GI side effects. These symptoms resolved completely with time. Androgen deprivation was quite tolerable. Hot flashes were minimal. The dramatic suppression of libido brought me to the powerful recognition, beyond any text description, of the power of the steroid molecules to imprint and drive behavior. I discontinued androgen deprivation after 6 months of therapy at which time my PSA has fallen to less than 0.02 ng/mL. This level was maintained over the next 3 years. Serum testosterone recovered and I truly felt that the clock had been reset and that my quality of life had been restored to the pre-hypogonadal state. Equipoise had been re-established and life was good. That is not to say that life had been previously bad. I only use this well-understood colloquialism to express my renewed state of well-being. However, 36 months after initiation of androgen deprivation and 33 months after completion of salvage radiation, the PSA began another series of rises. It is worth reflecting on the emotional impact of the first rise after radical prostatectomy and this second and subsequent rises. The first PSA rise after surgery brought home the fact that surgery had failed to remove all cancer and that "cure" (yes, I was in this thought mode) had not been achieved. There was significant anxiety and disappointment. The second PSA failure confirmed that I was in the story for the long haul. The alien remained in residence. Resolve replaced anxiety and disappointment. I was going to become a greater participant in the process and would need to turn my strategy from cancer elimination to delaying progression and living well with the situation. And it was now necessary to start thinking about the next step. I obtained serial PSA's

over the next 6 months with a progression to a PSA of 0.7 ng/mL (calculated doubling time of approximately 4 months). During this time I scanned for the possibilities of a clinical trial in lieu of androgen deprivation. Androgen deprivation was certainly going to play a role in the future but other clinical trial possibilities might be of benefit, and androgen deprivation would disqualify entry in these trials. Throughout the years I had encouraged patients to enter clinical trials and supervised many such patients on a number of a wide variety of Phase II and Phase III trials. Now it was my turn to practice what I had preached.

56.4 Search for Clinical Trial

Quite remarkable, in 2004, there was a paucity of clinical trials for a rising PSA in the hormone naïve population (since androgen deprivation was 3 years previous and my testosterone was normal, I was still in the naïve clinical state). One was a vaccine immunotherapy trial under the auspices of CALGB and another tyrosine kinase inhibitor trial under ECOG. Geography determined the trial in which I would enroll because the ECOG site was a short Southwest airlines flight away permitting 1 day travel to and return. I was most satisfied with the clinical care but personal experience with trials demonstrated that clinical trial entry and participation are every time intense and resource consumptive effort. In the absence of my position as a physician whereby I could determine blood draws and scan schedules, it would have been quite difficult to adhere to trial requirements. It would certainly impact on the earning power and professional responsibilities of the average citizen. Clearly a more friendly clinical trial process is necessary for the patient and physician. Clinical trialists have written convincingly in this regard. Streamlining will be necessary if the 2–3% enrolment is to be improved upon and if Level I evidence is to become available.[19]

While the experimental agent, (I received a dual tyrosine kinase inhibitor, which was recently approved for the use in recurrent breast cancer), slowed the rate of PSA rise, it nevertheless continued to progress to a level of 4 ng/mL. At this time I felt it was appropriate to once again pull the androgen deprivation trigger.

Parenthetically the final analysis of this ECOG trial is still pending as is the correlation of response with tissue Erb 2, and EGF levels, the receptors against which the dual tyrosine kinase inhibitor was directed. Information from clinical trials can be long delayed.

An interesting observation as a result of this trial process was the review of pathology as part of eligibility. Both the initial pathology and the trial review of pathology were reported by expert genitourinary pathologists. There was significant discrepancy in both the pathologic staging (PT 2, margin negative became PT 3A margin positive) and Gleason grade (4+4 with tertiary pattern of 5 became 3+4). Clearly comparing results of one institutional series to another is problematic due to the subjective nature of pathology examination and variability of institutional definitions. And add to all of this the variables with specimen processing.

56.5 The Rest of the Story

If I was to initiate androgen deprivation, I made the decision to employ combined androgen blockade, a combination of Lh/Rh agonists, anti-androgen, and 5-alpha reductase inhibitor. While the PSA fell, it did so somewhat sluggishly and after reaching a PSA nadir of 0.2 ng/mL began rising at 9 months post-initiation of therapy. At 0.4 ng/mL anti-androgens were withdrawn without response. There is ample data that a PSA nadir is a prognostic factor with regard to subsequent outcome[20] and some recent intriguing data would suggest that PSA lower than 0.2 ng/mL, and into the ultrasensitive undetectable level of less than 0.05 ng/mL, is desirable.[21] I decided to participate further into the field of secondary hormonal therapy based on the accumulating evidence of persistent androgen receptor activity in what is now termed the castrate resistant rather than the androgen independent or hormone refractory state. The term "castrate resistant" may need further refinement definition. What is a castrate T level? Traditionally 50 ng/mL has been the cutpoint to identify the castrate state and is the FDA requirement for approval of agents for medical castration. This is only because radioimmune assays have been limited in their ability to a lower level reliability. Newer chemoluminescent methodology permits serum T level assessment to levels < 0.1 ng/mL. Furthermore ample evidence now exists that serum T does not reflect tissue T because cellular benign and

especially malignant enzymatic activity produces T sufficient to drive the androgen receptor. All these findings extend the window of opportunity for AR receptor modulation and secondary hormonal therapy prior to cytotoxic therapy. I believe in the future we will need to redefine the serum testosterone level which identifies the castrate-resistant state. And we will need to recognize that tissue androgens and the steriodogenic enzymes to produce them reside in the prostate cancer cell even while serum testosterone registers a castrate level.

I began a transdermal estradiol patch,[22] ketoconazole, and hydrocortisone[23] and based on some interesting but oft not utilized therapy, a brief course of GMCSF.[24] All have been tolerated with negligible side effects. Estradial has eliminated the hot flushes and is maintaining bone health. Recall that the VAURG studies demonstrated that DES 5.0 mg was associated with an excellent cancer-specific survival – superior to orchiectomy – an observation overwhelmed by the higher all cause mortality secondary to an excess of cardiovascular deaths. Transdermal absorption side steps the cardiovascular side effects by avoiding the first pass risk of oral therapy. My PSA level reversed and stabilized at 0.2–0.4 ng/mL. Muscle mass has certainly suffered, although I have managed to avoid weight gain by adhering to a home-based diet of soy burgers, fish, beans, and rice (meetings and events provide a brief respite).

I am happy to be on statins for heart health and Celebrex to combat arthritis. Both are associated with data to support activity against prostate cancer. I take Vitamin D to keep my serum level >32 ng/mL. This requires 4,000 IU cholecalciferol D3 daily. Yes, I take lycopene and low-dose selenium* and three omega fatty acid supplements. And since all medicine needs to go down, I take the opportunity to use green tea and pomegranate juice to provide the vehicle.[25]

I also look forward to the advances that promise new therapeutic options. Sipuleucel-T[26] has demonstrated a survival benefit and opens a fourth modality immunotherapy for the treatment of prostate cancer and hopefully other cancers as well. Abiraterone, which is very effective in lowering serum and likely tissue androgens has shown promise in Phase II trials

----

* Selenium has been discontinued based on SELECT trial data.

and is currently being tested in large Phase III RCTs.[27] MDV 3100, a novel anti-androgen which not only inhibits ligand binding but also inactivates and abrogates the receptor, has also shown promise in Phase II trials and is undergoing testing in Phase III RCT.[28]

In conclusion, prostate cancer is often not cured or completely eradicated but can be reduced to a chronic disease which may be controlled for a prolonged period of time. Philosophically it can be said to mimic life by its slow pace of attrition. Patients can be considered participants and partners in the process of the therapeutic efforts to slow attrition. Finally I paraphrase a physician author Wendy Harpham who described her reaction to the news that her hematologic malignancy had returned after a period of remission. She wrote as follows – my cancer didn't make life uncertain but exposed me to the uncertainties of life. In losing my sense of tomorrow, its concerns, its uncertainties, I began to appreciate the time I had – and a way never before possible – I found today. So I continue to participate and life is good.

References

1. Gann PH, Hennekens CH, Stampfer MJ. A prospective evaluation of plasma prostate-specific antigen for detection of prostatic cancer. *JAMA*. January 25, 1995;273(4):289–294.
2. Messing EM, Manola J, Yao J, et al. Eastern cooperative oncology group study EST 3886. Immediate versus deferred androgen deprivation treatment in patients with node-positive prostate cancer after radical prostatectomy and pelvic lymphadenectomy. *Lancet Oncol*. June, 2006;7(6):472–479.
3. Thompson IM, Tangen CM, Paradelo J, et al. Adjuvant radiotherapy for pathological T3N0M0 prostate cancer significantly reduces risk of metastases and improves survival: long-term followup of a randomized clinical trial. *J Urol*. March, 2009;181(3):956–962.
4. Thompson I, Thrasher JB, Aus G, et al. AUA prostate cancer clinical guideline update panel. Guideline for the management of clinically localized prostate cancer: 2007 update. *J Urol*. June, 2007;177(6):2106–2131.
5. Wilt TJ, Shamliyan T, Taylor B, et al. Comparative effectiveness of therapies for clinically localized prostate cancer. Comparative Effectiveness Review No. 13. (Prepared by Minnesota Evidence-based Practice Center under Contract No. 290-02-00009.) Rockville, MD: Agency for Healthcare Research and Quality. February, 2008.
6. Schild SE, Wong WW, Grado GL, et al. The result of radical retropubic prostatectomy and adjuvant therapy for pathologic stage c prostate cancer. *Int J Radiat Oncol Biol Phys*. February 1, 1996;34(3):535–541.
7. Stephenson AJ, Scardino PT, Kattan MW, et al. Predicting the outcome of salvage radiation therapy for recurrent prostate cancer after radical prostatectomy. *J Clin Oncol*. September 10, 2007;25(26):4153.
8. Spiotto MT, Hancock SL, King CR. Radiotherapy after prostatectomy: improved biochemical relapse-free survival with whole pelvic compared with prostate bed only for high-risk patients. *Int J Radiat Oncol Biol Phys*. September 1, 2007;69(1):54–61.
9. Mehta SS, Lubeck DP, Sadetsky N, Pasta DJ, Carroll PR. Patterns of secondary cancer treatment for biochemical failure following radical prostatectomy: data from capsure. *J Urol*. January, 2004;171(1):215–219.
10. Lightner DJ, Lange PH, Reddy PK, Moore L. Prostate specific antigen and local recurrence after radical prostatectomy. *J Urol*. October, 1990;144(4):921–926.
11. Koppie TM, Grossfeld GD, Nudell DM, Weinberg VK, Carroll PR. Is anastomotic biopsy necessary before radiotherapy after radical prostatectomy? *J Urol*. 2001;166(1):111–115.
12. Swanson GP, Hussey MA, Tangen CM, et al. Predominant treatment failure in postprostatectomy patients is local: analysis of patterns of treatment failure in SWOG 8794. *J Clin Oncol*. June 1, 2007;25(16):2225–2229.
13. Bill-Axelson A, Holmberg L, Ruutu M, et al. Radical prostatectomy versus watchful waiting in early prostate cancer. *N Engl J Med*. May 12, 2005;352(19):1977–1984.
14. Lecouvet FE, Geukens D, Stainier A, et al. Magnetic resonance imaging of the axial skeleton for detecting bone metastases in patients with high-risk prostate cancer: diagnostic and cost-effectiveness and comparison with current detection strategies. *J Clin Oncol*. 2007;25:3281–3287.
15. Morgan TM, Lange PH, Porter MP, et al. Disseminated tumor cells in prostate cancer after radical prostatectomy and without evidence of disease predicts biochemical recurrence. *Clin Can Res*. January 15, 2009;15(2):677–683.
16. James ND, Sydes MR, Clarke NW, et al. Systemic therapy for advancing or metastatic prostate cancer (STAMPEDE): a multi-arm, multistage randomized controlled trial. *BJU Int*. 2009;103(4):464–469. [Epub October 8, 2008]. Accessed February, 2009.
17. Stephenson AJ, Kattan MW, Eastham JA, et al. Defining biochemical recurrence of prostate cancer after radical prostatectomy: a proposal for a standardized definition. *J Clin Oncol*. 2006;24(24):3973–3978.
18. Cookson MS, Aus G, Burnett AL, et al. Variation in the definition of biochemical recurrence in patients treated for localized prostate cancer: the American urological association prostate guidelines for localized prostate cancer update panel report and recommendations for a standard in the reporting of surgical outcomes. *J Urol*. 2007;177(2):540–545.
19. Steensma DP. The ordinary miracle of cancer clinical trials. *J Clin Oncol*. April 10, 2009;27(11):1761–1766.
20. Hussain M, Tangen CM, Higano C, et al. Southwest oncology group trial 9346 (INT-0162). Absolute prostate-specific antigen value after androgen deprivation is a strong independent predictor of survival in new metastatic prostate cancer: data from southwest oncology Group Trial 9346 (INT-0162). *J Clin Oncol*. August 20, 2006;24(24):3984–3990.

21. Scholz M, Lam R, Strum S, Jennrich R, Johnson H, Trilling T. Prostate-cancer-specific survival and clinical progression-free survival in men with prostate cancer treated intermittently with testosterone-inactivating pharmaceuticals. *Urology*. September, 2007;70(3):506–510.

22. Ockrim JL, Lalani EN, Laniado ME, Carter SS, Abel PD. Transdermal estradiol therapy for advanced prostate cancer – forward to the past? *J Urol*. May, 2003;169(5):1745–1746.

23. Small EJ, Baron A, Bok R. Simultaneous antiandrogen withdrawal and treatment with ketoconazole and hydrocortisone in patients with advanced prostate carcinoma. *Cancer*. 1997;80(9):1755–1759.

24. Rini BI, Weinberg V, Bok R, Small EJ. Prostate-specific antigen kinetics as a measure of the biologic effect of granulocyte-macrophage colony-stimulating factor in patients with serologic progression of prostate cancer. *J Clin Oncol*. January 1, 2003;21(1):99–105.

25. Hong MY, Seeram NP, Heber D. Pomegranate polyphenols down-regulate expression of androgen-synthesizing genes in human prostate cancer cells overexpressing the androgen receptor. *J Nutr Biochem*. 2008;19(12):848–855. [Epub May 13, 2008]. Accessed December, 2008.

26. Higano CS, Schellhammer PF, Small EJ, Burch PA, Nemunaitis J, Yuh L, Provost N, Frohlich MW. Integrated data from 2 randomized, double-blind, placebo-controlled, phase 3 trials of active cellular immunotherapy with sipuleucel-T in advanced prostate cancer. *Cancer*. August 15, 2009;115(16):3670–3679.

27. Attard G, Reid AH, A'Hern R, Parker C, Oommen NB, Folkerd E, Messiou C, Molife LR, Maier G, Thompson E, Olmos D, Sinha R, Lee G, Dowsett M, Kaye SB, Dearnaley D, Kheoh T, Molina A, de Bono JS. Selective inhibition of CYP17 with abiraterone acetate is highly active in the treatment of castration-resistant prostate cancer. *J Clin Oncol*. August 10, 2009;27(23):3742–3748. [Epub May 26, 2009].

28. Tran C, Ouk S, Clegg NJ, et al. Development of a second-generation antiandrogen for treatment of advanced prostate cancer. *Science*. 2009;324(5928):787–790. [Epub April 9, 2009]. Accessed May 9, 2009.

Chapter 57

My Prostate Cancer

John M. Barry

57.1 Introduction

On March 6, 2007, I had a robotic-assisted radical prostatectomy and pelvic lymph node dissection for a pT2C, N0, M0, Gleason 3 + 4 adenocarcinoma of the prostate. At my 3-year follow-up, I was disease-free, continent of urine, and as potent as I wanted to be. This is my story.

57.2 Diagnosis and Treatment Plan

My serum prostate-specific antigen (PSA) level was elevated to 6.81 ng/mL on October 9, 2006. I was 66 years old. My prostate was normal on digital rectal examination. All of my previous PSA determinations had been normal, and I didn't have time to deal with the issue. There were two meetings coming up, the Western Section of the American Urological Association (AUA) and the Northwest Urological Society (NWUS), and I wanted to spend Christmas with my mother who was dying in a nursing home in Winona, MN, 2,000 miles away. At the section meeting, I was nominated to be the President of the AUA. After the NWUS meeting in early December, I spent Christmas with my mother, and then returned to Portland for a determination of my total and free PSA. On December 27, 2006, they were 6.7 ng/mL and 10%, respectively.

J.M. Barry (✉)
Division of Urology, Oregon Health and Science University,
Portland, OR, USA
e-mail: barryj@ohsu.edu

I plotted my data on two nomograms and determined that the probability of a positive biopsy was about 0.85.

I stopped taking a baby aspirin a day, which I had been doing for no good reason, calculated my International Prostate Symptom Score (IPSS) and Sexual Health in Men (SHIM) score (they were 7 and 21, respectively), and made two telephone calls: one to Dr. Mark Garzotto, one of our three urologic oncologists, and one to Karen Gates, RN who had been in our urology clinic nurse for over two decades. After my lower colon prep and an oral dose of a fluroquinolone, the three of us met in the procedure room of our urology clinic at 7:00 AM, Wednesday, January 3, 2007, where Mark did a digital rectal exam, a transrectal ultrasound (TRUS)-guided prostatic local anesthetic block, and 10 needle core biopsies. I developed a vasovagal reaction with the first biopsy, spent a few minutes in the head-down position until my blood pressure and pulse returned to normal, and nine more samples were taken. My prostatic apex was not numb.

At 8:00 AM, right after the biopsies, I did my morning general urology clinic, finished it shortly after noon, and then took the tram up the hill to the other campus to do the kidney transplant candidate clinic with the transplant nephrology staff and residents.

Dr. Chris Corless, genitourinary pathologist, read the slides later that day, and Mark Garzotto called and said that he and I needed to discuss the results. We met at the conclusion of the afternoon renal transplant candidate clinic and reviewed the results (Table 57.1). We agreed on the necessity of treatment of this intermediate risk prostate cancer and reviewed the options of surgery, radiation, cryosurgery, and high-intensity focused ultrasound (HIFU). We decided that the best therapy for this curable lesion was a

Table 57.1 Prostate biopsy results

Site	Right	(% of core)	Left	(% of core)
Base	3 + 3	<5	PIN	
Upper mid	3 + 4	10	3 + 4	10
Lower mid	3 + 3	20	3 + 3	5
Apex	3 + 3	20	Benign	
Transition zone			PIN	3 + 3

radical prostatectomy, probably unilateral nerve sparing on the left. The questions were, "Where and by whom?" I started my Kegel's exercises.

After input from many sources, including three of my friends who were experienced open prostatectomy surgeons and had become robotic prostatectomy surgeons, I decided to have a robotic-assisted laparoscopic radical prostatectomy by my friend of 25 years, Dr. Mani Menon, at the Vattikuti Urologic Institute of the Henry Ford Health System (HFHS) in Detroit. As he and I chatted on the telephone, I felt my anxieties melt away, and I knew the decision was correct.

57.3 Recovery from the Biopsies

Initial gross hematuria started the day after the biopsies and resolved, for the first time, 4 days later, just before my wife, Toni, and I went to the Oregon Governor's Inaugural Ball at the Convention Center. Hematuria returned on Monday, January 8, 2007, right after the resident, Dr. Lisa Bland, and I finished bilateral nephrectomies and a kidney transplant. It resolved 11 days after the biopsies.

The prostatic soreness required regular dosing with acetaminophen for 4 days. It recurred from time to time after that and it always responded to acetaminophen.

The lower urinary tract symptoms (LUTS) initially resolved 4 days after the biopsies, only to recur at decreasing intervals. By January 17, 2 weeks after the biopsy, the LUTS were gone.

A sleep disturbance began the day of the biopsies and required some help from my primary care physician, Dr. Donald Girard. He prescribed a short-acting hypnotic (zaleplon), which I took when I was awakened by thoughts about prostate cancer between 1:00 AM and 3:00 AM each night. The night of January 13, 10 days after the biopsies, sleep was finally undisturbed by my ruminations about prostate cancer.

My first ejaculate, a week after the biopsies, was like crank case oil (or hot fudge sauce, depending on one's frame of reference). A week later, it had changed to the color of caramel sauce, and then finally became clear.

January 11–26 was spent surfing, first in The Cove on Maui, and then on the North Shore of Oahu.

On January 13, 10 days after the biopsies, my thoughts changed from, "I'm going to miss my prostate" to "I want it out."

57.4 Detroit

Toni and I flew coach on Northwest Airlines from Portland, OR, to Detroit on Sunday, March 4. We were met in the baggage claim area by a driver with a Lincoln Town Car and taken to the Ritz-Carlton Hotel in Dearborn. We arrived at the hotel at about 7:00 PM. We stayed in a suite with Club Floor privileges and the Vattikuti Comfort and Care Package.

We were driven in a Town Car to the HFHS campus for our visit with Dr. Mani Menon's team and the Department of Anesthesiology on Monday, March 5. That evening, it was a soft diet and a bisacodyl suppository. Shameem, Mani's wife, called to see how I was doing, and I told her that I hadn't quite started bouncing off the walls, but I was close to doing so. My daughter, Dr. Michelle Barry, checked into the adjacent room very late that night.

57.5 Radical Robotic Prostatectomy + Bilateral Pelvic Lymphadenectomies

The three of us were up at 3:30 AM to get ready to take a Town Car back to the Henry Ford Hospital and its preoperative area. After I stripped and got into a hospital gown, Nurse Christine started an IV in my right hand, gave me heparin 5,000 subcutaneously, and hung the IV antibiotic, a cephalosporin. Pam, a big black woman, came in and shaved my anterior thighs and ticklish abdomen. Dan Eun, one of the urology residents, introduced himself, and Mani came by to say, "Hello." My anxiety level peaked. I started thinking about Saddam Hussein's execution and criminals who were getting prepared for lethal injection. Then I was wheeled out of the preoperative area, down the hall, and into OR 21. The anesthesiologist met me at the doorway, and in we went. It was the same room where I'd watched Mani do a robotic prostatectomy 17 months earlier when I was a Vattikuti Visiting Professor. I transferred to the OR table, and that's the last thing I remembered until we were on our way from the recovery room to my private room, 21A, on B-3. Michelle and Toni were with me. My calf squeezers were working, ketorolac was given IV every 6 h, and I was getting heparin 5,000 units subcutaneously every 8 h. The 20 Fr. 5 cc Bard 0165v20s Silastic-coated Foley catheter with 20 cc in the balloon was taped to my left thigh and drained into a bag off the left side of the bed.

I was euphoric! The prostate was out, and I was alive.

The evening of surgery, I was up, walking in the hall, and chatting with patients and their families. I even invited the wife and daughter of the man across the hall to come over and chat. He had undergone his radical prostatectomy that same day. I called my wife at the hotel and asked her to bring my laptop computer and thumb drives so I could give a talk the next morning.

The next morning, it was a liquid diet, an inspection of the six port sites, the left peri-umbilical one of which was the extraction site, and off to give my 7:00 AM Urology Grand Rounds talk, "Time Management for Urologists," in my purple Vattikuti Instititute robe and hooked to my Jackson-Pratt drain, IV, and urine drainage bag. This was followed by a short case presentation of a woman with end stage renal disease, chronic pyelonephritis and an ileal conduit. I gave a Society for the Prevention of Cruelty to the Prostate (SPCP) necktie to each of the three residents, Michael Fumo, Daniel Eun, and James Lewis, who had participated in my surgery. Then I returned to my room to wait for the discharge/outpatient care class. The nurse suggested that I take a couple of acetaminophen + codeine tablets to deal with any discomfort during the class. This turned out to be the only narcotic I took in the entire postoperative period. Brad Baize, a nurse with an injured hand, gave an excellent presentation about the expected postoperative course and how to manage the bladder drainage catheter and deal with potential problems. I was disappointed that many of the patients said that their urologists at home refused to provide follow-up care unless the procedure had been done by them or in their medical community. When I returned to my hospital room, I received my last dose of ketorolac, my last dose of heparin, my drain was removed, my IV was pulled, the catheter tape was removed and replaced with an elastic Velcro strap, I changed the overnight bag for a leg bag, and I got dressed in my navy blue suit, white shirt, and necktie. We called for a Town Car and the three of us returned to the Ritz-Carlton.

57.6 Postop Days 1–6

The afternoon of postoperative day 1, we walked from the hotel to the mall, which was about a quarter of a mile away, and back, and spent about an hour in the club on the 10th floor. That evening, I took a bisacodyl suppository and had a loose, incomplete bowel movement. That night, I streaked the sheets with a small amount of stool. After that, I used a pad on the sheets every night until we left the hotel. Fortunately, I never needed one after that first night. The next day, we walked to the mall and spent some time with Michelle who left for Albuquerque in the early afternoon.

Friday, we saw the movie, "300," by mistake. It was good.

Saturday, I had a normal bowel movement, and we went to see the movie, "Dreamgirls." It was good.

Sunday, we visited the mall and relaxed. That evening, Mani and Shameem picked us up, and we went to dinner at an excellent Lebanese restaurant, Le Sheesh. I came to the conclusion that the back seat of a Lincoln Town Car was more comfortable than the back seat of a sport-utility vehicle (SUV).

Monday, we went to the Henry Ford Museum, and I revised the VIP discharge patient instructions. I went by Town Car to the Henry Ford Hospital (HFH) where I was assigned an office next to Mani's. I saw two pre-op patients to whom I described my experience. I illustrated my leg bag to the second one. Afterward, I met with the residents and some of the staff for a presentation of the day's inpatients. Then we made hospital rounds. I was pleased to be the "Poster Boy" for the VIP program. After a return to the hotel, I started trimethoprim/sulfa (TMP/S) in preparation for a cystogram and, hopefully, catheter removal the next day.

57.7 One-Week Follow-up

Tuesday, 1 week after surgery, we loaded the carry-on bag with urinary incontinence supplies, books, and two daily newspapers. We were driven to HFH for our 10:50 AM appointment. The cystogram was negative for a leak, and the physician assistant, Folusho Ogunfiditimi, removed the catheter a few minutes later. Mani, Folusho, Toni, and I reviewed the pathology reports for both the intraoperative frozen sections and the surgical specimen permanent sections. The specimen weighed 38.3 g. The intraoperative frozen section margins were negative for tumor. The final stage was pT2C, N0, M0. The final Gleason grade was $3 + 4$. We discussed penile rehabilitation with a 5-phosphodiesterase inhibitor and injections of Bimix, a combination of papaverine and phentolamine. I signed up. One-half hour later, I felt the urge to void, and went into the rest room where I voided clear urine with a good stream. There was a twinge of perineal pain at the very end of the void, and I had difficulty shutting it off. Thirty minutes later, I went again and noticed that my pad and briefs were wet. I had brought extra pads, but had forgotten to bring an extra pair of briefs. So, it was back to the hotel and a call to Mani's office to cancel my participation in the VIP web site revision, case reviews with the residents, and rounds on the robotic prostatectomy patients done that day.

Wednesday morning, it was up at 6:30 AM, a Town Car ride to the HFH where I gave Urology Grand Rounds on "The Urinary Tract in Renal Transplantation." After that, I made rounds with the residents and Mani, revised the Vattikuti web site with a webmeister, Pam Landis, went to the off-site clinic to see patients with Mani, and talked on the telephone with a mutual friend who, unfortunately, had a recurrence of his leukemia. I saw pre-prostatectomy patients until about 2 PM. Then I returned to the hotel by Town Car and took a nap. That evening, we had dinner with Mani and Shameem in the restaurant at the Ritz-Carlton.

Thursday morning, we had breakfast on the club floor and took the hotel's courtesy SUV to the Greenfield Village, which, unfortunately, was closed. So, we did a second visit to the Henry Ford Museum. The pads and I were becoming well acquainted. I found that if I folded a towel from a towel dispenser in a men's room, it would fit inside a pad and soak up a few milliliter of urine so I could just toss or replace the paper towel and not have to change the pad.

Friday morning, after breakfast on the club floor, we walked over to the mall and saw a bad movie, "Wild Hogs." That evening, we returned to the mall and went to a sports bar called "Strikers." Toni had a giant salad topped with chicken, and I had 1/2 rack of St. Louis style baby back ribs with mashed potatoes and a beer. Ah, real food.

On the 11th post-operative day, we went to the Club Floor for our last breakfast and packed for the long trip home. Our hotel bill for the 13 days was about $6,700. It was worth every penny. We were driven by Town Car to the airport; checked our bags; and ate a great lunch of shrimp, bean soup, and tuna sashimi at the restaurant in the Airport Westin Hotel. Then we flew home First Class on Northwest Airlines with a change of planes in Minneapolis. Toni's parents and Cody, our dog, met us at the airport. We were home in bed by 10 PM.

57.8 The First 3 Months

Sunday, March 18, was grocery shopping, pad shopping, and relaxation by reading the Sunday Oregonian and watching some of the NCAA men's basketball tournament games on TV. That evening, we took chicken soup and cocktail fixings to Duane and Christie's house where we had dinner and played with the dogs.

On postoperative day 13, Toni went back to work and I went into the urology office at the Oregon Health Sciences University (OHSU) Center for Health and Healing (CHH) to pick up some files. Then I visited the laundry, picked up the mail, talked to the Lake Winona Manor health-care team about my mother's deteriorating health, chatted with Jim, my brother, on the telephone, and made a list of things-to-do for the first part of the week. Things were getting back to normal.

On postoperative day #16, I did office work that included revision of our urology web site and the chairing the Renal Transplant Selection Conference.

Friday, I gave myself the first of the biweekly injections of Bimix (papaverine and phentolamine). It resulted in a three of five erection.

Saturday, we went to the beach for a 24-h stay that included two long walks. The urinary control was slowly getting better. Pads + toilet paper or another paper liner were still required, and I was down from three or four pads a day to one or two.

Sunday was shopping for the week, paying bills, Kegel's exercises, and resting at home.

Monday, March 26, postoperative day #20 was to be another short day in the office. I met with the Portland Veterans Affairs Medical Center Renal Transplant Program Administrator and transplant nephrologists in the morning, and gave a medical student lecture at 4 PM on male external genitalia. In between, I met with the nurse coordinators who gave me a "Welcome Home" basket full of goodies.

Tuesday, March 27, 3 weeks after prostatectomy, a pleasant orgasm without ejaculation was induced.

Wednesday, I worked in the office from 7:00 AM until 12:30 PM.

Thursday, I worked in the office from 7:45 AM until 5:00 PM. The Vattikuti website editing was completed and mailed to Pam.

Friday was a day off, the first dose of tadalifil, the second postoperative orgasm, a movie ("The Shooter") with one of my daughters, Wendy, and a visit to the gym with care not to lift more than the prescribed 20 pounds. The pad count was three for 24 h because of the exercise routine.

Saturday was an early visit to the gym, breakfast with Toni's family, and completion of the tax preparation packet for our accountant, Maurice Williams. Tadalafil 10 mg caused a stomach cramp that lasted for 2 days.

Sunday evening my painful perineum, blood-tinged urine, and relatively poor urine control reminded me that I had done too much at the gym Friday, Saturday, and Sunday.

The week of April 2 was my first full week back at work. Monday was 7:00 AM–4:00 PM. Tuesday was 7:00 AM–12:30 PM, Wednesday was 7:00 AM–4:30 PM, and Thursday was 6:30 AM–7:00 PM, a day that was too long. Urinary continence was good until about 12:30 PM each day. Walking and running for the tram resulted in pelvic pain and initial hematuria. I had to take ibuprofen Thursday night for the first time since post-op day 10. Friday, April 6, was the 1-month anniversary of the robotic prostatectomy and my first living donor renal transplant since surgery. It went well. I was continent for the $4\frac{1}{2}$ h it took, but initial hematuria began to plague me. Friday night I had pelvic discomfort. Saturday morning we had breakfast

with Toni's sister and her husband at a local café. Part of Saturday was cleaning house and shopping in preparation for cocktails at 5:00 PM with Dr. Ja-Hong Kim, a urology chief resident from the Cleveland Clinic, her husband, and a woman friend of hers. Saturday night was spent forcing oral fluids, passing clots at the beginning of each void, and taking acetaminophen for pelvic soreness. The initial hematuria had cleared by dawn. I had done too much. Urinary continence was best when I wasn't very active, and Sunday was a one-pad day.

Monday, April 9, was to be a usual full day. Monday included the residents' conference at CHH, the VA for a renal transplant meeting, and back to CHH where I had the first postoperative PSA blood draw. The result was a very reassuring 0.05 ng/mL. Tuesday was a very light day. Wednesday was the usual 6:45 AM–5:30 PM. After work, Dr. Susan Orloff, a liver transplant surgeon, and I shared a bottle of wine with some cheese and bread while we discussed the future of transplantation at OHSU. My urine control faded as the day progressed. Thursday was the usual 6:45–7:00 PM. Friday was two cases in the OR, the second of which was a living, genetically related donor renal transplant. Bloody spotting of my pads was apparent at the end of the case and there was a little gross hematuria. Perineal discomfort was present while I made rounds at University Hospital, the Veterans Affairs Hospital, and Doenbecher's Children's Hospital before I head back to the tram for the ride to the office to finish the workday. Friday night, I passed two eraser-sized dark clots. Saturday morning was breakfast with Toni's family and some light shopping. That evening, while Toni was at her dental school class reunion, I had an enjoyable dinner at Jake's with Nadir Monis, a former Afghani, who has returned to work for Novartis. Sunday was without incident, and I started practicing my pop-ups on the bedroom floor that morning in anticipation of a return to surfing.

Monday, April 16, I drove to the clinic, parked my car, and took a streetcar to the Governor Hotel where I was one of the faculty members for the Liver and Renal Transplant Seminar. I was dry all day. Tuesday was the 6-week mark, and I was dry nearly all day. I've continued with the 5-PDE inhibitor pills and the Bimix penile injection protocol. There was a persistent area of numbness on my upper, inner left thigh in the distribution of a branch of the genitofemoral nerve. I suspect the nerve was cut, burned, or stretched during the pelvic lymphadenectomy. Tuesday was spent in the office, making resident rounds and preparing for adoption of the electronic medical record system to the inpatient services. Wednesday, Toni and I flew by Southwest Airlines to Phoenix to attend the American Association of Genitourinary Surgeons meeting. Although there was no more hematuria, urinary leakage would occur late in the day and with sudden increases in abdominal pressure. It was a good meeting. I went swimming for the first time since the surgery, and met with friends, including Mani Menon, my surgeon. I sat next to a friend from the Cleveland Clinic at the banquet, and we revisited our radical prostatectomy experiences. Toni and I returned home Saturday evening.

The week of April 23 was a full-time work week. The surgeries were two cases of bilateral nephrectomies for polycystic kidney disease with renal transplantation, and one kidney transplant into a morbidly obese diabetic man. Saturday, I tried a penile injection 20 µg of prostaglandin E1. It resulted in a 10 of 10 painful erection. The erection lasted for about 30 min. The pain lasted for about 2 h. Urinary continence continued to slowly improve. A pad was still necessary. I didn't leak during the hours of surgery, but I took a bladder break every 2–3 h and I had a spot of blood on the pad liner after standing at the operating room table for several hours. Sunday, I returned to the gym and did two sets of three upper body exercises and three pop-ups with leg flexion exercises. There was no hematuria afterward and no incontinence during the workout.

The weeks of April 30 and May 7 were both full work weeks. I was totally continent of urine until mid-afternoon, and then minimal to mild stress incontinence appeared. I wore a pad all day. The triangular pads were more comfortable than the uniform width pads. I was hoping that erections without chemical enhancement would arrive one of these months. The left upper inner thigh numbness persisted.

Saturday, May 19, Room 6,323 at the Disney Grand Californian Hotel during the AUA Annual Meeting was our first attempt at intercourse since the prostatectomy. It was successful in the sense that the 10 µg PGE1-enhanced erection was adequate for penetration, and the orgasm was as pleasant as before. Instead of ejaculate, however, there was urine even though I'd emptied my bladder just before bed. The PGE1 erection lasted for about 30 more minutes and the penile pain lasted for another 3 h. Minor perirectal pain persisted for a few hours and responded to 1 g

of acetaminophen. Urinary continence continued to slowly improve. The left upper inner thigh numbness was replaced at times by an inappropriate sensation of coldness. Monday night, masturbation produced no urine leakage.

June 1 was another long case of bilateral nephrectomies and a renal transplant. I was totally dry during a long case, but still wear a pad for security. I tended to leak a bit late in the day. That weekend, I started practicing my long board pop-ups in the swimming pool.

57.9 Three Months

The pelvic soreness with exercise and bowel movements resolved. The hematuria had resolved several weeks ago. Erections were not present without chemical enhancement. Orgasm was accompanied by ejaculation of clear urine. This could be reduced with an empty bladder, controlled with a conscious effort to contract the external sphincter at the time of orgasm or by using a condom, and eliminated if the orgasm took place when supine. The combination of papaverine and phentolamine worked, prostaglandin E1 in lidocaine worked very well, but was painful, and the combination of a vacuum erection device and penile injection worked well. Oral tadalafil 10 mg didn't work. A "Pocket Rocket" vibrator was a good addition to the penile rehabilitation program.

I wore one pad per 24 h for occasional urinary leakage. Leakage would occur late in the day when I was tired, broke wind, or laughed with a full bladder. The left femoral branch of the genitofemoral sensory neuropathy was slowly improving.

It wasn't unusual to go for 48 h without a bowel movement, and glycerin suppositories were helpful.

The serum PSA on July 2 was <0.05 ng/mL.

August 9–12. I returned to surfing for the first time since the surgery. I was a little rusty, but Toni and I caught several waves at San Onofre, Cardiff Beach, and Cardiff Reef in Sothern California.

57.10 Six Months

My IPSS was 4 (low) with a bother, or quality of life, score of 2. In retrospect, I had urinary urgency before the radical prostatectomy and that had completely resolved. The SHIM score without treatment was 5 (severe impotence). With treatment, specifically penile injection with a vasodilating agent, the SHIM score was 27.

September 19, 2007, Toni and I traveled to Chicago where we spent two and a half days with three members of the AUA staff doing a site visit for the 2009 AUA Annual Meeting. I was dry, but wore a panty liner for security.

The PSA on October 2 was <0.05 ng/mL. I let Drs. Menon and Garzotto know the good news.

57.11 Nine Months

December 6 found us on our way to the Northwest Urological Society where I read the paper, "Ten things your urologist may not have told you about your radical prostatectomy." The paper was well received, and we had a good time at the meeting. I still wore a panty liner a day for security.

57.12 One Year

I was cancer free by PSA determinations, continent of urine, but wore a panty liner for security at work or when I wore light-colored slacks; erections were adequate with penile injection of PGE1, papaverine, and phentolamine or Triple P, and the left inner thigh numbness and dysesthesia were hardly noticeable.

On May 23, 2008, we had just returned from the AUA Annual Meeting in Orlando. I was now President of the AUA. I didn't have to wear a pad at any time. The left anterior thigh numbness and dysesthesia continued to slowly resolve. Every now and then, there was about a 2.5 of 5 spontaneous erection that was not quite "stuffable."

June 6, 2008, I was dry. ED required treatment. The left genitofemoral neuropathy was ~95% resolved, scrotal muscle tone was returning to normal, and the scars were almost unnoticeable.

June 28, 2008, was my real return to surfing. We were at Short Sands Beach on the Oregon coast about 2 h from home. With a hood, 4/3 wetsuit, gloves, booties, a 12 ft long board, and perfect swells on a high tide, I had eight rides, one after the other. It was perfect. In August, we surfed at Turtles in Southern California.

57.13 Eighteen Months

On October 8, 2008, my PSA was 0.01 ng/mL.

57.14 Two Years

On March 10, 2009, my PSA was <0.05 ng/mL, I had pad-free urinary continence, no bowel dysfunction, and I was as potent as I wanted to be with intracavernous injections. The left genitofemoral nerve numbness had resolved.

57.15 Three Years

On March 5, 2010, my PSA was 0.01 ng/ml, and my urinary control, bowel function and erectile function were unchanged from the 2-year follow-up.

57.16 Afterthought

Would I do it again? Yes, in a heartbeat.

Part IX
Future Perspectives

Chapter 58

Telementoring and Telesurgery in Urology

Ben Challacombe and Prokar Dasgupta

58.1 Introduction

Since the initial development of telegraphy by Sir Charles Wheatstone in 1837 and the subsequent invention of the telephone by Alexander Graham Bell in 1875, doctors have been able to convey medical information to each other across great distances. The term "telemedicine" derives from the Greek word "*tele*" meaning "at a distance" and the modern word "medicine" which itself derives from the Latin "*mederi*" meaning "healing." Although the word telemedicine has a number of definitions, it was first used in the 1970s by Thomas Bird, who referred to a system of health-care delivery where doctors could examine patients at a distance through the use of telecommunications technologies. It is currently taken to mean the rapid access to shared and remote medical expertise by means of telecommunications and information technologies, no matter where the patient or relevant information is located. It incorporates the real-time communication of medical information between physicians in different locations. The communication medium was initially voice, but more recently ISDN, email, and the Internet have enabled the transmission of images.

Telemedicine as a concept has existed for many decades, being regularly mentioned in science-fiction books and films, and there is an early reference in a novel by Michael Crichton in 1969.[1] Within this true account of his time spent at the Massachusetts General Hospital, he recalls how physicians at this hospital would take a history and examine patients at the medical station in Boston International airport via a video link.

Prior to this in the 1920s, medicine, aviation, and radio were combined to bring health care to the people who live, work, and travel in the more remote areas of Australia as the Royal Flying Doctor Service (RFDS) of Australia which was officially launched in 1928. This service provided not only emergency medical aid to the people of inland Australia, but also a comprehensive health care and community service via one of the earliest means of telemedicine communication, the pedal-driven radio designed by Adelaide engineer, Alf Traeger in 1927 (Fig. 58.1).

Perhaps the greatest regular user of telemedicine today remains the aviation industry, where most commercial airliners now routinely carry global emergency telemedicine equipment. This includes remote vital-sign monitors (e.g., MedAireTM) that send diagnostic information instantaneously back to ground-based doctors who subsequently give medical advice to on-board caregivers.[2]

During the 1990s the development and application of minimally invasive technology, particularly laparoscopy, revolutionized surgery[3] and opened the way for remote operating, once a mechanical way of controlling the instruments had been developed. This appeared in the form of robots modified for medical use. Robots, originally from the Czech word for worker, have been used in surgical practice since the 1980s, when they were introduced to assist with orthopedic and neurosurgical procedures.[4]

With the ever-increasing number of minimally invasive surgical techniques, including laparoscopic and

B. Challacombe (✉)
The Urology Centre, Guy's Hospital, London, UK
e-mail: benchallacombe@doctors.net.uk

A.K. Hemal, M. Menon (eds.), *Robotics in Genitourinary Surgery*,
DOI 10.1007/978-1-84882-114-9_58, © Springer-Verlag London Limited 2011

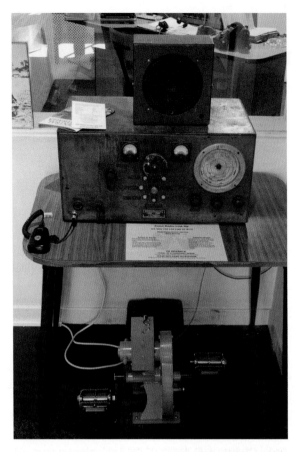

Fig. 58.1 The original 1927 Traeger pedal-driven radio receiver at the RFDS station in Alice Springs, Australia

viewed by means of a television or monitor are ideally suited to the transmission of video images to other sites. In addition, minimally invasive surgery, when performed by experienced surgeons, provides benefits for the patients themselves, the hospital, and the operating surgeons. Patients could potentially benefit by receiving treatment from experts who they would not normally have access to, resulting in reduced length of hospital stay, earlier return to full activity, improved cosmetic results, and a more precise surgical procedure (Fig. 58.2).

Telecommunication involves providing advice and no specialist equipment is required. Telementoring requires a telelink, but still primarily involves offering advice and guidance. Telesurgery requires specialist surgical robots and involves the surgeon conducting a procedure remotely.

58.2 Components of a Telemedicine Link

The telecommunication technology may incorporate a number of differing methods for the transfer of data by electromagnetic means. This includes analogue or digital telephones, telegraphy, radio, and television and includes any system combining a transmitter, transmission channel, and a receiver. The transmission channel may be a wire, an optical fiber, a radio or infrared wave, or satellite signal.

In the 1990s most telemedicine connections were via integrated services digital network (ISDN) lines.

robotically assisted surgery, there is huge potential to further incorporate telemedicine techniques within this field. Procedures in which the internal organs are

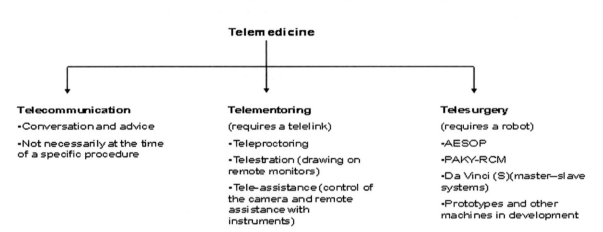

Fig. 58.2 The three subdivisions of telemedicine (Abbreviations: AESOP®, Automated Endoscopic System for Optimal Positioning; PAKY-RCM, Percutaneous Access to the Kidney Remote Center of Motion)

With ISDN, voice and data are carried by bearer channels (B channels) occupying a bandwidth of 64 kb/s (bits per second). There are variations in the potential bandwidths from 64 kb/s up to 512 kb/s (equivalent of 8 basic calls, 4 × B channels) with the broader bandwidths offering superior audio and visual resolution but incurring significant extra costs. At both the local and the remote stations a teleconferencing system is needed to convert the data onto the output devices (PC monitor and speakers).

The introduction of broadband Internet services, such as xDSL, ADSL, and Cable Modem service, has improved many telemedicine connections. These services are faster, less expensive, and easier to set up and maintain than ISDN, but are subject to failure at times of peak usage and are potentially not as secure as ISDN.

Asynchronous transfer mode networks (ATM) are also superior to ISDN lines as robot commands, audio, visual, and medical images can be merged into a single stream of fixed-size ATM data packets, and the network is thought to be reliable and safe.[5] ATM networks are interconnected through a high-speed terrestrial fiber optic system that transports data through virtual connections dedicated to each customer with a data transfer speed of 25,000–155,000 kb/s. However, ATM connections are significantly more expensive than ISDN with annual line rentals of over $100,000.

The new third generation of video mobile phones can now bring telemedicine to huge numbers of doctors who may be able to ask for detailed advice by simply relaying images on their phones.[6] In addition digital cameras can produce both still images and movie clips that can be distributed between doctors in teleconsultation.

To date only the Lindbergh trial, which used a 10 mb/s bandwidth, transmitted images of today's true high-definition quality.[7] This lack of bandwidth and consequent reduction in image quality might partially explain the slow acceptance of this technology worldwide. An amplified audio connection is also required and sound quality is improved if the operating surgeon wears a headset microphone. Improved connections can allow the use of PACS (Picture Archiving and Communication System) images and other patient images while telementoring. Other links use an asynchronous transfer mode link which is faster than standard ISDN.

Security of the connection is vital, and encryption, which is now an established technology, is required for all systems, in addition to firewalls, within hospital LANs. Security measures, such as firewalls, will prevent hackers from entering the network and mean that acquiring direct access to the video stream is only theoretically possible. The use of firewalls is a matter of debate; some authors think that, rather than assisting in making telemedicine more secure, firewalls can present a barrier to telementoring.

58.3 Early Telemedicine

For many years telemedicine existed in its most basic form of *teleconsultation*, where one doctor asked the advice of another via audio or written text connections using telephones, telex, fax, or even Morse code. With ever increasing technology and the introduction of video links, high-speed ISDN lines, and satellite transmission, truly interactive telemedicine has evolved. A number of medical conferences, meetings, and lectures are now regularly broadcast to local and remote hospital locations via teleconferencing links. A live link was first used in the UK between the Middlesex Hospital and the Royal College of Physicians in 1981. The first conference to promote Internet-based poster presentation was the Society for Medical Innovation and Technology (SMIT, previously Society for Minimally Invasive Therapy) meeting in London in 1998 and this is now commonplace. By 1985 SMIT was regularly performing telelinks during their meetings, and in 1991 three operating theaters transmitted live images to 36 European centers. Indeed, the highlight of most major international urological conferences today is the "live telesurgery" which enables large numbers of delegates to observe, listen, and interact by asking questions of an expert performing a specific, usually robotic, procedure. In this way operative nuances and novel techniques can be disseminated widely to surgical communities. This technique uses specific software, cameras that can be controlled remotely, and microphones to relay sound and vision in almost real time. Some hospitals are developing local area network (LAN) systems that will allow audiovisual links to be made from almost every clinical area. Most surgical national and international meetings now provide a live-surgery link to an operating theater in a nearby hospital allowing delegates to see, hear, and interact via questions with the surgical team.

58.4 Telementoring

Telementoring, as opposed to a live telelink where groups only observe a procedure, is an active process and comprises the ability to guide, direct, and interact with another health-care professional (in this case a surgeon) in a different location during an operation or clinical episode. The level of interaction from the mentor can be as simple as verbal guidance while watching a transmitted real-time video of the operation. In its more complex forms it can involve indicating target areas on the local monitor screen (telestration), controlling the camera, or taking over as the assistant by controlling retractors and instruments via a robotic arm.

Telementoring requires a secure high-speed connection with sufficient bandwidth to give a good picture quality at the mentor's station. The connection must transmit both sound and vision in both directions. It has been shown that surgeons are generally able to compensate for delays of up to 700 m/s but delays over 500 m/s (half a second) are quite noticeable.[8] If using an integrated services digital network (ISDN) connection, a bandwidth of 384 kb/s (six lines) is generally needed to give sufficient picture quality for accurate interpretation by the mentor, although clinical work has been carried out using bandwidths as low as 128 kb/s.[9] An amplified audio connection is also required and sound quality is improved if the operating surgeon wears a headset microphone. More modern links use an Asynchronous Transfer Mode (ATM) link which is faster than standard ISDN.

One early use of telementoring was between the USS Abraham Lincoln Aircraft Carrier Battle group cruising the Pacific Ocean and locations in Maryland and California, forming the Battle Group Telemedicine (BGTM) system.[10] Five laparoscopic inguinal hernia repairs were successfully completed under telementoring guidance from land-based surgeons thousands of miles away. This work illustrated the potential for telementoring in the extreme environments of warfare and potentially in space. In 1996 the group from Johns Hopkins successfully used an experienced mentor to supervise an inexperienced surgeon 1,000 ft away. A robotic arm was used to control the video endoscope, and a telestrator indicated important features on the surgeon's screen.[11] They concluded that operative times compared between telementored and traditionally mentored procedures were not statistically different for basic procedures but were longer for advanced cases.

At a similar time, assessment of training in laparoscopic colonic resections and Nissen fundoplication was compared between locally and telementored groups with no difference in performance outcome.[12] To illustrate the potential of telementoring in remote environments a laparoscopic cholecystectomy was successfully telementored from the department of surgery at Yale University School of Medicine to the mobile surgery unit in Ecuador.[9] The Hopkins group have collaborated with an Italian group resulted in successful telementoring of remote surgeons in procedures as advanced as laparoscopic nephrectomy.[3]

More recently a renal transplant surgeon who was a relative novice at laparoscopy was able to initiate independent hand-assisted laparoscopic donor nephrectomy by means of international telementoring from an expert in the field. Early results appeared to show that telementoring can significantly shorten the learning curve and the mentored unit has now built an independent practice.[13] This telementoring program indicated the simplicity, effectiveness, and value for money associated with this technology as for only US$10,000 and 20 h of mentoring an entire program was established with subsequent training of three other surgeons and several fellows.

The da Vinci S HD is ideally suited for training due to the capability for telestration, whereby an instructing surgeon can draw on a monitor with the resulting image transmitted to the console where the mentee is able to view this image superimposed on the screen. This feature could be easily translated to remote telementoring to indicate appropriate tissue planes or specific lines of incision during urological procedures. The most recent da Vinci Si HD dual console system is further aimed at enhanced training as the system has dual controls enabling the mentor to take over to illustrate key points of technique.

58.4.1 Telesurgical Telementoring

After their initial success with telementoring, the Hopkins Urobotics group increased the distance to their remote site to 3.5 miles while incorporating controls to a robotic arm that manipulated the laparoscope and access to electrocautery for tissue cutting or hemostasis during the telementored cases. They named this "telesurgical mentoring."[14] Using a similar setup, the first international telesurgical mentoring occurred between Baltimore and Innsbruck, Austria (laparoscopic adrenalectomy), and subsequently between Baltimore and Singapore (laparoscopic varicocelectomy) using three ISDN lines and a bandwidth of 384 kb/s and a 1 s delay.[15]

With this equipment the Hopkins group have successfully telementored a laparoscopic bilateral varicocelectomy and a percutaneous renal access for a percutaneous nephrolithotomy between Baltimore and Sao Paulo, Brazil.[16] The remote surgeon controlled the laparoscope via an ASEOP 3000 (Computer Motion Inc.). This group have now carried out telesurgical telementoring in over 17 cases[17] using ASEOP or the Percutaneous Access to the Kidney (PAKY) robot.

58.5 Telesurgery

The next logical progression from telesurgical telementoring (the mentor controls the laparoscopic camera and/or a laparoscopic retractor but is not the primary surgeon) was to the true telesurgery that is mainly or entirely controlled by a surgeon at a remote site. The first published example of this was a trans-rectal ultrasound (TRUS) guided prostate biopsy performed by Professor Rovetta. In this case a SR 8438 Sankyo Scara robot mimicked manual handling of TRUS biopsy device in the patient's rectum, in a telesurgery scenario.[18] This system did not gain popularity as the benefits of telesurgery were outweighed by the increased cost and complexity of the robotic procedure, although it was the first evidence of the feasibility of telesurgery.

The US military were next to explore the potential of remote surgery and developed a prototype remote telepresence surgery system with the aim of bringing acute surgical care to wounded soldiers in the combat zone.[19] This concept was supported by Professor Rick Satava who foresaw a Mobile Advance Surgical Hospital (MASH) with the capability for remote telepresence surgery.[20]

In 2002 collaboration between Johns Hopkins and Guy's Hospital, London, resulted in the first randomized controlled trial of telerobotic surgery.[21] They compared human with robotic and trans-Atlantic

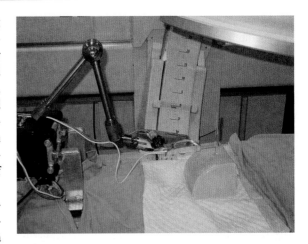

Fig. 58.3 The PAKY-RCM robot during the first randomised controlled trial of telerobotic surgery

telerobotic percutaneous needle access using a validated kidney model into which a Kellet™ needle was inserted 304 times. Half the insertions were performed by a robotic arm and the other half by urological surgeons. Order was decided randomly except for a subgroup of 30 trans-Atlantic robotic procedures that were controlled by a team at Johns Hopkins, Baltimore, via four ISDN lines. The robot was slower than the human to complete insertions, but was more accurate both locally and remotely compared to human operators as it made less attempts for successful needle insertion.[22] In a second "cross-over" trial the telerobotic procedures were reversed with the robot in Baltimore and the operators in London with equivalent results for both time and accuracy (Fig. 58.3).

58.5.1 Telesurgery Using Master–Slave Devices

With the introduction of the da Vinci and Zeus robots in the late 1990s (Intuitive Surgical, Sunnyvale, CA, USA) the possibility of true telesurgery arrived. These master–slave systems have the surgeon sitting at a console several feet away from the robotic arms themselves. The Zeus robot has been phased out after company takeover but the da Vinci system has proliferated around the world and is the premier operating robot today. The da Vinci system itself is often referred to as a "telerobotic" system as the console is usually several feet from the patient. Generally the console is situated adjacent to the patient in the same room. This system ideally lends itself to genuine remote telesurgical operating. The huge range of procedures possible with the da Vinci platform means that remote surgeons have the ability to assist, intervene, and carry out a range of operations.

The first true (remote) telesurgical operation was the Lindbergh procedure, named after Charles Lindbergh's first trans-Atlantic flight from New York to Paris, a laparoscopic cholecystectomy, which was successfully carried out using the Zeus robot with the surgeon in New York and the patient in Strasbourg, France.[7] French Telecom provided the trans-Atlantic connection gratis, the operation lasted 45 min and the patient had no postoperative complications. The transmission delay was reduced to 150 ms over the 13,000 km distance, thus greatly facilitating the operator's movements.

In 2005, Colonel Noah Schenkman of the Walter Reed Army Medical Center performed live telesurgery on two pigs at the American Telemedicine Association event. This was the first telesurgery using the da Vinci®[23] surgical system, the first procedure to use stereoscopic surgical video streaming, and the first telesurgery over the Internet. Telesurgery with the da Vinci system has also been trialed using a pig model up to 2,400 miles away with round trip time delays of up to 900 ms.[24] Both telementoring and telesurgical approaches were used in this trial, with residents at the console adjacent to the swine, and attending surgeons simultaneously operating at second console. All four procedures were successful with round-trip delays of 450–900 ms. Blood loss was minimal and there were no intra-operative complications.

A team from Canada has perhaps the largest and most extensive experience with remote telementoring at present. Mehran Anvari's group have established a remote surgical service between his hospital in Hamilton, Ontario, and North Bay General Hospital, some 400 km away.[25] Using a ZEUS system communicating through a redundant Internet Protocol Virtual Private Network at a bandwidth of up to 15 mb/s, he has reported on 21 cases including Nissen fundoplications, anterior resections, and inguinal hernia repairs. The transmission latency was 140 ms and the surgeon adapted to this easily. More recently, the da Vinci system has been modified and enabled for use over the Internet as well. A surgeon is present on the patient side as an assistant and the surgeons were able to switch primary surgeon responsibilities

back and forth depending on need. They reported good patient outcomes for the procedures and there have been no conversions, no significant complications, and outcomes have been similar to standard laparoscopic surgery. In some cases, the patient-side surgeon did not need to interact aside from placing the ports and robotic arms. There were no issues concerning quality or loss of signal and they concluded that telerobotic assistance was a significant enabling tool for this type of surgery.[26] This group have also investigated the effect of differing time delays on surgical performance and have found that errors and task completion times increase with delays above 500 m/s[27] and this supports the previous work of Fabrizio and colleagues[8] (Fig. 58.4a, b).

Another Canadian group have also assessed the potential role on the da Vinci system using a bandwidth of 17 mb/s bandwidth over a VPNe network spanning 2,848 km round-trip landline distance.[28] The observed latency was 370 ms, with 140 ms due to transport delay, and the team were able to perform

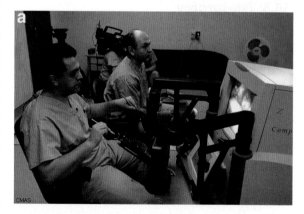

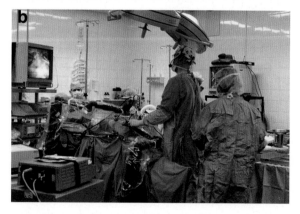

Fig. 58.4 **a** Dr. Anvari at the Zeus TS robotic platform. **b** The remote patient (Courtesy of M. Anvari, MB, BS, PhD.)

robotic-assisted pyeloplasty with a respectable average anastomotic times of 20.7 ± 4.7 min.

58.6 Benefits

The advantages of telemedicine in the areas of telementoring and telerobotics are potentially huge but at present remain mainly undiscovered. Remote surgeons/mentors can facilitate procedures that would otherwise not be attempted due to complexity, difficulty, and lack of local surgeon experience. They can also give guidance when unexpected operative findings are discovered and assist in emergencies due to their previous experiences of similar situations. In a similar manner to the recent protocols aimed at a reduction in intra-operative errors from wrong site/patient surgery we should follow the lead of the aviation industry in introducing a network of telementoring centers to improve performance in general. The potential for litigation may decrease if surgeons have rapid access to advice from world experts in times of trouble as well as providing reassurance and back up to surgeons on their learning curves. It is likely that the learning curve when commencing a new procedure will be reduced by telementoring and that subsequently operating times will fall more quickly than by local surgeons struggling on independently.

Developed countries with remote populations such as Australia and Canada are ideal for telesurgical operating as a robotic system can be installed locally and an on-site team taught how to set up and dock the system. An expert remote surgeon can then take over and perform complex surgery. As the da Vinci system is introduced into a wider variety of countries with little traditional background in advanced surgical techniques the ability to access high-class telementoring becomes ever more important.

58.7 Problems

A number of significant external issues are raised by the continued development of telementoring and telesurgery where surgical control or direction is remote to the patient. At present medical qualifications from the European Union are not recognized in the United States and vice versa while surgical insurance policies are usually specific to a country or even a region or state. This gives rise to major ethical and potential medico-legal issues when a surgeon in one country operates on a patient in another. In the Lindbergh operation, the surgeon took consent from the patient locally in France before traveling to the USA to carry out the procedure telerobotically.[7] For international telerobotic surgery to become commonplace, special arrangements would need to be in place for patient responsibility and the remote surgeon would have to take liability for the peri-operative welfare of patients.

The security of the telecommunication link is vital and nonhard-wired methods such as the Internet run the potential risk of deliberate hacking and subsequent interruption or even interference during telesurgical procedures. There is also the issue of reliability of the link itself as it could be potentially disastrous to lose a connection at a critical operative stage. ISDN incorporates a secure hard-wired system as does SDSL thus reducing the risk of interruptions to the connection but both require installation of specific cabling into the operating theater which consequently will drive up costs. The cost of buying a telecommunication system and installing cabling for hard-wired connection currently stands at approximately $20,000. However, the operative line rental from the telecom companies for the subsequent cases soon exceeds this initial outlay. It would be logical for the local center to foot the bill for the telesurgical link but this may financially prohibit exactly the smaller remote medical centers that stand to benefit most from such systems.

58.8 The Future

As hospitals are modernized, it should be possible to install high-speed communication links or Internet connections in all operating suites. This will provide a readymade local area network in each hospital. It will also be possible to expand this to a wide area network for regional or international connections.

As links between institutions grow an internationally recognized telementoring pathway may result in an accredited qualification in surgical telementoring. The operating room of the future is likely to involve robotic telemanipulation as one of the range of advances including robots, miniaturization, biosurgery, and "intelligent" instruments.[29]

The ability of the remote surgeon to appreciate haptic force feedback will improve the ability to discriminate tissue abnormalities at a remote location. Bhattacharjee and colleagues have investigated such a unit where the slave can very accurately track the position of the master device with negligible error.[30]

In addition to standardized telesurgical techniques the recent advances in natural orifice trans-esophageal surgery (NOTES) and other associated minimally invasive platforms including telemicrosurgery make these areas adaptable for remote operating.[31]

In an attempt to improve the speed and reliability of transmission between the surgeon and the patient site in telesurgery one group have proposed the SURGNET.[32] This system can reduce information disrupted by packet loss and delay jitter using algorithms include adaptive packet prediction and buffer time adjustment techniques, to significantly improve performance. Another new robotic interface is the RoboConsultant (RemotePresence-7; InTouch Health, Sunnyvale, CA), a mobile robotic telementoring system controlled by a portable laptop control station linked via broadband Internet connection.[33] This has been used intraoperative telementoring and consultation by a senior surgeon during five laparoscopic and endoscopic urologic procedures. The authors found that this system provided clear, real-time, and effective telementoring and telestration that allowed the mentor to experience remote presence in the operating room environment.

Just as true robotic surgery is independent of human control, true telerobotic surgery is also performed by the robot itself unassisted but distant from the overseeing team. This concept has also been recently realized as Carlo Pappone, an Italian surgeon, has developed a robot and software program that uses data collected from several surgeons and thousands of different operations to perform remote cardiac surgery without human intervention. In 2006 over 50 min he monitored a cardiac ablation on a 34-year-old patient suffering from atrial fibrillation in a Milanese hospital. The operation was conducted from Boston, USA, by a PC monitored by Dr Pappone. This paves the way for further independent telerobotic operating where the robot is autonomous and can adapt to different clinical scenarios.[34]

An ethical appraisal has been investigated to assess the unique patient–physician relationship that occurs as a result of telesurgery.[35] They proposed that if the inherent danger of technology in health care is reducing the patient to an object, it follows that using the distant surgeon to complement the patient–physician relationship and not the primary care taker is the manner in which the threat of patient objectification may be overcome. In other words the patient's clinical good is served by the remote surgeon while the on-site surgeon satisfies all other aspects of the patient's good; essentially augmenting both the quality and the quantity of care.

58.9 Conclusions

As the complexity of the available surgical technology continues to advance unabatedly, the costs of hardware, software, and the telecommunication link itself will fall. The world is becoming relatively smaller as a result of increased access to the Internet and global travel while patient expectations are rising. The field of international telementoring has steadily expanded rather than exploded over recent years. This is likely to be due to ethical considerations and differences in both software and hardware capabilities between individual countries. Telemedicine is ideally suited to use in developed countries with remote communities (e.g., Canada, Australia). Within health-care systems, it is logical to make use of all available resources and surgical knowledge is a key resource. Telementoring will allow dissemination of skills both nationally and internationally.

Disappointingly, despite the technology having been available for several years, there has not been the rush to take up telesurgery and, in particular, telementoring that many expected would happen. Surgeons may need to look at their colleagues in other specialities who have grasped telemedicine more completely as examples to follow in this direction. There can be no excuse in the present day for a surgeon experiencing difficulties during his/her learning not taking the opportunity to liaise with an experienced colleague wherever they are located. We are never too old or good to learn from others and perhaps surgeons are guilty of overlooking that on occasion.

As links between institutions grow, an internationally recognized telementoring pathway may result in an accredited qualification in surgical telementoring. The operating room of the future is likely to involve robotic telemanipulation as one of the range of advances including robots, miniaturization, biosurgery, and "intelligent" instruments.[29] All that remains is for urologists to fully embrace these technologies that they have already been pivotal in developing. The eventual goal is to have the world's best surgeons performing specialist procedures remotely using robotic control, wherever they or the patient are geographically. Remote surgical control is still not commonplace due to many of the issues stated above but the potential for active telementoring is enormous. It remains to be seen whether true remote surgery will have a role in future civilian life, but it is certainly an exciting prospect.

Acknowledgments Prokar Dasgupta acknowledges financial support from the Department of Health via the National Institute for Health Research (NIHR) comprehensive Biomedical Research Centre award to Guy's & St Thomas' NHS Foundation Trust in partnership with King's College London and King's College Hospital NHS Foundation Trust.

References

1. Crichton M. *Five Patients*. London: Arrow Publishers; 1995;119–161.
2. Garrett JS. MedAire: peace of mind in the skies – a flight nurse's dream come true. Interview by Marlene Jezierski. *J Emerg Nurs*. 1998;24:71–73.
3. Micali S, et al. Feasibility of telementoring between Baltimore (USA) and Rome (Italy): the first five cases. *J Endourol*. 2000;14:493–496.
4. Dasgupta P. Robotics in urology. *BJU Int*. (2001);88:300.
5. Eadie LH, Seifalian AM, Davidson BR. Telemedicine in surgery. *Br J Surg*. 2003;90:647–658.
6. Carter J, Bridle C. Telemedicine. *BMJ*. 2003;327:1458.
7. Marescaux J, et al. Transatlantic robot-assisted telesurgery. *Nature*. 2001;413:379–380.
8. Fabrizio MD, et al. Effect of time delay on surgical performance during telesurgical manipulation. *J Endourol*. 2000;14:133–138.
9. Rosser JC Jr, et al. Use of mobile low-bandwidth telemedical techniques for extreme telemedicine applications. *J Am Coll Surg*. 1999;189:397–404.
10. Cubano M, et al. Long distance telementoring. A novel tool for laparoscopy aboard the USS Abraham Lincoln. *Surg Endosc*. 1999;13:673–678.
11. Moore RG, et al. Telementoring of laparoscopic procedures: initial clinical experience. *Surg Endosc*. 1996;10:107–110.
12. Rosser J Jr, et al. Telementoring: pushing the telemedicine envelope. *J Assoc Acad Minor Phys*. 1997;8:11–15.
13. Challacombe B, et al. Telementoring facilitates independent hand-assisted laparoscopic living donor nephrectomy. *Transplant Proc*. 2005;37:613–616.
14. Schulam PG, et al. Telesurgical mentoring. Initial clinical experience. *Surg Endosc*. 1997;11:1001–1005.
15. Lee BR, et al. International surgical telementoring: our initial experience. *Stud Health Technol Inform*. 1998;50:41–47.
16. Rodrigues Netto N Jr, et al. Telementoring between Brazil and the United States: initial experience. *J Endourol*. 2003;17:217–220.
17. Bove P, et al. Is telesurgery a new reality? Our experience with laparoscopic and percutaneous procedures. *J Endourol*. 2003;17:137–142.
18. Rovetta A, Sala R. Execution of robot assisted biopsies within the clinical context. *J Image Guid Surg*. 1995;1:280–287.
19. Jensen JF, Hill JW. Advanced telepresence surgery system development. *Stud Health Technol Inform*. 1996;29:107–117.
20. Satava RM. Virtual reality and telepresence for military medicine. *Ann Acad Med Singapore*. 1997;26:118–120.
21. Challacombe BJ, et al. Trans-oceanic telerobotic surgery. *BJU Int*. 2003;92:678–680.
22. Challacombe B, Patriciu A, Glass J, et al. A randomized controlled trial of human versus robotic and telerobotic access to the kidney as the first step in percutaneous nephrolithotomy. *Comput Aided Surg*. 2005;10:165–171.
23. Hanly RJ, Miller B, Herman BC, et al. Stereoscopic robotic surgical telementoring: feasibility and future applications. *Telemed and E Health*. 2005;11(2):247.
24. Sterbis JR, Hanly EJ, Herman BC, et al. Transcontinental telesurgical nephrectomy using the da Vinci robot in a porcine model. *Urology*. 2008;71(5):971–973.
25. Anvari M, McKinley C, Stein H. Establishment of the world's first telerobotic remote surgical service for provision of advanced laparoscopic surgery in a rural community. *Ann Surg*. 241:460–464.
26. Sebajang H, et al. The role of telementoring and telerobotic assistance in the provision of laparoscopic colorectal surgery in rural areas. *Surg Endosc*. 2006;20:1389–1393.
27. Anvari M, Broderick T, Stein H, et al. The impact of latency on surgical precision and task completion during robotic-assisted remote telepresence surgery. *Comput Aided Surg*. 2005;10:93–99.
28. Nguan C, Miller B, Patel R. Pre-clinical remote telesurgery trial of a da Vinci telesurgery prototype. *Int J Med Robotics Comput Assist Surg*. 2008;4:304–309.
29. Satava RM. Future trends in the design and application of surgical robots. *Semin Laparosc Surg*. 11:129–135.
30. Bhattacharjee T, Son HI, Lee DY. Haptic control with environment force estimation for telesurgery. *Conf Proc IEEE Eng Med Biol Soc*. 2008:3241–3244.
31. Swanstrom LL, et al. Development of a new access device for transgastric surgery. *J Gastrointest Surg*. 9:1129–1136.
32. Natarajan S, Ganz A. SURGNET: an integrated surgical data transmission system for telesurgery. *Int J Telemed Appl*. (2009);435849. Epub 2009.

33. Agarwal R, Levinson AW, Allaf M, et al. The RoboConsultant: telementoring and remote presence in the operating room during minimally invasive urologic surgeries using a novel mobile robotic interface. *Urology.* 70:970–974.

34. Pappone C, Vicedomini G, Manguso F, et al. Robotic magnetic navigation for atrial fibrillation ablation. *J Am Coll Cardiol.* 47:1390–1400.

35. van Wynsberghe A, Gastmans C. Telesurgery: an ethical appraisal. *J Med Ethics.* 2008;34(10):e22.

Chapter 59

Robotic Systems: Past, Present, and Future

Shadie R. Badaan and Dan Stoianovici

59.1 Introduction

In the last decades we have witnessed the emergence of robotic surgery. The concept of "Medical Robotics" took time to become feasible and accepted by the medical community. A promoting factor for the development of these advanced medical instruments has also been the preceding development of minimally invasive surgery methods and laparoscopy in general surgery.

A robot, as defined by the American Society of Robotics, "is a reprogrammable, multifunctional device designed to manipulate and/or transport material through variable programmed motions for the performance of a variety of tasks." Thus a Robot must exhibit three key components:

1. Programmability; implies computerized or symbol-manipulating ability.
2. Mechanical capability; enabling it to act on its own environment.
3. Flexibility; can manipulate/transport in a variety of way.

Potential advantages of robotics in medical applications include remote, scaled, digital manipulation with precise and accurate positioning. Their ability to improve dexterity in minimally invasive approaches and perform operations remotely to reduce physician's radiation exposure has been an important factor in demonstrating the potential value of these technologies.

D. Stoianovici (✉)
Urology Robotics Laboratory, James Buchannan Brady
Urological Institute, Johns Hopkins Medicine, Baltimore,
MD, USA
e-mail: dss@jhu.edu

Robotic assistance in minimal invasive surgery is currently showing benefits to the patient with regard to length of hospital stay, return to full activity, and cosmetics. Despite the current cost of the robotic instruments several studies have shown that these may also become a cost-effective option. On the other hand there have been major concerns about their difficult compatibility with standard instrumentation, being technically demanding about safety, the loss of tactile feedback, and the lack of irrefutable clinical effectiveness.

Although, a robot has become a must have in every medical center involved in minimal invasive surgery, these technologies are still in their infancy and time only will show if these will become integral part of everyday practice as "the standard of care." In this chapter we will discuss the evolvement of medical robots, their current status, and give a perspective view of the ideas and projects currently under development.

59.2 History

The word "robot" was introduced by the Czech writer Karel Čapek in his satirical play "Rossum's Universal Robots" which premiered in 1921. The name was suggested by his brother Josef Čapek and was taken from the word "robota" meaning literally work or "slave labor." The term *robotic* was presented by Isaac Asimov in the year 1950 in his novel *Runaround*. Several years later, Asimov defined three novelistic laws of robotics: a robot cannot hurt a human being, it must obey the orders given to it by a human being, and a robot must protect its own existence without infringing the first two laws.[1]

Although the term is relatively recent, the idea of an intelligent machine dates back to antiquity, as in Song XVIII of the Iliad, Hephaestus, the God of Fire, builds three-legged tables fitted with casters that are able to go back and forth on their own in the palaces of the Gods.

The first programmable industrial manipulator was developed in the 1940s. George Devol, who is credited as the father of robotics, developed a magnetic process controller that could be used to manage these first robotic machines.

The beginning of the robotic age was marked by the development and integration of computers, when in 1954 the first robot used play back memory. The first master–slave robotic system was used to manipulate radioactive substances, invented in 1954 by R. Goertz.[2] The first industrial robot, called Unimate, was invented by G. Deroe and J. Engelberger in 1961 and consisted of an articulated arm with hydraulic motorization used in the automobile industry.[3]

Since then, robots have been used in industry for nearly everything, from the processing and assembling of microprocessors to the manufacturing of large-scale industrial machinery.

In the late 1980s we witnessed the development of minimally invasive surgical techniques including laparoscopy. This brought the idea that surgeons may no longer need to directly handle tissue to perform an operation.

Minimally invasive surgery (MIS) revolutionized the concept of surgery. In MIS, special slender instruments are inserted through small skin incisions. Although MIS brought substantial advantages including the reduction of surgical trauma, patient recovery time, and improvement in cosmetics it also introduced new substantial difficulties. These include the loss of wrist articulation, touch feedback, 3-dimensional (3D) vision, eye–hand coordination, and typically poor ergonomics of the tools. These limitations made procedures requiring delicate dissections difficult and technically demanding if not impossible. As such, the range of minimal procedures that could be performed with MIS was limited. This has shown the potential advantages of using more advanced instrumentation for MIS, such as robots especially developed for surgery. Satava,[4] Ballantyne, and Moll[5] have suggested that laparoscopic surgery is a "transitional" technology leading to robotic surgery.

59.3 Classification of Medical Robots

A wide variety of surgical robots have been developed over the last decades. One classification method suggested by Taylor[6] would be based on *technology*, *application*, or *role*. A technology-based taxonomy might have categories such as autonomous and teleoperated robots, whereas an application-based taxonomy might have categories such as cardiology and urology. The problem with these two approaches is that, on either side, classifications may become quite esoteric and lose meaning for those outside the involved community. Furthermore, this is an artificial decoupling because the application that defines the problem is divorced from the technology that provides the solution.

Role-based classifications can be more useful because they are far-reaching and speak to technology developers as well as end-users. Such taxonomy can be a means of communication among all interested groups in describing needs, requirements, performance, and specifications.

A procedural role-based classification was suggested by Camarillo et al.[7] that can be divided into three discrete categories:

1. Passive role: The role of the robot is limited in scope or its involvement is largely low risk.
2. Restricted role: The robot is responsible for more invasive tasks with higher risk, but is still restricted from essential portions of the procedure.
3. Active role: The robot is intimately involved in the procedure and carries high responsibility and risk.

We suggest the use of a classification based on two criteria:

First, the operational point of view: (a) Remotely controlled, (b) Synergistic, and (c) automated or semi-automated robots. In the first two types, the physician has direct real-time control of the robotic instrument either from a console or by handling the instrument itself. The best-known remote system is the da Vinci (Intuitive Surgical, Inc.), and examples of the synergetic class are the Mako orthopedics robot (Mako Surgical Corp.) or Acrobot system (Acrobot Company, Ltd). For the later class, the physician does not have to continuously control the motion of the robot, but rather define its task and monitor the execution. Image-guided robots are commonly operated under this mode, for example, the Innomotion robot (Innomedic, GmbH) and our AcuBot robot for CT-guided interventions.

Second, the localization method applied for the procedure: (a) visual (b) image guided; with the help of imaging equipment like magnetic resonance imaging (MRI), computed tomography (CT), ultrasound (US), or fluoroscopy.

59.4 Evolution of Medical Robots

Robots for medical applications have been initially derived from industrial robots. In 1985, the PUMA 560, the first medical robot was released by Kwoh et al. and was used to perform neurosurgical biopsies under Computed Topography guidance.[8] The robot was used to hold a fixture next to the patient's head to guide a biopsy instrument. Then it was locked in position, with power removed, while manually the surgeon used the fixture to orient drills and biopsy probes. Thus the robot was relegated to the role of a traditional stereotactic frame in neurosurgery. The procedure was performed with greater precision and took less time than the stereotactic brain surgery techniques used at the time. The Puma 560 was an improvement of the PUMA 200 produced by Unimation Limited and used for industrial purposes.

Despite its accuracy, the system did not appear adapted to surgery due to some drawbacks, such as safety, the time needed for the setup, and its limited workspace.

Three years later, Davies and his team performed a transurethral resection of the prostate (TURP) using the Puma 560. For this, it was necessary to add two frameworks onto the puma robot, mainly for safety considerations.[9] This was the first urologic use of medical robot.

Shortly after, Unimation Limited Company was sold to Westinghouse Limited, who refused to allow the use of the robot for surgery purposes on the basis that it was unsafe, since the industrial robot was designed to be used inside a barrier away from all contact with people.

Thus, in spite of the encouraging preliminary results, the work on the PUMA robot was ceased.

The robotic system used for TURP eventually led to the development of ProBot, an automated robot system designed specifically for transurethral resection of the prostate. It was designed by the team at the Imperial College in London 1991.[10,11] The system had a 7 degrees of freedom (DOF) coupled to a motorized component to automate transurethral resection of the prostate for benign prostatic hypertrophy. The coordinates for resection were based on pre-operative prostate volume and shape determined by transrectal ultrasound (TRUS) scans. This was the first time that an active robot had been single used to remove tissue from a patient.

However, the dependence of ProBot on pre-operative TRUS, the relative inaccuracies of the TRUS estimation, and the need for manual electrocautery for hemostasis hampered the widespread adoption of ProBot.

While ProBot was being developed, Integrated Surgical Systems (ISS), Inc. of Sacramento, CA, was clinically developing ROBODOC, a robotic system designed to machine the femur with greater precision in hip replacement surgeries. ROBODOC prototype was developed at IBM Research.[12]

The ROBODOC system allowed the surgeons to plan the procedure preoperatively by selecting and positioning an implant with respect to a preoperative computer tomography (CT) study and intraoperatively mill the corresponding canal in the femur with a high-speed tool controlled by a robotic arm. The ROBODOC system consists of an interactive preoperative planning system and a robotic system for intraoperative execution. ROBODOC has been tested internationally and has recently received Premarket Notification (510 k) from the Food and Drug Administration (FDA).

The introduction of these initial medical Robots, PUMA 560, ProBot, and ROBDOC, facilitated the acceptance of medical robots and gave a thrust for the development and adaption of a wider variety of robots.

The URobot system was developed in Singapore by Ng et al. The robot was designed to perform a transurethral and trans-perineal access to the prostate for laser resection in 2001[13] or brachytherapy,[14] respectively. At the Johns Hopkins University our team has developed several needle driving systems under various X-Ray-based guidance modalities and performed numerous clinical tests for urology applications.[15–20]

Simultaneously, other research teams worked on the concept of remote manipulation mostly for augmenting the performance of minimally invasive surgery.[21] The first system was named Artemis (Advanced Robotic Telemanipulator for Minimally Invasive Surgery).[22] Computer Motion Inc. (Santa Barbara, CA) was able to develop the first robotic arm approved by the FDA to hold an endoscope.[23] This system called AESOP (Automated Endoscopic System for Optimal Positioning) was a robotic arm with motorized joints controlled by the surgeon with hand and foot controls or through a speech recognition system. Early clinical use was reported[24] and the idea to use the same arm to drive surgical tools gave birth to the Zeus surgical system. This system consists of a surgeon's console and three separate robotic arms that are attached to the operating room table. The distance between the interface, by which the operator gives his instructions to the machine, and the patient can range from several meters to several thousand kilometers, opening the way to telesurgery and made possible the first intercontinental surgery, operation Lindberg.[25] Nevertheless, the Zeus was not FDA approved and another company, Intuitive Surgical, (Sunnyvale, CA), opened the field of robotic surgery with the da Vinci® Surgical System. The da Vinci robotic platform is a master–slave system with three or four arms allowing endowrist capabilities and a 3D visualization of the surgical field. Even though several drawbacks have been echoed about its functionality and possible improvements, this system popularized the concept and instrumentation of robotic surgery in several medical fields. The first radical prostatectomy was reported in 2000 by Abbou et al.[26] Some other applications in general surgery were explored,[27] but even though the system was not purposely designed for urology; prostatectomy appears to be its best-suited application.

59.5 Robots in Current Clinical Use

Currently, the da Vinci® platform is the main robotic system used in common practice with more than 1,200 robots installed worldwide. In large majority the robots are used for robotic-assisted laparoscopic radical prostatectomy (RALP).[28] Even if the review of published literature on RALP and open radical prostatectomy (ORP) is currently insufficient to favor one

surgical technique, it seems that short-term outcomes of RALP achieve equivalence to open surgery with regard to complications and functional results.[29] It is worth indicating that nearly half of the Radical Prostatectomy Procedures done in the USA are RALP. Applications to bladder cancer, renal cancer, ureteropelvic junction obstruction, and pelvic prolapse have also been explored.[30] The main technical improvement since the first release of the system was the addition of a fourth robotic arm, yet other features especially with respect to improved sensory feedback could significantly improve its performance and surgeon's acceptance.

The CyberKnife from Accuray (Sunnyvale, CA, USA) is a frameless robotic system for stereotactic radiosurgery. It uses image-guided radiotherapy (IGRT) and adaptive radiotherapy (ART) for stereotactic radiosurgery technique in the treatment of intra- and extracranial lesions and is being adapted for urologic prostate radiotherapy.[31]

In other fields of medicine, mainly orthopedic surgery, a number of operational systems have been developed and are being used but not as extensively as the da Vinci system. A new class of robots, synergistic,[32] is under evaluation mainly for orthopedic surgery. This Mako System robot (Mako Surgical Corp.) confines a bone cutting tool by hardware and software robotic means to a defined volume in space creating a "no-fly zone" defined by the surgeon based on pre-acquired images. Another orthopedic system is the Acrobot system (Acrobot Company, Ltd) which can be used for unicompartmental knee replacement[33] or hip resurfacing surgery.[34]

59.6 Future Directions

Generally speaking; developments aim at improving existing robotic systems and introducing new systems with decreased learning curves that would allow safer and more homogeneous outcomes with less variability depending on surgeon performance, as well as new tools to perform more autonomous tasks in a less invasive way at lower costs.

Thus future systems are expected to advance in the following two directions: improvements of remote manipulation robots for surgery, developments of image-guided robots for interventions, and possibly combining the two categories.

59.6.1 Remote Manipulation Robots

Although the da Vinci system proved to be a valuable tool in the surgery room, it still incorporates a number of drawbacks. The system is still bulky and hard to manipulate. Improvements in the system design making it smaller, lighter, and easier to move may prove helpful and new versions of the system are being developed.

Current surgical robotic research shows a trend of size reduction compared to the da Vinci system. For example, the NeuroArm (University of Calgary, Canada) proceeds with the development of a remotely controlled bilateral arm robot for neurosurgical operations. Part of the scope is to reduce its size to where the robot could be brought in the bore of an MRI scanner. Even though this is not yet possible, their current version is substantially smaller than the da Vinci, and has additional features such as force feedback.[35] Another example is the VickY system,[36] which is a very compact robot allowing to move a laparoscopic camera. Technical works to hold surgical tools on this platform are ongoing and commercial developments have been recently started by EndoControl company (Grenoble, France).

The lack of haptic feedback of the da Vinci robot is considered by the surgeons to be a major limitation. It is often the case that the sense of touch is a determinant factor in the localization of nearby structures

and controlling the margins of resection during RALP. In delicate balance with Neurovascular Bundle sparing, the part of the prostate to be resected is a crucial factor in the outcome of the operation. To overcome this, haptic feedback systems are being developed, several teams are pursuing additions to the existing system for augmenting sensory feedback[37] including modifying trocar instruments for allowing the measurement of manipulation forces.[38]

Another way to overcome the lack of feedback is by improving the localization of the robotic arms by better 3D visualization systems and the incorporation of intraoperative imaging systems. For example, the addition of Transrectal Ultrasound (TRUS) imaging during RALP may provide better comprehension of nearby organs including the neurovascular bundle (NVB).[39] A TRUS Robot was developed in our laboratory to provide a steady holding of the TRUS probe and allow remote manipulation (Fig. 59.1). Preliminary clinical study has shown the system as helpful in recognizing the NVB and nearby organs, and further research is being done in order to evaluate its assistance and navigational guidance to the surgeon during RALP.

Improved localization may be achieved also by the superimposition of 3D computerized reconstructed preacquired images over the real-time intraoperative laparoscopic view. This is referred to as Augmented Reality (AR).[40,41] It gives the surgeon a transparent visual anatomy of the internal structures or lesions through the overlying tissues. The source of the reconstructed images is based on pre-operative CT or MRI. These reconstructed images are then registered onto anatomic landmarks and tracked by the computer

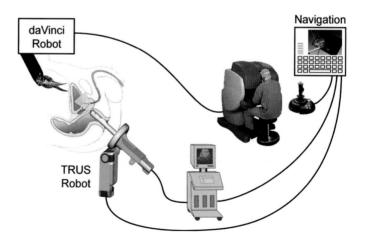

Fig. 59.1 Tandem robot-assisted laparoscopic radical prostatectomy system setup

according to the surgeon's dissection and camera movements.[40,41]

Better imaging can be achieved by image fusion from various imaging modalities, such as preoperative CT with laparoscopic images.[42] Fusion of fluoroscopic and ultrasound images has been proposed to couple the intraoperative guidance.[43] Real-time ultrasound can be fused with preoperative images with higher imaging capabilities like CT or MRI combining the advantages of different modalities.

Another novel approach is pursuing the development of tools to be deployed in the peritoneal cavity and controlled externally with magnetic fields for reducing the number of transabdominal trocars and for increasing the range of motion and accessibility.[44]

The development of natural orifice translumenal endoscopic surgery (NOTES) is potentially the next paradigm shift in minimally invasive surgery. The concept is to access to the peritoneal cavity without passing through the anterior abdominal wall. The first clinical case, performed in 2007, was a cholecystectomy in a woman via a transvaginal approach.[45] Nevertheless, NOTES procedures are performed using modified endoscopic tools with significant constraints. New tools are necessary to allow the surgeon to better visualize and dexterously manipulate within the surgical environment. This may be approached with help of newly designed robots specialized for NOTES. A two-armed dexterous miniature robot with stereoscopic vision capabilities is under development.[46] Snake like or serpentine robots are also being targeted toward this field, these robots will have multiple degrees of freedom, and will not fail if one joint locks/blocks and can be used trans-gastrically.[39] One such device is the CardioARM™ (Articulated Robotic MedProbe), a snake like surgical robot developed at Carnegie Mellon University, which hopes to allow cardiac surgeons to perform procedures through a single subxiphoid incision. The robot has a series of joints that automatically adjust to follow the course plotted by the robot's head, providing greater precision than the standard flexible endoscope can offer.[40] The same team is also developing a LaparoARM™, GastroARM™, and ArthroARM™ which will provide platforms for various endoscopic and laparoscopic procedures. These and other similar devices open the door for single incision or external scarless surgery.

59.6.2 Direct Image-Guided Robots

Image-guided robots have stringent requirements for imager compatibility, precision, sterility, safety, as well as size and ergonomics.[47] A robot's compatibility with a medical imager refers to the capability of the robot to safely operate within the confined space of the imager while performing its clinical function, without interfering with the functionality of the imager.[48]

The current research trend is to embed the robot with the imager (CT, MRI, ultrasound, fluoroscopy, etc.) for re-imaging during the intervention for relocalization, treatment planning updates, and quality control. We term these procedures Direct Image-Guided Interventions (DIGI). The performance of DIGI interventions is not new, in fact the routine TRUS biopsy is done under direct guidance; however, the new term is essential for distinguishing this important class of Image-Guided Intervention (IGI) from navigation based on pre-acquired imaging data.

Traditionally, image guidance and navigation of instruments have been performed manually based on pre-acquired images with the use of spatial localizers such as optical[49] and magnetic trackers.[50] However, robots have the potential to improve the precision, accuracy, and reliability of performance in image-guidance interventions because the tasks are done in a full digital way, from image to instrument manipulation.

Robots for interventions with needles or other slender probes or instruments can be connected to an imaging modality (CT, MRI, ultrasound, fluoroscopy, etc.). Targets and paths are defined in the image based on planning algorithms and the robot aligns and may insert the needle accordingly. The true potential of needle delivery mechanisms relies on their ability to operate with, be guided by, and use feedback from medical imaging equipment. This may compensate for organ reposition during the procedure caused by patient movement or by simple breathing.

Moreover, robots can do complex movements, impossible to perform by a human to limit tissue displacement and needle deformations during the insertion. Indeed, mechanical laws dictate that the reduction of needle insertion force diminishes tissue deformations and target deflection.

Decreasing the force of needle insertion has been proposed with special movements for increasing the accuracy to reach a target. Abolhassani[51] describes an interesting approach during the puncture of a prostate phantom. The deflection of the needle is estimated using online force/moment measurements at the needle base and to compensate for the needle deflection, the needle is axially rotated through 180°. Results were encouraging with reduction of nearly 90% of the deflection. Nevertheless, applying just a rotation of the needle at the rate of 50 rpm is less complex and the results were similar.[52] Podder et al.[53] proposed a system designed to insert multiple needles simultaneously for prostate therapies. Rotation was also used for reducing insertion forces.

Professor Brian Davies of the Imperial College in London, who pioneered the robotics filed in urology with the Probot,[54] has also reported the development of a simple robot that performs similar to the brachytherapy template.[55] Rotation about the axis of the needle is added in order to reduce needle deflections. The system uses 2D TRUS guidance and the report describes successful preclinical testing.

In the Robarts Research Institute (London, Canada)[56] and in the Nanyang Technological University (Singapore),[57] 3D reconstruction from a regular 2D TRUS probe has been investigated by sweeping the probe about its axis. This was integrated with a robot in a system for prostate brachytherapy or biopsy. Mockup tests demonstrated a precision on the order of 1 mm and a clinical study for biopsy is ongoing in Singapore.

Our URobotics laboratory at Johns Hopkins has also developed several versions of a CT-guided robots.[15] Recently, the AcuBot robot was instrumented with a new end-effecter, the Revolving Needle Driver (RND). The RND is a fully actuated driver for needle insertion, spinning, release, and force measurement (Fig. 59.2). The driver supports the needle from its head and provides an additional needle support guide in close proximity of the skin entry point. This is similar to holding the needle with two finger-like grippers, one from its head and one from its barrel next to the skin. The top one pushes the needle in and out, while the lower holds the guide to support the direction of the needle as close as possible to the skin. Both grippers can simultaneously release the needle automatically. Finally, the new driver is also equipped with a set of force sensors to measure the interaction of the nozzle with the patient and the force of needle insertion.[58,59]

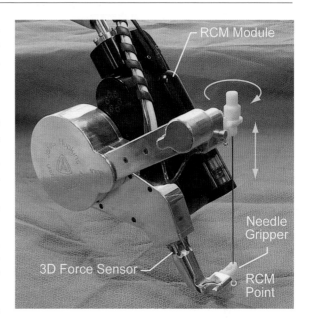

Fig. 59.2 Revolving needle driver on the AcuBot robot

59.6.3 MRI-Compatible Robots

Among all types of imagers, the MRI is the most demanding and the development of MRI-compatible robots is a very challenging engineering task.[60] But, this also makes MRI compatible robots to be multi-imager compatible, if care is taken for the selection of radiolucent materials for the components in immediate proximity of the imaging site.[48] Due to the strong requirements needed to build a MRI-compatible robot, the following description of many robots under development is presented with respect to their capabilities of operation leading up to those used in conjunction with MRI.

The earliest work for MRI-guided prostate intervention robots was performed at the Brigham and Women's Hospital (BWH), Boston, MA, in collaboration with AIST-MITI, Japan.[61] A robotic intervention assistant was constructed for open MRI to provide a guide for needles and probes.[62] To minimize image interference from motors, the robot had to be located distally, at the top of the imager between the vertical coils of the MRI. To operate at the isocenter, long arms had to be extended, which made them flexible. The system assists the physician by positioning a needle guide for manual needle intervention. Applications included prostate biopsy and brachytherapy.[63,64]

The Institute for Medical Engineering and Biophysics (IMB), Karlsruhe, Germany, reported several versions of a robotic system for breast lesion biopsy and therapy under MR guidance.[65,66] Their last version used a cylinder for driving an end-effector axis,[67] and their report gives a well-reasoned presentation of these advantages. This German institute is no longer active, but fortunately a spin-off company was created. The company (Innomedic, Germany) is developing a pneumatic robot for general CT or MRI-guided needle procedures.[68] The robot orients the needle about the axial–sagittal planes for interventions targeting abdominal organs. However, a group from Frankfurt, Germany, has recently used the Innomedic system for targeting the prostate.[69,70] The limitations of the robot restricted the access to the transgluteal path (prone patient with needle pointing down) for which the needle path is much deeper than normal (~14 cm reported in the cadaver experiment). A 15 Ga needle was used to prevent deflections. Manual needle insertion was performed through the guide after retracting the table from the scanner. Even though the Innomedic system is not FDA approved and its designed application range does not include the prostate, it is approved for clinical use in Europe and is a commercial DIGI robot.

TIMC laboratory in France reported a lightweight MRI-compatible robot for abdominal and thoracic percutaneous procedures.[71] This robot, named LPR (acronym for Light Puncture Robot), has an original compact (15 × 23 cm) body-supported architecture, which is naturally able to follow the patient body surface respiratory movements. It is entirely made of plastic, and uses MR-compatible pneumatic actuators powered by compressed air. The needle-holder puncture part includes clamps used to grasp the needle and a translation unit (a fast linear pneumatic actuator), which are able to perform a fast puncture in a single motion (above 9 cm/s) to perforate the skin or organs walls. Mockup experiments are on going to measure system accuracy in the MRI.

Our group at Johns Hopkins has also developed an MRI-compatible robot for prostate access.[72] MrBot, was constructed to be multi-imager compatible, which includes compatibility with all classes of medical imaging equipment (ultrasound, X-Ray, and MR based imagers).[48] All robotic components are constructed of nonmagnetic and dielectric materials. To overcome MRI incompatibilities a new type of motor was purposely designed for the robot. This, PneuStep,[73] is a pneumatic motor using optical feedback with fail safe operation and it is the only fully MRI compatible motor.

The robot presents 6 DOF, 5 for positioning and orienting the injector, and 1 for setting the depth of needle insertion. Various needle drivers can be mounted in the robot for performing various needle interventions. The first driver was developed for fully automated low dose (seed) brachytherapy[74–77] (Fig. 59.3).

Compared with the classic template of needle guide holes, commonly used in TRUS interventions, the robot gives additional freedom of motion for better targeting. For example, the skin entry point may be chosen ahead of time and targeting can be performed with angulations, which is impossible with the template. As such, multiple needle insertions can be performed through the same skin entry point. Moreover, angulations also allow for reducing pubic arch interference, thus allowing for targeting otherwise inaccessible regions of the prostate.

The robot is controlled from a unit remotely located outside the imager's room, either in the control room of the imager or in other proximal space. The robot is connected to the control cabinet by a bundle of hoses. This allows for all MRI-incompatible components of the system to be located outside the MRI room.

Precision tests in tissue mock-ups yielded a mean seed placement error of 0.72 ± 0.36 mm.[76] With different needle drivers, the MrBot applies to various automated DIGI, such as biopsy, therapy injections,

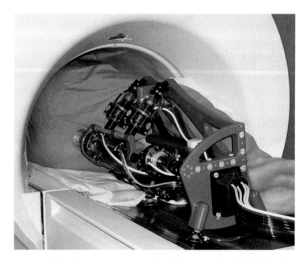

Fig. 59.3 MrBot robot for MRI-guided prostate interventions

and thermal or radiofrequency ablations. The system is presently in preclinical testing with cadaver and animal experiments, but tests show very promising results and clinical trials are expected soon.

59.6.4 Image-Augmented Remote Manipulation Robots

The combination of the two classes presented above, remote manipulation and image-guided robots, is a very likely, highly promising direction of future developments. Augmenting guidance from medical imagers to surgical procedures could substantially improve the way that operations are being performed and would give a clear undisputable advantage for using robotic technologies in surgery.

The NeuroArm robot under development in Canada is a good example of these technologies.[35] Even though it may not yet operate inside the MRI scanner as planned, this may operate next to the MRI scanner and take advantage of recently acquired images to guide the surgery. This does not qualify as MRI safe and compatible, but is a "mini da Vinci" with force feedback. Image processing algorithms used in robotic surgery could also improve the localization of the surgical tools[78] and intraoperative analyses.[79]

59.7 Conclusion

As described above, substantial advances have been made in urology robotics since the first adoption in surgery. This field has become one of the most active areas of applied research. Medical robotic developments span across several scientific fields and disciplines: mechanical and electrical engineering, computer science, and medicine. The delicate process of robot advance has to take into consideration and satisfy all contributing developers that, in addition to the particularities of the field such as sterilization, medical safety, and imager compatibility, make it a very challenging and highly demanding research activity. On the other hand, there is enormous demand from patients and surgeons for less invasive surgical techniques that include medical robots.

We expect that the demand for medical robots will continue to expand, leading to the development and adoption of a wider variety of systems with better performance and cost-effectiveness that can apply to a larger population base. Hopefully, robot advances that we now experience will soon reflect in substantially better clinical outcomes and improved quality of life for the patients.

Acknowledgments The research presented in this publication from the Urology Robotics Laboratory at Johns Hopkins Medicine has been partially supported by grants R21CA088232, R21CA141835 from the National Cancer Institute (NCI), the Prostate Cancer Research Program of the Department of Defense (PCRP) grant W81XWH0810221, and RC1EB010936 from the National Institute of Biomedical Imaging and Bioengineering (NIBIB). The contents are solely the responsibility of the authors and do not necessarily represent the official views of NCI, PCRP, or the NIBIB.

References

1. Asimov I. *Runaround.* 1942.
2. Goertz RC, Thompson WM. Electronically controlled manipulator. *Nucleonics.* 1954;12(11):46–47.
3. Devol J. Programmed article transfer. *USA Patent.* 1954.
4. Satava RM. Emerging technologies for surgery in the 21st century. *Arch Surg.* November, 1999;134(11):1197–1202.
5. Ballantyne GH, Moll F. The da Vinci telerobotic surgical system: the virtual operative field and telepresence surgery. *Surg Clin North Am.* December, 2003;83(6):1293–1304.
6. Taylor R. Robots as surgical assistants: where we are, wither we are tending, and how to get there. *Lect Notes Artif Intell.* 1997;(1211):3–11.
7. Camarillo DB, Krummel TM, Salisbury JK Jr.. Robotic technology in surgery: past, present, and future. *Am J Surg.* October, 2004;188(Suppl 4A):2S–15S.
8. Kwoh YS, Hou J, Jonckheere EA, Hayati S. A robot with improved absolute positioning accuracy for CT guided stereotactic brain surgery. *IEEE Trans Biomed Eng.* February, 1988;35(2):153–160.
9. Davies BL, Hibberd RD, Coptcoat MJ, Wickham JE. A surgeon robot prostatectomy–a laboratory evaluation. *J Med Eng Technol.* November–December, 1989;13(6):273–277.
10. Davies BL, Hibberd RD, Ng WS, Timoney AG, Wickham JE. The development of a surgeon robot for prostatectomies. *Proc Inst Mech Eng H.* 1991;205(1):35–38.
11. Harris SJ, Arambula-Cosio F, Mei Q, et al. The Probot–an active robot for prostate resection. *Proc Inst Mech Eng H.* 1997;211(4):317–325.
12. Taylor RH, Joskowicz L, Williamson B, et al. Computer-integrated revision total hip replacement surgery: concept and preliminary results. *Med Image Anal.* September, 1999;3(3):301–319.

13. Ho G, Ng WS, Teo MY, Kwoh CK, Cheng WS. Experimental study of transurethral robotic laser resection of the prostate using the LaserTrode lightguide. *J Biomed Opt.* April, 2001;6(2):244–251.

14. Ng WS, Chung VR, Vasan S, Lim P. Robotic radiation seed implantation for prostatic cancer. *Eng Med Biol Soc.* 1996;1:231–233.

15. Stoianovici D, Cleary K, Patriciu A, et al. Robot for radiological interventions. *IEEE Trans Robot Autom.* October, 2003;19(5):926–930.

16. Solomon SB, Patriciu A, Stoianovici DS. Tumor ablation treatment planning coupled to robotic implementation: a feasibility study. *J Vasc Interv Radiol.* May, 2006;17(5):903–907.

17. Su LM, Stoianovici D, Jarrett TW, et al. Robotic percutaneous access to the kidney: comparison with standard manual access. *J Endourol.* September, 2002;16(7):471–475.

18. Solomon SB, Patriciu A, Bohlman ME, Kavoussi LR, Stoianovici D. Robotically driven interventions: a method of using CT fluoroscopy without radiation exposure to the physician. *Radiology.* October, 2002;225(1):277–282.

19. Stoianovici D, Whitcomb LL, Anderson JH, Taylor RH, Kavoussi LR. A modular surgical robotic system for image guided percutaneous procedures. *Lect Notes Comp Sci.* 1998;1496:404–410.

20. Stoianovici D, Cadeddu JA, Demaree RD, et al. An efficient needle injection technique and radiological guidance method for percutaneous procedures. *Lect Notes Comp Sci.* 1997;1205:295–298.

21. Challacombe B, Kavoussi L, Patriciu A, Stoianovici D, Dasgupta P. Technology insight: telementoring and telesurgery in urology. *Nat Clin Pract Urol.* November, 2006;3(11):611–617.

22. Schurr MO, Buess G, Neisius B, Voges U. Robotics and telemanipulation technologies for endoscopic surgery. A review of the ARTEMIS project. Advanced Robotic Telemanipulator for Minimally Invasive Surgery. *Surg Endosc.* April, 2000;14(4):375–381.

23. Unger SW, Unger HM, Bass RT. AESOP robotic arm. *Surg Endosc.* September, 1994;8(9):1131.

24. Kavoussi LR, Moore RG, Partin AW, Bender JS, Zenilman ME, Satava RM. Telerobotic assisted laparoscopic surgery: initial laboratory and clinical experience. *Urology.* July, 1994;44(1):15–19.

25. Marescaux J, Leroy J, Gagner M, et al. Transatlantic robot-assisted telesurgery. *Nature.* September 27, 2001;413(6854):379–380.

26. Abbou CC, Hoznek A, Salomon L, et al. Remote laparoscopic radical prostatectomy carried out with a robot. Report of a case. *Prog Urol.* September, 2000;10(4):520–523.

27. Cadiere GB, Himpens J, Germay O, et al. Feasibility of robotic laparoscopic surgery: 146 cases. *World J Surg.* November, 2001;25(11):1467–1477.

28. Badani KK, Kaul S, Menon M. Evolution of robotic radical prostatectomy: assessment after 2766 procedures. *Cancer.* November 1, 2007;110(9):1951–1958.

29. Rassweiler J, Hruza M, Teber D, Su LM. Laparoscopic and robotic assisted radical prostatectomy–critical analysis of the results. *Eur Urol.* April, 2006;49(4):612–624.

30. Dasgupta P. Robotics in urology. *Int J Med Robot.* March, 2008;4(1):1–2.

31. Morgia G, De Renzis C. CyberKnife in the treatment of prostate cancer: a revolutionary system. *Eur Urol.* February 23, 2009.

32. Troccaz J, Peshkin M, Davies B. Guiding systems for computer-assisted surgery: introducing synergistic devices and discussing the different approaches. *Med Image Anal.* June, 1998;2(2):101–119.

33. Cobb J, Henckel J, Gomes P, et al. Hands-on robotic unicompartmental knee replacement: a prospective, randomised controlled study of the acrobot system. *J Bone Joint Surg Br.* February, 2006;88(2):188–197.

34. Barrett AR, Davies BL, Gomes MP, et al. Computer-assisted hip resurfacing surgery using the acrobot navigation system. *Proc Inst Mech Eng [H].* October, 2007;221(7):773–785.

35. Sutherland GR, Latour I, Greer AD. Integrating an image-guided robot with intraoperative MRI: a review of the design and construction of neuroArm. *IEEE Eng Med Biol Mag.* May–June, 2008;27(3):59–65.

36. Long JA, Cinquin P, Troccaz J, et al. Development of miniaturized light endoscope-holder robot for laparoscopic surgery. *J Endourol.* August, 2007;21(8):911–914.

37. Reiley CE, Akinbiyi T, Burschka D, Chang DC, Okamura AM, Yuh DD. Effects of visual force feedback on robot-assisted surgical task performance. *J Thorac Cardiovasc Surg.* January, 2008;135(1):196–202.

38. Zemiti N, Morel G, Ortmaier T, Bonnet N. Mechatronic design of a new robot for force control in minimally invasive surgery. *Mechatron, IEEE/ASME Trans.* 2007;12(2):143–153.

39. Ukimura O, Gill IS, Desai MM, et al. Real-time transrectal ultrasonography during laparoscopic radical prostatectomy. *J Urol.* July, 2004;172(1):112–118.

40. Tang SL, Kwoh CK, Teo MY, Sing NW, Ling KV. Augmented reality systems for medical applications. *IEEE Eng Med Biol Mag.* May–June, 1998;17(3):49–58.

41. Shuhaiber JH. Augmented reality in surgery. *Arch Surg.* February, 2004;139(2):170–174.

42. Ukimura O, Gill IS. Imaging-assisted endoscopic surgery: Cleveland Clinic experience. *J Endourol.* April, 2008;22(4):803–810.

43. Mozer P, Conort P, Leroy A, et al. Aid to percutaneous renal access by virtual projection of the ultrasound puncture tract onto fluoroscopic images. *J Endourol.* May, 2007;21(5):460–465.

44. Zeltser IS, Cadeddu JA. A novel magnetic anchoring and guidance system to facilitate single trocar laparoscopic nephrectomy. *Curr Urol Rep.* January, 2008;9(1):62–64.

45. Marescaux J, Dallemagne B, Perretta S, Wattiez A, Mutter D, Coumaros D. Surgery without scars: report of transluminal cholecystectomy in a human being. *Arch Surg.* September, 2007;142(9):823–826.

46. Lehman AC, Dumpert J, Wood NA, Visty AQ, Farritor SM, Oleynikov D. In vivo robotics for natural orifice transgastric peritoneoscopy. *Stud Health Technol Inform.* 2008;132:236–241.

47. Taylor RH, Stoianovici D. Medical robotics in computer-integrated surgery. *IEEE Trans Robot Autom.* October, 2003;19(5):765–781.

48. Stoianovici D. Multi-imager compatible actuation principles in surgical robotics. *Int J Med Robot Comp Assist Surg.* January 15, 2005;1(2):86–100.

49. Bucki M, Dauliac B, Daanen V, Moalic R, Descotes J-L, Troccaz J. PRONAV: a navigation software for prostate biopsies. *Surgeticaâ€^TM2005*: Sauramps Medical. 2005;479–483.

50. Xu S, Kruecker J, Guion P, et al. Closed-loop control in fused MR-TRUS image-guided prostate. *Biopsy.* 2007;10(Pt 1):128–135.

51. Abolhassani N, Patel RV, Ayazi F. Minimization of needle deflection in robot-assisted percutaneous therapy. *Int J Med Robot.* June, 2007;3(2):140–148.

52. Meltsner MA, Ferrier NJ, Thomadsen BR. Observations on rotating needle insertions using a brachytherapy robot. *Phys Med Biol.* 2007;52(19):6027–6037.

53. Podder TK, Ng WS, Yu Y. Multi-channel robotic system for prostate brachytherapy. *IEEE MBS Int.* 2007;1:1233–1236.

54. Davies BL, Hibberd RD, Ng WS, Timoney AG, Wickham JE. The development of a surgeon robot for prostatectomies. *Proc Inst Mech Eng [H].* 1991;205(1): 35–38.

55. Davies BL, Harris SJ, Dibble E. Brachytherapy – an example of a urological minimally invasive robotic procedure. *Int J Med Robot Comp Assist Surg.* 2004;(1):88–96.

56. Wei Z, Wan G, Gardi L, Mills G, Downey D, Fenster A. Robot-assisted 3D-TRUS guided prostate brachytherapy: system integration and validation. *Med Phys.* March, 2004;31(3):539–548.

57. Yu Y, Podder T, Zhang Y, et al. Robot-assisted prostate brachytherapy. *Med Image Comput Comput Assist Interv.* 2006;9(Pt 1):41–49.

58. Shah S, Kapoor A, Ding J, et al. Robotically assisted needle driver: evaluation of safety release, force profiles, and needle spin in a swine abdominal model. *Int J Comp Assist Radiol Surg.* May 21, 2008;3:173–179.

59. Petrisor D, Mozer P, Vigaru B, Cleary K, Stoianovici D. Rotating needle driver for robotic interventions. 2008;22.

60. Gassert R, Yamamoto A, Chapuis D, Dovat L, Bleuler H, Burdet E. Actuation methods for applications in MR environments. *Concepts Magn Reson Part B-Magn Reson Eng.* October, 2006;29B(4):191–209.

61. Chinzei K, Hata N, Jolesz FA, Kikinis R. MR compatible surgical assist robot: System integration and preliminary feasibility study. *Med Image Comput Comp-Assist Interv – Miccai 2000.* 2000;1935:921–930.

62. Chinzei K, Miller K. Towards MRI guided surgical manipulator. *Med Sci Monit.* January–February, 2001;7(1):153–163.

63. Koseki Y, Koyachi N, Arai T, Chinzei K. Remote actuation mechanism for MR-compatible manipulator using leverage and parallelogram – workspace analysis, workspace control, and stiffness evaluation. *ICRA.* 2003;1:652–657.

64. Koseki Y, Kikinis R, Jolesz FA, Chinzei K. Precise evaluation of positioning repeatability of MR-compatible manipulator inside MRI. *Med Image Comput Comp-Assist Interv – Miccai 2004, Pt 2, Proc.* 2004;3217:192–199.

65. Kaiser WA, Fischer H, Vagner J, Selig M. Robotic system for biopsy and therapy of breast lesions in a high-field whole-body magnetic resonance tomography unit. *Invest Radiol.* August, 2000;35(8):513–519.

66. Felden A, Vagner J, Hinz A, et al. ROBITOM-robot for biopsy and therapy of the mamma. *Biomed Tech (Berl).* 2002;47(Suppl 1 Pt 1):2–5.

67. Hempel E, Fischer H, Gumb L, et al. An MRI-compatible surgical robot for precise radiological interventions. *Comput Aided Surg.* 2003;8(4):180–191.

68. Cleary K, Melzer A, Watson V, Kronreif G, Stoianovici D. Interventional robotic systems: applications and technology state-of-the-art. *Minim Invasive Ther.* 2006;15(2):101–113.

69. Zangos S, Eichler K, Thalhammer A, et al. MR-guided interventions of the prostate gland. *Minim Invasive Ther Allied Technol.* 2007;16(4):222–229.

70. Zangos S, Herzog C, Eichler K, et al. MR-compatible assistance system for puncture in a high-field system: device and feasibility of transgluteal biopsies of the prostate gland. *Eur Radiol.* April, 2007;17(4):1118–1124.

71. Bricault I, Zemiti N, Jouniaux E, et al. Light puncture robot for CT and MRI interventions: designing a new robotic architecture to perform abdominal and thoracic punctures. *IEEE Eng Med Biol Mag.* May–June, 2008;27(3):42–50.

72. Stoianovici D, Song D, Petrisor D, et al. "MRI Stealth" robot for prostate interventions. *Minim Invasive Ther Allied Technol.* 2007;16(4):241–248.

73. Stoianovici D, Patriciu A, Mazilu D, Petrisor D, Kavoussi L. A new type of motor: pneumatic step motor. *IEEE/ASME Trans Mechatron.* February, 2007;12(1):98–106.2008.

74. Muntener M, Ursu D, Patriciu A, Petrisor D, Stoianovici D. Robotic prostate surgery. *Expert Rev Med Devices.* September, 2006;3(5):575–584.

75. Muntener M, Patriciu A, Petrisor D, et al. Transperineal prostate intervention: robot for fully automated MR imaging–system description and proof of principle in a canine model. *Radiology.* May, 2008;247(2):543–549.

76. Muntener M, Patriciu A, Petrisor D, et al. Magnetic resonance imaging compatible robotic system for fully automated brachytherapy seed placement. *Urology.* December, 2006;68(6):1313–1317.

77. Patriciu A, Petrisor D, Muntener M, Mazilu D, Schar M, Stoianovici D. Automatic brachytherapy seed placement under MRI guidance. *IEEE Trans Biomed Eng.* August, 2007;54(8):1499–1506.

78. Voros S, Long JA, Cinquin P. Automatic localization of laparoscopic instruments for the visual serving of an endoscopic camera holder. *Med Image Comput Comput Assist Interv.* 2006;9(Pt 1):535–542.

79. Reiley CE, Lin HC, Varadarajan B, et al. Automatic recognition of surgical motions using statistical modeling for capturing variability. *Stud Health Technol Inform.* 2008;132:396–401.

Index

Note: The letters 'f' and 't' following the locators refer to figures and tables respectively.